Pharmacology

THIRD EDITION

DISCARD

Pharmacology

THIRD EDITION

George M. Brenner, Ph.D.

Chair and Professor Emeritus of Pharmacology
Oklahoma State University
Center for Health Sciences
Tulsa, Oklahoma

Craig W. Stevens, Ph.D.

Chair and Professor of Pharmacology
Oklahoma State University
Center for Health Sciences
Tulsa, Oklahoma

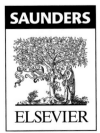

SAUNDERS

ELSEVIER

SAUNDERS
ELSEVIER

1600 John F. Kennedy Blvd.
Ste 1800
Philadelphia, PA 19103-2899

PHARMACOLOGY, THIRD EDITION

ISBN: 978-1-4160-6627-9

Notice

Knowledge and best practice in this field are constantly changing. As new research and experience broaden our knowledge, changes in practice, treatment and drug therapy may become necessary or appropriate. Readers are advised to check the most current information provided (i) on procedures featured or (ii) by the manufacturer of each product to be administered, to verify the recommended dose or formula, the method and duration of administration, and contraindications. It is the responsibility of the practitioner, relying on their own experience and knowledge of the patient, to make diagnoses, to determine dosages and the best treatment for each individual patient, and to take all appropriate safety precautions. To the fullest extent of the law, neither the Publisher nor the Authors assume any liability for any injury and/or damage to persons or property arising out of or related to any use of the material contained in this book.

The Publisher

Previous editions copyrighted 2000, 2006

Library of Congress Cataloging-in-Publication Data
Brenner, George M.
Pharmacology/George M. Brenner, Craig W. Stevens. — 3rd ed.
P. ; cm.
Includes bibliographical references and index.
ISBN 978-1-4160-6627-9
1. Pharmacology. I. Stevens, Craig W. II. Title.
[DNLM: 1. Pharmacology—methods. 2. Drug Therapy. 3. Pharmaceutical Preparations. QV 4 B838p 2010]

RM300.B74 2010
615'.1—dc22

2008043220

Acquisitions Editor: Kate Dimock
Developmental Editor: Nicole DiCicco
Production Manager: David M. Saltzberg
Design Direction: Karen O'Keefe Owens

Printed in China
Last digit is the print number: 9 8 7 6 5 4 3 2 1

CONTENTS

PREFACE

Medical pharmacology is primarily concerned with the mechanisms by which drugs relieve symptoms and counteract the pathophysiological manifestations of disease. It is also concerned with the factors that determine the time course of drug action, including drug absorption, distribution, biotransformation, and excretion. Students are often overwhelmed by the vast amount of pharmacologic information available today. This textbook provides the essential concepts and information that students need to be successful in their courses without an overwhelming amount of detail.

This text is primarily intended for students who are taking their first course in pharmacology, but it will also be useful for those who are preparing to take medical board or licensing examinations. Because of the large number of drugs available today, this text emphasizes the general properties of drug categories and prototypical drugs. Chapters begin with a drug classification box to familiarize students with drug categories, subcategories, and specific drugs to be discussed in the chapter.

Throughout the book, pharmacologic information is organized in the same format, with sections on mechanisms of action, physiologic effects, pharmacokinetic properties, adverse effects and interactions, and clinical uses for each drug category. Numerous illustrations are used to depict drug mechanisms and effects, while well-organized tables compare the specific properties of drugs within a therapeutic category. At the end of each chapter, a summary of important points is provided to reinforce concepts and clinical applications that are crucial for students to remember. Review questions and selected readings are also included to test the reader's comprehension and lead to further study.

Several changes have been incorporated into the third edition of this text. We have revised each chapter to incorporate new drugs and drug categories, as well as to update new findings from the pharmacology literature on the mechanisms of action and therapeutic use. Importantly, approved drugs that were taken off the market are highlighted, as well as revised warnings of existing drugs added to prescription guidelines since the last edition.

This book would not have been possible without the advice and encouragement of mentors, colleagues, and editorial personnel. We are especially thankful for the time and effort made by John R. Brenner, DO, and Vivian M. Stevens, PhD, in reviewing parts of the revised text. Finally, we are particularly appreciative to Kate Dimock and Nicole DiCicco at Elsevier Inc. for their helpful assistance and support throughout the production of this book.

George M. Brenner, Ph.D.
Craig W. Stevens, Ph.D.

PRINCIPLES OF PHARMACOLOGY

CHAPTER 1

Introduction to Pharmacology

PHARMACOLOGY AND RELATED SCIENCES

Pharmacology is the study of drugs and their effects on life processes. It is a fundamental science that sprang to the forefront of modern medicine with demonstrated success in treating disease and saving lives. It is also a discipline that drives the international pharmaceutical industry to billion-dollar profits. This chapter reviews the history and subdivisions of pharmacology and discusses, in detail, the types of drugs, formulations, and routes of administration.

History and Role of Pharmacology

Since the beginning of the species, people have treated pain and disease with substances derived from plants, animals, and minerals. However, the science of pharmacology is less than 150 years old, ushered in by the ability to isolate pure compounds and the establishment of the scientific method. Historically, the selection and use of drugs were based on superstition or on experience (empiricism).

In the first or earliest phase of drug usage, noxious plant and animal preparations were administered to a diseased patient to rid the body of the evil spirits believed to cause illness. The Greek word *pharmakon,* from which the term *pharmacology* is derived, originally meant a magic charm for treating disease. Later, *pharmakon* came to mean a remedy or drug.

In the second phase of drug usage, experience enabled people to understand which substances were actually beneficial in relieving particular disease symptoms. The first effective drugs were probably simple external preparations, such as cool mud or a soothing leaf, and the earliest known prescriptions from 2100 BCE included salves containing thyme. Over many centuries, people learned the therapeutic value of natural products through trial and error. By 1500 BCE, Egyptian prescriptions called for castor oil, opium, and other drugs that are still used today. In China, ancient scrolls from this time listed prescriptions of herbal medicines for more than 50 diseases. Dioscorides, a Greek army surgeon who lived in the 1st century, described more than 600 medicinal plants that he collected and studied as he traveled with the Roman army. Susruta, a Hindu physician, described the principles of Ayurvedic medicine in the 5th century. During the Middle Ages, Islamic physicians (most famously Avicenna) and Christian monks cultivated and studied the use of herbal medicines.

The third phase of drug usage, the rational or scientific phase, gradually evolved with important advances in chemistry and physiology that gave rise to the new science of pharmacology. At the same time, a more rational understanding of disease mechanisms provided a scientific basis for using drugs whose physiologic actions and effects were understood.

The advent of pharmacology was particularly dependent on the isolation of pure drug compounds from natural sources and on the development of experimental physiology methods to study these compounds. The **isolation of morphine** from opium in 1804 was rapidly followed by the extraction of many other drugs from plant sources, providing a diverse array of pure drugs for pharmacologic experimentation. Advances in physiology allowed pioneers, such as François Magendie and Claude Bernard, to conduct some of the earliest pharmacologic investigations, including studies that localized the site of action of curare to the neuromuscular junction. The first medical school pharmacology laboratory was started by Rudolf Büchheim in Estonia. Büchheim and one of his students, Oswald Schmiedeberg, trained many other pharmacologists, including John Jacob Abel, who established the first pharmacology department at the University of Michigan in 1891 and is considered the father of American pharmacology.

The goal of pharmacology is to understand the mechanisms by which drugs interact with biological systems to enable the rational use of effective agents in the diagnosis and treatment of disease. The success of pharmacology in this task has led to an explosion of new drug development, particularly in the past 50 years. Twentieth-century developments include the isolation and use of insulin for diabetes, the discovery of antimicrobial and antineoplastic drugs, and the advent of modern psychopharmacology. Recent advances in molecular biology, genetics, and drug design suggest that new drug development and pharmacologic innovations will provide even greater advances in the treatment of medical disorders in this century.

The history of many significant events in pharmacology, as highlighted by selected Nobel Prize recipients, is presented in Table 1–1.

TABLE 1-1. The Nobel Prize and the History of Pharmacology*	
Person(s) and Year Awarded	**Significant Discovery in Pharmacology**
Elie Metchnikoff, Paul Ehrlich (1908)	First antimicrobial drugs ("magic bullet")
Frederick Banting, John Macleod (1923)	Isolation and discovery of insulin and its application in the treatment of diabetes
Sir Henry Dale, Otto Loewi (1936)	Chemical transmission of nerve impulses
Ernst Chain, Sir Alexander Fleming, Sir Howard Florey (1945)	Discovery of penicillin and its curative effect in various infectious diseases
Edward Kendall, Tadeus Reichstein, Philip S. Hench (1950)	Hormones of the adrenal cortex, their structure and biological effects
Daniel Bovet (1957)	Antagonists that block biologically active amines, including the first antihistamine
Julius Axelrod, Sir Bernard Katz, Ulf von Euler (1970)	Transmitters in the nerve terminals and the mechanism for storage, release, and inactivation
Earl Sutherland, Jr. (1971)	Mechanisms of the action of hormones with regard to inhibition and stimulation of cyclic AMP
Sune Bergström, Bengt Samuelsson, John R. Vane (1982)	Discovery of prostaglandins and the mechanism of action of aspirin which inhibits prostaglandin synthesis
Sir James W. Black, Gertrude B. Elion, George H. Hitchings (1988)	Development of the first beta-blocker, propranolol, and anticancer agents that block nucleic acid synthesis
Alfred Gilman, Martin Rodbell (1994)	Discovery of G proteins and the role of these proteins in signal transduction in cells
Robert Furchgott, Louis Ignarro, Ferid Murad (1998)	Recognition of nitric oxide as a signaling molecule in the cardiovascular system
Arvid Carlsson, Paul Greengard, Eric Kandel (2000)	Role of dopamine in schizophrenia and signal transduction in the nervous system leading to long-term potentiation

*Selected from the list of recipients of the Nobel Prize for Physiology or Medicine; note that many other discoveries pertinent to pharmacology were made by other Nobel Prize winners in this field and in the field of chemistry and that the original discovery was often made many years before the Nobel Prize was awarded.

AMP = adenosine monophosphate.

Pharmacology and Its Subdivisions

Pharmacology is the biomedical science concerned with the interaction of chemical substances with living cells, tissues, and organisms. It is particularly concerned with the mechanisms by which drugs counteract the manifestations of disease and affect fertility. Pharmacology is not primarily focused on the methods of synthesis or isolation of drugs, or with the preparation of pharmaceutical products. The disciplines that deal with these subjects are described below.

Pharmacology is divided into two main subdivisions, **pharmacokinetics** and **pharmacodynamics**. The relationship between these subdivisions is shown in Figure 1–1. Pharmacokinetics is concerned with the processes that determine the concentration of drugs in body fluids and tissues over time, including **drug absorption, distribution, biotransformation** (**metabolism**), and **excretion**. Pharmacodynamics is the study of the actions of drugs on target organs. A shorthand way of thinking about it is that pharmacodynamics is what the drug does to the body, and pharmacokinetics is what the body does to the drug. Modern pharmacology is focused on the biochemical and molecular mechanisms by which drugs produce their physiologic effects and with the **dose-response relationship**, defined as the relationship between the concentration of a drug in a tissue and the magnitude of the tissue's response to that drug. Most drugs produce their effects by binding to protein **receptors** in target tissues, a process that activates a cascade of events known as **signal transduction**. Pharmacokinetics and pharmacodynamics are discussed in greater detail in Chapters 2 and 3.

Toxicology

Toxicology is the study of **poisons** and **organ toxicity**. It focuses on the harmful effects of drugs and other chemicals, and on the mechanisms by which these agents produce pathologic changes, disease, and death. As with pharmacology, toxicology is concerned with the relationship between the dose of an agent and the resulting tissue concentration and biologic effects that the agent produces. Most drugs have toxic effects at high enough doses and may have **adverse effects** related to toxicity at therapeutic doses.

Pharmacotherapeutics

Pharmacotherapeutics is the medical science concerned with the use of drugs in the treatment of disease. Pharmacology provides a rational basis for pharmacotherapeutics by explaining the mechanisms and effects of drugs on the body and the relationship between dose and drug response. Human studies known as **clinical trials** are then used to determine the efficacy and safety of drug therapy in human subjects. The purpose, design, and evaluation of human drug studies are discussed in Chapter 4.

Pharmacy and Related Sciences

Pharmacy is the science and profession concerned with the preparation, storage, dispensing, and proper use of drug products. Related sciences include pharmacognosy, medicinal chemistry, and pharmaceutical chemistry. **Pharmacognosy** is the study of drugs isolated from natural sources, including plants, microbes, animal tissues, and

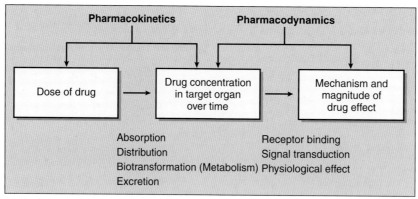

Figure 1-1. Relationship between pharmacokinetics and pharmacodynamics.

minerals. **Medicinal chemistry** is a branch of organic chemistry that specializes in the design and chemical synthesis of drugs. **Pharmaceutical chemistry,** or **pharmaceutics,** is concerned with the formulation and chemical properties of pharmaceutical products, such as tablets, liquid solutions and suspensions, and aerosols.

DRUG SOURCES AND PREPARATIONS

A **drug** can be defined as a natural product, chemical substance, or pharmaceutical preparation intended for administration to a human or animal to diagnose or treat a disease. The word *drug* is derived from the French *drogue*, which originally meant dried herbs and was applied to herbs in the marketplace used for cooking rather than for any medicinal reason. Ironically, the medical use of the drug marijuana, a dried herb, is hotly debated in many societies today. **Medication,** and less frequently, **medicament** are terms that are synonymous with the word *drug*.

Natural Sources of Drugs

Drugs have been obtained from plants, microbes, animal tissues, and minerals. Among the various types of drugs derived from plants are **alkaloids**, which are substances containing nitrogen groups and give an alkaline reaction in aqueous solution. Examples of alkaloids include morphine, cocaine, atropine, and quinine. **Antibiotics** have been isolated from numerous microorganisms, including *Penicillium* and *Streptomyces* species. **Hormones** are the most common type of drug obtained from animals, whereas **minerals** have yielded a few useful therapeutic agents, including the lithium compounds used to treat bipolar mental illness.

Synthetic Drugs

Modern chemistry in the 19th century enabled scientists to synthesize new compounds and to modify naturally occurring drugs. Aspirin, barbiturates, and local anesthetics (e.g., procaine) were among the first drugs to be synthesized in the laboratory. Semisynthetic derivatives of naturally occurring compounds have led to new drugs with different properties, such as the morphine derivative **oxycodone.**

In some cases, new drug uses were discovered by accident when drugs were used for another purpose, or by actively screening a huge number of related molecules for a specific pharmacologic activity. Medicinal chemists now use molecular modeling software to discern the **structure-activity relationship**, which is the relationship between the drug molecule, its target receptor, and the resulting pharmacologic activity. In this way, a virtual model for the receptor of a particular drug is created, and drug molecules that best fit the three-dimensional conformation of the receptor are synthesized. This approach has been used, for example, to design agents that inhibit angiotensin synthesis, treat hypertension, and inhibit the maturation of the human immunodeficiency virus in AIDS patients.

Drug Preparations

Drug preparations include **crude drug** preparations obtained from natural sources, **pure drug** compounds isolated from natural sources or synthesized in the laboratory, and **pharmaceutical preparations** of drugs intended for administration to patients. The relationship between these types of drug preparations is illustrated in Figure 1–2.

Crude Drug Preparations

Some crude drug preparations are made by drying or pulverizing a plant or animal tissue. Others are made by extracting substances from a natural product with the aid of hot water or a solvent such as alcohol. Familiar examples of crude drug preparations are coffee and tea, made from distillates of the beans and leaves of *Coffea arabica* and *Camellia sinensis* plants, and opium, which is the dried juice of the unripe poppy capsule of the plant, *Papaver somniferum*.

Pure Drug Compounds

It is difficult to identify and quantify the pharmacologic effects of crude drug preparations because these products contain multiple ingredients, the amounts of which may vary from batch to batch. Hence, the development of methods to isolate pure drug compounds from natural sources was an important step in the growth of pharmacology and rational therapeutics. Frederick Sertürner, a German apothecary, isolated the first pure drug from a natural source

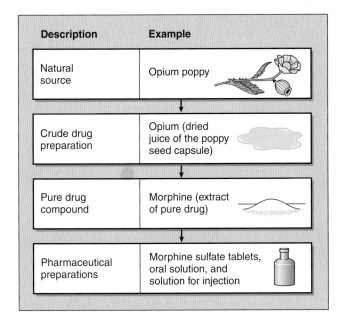

Description	Example
Natural source	Opium poppy
Crude drug preparation	Opium (dried juice of the poppy seed capsule)
Pure drug compound	Morphine (extract of pure drug)
Pharmaceutical preparations	Morphine sulfate tablets, oral solution, and solution for injection

Figure 1–2.   Types of drug preparations. A crude drug preparation retains most or all of the active and inactive compounds contained in the natural source from which it was derived. After a pure drug compound (e.g., morphine) is extracted from a crude drug preparation (in this case, opium), it is possible to manufacture pharmaceutic preparations that are suitable for administration of a particular dose to the patient.

when he extracted a potent **analgesic** agent from opium in 1804 and named it **morphine**, from Morpheus, the Greek god of dreams. The subsequent isolation of many other drugs from natural sources provided pharmacologists with a number of pure compounds for study and characterization. One of the greatest medical achievements of the early 20th century was the isolation of insulin from the pancreas. This achievement by Frederick Banting and Charles Best led to the development of **insulin** preparations for treating **diabetes mellitus**.

Pharmaceutical Preparations

Pharmaceutical preparations or dosage forms are drug products suitable for administration of a specific dose of a drug to a patient by a particular route of administration. Most of these preparations are made from pure drug compounds, but a few are made from crude drug preparations and sold as herbal remedies.

TABLETS AND CAPSULES. Tablets and capsules are the most common preparations for oral administration because they are suitable for mass production, are stable and convenient to use, and can be formulated to release the drug immediately after ingestion or to release it over a period of hours.

In the manufacture of tablets, a machine with a punch and die mechanism compresses a mixture of powdered drug and inert ingredients into a hard pill. The **inert ingredients** include specific components that provide bulk, prevent sticking to the punch and die during manufacture, maintain tablet stability in the bottle, and facilitate solubilization of the tablet when it reaches gastrointestinal fluids. These ingredients are called **fillers, lubricants, adhesives**, and **disintegrants**, respectively.

A tablet must disintegrate after it is ingested, and then the drug must dissolve in gastrointestinal fluids before it can be absorbed into the circulation. Variations in the rate and extent of tablet disintegration and drug dissolution can give rise to differences in the oral bioavailability of drugs from different tablet formulations (see Chapter 4).

Tablets may have various types of coatings. **Enteric coatings** consist of polymers that will not disintegrate in gastric acid but will break down in the more basic pH of the intestines. Enteric coatings are used to protect drugs that would otherwise be destroyed by gastric acid and are also to slow the release and absorption of a drug when a large dose is given at one time, for example, in the formulation of the antidepressant, fluoxetine, called PROZAC WEEKLY.

Sustained-release products, or **extended-release products**, release the drug from the preparation over many hours. The two methods used to extend the release of the drug are **controlled diffusion** and **controlled dissolution.** With controlled diffusion, release of the drug from the pharmaceutical product is regulated by a rate-controlling membrane. Controlled dissolution is done by inert polymers that gradually break down in body fluids. These polymers may be part of the tablet matrix, or they may be used as coatings over small pellets of drug enclosed in a capsule. In either case, the drug is gradually released into the gastrointestinal tract as the polymers dissolve.

Some products use **osmotic pressure** to provide a sustained release of a drug. These products contain an osmotic agent that attracts gastrointestinal fluid at a constant rate. The attracted fluid then forces the drug out of the tablet through a small laser-drilled hole (Fig. 1–3A).

Capsules are hard or soft gelatin shells enclosing a powdered or liquid medication. **Hard capsules** are used to enclose powdered drugs, whereas **soft capsules** enclose a drug in solution. The gelatin shell quickly dissolves in gastrointestinal fluids to release the drug for absorption into the circulation.

SOLUTIONS AND SUSPENSIONS. Drug solutions and particle suspensions, the most common **liquid** pharmaceutical preparations, can be formulated for oral, parenteral, or other routes of administration. Solutions and suspensions provide a convenient method for administering drugs to pediatric and other patients who cannot easily swallow pills or tablets. They are less convenient than solid dosage forms, however, because the liquid must be measured each time a dose is given.

Solutions and suspensions for oral administration are often sweetened and flavored to increase palatability. Sweetened aqueous solutions are called **syrups**, whereas sweetened aqueous–alcoholic solutions are known as **elixirs.** Alcohol is included in elixirs as a solvent for drugs that are not sufficiently soluble in water alone.

Sterile solutions and suspensions are available for **parenteral** administration with a needle and syringe, or with an intravenous infusion pump. Many drugs are formulated as sterile powders for reconstitution with sterile liquids at the time the drug is to be injected, because the drug is not stable for long periods of time in solution. Sterile ophthalmic solutions and suspensions are suitable for administration with an eyedropper into the conjunctival sac.

SKIN PATCHES. Transdermal skin patches are drug preparations in which the drug is slowly released from the patch for absorption through the skin into the circulation. Most skin patches use a **rate-controlling membrane** to regulate the diffusion of the drug from the patch (Fig. 1–3B). Such devices are most suitable for **potent** drugs, which are therefore effective at relatively low dosages, and have sufficient **lipid solubility** to enable skin penetration.

AEROSOLS. Aerosols are a type of drug preparation administered by **inhalation** through the nose or mouth. They are particularly useful for treating respiratory disorders because they deliver the drug directly to the site of action and may thereby minimize the risk of systemic side effects. Some aerosol devices contain the drug dispersed in a pressurized gas and are designed to deliver a precise dosage each time they are activated by the patient. **Nasal sprays**, another type of aerosol preparation, can be used either to deliver drugs that have a localized effect on the nasal mucosa or to deliver drugs that are absorbed through the mucosa and exert an effect on another organ. For example, **butorphanol**, an opioid analgesic, is available as a nasal spray (STADOL **NS**) for the treatment of pain.

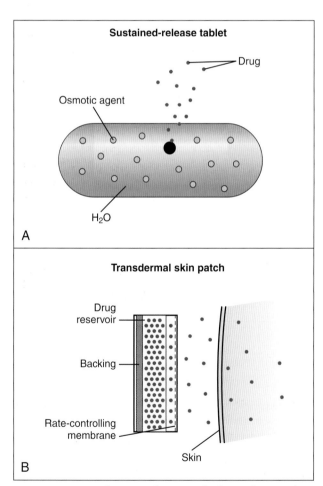

Figure 1–3. Mechanisms of sustained-release drug products. In the sustained-release tablet (A), water is attracted by an osmotic agent in the tablet, and this forces the drug out through a small orifice. In the transdermal skin patch (B), the drug diffuses through a rate-controlling membrane and is absorbed through the skin into the circulation.

OINTMENTS, CREAMS, LOTIONS, AND SUPPOSITORIES. Ointments and creams are semisolid preparations intended for **topical application** of a drug to the skin or mucous membranes. These products contain an active drug that is incorporated into a vehicle (e.g., polyethylene glycol or petrolatum), which enables the drug to adhere to the tissue for a sufficient length of time to exert its effect. Lotions are liquid preparations often formulated as oil-in-water emulsions and are used to treat dermatologic conditions. Suppositories are products in which the drug is incorporated into a **solid base** that melts or dissolves at body temperature. Suppositories are used for **rectal**, **vaginal**, or **urethral** administration and may provide either localized or systemic drug therapy.

ROUTES OF DRUG ADMINISTRATION

Some routes of drug administration, such as the **enteral** and common **parenteral** routes compared in Table 1–2, are intended to elicit systemic effects and are therefore called **systemic routes**. Other routes of administration, such as the inhalational route, can elicit either localized effects or systemic effects, depending on the drug being administered.

Enteral Administration

The enteral routes of administration are those in which the drug is absorbed from the gastrointestinal tract. These include **sublingual**, **buccal**, **oral**, and **rectal** routes.

In **sublingual administration**, a drug product is placed under the tongue. In **buccal administration**, the drug is placed between the cheek and the gum. Both sublingual and buccal administrations enable the rapid absorption of certain drugs and are not affected by first-pass drug metabolism in the liver. Drugs for sublingual and buccal administration are given in a relatively low dosage and must have good solubility in water and lipid membranes. Larger doses might be irritating to the tissue and would likely be washed away by saliva before the drug would be absorbed. Two examples of drugs available for sublingual administration are **nitroglycerin** for treating ischemic heart disease and **hyoscyamine** for treating bowel cramps. **Fentanyl**, a potent opioid analgesic, is available in an oral transmucosal formulation (ACTIQ) like a lollypop for rapid absorption from the buccal mucosa in the treatment of breakthrough cancer pain.

In medical orders and prescriptions, **oral administration** is designated as *per os* (PO), which means to administer 'by mouth'. The medication is swallowed, and the drug is absorbed from the stomach and small intestines. Because the oral route of administration is convenient and relatively safe and economical, it is the **most commonly used route**. It does have some disadvantages, however. Absorption of orally administered drugs can vary widely because of the interaction of drugs with food and gastric acid and the varying rates of gastric emptying, intestinal transit, and tablet disintegration and dissolution. Moreover, some drugs are inactivated by the liver following their absorption from the gut, called **first-pass metabolism**, and oral administration is not suitable for use by patients who are sedated, comatose, or suffering from nausea and vomiting.

TABLE 1-2. **Advantages and Disadvantages of Four Common Routes of Drug Administration**

Route	Advantages	Disadvantages
Oral	Convenient, relatively safe, and economical.	Cannot be used for drugs that are inactivated by gastric acid, for drugs with a large first-pass effect, or for drugs that irritate the gut.
Intramuscular	Suitable for suspensions and oily vehicles. Absorption is rapid from solutions and is slow and sustained from suspensions.	May be painful. Can cause bleeding if the patient is receiving an anticoagulant.
Subcutaneous	Suitable for suspensions and pellets. Absorption is similar to the intramuscular route but is usually somewhat slower.	Cannot be used for drugs that irritate cutaneous tissues or for drugs that must be given in large volumes.
Intravenous	Bypasses absorption to give an immediate effect. Allows for rapid titration of dosage. Has 100% bioavailability.	Poses more risks for toxicity and tends to be more expensive than other routes.

Rectal administration of drugs in suppository form can result in either a localized effect or a systemic effect. Suppositories are useful when patients cannot take medications by mouth, such as in the treatment of nausea and vomiting. They can also be administered for localized conditions such as hemorrhoids. Drugs absorbed from the lower rectum undergo relatively little first-pass metabolism in the liver.

Parenteral Administration

Parenteral administration refers to drug administration with a needle and syringe, or with an intravenous infusion pump. The most commonly used parenteral routes are the **intravenous**, **intramuscular**, and **subcutaneous** routes.

Intravenous administration bypasses the process of drug absorption and provides the greatest reliability and control over the dose of drug reaching the general circulation. It is often preferred for administration of drugs with short half-lives and drugs whose dosage must be carefully titrated to the physiologic response, such as agents used to treat hypotension, shock, and acute heart failure. The intravenous route is widely used to administer antibiotics and antineoplastic drugs to critically ill patients, as well as to treat various types of medical emergencies. The intravenous route is potentially the **most dangerous**, because rapid administration of drugs by this route can cause serious toxicity.

Intramuscular and **subcutaneous administration** is suitable for treatment with drug solutions and particle suspensions. Solutions are absorbed more rapidly than particle suspensions, so suspensions are often used to extend the duration of action of a drug over many hours or days. Most drugs are absorbed more rapidly after intramuscular than after subcutaneous administration because of the greater circulation of blood to the muscle.

Intrathecal administration refers to injection of a drug through the thecal covering of the spinal cord and into the subarachnoid space. In cases of meningitis, the intrathecal route is useful in administering antibiotics that do not cross the blood-brain barrier. **Epidural administration**, common in labor and delivery, targets analgesics into the space above the dura membranes of the spinal cord.

Other less common parenteral routes include **intraarticular administration** of drugs used to treat arthritis, **intradermal** for allergy tests, and **insufflation** (**intranasal**) for sinus medications.

Transdermal Administration

Transdermal administration is the application of drugs to the skin for absorption into the circulation. Application can be via a **skin patch** or, less commonly, via an ointment. Transdermal administration, which bypasses first-pass metabolism, is a reliable route of administration for drugs that are effective when given in a relatively low dosage and that are highly soluble in lipid membranes. Transdermal skin patches slowly release medication for periods of time that typically range from one to seven days. Two examples of transdermal preparations are the skin patches called **fentanyl transdermal** (DURAGESIC) used to treat severe chronic pain, and **nitroglycerin** ointment that is used to treat heart failure and angina pectoris.

Inhalational Administration

Inhalational administration can be used to produce either a localized or a systemic drug effect. A localized effect on the respiratory tract is obtained with drugs used to treat **asthma** or **rhinitis**, whereas a systemic effect is observed when a general anesthetic, such as **halothane**, is inhaled.

Topical Administration

Topical administration refers to the application of drugs to the **surface** of the body to produce a localized effect. It is often used to treat disease and trauma of the skin, eyes, nose, mouth, throat, rectum, and vagina.

DRUG NAMES

A drug often has several names, including a **chemical** name, a **nonproprietary** (**generic**) name, and a **proprietary** name (or **trade** or **brand** name).

The **chemical name**, which specifies the chemical structure of the drug, uses standard chemical nomenclature. Some chemical names are short and easily pronounceable, for example the chemical name of aspirin is acetylsalicylic acid. Others are long and hard to pronounce due to the size and complexity of the drug molecule. For most drugs, the chemical name is used primarily by medicinal chemists.

The **nonproprietary name**, or **generic name**, is the type of drug name most suitable for use by health care professionals. In the United States, the preferred nonproprietary names are the **United States Adopted Names (USAN)** designations. These designations, which are often derived from the chemical names of drugs, provide some indication of the class to which a particular drug belongs. For example, oxacillin can be easily recognized as a type of penicillin. The designations are selected by the USAN Council, which is a nomenclature committee representing the medical and pharmacy professions and the United States Pharmacopeia (see Chapter 4), with advisory input from the U.S. Food and Drug Administration. The USAN is often the same as the **International Nonproprietary Name** and the **British Approved Name**. International generic names for drugs can vary with the language in which they are used.

The **proprietary name, trade name**, or **brand name** for a drug is the registered trademark belonging to a particular drug manufacturer and used to designate a drug product marketed by that manufacturer. Many drugs are marketed under two or more brand names, especially after the manufacturer loses patent exclusivity. For example, ibuprofen (generic name) is marketed in the United States with the brand names of ADVIL, MOTRIN, and MIDOL. Drugs can also be marketed under their USAN designation. For these reasons, it is often less confusing and more precise to use the USAN rather than a brand name for a drug. However, the brand name may provide a better indication of the drug's pharmacologic or therapeutic effect. For example, DIURIL is a brand name for **chlorothiazide**, a diuretic; FLOMAX for **tamsulosin**, a drug used to increase urine flow; and MAXAIR is the brand name for **pirbuterol**, a drug used to treat asthma. In this textbook the generic name of a drug is given in normal font and its brand name(s) in SMALL CAPS font.

SUMMARY OF IMPORTANT POINTS

■ The development of pharmacology was made possible by important advances in chemistry and physiology that enabled scientists to isolate and synthesize pure chemical compounds (drugs) and to design methods for identifying and quantifying the physiologic actions of the compounds.

■ Pharmacology has two main subdivisions. Pharmacodynamics is concerned with the mechanisms of drug action and the dose-response relationship, whereas pharmacokinetics is concerned with the relationship between the drug dose and the plasma drug concentration over time.

■ The sources of drugs are natural products (including plants, microbes, animal tissues, and minerals) and chemical synthesis. Drugs can exist as crude drug preparations, pure drug compounds, or pharmaceutical preparations used to administer a specific dose to a patient.

■ The primary routes of administration are enteral (e.g., oral ingestion), parenteral (e.g., intravenous, intramuscular, and subcutaneous injection), transdermal, inhalational, and topical. Most routes produce systemic effects. Topical administration produces a localized effect at the site of administration.

■ All drugs (pure compounds) have a nonproprietary name (or generic name, such as a USAN designation) as well as a chemical name. Some drugs also have one or more proprietary names (trade names or brand names) under which they are marketed by their manufacturer.

Review Questions

1. Which route of drug administration is used with potent and lipophilic drugs in a patch formulation and avoids first-pass metabolism?
   (A) topical
   (B) sublingual
   (C) rectal
   (D) oral
   (E) transdermal

2. Which one of the following routes of administration does not have an absorption phase?
   (A) subcutaneous
   (B) intramuscular
   (C) intravenous
   (D) sublingual
   (E) inhalation

3. Which of the following correctly describes the intramuscular route of parenteral drug administration?
   (A) drug absorption is erratic and unpredictable
   (B) used to administer drug suspensions that are slowly absorbed
   (C) bypasses the process of drug absorption to give an immediate effect
   (D) cannot be used for drugs that undergo a high degree of first-pass metabolism
   (E) poses more risks than intravenous administration

4. An elderly patient has problems remembering to take her medication three times a day. Which one of the drug formulations might be particularly useful in this case?
   (A) extended-release
   (B) suspension
   (C) suppository
   (D) skin-patch
   (E) enteric-coated

5. Which form of a drug name is most likely known by patients from exposure to drug advertisements?
   (A) nonproprietary name
   (B) British Approved Name
   (C) chemical name
   (D) generic name
   (E) proprietary name

Answer and Explanations

1. **The answer is E:** transdermal. The topical, sublingual, rectal (suppositories), and transdermal routes of administration all avoid first-pass hepatic drug metabolism; however, only the transdermal formulation uses a patch with potent and lipophilic drugs. Orally administered drugs have the highest exposure to first-pass metabolism.

2. **The answer is C:** intravenous administration. Drug absorption refers to the process by which drugs get into the bloodstream. With subcutaneous, intramuscular, sublingual, and inhalation routes of administration, drug molecules have to cross membranes to get into the blood. Direct delivery of drug into the blood by intravenous administration therefore has no absorption phase.

3. **The answer is B:** used to administer drug suspensions that are slowly absorbed. After intramuscular injection of a suspension of drug particles, the particles slowly dissolve in interstitial fluid to provide sustained drug absorption over many hours or days. When a drug solution is injected intramuscularly, the drug is usually absorbed rapidly and completely.

4. **The answer is A:** extended-release. Using an extended-release tablet or capsule, the patient could most likely reduce the schedule of medication from three times a day to once a day. A suspension, for oral administration, would not likely reduce the schedule; a suppository would be difficult and reduce patient compliance; and a skin-patch for transdermal administration would only work in a few cases with potent and highly lipophilic drugs. Enteric-coated may help absorption or drug stability but would not reduce the schedule of medication.

5. **The answer is E:** proprietary name. The proprietary name, also known as the trade name or the brand name, is the name trademarked by the manufacturer and promoted on television, radio, and print ads. The chemical name is rarely seen, being tedious and descriptive only to medicinal chemists, whereas the generic name may be seen in the fine print of the ad but is not usually promoted as highly as the proprietary name. The nonproprietary name is the same thing as the generic name, and the British Approved Name is an official name that is usually the same as the generic name.

SELECTED READINGS

Huxtable, R.J., and Schwartz, S.K.W. The isolation of morphine: first principles in science and ethics. Mol Interv 1:189–191, 2001.

Loudon, I., ed. Western Medicine: An Illustrated History. Oxford, Oxford University Press, 1997.

Rubin, R.P. A brief history of great discoveries in pharmacology: in celebration of the centennial anniversary of the founding of the American Society of Pharmacology and Experimental Therapeutics. Pharmacol Rev 59:289–359, 2007.

United States Pharmacopeial Convention. USP Dictionary of USAN and International Drug Names. Rockville, Md., United States Pharmacopeia, 2004.

CHAPTER 2

Pharmacokinetics

OVERVIEW

Pharmacokinetics is the study of drug disposition in the body and focuses on the changes in **drug plasma concentration**. For any given drug and dose, the plasma concentration of the drug will rise and fall according to the rates of three processes: **absorption, distribution**, and **elimination.** Absorption of a drug refers to the movement of drug into the bloodstream, with the rate dependent on the physical characteristics of the drug and its formulation. Distribution of a drug refers to the process of a drug leaving the bloodstream and going into the organs and tissues. Elimination of a drug from the blood relies on two processes: **biotransformation (metabolism)** of a drug to one or more metabolites, primarily in the liver; and the **excretion** of the parent drug or its metabolites, primarily by the kidneys. The relationship between these processes is shown in Figure 2–1.

DRUG ABSORPTION

Drug absorption refers to the **passage of drug molecules** from the site of administration into the circulation. The process of drug absorption applies to all routes of administration, except for the topical route, where drugs are applied directly on the target tissue, and intravenous administration, where the drug is already in the circulation. Drug absorption requires that drugs cross one or more layers of cells and cell membranes. Drugs injected into the subcutaneous tissue and muscle bypass the epithelial barrier and are more easily absorbed through spaces between capillary endothelial cells. In the gut, lungs, and skin, drugs must first be absorbed through a layer of epithelial cells that have tight junctions. For this reason, drugs face a greater **barrier** to absorption after oral administration than after parenteral administration.

Processes of Absorption

Most drugs are absorbed by **passive diffusion** across a biologic barrier and into the circulation. The rate of absorption is proportional to the drug concentration gradient across the barrier and the surface area available for absorption at that site, known as **Fick's Law**. Drugs can be absorbed passively through cells either by lipid diffusion or by aqueous diffusion. **Lipid diffusion** is a process in which the drug dissolves in the lipid components of the cell membranes. This process is facilitated by a high degree of lipid solubility of the drug. **Aqueous diffusion** occurs by passage through aqueous pores in cell membranes. Because aqueous diffusion is restricted to drugs with low molecular weights, many drugs are too large to be absorbed by this process.

A few drugs are absorbed by **active transport** or by **facilitated diffusion.** Active transport requires a **carrier molecule** and a form of **energy**, provided by hydrolysis of the terminal high-energy phosphate bond of ATP. Active transport can transfer drugs against a concentration gradient. For example, the antineoplastic drug, **5-fluorouracil**, undergoes active transport. Facilitated diffusion also requires a carrier molecule, but no energy is needed. Thus drugs or substances cannot be transferred against a concentration gradient but diffuse faster than without a carrier molecule present. Some cephalosporin antibiotics, such as **cephalexin**, undergo facilitated diffusion by an oligopeptide transporter protein located in intestinal epithelial cells.

Effect of pH on Absorption of Weak Acids and Bases

Many drugs are weak acids or bases that exist in both ionized and non-ionized forms in the body. Only the **non-ionized form** of these drugs is sufficiently soluble in membrane lipids to cross cell membranes (Box 2–1). The ratio of the two forms at a particular site influences the **rate of absorption** and is also a factor in distribution and elimination.

The protonated form of a weak acid is non-ionized, whereas the protonated form of a weak base is ionized. The ratio of the protonated form to the nonprotonated form of these drugs can be calculated using the **Henderson-Hasselbalch equation** (see Box 2–1). The pKa is the negative log of the ionization constant, particular for each acidic or basic drug. At a pH equal to the pK_a, **equal** amounts of the protonated and nonprotonated forms are present. If the pH is less than the pK_a, the protonated form predominates. If the pH is greater than the pK_a, the nonprotonated form predominates.

In the stomach, with a pH of 1, weak acids and bases are highly protonated. At this site, the non-ionized form of weak acids (pK_a = 3–5) and the ionized form of weak bases

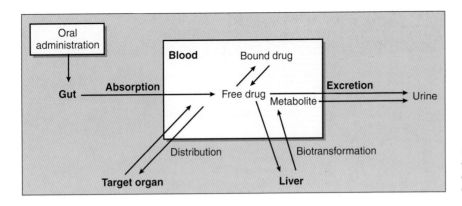

Figure 2-1. The absorption, distribution, biotransformation (metabolism), and excretion of a typical drug after its oral administration.

(pK_a = 8–10) will predominate. Hence, weak acids are more readily absorbed from the stomach than are weak bases. In the intestines, with a pH of 7, weak bases are also mostly ionized, but much less so than in the stomach, and weak bases are absorbed more readily from the intestines than from the stomach.

However, weak acids can also be absorbed more readily from the intestines than from the stomach, despite their greater ionization in the intestines, because the intestines have a greater surface area than the stomach for absorption of the non-ionized form of a drug, and this outweighs the influence of greater ionization in the intestines.

DRUG DISTRIBUTION

Drugs are distributed to organs and tissues via the circulation, diffusing into interstitial fluid and cells from the circulation. Most drugs are not uniformly distributed throughout total body water, and some drugs are restricted to the extracellular fluid or plasma compartment. Drugs with sufficient lipid solubility can simply diffuse through membranes into cells. Other drugs are concentrated in cells by the phenomenon of **ion trapping**, which is described further below. Drugs can also be actively transported into cells. For example, some drugs are actively transported into hepatic cells, where they may undergo enzymatic biotransformation. In the intestines, drug transport by **P-glycoprotein (Pgp)** in the blood-to-lumen direction leads to a secretion of various drugs into the intestinal tract, thereby serving as a detoxifying mechanism. The Pgp proteins also remove many drugs from tissues throughout the body, including anticancer agents. Inhibition of Pgp by amiodarone, erythromycin, propranolol, and other agents can increase tissue levels of these drugs and augment their pharmacologic effects.

Factors Affecting Distribution

Organ Blood Flow

The rate at which a drug is distributed to various organs after a drug dose is administered depends largely on the proportion of **cardiac output** received by the organs. Drugs are rapidly distributed to highly perfused tissues, namely the brain, heart, liver, and kidney, and this enables a rapid onset of action of drugs affecting these tissues. Drugs are distributed more slowly to less perfused tissues such as skeletal muscle and even more slowly to those with the lowest blood flow, such as skin, bone, and adipose tissue.

Plasma Protein Binding

Almost all drugs are reversibly bound to plasma proteins, primarily **albumin**, but also lipoproteins, glycoproteins, and β globulins. The extent of binding depends on the affinity of a particular drug for protein-binding sites and ranges from less than 10% to as high as 99% of the plasma concentration. As the free (unbound) drug diffuses into interstitial fluid and cells, drug molecules dissociate from plasma proteins to maintain the equilibrium between free drug and bound drug. In general, acid drugs bind to albumin and basic drugs to glycoproteins and β globulins.

Plasma protein binding is **saturable**, and a drug can be displaced from binding sites by other drugs that have a high affinity for such sites. However, most drugs are not used at high enough plasma concentrations to occupy the vast number of plasma protein binding sites. There are a few agents that may cause drug interactions by competing for plasma protein binding sites, as highlighted in Chapter 4.

Molecular Size

Molecular size is a factor affecting the distribution of extremely large molecules, such as those of the anticoagulant **heparin**. Heparin is largely confined to the plasma compartment, although it does undergo some biotransformation in the liver.

Lipid Solubility

Lipid solubility is a major factor affecting the extent of drug distribution, particularly to the brain, where the **blood-brain barrier** restricts the penetration of polar and ionized molecules. The barrier is formed by tight junctions between the capillary endothelial cells and also by the glial cells that surround the capillaries, which inhibit the penetration of polar molecules into brain neurons.

DRUG BIOTRANSFORMATION

Drug **biotransformation** and **excretion** are the two processes responsible for the decline of the plasma drug concentration over time. Both of these processes contribute to the

BOX 2–1. EFFECT OF pH ON THE ABSORPTION OF A WEAK ACID AND A WEAK BASE

Weak **acids** (HA) donate a proton (H^+) to form anions (A^-), whereas **weak bases** (B) accept a proton to form cations (HB^+).

HA	⇌	$H^+ + A^-$	For weak acids, the protonated form is nonionized.
$B + H^+$	⇌	HB^+	For weak bases, the protonated form is ionized.

Only the **non-ionized form** of a drug can readily penetrate cell membranes.

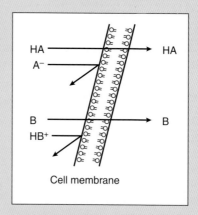

Cell membrane

The **pK$_a$** of a weak acid or weak base is the **pH** at which there are equal amounts of the protonated form and the nonprotonated form. The **Henderson-Hasselbalch equation** can be used to determine the ratio of the two forms:

$$\log \frac{[\text{protonated form}]}{[\text{Nonprotonated form}]} = pK_a - pH$$

For **salicylic acid**, which is a weak acid with a pK$_a$ of 3, log [HA]/[A$^-$] is 3 minus the pH. At a pH of 2, then, log [HA]/[A$^-$] = 3 − 2 = 1. Therefore, [HA]/[A$^-$] = 10/1.

COOH / OH (Protonated)	⇌	COO$^-$ / OH + H^+ (Nonprotonated)

For **amphetamine**, which is a weak base with a pK$_a$ of 10, log [HB$^+$]/[B] is 10 minus the pH. At a pH of 8, then, log [HB$^+$]/[B] = 10 − 8 = 2. Therefore, [HB$^+$]/[B] = 100/1.

$CH_2 - CH - NH_2$ / CH_3 + H^+ (Nonprotonated)	⇌	$CH_2 - CH - NH_3^+$ / CH_3 (Protonated)

(Continued)

BOX 2–1. EFFECT OF pH ON THE ABSORPTION OF A WEAK ACID AND A WEAK BASE—cont'd

The following are the ratios of the protonated form to the nonprotonated form at different pH levels:

		Salicylic acid					Amphetamine			
Protonated		10	1	1	1	1	1000	100	10	1
pH		2	3	4	5	6	7	8	9	10
Nonprotonated		1	1	10	100	1000	1	1	1	1

elimination of active drug from the body, and as discussed later in the chapter, **clearance** is a measure of the rate of elimination. Biotransformation, or **drug metabolism**, is the enzyme-catalyzed conversion of drugs to their metabolites. Most drug biotransformation takes place in the liver, but drug-metabolizing enzymes are found in many other tissues, including the gut, kidneys, brain, lungs, and skin.

Role of Drug Biotransformation

The fundamental role of drug-metabolizing enzymes is to **inactivate and detoxify** drugs and other foreign compounds (xenobiotics) that can harm the body. Drug metabolites are usually more water soluble than is the parent molecule and, therefore, they are more readily excreted by the kidneys. No particular relationship exists between biotransformation and pharmacologic activity. Some drug metabolites are active, whereas others are inactive. Many drug molecules undergo attachment of polar groups, a process called **conjugation,** for more rapid excretion. As a general rule, most conjugated drug metabolites are inactive, but a few exceptions exist.

Formation of Active Metabolites

Many pharmacologically active drugs, such as the sedative-hypnotic agent **diazepam** (VALIUM), are biotransformed to active metabolites. Some agents, known as **prodrugs,** are administered as inactive compounds and then biotransformed to active metabolites. This type of agent is usually developed because the prodrug is better absorbed than its active metabolite. For example, the antiglaucoma agent **dipivefrin** (PROPINE) is a prodrug that is converted to its active metabolite, epinephrine, by corneal enzymes after topical ocular administration. Orally administered prodrugs, such as the antihypertensive agent **enalapril** (VASOTEC), are converted to their active metabolite by hepatic enzymes during their first pass through the liver.

First-Pass Biotransformation

Drugs that are absorbed from the gut reach the liver via the hepatic portal vein before entering the systemic circulation (Fig. 2–2). Many drugs, such as the antihypertensive agent felodipine (PLENDIL), are extensively converted to inactive metabolites during their first pass through the gut wall and liver, and have low **bioavailability** (see below) after oral administration. This phenomenon is called the **first-pass effect**. Drugs administered by the sublingual or rectal route undergo less first-pass metabolism and have a higher degree of bioavailability than do drugs administered by the oral route.

Phases of Drug Biotransformation

Drug biotransformation can be divided into two phases, each carried out by unique sets of metabolic enzymes. In many cases, phase I enzymatic reactions create or unmask a chemical group required for a phase II reaction. In some cases, however, drugs bypass phase I biotransformation and go directly to phase II. Although some phase I drug metabolites are pharmacologically active, most phase II drug metabolites are inactive.

Phase I Biotransformation

Phase I biotransformation includes oxidative, hydrolytic, and reductive reactions (Fig. 2–3).

OXIDATIVE REACTIONS. Oxidative reactions are the most common type of phase I biotransformation. They are catalyzed by enzymes isolated in the microsomal fraction of liver homogenates (the fraction derived from the endoplasmic reticulum) and by cytoplasmic enzymes.

The **microsomal cytochrome P450 (CYP) monooxygenase system** is a family of enzymes that catalyzes the biotransformation of drugs with a wide range of chemical structures. The microsomal **monooxygenase reaction** requires the following: CYP (a hemoprotein); a flavoprotein that is reduced by nicotinamide adenine dinucleotide phosphate (NADPH), called NADPH CYP reductase; and membrane lipids in which the system is embedded. In the drug-oxidizing reaction, one atom of oxygen is used to form a hydroxylated metabolite of a drug, as shown in Figure 2–4, whereas the other atom of oxygen forms water when combined with electrons contributed by NADPH. The hydroxylated metabolite may be the end product of the reaction or serve as an intermediate that leads to the formation of another metabolite.

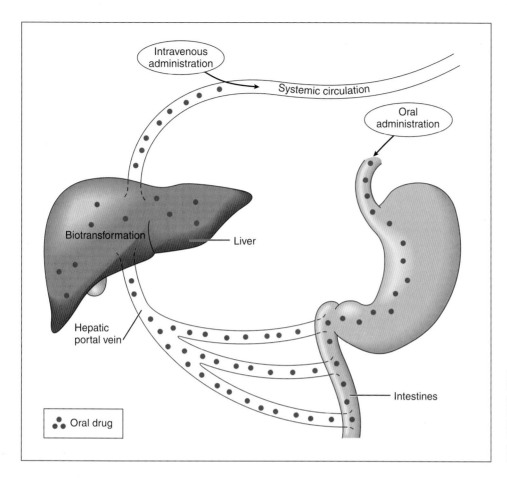

Figure 2-2. First-pass drug biotransformation. Drugs that are absorbed from the gut can be biotransformed by enzymes in the gut wall and liver before reaching the systemic circulation. This process lowers their degree of bioavailability.

The most common chemical reactions catalyzed by CYP enzymes are aliphatic hydroxylation, aromatic hydroxylation, N-dealkylation, and O-dealkylation.

Many **CYP isozymes** have been identified and cloned, and their role in metabolizing specific drugs elucidated. Each isozyme catalyzes a different but overlapping spectrum of oxidative reactions. Most drug biotransformation is catalyzed by three CYP families named CYP1, CYP2, and CYP3. The different CYP families are likely related by gene duplication and each family is divided into subfamilies, also clearly related by homologous protein sequences. The **CYP3A** subfamily catalyzes more than half of all microsomal drug oxidations.

Many drugs alter drug metabolism by inhibiting or inducing CYP enzymes, and **drug interactions** can occur when these drugs are administered concurrently with other drugs that are metabolized by CYP (see Chapter 4). Two examples of **inducers of CYP** are the barbiturate, **phenobarbital**, and the antitubercular drug, **rifampin**. The inducers stimulate the transcription of genes encoding CYP enzymes, resulting in increased messenger RNA (mRNA) and protein synthesis. Drugs that induce CYP enzymes activate the binding of **nuclear receptors** to enhancer domains of CYP genes, increasing the rate of gene transcription.

A few drugs are oxidized by **cytoplasmic enzymes.** For example, **ethanol** is oxidized to aldehyde by alcohol dehydrogenase, and **caffeine** and the bronchodilator **theophylline** are metabolized by xanthine oxidase. Other cytoplasmic

oxidases include **monoamine oxidase**, a site of action for some psychotropic medications.

HYDROLYTIC REACTIONS. Esters and amides are hydrolyzed by a variety of enzymes. These include cholinesterase and other plasma esterases that inactivate choline esters, local anesthetics, and drugs such as **esmolol** (BREVIBLOC), an agent for the treatment of tachycardia that blocks cardiac β_1-adrenoceptors. There are few CYP enzymes that carry out hydrolytic reactions.

REDUCTIVE REACTIONS. Reductive reactions are less common than are oxidative and hydrolytic reactions. **Chloramphenicol**, an antimicrobial agent, and a few other drugs are partly metabolized by a hepatic nitro reductase, and this process involves CYP enzymes. **Nitroglycerin**, a vasodilator, undergoes reductive hydrolysis catalyzed by glutathione-organic nitrate reductase.

Phase II Biotransformation

In phase II biotransformation, drug molecules undergo **conjugation reactions** with an endogenous substance such as **acetate, glucuronate, sulfate,** or **glycine** (Fig. 2–5). Conjugation enzymes, which are present in the liver and other tissues, join various drug molecules with one of these endogenous substances to form water-soluble metabolites that are more easily excreted. Except for microsomal **glucuronosyltransferases**, these enzymes are located in the

Description	Reaction	Examples
Oxidative reactions		
Aliphatic hydroxylation	$R-CH_2CH_3 \longrightarrow R-\overset{\overset{\displaystyle OH}{\mid}}{C}HCH_3$	Ibuprofen, pentobarbital, and tolbutamide
Aromatic hydroxylation	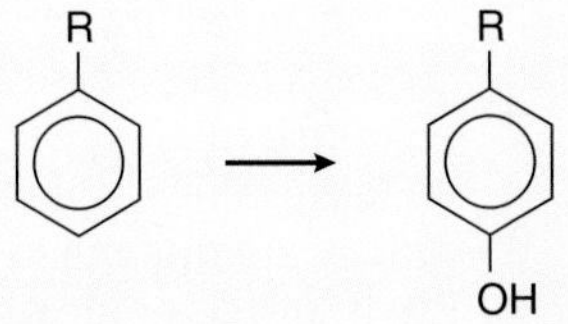	Phenobarbital, phenytoin, and propranolol
N-Dealkylation	$R-NHCH_3 \longrightarrow R-NH_2 + CH_2O$	Codeine, imipramine, and theophylline
O-Dealkylation	$R-OCH_3 \longrightarrow R-OH + CH_2O$	Codeine, dextromethorphan, and indomethacin
Deamination	$R-\overset{\overset{\displaystyle }{\mid}}{C}HCH_3 \longrightarrow R-C-CH_3 \longrightarrow R-C-CH_3 + NH_2$	Amphetamine and diazepam
N-Oxidation	$\begin{matrix}R_1\\ \quad NH\\R_2\end{matrix} \longrightarrow \begin{matrix}R_1\\ \quad N-OH\\R_2\end{matrix}$	Chlorpheniramine
S-Oxidation	$\begin{matrix}R_1\\ \quad S\\R_2\end{matrix} \longrightarrow \begin{matrix}R_1\\ \quad S=O\\R_2\end{matrix}$	Chlorpromazine and cimetidine
Hydrolytic reactions		
Amide hydrolysis	$R_1-\overset{\overset{\displaystyle O}{\parallel}}{C}NR_2 \longrightarrow R_1-COOH + R_2-NH_2$	Lidocaine and procainamide
Ester hydrolysis	$R_1-\overset{\overset{\displaystyle O}{\parallel}}{C}OR_2 \longrightarrow R_1-COOH + R_2-OH$	Aspirin, esmolol, and procaine
Reductive reactions		
Nitro reduction	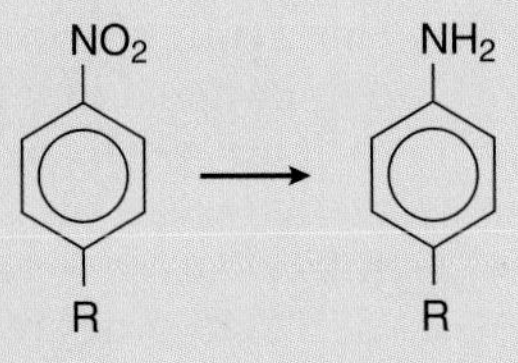	Chloramphenicol
Reductive hydrolysis	$R-ONO_2 \longrightarrow R-OH + NO_2^-$	Nitroglycerin

Figure 2-3. Phase I drug biotransformation. Many drugs are biotransformed by oxidative, hydrolytic, or reductive reactions and then undergo conjugation with endogenous substances. A few drugs bypass phase I reactions and directly enter phase II biotransformation.

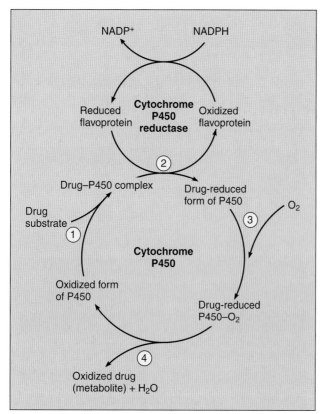

Figure 2-4. The CYP reductase mechanism for drug oxidation. Four steps are involved in the CYP reaction: First, the drug substrate binds to the oxidized form of P450 (i.e., Fe^{3+}). Second, the drug P450 complex is reduced by CYP reductase, using electrons donated by the reduced form of NADPH. Third, the drug-reduced form of P450 (i.e., Fe^{2+}) interacts with oxygen. Fourth, the oxidized drug (metabolite) and water are produced.

cytoplasm. Most conjugated drug metabolites are pharmacologically inactive.

GLUCURONIDE FORMATION. Glucuronide formation, the most common conjugation reaction, utilizes glucuronosyltransferases to conjugate a glucuronate molecule with the parent drug molecule.

ACETYLATION. Acetylation is accomplished by **N-acetyltransferase** enzymes that utilize acetyl coenzyme A (**acetyl CoA**) as a source of the acetate group.

SULFATION. Sulfotransferases catalyze the conjugation of several drugs, including the vasodilator **minoxidil** and the potassium-sparing diuretic **triamterene**, whose sulfate metabolites are pharmacologically active.

Pharmacogenomics

Since the completion of the human genome, it is now fully realized that there is a great degree of individual variation, called **polymorphism**, in the genes coding for drug-metabolizing enzymes. Modern genetic studies were triggered by rare fatalities in children being treating for leukemia using the thiopurine agent, 6-mercaptopurine (6-MP). It was discovered that the children died as a result of drug toxicity

because they expressed a faulty variant of thiopurine methyltransferase, the enzyme that metabolizes 6-MP.

Variations in Acetyltransferase Activity

Individuals exhibit slow or fast acetylation of some drugs because of genetically determined differences in N-acetyltransferase. Slow acetylators (SAs) were first identified by neuropathic effects of **isoniazid**, a drug to treat tuberculosis. These patients had higher plasma levels of isoniazid compared to other patients classified as rapid acetylators (RAs). The SA phenotype is autosomal recessive, although there are more than 20 allelic variants of the gene for N-acetyltransferase identified. In individuals with one wild-type enzyme and one faulty variant, an intermediate phenotype is observed. The **distribution** of these phenotypes varies from population to population. About 15% of Asians, 50% of Caucasians and Africans, and more than 80% of Mideast populations have the SA phenotype. Other drugs that may cause toxicity in the SA patient are **sulfonamide antibiotics**, the antiarrhythmic agent **procainamide**, and the antihypertensive agent **hydralazine.**

Variations in CYP2D6 and CYP2C19 Activity

Variations in oxidation of some drugs have been attributed to genetic differences in certain CYP enzymes. Genetic polymorphisms of CYP2D6 and CYP2C19 enzymes are well characterized, and human populations of "extensive metabolizers" and "poor metabolizers" have been identified. These differences are caused by more than 70 identified variants in the CYP2D6 gene and more than 25 variants of the CYP2C19 genes, resulting from point mutations, deletions, or additions; gene rearrangements; or deletion or duplication of the entire gene. This gives rise to an increase, reduction, or complete loss of enzyme activity and to different levels of enzyme expression that result in **altered rates** of enzymatic reactions.

Most individuals are extensive metabolizers of CYP2D6 substrates, but 10% of Caucasians and a smaller fraction of Asians and Africans are poor metabolizers of substrates for CYP2D6. Psychiatric patients who are poor metabolizers of CYP2D6 drugs have been found to have a higher rate of adverse drug reactions than do those who are extensive metabolizers because of higher psychotropic drug plasma levels. In addition, poor metabolizers of CYP2D6 drugs have a reduced ability to metabolize **codeine** to morphine sufficiently to obtain adequate pain relief when codeine is administered for analgesia.

Poor metabolizers of CYP2C19 substrates have higher plasma levels of proton pump inhibitors, such as **omeprazole** (PRILOSEC), whereas some extensive metabolizers of CYP2C19 drugs require larger doses of omeprazole to treat peptic ulcer.

Other Variations in Drug Metabolism Enzymes

About 1 of 3000 individuals exhibits a familial **atypical cholinesterase** that will not metabolize succinylcholine, a neuromuscular blocking agent, at a normal rate. Affected individuals are subject to prolonged apnea after receiving the usual dose of the drug. For this reason, patients should be screened for atypical cholinesterase before receiving succinylcholine.

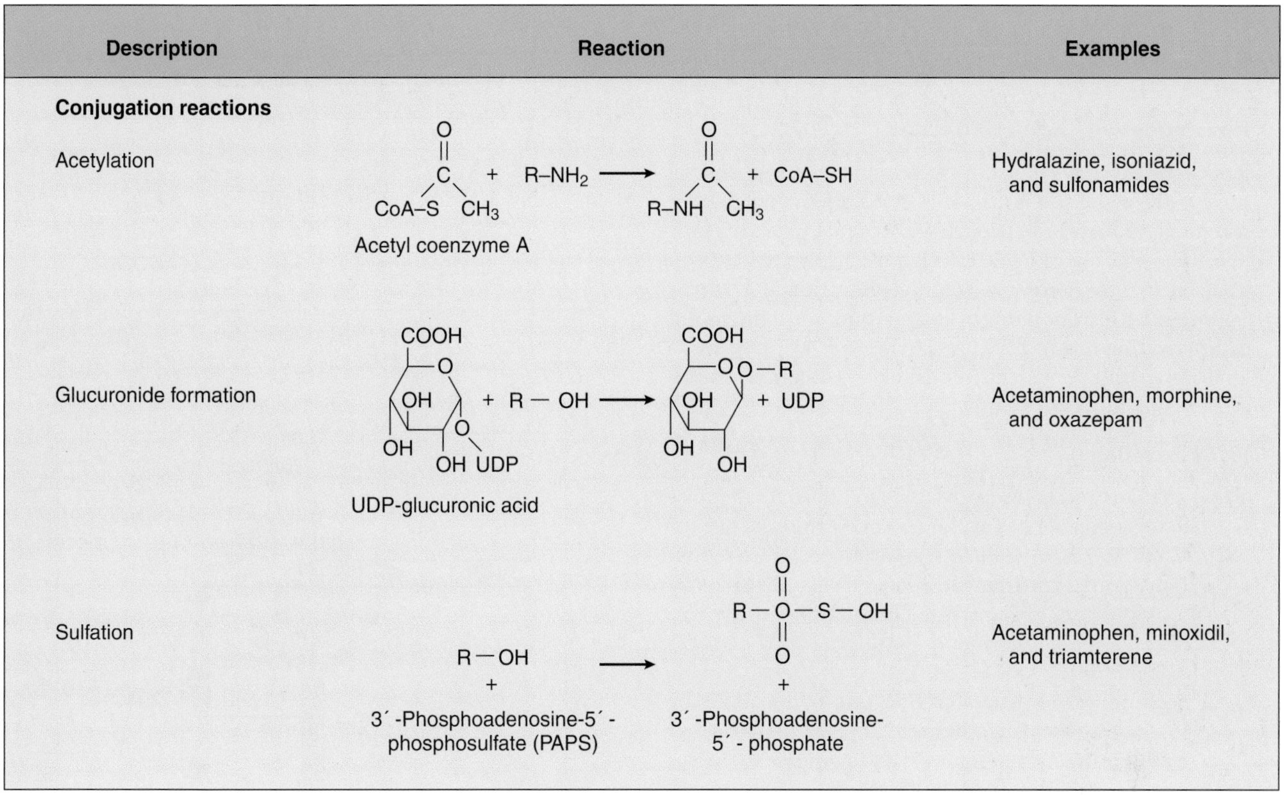

Description	Reaction	Examples
Conjugation reactions		
Acetylation	$\underset{\text{Acetyl coenzyme A}}{\underset{\text{CoA–S}}{\overset{\text{O}}{\underset{\text{CH}_3}{\|}}\text{C}} + \text{R–NH}_2 \longrightarrow \underset{\text{R–NH}}{\overset{\text{O}}{\underset{\text{CH}_3}{\|}}\text{C}} + \text{CoA–SH}}$	Hydralazine, isoniazid, and sulfonamides
Glucuronide formation	UDP-glucuronic acid $+ \text{R—OH} \longrightarrow + \text{UDP}$	Acetaminophen, morphine, and oxazepam
Sulfation	$\text{R—OH} + \text{3'-Phosphoadenosine-5'-phosphosulfate (PAPS)} \longrightarrow \underset{\text{O}}{\overset{\text{O}}{\text{R—O—S—OH}}} + \text{3'-Phosphoadenosine-5'-phosphate}$	Acetaminophen, minoxidil, and triamterene

Figure 2-5. Phase II drug biotransformation. UDP = uridine diphosphate.

There are many more polymorphisms in both phase I and phase II metabolic enzymes. With more than 30 families of drug-metabolizing enzymes, all with genetic variants, a major development in pharmacotherapy will be the individual tailoring of drug and dose to each patient's genomic identity.

DRUG EXCRETION

Excretion is the removal of drug from body fluids and occurs primarily in the **urine**. Other routes of excretion from the body include in bile, sweat, saliva, tears, feces, breast milk, and exhaled air.

Renal Drug Excretion

Most drugs are excreted in the urine, either as the parent compound or as a drug metabolite. Drugs are handled by the kidneys in the same manner as are endogenous substances, undergoing processes of glomerular filtration, active tubular secretion, and passive tubular reabsorption. The amount of drug excreted is the sum of the amounts filtered and secreted minus the amount reabsorbed. The relationship between these processes, the rate of drug excretion, and renal clearance is shown in Box 2–2.

Glomerular Filtration

Glomerular filtration is the first step in renal drug excretion. In this process, the free drug enters the renal tubule as a dissolved solute in the plasma filtrate (see Box 2–2). If a drug has a large fraction bound to plasma proteins, as is the case with the anticoagulant **warfarin**, it will have a low rate of glomerular filtration.

Active Tubular Secretion

Some drugs, particularly weak acids and bases, undergo active tubular secretion by transport systems located primarily in proximal tubular cells. This process is competitively inhibited by other drugs of the same chemical class. For example, the secretion of penicillins and other weak acids is inhibited by **probenecid**, an agent used to treat gout.

Active tubular secretion is not affected by plasma protein binding. This is due to the equilibrium of free drug and bound drug such that when free drug is actively transported across the renal tubule, this fraction of free drug is replaced by a fraction that dissociates from plasma proteins.

Passive Tubular Reabsorption

The extent to which a drug undergoes passive reabsorption across renal tubular cells and into the circulation depends on the **lipid solubility** of the drug. Drug biotransformation facilitates drug elimination by forming polar drug metabolites that are not as readily reabsorbed as the less-polar parent molecules.

Most nonelectrolytes, including **ethanol**, are passively reabsorbed across tubular cells. Ionized weak acids and bases are not reabsorbed across renal tubular cells, and they are more rapidly excreted in the urine than are non-ionized drugs that undergo passive reabsorption. The proportion of ionized and non-ionized drugs is affected by **renal tubular**

BOX 2–2. THE RENAL EXCRETION AND CLEARANCE OF A WEAK ACID, PENICILLIN G

Description and Chemical Structure

Penicillin G (benzylpenicillin) is an example of a weak acid. It has a pK_a of 2.8 and is primarily excreted via renal tubular secretion. About 60% of penicillin G is bound to plasma proteins. The pharmacokinetic calculations below are based on a urine **pH** of 5.8, a **plasma drug concentration** of 3 μg/mL, a **glomerular filtration rate** of 100 mL/min, and a **measured drug excretion rate** of 1200 μg/min. Because 40% of penicillin G is free (unbound), the **free drug plasma concentration** is 0.4 × 3 μg/mL = 1.2 μg/mL.

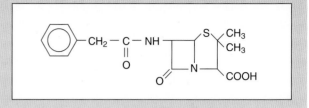

Renal Excretion

The discussion and accompanying figure illustrate the relationship between the rates of glomerular filtration, active tubular secretion, passive tubular reabsorption, and excretion.

1. **Filtration.** The **drug filtration rate** is calculated by multiplying the glomerular filtration rate by the free drug plasma concentration: 100 mL/min × 1.2 μg/mL = 120 μg/min.
2. **Secretion.** The **drug secretion rate** is calculated by subtracting the drug filtration rate from the drug excretion rate: 1200 μg/min − 120 μg/min = 1080 μg/min. This amount indicates that 90% of the drug's excretion occurs by the process of tubular secretion.
3. **Reabsorption.** The ratio of the non-ionized form to the ionized form of the drug in the urine is equal to the antilog of the pK_a minus the pH: antilog of 2.8 − 5.8 = antilog of −3 = 1:1000. Because most of the drug is ionized in the urine, the **drug reabsorption rate** is probably <1 μg/min.
4. **Excretion.** The drug excretion rate was initially given as 1200 μg/min. It was determined by measuring the drug concentration in urine and multiplying it by the urine flow rate. Note that the drug excretion rate is equal to the drug filtration rate (120 μg/min) plus the drug secretion rate (1080 μg/min) minus the drug reabsorption rate (<1 μg/min).

Renal Clearance

Renal clearance is calculated by dividing the excretion rate (1200 μg/min) by the plasma drug concentration (3 μg/mL). The result is 400 mL/min, which is equal to 24 L/h.

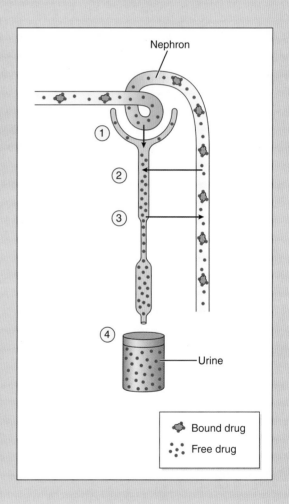

---

pH, which can be manipulated to increase the excretion of a drug after a drug overdose (Box 2–3).

Biliary Excretion and Enterohepatic Cycling

Many drugs are excreted in the bile as the parent compound or a drug metabolite. Biliary excretion favors compounds with molecular weights that are higher than 300 and with both polar and lipophilic groups; smaller molecules are excreted only in negligible amounts. Conjugation, particularly with **glucuronate**, increases biliary excretion.

Numerous conjugated drug metabolites, including both the glucuronate and sulfate metabolites of steroids, are excreted in the bile. After the bile empties into the intestines, a fraction of the drug may be reabsorbed into the circulation and eventually return to the liver. This phenomenon is called **enterohepatic cycling** (Fig. 2–6). Excreted conjugated drugs can be hydrolyzed back to the parent drug by intestinal bacteria, and this facilitates the drug's reabsorption. Thus, biliary excretion eliminates substances from the body only to the extent that enterohepatic cycling is incomplete, that is, when some of the excreted drug is not reabsorbed from the intestine.

If a drug or other compound is a weak acid or base, its degree of ionization and rate of renal excretion will depend on its pK_a and on the pH of the renal tubular fluid. The rate of excretion of a **weak acid** can be accelerated by **alkalinizing the urine**, whereas the rate of excretion of a **weak base** can be accelerated by **acidifying the urine.** These procedures have been used to enhance the excretion of drugs and poisons, but they are not without risk to the patient, and their benefits have been established for only a few drugs.

To make manipulation of the urine pH worthwhile, a drug must be excreted to a large degree by the kidneys. The short-acting barbiturates (e.g., secobarbital) are eliminated almost entirely via biotransformation to inactive metabolites, so modification of the urine pH has little effect on their excretion. In contrast, phenobarbital is excreted to a large degree by the kidneys, so urine alkalinization is useful in treating an overdose of this drug. Urine acidification to enhance the elimination of weak bases (e.g., amphetamine), has been largely abandoned because it does not significantly increase the elimination of these drugs and poses a serious risk of metabolic acidosis.

In cases involving an overdose of aspirin or other salicylate, alkalinization of the urine produces the dual benefits of increasing drug excretion and counteracting the metabolic acidosis that occurs with serious aspirin toxicity. For patients suffering from phenobarbital overdose or from herbicide 2,4-dichlorophenoxyacetic acid poisoning, alkalinization of the urine is also helpful: this is accomplished by administering sodium bicarbonate intravenously every 3 to 4 hours to increase the urinary pH to 7–8.

Other Routes of Excretion

Sweat and saliva represent minor routes of excretion for some drugs. In pharmacokinetic studies, saliva measurements are sometimes used because the saliva concentration of a drug often reflects the intracellular concentration of the drug in target tissues.

QUANTITATIVE PHARMACOKINETICS

To derive and use expressions for pharmacokinetic parameters, the first step is to establish a mathematical model that accurately relates the plasma drug concentration to the rates of drug absorption, distribution, and elimination. The **one-compartment model** is the simplest model of drug disposition, but the **two-compartment model** provides a more accurate representation of the pharmacokinetic behavior of many drugs (Fig. 2–7). With the one-compartment model, drug undergoes absorption into the blood according to the rate constant, k_a, and elimination from the blood with a rate constant, k_e. In the two-compartment model, drugs are absorbed into the central compartment (blood), distributed from the central compartment to the peripheral compartment (the tissues), and eliminated from the central compartment. Regardless of the model used, rate constants can be determined for each process and used to derive expressions for other pharmacokinetic parameters, such as the **elimination half-life ($t_{1/2}$)** of a drug. In this section, the most important parameters of pharmacokinetics are explained in greater detail.

Drug Plasma Concentration Curves

Figure 2–8A shows a standardized **drug plasma concentration curve** over time after oral administration of a typical drug. The Y-axis is a linear scale of drug plasma

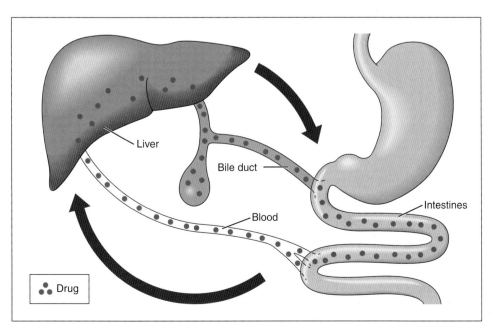

Figure 2-6. Enterohepatic cycling. Drugs and drug metabolites with molecular weights higher than 300 may be excreted via the bile, stored in the gallbladder, delivered to the intestines by the bile duct, and then reabsorbed into the circulation. This process reduces the elimination of a drug and prolongs its half-life and duration of action in the body.

Liver

Bile duct

Blood

Intestines

Drug

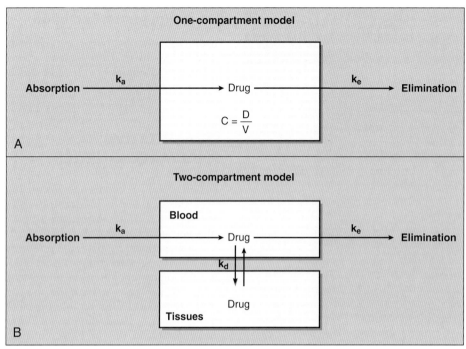

Figure 2-7. **Two models of the processes of drug absorption, distribution, and elimination.** k_a, k_d, and k_e are the rate constants, representing the fractional completion of each process per unit of time. (A) In the one-compartment model, the drug concentration at any time, C, is the amount of drug in the body at that time, D, divided by the volume of the compartment, V. Thus, D is a function of the dose administered and the rates of absorption and elimination represented by k_a and k_e, respectively. (B) In the two-compartment model, the drug concentration in the central compartment (the blood) is a function of the dose administered and the rates of drug absorption, distribution to the peripheral compartment (the tissues), and elimination from the central compartment.

concentration, often in μg/mL or mg/L, and the X-axis is a time scale, usually in hours. Parameters of the plasma drug concentration curve are the **maximum concentration** (C_{max}), the time needed to reach the maximum (T_{max}), the **minimum effective concentration** (**MEC**), and the **duration of action**. A measure of the total amount of drug during the time course is given by the **area under the curve** (**AUC**). These measures are useful for comparing the **bioavailability** of different pharmaceutical formulations or of drugs given by different routes of administration.

Bioavailability (F)

Bioavailability is defined as the **fraction** (**F**) of the administered dose of a drug that reaches the systemic circulation in an active form. As shown in Figure 2–8B, the oral bioavailability of a particular drug is determined by dividing the AUC of an orally administered dose of the drug (AUC_{oral}) by the AUC of an intravenously administered dose of the same drug (AUC_{IV}). By definition, an intravenously administered drug has 100% bioavailability. The bioavailability of drugs administered intramuscularly or via other routes can be determined in the same manner as the bioavailability of drugs administered orally.

The bioavailability of orally administered drugs is of particular concern because it can be reduced by many pharmaceutical and biologic factors. Pharmaceutical factors include the rate and extent of tablet disintegration and drug dissolution. Biologic factors include the effects of food, which can sequester or inactivate a drug; the effects of gastric acid,

which can inactivate a drug; and the effects of gut and liver enzymes, which can metabolize a drug during its absorption and first pass through the liver. The CYP3A4 isozyme found in intestinal enterocytes and hepatic cells is a particularly important catalyst of first-pass drug metabolism. CYP3A4 works in conjunction with Pgp (described in the section titled "Drug Distribution") as the 3A4 isozyme located in enterocytes inactivates drugs transported into the intestinal lumen by Pgp.

Volume of Distribution

The volume of distribution (V_d) is defined as the volume of fluid in which a drug would need to be dissolved to have the **same concentration** as it does in plasma. The V_d does not represent the volume in a particular body fluid compartment (Fig. 2–9A); instead, as shown in Figure 2–9B, it is an apparent volume that represents the relationship between the dose of a drug and the resulting plasma concentration of the drug.

Calculation of V_d

After intravenous drug administration, the plasma drug concentration falls rapidly at first, as the drug is distributed from the central compartment to the peripheral compartment. The V_d is calculated by dividing the dose of a drug given intravenously by the plasma drug concentration immediately after the distribution phase (α). As shown in Figure 2–9C, this drug concentration can be determined by extrapolating the plasma drug concentration back to time

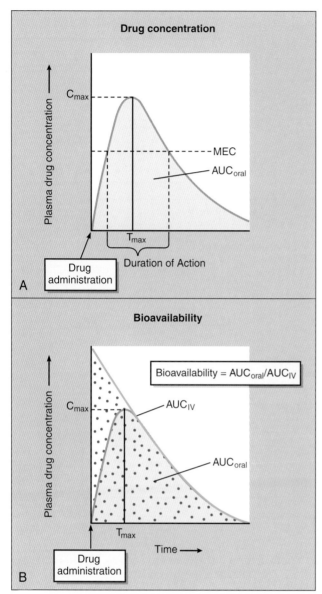

Figure 2-8. Plasma drug concentration and drug bioavailability. The plasma drug concentration curve for a single dose of a drug given orally (A) shows C_{max}, t_{max}, MEC, the duration of action, and AUC. (B) To determine bioavailability, F, the AUC of the AUC_{oral}, is divided by the AUC of the intravenously administered drug, AUC_{IV}.

zero from the linear part of the elimination phase (β). Note that the Y-axis in this case is plotted on a **log scale** so that the exponential elimination phase is converted to a straight line. The plasma drug concentration at time zero (C_0) represents the plasma concentration of a drug that would be obtained if it were instantaneously dissolved in its V_d. The equation for calculating V_d is rearranged to determine the dose of a drug that is required to establish a specified plasma drug concentration (see Box 2–4).

Interpretation of V_d

Although the V_d does not correspond to an actual body fluid compartment, it does provide a measure of the extent of distribution of a drug. A low V_d that approximates plasma

volume or extracellular fluid volume usually indicates that the drug's distribution is restricted to a particular compartment (the plasma or extracellular fluid). The anticoagulant **warfarin** has a V_d of about 8 L, which reflects a high degree of plasma protein binding. When the V_d of a drug is equivalent to total body water (about 40 L, as occurs with ethanol), this usually indicates that the drug has reached the intracellular fluid as well.

Some drugs have a V_d that is much larger than total body water. A large V_d may indicate that the drug is concentrated intracellularly, with a resulting low concentration in the plasma. Many weak bases, such as the antidepressant **fluoxetine** (PROZAC), have a large V_d (40–55 L) because of the phenomenon of intracellular **ion trapping.** Weak bases are less ionized within plasma than they are within cells because intracellular fluid usually has a lower pH than extracellular fluid. After a weak base diffuses into a cell, a larger fraction is ionized in the more acidic intracellular fluid. This restricts its diffusion out of a cell and results in a large V_d.

A large V_d may also result from sequestration into fat tissue, such as occurs with the antimalarial agent **chloroquine.**

Drug Clearance

Clearance (**Cl**) is the most fundamental expression of drug elimination. It is defined as the volume of body fluid (blood) from which a drug is removed per unit of time. Whereas the clearance of a particular drug is **constant**, it is important to note that the amount of drug contained in the clearance volume will **vary** with the plasma drug concentration.

RENAL CLEARANCE. Renal clearance can be calculated as the renal excretion rate divided by the plasma drug concentration (see Box 2–2). Drugs that are eliminated primarily by glomerular filtration, with little tubular secretion or reabsorption, will have a renal clearance that is approximately equal to the creatinine clearance, which is normally about 100 mL/min in an adult. A renal drug clearance that is higher than the creatinine clearance indicates that the drug is a substance that undergoes tubular secretion. A renal drug clearance that is lower than the creatinine clearance suggests that the drug is highly bound to plasma proteins or that it undergoes passive reabsorption from the renal tubules.

HEPATIC CLEARANCE. Hepatic clearance is more difficult to determine than renal clearance. This is because hepatic drug elimination includes the biotransformation and biliary excretion of parent compounds. For this reason, hepatic clearance is usually determined by multiplying hepatic blood flow by the arteriovenous drug concentration difference.

SINGLE DOSE PHARMACOKINETICS

First-Order Kinetics

Most drugs exhibit **first-order kinetics**, in which the rate of drug elimination (amount of drug eliminated per unit time) is proportional to the plasma drug concentration and follows an exponential decay function. Note that the rate of

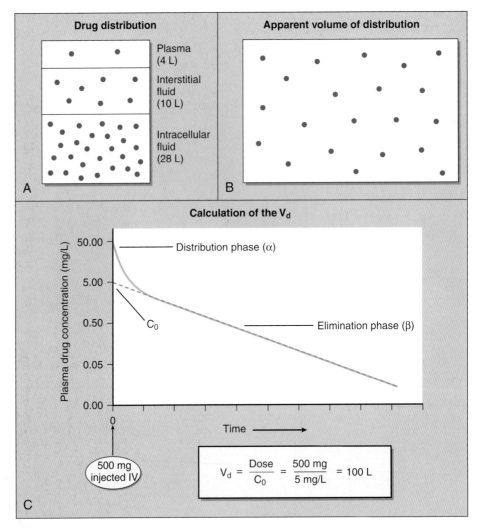

Figure 2–9. Calculating the volume of distribution (V_d) of a drug. Unlike the physiologic distribution of a drug (A), the calculated V_d of a drug is an apparent volume that can be defined as the volume of fluid in which a drug would need to be dissolved to have the same concentration in that volume as it does in the plasma (B). The graph (C) provides an example of how the V_d is calculated. In this example, a dose of 500 mg was injected intravenously at time zero, and plasma drug concentrations were measured over time. The terminal elimination curve (β) was extrapolated back to time zero to determine that the plasma drug concentration at time zero, C_0, was 5 mg/L. Then the V_d was calculated by dividing the dose by the C_0. In this case, the result was 100 L.

drug elimination is not the same as the elimination rate constant, k_e (fraction of drug eliminated per unit time). A few drugs (e.g., ethanol) exhibit **zero-order kinetics**, in which the rate of drug elimination is constant and independent of plasma drug concentration (see Fig. 2–10B).

For drugs that exhibit first-order kinetics, the plasma drug concentration can be determined from the dose of a drug and its clearance. Because the plasma drug concentration is often correlated with the magnitude of a drug's effect, it is possible to use pharmacokinetic expressions to determine and adjust drug dosages to achieve a desired therapeutic effect (see Box 2–4).

The following principles pertain to first-order kinetics: A drug's rate of elimination is equal to the plasma drug concentration multiplied by the drug clearance; the elimination rate declines as the plasma concentration declines (see Fig. 2–10A); and the half-life and clearance of the drug remain constant as long as renal and hepatic function do not change.

Elimination Half-Life ($t_{1/2}$)

Elimination half-life ($t_{1/2}$) is the time required to reduce the plasma drug concentration by 50%. It can be calculated from the elimination rate constant, but it is usually

determined from the plasma drug concentration curve (Fig. 2–11). The half-life can also be expressed in terms of the drug's clearance and volume of distribution, indicating that the drug's half-life will change when either of these factors is altered. The formula for relating half-life to clearance and volume of distribution is given in the legend of Figure 2–11. Disease, age, and other physiologic variables can alter drug clearance or volume of distribution and thereby change the elimination half-life (see Chapter 4).

Zero-Order Kinetics

The following principles pertain to zero-order kinetics: The rate of drug elimination is constant (see Fig. 2–10B); the drug's elimination half-life is **proportional** to the plasma drug concentration; the clearance is **inversely proportional** to the drug concentration; and a small increase in dosage can produce a disproportionate increase in the plasma drug concentration.

In many cases, the reason that the rate of drug elimination is constant is that the elimination process becomes **saturated**. This occurs, for example, at most plasma concentrations of **ethanol**. In some cases, drugs exhibit zero-order elimination when high doses are administered, which occurs, for example, with **aspirin** and the anticonvulsant

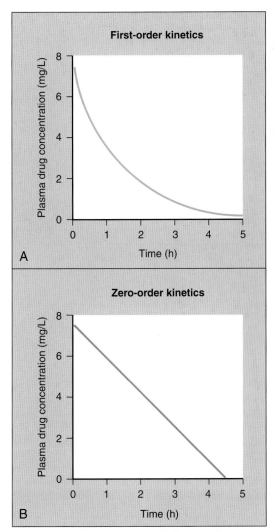

Figure 2-10. The kinetic order of drugs. In first-order kinetics (A), the rate of drug elimination is proportional to the plasma drug concentration. In zero-order kinetics (B), the rate of drug elimination is constant. The kinetic order of a drug is derived from the exponent, n, in the following expression:

$$\Delta[\text{Drug}]/\Delta t = - k_e [\text{Drug}]^n$$

where Δ represents change, [Drug] represents the plasma drug concentration, and t is time. If n is 1, then $\Delta[\text{Drug}]/\Delta t$ is proportional to [Drug]. If n is 0, then $\Delta[\text{Drug}]/\Delta t$ is constant (k_e), because $[\text{Drug}]0$ equals 1.

phenytoin (DILANTIN) or when a hepatic or renal disease has impaired the drug elimination processes.

CONTINUOUS DOSE AND MULTIPLE DOSE KINETICS

Drug Accumulation and the Steady-State Principle

When a drug that exhibits first-order pharmacokinetics is administered to a patient continuously or intermittently, the drug will accumulate until it reaches a plateau or steady-state plasma drug concentration.

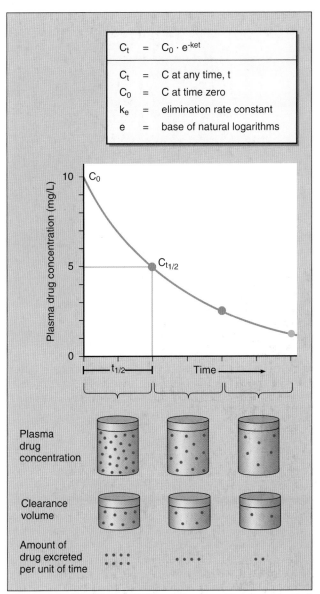

Figure 2-11. Drug half-life and clearance. The elimination half-life ($t_{1/2}$) is the time required to reduce the plasma drug concentration (C) by 50%. The formula is as follows:

$$t_{1/2} = 0.693/k_e$$

where 0.693 is the natural logarithm of 2, and k_e is the elimination rate constant. The half-life is often determined from the plasma drug concentration curve shown here. The clearance (Cl) is the volume of fluid from which a drug is eliminated per unit of time. It can be calculated as the product of the volume of distribution, V_d, and k_e. If $0.693/t_{1/2}$ is substituted for ke, the equation is as follows:

$$Cl = 0.693\, V_d/t_{1/2}$$

Thus, a drug's clearance is directly proportional to its volume of distribution and is inversely proportional to its half-life.

The basis for this accumulation to a steady state is shown in Figure 2–12. When the drug is first administered, the rate of administration is much greater than the rate of elimination, because the plasma concentration is so low. As the drug continues to be administered, the rate of drug elimination gradually increases, whereas the rate of administration

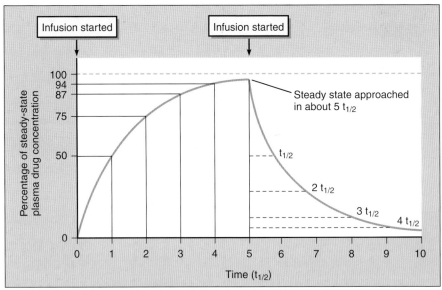

Figure 2–12. Drug accumulation to the steady state. The time required to reach the steady state depends on the half-life ($t_{1/2}$); it does not depend on the dose or dose interval. The steady-state drug concentration depends on the drug dose administered per unit of time and on the drug's clearance or half-life.

remains constant. Eventually, as the plasma concentration rises sufficiently, the rate of drug elimination equals the rate of drug administration. At this point, the **steady-state equilibrium** is achieved.

Time Required to Reach the Steady-State Condition

Drug accumulation to a steady state is a first-order process and therefore obeys the rule that half of the process is completed in a defined time. Because the time to reach the steady state is dependent on the time it takes for the rate of drug elimination to equal to the rate of drug administration, the time to reach the steady state is a function of the elimination half-life of the drug. Any first-order process requires about five half-lives to be completed; thus the time to reach the steady-state drug concentration is about five drug half-lives. If the half-life of a drug changes, then the time required to reach the steady-state also changes. Note that the time required to reach the steady state is independent both of the drug dose and the rate or frequency of drug administration.

Steady-State Drug Concentration

The steady-state drug concentration depends on the drug dose administered per unit of time and on the half-life of the drug. Figure 2–13 illustrates typical plasma concentration curves after drugs are administered continuously or intermittently. If the dose is doubled, the steady-state concentration is also doubled (Fig. 2–13A). Likewise, if the half-life is doubled, the steady-state concentration is doubled (Fig. 2–13B).

A drug administered intermittently will accumulate to a steady state at the same rate as a drug given by continuous infusion, but the plasma drug concentration will fluctuate as each dose is absorbed and eliminated. The average steady-state plasma drug concentration with intermittent intravenous administration will be the same as if the equivalent dose were administered by continuous infusion (Fig. 2–13C). A comparison of the steady-state drug levels following continuous intravenous infusion, multiple oral doses, and a single oral dose is shown in Figure 2–13D. With intermittent oral administration, the bioavailability of the drug will also influence the steady-state plasma concentration.

Dosage Calculations

The methods for calculating both the loading dose and the maintenance dose are given in Box 2–4.

Loading Dose

A loading dose, or **priming dose**, is given to rapidly establish a therapeutic plasma drug concentration. The loading dose can be calculated by multiplying the volume of distribution by the desired plasma drug concentration. The loading dose, which is larger than the maintenance dose, is generally administered as a single dose, but it can be divided into fractions that are given over several hours. A **divided loading dose** is sometimes used for drugs that are more toxic, for example, **digitalis glycosides** used to treat congestive heart failure.

Maintenance Dose

A maintenance dose is given to establish or maintain the **desired steady-state** plasma drug concentration. For drugs given intermittently, the maintenance dose is one of a series of doses administered at regular intervals. The amount of drug to be given is based on the principle that at the steady state, the rate of drug administration equals the rate of drug elimination. To determine the rate of drug elimination, the drug clearance is multiplied by the average steady-state plasma drug concentration. The maintenance dose is then calculated as the rate of drug elimination multiplied by the dosage intervals. If the drug is administered orally, its bioavailability must also be included in the equation.

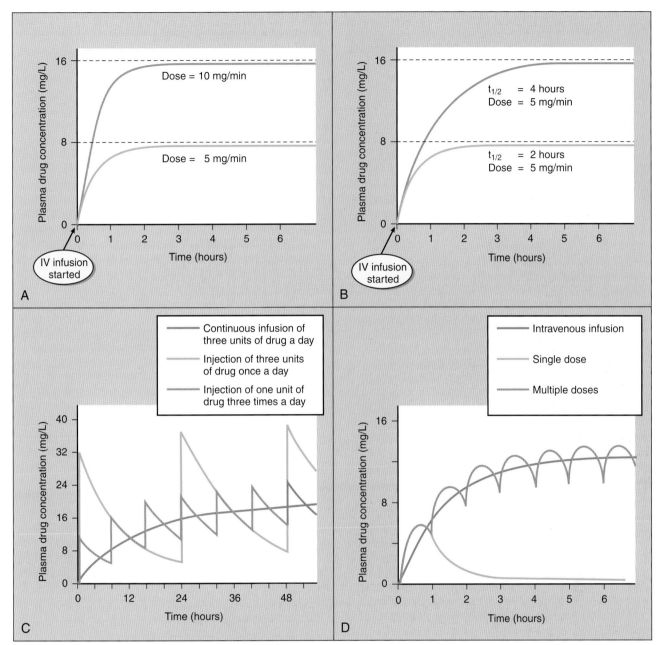

Figure 2-13. Plasma drug concentrations after continuous or intermittent drug administration. (A) The steady-state plasma drug concentration is proportional to the dose administered per unit of time. (B) The steady-state plasma drug concentration is directly proportional to the half-life (and is inversely related to clearance). (C) The average steady-state concentration is the same for intermittent infusion as it is for continuous infusion. With intermittent drug administration, however, the plasma concentrations fluctuate between doses, and the size of fluctuations increases as the dosage interval increases. (D) Plasma drug concentrations after intermittent oral administration are affected by the rates of drug absorption, distribution, and elimination. If only one dose is given, the peak in plasma drug concentration is followed by a continuous decline in the curve.

BOX 2–4. DRUG DOSAGE CALCULATIONS

Loading Dose

The loading dose, or priming dose, of a drug is determined by multiplying the **volume of distribution** (V_d) of the drug by the **desired plasma drug concentration** (desired C). (This information can be found in the medical literature.) For theophylline, for example, the estimated V_d for an adult weighing 70 kg is 35 L, and the desired C is 15 mg/L. The calculation is as follows:

$$\text{Loading dose} = V_d \times C$$
$$= 35L \times 15\,mg/L$$
$$= 525\,mg$$

As is discussed in Chapter 4 (see Table 4–5), the patient's age can affect the V_d and, therefore, should be considered in determining the appropriate loading dose for a particular patient.

Maintenance Dose

Calculations of the maintenance dose must take into consideration the **intended frequency of drug administration.** With intermittent administration, the fluctuations in C increase as the dosage interval increases. A twofold fluctuation in C will occur when the dosage interval is equal to the drug's half-life. This is because the C will fall 50% between doses. For many drugs, the half-life is a convenient and acceptable dosage interval.

The maintenance dose is designed to establish or maintain a **desired steady-state C.** The amount of drug to be given is based on the principle that at the steady state, the rate of drug administration equals the rate of drug elimination. The rate of elimination is equal to the clearance multiplied by the steady-state drug concentration. For example, if the steady-state gentamicin concentration is 2 mg/L and the clearance for gentamicin is 100 mL/min (0.1 L/min), then the elimination rate is 0.1 L/min × 2 mg/L = 0.2 mg/min. If the drug is to be administered every 8 hours, then the dosage would be calculated as follows:

$$\text{Maintenance dose} = \text{Hourly rate}$$
$$\times \text{dosage interval in hours}$$
$$= 0.2\,mg/min$$
$$\times 60\,\text{minutes in an hour}$$
$$\times 8\,\text{hours}$$
$$= 96\,mg\,\text{every 8 hours}$$

If a drug is to be administered orally, the calculated dose must be divided by the fractional bioavailability to determine the administered dose.

Dosage Adjustment Using Pharmacokinetic Values

First, choose the target C and administer the initial dose on the basis of the standard published values (general population values) for clearance or V_d. Second, measure the patient's plasma drug levels and calculate the patient's V_d and clearance. Third, revise the dosage based on the patient's V_d and clearance.

SUMMARY OF IMPORTANT POINTS

■ Most drugs are absorbed by passive diffusion across or between cells. The rate of passive diffusion of a drug across cell membranes is proportional to the drug's lipid solubility and the surface area available for absorption. Only the non-ionized form of weak acids and bases is lipid soluble.

■ The ratio of the ionized form to the non-ionized form of a weak acid or base can be determined from the pK_a of the drug and the pH of the body fluid in which the drug is dissolved.

■ The distribution of a drug is influenced by organ blood flow and by the plasma protein binding, molecular size, and lipid solubility of the drug. Only drugs with high lipid solubility can penetrate the blood-brain barrier.

■ The volume of distribution is the volume of fluid in which a drug would need to be dissolved to have the same concentration in that volume as it does in plasma. It is calculated by dividing the drug dose by the plasma drug concentration at time zero.

■ Many drugs are biotransformed before excretion. Drug metabolites can be pharmacologically active or inactive. Phase I reactions include oxidative, reductive, and hydrolytic reactions, whereas phase II reactions conjugate a drug with an endogenous substance. The CYP enzymes located in the endoplasmic reticulum of liver cells are the most important oxidative metabolic enzymes.

■ Most drugs are excreted in the urine, either as the parent compound or as drug metabolites, and undergo the processes of glomerular filtration, active tubular secretion, and passive tubular reabsorption. The renal clearance of a drug can be calculated by dividing the renal excretion rate by the plasma drug concentration.

■ Most drugs exhibit first-order kinetics, in which the rate of drug elimination is proportional to the plasma drug concentration at any given time. If drug elimination mechanisms (biotransformation and excretion) become saturated, a drug can exhibit zero-order kinetics, in which the rate of drug elimination is constant.

■ In first-order kinetics, a drug's half-life and clearance are constant as long as physiologic elimination processes are constant. The half-life is the time required for the plasma drug concentration to decrease by 50%. The clearance is the volume of plasma from which a drug is eliminated per unit of time.

■ The oral bioavailability of a drug is the fraction of the administered dose that reaches the circulation in an active form. It is determined by dividing the AUC after oral administration by the AUC after intravenous administration. Factors that reduce bioavailability include incomplete tablet disintegration and first-pass and gastric inactivation of a drug.

■ With continuous or intermittent drug administration, the plasma drug concentration increases until it reaches a steady-state condition, in which the rate of drug elimination is equal to the rate of drug administration. It takes about four to five drug half-lives to achieve the steady-state condition.

■ The steady-state drug concentration can be calculated as the dose per unit of time divided by the clearance, and this equation can be rearranged to determine the dose per unit of time required to establish a specified steady-state drug concentration.

■ A loading dose is a single or divided dose given to rapidly establish a therapeutic plasma drug concentration. The dose can be calculated by multiplying the volume of distribution by the desired plasma drug concentration.

Review Questions

1. If food decreases the rate but not the extent of the absorption of a particular drug from the gastrointestinal tract, then taking the drug with food will result in a smaller
   (A) area under the plasma drug concentration time curve
   (B) maximal plasma drug concentration
   (C) time at which the maximal plasma drug concentration occurs
   (D) fractional bioavailability
   (E) total clearance

2. If a drug exhibits first-order elimination, then
   (A) the elimination half-life is proportional to the plasma drug concentration
   (B) the drug is eliminated at a constant rate
   (C) hepatic drug metabolizing enzymes are saturated
   (D) drug clearance will increase if the plasma drug concentration increases
   (E) the rate of drug elimination (mg/min) is proportional to the plasma drug concentration

3. After a person ingests an overdose of an opioid analgesic, the plasma drug concentration is found to be 32 mg/L. How long will it take to reach a safe plasma concentration of 2 mg/L if the drug's half-life is 6 hours?
   (A) 12 hours
   (B) 24 hours
   (C) 48 hours
   (D) 72 hours
   (E) 1 week

4. What dose of a drug should be injected intravenously every 8 hours to obtain an average steady-state plasma drug concentration of 5 mg/L if the drug's volume of distribution is 30 L and its clearance is 8 L/h?
   (A) 40 mg
   (B) 80 mg
   (C) 160 mg
   (D) 320 mg
   (E) 400 mg

5. The volume of distribution of a drug will be greater if the drug
   (A) is more ionized inside cells than in plasma
   (B) is administered very rapidly
   (C) is highly ionized in plasma
   (D) has poor lipid solubility
   (E) has a high molecular weight

Answers and Explanations

1. **The answer is B:** the maximal plasma drug concentration. If the rate of drug absorption is reduced, then the maximal plasma drug concentration will be less because more time will be available for drug distribution and elimination while the drug is being absorbed. Moreover, the time at which the maximal plasma drug concentration occurs will increase. If the extent of drug absorption (fraction absorbed) does not change, then the area under the curve and fractional bioavailability will not change.

2. **The answer is E:** the rate of drug elimination (mg/min) is proportional to the plasma drug concentration. In first-order elimination, drug half-life and clearance do not vary with the plasma drug concentration, but the rate of drug elimination (quantity per time) is proportional to plasma drug concentration at any time.

3. **The answer is B:** 24 hours. The half-life is the time required to reduce the plasma drug concentration 50%. In this case, it will take four drug half-lives, or 24 hours, to reduce the plasma level from 32 to 2 mg/L.

4. **The answer is D:** 320 mg. The dose required to establish a target plasma drug concentration is calculated by multiplying the clearance by the target concentration and dosage interval. In this case, it is 5 mg/L × 8 L/h × 8 hours = 320 mg.

5. **The answer is A:** is more ionized inside cells than in plasma. When a drug is more ionized inside cells, the drug becomes sequestered in the cells and the volume of distribution can become quite large. This is called ion-trapping.

SELECTED READINGS

Birkett, D.J. Pharmacokinetics Made Easy, 2nd ed. Roseville, Australia, McGraw-Hill Australia, 2002.

Guengerich, F.P. Cytochromes P450, drugs, and diseases. Mol Interv 3: 194–204, 2003.

Handschin, C., and U.A. Meyer. Induction of drug metabolism: the role of nuclear factors. Pharmacol Rev 55:649–673, 2003.

Levine, R.R. Pharmacology: Drug Actions and Reactions, 6th ed. New York, Parthenon, 2000.

Weinshilboum, R.M., and L. Wang. Pharmacogenetics and pharmacogenomics: development, science, and translation. Annu Rev Genomics Hum Genet 7:223–245, 2006.

CHAPTER 3

Pharmacodynamics

OVERVIEW

Pharmacodynamics is the study of the detailed **mechanism of action** by which drugs produce their pharmacological effects. This study starts at the binding of a drug to its target receptor or enzyme, continues through a **signal transduction** pathway by which the receptor activates **second messenger** molecules, and ends with the ultimate description of intracellular processes altered by the impact of the drug. There is also a quantitative aspect to pharmacodynamics in characterizing the **dose-response curve**, which is the relationship between drug dose and the magnitude of the pharmacological effect. Pharmacodynamics provides a scientific basis for the selection and use of drugs to counteract specific pathophysiologic changes due to disease or trauma.

NATURE OF DRUG RECEPTORS

Drugs produce their effects by interacting with specific cell molecules called receptors. By far, most **ligands** (drugs or neurotransmitters) bind to **protein** molecules, although some agents act directly on DNA or membrane lipids (Table 3–1).

Types of Drug Receptors

The largest family of receptors for pharmaceutical agents is **G protein–coupled receptors,** (**GPCRs**). These membrane-spanning proteins consist of four extracellular, seven transmembrane, and four intracellular domains (Fig. 3–1). Extracellular domains and, to some extent, transmembrane regions determine ligand binding and selectivity. Intracellular loops, especially the third one, mediate the receptor interaction with its **effector molecule**, a **guanine nucleotide binding protein (G protein)**.

A number of ligands inhibit the function of specific **enzymes** by competitive or noncompetitive inhibition. A ligand that binds to the same active, catalytic site as the endogenous substrate is a **competitive inhibitor.** Ligands that bind at a different site on the enzyme and alter the shape of the molecule, thereby reducing its catalytic activity, are called **noncompetitive inhibitors.**

Drugs also target **membrane transport proteins,** including ligand- and voltage-gated ion channels and neurotransmitter transporters. At ligand-gated ion channels, drugs can bind at the same site as the endogenous ligand and directly compete for the receptor site. Drugs can also bind at a different site, an **allosteric site**, that alters the response of the endogenous ligand binding to the ligand-gated ion channel and increase or decrease the flow of ions. Some drugs directly bind and inactivate **voltage-gated ion channels**; these are ion channel proteins that do not have an endogenous ligand (as ligand-gated ion channels do) but open or close as a function of the membrane voltage potential. **Neurotransmitter transporter proteins** are large, 12-transmembrane domain proteins that transfer neurotransmitter molecules out of the synapse and back into the neuron. A large group of agents, known generally as **re-uptake inhibitors**, target these transport proteins.

Steroid hormone receptors are intracellular proteins that translocate to the nucleus upon ligand (steroid) binding. In the nucleus, the steroid-receptor complex alters the transcription rate of specific genes. DNA is also a receptor site for ligands that bind directly to **nucleic acids**, most notably the antineoplastic agents. Other macromolecules that serve as receptors include the various lipids and phospholipids that make up the membrane. Some of the effects of general anesthetics and alcohol are due to interaction with membrane lipids.

Receptor Classification

Drug receptors are classified according to **drug specificity, tissue location,** and, more recently, by their **primary amino acid sequence**. For example, adrenoceptors were initially divided into two types (α and β), based on their affinity for norepinephrine, epinephrine, and other agents in different tissues. Subsequently, the distinction between the types was confirmed by the development of selective antagonists that blocked either α-adrenoceptors or β-adrenoceptors. Later, the two types of receptors were divided into subtypes, based on more subtle differences in agonist potency, tissue distribution, and varying effects.

At present, most receptors for drug targets and endogenous ligands are cloned and their amino acid sequences determined. There are also numerous other receptor-like proteins predicted from the human genome for which an endogenous ligand is not identified, called **orphan receptors.**

The orphan receptors are of great interest to pharmaceutical companies as they represent targets for the development of new drugs. Families of receptors types are grouped by their sequence similarity using bioinformatics and this classification supports results from earlier in vivo and in vitro functional studies. In many cases, each type of receptor corresponds to a single, unique gene with subtypes of receptors arising from different transcripts of the same gene by the process of **alternative splicing.**

DRUG-RECEPTOR INTERACTIONS

Receptor Binding and Affinity

To initiate a cellular response, a drug must first bind to a receptor. In most cases, drugs bind to their receptor by forming **hydrogen, ionic,** or **hydrophobic** (Van der Waals) bonds with a receptor site (Fig. 3–2). These weak bonds are reversible and enable the drug to dissociate from the receptor as the tissue concentration of the drug declines. The binding of drugs to receptors often exhibits **stereospecificity,** so that only one of the stereoisomers will form a three-point attachment with the receptor. In a few cases, drugs form relatively permanent covalent bonds with a specific receptor. This occurs, for example, with antineoplastic drugs that bind to DNA and with drugs that irreversibly inhibit the enzyme cholinesterase.

The tendency of a drug to combine with its receptor is called **affinity,** which is a measure of the strength of the drug-receptor complex. According to the **law of mass action,** the number of receptors $[R]$ occupied by a drug depends on the drug concentration $[D]$ and the drug-receptor association and dissociation rate constants (k_1 and k_2):

$$[D] + [R] \underset{k_2}{\overset{k_1}{\rightleftharpoons}} [D\text{-}R] \longrightarrow \text{Effect}$$

The ratio of k_2 to k_1 is known as the K_D and represents the drug concentration required to saturate 50% of the receptors. The lower the K_D is, the greater is the drug's affinity for the receptor. Most drugs have a K_D in the micromolar to nanomolar (10^{-6} to 10^{-9} M) range of drug concentrations.

TABLE 3–1. Drug Receptors

Types of Drug Receptors	Examples of Drugs that Bind Receptors
Hormone and Neurotransmitter Receptors	
Adrenoceptors	Epinephrine and propranolol
Histamine receptors	Cimetidine and diphenhydramine
5-Hydroxytryptamine (serotonin) receptors	LSD and sumatriptan
Insulin receptors	Insulin
Muscarinic receptors	Atropine and bethanechol
Opioid receptors	Morphine and naltrexone
Steroid receptors	Cortisol and tamoxifen
Enzymes	
Carbonic anhydrase	Acetazolamide
Cholinesterase	Donepezil and physostigmine
Cyclooxygenase	Aspirin and celecoxib
DNA polymerase	Acyclovir and zidovudine
DNA topoisomerase	Ciprofloxacin
Human immunodeficiency virus (HIV) protease	Indinavir
Monoamine oxidase	Phenelzine
Na⁺-K⁺-adenosine triphosphatase	Digoxin
Xanthine oxidase	Allopurinol
Membrane Transport Proteins	
Ligand-gated ion channels	Diazepam and ondansetron
Voltage-gated ion channels	Lidocaine and verapamil
Ion transporters	Furosemide and hydrochlorothiazide
Neurotransmitter transporters	Fluoxetine and cocaine
Other Macromolecules	
Membrane lipids	Alcohol and amphotericin B
Nucleic acids	Cyclophosphamide and doxorubicin

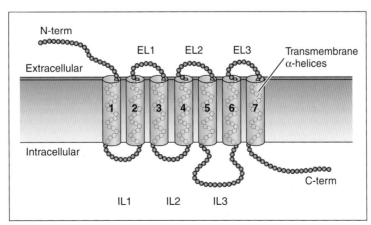

Figure 3–1. Structure of a typical GPCR. All GPCRs consist of a long polypeptide chain of amino acids threaded through the cell membrane with seven transmembrane (TM) domains. These TM domains are arranged in α-helices composed of hydrophobic residues. The N-terminal of the receptor protein is outside the cell and the C-terminal is on the inside. Three extracellular loops (ELs) and three intracellular loops (ILs) are formed by this configuration. The protein in the cell membrane forms a circle with TM1 and TM7 in close proximity but is shown here in a two-dimensional view for clarity.

As discussed below, receptor **affinity** is the primary determinant of drug **potency**.

Signal Transduction

Signal transduction describes the pathway from ligand binding to conformational changes in the receptor, receptor interaction with an effector molecule (if present), and other downstream molecules called second messengers. This cascade of receptor-mediated biochemical events ultimately leads to a physiologic effect (Table 3–2).

G PROTEIN–COUPLED RECEPTORS (GPCRS). The signal transduction pathway for GPCRs is well understood. These receptors constitute a superfamily of receptors for many endogenous ligands and drugs, including receptors for acetylcholine, epinephrine, histamine, opioids, and serotonin. Figure 3–3 illustrates **signal transduction** for a receptor that is coupled with G proteins.

The **heterotrimeric** G proteins have three subunits, known as G_α, G_β, and G_γ. The G_α subunit serves as the site of guanosine triphosphate (GTP) hydrolysis, a process catalyzed by innate GTPase activity, which acts to terminate the signal (see Fig. 3–3). Several types of G_α subunits exist, each of which determines a specific cellular response. For example, the $\mathbf{G_{\alpha s}}$ (stimulating) subunit **increases** adenylyl cyclase activity and thereby stimulates the production of cyclic adenosine monophosphate (**cyclic AMP**, or **cAMP**). The $\mathbf{G_{\alpha i}}$ (inhibitory) subunit **decreases** adenylyl cyclase activity and inhibits the production of cAMP. Another G protein ($\mathbf{G_{\alpha q}}$) **activates phospholipase C** and leads to the formation of **inositol triphosphate** ($\mathbf{IP_3}$) and **diacylglycerol** (**DAG**) from membrane phospholipids. IP_3 and DAG further cause an **elevation of Ca^{+2} ions** inside the cell. Several other types of G_α subunits are also present in cells and activated by receptors. The G_β, and G_γ subunits are so tightly bound together that they do not dissociate and are therefore written as $\mathbf{G_{\beta\gamma}}$. The $G_{\beta\gamma}$ also has signaling function when separated from G_α upon ligand-receptor activation, for example, by altering K^+ or Ca^{+2} channel conductance.

The **second messengers** cAMP, IP_3, DAG, and Ca^{+2} activate or inhibit unique cellular enzymes in each target cell. Cyclic AMP activates a number of tissue-specific **cAMP-dependent protein kinases**. These kinases **phosphorylate** other enzymes or proteins that ultimately affect intracellular processes such as ion channel activity, release of neurotransmitter, regulation of transcription, and numerous other processes. For example, one of the best studied kinases, **protein kinase A**, is activated by the increase of cAMP produced by epinephrine binding to β_2-adrenoceptors in muscle. Protein kinase A phosphorylates the enzyme **glycogen phosphorylase**, which then increases the breakdown of glycogen to free glucose, providing the fuel needed by the muscles to respond to the event that initiated the release of epinephrine.

IP_3 and DAG evoke the release of calcium from intracellular storage sites and thereby augment calcium-mediated processes such as **muscle contraction**, **glandular secretion**, and **neurotransmitter release**. The increased intracellular Ca^{+2} ions also activate calcium-dependent **kinases** and a number of other enzyme cascades.

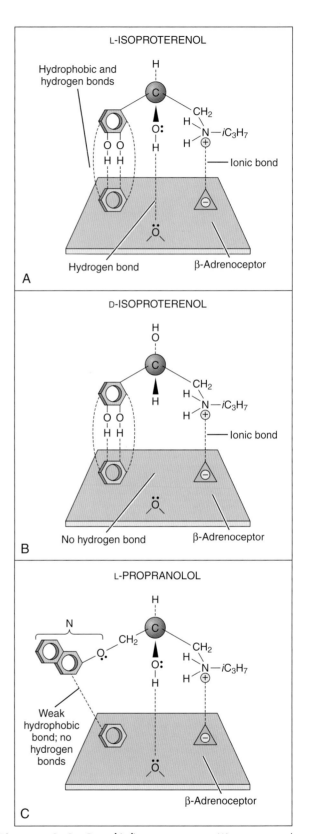

Figure 3–2. Drug binding to receptors. (A) L-isoproterenol, a β-adrenoceptor agonist, forms hydrogen, ionic, and hydrophobic (Van der Waals) bonds with three sites on the β-adrenoceptor. (B) D-isoproterenol binds to two sites on the β-adrenoceptor but is unable to bind with the third site. (C) L-Propranolol, a β-adrenoceptor antagonist, binds to two sites on the receptor in the same way that L-isoproterenol does. The naphthyloxy group (N) forms weak bonds with the third receptor site, but these are not sufficiently strong for the drug to have intrinsic (agonist) activity. iC_3H_7 = isopropyl.

TABLE 3-2. **Examples of Receptors and Signal Transduction Pathways**

Family and Type of Receptor	Mechanism of Signal Transduction	Example of Effect in Tissue or Cell
G Protein–Coupled Receptors		
α_1-Adrenoceptor	Activation of phospholipase C	Vasoconstriction
α_2-Adrenoceptor	Inhibition of adenylyl cyclase	Release of norepinephrine decreased
β-Adrenoceptor	Stimulation of adenylyl cyclase	Heart rate increased
Muscarinic receptor	Activation of phospholipase C	Glandular secretion increased
Ligand-Gated Ion Channels		
$GABA_A$ receptors	Chloride ion flux	Hyperpolarization of neuron
Nicotinic receptors	Sodium ion flux	Skeletal muscle contraction
Membrane-Bound Enzymes		
Atrial natriuretic factor receptors	Stimulation of guanylyl cyclase	Sodium excretion increased
Insulin receptors	Activation of tyrosine kinase	Glucose uptake stimulated
Nuclear Receptors		
Steroid receptors	Activation of gene transcription	Reduced cytokine production
Thyroid hormone receptors	Activation of gene transcription	Oxygen consumption increased

GABA = γ-aminobutyric acid.

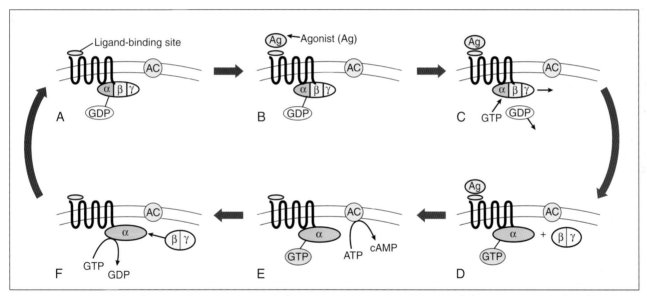

Figure 3-3. Signal transduction with a G protein–coupled receptor. (A) A typical G protein–coupled receptor contains a ligand-binding site on the external surface of the plasma membrane and a G protein–binding site on the internal surface. In the inactive state, guanosine diphosphate (GDP) is bound to the G_α subunit of the G protein. (B) and (C) When the agonist (Ag) binds to the receptor, guanosine triphosphate (GTP) binds to the G protein and causes the dissociation of GDP. (D) Activation of the G_α subunit by GTP causes the dissociation of the G_β and G_γ subunits. (E) The G_α subunit is then able to activate adenylyl cyclase (AC) and thereby stimulate the conversion of adenosine triphosphate (ATP) to cyclic adenosine monophosphate (cAMP). (F) GTP hydrolysis, catalyzed by G_α subunit GTPase, leads to reassociation of the G_α and the G_β and G_γ subunits.

LIGAND-GATED ION CHANNELS. Ligand-gated ion channels are a large class of membrane proteins that share similar subunit structure and are assembled in tetrameric or pentameric structures. Drugs that bind to ligand-gated ion channels alter the **conductance (g)** of ions through the channel protein. In this case there are no second messengers directly activated by the drug binding to a ligand-gated ion channel, but the resulting changes in intracellular ion concentrations may regulate other enzyme signaling cascades.

MEMBRANE-BOUND ENZYMES. Membrane-bound enzymes that serve as receptors for various endogenous substances and drugs are classified into five types: receptor **guanylyl cyclases,**

receptor **tyrosine kinases, tyrosine-kinase–associated** receptors, receptor **tyrosine phosphatases,** and receptor **serine/ threonine kinases.** The first type, receptor **guanylyl cyclases,** is the target for **atrial natriuretic factor** (ANF) and related peptides, and consists of a single transmembrane domain protein with an extracellular domain that is the binding site for ANF and intracellular domain that has guanylyl cyclase activity. Binding of ANF produces direct activation of guanylyl cyclase and increase of intracellular cyclic guanosine monophosphate (cGMP), which, like cAMP signaling, activates specific cGMP-dependent kinases.

The second type of membrane-bound enzyme receptors is the class of receptor **tyrosine kinases.** There are a large number of ligands that activate these receptors including epidermal growth factor, nerve growth factor, and insulin. These receptors are composed of a single transmembrane protein, with an extracellular binding domain, and in this case, an intracellular domain with **tyrosine kinase** activity. When a growth factor or insulin binds to its receptor, kinase activity phosphorylates tyrosine residues of the receptor protein itself, causing **dimerization** of two receptors. The dimerized receptor then goes on to phosphorylate a number of intracellular enzymes and proteins at tyrosine residues and alters the activity of resulting enzyme cascades.

The other types of membrane-bound enzyme receptors initiate signaling in much the same way but have different ligands and different substrates as their signaling targets.

NUCLEAR RECEPTORS. The nuclear receptor family consists of **two types** of receptors that have similar protein structure. Parts of the receptor protein, called **domains**, are homologous (contain similar amino acid sequence) among all nuclear receptor family members and include an N-terminal variable domain, a DNA binding domain, a hinge region, and a C-terminal hormone binding domain. **Type I nuclear receptors** include targets for sex hormones (androgen, estrogen, and progesterone receptors), glucocorticoid receptors, and mineralocorticoid receptors. These steroid receptors are located inside the cell, bound to accessory **heat-shock proteins** and activated by steroids that diffuse through the cell membrane. Upon activation, the heat-shock protein dissociates and two steroid-receptor proteins **dimerize** and **translocate** to the nucleus. **Type II nuclear receptors** include receptors for nonsteroid ligands including thyroid hormone, vitamin A and D receptors, and retinoid receptors. These receptors are already present in the nucleus and are activated by the ligand entering the nucleus through nuclear pores.

Once activated, both types of receptors bind to specific DNA sequences upstream of genes and initiate transcription. A schematic of **steroid hormone signaling** is shown in Figure 3–4.

Efficacy

The ability of a drug to initiate a cellular effect is called **intrinsic activity** or **efficacy**. Efficacy is not directly related to receptor affinity and differs among various drugs that bind to a receptor and start the signal transduction pathway. Drugs that have both receptor affinity and efficacy are called **agonists**, whereas drugs that have receptor affinity but lack efficacy are called **antagonists**. With a few classes of drugs, such as agonists and antagonists at the β-adrenoceptor, the specific molecular structures responsible for affinity and efficacy are identified. Both agonists and antagonists have common components sufficient for receptor affinity, but only agonists have the structure required for efficacy (see Fig. 3–2).

There are three types of agonists. **Full agonists** can produce the maximal response obtainable in a tissue and therefore have maximal efficacy. **Partial agonists** can produce only a submaximal response. In the presence of a full agonist, a partial agonist will act like an antagonist because it will prevent the full agonist from

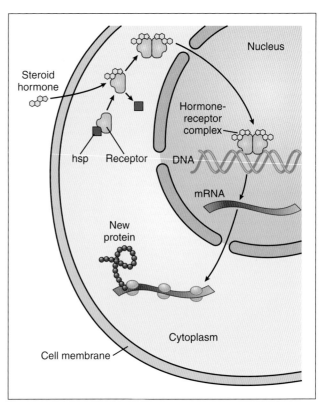

Figure 3–4. **Signal transduction with a steroid hormone receptor.** Steroid hormones diffuse through the cell membrane and bind to steroid receptors in the cytoplasm. Binding of the steroid ligand displaces accessory heat-shock proteins (hsp) and allows steroid receptor dimerization. The dimerized steroid hormone–receptor complex is translocated to the nucleus and binds to specific sequences on the DNA upstream of a gene, leading to increased transcription of a gene, mRNA, and translation of proteins.

binding the receptor and exerting a maximal response. **Inverse agonists**, which are also called **negative antagonists**, are involved in a special type of drug-receptor interaction. The effect of inverse agonists is based on the finding, in some cases, that signal transduction proceeds at a basal rate in the absence of any ligand binding to the receptor. A **full agonist increases** the rate of signal transduction when it binds to the receptor, whereas an **inverse agonist decreases** the rate of signal transduction. Only a few inverse agonists are identified, and some drugs that bind to the GABA$_A$ receptor located in the central nervous system are examples (see Chapter 19). Antagonists can prevent the action of agonists and inverse agonists by occupying binding sites on the receptor. **Competitive antagonists** bind to the same site as the agonist on the receptor but are reversibly bound. **Noncompetitive antagonists** block the agonist site irreversibly, usually by forming a covalent bond.

Receptor Regulation and Drug Tolerance

Receptors can undergo dynamic changes with respect to their **density** (number per cell) and their **affinity** for drugs and other ligands. The continuous or repeated exposure to agonists can desensitize receptors, usually by phosphorylating serine or threonine residues in the C-terminal domain of GPCRs. Phosphorylation of the receptor reduces the G protein–coupling efficiency and alters their binding affinity. This short-term effect of agonist exposure is called **desensitization** or **tachyphylaxis. Phosphorylation** also signals the cell to internalize the membrane receptor. By **internalization** and regulation of the receptor gene, the number of receptors on the cell membrane decreases. This longer-term adaptation is called **down-regulation**. In contrast, continuous or repeated exposure to antagonists initially can increase the response of the receptor, called **supersensitivity**. With chronic exposure to antagonists, the number of receptors on the membrane surface (density) increases via **up-regulation**.

Drug tolerance is seen when the same dose of drug given repeatedly loses its effect or when greater doses are needed to achieve a previously obtained effect. Receptor down-regulation is often responsible for **pharmacodynamic tolerance**, which describes adaptations to chronic drug exposure at the tissue and receptor level. Pharmacodynamic tolerance is distinct from **pharmacokinetic tolerance** in that the latter is caused by accelerated drug elimination, usually due to an up-regulation of the enzymes that metabolize the drug.

Disease states can alter the number and function of receptors and thereby affect the response to drugs. For example, **myasthenia gravis** is an autoimmune disorder in which antibodies destroy the nicotinic receptors in skeletal muscle, leading to impaired neurotransmission and muscle weakness. This condition is treated by administration of nicotinic receptor agonists (see Chapter 6).

DOSE-RESPONSE RELATIONSHIPS

In pharmacodynamic studies, different doses of a drug can be tested in a group of subjects or in isolated organs, tissues, or cells. The relationship between the concentration of a drug at the receptor site and the magnitude of the response is called the **dose–response relationship**. Depending on the purpose of the studies, this relationship can be described in terms of a **graded** (continuous) response or a **quantal** (all-or-none) response.

Graded Dose-Response Relationships

In graded dose-response relationships, the response elicited with each dose of a drug is described in terms of a percentage of the **maximal response** and is plotted against the **log dose** of the drug (Fig. 3–5). Graded dose-response curves illustrate the relationship between drug dose, receptor occupancy, and the magnitude of the resulting physiologic effect. For a given drug, the maximal response is produced when all of the receptors are occupied, and the half-maximal response is produced when 50% of the receptors are occupied. In some cases, fewer than 50% of total receptors will be occupied but still give the half-maximal response. This is because only a fraction of the total receptors are needed to produce the maximal response. The remaining unbound receptors are considered to be **spare receptors**.

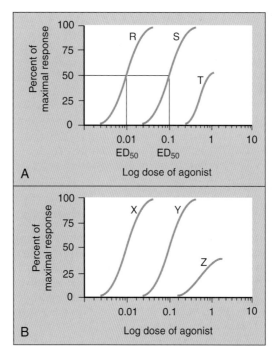

Figure 3–5. Graded dose-response relationships. (A) The dose-response curves of three agonists (R, S, and T) are compared. Drugs R and S are full agonists. Both have maximal efficacy, but R is more potent than S. Drug T is a partial agonist and, therefore, is incapable of producing the same magnitude of effect as a full agonist. T is also less potent than R and S. ED_{50} = median effective dose. (B) The effects that antagonists have on an agonist's dose-response curve are compared. X = agonist alone; Y = agonist in the presence of a competitive antagonist; Z = agonist in the presence of a noncompetitive antagonist.

Potency is a characteristic of drug action useful for comparing different pharmacologic agents. It is usually expressed in terms of the **median effective dose (ED_{50})**, which is the dose that produces 50% of the maximal response. For in vitro experiments, this value may also be expressed as EC_{50} (effective concentration for 50% effect). The potency of a drug varies inversely with ED_{50} of a drug, so that a drug with an ED_{50} of 4 mg is 10 times more potent than a drug whose ED_{50} is 40 mg. Potency is largely determined by the affinity of a drug for its receptor, because drugs with greater affinity require a lower dose to occupy 50% of the functional receptors (or less if spare receptors are present).

The maximal response produced by a drug is known as its **efficacy**. A **full agonist** has maximal efficacy, whereas a **partial agonist** has less than maximal efficacy and is incapable of producing the same magnitude of effect as a full agonist, even at the very highest doses (see Fig. 3–5A). When a partial agonist is administered with an agonist, the partial agonist may act as an antagonist by preventing the agonist from binding to the receptor and thereby reducing its effect. An antagonist, by definition, has no efficacy in this sense but can be an effective medication, as in the use of a β-adrenoceptor antagonist (β-blocker) to treat hypertension.

The effect that an **antagonist** has on the dose-response curve of an agonist depends on whether the antagonist is competitive or noncompetitive (see Fig. 3–5B).

A **competitive antagonist** binds reversibly to a receptor, and its effects are surmountable if the dose of the agonist is increased sufficiently. A competitive antagonist shifts the agonist's dose-response curve to the right, but it does not reduce the maximal response. Although a **noncompetitive antagonist** also shifts the agonist's dose-response curve to the right, it binds to the receptor in a way that reduces the ability of the agonist to elicit a response. The amount of reduction is in proportion to the dose of the antagonist. The effects of a noncompetitive antagonist cannot be overcome or surmounted with greater doses of an agonist.

Quantal Dose-Response Relationship

In quantal dose-response relationships, the response elicited with each dose of a drug is described in terms of the cumulative percentage of subjects exhibiting a defined **all-or-none effect** and is plotted against the **log dose** of the drug (Fig. 3–6). An example of an all-or-none effect is sleep or not-asleep when a sedative-hypnotic agent is given. With quantal dose-response curves, the ED_{50} is the dose that produces the observed effect in 50% of the experimental subjects.

Quantal relationships can be defined for both toxic and therapeutic drug effects to allow calculation of the **therapeutic index (TI)** and the **certain safety factor (CSF)** of a drug. The TI and CSF are based on the difference between the toxic dose and the therapeutic dose in a population of subjects. The TI is defined as the ratio between the median lethal dose (LD_{50}) and the ED_{50}. It provides a general indication of the margin of safety of a drug, but the CSF is a more realistic estimate of drug safety (see Fig. 3–6). The CSF is defined as the ratio between the dose that is lethal in 1% of subjects (LD_1) and the dose that produces a therapeutic effect in 99% of subjects (ED_{99}). When phenobarbital was tested in animals, for example, it was found to have a TI of 10 and a CSF of 2. Because the dose that will kill 1% of animals is twice the dose that is required to produce the therapeutic effect in 99% of animals, the drug has a good margin of safety.

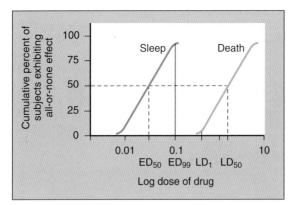

Figure 3–6. Quantal dose-response relationships. The dose-response curves for a therapeutic effect (sleep) and a toxic effect (death) of a drug are compared. The ratio of the LD_{50} to the ED_{50} is the therapeutic index. The ratio of the LD_1 to the ED_{99} is the certain safety factor. ED = effective dose; LD = lethal dose.

SUMMARY OF IMPORTANT POINTS

■ Most drugs form reversible, stereospecific bonds with macromolecular receptors located in target cells.

■ The tendency of a drug to bind to a receptor, called affinity, is directly related to potency. The affinity of a drug is often expressed as the K_D, which is the drug concentration required to saturate 50% of the functional receptors.

■ The ability of a drug to initiate a response is called intrinsic activity or efficacy. Agonists have both affinity and efficacy, whereas antagonists only have receptor affinity.

■ Graded dose-response curves show the relationship between the dose and the magnitude of the drug effect in a group of subjects or in a particular tissue, organ, or type of cell. The median effective dose (ED_{50}) produces 50% of the maximal response.

■ Both a competitive antagonist and a noncompetitive antagonist will cause a rightward shift in the dose-response curve of an agonist, but only a noncompetitive antagonist will reduce the maximal response of the agonist.

■ Quantal dose-response curves show the relationship between the dose and the cumulative percentage of subjects exhibiting an all-or-none effect. The ratio of the median lethal dose (toxic dose) to the median effective dose (therapeutic dose) is called the therapeutic index, which is an indication of the margin of safety of a drug.

Review Questions

1. The description of molecular events initiated with the ligand binding and ending with a physiologic effect is called
   (A) receptor down-regulation
   (B) signal transduction pathway
   (C) ligand-receptor binding
   (D) law of mass action
   (E) intrinsic activity or efficacy

2. G protein–coupled receptors that activate an inhibitory G_α subunit alter the activity of adenylyl cyclase to
   (A) increase the coupling of receptor to G protein
   (B) block the ligand from binding
   (C) initiate the conversion of GTP to GDP
   (D) generate intracellular inositol triphosphate
   (E) decrease the production of cAMP

3. The law of mass action explains the relationship between
   (A) dose of drug and physiologic response
   (B) the concentration of drug and the association or dissociation of drug-receptor complex
   (C) receptors and the rate of signal transduction
   (D) an enzyme and ligands that inhibit the enzyme
   (E) graded and quantal dose-response curves

4. In a log dose–response plot, drug efficacy is determined by the maximal height of the measured response on the effect axis, whereas drug potency is determined by
   (A) number of animals exhibiting an all-or-none response
   (B) signal transduction pathway
   (C) formula, including the affinity of the drug and the number of drug receptors
   (D) position of the curve along the log-dose axis
   (E) steepness of the dose-response curve

5. A partial agonist is best described as an agent that
   (A) has low potency but high efficacy
   (B) acts as both an agonist and antagonist
   (C) interacts with more than one receptor type
   (D) cannot produce the full effect, even at high doses
   (E) blocks the effect of the antagonist

Answers and Explanations

1. **The correct answer is B:** the signal transduction pathway. Pharmacodynamics is the study of the detailed molecular pathway starting from the drug (ligand) binding to its receptor, the activation of effector molecules (e.g., G proteins), and the generation of second messengers, which ultimately produce an effect that can be measured at the cell, tissue, or whole animal level. This process is called the signal transduction pathway.

2. **The correct answer is E:** decrease the production of cAMP. Adenylyl cyclase is an enzyme that converts ATP to cyclic AMP (cAMP). GPCRs that activate inhibitory (G_α) subunits are known to inhibit adenylyl cyclase and, therefore, reduce the generation of cAMP. cAMP is the second messenger in this system, even though in this case its levels are decreased. Activated G_α subunits also have direct effects on ion channels.

3. **The correct answer is B:** the relationship of the concentration of drug and the association or dissociation of drug-receptor complex. The law of mass action is used to derive the affinity of a drug for its receptor and is noted as the K_D. The K_D, which is the equilibrium dissociated constant, comes from the kinetic rate (k_2) of drug-receptor dissociation divided by the rate (k_1) of drug-receptor association.

4. **The correct answer is D:** the position of the curve along the log-dose axis. Potency and efficacy can be determined from a graph of the log dose–response curve by visual inspection. The height of the curve along the effect or y-axis is a measure of efficacy. The placement of the curve along the log-dose axis or x-axis determines potency such that curves to the left represent more potent drugs than curves to the right. This is because curves to the left give rise to smaller doses of a drug needed to reach 50% effect, or ED_{50}. The ED_{50} is a measure of the drug's potency but says nothing of efficacy. Whereas some agents are potent and efficacious, these two characteristics of drug action are not necessarily correlated. It is possible to have an agent that is highly potent but does not have great efficacy.

5. **The correct answer is D:** cannot produce the full effect, even at high doses. An agonist acts at its receptor to activate the signal transduction pathway and produce an effect. An antagonist binds to its receptor, produces no effect at the receptor but rather blocks the receptor so that agonists cannot bind and produce an effect. A partial agonist binds to the receptor and activates the signal transduction pathway, but not to the maximal degree. Because the degree that a ligand activates its receptor is called its efficacy, it is clear that partial agonists do not have full efficacy.

SELECTED READINGS

Acconcia, F., and R. Kumar. Signaling regulation of genomic and nongenomic functions of estrogen receptors. Cancer Lett 238:1–14, 2006.

Fredriksson, R., M.C. Lagerström, L.G. Lundin, and H.B. Schiöth. The G-protein-coupled receptors in the human genome form five main families: phylogenetic analysis, paralogon groups, and fingerprints. Mol Pharmacol 63:1256–1272, 2003.

Gainetdinov, R.R., R.T. Premont, L.M. Bohm, R.J. Lefkowitz, and M.G. Caron. Desensitization of G protein-coupled receptors and neuronal functions. Annu Rev Neurosci 27:107–144, 2004.

Landry, Y., and J.P.Gies. Drugs and their molecular targets: an updated overview. Fundam Clin Pharmacol 22:1–18, 2008.

Oldham, W.M., and H.E. Hamm. Heterotrimeric G protein activation by G-protein-coupled receptors. Nat Rev Mol Cell Biol 9:60–71, 2008.

CHAPTER 4

Drug Development and Safety

OVERVIEW

The arrival of a new drug launched with a massive advertisement campaign and clever commercials does little to illuminate the highly regulated process that drugs go through to make it to the market. The overwhelming success in modern pharmacotherapy in treating disease states attests to the safety and efficacy of prescribed agents. However, drugs can also be poisons causing unwanted **adverse effects**, and drugs can kill. This chapter begins with a description of drug development and the processes for evaluating drug safety and efficacy and then discusses the various types of adverse effects and interactions that are caused by drugs. Considerations for specific populations, such as the neonate and the elderly, are highlighted, and the laws relating to drug use and abuse are briefly reviewed.

DRUG DEVELOPMENT

Drug development in most countries has many features in common, beginning with the discovery and characterization of a new drug and proceeding through the clinical investigations that ultimately lead to regulatory approval for marketing the drug. Steps in the process of drug development in the United States are depicted in Figure 4–1.

Discovery and Characterization

New drug compounds are either synthesized *de novo*, isolated from a natural product, or a combination of the two as in semi-synthetic compounds. Synthetic drugs may be patterned after other drugs with known pharmacologic activity, or their structure may be designed to bind a particular receptor and based on computer modeling of the drug and receptor. Because the likely activity of some new compounds is relatively uncertain, they must be submitted to a battery of screening tests to determine their effects. There are cases in which a particular pharmacologic activity of a drug was discovered accidentally after the drug was administered to patients for other purposes. For example, the antihypertensive effect of clonidine was discovered when tested for treatment of nasal congestion

and a profound hypotensive episode ensued. This led to the subsequent development of clonidine for treating hypertension.

Preclinical Studies

Before a new drug is administered to humans, its pharmacologic effects are thoroughly investigated in studies involving animals, called **preclinical testing**. The studies are designed to (a) ascertain whether the new drug has any harmful or beneficial effects on vital organ function, including cardiovascular, renal, and respiratory function; (b) elucidate the drug's mechanisms and therapeutic effects on target organs; and (c) determine the drug's pharmacokinetic properties, thereby providing some indication of how the drug would be handled by the human body. Although a few people object to using animals, there are even fewer willing to refuse all medical treatment and pharmacotherapy that result from animal testing.

Federal regulations require that extensive toxicity studies in animals be conducted to predict the risks that will be associated with administering the drug to healthy human subjects and patients. The value of the preclinical studies is based on the proven correlation between drug toxicity in animals and humans. As outlined in Table 4–1, the studies involve short-term and long-term administration of the drug and are designed to determine the risk of **acute, subacute,** and **chronic toxicity**, as well as the risk of **teratogenesis, mutagenesis,** and **carcinogenesis.** After animals are treated with the new drug, their behavior is assessed and their blood samples are analyzed for indications of tissue damage, metabolic abnormalities, and immunologic effects. Tissues are removed and examined for gross and microscopic pathologic changes. Offspring also are studied for adverse effects.

Studies in animals may not reveal all of the adverse effects that will be found in human subjects, either because of the low incidence of particular effects or because of differences in susceptibility among species. This means that some adverse reactions may not be detected until the drug is administered to humans. However, because studies of chronic toxicity of new drugs in animals may require years for completion, it is usually possible to begin human studies while animal studies

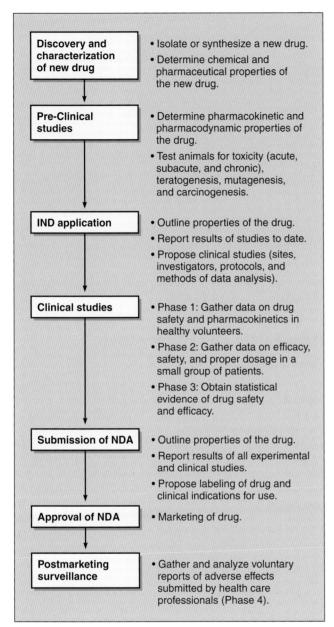

Discovery and characterization of new drug	• Isolate or synthesize a new drug. • Determine chemical and pharmaceutical properties of the new drug.
Pre-Clinical studies	• Determine pharmacokinetic and pharmacodynamic properties of the drug. • Test animals for toxicity (acute, subacute, and chronic), teratogenesis, mutagenesis, and carcinogenesis.
IND application	• Outline properties of the drug. • Report results of studies to date. • Propose clinical studies (sites, investigators, protocols, and methods of data analysis).
Clinical studies	• Phase 1: Gather data on drug safety and pharmacokinetics in healthy volunteers. • Phase 2: Gather data on efficacy, safety, and proper dosage in a small group of patients. • Phase 3: Obtain statistical evidence of drug safety and efficacy.
Submission of NDA	• Outline properties of the drug. • Report results of all experimental and clinical studies. • Propose labeling of drug and clinical indications for use.
Approval of NDA	• Marketing of drug.
Postmarketing surveillance	• Gather and analyze voluntary reports of adverse effects submitted by health care professionals (Phase 4).

Figure 4–1. Steps in the process of drug development in the United States. IND = investigational new drug; NDA = new drug application.

are being completed if the acute and subacute toxicity studies have not revealed any abnormalities in animals.

THE INVESTIGATIONAL NEW DRUG (IND) APPLICATION

The **Food and Drug Administration (FDA)** must approve an application for an **investigational new drug (IND)** before the drug can be distributed for the purpose of conducting studies in human subjects. The IND application includes a complete description of the drug, the results of all preclinical studies completed to date, and a description of the design and methods of the proposed clinical studies and the qualifications of the investigators.

Clinical Trials

Phase I clinical trials seek to determine the pharmacokinetic properties and safety of an IND in healthy human subjects. In the past, most of the subjects were men. Today, women are included in Phase I studies to determine if gender has any influence on the properties of the IND. The subjects typically undergo a complete history and physical examination, diagnostic imaging studies, and chemical and pharmacokinetic analyses of samples of blood and other bodily fluids. The pharmacokinetic analyses provide a basis for estimating doses to be employed in the next phase of trials, and the other examinations seek to determine if the drug is safe for use in humans.

Phase II clinical trials are the first studies to be performed in human subjects who have the particular disease for which the IND is targeting. These studies use a small number of patients to obtain a preliminary assessment of the drug's efficacy and safety in diseased individuals and to establish a dosage range for further clinical studies.

Phase III clinical trials are conducted to compare the safety and efficacy of the IND with that of another substance or treatment approach. Phase III studies employ a larger group of subjects, often consisting of hundreds or even thousands of patients and involving multiple clinical sites and investigators. Phase III clinical trials are rigorously designed to prevent investigator bias and include **double-blind** and **placebo-control** procedures. In a double-blind study, neither the investigator nor the patient knows if the patient is receiving the new drug or another substance. Placebo control design includes a group receiving an identical formulation but with no active ingredients. With some diseases, it is unethical to administer a placebo because of the proven benefits of standard drug therapy. In such cases, the new drug is compared with the standard drug for treatment of that disease. Phase III trials often involve **crossover studies**, in which the patients receive one medication or placebo for a period of time and then are switched, after a washout period, to the other medication or placebo.

In many cases, the data are analyzed statistically at various points to determine whether the IND is sufficiently effective or toxic to justify terminating a clinical trial. For example, if a statistically significant greater therapeutic effect can be demonstrated after 6 months in the group of patients who are receiving the new drug, it is unethical to continue giving a placebo or a standard drug to the control group, the members of which could also benefit from receiving the new drug. A clinical trial is also stopped if the new drug causes a significant increase in rate of mortality or serious toxicity.

The New Drug Application (NDA) and Its Approval

After Phase III clinical trials are completed and analyzed, the drug developer may submit a **new drug application (NDA)** to the FDA to request approval to market the drug. This application includes the results of all preclinical and

TABLE 4–1.	Drug Toxicity Studies in Animals	
Type of Study	**Method**	**Observations**
Acute toxicity	Administer a single dose of the drug in two species via two routes.	Behavioral changes, LD_{50},* and mortality.
Subacute toxicity	Administer the drug for 90 days in two species via a route intended for humans.	Behavioral and physiologic changes, blood chemistry levels, and pathologic findings in tissue samples.
Chronic toxicity	Administer the drug for 6–24 months, depending on the type of drug.	Behavioral and physiologic changes, blood chemistry levels, and pathologic findings in tissue samples.
Teratogenesis	Administer the drug to pregnant rats and rabbits during organogenesis.	Anatomic defects and behavioral changes in offspring.
Mutagenesis	Perform the Ames test in bacteria. Examine cultured mammalian cells for chromosomal defects.	Evidence of chromosome breaks, gene mutations, chromatid exchange, trisomy, or other defects.
Carcinogenesis	Administer the drug to rats and mice for their entire lifetime.	Higher than normal rate of malignant neoplasms.

*The LD_{50} (the median lethal dose) is the dose that kills half of the animals in a 14-day period after the dose is administered.

clinical studies, as well as the proposed labeling and clinical indications for the drug. The NDA typically constitutes an enormous amount of written material.

The FDA often requires a number of months to review the NDA before deciding whether to permit the drug to be marketed. Approved drugs are labeled for **specific indications** based on the data submitted to the FDA. Some drugs are found to have other clinical uses after the drug has been introduced to the market. These indications are known as unlabeled or "off-label" uses. For example, **gabapentin** (NEURONTIN) was initially approved for treating partial seizures but was used "off label" for preventing migraine headaches and treating chronic pain. In some cases, manufacturers will seek a revised labeling of an approved drug for another indication and establish a new trade name. This was done for the antidepressant **bupropion**, the exact same drug marketed as WELLBUTRIN for treating depression and ZYBAN for use in smoking cessation.

Postmarketing Surveillance

If a drug is approved for marketing, its safety in the general patient population is monitored by a procedure known as postmarketing surveillance, also considered **Phase IV**. The FDA seeks voluntary reporting of adverse drug reactions from health care professionals through its MedWatch program, and standard forms for this purpose are disseminated widely. Postmarketing surveillance is particularly important for detecting drug reactions that are uncommon and are therefore unlikely to be found during clinical trials.

FEDERAL DRUG LAWS AND REGULATIONS IN THE UNITED STATES

There are two major types of legislation pertaining specifically to drugs. One type concerns **drug safety and efficacy** and regulates the processes by which drugs are evaluated, labeled, and marketed. The other type focuses on the **prevention of drug abuse**. In both cases, the laws and regulations reflect the concern of society with minimizing the harm that may result from drug use while permitting the therapeutic use of safe and beneficial agents.

Drug Safety and Efficacy Laws

Pure Food and Drug Act

The Pure Food and Drug Act of 1906 was the first federal legislation concerning drug product safety and efficacy in the United States. The Act was passed in response to the sale of patent medicines, often by so-called snake-oil salesmen, which contained toxic or habit-forming ingredients. The legislation required **accurate labeling** of the ingredients in drug products and sought to prevent the adulteration of products through the substitution of inactive or toxic ingredients for the labeled ingredients. Because the Act did not regulate fraudulent advertising, the legislation was only partially successful in eliminating unsafe drug products.

Food, Drug, and Cosmetic Act

The Food, Drug, and Cosmetic (FD&C) Act of 1938 came in response to a tragic incident in which over 100 people died after ingesting an elixir that contained sulfanilamide, used to treat streptococcal infections, in a solution of ethylene glycol. The legislation, which is still in force today, made major strides by requiring evidence of drug safety before a drug product could be marketed, by establishing the FDA to enforce this requirement, and by giving legal authority to the drug product standards contained in the **United States Pharmacopeia** (**USP**).

First compiled in 1820, the USP has been updated and published at regular intervals by a private organization that is called the **United States Pharmacopeial Convention** and is composed of representatives of medical and pharmacy colleges and societies from each state. The USP contains information on the chemical analysis of drugs and indicates how much variance in drug content is allowable for each drug product. For example, the USP states that aspirin tablets must contain not less than 90% and not more than 110% of the labeled amount of $C_9H_8O_4$ (aspirin). In addition, the USP outlines **standards** for tablet disintegration and many other aspects of drug product composition and analysis.

PROVISIONS OF THE FOOD, DRUG, AND COSMETIC ACT. The FD&C Act prohibits the distribution of drug products that are **adulterated**, **misbranded** (mislabeled), or that do not have an **approved NDA**. The Act requires that drug product labels contain the name, dosage, and quantity of ingredients, as well as warnings against unsafe use in children or in persons with medical conditions for whom use of the drug might be dangerous. A drug product is said to be adulterated if it does not meet USP standards or if it is not manufactured according to defined "good manufacturing practices."

AMENDMENTS TO THE FOOD, DRUG, AND COSMETIC ACT. The FD&C Act has been amended many times. The **Durham-Humphrey Amendment** was passed in 1952 and created a legal distinction between nonprescription and prescription drugs. **Prescription drugs** are labeled "Rx Only." Agents that are classified as prescription drugs are those that are determined to be unsafe for use without the supervision of a designated health care professional. After a new drug has been marketed for a period of time or if it is found to be safe enough to be used without physician supervision, the FDA may reclassify the drug as a nonprescription drug, known as an **over-the-counter (OTC) drug.** For example, topical cortisone products, antifungal drugs for treating candidiasis, proton pump inhibitors for treating acid reflux such as **omeprazole** (PRILOSEC), and antihistamines such as **loratadine** (CLARITIN) were originally classified as prescription drugs but are now classified as nonprescription drugs.

The **Kefauver-Harris Amendments** were passed in 1962, largely in response to reports of severe malformations in the offspring of women in Europe who took **thalidomide**, for sedation, during their pregnancy. In fact, thalidomide had not been marketed in the United States, because a female scientist at the FDA, Frances Kelsey, held up approval of thalidomide. Nevertheless, the shocking pictures from Europe of deformed babies spurred Congress to more strongly regulate drug development; as a result, Congress passed amendments that required the demonstration of both **safety** and **efficacy** in studies involving animals and humans before a drug product could be marketed. Although the processes of new drug development and testing have not changed substantially since this amendment was passed, the FDA review of new drugs has been streamlined in recent years.

The **Orphan Drug Amendments** were passed in 1983 to provide tax benefits and other incentives for drug manufacturers to test and produce drugs that are used in the treatment of rare diseases and are therefore unlikely to generate large profits. The Act appears to have been successful, as several hundred orphan drugs are now available. Examples are drugs used for the treatment of urea cycle enzyme deficiencies, Gaucher's disease, homocystinuria, and other rare metabolic disorders.

Drug Price Competition and Patent Restoration Act

The **Drug Price Competition and Patent Restoration Act** of 1984 extended the patent life of drug products (which at that time was 17 years) by adding the amount of time required for regulatory review of an NDA. It also accelerated the approval of **generic drug products** by allowing investigators to submit an **abbreviated NDA** in which the generic product is shown to be therapeutically equivalent to an approved brand name product. Therapeutic equivalence is demonstrated on the basis of a single-dose oral **bioavailability** study that compares the generic drug with the brand name drug. If the variance is within a specified range (usually ±20%), the generic drug may be approved for marketing. The cost of such a study is relatively small compared with the millions of dollars required for the development of a completely new drug.

In 1992, **accelerated drug approval** was authorized for **new drugs to treat life-threatening conditions** such as acquired immunodeficiency syndrome (AIDS) and cancer. Under the new regulations, patients with these conditions can be treated with an investigational drug before clinical trials have been completed.

Drug Abuse Prevention Laws

Harrison Narcotics Act

The Harrison Narcotics Act of 1914 was the **first major drug abuse legislation** in the United States. It was prompted by the growing problem of heroin abuse, which followed the synthesis of this potent and rapid-acting derivative of morphine. The Act sought to control narcotics through the use of tax stamps on legal drug products, a practice similar to the use of tax stamps on alcoholic beverages today. The Harrison Narcotics Act had a profound and controversial effect on the treatment of substance abuse in that it prohibited physicians from administering opioid drugs to drug-dependent patients as part of their treatment program.

Comprehensive Drug Abuse Prevention and Control Act

During the 1960s, the **prevalence of drug abuse increased**, especially among adolescents and young adults, who were using a wide range of drugs that included prescription sedatives and stimulants as well as substances such as lysergic acid diethylamide (LSD), marijuana, and other hallucinogens. Believing that the drug abuse problem required a new approach, members of Congress passed the Comprehensive Drug Abuse Prevention and Control Act of 1970. This law is often called the **Controlled Substances Act (CSA)**.

The CSA classified drugs with abuse potential into five schedules, based on their degree of potential for abuse and their clinical usage. **Schedule I drugs** were classified as high abuse potential and no legitimate medical use, and their distribution and possession are prohibited. **Schedule II drugs** have high abuse potential but a legitimate medical use, and their distribution is highly controlled through requirements for inventories and records and through restrictions on prescriptions. **Schedule III, IV, and V drugs** have lower abuse potential and decreasingly fewer restrictions on distribution. The CSA requires that all manufacturers, distributors, physicians, and medical researchers using controlled drugs register with the **Drug Enforcement Agency**, which is responsible for enforcing the Act.

ADVERSE EFFECTS OF DRUGS

Adverse effects, or **side effects**, can be classified with respect to their mechanisms of action and predictability. Those due to excessive pharmacologic activity are the most predictable and are often the easiest to prevent or counteract. Organ toxicity caused by other mechanisms is often unpredictable, because its occurrence depends on the drug susceptibility of the individual patient, the drug dosage, and numerous other factors. Hypersensitivity reactions are responsible for a large number of adverse organ system effects. These reactions occur frequently with some drugs but only rarely with others.

Excessive Pharmacologic Effects

Drugs often produce adverse effects by the **same mechanism** that is responsible for their therapeutic effect on the target organ. For example, **atropine** may cause dry mouth and urinary retention by the same mechanism that reduces gastric acid secretion in the treatment of peptic ulcer, namely, by muscarinic receptor antagonism. This type of adverse effect may be managed by reducing the drug dosage or by substituting a drug that is more selective for the target organ.

Hypersensitivity Reactions

Hypersensitivity reactions, or **drug allergies**, are responsible for a large number of organ toxicities that range in severity from a mild skin rash to major organ system failure. An allergic reaction occurs when the drug, acting as a **hapten**, combines with an endogenous protein to form an antigen that induces antibody production. The antigen and antibody subsequently interact with body tissues to produce a wide variety of adverse effects.

In the **Gell and Coombs classification system**, allergic reactions are divided into four general types, each of which can be produced by drugs. **Type I reactions** are **immediate hypersensitivity** reactions that are mediated by immunoglobulin E (IgE) antibodies. Examples of these reactions are urticaria (hives), atopic dermatitis, and **anaphylactic shock**. **Type II reactions** are **cytolytic reactions** that involve immune complement and are mediated by immunoglobulins G and M. Examples are hemolytic anemia, thrombocytopenia, and drug-induced lupus erythematosus. **Type III reactions** are mediated by **immune complexes**. The deposition of antigen-antibody complexes in vascular endothelium leads to inflammation, lymphadenopathy, and fever (serum sickness). An example is the severe skin rash seen in patients with a life-threatening form of drug-induced immune vasculitis that is known as **Stevens-Johnson syndrome**. **Type IV reactions** are **delayed hypersensitivity** reactions that are mediated by sensitized lymphocytes. An example is the ampicillin-induced skin rash that occurs in patients with viral mononucleosis.

Adverse Effects on Organs

In some cases, the adverse effects and therapeutic effects of a drug are caused by different mechanisms. For example, in patients taking **aspirin**, the adverse reaction such as hyperventilation that leads to respiratory alkalosis is caused by adverse effects that do not appear to be mediated by the drug's primary mechanism of action, which is inhibition of prostaglandin synthesis. A variety of drugs (Table 4–2) produce toxicity of the liver, kidneys, or other vital organs, and this toxicity may not be readily apparent until significant organ damage has occurred. Patients receiving these drugs should be monitored with appropriate laboratory tests. For example, **hepatotoxicity** may be detected by monitoring serum transaminase levels, while **hematopoietic toxicity** may be detected by periodically performing blood cell counts.

Hematopoietic Toxicity

Bone marrow toxicity, one of the most frequent types of drug-induced toxicity, may present as **agranulocytosis, anemia, thrombocytopenia**, or a combination of these

TABLE 4-2. Drug-Induced Organ Toxicities		
Organ Toxicity	**Examples of Adverse Effects**	**Examples of Drugs**
Cardiotoxicity	Cardiomyopathy	Daunorubicin, doxorubicin, and idarubicin,
Hematopoietic toxicity	Agranulocytosis*	Captopril, chlorpromazine, chlorpropamide, clozapine, and propylthiouracil
	Aplastic anemia*	Chloramphenicol and phenylbutazone
	Hemolytic anemia*	Captopril, levodopa, and methyldopa
	Thrombocytopenia*	Quinidine, rifampin, and sulfonamides
Hepatotoxicity	Cholestatic jaundice*	Erythromycin estolate and phenothiazines
	Hepatitis*	Amiodarone, captopril, isoniazid, phenytoin, and sulfonamides
Nephrotoxicity	Acute tubular necrosis	Aminoglycoside antibiotics, amphotericin B, and vancomycin
	Interstitial nephritis*	Nonsteroidal anti-inflammatory drugs (NSAIDs) and penicillins (especially methicillin)
Ototoxicity	Vestibular and cochlear disorders	Aminoglycoside antibiotics, furosemide, and vancomycin
Pulmonary toxicity	Inflammatory fibrosis	Methysergide
	Pulmonary fibrosis	Amiodarone, bleomycin, busulfan, and nitrofurantoin
Skin toxicity	All forms of skin rash*	Antibiotics, diuretics, phenytoin, sulfonamides, and sulfonylureas

*Immunologic mechanisms known or suspected.

(**pancytopenia**). The effects are often reversible when the drug is withdrawn, but they may have serious consequences before toxicity can be detected. For example, patients who develop **agranulocytosis** may succumb to a fatal infection before the problem is recognized.

Many drugs, such as **chloramphenicol**, are believed to cause hematopoietic toxicity by triggering hypersensitivity reactions directed against the stem cells in bone marrow or their derivatives. Chloramphenicol also produces a reversible form of anemia by blocking the action of the enzyme ferrochelatase and thereby preventing the incorporation of iron into heme.

The most serious form of hematopoietic toxicity is **aplastic anemia**, which may be associated with several types of blood cell deficiencies and lead to **pancytopenia**. Aplastic anemia is probably due to a hypersensitivity reaction and is often irreversible, although it has recently been treated by administration of **hematopoietic growth factors** (see Chapter 17).

Hepatotoxicity

A large number of drugs produce liver toxicity, either via an immunologic mechanism or via their direct effect on the hepatocytes. Liver toxicity can be classified as cholestatic or hepatocellular. **Cholestatic hepatotoxicity** is often caused by a hypersensitivity mechanism producing inflammation and stasis of the biliary system. **Hepatocellular toxicity** is sometimes caused by a toxic drug metabolite. For example, acetaminophen and isoniazid have toxic metabolites that may cause hepatitis. With many hepatotoxic drugs, elevated **serum transaminase** levels may provide an early indication of liver damage and levels should be monitored during the first 6 months of therapy and at longer intervals thereafter. Many authorities believe that if transaminase levels exceed 2 times the upper normal limit, a physician should consider alternative drug therapy or frequent monitoring of enzyme levels. If transaminase levels exceed 3 times the upper normal limit, the drug should be discontinued. Unfortunately, some patients have developed acute hepatic failure even when serum transaminase levels have been monitored appropriately. In recent years, several drugs such as **troglitazone**, used to treat diabetes, were removed from the market as a result of excessive cases of fatal hepatic failure.

Nephrotoxicity

Renal toxicity is caused by various drugs, including several groups of antibiotics. The forms of renal toxicity can be classified according to site and mechanism and include **interstitial nephritis, renal tubular necrosis**, and **crystalluria** (the precipitation of insoluble drug in the renal tubules). Nephrotoxicity often reduces drug **clearance**, thereby elevating plasma drug concentrations and leading to greater toxicity. With some drugs that routinely cause renal toxicity, such as the antineoplastic agent cisplatin, the kidneys can be protected by means of forced diuresis, in which the drug is administered with large quantities of intravenous fluid so as to lower the drug concentration in the renal tubules.

Bladder toxicity is less common than renal toxicity, but it may occur as an adverse effect of a few drugs. One example is cyclophosphamide, an antineoplastic drug whose metabolite causes **hemorrhagic cystitis**. This disorder can be prevented by administering **mesna**, a sulfhydryl-releasing agent that conjugates the toxic metabolite in the urine.

Other Organ Toxicities

Pulmonary toxicity occurs through a variety of mechanisms. Some drugs, such as **opioid analgesics,** cause **respiratory depression** via their effects on the brain stem respiratory centers. The drugs bleomycin and amiodarone produce **pulmonary fibrosis**, so patients who are being treated with these agents should have periodic chest x-rays and blood gas measurements to detect early signs of fibrosis.

Relatively few drugs produce **cardiotoxicity.** Anthracycline anticancer drugs, such as **doxorubicin** (ADRIAMYCIN), produce adverse cardiac effects that resemble congestive heart failure. HMG-CoA (3-hydroxy-3-methylglutaryl–coenzyme A) reductase inhibitors such as **lovastatin** (MEVACOR) may cause **skeletal muscle damage** evidenced by muscle pain and sometimes leading to rhabdomyolysis.

Skin rashes of all varieties, including macular, papular, maculopapular, and urticarial rashes, may be produced by drug hypersensitivity reactions. A mild skin rash may disappear with continued drug administration. Nevertheless, because rashes may lead to more serious skin or organ toxicity, they should be monitored carefully.

Idiosyncratic Reactions

Idiosyncratic reactions are unexpected drug reactions caused by a genetically determined susceptibility. For example, patients who have glucose-6-phosphate dehydrogenase deficiency may develop hemolytic anemia when they are exposed to an oxidizing drug such as primaquine or to a sulfonamide.

DRUG INTERACTIONS

A drug interaction is defined as a change in the pharmacologic effect of a drug that results when it is given concurrently with another drug or with food. Drug interactions may be caused by changes in the pharmaceutical, pharmacodynamic, or pharmacokinetic properties of the affected drug (Table 4–3).

Pharmaceutical Interactions

Pharmaceutical interactions are due to a chemical reaction between drugs prior to their administration or absorption. Pharmaceutical interactions occur most frequently when drug solutions are combined before they are given intravenously. For example, if a penicillin solution and an aminoglycoside solution are mixed, they will form an insoluble precipitate, because penicillins are negatively charged and aminoglycosides are positively charged. Many other drugs are incompatible and should not be combined before they are administered.

TABLE 4-3. Types and Mechanisms of Drug Interactions

Type	Mechanism
Drug Interactions with Food	Altered drug absorption
Pharmaceutical Interactions (Drug Incompatibilities)	Chemical reaction between drugs prior to their administration or absorption
Pharmacodynamic Interactions	Additive, synergistic, or antagonistic effects on a microbe or tumor cells
	Additive, synergistic, or antagonistic effects on a tissue or organ system
Pharmacokinetic Interactions	
Altered drug absorption	Altered gut motility or secretion
	Binding or chelation of drugs
	Competition for active transport
Altered drug distribution	Displacement from plasma protein–binding sites
	Displacement from tissue-binding sites
Altered drug biotransformation	Altered hepatic blood flow
	Enzyme induction
	Enzyme inhibition
Altered drug excretion	Altered biliary excretion or enterohepatic cycling
	Altered urine pH
	Drug-induced renal impairment
	Inhibition of active tubular secretion

Pharmacodynamic Interactions

Pharmacodynamic interactions occur when two drugs have additive, synergistic, or antagonistic effects on a tissue, organ system, microbe, or tumor cells. An **additive effect** is equal to the sum of the individual drug effects, whereas a **synergistic effect** is greater than the sum of the individual drug effects. Some pharmacodynamic interactions occur when two drugs act on the same receptor, and others occur when the drugs affect the same physiologic function through actions on different receptors. For example, epinephrine and histamine affect the same function but have **antagonistic effects.** Epinephrine activates adrenergic receptors to cause bronchial smooth muscle relaxation, whereas histamine activates histamine receptors to produce bronchial smooth muscle contraction.

Pharmacokinetic Interactions

In pharmacokinetic interactions, a drug alters the absorption, distribution, biotransformation, or excretion of another drug or drugs. Mechanisms and examples of pharmacokinetic interactions are provided in Tables 4-3 and 4-4.

Altered Drug Absorption

There are several mechanisms by which a drug may affect the absorption and bioavailability of another drug. One mechanism involves binding to another drug in the gut and preventing its absorption. For example, **cholestyramine,** a bile acid sequestrant, binds to **digoxin** and prevents its absorption. Another mechanism involves altering gastric or intestinal motility so as to affect the absorption of another drug. Drugs tend to be absorbed more rapidly from the intestines than from the stomach. Therefore, a drug that slows gastric emptying, such as atropine, often delays the absorption of another drug. A drug that increases intestinal motility, such as a laxative, may reduce the time available for the absorption of another drug, thereby causing its incomplete absorption.

Altered Drug Distribution

Many drugs displace other drugs from plasma proteins and thereby increase the plasma concentration of the free (unbound) drug, but the magnitude and duration of this effect are usually small. As the free drug concentration increases, so does the drug's rate of elimination, and any change in the drug's effect on target tissues is usually short-lived.

The enterohepatic cycling of some drugs is dependent on intestinal bacteria that hydrolyze drug conjugates excreted by the bile and thereby enable the more lipid-soluble parent compound to be reabsorbed into the circulation. Antibiotics administered concurrently with these drugs may kill the bacteria and reduce the enterohepatic cycling and plasma drug concentrations. When antibiotics are taken concurrently with oral contraceptives containing estrogen, for example, they may reduce the plasma concentration of estrogen and cause contraceptive failure (Fig. 4–2).

Altered Drug Biotransformation

In some cases, biotransformation is affected by drugs that alter hepatic blood flow. In many cases, it is affected by drug interactions that either induce or inhibit drug-metabolizing enzymes (see Table 4–4).

Inducers of cytochrome P450 enzymes include barbiturates, carbamazepine, and rifampin, which bind to regulatory domains of cytochrome P450 (CYP) genes and increase gene transcription. These agents induce the CYP1A2, CYP2C9, CYP2C19, and CYP3A4 isozymes, whereas the CYP2D6 and CYP2E1 isozymes are not readily induced by commonly used drugs. The rate of induction depends on the dose and frequency of administration. Enzyme induction is usually maximal after several days of continuing drug administration. Enzyme induction increases the clearance and reduces the half-life of drugs biotransformed by the enzyme. When the inducing drug is discontinued, the synthesis of P450 enzymes gradually returns to the pretreatment level.

A large number of drugs bind to and **inhibit CYP** isozymes. CYP3A4 is selectively inhibited by erythromycin, itraconazole, and doxycycline, whereas other drugs such as cimetidine, ketoconazole, and fluoxetine inhibit several CYP isozymes. Significant interactions occur when these drugs reduce the clearance and increase the plasma concentration of other drugs. For example, itraconazole inhibits the biotransformation of HMG-CoA reductase inhibitors, such as lovastatin and atorvastatin, by CYP3A4. This inhibition increases plasma levels several fold, sometimes leading to severe muscle inflammation and lysis (rhabdomyolysis). **Grapefruit juice** has been found to contain bioflavonoid compounds that inhibit CYP3A4 and thereby elevate

TABLE 4–4. Management of Clinically Significant Pharmacokinetic Drug Interactions

Examples of Inducers or Inhibitors	Examples of Affected Drugs	Management
Inducers of Drug Biotransformation		
Barbiturates, carbamazepine, and rifampin	Warfarin	Increase warfarin dosage as indicated by prothrombin time (international normalized ratio).
Carbamazepine	Theophylline	Monitor plasma theophylline concentration and adjust dosage as needed.
Rifampin	Phenytoin	Monitor plasma phenytoin concentration and adjust dosage as needed.
Inhibitors of Drug Absorption		
Aluminum, calcium, and iron	Tetracycline	Give tetracycline 1 hour before or 2 hours after giving the other agent.
Cholestyramine	Digoxin and warfarin	Give digoxin or warfarin 1 hour before or 2 hours after giving cholestyramine.
Inhibitors of Drug Biotransformation		
Cimetidine	Benzodiazepines, lidocaine, phenytoin, theophylline, and warfarin	Instead of giving cimetidine, substitute a histamine blocker that does not inhibit drug metabolism.
Disulfiram	Ethanol	Make sure the patient understands that disulfiram is used therapeutically to promote abstinence from alcohol (ethanol).
Erythromycin	Carbamazepine and theophylline	Lower the dose of the affected drug during erythromycin therapy.
Erythromycin, itraconazole, and ketoconazole	Lovastatin and atorvastatin	Avoid concurrent therapy and thereby avoid myopathy.
Monoamine oxidase inhibitors	Levodopa and sympathomimetic drugs	Avoid concurrent therapy, if possible; otherwise, give a subnormal dose of the affected drug.
Inhibitors of Drug Clearance		
Diltiazem, quinidine, and verapamil	Digoxin	Give a subnormal dose of digoxin and monitor the plasma drug concentration.
Probenecid	Cephalosporins and penicillin	Advise the patient that the combination of drugs is intended to increase the plasma concentration of the antibiotic.
Thiazide diuretics	Lithium	Give a subnormal dose of lithium and monitor the plasma drug concentration.

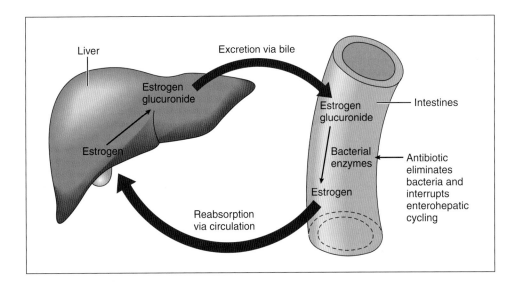

Figure 4–2. Interaction of antibiotics with estrogens found in oral contraceptives. Estrogen is conjugated with glucuronate and sulfate in the liver, and the conjugates are excreted via the bile into the intestines. Intestinal bacteria hydrolyze the conjugates, and estrogen is reabsorbed into the circulation. The enterohepatic cycling is interrupted if concurrently administered antibiotics destroy the intestinal bacteria. Contraceptive failure may result.

concentrations of drugs such as **felodipine** (PLENDIL) that are metabolized by this enzyme.

Altered Drug Excretion

Drugs can alter the renal or biliary excretion of other drugs by several mechanisms. A few drugs, such as **carbonic anhydrase inhibitors**, alter the renal pH. This in turn can change the ratio of another drug's ionized form to its non-ionized form and affect its renal excretion. **Probenecid** competes with other organic acids, such as penicillin, for the active transport system in renal tubules. **Quinidine** and **verapamil** decrease the biliary clearance of digoxin and thereby increase serum digoxin levels. Potentially nephrotoxic drugs, such as the **aminoglycoside antibiotics**, may impair the renal excretion of other drugs via their effect on renal function.

Clinical Significance of Drug Interactions

The clinical significance of drug interactions varies widely. In some cases, toxicity is severe and can be prevented only by avoiding the concurrent administration of drugs. In other cases, toxicity can be avoided by proper dosage adjustment and other measures (see Table 4–4). For example, when quinidine and digoxin are administered concurrently, a subnormal dose of digoxin should be used to prevent adverse effects. Fortunately, many drug interactions are of minor significance, and the interacting drugs can usually be administered concurrently without affecting their efficacy or the patient's safety. Drug interactions are more likely to occur if the affected drug has a low therapeutic index or is being used to treat a critically ill patient. However, **polypharmacy**, which refers to the use of multiple medications by a patient, is linked to many adverse effects and toxicity due to drug interactions in the elderly.

FACTORS AFFECTING DRUG SAFETY AND EFFICACY

Age, disease, pregnancy, and lactation are important biologic variables that can alter the response to drugs in particular patients.

Age

Factors affecting drug disposition in different age populations are summarized in Table 4–5.

In neonates, and especially in premature infants, the capacity to metabolize and excrete drugs is often greatly **reduced** because of low levels of drug biotransformation enzymes. Oxidative reactions and glucuronate conjugation occur at a lower rate in neonates than in adults, whereas sulfate conjugation is well developed in neonates. Consequently, some drugs that are metabolized primarily by glucuronate conjugation in adults (drugs such as acetaminophen) are metabolized chiefly by sulfate conjugation in neonates. Nevertheless, the overall rate of biotransformation of most drugs is lower in neonates and infants than it is in adults.

In comparison with children and young adults, elderly adults also tend to have a **reduced** capacity to metabolize drugs. Biotransformation via oxidative reactions usually declines more than biotransformation via drug conjugation. Therefore, it may be safer to use drugs that are conjugated when the choice is available. For example, benzodiazepines that are metabolized by conjugation, such as **lorazepam** and **temazepam**, are believed to be safer for treatment of the elderly than are benzodiazepines that undergo oxidative biotransformation (e.g., diazepam).

Renal function is lower in neonates and elderly adults than it is in young adults, and this affects the renal excretion of many drugs. For example, the half-lives of aminoglycoside antibiotics are greatly prolonged in neonates. Glomerular filtration declines 35% between the ages of 20 and 90 years, with a corresponding reduction in the renal elimination of many drugs.

Because the very young and the very old tend to have increased sensitivity to drugs, the dosage per kilogram of body weight should be reduced when most drugs are used in the treatment of these populations.

Disease

Hepatic and renal disease may reduce the capacity of the liver and kidneys to biotransform and excrete drugs, thereby **reducing drug clearance** and necessitating a dosage reduction to avoid toxicity. Heart failure and other conditions that reduce hepatic blood flow may also reduce drug biotransformation. Oxidative drug metabolism is usually impaired in patients with hepatic disease, whereas conjugation processes may be little affected.

Guidelines for dosage adjustment in patients with hepatic or renal disease are available and can be found in clinical references. Dosage adjustments are made by reducing the dose, increasing the interval between doses, or both. Adjustments for individual patients are usually based on laboratory measurements of renal or hepatic function and on plasma drug concentration.

Pregnancy and Lactation

Drugs taken by a woman during pregnancy or lactation can cause adverse effects in the fetus or infant.

TABLE 4–5.   Factors Affecting Drug Disposition in Different Age Populations

Process of Drug Disposition	POPULATION		
	Neonates and Infants	**Children**	**Elderly Adults**
Absorption	Altered absorption of some drugs.	No major changes, but first-pass inactivation may be increased.	No major changes.
Distribution	Incomplete blood-brain barrier; higher volumes of distribution for water-soluble drugs.	No major changes.	Higher volumes of distribution for fat-soluble drugs.
Biotransformation	Lower rate of oxidative reactions and glucuronate conjugation.	Biotransformation rate for some drugs higher than in adults.	Reduced oxidative metabolism; relatively unchanged conjugation metabolism.
Excretion	Reduced capacity to excrete drugs.	No major changes.	Reduced capacity to excrete drugs.

The risk of drug-induced developmental abnormalities known as **teratogenic effects** is the greatest during the period of organogenesis from the 4th to the 10th week of gestation. After the 10th week, the major risk is to the development of the brain and spinal cord. An estimated 1% to 5% of fetal malformations are attributed to drugs. Although only a few drugs have been proven to cause teratogenic effects (Table 4–6), the safety of many other drugs has not yet been determined.

The FDA has divided drugs into five categories, based on their **safety in pregnant women**. Drugs in Categories A and B are relatively safe. Drugs in Category A have been shown in clinical studies to pose no risk to the fetus, whereas those in Category B may have shown risk in animal studies but not in human studies. For drugs in Category C, adverse effects on the fetus have been demonstrated in animals, but there is insufficient data in pregnant women, so risk to the fetus cannot be ruled out. Drugs in Category D show positive evidence of risk to the fetus, and drugs in Category X are **contraindicated** during pregnancy.

Drugs of choice for pregnant women are listed in clinical references and are selected on the basis of their safety to the fetus as well as their therapeutic efficacy. For example, penicillin, cephalosporin, and macrolide antibiotics (all Category B drugs) are preferred for treating many infections in pregnant women, whereas tetracycline antibiotics (Category D) should be avoided. Acetaminophen (Category B) is usually the analgesic of choice in pregnancy, but ibuprofen and related drugs are also in Category B and may be used when required. For the treatment of nausea and vomiting of pregnancy, the combination of pyridoxine (Category A) in combination with doxylamine (Category B) is the only medication specifically labeled for this indication by the FDA. Other drugs considered relatively safe for use in pregnancy include insulin and metformin (GLUCOPHAGE) for treating diabetes mellitus (both Category B drugs), famotidine (PEPCID) and omeprazole (PRILOSEC) for reducing gastric acidity (Category B drugs), diphenhydramine (BENADRYL) for treating allergic reactions (Category B), and tricyclic antidepressants such as desipramine (NORPRAMIN) for treating mood depression (Category B). Most antiepileptic drugs pose some risk to the fetus, and the selection of drugs for treating epilepsy in pregnant women requires careful consideration of the risks and benefits of such medication.

Some drugs can be taken by lactating women without posing a risk to their breast-fed infants. Other drugs place the infant at risk for toxicity. As a general rule, breast-feeding should be avoided if a drug taken by the mother would cause the infant's plasma drug concentration to be greater than 50% of the mother's plasma concentration. Clinical references provide guidelines on the use of specific drugs by lactating women.

TABLE 4-6. Examples of Teratogenic Drugs and Their Effects on the Fetus or Newborn Infant*

Drug	Adverse Effects
Alkylating agents and antimetabolites (anticancer drugs)	Cardiac defects; cleft palate; growth retardation; malformation of ears, eyes, fingers, nose, or skull; and other anomalies.
Carbamazepine	Abnormal facial features; neural tube defects, such as spina bifida; reduced head size; and other anomalies.
Coumarin anticoagulants	Fetal warfarin syndrome (characterized by chondrodysplasia punctata, malformation of ears and eyes, mental retardation, nasal hypoplasia, optic atrophy, skeletal deformities, and other anomalies).
Diethylstilbestrol (DES)	Effects in female offspring: clear cell vaginal or cervical adenocarcinoma; irregular menses; and reproductive abnormalities, including decreased rate of pregnancy and increased rate of preterm deliveries. Effects in male offspring: cryptorchidism, epididymal cysts, and hypogonadism.
Ethanol	Fetal alcohol syndrome (characterized by growth retardation, hyperactivity, mental retardation, microcephaly and facial abnormalities, poor coordination, and other anomalies).
Phenytoin	Fetal hydantoin syndrome (characterized by cardiac defects; malformation of ears, lips, palate, mouth, and nasal bridge; mental retardation; microcephaly; ptosis; strabismus; and other anomalies).
Retinoids (systemic)	Spontaneous abortions. Hydrocephaly; malformation of ears, face, heart, limbs, and liver; microcephaly; and other anomalies.
Tetracycline	Hypoplasia of tooth enamel and staining of teeth.
Thalidomide	Deafness, heart defects, limb abnormalities (amelia or phocomelia), renal abnormalities, and other anomalies.
Valproate	Cardiac defects, central nervous system defects, lumbosacral spina bifida, and microcephaly.

*Other substances known to be teratogenic include lead, lithium, methyl mercury, penicillamine, polychlorinated biphenyls, and trimethadione. Other drugs that should be avoided during the second and third trimester of pregnancy are angiotensin-converting enzyme inhibitors, chloramphenicol, indomethacin, prostaglandins, sulfonamides, and sulfonylureas. Other drugs that should be used with great caution during pregnancy include antithyroid drugs, aspirin, barbiturates, benzodiazepines, corticosteroids, heparin, opioids, and phenothiazines.

SUMMARY OF IMPORTANT POINTS

■ The process of drug development includes chemical and pharmacologic characterization, experimental studies to test for toxicity in animals, and clinical studies to determine efficacy and safety in humans.

■ Drug development is regulated by the FDA. An IND application must be completed before clinical studies can be started, and an NDA must be submitted and approved before the drug can be marketed.

■ Phase I studies provide data about drug safety and pharmacokinetics in healthy subjects; Phase II studies provide data about the proper dosage and potential efficacy in a small group of patients; and Phase III studies provide statistical evidence of efficacy and safety in a controlled clinical trial.

■ The Food, Drug, and Cosmetic Act established the FDA to regulate the development, manufacturing, distribution, and usage of drugs. Amendments have established the prescription class of drugs, stricter requirements for human drug testing, incentives for developing orphan drugs for rare diseases, and abbreviated procedures for marketing generic drug products.

■ The Comprehensive Drug Abuse Prevention and Control Act, also called the Controlled Substances Act (CSA), classifies potentially abused drugs in five categories (Schedules I–V), requires registration of legitimate drug distributors and health care professionals, and limits the prescription and distribution of controlled substances.

■ The adverse effects of drugs may be due to excessive pharmacologic effects, hypersensitivity reactions, or other mechanisms responsible for organ toxicities. The bone marrow, liver, kidney, and skin are frequent sites of drug toxicity.

■ Drug interactions occur when one drug alters the pharmacologic properties of another drug. Most interactions are due to pharmacokinetic effects, particularly inhibition or induction of drug biotransformation.

■ Age, disease, pregnancy, and lactation are factors that must be considered in drug selection and dosage. The very young and the very old tend to have an increased sensitivity to therapeutic agents, usually because of a reduced capacity to eliminate drugs. Target organs may also be more sensitive to drugs in these populations.

Review Questions

1. An advertisement in a local newspaper seeks to enroll 20 patients with arthritis in a medical study that would be the first time that a new drug would be tested in persons with this disease. The study would therefore be classified as a
   (A) Phase I clinical study
   (B) Phase II clinical study
   (C) Phase III clinical study
   (D) Phase IV clinical study
   (E) Phase V clinical study

2. Which one of the following schedules of controlled substances is for drugs with the highest abuse potential that have a legitimate medical use?
   (A) Schedule I
   (B) Schedule II
   (C) Schedule III
   (D) Schedule IV
   (E) Schedule V

3. The 4th to the 10th week of gestation is the period of time when there is the greatest concern about drug-induced
   (A) fetal cardiac arrest
   (B) fetal hemorrhage
   (C) fetal malformations
   (D) labor
   (E) fetal jaundice

4. Which of the following drug interaction mechanisms is most likely to lead to sustained elevations of plasma drug concentrations and drug toxicity?
   (A) induction of CYP2C19
   (B) inhibition of CYP3A4
   (C) displacement of a drug from plasma albumin binding sites
   (D) inhibition of the P-glycoprotein carrier protein
   (E) acceleration of gastric emptying by a "prokinetic" drug

5. Elderly persons may have altered drug disposition because of
   (A) markedly reduced absorption of many drugs
   (B) higher volumes of distribution for water-soluble drugs
   (C) accelerated renal excretion of ionized drugs
   (D) increased permeability of the blood-brain barrier
   (E) reduced capacity to oxidize drugs

Answers and Explanations

1. **The answer is B:** Phase II study. Phase II studies are done in a small group of test subjects that have the disease state targeted by the new drug. Phase I studies are done to establish safety and pharmacokinetics in healthy subjects, often students in the health professions. Phase III studies are large, multicenter studies in patients with the disease state. Phase IV studies are post-marketing surveillance, in which physicians report adverse effects to the FDA. There is no Phase V in the drug development process.

2. **The answer is B:** Schedule II. Schedule II controlled drugs have a high degree of abuse potential but are still used by the medical profession. These drugs may still be abused by diversion, the act of illegally obtaining prescription drugs by sale or theft. Schedule I lists the most abused and illegal drugs, including marijuana, mescaline, LSD, and MDMA ("ecstasy"). Note that cocaine, although much abused in the form of powder ("coke") and free base ("crack") is listed as Schedule II as it does have a limited medical use, as a local anesthetic and vasoconstricting agent in ear, nose, and throat procedures. Schedules III–V controlled drugs have some degree of abuse potential but less than those of Schedule II.

3. The answer is C: fetal malformations. The 4th to 10th week of gestation is the period when fetal organs are developed. Teratogenic drugs may cause fetal malformations if taken by a pregnant woman during this interval. These malformations include cleft palate, malformation of fingers and toes, heart defects, facial abnormalities, and skeletal deformities. Drug-induced labor or jaundice is primarily of concern during the last trimester of pregnancy. Drug-induced cardiac arrest and hemorrhage are not specifically associated with the 4th to 10th week of gestation.

4. The answer is B: inhibition of CYP3A4. Inhibition of drug-metabolizing enzymes will increase the half-life and plasma concentrations of affected drugs, thereby posing a risk of toxicity. Induction of these enzymes will reduce half-life and plasma levels. Displacement of a drug from plasma proteins or inhibition of P-glycoprotein might increase plasma levels temporarily until the rate of elimination increases. Acceleration of gastric emptying might increase the rate of drug absorption but would not permanently increase plasma drug levels.

5. The answer is E: reduced capacity to oxidize drugs. Conjugative metabolism is relatively unchanged in the elderly, but oxidative drug metabolism is usually reduced. The elderly tend to have a higher percentage of body fat than younger adults and therefore have increased volumes of distribution of fat-soluble drugs. Drug absorption is not typically altered in the elderly, and their blood-brain barrier is not noticeably impaired in most cases.

SELECTED READINGS

Bahna, S.L., and B. Khalili. New concepts in the management of adverse drug reactions. Allergy Asthma Proc 28:517–524, 2007.

Gee, D. Establishing evidence for early action: the prevention of reproductive and developmental harm. Basic Clin Pharmacol Toxicol 102: 257–266, 2008.

Hajjar, E.R., A.C. Cafiero, and J.T. Hanlon. Polypharmacy in elderly patients. Am J Geriatr Pharmacother 5:345–351, 2007.

Sakata, T., and E.A. Winzeler. Genomics, systems biology and drug development for infectious diseases. Mol Biosyst 3:841–848, 2007.

Zwillich, T. US lawmakers tackle safety reforms at the FDA. Lancet 369:1989–1990, 2007.

AUTONOMIC AND NEUROMUSCULAR PHARMACOLOGY

CHAPTER 5

Introduction to Autonomic and Neuromuscular Pharmacology

OVERVIEW

The nervous system consists of the central and peripheral nervous systems. The **central nervous system** includes the brain and spinal cord, whereas the **peripheral nervous system** includes the autonomic nervous system and the somatic nervous system.

Drugs alter nervous system function primarily by affecting **neurotransmitters** or their **receptors**. In some cases, drugs affect the synthesis, storage, release, inactivation, or neuronal reuptake of neurotransmitters. In other cases, they activate or block neurotransmitter receptors. Most drugs are relatively specific for a particular neurotransmitter or receptor. The spectrum of effects produced by a drug depends on the distribution of the affected neurotransmitters in the central and peripheral nervous systems. The actions of some drugs are localized to either the central or the peripheral nervous system, whereas the actions of other drugs (e.g., cocaine and amphetamine) affect both central and peripheral functions.

This chapter reviews the anatomy and physiology of the peripheral nervous system and provides an overview of the mechanisms by which drugs affect nervous system function. Drugs that act primarily on the central nervous system are discussed in the chapters of Section IV.

ANATOMY AND PHYSIOLOGY OF THE PERIPHERAL NERVOUS SYSTEM

The **autonomic nervous system** involuntarily regulates the activity of smooth muscles, exocrine glands, cardiac tissue, and certain metabolic activities, whereas the **somatic nervous system** activates skeletal muscle contraction, thereby enabling voluntary body movements. Both autonomic and somatic nervous systems are part of the peripheral nervous system, but they are controlled by the central nervous system. The autonomic nervous system is regulated by brain stem centers responsible for cardiovascular, respiratory, and other visceral functions. The somatic nervous system

is activated by corticospinal tracts, which originate in the motor cortex, and by spinal reflexes.

Autonomic Nervous System

The autonomic nervous system consists of sympathetic and parasympathetic divisions. In the **sympathetic nervous system**, nerves arise from the thoracic and lumbar spinal cord and have a short preganglionic fiber and a long postganglionic fiber. Most of the ganglia are located in the paravertebral chain adjacent to the spinal cord, but a few prevertebral ganglia (the celiac, splanchnic, and mesenteric ganglia) are located more distally to the spinal cord. The **parasympathetic nervous system** includes portions of cranial nerves III, VII, IX, and X (the oculomotor, facial, glossopharyngeal, and vagus nerves, respectively) and some of the nerves originating from the sacral spinal cord. The parasympathetic nerves have long preganglionic fibers and short postganglionic fibers, with the ganglia often located in the innervated organs.

The origins, neurotransmitters, and receptors of the sympathetic and parasympathetic systems are shown in Figure 5–1. The sympathetic nervous system tends to discharge as a unit, producing a diffuse activation of target organs. Preganglionic, sympathetic neurons synapse with a large number of postganglionic neurons, which contributes to widespread activation of the organs during sympathetic stimulation. In addition, the release of epinephrine and norepinephrine from the adrenal medulla into the circulation enables the activation of target tissues throughout the body, including some tissues not directly innervated by sympathetic nerves. In contrast to the sympathetic system, the parasympathetic system can discretely activate specific target tissues. For example, it is possible for parasympathetic nerves to slow the heart rate without simultaneously stimulating gastrointestinal or bladder function. This is partly because a low ratio exists of postganglionic fibers to preganglionic fibers in the parasympathetic system.

As shown in Figure 5–2, the sympathetic and parasympathetic nervous systems often have opposing effects on organ function. Activation of the sympathetic system produces the **"fight or flight"** response, which enables

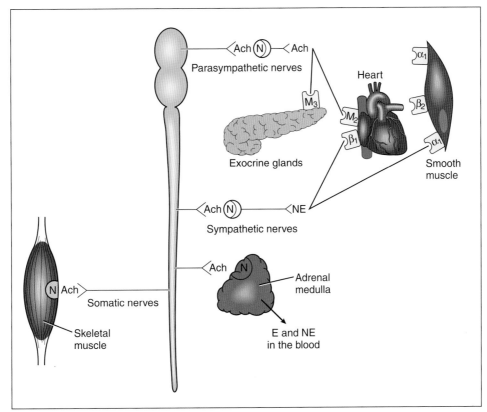

Figure 5-1. **Neurotransmission in the autonomic and somatic nervous systems.** The parasympathetic nervous system consists of cranial and sacral nerves with long preganglionic and short postganglionic fibers. The sympathetic nervous system consists of thoracic and lumbar nerves with short preganglionic and long postganglionic fibers. The sympathetic system includes the adrenal medulla, which releases norepinephrine and epinephrine into the blood. The somatic nervous system consists of motor neurons to the skeletal muscle. α = α-adrenoceptors; ACh = acetylcholine; β = β-adrenoceptors; E = epinephrine; N = nicotinic receptors; NE = norepinephrine; M = muscarinic receptors.

a person to respond to threatening situations. During this response, cardiovascular stimulation provides skeletal muscles with the oxygen and energy substrates required to support vigorous physical activity. Increases in glycogenolysis and lipolysis also help provide the required energy fuels. The parasympathetic system is sometimes called the **"rest and digest" system,** because it slows the heart rate and promotes more vegetative functions, such as digestion, defecation, and micturition. Many parasympathetic effects (including pupillary constriction, bronchoconstriction, and stimulation of gut and bladder motility) are caused by smooth muscle contraction.

Somatic Nervous System

The somatic nervous system consists of the motor neurons to the skeletal muscle. These neurons have a single nerve fiber that releases acetylcholine at the neuromuscular junction.

Enteric Nervous System

The enteric nervous system (ENS) is sometimes called the third division of the autonomic nervous system. The ENS consists of a network of autonomic nerves that are located in the gut wall and regulate gastrointestinal motility and secretion. The ENS, which includes the submucosal,

myenteric, and subserosal plexuses, receives innervation from the sympathetic and parasympathetic nervous systems. The ENS has afferent fibers and efferent fibers, and it integrates input received from autonomic nerves with localized reflexes to synchronize the waves of peristalsis (the propulsive contractions of gut muscle). Parasympathetic stimulation activates the ENS, whereas sympathetic stimulation inhibits the ENS. The ENS can function independently of autonomic innervation following autonomic denervation.

NEUROTRANSMITTERS AND RECEPTORS

Neurotransmitters

The primary neurotransmitters found in the autonomic and somatic nervous systems are **acetylcholine** and **norepinephrine** (see Fig. 5–1). The terms *adrenergic* and *cholinergic* refer to neurons that release norepinephrine or acetylcholine, respectively.

Acetylcholine is the transmitter at all autonomic ganglia, at parasympathetic neuroeffector junctions, and at somatic neuromuscular junctions. It is also the transmitter at a few sympathetic neuroeffector junctions, including the junctions of nerves in sweat glands and vasodilator fibers

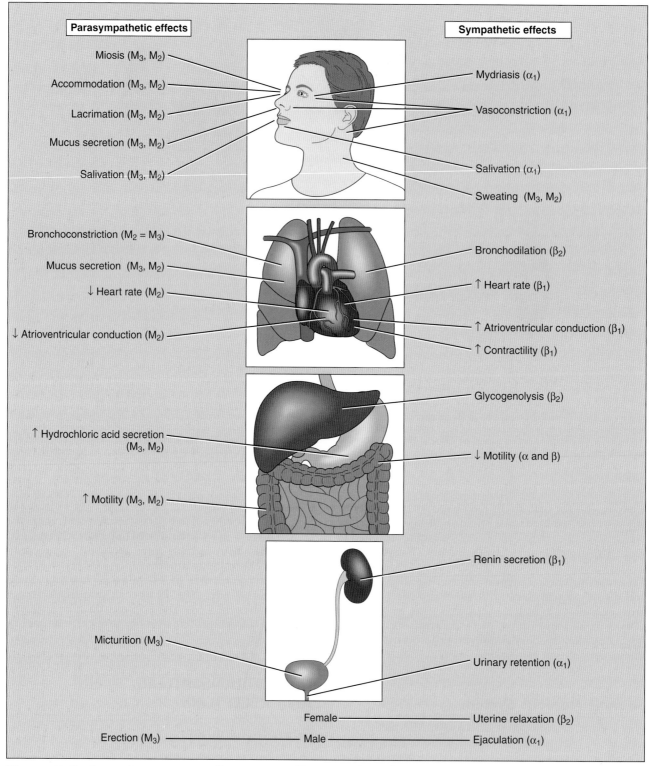

Figure 5-2. **Autonomic nervous system effects on organs.** All parasympathetic effects are mediated by muscarinic receptors. Sympathetic effects are mediated by α-adrenoceptors (a), β-adrenoceptors (β), or muscarinic receptors (M).

in skeletal muscle. The presence of acetylcholine in several types of autonomic and somatic synapses contributes to the lack of specificity of drugs acting on acetylcholine neurotransmission.

Although norepinephrine (noradrenaline) is the primary neurotransmitter at most sympathetic postganglionic

neuroeffector junctions, **epinephrine** (adrenaline) is the principal catecholamine released from the adrenal medulla in response to activation of the sympathetic nervous system.

A number of other neurotransmitters have been identified in autonomic nerves of the ENS of the gastrointestinal tract, as well as in the genitourinary tract and certain blood vessels. The transmitters released by these neurons include **neuropeptide Y**, **vasoactive intestinal polypeptide**, **enkephalin**, **substance P**, **serotonin** (5-hydroxytryptamine), **adenosine triphosphate**, and **nitric oxide**. In some tissues, adenosine triphosphate released by these neurons is converted to **adenosine**, which can then activate adenosine receptors in a number of tissues (see Chapter 27). Nitric oxide is an important neurotransmitter that produces vasodilatation in a many vascular beds and is also found in the ENS.

Receptors for Acetylcholine, Norepinephrine, and Epinephrine

The **acetylcholine receptors** have been divided into two types, based on their selective activation by one of two plant alkaloids. **Muscarinic (M) receptors**, which are acetylcholine receptors activated by muscarine, are primarily located at parasympathetic neuroeffector junctions. **Nicotinic receptors**, which are acetylcholine receptors activated by nicotine, are found in all autonomic ganglia, at somatic neuromuscular junctions, and in the brain. Muscarinic receptors are subdivided based on molecular and pharmacologic criteria. Activation of the M_3 receptor produces smooth muscle contraction (except sphincters) and gland secretion. Activation of the M_2 receptor mediates cardiac slowing. The M_1 receptor is primarily concerned with modulation of neurotransmission at central and peripheral sites. Activation of nicotinic receptors in autonomic ganglia excites neurotransmission, whereas activation of these receptors in skeletal muscle causes muscle contraction.

The receptors for norepinephrine and epinephrine at sympathetic neuroeffector junctions are called ***adrenoceptors***, a term which is derived from adrenaline, another name for epinephrine. Two types of adrenoceptors, called **α-adrenoceptors** and **β-adrenoceptors**, are distinguished on the basis of their selective activation and blockade by adrenoceptor agonists and antagonists. These receptors have been further divided into several subtypes. The α_1-adrenoceptors mediate smooth muscle contraction, whereas β_2-adrenoceptors mediate smooth muscle relaxation. Activation of β_1-adrenoceptors produces cardiac stimulation.

NEUROTRANSMISSION AND SITES OF DRUG ACTION

Cholinergic and adrenergic neurotransmission have many basic similarities. In both cases, the neurotransmitter is synthesized in nerve terminals, stored in membrane-bound vesicles, and released into the synapse in response to nerve stimulation. After the neurotransmitter activates postjunctional receptors to initiate a physiologic effect, neurotransmitter action is terminated either by metabolism or neuronal reuptake. Various drugs exert their effects at specific steps in the process.

Examples and sites of action for drugs that affect autonomic neurotransmission are shown in Figure 5–3, and the mechanisms of action are listed in Table 5–1.

Cholinergic Neurotransmission

Acetylcholine is synthesized from choline and acetate in the neuronal cytoplasm by choline acetyltransferase, and then it is stored in vesicles. When parasympathetic nerve is stimulated, the action potential induces calcium influx into the neuron, and calcium mediates release of the neurotransmitter by a process called exocytosis. During exocytosis, the vesicle membrane and plasma membrane fuse, and the neurotransmitter is released into the synapse through an opening in the fused membranes. After acetylcholine activates postsynaptic acetylcholine receptors, it is rapidly hydrolyzed by the enzyme cholinesterase to form choline and acetate. Choline is recycled through the process of reuptake by the presynaptic neuron. This process is mediated by a membrane protein that transports choline into the neuron. Acetylcholine can also activate presynaptic autoreceptors, which inhibits further release of the neurotransmitter by the neuron.

Drugs Affecting Cholinergic Neurotransmission

Figure 5–3A shows the sites of various agents that affect cholinergic neurotransmission.

Hemicholinium blocks choline transport into the neuron and thereby inhibits the synthesis of acetylcholine, whereas **vesamicol** prevents the vesicular storage of acetylcholine. Neither of these drugs has any current medical use.

Several toxins affect the release of acetylcholine. One example, **black widow spider venom** containing **α-latrotoxin** has been found to markedly stimulate vesicular release of acetylcholine producing excessive activation of acetylcholine receptors. A black widow spider bite often causes severe contraction and pain in local muscles, which then spreads to regional muscles and throughout the body. Abdominal pains are usually the most severe, mimicking appendicitis or food poisoning. Salivation, lacrimation, sweating, changes in heart rate, high blood pressure, shock, and coma may occur, though death from black widow spider bite is rare.

Botulinum toxin A, which is produced by *Clostridium botulinum*, blocks the exocytotic release of acetylcholine and inhibits neuromuscular transmission. Botulinum toxin is being used for an increasing number of medical and cosmetic conditions. It is used to treat localized spasms of various muscles, including those of the eyes, face, and hands, and it is employed in treating tremor, dystonia, excessive salivation, and other symptoms of Parkinson's disease. In these applications, botulinum toxin is injected directly into the muscle, where it causes muscle relaxation. Injections of a preparation of this toxin known as BOTOX have been shown to reduce facial wrinkles and have been widely utilized for cosmetic purposes. More recently, botulinum toxin has been used to treat excessive sweating (hyperhidrosis) of the palms and soles, and botulinum toxin is being studied as an alternative to acetylcholine receptor antagonists in the treatment of overactive urinary bladder. The most common side effects of botulinum toxin injections are dry mouth and dysphagia.

After acetylcholine is released, it can activate postsynaptic muscarinic or nicotinic receptors. Many drugs, including

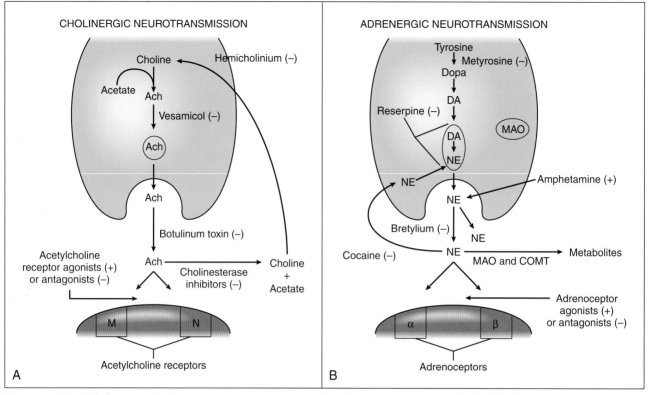

Figure 5–3. Cholinergic and adrenergic neurotransmission and sites of drug action. (A) Acetylcholine (ACh) is synthesized from choline and acetate, stored in neuronal vesicles, and released into the synapse by nerve stimulation. Hemicholinium blocks choline uptake by the neuron and inhibits ACh synthesis. Vesamicol blocks ACh storage, and botulinum toxin blocks ACh release. ACh breakdown is inhibited by cholinesterase inhibitors such as physostigmine. Postjunctional acetylcholine receptors are activated or blocked by acetylcholine receptor agonists or antagonists, respectively. (B) Norepinephrine (NE) is synthesized from tyrosine in a three-step reaction: tyrosine to dopa (dihydroxyphenylalanine), dopa to dopamine (DA), and dopamine to NE. The conversion of tyrosine to dopa is inhibited by metyrosine. The vesicular storage of DA and NE is blocked by reserpine, and the release of NE in response to nerve stimulation is blocked by bretylium. After activating postsynaptic receptors, NE is sequestered by neuronal reuptake, a process blocked by cocaine. Amphetamine indirectly increases the transport of NE into the synapse. Postsynaptic adrenoceptors are activated or blocked by adrenoceptor agonists or antagonists, respectively. α = α-adrenoceptors; β = β-adrenoceptors; COMT = catechol-O-methyltransferase; M = muscarinic receptors; MAO = monoamine oxidase; N = nicotinic receptors; (–) = inhibits; (+) = stimulates.

TABLE 5–1. Examples of Drugs Affecting Autonomic Neurotransmission

Mechanism of Action	Drugs Affecting Acetylcholine Neurotransmission	Drugs Affecting Sympathetic Neurotransmission
Inhibit synthesis of neurotransmitter	Hemicholinium*	Metyrosine (alpha-methyl-para-tyrosine)
Prevent vesicular storage of neurotransmitter	Vesamicol*	Reserpine
Inhibit release of neurotransmitter	Botulinum toxin	Bretylium
Increase release of neurotransmitter	Black widow spider venom (α-latrotoxin)*	Amphetamine
Inhibit reuptake of neurotransmitter	—	Cocaine
Inhibit metabolism of neurotransmitter	Cholinesterase inhibitors (physostigmine)	Monoamine oxidase inhibitors (phenelzine)
Activate postsynaptic receptors	Acetylcholine, bethanechol, and pilocarpine	Albuterol, dobutamine, and epinephrine
Block postsynaptic receptors	Atropine and tubocurarine (block muscarinic and nicotinic receptors, respectively)	Phentolamine and propranolol (block α- and β-adrenoceptors, respectively)

*These agents have no current medical use.

choline esters such as **bethanechol** and plant alkaloids such as **pilocarpine**, mimic the effect of acetylcholine at these same receptors. These drugs are called **direct-acting acetylcholine receptor agonists** because they directly bind and activate acetylcholine receptors.

Another group of drugs, the **cholinesterase inhibitors** such as physostigmine, prevent the breakdown of acetylcholine

and thereby increase the synaptic concentration of acetylcholine. Because this action leads to an increase in the activation of acetylcholine receptors by acetylcholine, these drugs are called **indirect-acting acetylcholine receptor agonists** (see Chapter 6).

The most important group of drugs that inhibit cholinergic neurotransmission contains the **acetylcholine receptor**

antagonists. The group is divided into two subgroups. The first consists of **muscarinic receptor antagonists** and includes drugs such as atropine, whereas the second consists of **nicotinic receptor antagonists** and includes **ganglionic blocking agents** (e.g., trimethaphan) and **neuromuscular blocking drugs** (e.g., tubocurarine).

Sympathetic Neurotransmission

Norepinephrine is synthesized via the following steps: tyrosine → dopa → dopamine → norepinephrine. This pathway is illustrated in Figure 18–3.

First, the amino acid tyrosine is converted to dopa (dihydroxyphenylalanine) by tyrosine hydroxylase, the rate-limiting enzyme in the pathway. Dopa is then converted to dopamine by L-aromatic amino acid decarboxylase (dopa decarboxylase). At this point, dopamine is accumulated by neuronal storage vesicles. Inside the vesicles, dopamine is converted to norepinephrine by dopamine-β-hydroxylase.

As with acetylcholine, norepinephrine is released into the synapse by calcium-mediated exocytosis in response to nerve stimulation. Once in the synapse, norepinephrine activates postjunctional α- and β-adrenoceptors. It also activates prejunctional autoreceptors that exert negative feedback and inhibit further release of norepinephrine.

Norepinephrine is removed from the synapse primarily by neuronal reuptake via a transport protein known as the catecholamine transporter that is localized in the presynaptic neuronal membrane. The reuptake of norepinephrine limits the duration of presynaptic and postsynaptic receptor activation and enables the neurotransmitter to be used again for neurotransmission. Once inside the neuron, norepinephrine is sequestered in storage vesicles and is recycled by adrenergic neurons in a manner similar to that used by cholinergic neurons to recycle choline. The catecholamine transporter can also sequester epinephrine and other catecholamines.

The enzymes catechol-O-methyltransferase (COMT) and monoamine oxidase (MAO) primarily serve to inactivate norepinephrine that is not sequestered by presynaptic neurons. These enzymes are found in many tissues, including the liver and gut. MAO is also located inside neuronal mitochondria and degrades cytoplasmic norepinephrine that is not accumulated by storage vesicles.

Drugs Affecting Adrenergic Neurotransmission

Figure 5–3B shows the sites of various agents that affect adrenergic neurotransmission.

The synthesis of norepinephrine is inhibited by **metyrosine** (DEMSER), a drug that is a competitive inhibitor of tyrosine hydroxylase. Metyrosine can be used to inhibit norepinephrine and epinephrine synthesis in persons with an adrenal medullary tumor (pheochromocytoma) that secretes large amounts of these substances and thereby causes severe hypertension. The drug has also been studied as a treatment for dystonia or dyskinesia in persons being treated with neuroleptic (antipsychotic) drugs.

The storage of norepinephrine in neuronal vesicles is blocked by **reserpine**, a drug that inhibits the transporter for amines located in the vesicular membrane. Bretylium blocks the release of norepinephrine in response to nerve stimulation. Drugs that block the synthesis, storage, or release of norepinephrine are called **neuronal blocking agents**.

Some endogenous substances and synthetic compounds directly activate α- or β-adrenoceptors and, therefore, are called **direct-acting adrenoceptor agonists**. Examples include **albuterol**, **dobutamine**, and **epinephrine**. Other drugs indirectly increase the activation of adrenoceptors by increasing the synaptic concentration of norepinephrine. These drugs are called **indirect-acting adrenoceptor agonists**, and examples include **amphetamine** and **cocaine**. The indirect-acting agonists require the presence of a functional postganglionic neuron to exert their effects. Cocaine binds to and competitively inhibits the catecholamine transporter located in the presynaptic nerve terminal, thereby increasing the duration of action of norepinephrine at the synapse. Amphetamine and related drugs are substrates for the transporter, which transports the drugs into the presynaptic neuron where they inhibit the storage of norepinephrine by synaptic vesicles, leading to reverse transport of norepinephrine into the synapse by the catecholamine transporter. These actions serve to increase the synaptic concentration of norepinephrine and its activation of adrenoceptors.

Another group of drugs act by inhibiting the breakdown of norepinephrine by COMT or MAO. As discussed in Chapters 22 and 24, these **catechol-O-methyltransferase inhibitors** and **monoamine oxidase inhibitors** primarily exert their effects on the central nervous system.

Drugs that inhibit sympathetic stimulation of target organs include the neuronal blocking agents (described earlier in this section) and the **adrenoceptor antagonists**. Examples of the latter are **phentolamine**, which selectively blocks α-adrenoceptors; **propranolol**, which selectively blocks β-adrenoceptors; and **labetalol**, which blocks both receptor types.

Drugs Modulating the Baroreceptor Reflex

In addition to exerting their primary pharmacologic actions, a number of adrenoceptor agonists and antagonists modulate the baroreceptor reflex (Fig. 5–4).

When a drug or a physiologic action increases blood pressure, this activates stretch receptors (mechanoreceptors) located in the aortic arch and in the carotid sinus at the bifurcation of the carotid artery. Receptor activation initiates impulses that travel via afferent nerves to the brain stem vasomotor center. Stimulation of the vagal motor nucleus (via nerves from the solitary tract nucleus) leads to an increase in vagal (parasympathetic) outflow, a decrease in heart rate, and a decrease in the sympathetic nerve outflow from the vasomotor center. The effect on the heart rate is called reflex bradycardia.

If a drug lowers the blood pressure sufficiently, it may reduce the baroreceptor tone and thereby produce an acceleration of the heart rate and activation of sympathetic vasoconstriction. In this case, the effect on the heart rate is called reflex tachycardia.

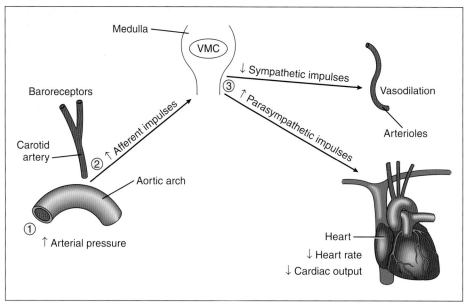

Figure 5–4. The baroreceptor reflex. (A) Increased arterial pressure activates stretch receptors in the aortic arch and carotid sinus. (B) Receptor activation initiates afferent impulses to the brain stem vasomotor center (VMC). (C) Via solitary tract fibers, the VMC activates the vagal motor nucleus, which increases vagal (parasympathetic) outflow and slows the heart. At the same time, the VMC reduces stimulation of spinal intermediolateral neurons that activate sympathetic preganglionic fibers, and this decreases sympathetic stimulation of the heart and blood vessels. By this mechanism, drugs that increase blood pressure produce reflex bradycardia. Drugs that reduce blood pressure attenuate this response and cause reflex tachycardia.

SUMMARY OF IMPORTANT POINTS

■ The sympathetic and parasympathetic divisions of the autonomic nervous system have opposing effects in many tissues. Drugs that activate one division often have the same effects as drugs that inhibit the other division.

■ Acetylcholine is the primary neurotransmitter at parasympathetic and somatic neuroeffector junctions, and norepinephrine is the transmitter at most sympathetic junctions. In the autonomic nervous system there are several nonadrenergic-noncholinergic neurotransmitters, including peptides, nitric oxide, and serotonin.

■ Most autonomic drugs activate or block receptors for acetylcholine or norepinephrine in smooth muscle, cardiac tissue, and glands. Activation of muscarinic and α-adrenoceptors produces smooth muscle contraction, whereas activation of β-adrenoceptors produces smooth muscle relaxation and cardiac stimulation.

■ Some drugs have effects on neurotransmitter synthesis, storage, release, or metabolism. These are called indirect-acting drugs.

■ Indirect-acting agonists increase the concentration of a neurotransmitter at synapses, either by inhibiting transmitter inactivation (cholinesterase inhibitors), increasing transmitter release (amphetamine and tyramine), or blocking transmitter reuptake (cocaine).

Review Questions

1. A woman with facial muscle spasms is treated with an agent that inhibits the release of acetylcholine. Which side effect is most likely to occur in this patient?
(A) bradycardia
(B) urinary incontinence
(C) dry mouth
(D) diarrhea
(E) constriction of the pupils

2. A man receives an injection of epinephrine to treat an allergic reaction. Which effect would result from this treatment?
(A) increased glucose absorption from the gut
(B) increased hepatic output of glucose
(C) increased uptake of glucose by skeletal muscle
(D) increased formation of glycogen
(E) increased conversion of glucose to fat

3. Which property is characteristic of the sympathetic nervous system?
(A) discrete activation of specific organs
(B) long preganglionic neurons
(C) action terminated by cholinesterase
(D) inhibits the enteric nervous system
(E) activated by increased arterial blood pressure

4. A man is arrested while using a substance that inhibits the neuronal catecholamine transporter. Which sign would most likely be observed in this person?
(A) excessive sweating
(B) dilation of the pupils
(C) involuntary muscle contractions

(D) flushing of the skin
(E) sedation

5. A woman with acute high blood pressure is given a drug that inhibits formation of dihydroxyphenylalanine. Which response would result from this treatment?
(A) diarrhea
(B) bronchodilation
(C) renin secretion
(D) decreased heart rate
(E) salivation

Answers and Explanations

1. The answer is C: dry mouth. Botulinum toxin inhibits the release of acetylcholine from cholinergic neurons, and it is used to inhibit neuromuscular transmission in persons with dystonia. The drug may also inhibit acetylcholine release from parasympathetic nerves and cause dry mouth and dysphagia, particularly when it is administered to the head and neck. Bradycardia, urinary incontinence, diarrhea, and miosis are effects that would be caused by increased release of acetylcholine from parasympathetic nerves.

2. The answer is B: increased hepatic output of glucose. Epinephrine activates β_2-adrenoceptors and thereby increases the formation of glucose from glycogen (glycogenolysis). Epinephrine does not increase glucose absorption (Option A), glucose utilization (Option C), glycogen formation (Option D), or conversion of glucose to fat (Option E).

3. The answer is D: inhibits the enteric nervous system. Options A, B, C, and E (discrete activation of specific organs, long preganglionic neurons, action terminated by cholinesterase, activated by increased arterial blood pressure) are attributes of the parasympathetic nervous system.

4. The answer is B: dilation of the pupils. Cocaine inhibits the catecholamine transporter and increases synaptic concentrations of norepinephrine, leading to the activation of adrenoceptors in peripheral tissues and the central nervous system. Norepinephrine activates α_1-adrenoceptors in the iris dilator muscle, thereby causing muscle contraction and pupillary dilation. Excessive sweating (Option A) would result from activation of muscarinic receptors in sweat glands, whereas involuntary muscle contractions (Option C) would result from nicotinic receptor stimulation. Flushing of the skin (Option D) and sedation (Option E) are not typically caused by adrenoceptor or acetylcholine receptor activation.

5. The answer is D: decreased heart rate. Metyrosine inhibits tyrosine hydroxylase and norepinephrine synthesis, thereby decreasing sympathetic tone and reducing activation of β_1-adrenoceptors in cardiac tissue. Bronchodilation (Option B) and renin secretion (Option C) result from increased activation of β_2- and β_1-adrenoceptors, respectively. Diarrhea (Option A) and salivation (Option E) primarily result from muscarinic receptor activation.

SELECTED READINGS

Akenman, R., and M.F. Salvatore. Low dose alpha-methyl-para-tyrosine in the treatment of dystonia and dyskinesia. J Neuropsychiatry Clin Neurosci 19:65–69, 2007.

Glaser, D.A., A.A. Hebert, D.M. Pariser, and N. Solish. Palmar and plantar hyperhidrosis: best practice recommendations and special considerations. Cutis 79:18–28, 2007.

Samuels, M.A. The brain-heart connection. Circulation 116:77–84, 2007.

Sellers, D.J., and N. McKay. Developments in the pharmacotherapy of overactive bladder. Curr Opin Urol 17:223–230, 2007.

Sheffield, J.K., and J. Jankovic. Botulinum toxin in the treatment of tremors, dystonias, sialorrhea, and other symptoms associated with Parkinson's disease. Expert Rev Neurother 7:637–647, 2007.

CHAPTER 6

Acetylcholine Receptor Agonists

CLASSIFICATION OF ACETYLCHOLINE RECEPTOR AGONISTS

Direct-Acting Acetylcholine Receptor Agonists
Choline esters
- Acetylcholine
- Bethanechol (URECHOLINE)
- Carbachol

Plant alkaloids
- Muscarine
- Nicotine
- Pilocarpine (SALAGEN)

Other drugs
- Cevimeline (EVOXAC)
- Varenicline (CHANTIX)

Indirect-Acting Acetylcholine Receptor Agonists
Drugs that inhibit cholinesterase
Reversible cholinesterase inhibitors
- Donepezil (ARICEPT)*
- Edrophonium (TENSILON)
- Neostigmine
- Physostigmine
- Pyridostigmine (MESTINON)

Irreversible cholinesterase inhibitors
- Echothiophate
- Isoflurophate
- Malahtion

Drugs that augment acetylcholine
- Sildenafil (VIAGRA)†

*Also rivastigmine (EXELON) and galantamine (REMINYL).
†Also tadalafil (CIALIS) and vardenafil (LEVITRA).

OVERVIEW OF CHOLINERGIC PHARMACOLOGY

Acetylcholine Receptors

Acetylcholine receptors (cholinergic receptors) are divided into two types, **muscarinic receptors** and **nicotinic receptors**, based on their selective activation by the alkaloids muscarine and nicotine.

Muscarinic Receptors

Muscarinic receptors are found in smooth muscle, cardiac tissue, and glands at parasympathetic neuroeffector junctions. They are also found in the central nervous system, on presynaptic sympathetic and parasympathetic nerves, and at autonomic ganglia. Activation of muscarinic receptors on presynaptic autonomic nerves inhibits further neurotransmitter release. The presence of muscarinic receptors on sympathetic nerve terminals provides for interaction between the parasympathetic and sympathetic nervous systems: the release of acetylcholine from parasympathetic nerves inhibits the release of norepinephrine from sympathetic nerves.

Muscarinic receptors are divided into five subtypes, M_1 through M_5, based on their pharmacologic properties and molecular structures. The principal subtypes found in most tissues are M_1, M_2, and M_3 receptors (Table 6–1). Muscarinic receptor stimulation leads to the activation of guanine nucleotide–binding proteins (G proteins), which increases or decreases the formation of other second messengers (see Chapter 3). The M_1, M_3, and M_5 receptors are coupled with Gq proteins and their activation stimulates phospholipase C, leading to the formation of inositol triphosphate (IP_3) and diacylglycerol from membrane phospholipids. In smooth muscles, IP_3 increases calcium release from the sarcoplasmic reticulum and increases muscle contraction. In exocrine glands, IP_3 causes calcium release and glandular secretion.

The M_2 and M_4 receptors are coupled with $G\alpha_i$ proteins and their activation decreases cyclic adenosine monophosphate (cyclic AMP, or cAMP) levels, by inhibiting adenylate cyclase, or increases potassium efflux. The effects produced by activation of muscarinic receptors are summarized in Table 6–1.

The acetylcholine receptor agonists that are currently available for clinical use do not selectively activate subtypes

BOX 6–1. TREATMENT OF CHRONIC OPEN-ANGLE GLAUCOMA

In the normal eye, aqueous humor is secreted by the ciliary processes and flows through the pupillary aperture of the iris and into the anterior chamber. It then drains through the trabecular meshwork in Schlemm's canal. In patients with open-angle glaucoma, persistently elevated intraocular pressure is associated with narrowing of the anterior chamber angle, a decrease in the rate of aqueous outflow, and the gradual loss of peripheral vision. Various types of drugs can be used to reduce intraocular pressure before irreversible optic nerve damage occurs. The sites of action of these drugs are shown below.

Some types of drugs act by enhancing the drainage of aqueous humor. **Muscarinic receptor agonists** (e.g., **pilocarpine**) stimulate the contraction of meridional ciliary muscle fibers that insert near the trabecular meshwork. Contraction of these fibers opens the trabecular spaces so

that aqueous humor drains more easily. **Prostaglandins** (e.g., **latanoprost**) increase aqueous drainage through an alternative pathway known as the uveoscleral route. In this pathway, aqueous humor flows through the ciliary muscles into the suprachoroidal space.

Other types of drugs act by reducing the amount of aqueous humor produced by the ciliary processes. The **β-adrenoceptor blockers** (e.g., **timolol**) and the **α₂-adrenoceptor agonists** (e.g., **apraclonidine**) reduce the formation of cyclic AMP, a substance that stimulates aqueous humor production. **Carbonic anhydrase inhibitors** (e.g., **dorzolamide**) block the formation of bicarbonate by carbonic anhydrase, an enzyme that is required for aqueous humor secretion. **Epinephrine** probably acts by reducing blood flow in the ciliary processes.

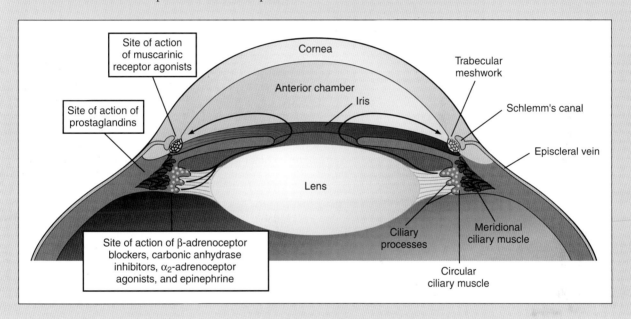

Other Drugs

Cevimeline is a synthetic direct-acting muscarinic receptor agonist that is administered orally to treat dry mouth and is undergoing investigation for the treatment of dry eyes. The drug is used to treat these conditions in patients who have had radiation therapy for head and neck cancer and in those with **Sjögren's syndrome** (dry eyes, dry mouth, and arthritis). Adverse effects include increased sweating, nausea, and visual disturbances caused by drug-induced miosis. As with other acetylcholine receptor agonists, cevimeline should be used cautiously in persons with asthma or cardiac arrhythmias.

Varenicline is a partial agonist at the nicotinic receptor subtype found in the brain that mediates the reinforcing effects of nicotine in smokers. The drug is used as an aid to smoking cessation and has been found to reduce both the craving and withdrawal effects caused by the absence of nicotine (see Chapter 25).

INDIRECT-ACTING ACETYLCHOLINE RECEPTOR AGONISTS

One group of indirect-acting agonists functions by inhibiting cholinesterase, whereas another group increases cyclic GMP levels and potentiates the vasodilative effects of acetylcholine.

Drugs that Inhibit Cholinesterase

The cholinesterase inhibitors prevent the breakdown of acetylcholine at all cholinergic synapses. The shorter-acting types are referred to as **reversible cholinesterase inhibitors**, whereas the longer-acting types are called **irreversible cholinesterase inhibitors.** The properties and clinical uses of inhibitors from each group are outlined in Table 6–3.

VASCULAR EFFECTS. Acetylcholine typically causes vasodilation, though vasoconstriction may occur under some conditions (see below). The **vasodilative effect** of acetylcholine is mediated by muscarinic M_3 receptors located in vascular endothelial cells, where muscarinic stimulation causes activation of nitric oxide synthetase and the formation of nitric oxide. Nitric oxide is a gas that diffuses into vascular smooth muscle cells and activates guanylyl cyclase to increase the formation of cyclic guanosine monophosphate (cyclic GMP), leading to vascular smooth muscle relaxation and vasodilation.

GASTROINTESTINAL AND URINARY TRACT EFFECTS. When muscarinic receptor agonists are taken, they stimulate salivary, gastric, and other secretions in the gastrointestinal tract. They also increase contraction of gastrointestinal smooth muscle (except sphincters) by stimulating the enteric nervous system located in the gut wall. This, in turn, increases gastrointestinal motility. Whereas muscarinic receptor agonists stimulate the bladder detrusor muscle, they relax the internal sphincter of the bladder, and these effects promote emptying of the bladder (micturition). Higher doses of these agonists, therefore, can produce excessive salivation and cause diarrhea, intestinal cramps, and urinary incontinence (the "all faucets turned on" syndrome).

Acetylcholine

CHEMISTRY AND PHARMACOKINETICS. Acetylcholine is the choline ester of acetic acid. It is rapidly hydrolyzed by cholinesterase and has an extremely short duration of action.

EFFECTS AND INDICATIONS. Because of its limited absorption, short duration of action, and lack of specificity for muscarinic or nicotinic receptors, acetylcholine has limited clinical applications.

An ophthalmic solution of acetylcholine available for intraocular use during **cataract surgery** produces miosis after extraction of the lens. The solution also can be used in other types of **ophthalmic surgery** that require rapid and complete miosis. Topical ocular administration of acetylcholine is not effective, because acetylcholine is hydrolyzed by corneal cholinesterase before it can penetrate to the iris and ciliary muscle.

In patients having **diagnostic coronary angiography**, acetylcholine can be administered by direct intracoronary injection to provoke coronary artery spasm. The **vasospastic effect** of acetylcholine is caused by stimulation of muscarinic M_3 receptors located on vascular smooth muscle that mediate smooth muscle contraction. In most situations, the vasodilative effect of acetylcholine is more pronounced than the vasoconstrictive effect. In patients with vasospastic angina pectoris, however, intracoronary injection of acetylcholine can provoke a localized vasoconstrictive response, and this helps establish the diagnosis of vasospastic angina.

Bethanechol and Carbachol

CHEMISTRY AND PHARMACOKINETICS. Bethanechol and carbachol are choline esters of carbamic acid. They are resistant to hydrolysis by cholinesterase, and their duration of action is relatively short, lasting for several hours after topical ocular or systemic administration.

EFFECTS AND INDICATIONS. Bethanechol selectively activates muscarinic receptors and can be used to stimulate bladder or gastrointestinal muscle without significantly affecting heart rate or blood pressure. Although it generally has been replaced by more effective treatments, bethanechol has been given postoperatively or postpartum to increase bladder muscle tone in patients who suffer from nonobstructive, neurogenic urinary retention after receiving anesthetics or other drugs administered during childbirth or surgery. Therapeutic doses of bethanechol given orally or subcutaneously have little effect on blood pressure, but the drug should never be administered intravenously, because this can cause hypotension and bradycardia.

Carbachol is effective in the treatment of **chronic open-angle glaucoma**, but it is usually used in cases in which a patient does not respond adequately to pilocarpine (see "Pilocarpine"). Carbachol can also be used to produce miosis during **ophthalmic surgery**.

Plant Alkaloids

The plant alkaloids include muscarine, nicotine, and pilocarpine.

Muscarine and Nicotine

SOURCE AND EFFECTS. Muscarine is found in mushrooms of the genera *Inocybe* and *Clitocybe*, and the consumption of these poisonous mushrooms can cause diarrhea, sweating, salivation, and lacrimation. Muscarine is also found in trace amounts in *Amanita muscaria*, the original source of muscarine, but the toxicity of this mushroom is largely due to its content of ibotenic acid. Nicotine is derived from *Nicotiana* plants and is contained in cigarettes and other tobacco products. The effects of nicotine dependence are discussed in Chapter 25.

INDICATIONS. Muscarine has no current medical use. Nicotine is available in chewing gum, transdermal patches, and other products designed for use in smoking cessation programs.

Pilocarpine

CHEMISTRY AND PHARMACOKINETICS. Pilocarpine is a tertiary amine alkaloid that is obtained from *Pilocarpus*, a small shrub. The drug is well absorbed after topical ocular and oral administration.

EFFECTS AND INDICATIONS. Pilocarpine, which has greater affinity for muscarinic receptors than for nicotinic receptors, can produce all of the effects of muscarinic receptor stimulation.

Pilocarpine is a second-line drug for the treatment of **chronic open-angle glaucoma**, in which it lowers intraocular pressure by increasing the outflow of aqueous humor (Box 6-1). It is also used in the treatment of **acute angle-closure glaucoma**, a medical emergency in which blindness can result if the intraocular pressure is not lowered immediately. The main side effects of ocular pilocarpine administration are decreased night vision, which is caused by miosis, and difficulty in focusing on distant objects, which occurs because the lens is accommodated for close vision.

In patients with **xerostomia** (dry mouth), pilocarpine is administered orally to stimulate salivary gland secretion. Low doses can be used to produce this effect with minimal side effects in many patients because of the high sensitivity of the salivary glands to muscarinic stimulation.

TABLE 6-2.   Properties and Clinical Uses of Direct-Acting Acetylcholine Receptor Agonists

Drug	Receptor Specificity	Hydrolyzed by Cholinesterase	Route of Administration	Clinical Use
Choline Esters				
Acetylcholine	Muscarinic and nicotinic	Yes	Intraocular	Miosis during ophthalmic surgery
			Intracoronary	Coronary angiography
Bethanechol	Muscarinic	No	Oral or subcutaneous	Gastrointestinal and urinary stimulation
Carbachol	Muscarinic and nicotinic	No	Topical ocular	Glaucoma
			Intraocular	Miosis during ophthalmic surgery
Plant Alkaloids				
Muscarine	Muscarinic	No	None	None
Nicotine	Nicotinic	No	Oral or transdermal	Smoking cessation programs
Pilocarpine	Muscarinic	No	Topical ocular	Glaucoma
			Oral	Xerostomia
Other Drugs				
Cevimeline	Muscarinic	No	Oral	Xerostomia
Varenicline	Nicotinic	No	Oral	Smoking cessation

Choline Esters

The choline esters include acetylcholine and synthetic acetylcholine analogues, such as bethanechol and carbachol.

General Properties

The choline esters are positively charged quaternary ammonium compounds that are poorly absorbed from the gastrointestinal tract and are not distributed to the central nervous system. Acetylcholine and carbachol activate both muscarinic and nicotinic receptors, whereas bethanechol activates only muscarinic receptors. Because of their lack of specificity for muscarinic receptor subtypes, the muscarinic receptor agonists cause a wide range of effects on many organ systems.

OCULAR EFFECTS. Muscarinic receptor agonists increase lacrimal gland secretion and stimulate contraction of the iris sphincter muscle and the ciliary muscles. Contraction of the iris sphincter muscle produces pupillary constriction (miosis), whereas contraction of the ciliary muscles enables accommodation of the lens to focus on close objects (Fig. 6–2).

RESPIRATORY TRACT EFFECTS. Stimulation of muscarinic receptors increases bronchial muscle contraction and causes an increase in the secretion of mucus throughout the respiratory tract. Because muscarinic receptor agonists can cause bronchoconstriction, they should be avoided or used with extreme caution in patients with asthma and other forms of obstructive lung disease.

CARDIAC EFFECTS. Muscarinic receptor agonists decrease impulse formation in the sinoatrial node by reducing the rate of diastolic depolarization. As a result, they slow the heart rate. In addition, they slow conduction of the cardiac action potential through the atrioventricular node, and this leads to an increased PR interval (time between the beginning of the P wave to the beginning of the QRS complex) on the electrocardiogram.

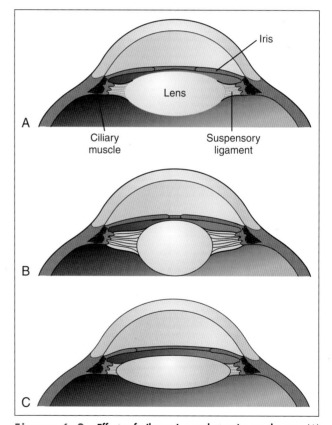

Figure 6-2. Effects of pilocarpine and atropine on the eye. (A) The relationship between the iris sphincter and ciliary muscle is shown in the normal eye. (B) When pilocarpine, a muscarinic receptor agonist, is administered, contraction of the iris sphincter produces pupillary constriction (miosis). Contraction of the ciliary muscle causes the muscle to be displaced centrally. This relaxes the suspensory ligaments connected to the lens, and the internal elasticity of the lens allows it to increase in thickness. As the lens thickens, its refractive power increases so that it focuses on close objects. (C) When atropine, a muscarinic receptor antagonist, is administered, the iris sphincter and ciliary muscles relax. This produces pupillary dilatation (mydriasis) and increases the tension on the suspensory ligaments so that the lens becomes thinner and focuses on distant objects.

TABLE 6–1. Properties of Acetylcholine Receptors

Type of Receptor	Principal Locations	Mechanism of Signal Transduction	Effects
Muscarinic			
M_1 ("neural")	Autonomic ganglia, presynaptic nerve terminals, and central nervous system	Increased IP_3	Modulation of neurotransmission
M_2 ("cardiac")	Cardiac tissue (sinoatrial and atrioventricular nodes)	Increased potassium efflux or decreased cAMP	Slowing of heart rate and conduction
M_3 ("glandular")	Smooth muscle and glands	Increased IP_3	Contraction of smooth muscles and stimulation of glandular secretions
	Vascular smooth muscle	Increased cGMP due to nitric oxide stimulation	Vasodilation
Nicotinic			
Muscle type	Neuromuscular junctions	Increased sodium influx	Muscle contraction
Ganglionic type	Autonomic ganglia	Increased sodium influx	Neuronal excitation
CNS type	Central nervous system	Increased sodium influx	Neuronal excitation

cAMP = cyclic adenosine monophosphate; cGMP = cyclic guanosine monophosphate; CNS = central nervous system; IP_3 = inositol triphosphate.

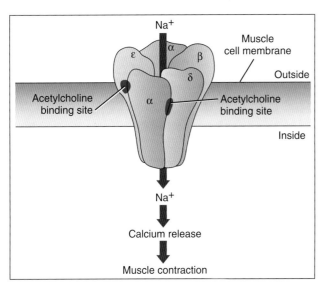

Figure 6–1. The nicotinic receptor is an acetylcholine-gated sodium channel. The channel is a polypeptide pentamer composed of varying combinations of α, β, δ, and ε subunits. In the muscle type of nicotinic receptor shown here, acetylcholine-binding sites are formed by pockets at the interface of the α and δ subunits and the α and ε subunits. Acetylcholine binding to the receptor causes sodium influx, membrane depolarization, release of calcium from the sarcoplasmic reticulum, and muscle contraction. Nicotinic receptors at autonomic ganglia and in the brain have a different subunit composition.

of muscarinic receptors, but an M_1 selective antagonist, pirenzepine, has been developed (see Chapter 7).

Nicotinic Receptors

Nicotinic receptors are found at all autonomic ganglia, at somatic neuromuscular junctions, and in the central nervous system. These receptors are acetylcholine-gated sodium channels whose activation leads to sodium influx and membrane depolarization. At autonomic ganglia, activation of nicotinic receptors produces excitation of postganglionic neurons leading to the release of neurotransmitters

at postganglionic neuroeffector junctions. At junctions of somatic nerves and skeletal muscle, activation of nicotinic receptors depolarizes the motor end plate and leads both to the release of calcium from the sarcoplasmic reticulum and to the contraction of muscles. In the brain, activation of nicotinic receptors causes excitation of presynaptic and postsynaptic neurons.

Nicotinic receptors are pentamers formed by the assembly of five transmembrane polypeptide subunits (Fig. 6–1). These subunits are divided into classes (alpha [α] through epsilon [ε]) according to their molecular structure. Each type of nicotinic receptor (muscle, ganglionic, brain) is composed of a unique combination of these subunits. All subunits appear to participate in the formation of acetylcholine-binding sites and influence the functional properties of the receptors, but a clear understanding of the unique roles of the different classes of subunits has not yet been obtained.

Classification of Acetylcholine Receptor Agonists

The acetylcholine receptor agonists can be classified as direct acting or indirect acting. The **direct-acting agonists** bind and activate acetylcholine receptors. Most **indirect-acting agonists** increase the synaptic concentration of acetylcholine by inhibiting cholinesterase, whereas others augment acetylcholine signal transduction.

DIRECT-ACTING ACETYLCHOLINE RECEPTOR AGONISTS

The direct-acting agonists include the **choline esters**, the **plant alkaloids**, and newer synthetic drugs called cevimeline and varenicline. These drugs all bind and activate acetylcholine receptors, but they differ with respect to their affinity for muscarinic and nicotinic receptors and their susceptibility to hydrolysis by cholinesterase (Table 6–2).

TABLE 6-2. Properties and Clinical Uses of Direct-Acting Acetylcholine Receptor Agonists

Drug	Receptor Specificity	Hydrolyzed by Cholinesterase	Route of Administration	Clinical Use
Choline Esters				
Acetylcholine	Muscarinic and nicotinic	Yes	Intraocular Intracoronary	Miosis during ophthalmic surgery Coronary angiography
Bethanechol	Muscarinic	No	Oral or subcutaneous	Gastrointestinal and urinary stimulation
Carbachol	Muscarinic and nicotinic	No	Topical ocular Intraocular	Glaucoma Miosis during ophthalmic surgery
Plant Alkaloids				
Muscarine	Muscarinic	No	None	None
Nicotine	Nicotinic	No	Oral or transdermal	Smoking cessation programs
Pilocarpine	Muscarinic	No	Topical ocular Oral	Glaucoma Xerostomia
Other Drugs				
Cevimeline	Muscarinic	No	Oral	Xerostomia
Varenicline	Nicotinic	No	Oral	Smoking cessation

Choline Esters

The choline esters include acetylcholine and synthetic acetylcholine analogues, such as bethanechol and carbachol.

General Properties

The choline esters are positively charged quaternary ammonium compounds that are poorly absorbed from the gastrointestinal tract and are not distributed to the central nervous system. Acetylcholine and carbachol activate both muscarinic and nicotinic receptors, whereas bethanechol activates only muscarinic receptors. Because of their lack of specificity for muscarinic receptor subtypes, the muscarinic receptor agonists cause a wide range of effects on many organ systems.

OCULAR EFFECTS. Muscarinic receptor agonists increase lacrimal gland secretion and stimulate contraction of the iris sphincter muscle and the ciliary muscles. Contraction of the iris sphincter muscle produces pupillary constriction (miosis), whereas contraction of the ciliary muscles enables accommodation of the lens to focus on close objects (Fig. 6–2).

RESPIRATORY TRACT EFFECTS. Stimulation of muscarinic receptors increases bronchial muscle contraction and causes an increase in the secretion of mucus throughout the respiratory tract. Because muscarinic receptor agonists can cause bronchoconstriction, they should be avoided or used with extreme caution in patients with asthma and other forms of obstructive lung disease.

CARDIAC EFFECTS. Muscarinic receptor agonists decrease impulse formation in the sinoatrial node by reducing the rate of diastolic depolarization. As a result, they slow the heart rate. In addition, they slow conduction of the cardiac action potential through the atrioventricular node, and this leads to an increased PR interval (time between the beginning of the P wave to the beginning of the QRS complex) on the electrocardiogram.

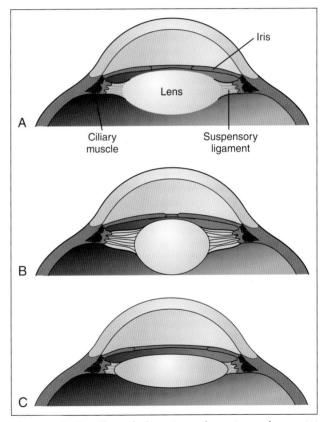

Figure 6-2. Effects of pilocarpine and atropine on the eye. (A) The relationship between the iris sphincter and ciliary muscle is shown in the normal eye. (B) When pilocarpine, a muscarinic receptor agonist, is administered, contraction of the iris sphincter produces pupillary constriction (miosis). Contraction of the ciliary muscle causes the muscle to be displaced centrally. This relaxes the suspensory ligaments connected to the lens, and the internal elasticity of the lens allows it to increase in thickness. As the lens thickens, its refractive power increases so that it focuses on close objects. (C) When atropine, a muscarinic receptor antagonist, is administered, the iris sphincter and ciliary muscles relax. This produces pupillary dilatation (mydriasis) and increases the tension on the suspensory ligaments so that the lens becomes thinner and focuses on distant objects.

TABLE 6-1. Properties of Acetylcholine Receptors

Type of Receptor	Principal Locations	Mechanism of Signal Transduction	Effects
Muscarinic			
M₁ ("neural")	Autonomic ganglia, presynaptic nerve terminals, and central nervous system	Increased IP₃	Modulation of neurotransmission
M₂ ("cardiac")	Cardiac tissue (sinoatrial and atrioventricular nodes)	Increased potassium efflux or decreased cAMP	Slowing of heart rate and conduction
M₃ ("glandular")	Smooth muscle and glands	Increased IP₃	Contraction of smooth muscles and stimulation of glandular secretions
	Vascular smooth muscle	Increased cGMP due to nitric oxide stimulation	Vasodilation
Nicotinic			
Muscle type	Neuromuscular junctions	Increased sodium influx	Muscle contraction
Ganglionic type	Autonomic ganglia	Increased sodium influx	Neuronal excitation
CNS type	Central nervous system	Increased sodium influx	Neuronal excitation

cAMP = cyclic adenosine monophosphate; cGMP = cyclic guanosine monophosphate; CNS = central nervous system; IP₃ = inositol triphosphate.

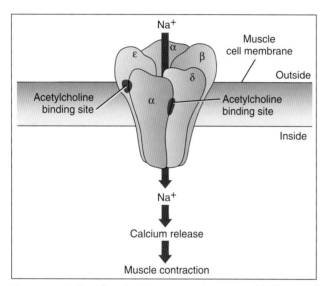

Figure 6-1. The nicotinic receptor is an acetylcholine-gated sodium channel. The channel is a polypeptide pentamer composed of varying combinations of α, β, δ, and ε subunits. In the muscle type of nicotinic receptor shown here, acetylcholine-binding sites are formed by pockets at the interface of the α and δ subunits and the α and ε subunits. Acetylcholine binding to the receptor causes sodium influx, membrane depolarization, release of calcium from the sarcoplasmic reticulum, and muscle contraction. Nicotinic receptors at autonomic ganglia and in the brain have a different subunit composition.

of muscarinic receptors, but an M₁ selective antagonist, pirenzepine, has been developed (see Chapter 7).

Nicotinic Receptors

Nicotinic receptors are found at all autonomic ganglia, at somatic neuromuscular junctions, and in the central nervous system. These receptors are acetylcholine-gated sodium channels whose activation leads to sodium influx and membrane depolarization. At autonomic ganglia, activation of nicotinic receptors produces excitation of postganglionic neurons leading to the release of neurotransmitters

at postganglionic neuroeffector junctions. At junctions of somatic nerves and skeletal muscle, activation of nicotinic receptors depolarizes the motor end plate and leads both to the release of calcium from the sarcoplasmic reticulum and to the contraction of muscles. In the brain, activation of nicotinic receptors causes excitation of presynaptic and postsynaptic neurons.

Nicotinic receptors are pentamers formed by the assembly of five transmembrane polypeptide subunits (Fig. 6–1). These subunits are divided into classes (alpha [α] through epsilon [ε]) according to their molecular structure. Each type of nicotinic receptor (muscle, ganglionic, brain) is composed of a unique combination of these subunits. All subunits appear to participate in the formation of acetylcholine-binding sites and influence the functional properties of the receptors, but a clear understanding of the unique roles of the different classes of subunits has not yet been obtained.

Classification of Acetylcholine Receptor Agonists

The acetylcholine receptor agonists can be classified as direct acting or indirect acting. The **direct-acting agonists** bind and activate acetylcholine receptors. Most **indirect-acting agonists** increase the synaptic concentration of acetylcholine by inhibiting cholinesterase, whereas others augment acetylcholine signal transduction.

DIRECT-ACTING ACETYLCHOLINE RECEPTOR AGONISTS

The direct-acting agonists include the **choline esters**, the **plant alkaloids**, and newer synthetic drugs called cevimeline and varenicline. These drugs all bind and activate acetylcholine receptors, but they differ with respect to their affinity for muscarinic and nicotinic receptors and their susceptibility to hydrolysis by cholinesterase (Table 6–2).

CHAPTER 7

Acetylcholine Receptor Antagonists

OVERVIEW

The acetylcholine receptor antagonists include drugs that selectively block either muscarinic or nicotinic receptors. Together, these drugs affect almost every organ system in the body and have a wide range of clinical applications. The muscarinic receptor blockers are used to relax smooth muscle, decrease gland secretions, and stimulate the heart, whereas the nicotinic receptor antagonists primarily consist of the neuromuscular blocking agents used to relax skeletal muscle. This chapter focuses on the pharmacologic properties, clinical use, and adverse effects of these two groups of drugs.

MUSCARINIC RECEPTOR ANTAGONISTS

The muscarinic receptor antagonists compete with acetylcholine for muscarinic receptors at parasympathetic neuroeffector junctions and thereby inhibit the effects of parasympathetic nerve stimulation. Because of these actions, the drugs are frequently called muscarinic receptor blockers or parasympatholytic drugs.

Some muscarinic receptor antagonists are belladonna alkaloids obtained from plants, whereas others are semisynthetic or synthetic drugs. The drugs in these two subgroups have similar effects on target organs, but they differ in their pharmacokinetic properties and clinical uses.

Belladonna Alkaloids

The belladonna alkaloids are extracted from a number of solanaceous plants found in temperate climates around the world, including *Atropa belladonna* (the deadly nightshade), *Datura stramonium* (jimson weed), and *Hyoscyamus niger*. Belladonna, which is Italian for "fair lady," originally referred to the pupillary dilatation produced by extracts of these plants, which was considered cosmetically attractive during the Renaissance.

Review Questions

1. A man complains of dry mouth after radiation therapy for throat cancer, and he is treated with cevimeline. Which mechanism produces the therapeutic effect of this drug?
   (A) activation of muscarinic M_2 receptors
   (B) increased formation of IP_3
   (C) increased cyclic AMP levels
   (D) increased cyclic GMP levels
   (E) increased potassium efflux

2. A woman in a smoking cessation program receives a drug that reduces craving and withdrawal effects. Which effect results from receptor activation by this drug?
   (A) sodium influx
   (B) potassium efflux
   (C) increased cyclic AMP
   (D) increased cyclic GMP
   (E) IP3 formation

3. A man receives a drug that increases cyclic GMP levels. Which adverse effect is most likely to result from this medication?
   (A) constipation
   (B) cough
   (C) dry mouth
   (D) sedation
   (E) headache

4. An agricultural worker is brought to the emergency department after abrupt onset of bowel and bladder incontinence and muscle weakness. He is given oxygen and antidotal drug treatments. Which drug mechanism would increase muscle strength in this patient?
   (A) blockade of muscarinic receptors
   (B) activation of nicotinic receptors
   (C) increased neurotransmitter degradation
   (D) induction of drug-metabolizing enzymes
   (E) increased urinary excretion of weak acids

Answers and Explanations

1. **The answer is B:** increased formation of IP_3. Cevimeline is a muscarinic receptor agonist. In salivary glands, muscarinic M_3 receptor activation leads to stimulation of phospholipase C and the formation of IP_3 and diacylglycerol. IP_3 releases intracellular calcium, which increases secretion of saliva.

2. **The answer is A:** sodium influx. The patient most likely received varenicline, a partial agonist at nicotinic receptors in brain. Nicotinic receptors are ligand-gated sodium channels and their activation leads to sodium influx. None of the other options is an effect of varenicline.

3. **The answer is E:** headache. Erectile dysfunction is treated with sildenafil and other drugs that inhibit breakdown of cyclic GMP by 5-PDE. These drugs cause vasodilation, which may lead to headache. Options A, B, C, and D (constipation, cough, dry mouth, and sedation) are unlikely to be caused by a phosphodiesterase inhibitor.

4. **The answer is C:** increased neurotransmitter degradation. The patient has signs and symptoms of organophosphate toxicity that are caused by inhibition of cholinesterase and excessive stimulation of muscarinic and nicotinic receptors by acetylcholine. The treatment of organophosphate intoxication includes administration of pralidoxime, which reactivates cholinesterase and leads to increased acetylcholine degradation. The patient's muscle weakness is due to prolonged depolarization of skeletal muscle. Activation of nicotinic receptors (Option B) would increase depolarization and muscle weakness.

SELECTED READINGS

Agrawal, A., A. Hila, R. Tutuian, I. Mainie, and D.O. Castell. Bethanechol improves smooth muscle function in patients with severe ineffective esophageal motility. J Clin Gastroenterol 41:366–370, 2007.

Kalamida D., K. Poulas, V. Avramopoulou, E. Fostieri, G. Lagoumintzis, et al. Muscle and neuronal nicotinic acetylcholine receptors. Structure, function, and pathogenicity. FEBS J 274:3799–3845, 2007.

Lam, S., and P.N. Patel. Varenicline: a selective alpha4beta2 nicotinic acetylcholine receptor partial agonist approved for smoking cessation. Cardiol Rev 15:154–161, 2007.

Uckert, S., M.E. Mayer, C.G. Stief, and U. Jonas. The future of the oral pharmacotherapy of male erectile dysfunction: things to come. Exp Opin Emerg Drugs 12:219–228, 2007.

Wess, J., R.M. Eglen, and D. Gautam. Muscarinic acetylcholine receptors: mutant mice provide new insights for drug development. Nature Rev Drug Discov 6:721–733, 2007.

BOX 7-1 A CASE OF DILATED PUPILS AND HALLUCINATIONS

CASE PRESENTATION: A 16-year-old boy was brought to the emergency department by his friends after he became highly agitated and experienced visual hallucinations, claiming that one of his friends had a mailbox for a head. His examination showed dry skin and mucous membranes, absent bowel sounds, and sinus tachycardia. His pupils were dilated, and his vision was blurred. The boy had ingested some seeds from plants growing in a vacant lot, but he denied use of alcohol or other substances. The plant material was collected and later identified as *Datura stramonium*. His laboratory findings were normal, and his blood alcohol level was zero. Gastric lavage was performed, and activated charcoal was administered to remove any unabsorbed substances. The patient became more agitated and delusional over time, and he was given an intravenous infusion of physostigmine. This treatment was repeated after 20 minutes, and his symptoms gradually subsided. Twelve hours later, the patient was much improved. He continued to improve over the next 36 hours and was discharged from hospital with normal vital signs and mental status.

CASE DISCUSSION: Jimson weed or locoweed (*Datura stramonium*) is a hallucinogenic plant containing belladonna alkaloids that is found throughout the United States. Ingestion or inhalation of any part of the plant can result in anticholinergic toxicity, with the clinical presentation resembling that seen in cases of atropine poisoning. Some fatalities have occurred from ingestion of this plant. Treatment is aimed at removing plant material from the gastrointestinal tract, keeping the patient safe, and counteracting severe anticholinergic effects with physostigmine, a cholinesterase inhibitor. Physostigmine increases levels of acetylcholine in peripheral tissues and the brain and thereby counteracts manifestations of atropine toxicity. Physostigmine should be reserved for persons with serious central nervous toxicity such as hallucinations and seizures.

Atropine, **scopolamine**, and **hyoscyamine** are examples of belladonna alkaloids. The belladonna alkaloids can be highly toxic and are sometimes the cause of accidental or intentional poisonings (Box 7–1). In fact, atropine was named after Atropos, one of the Fates in Greek mythology, who was responsible for cutting the thread of life.

Atropine and Scopolamine

CHEMISTRY AND PHARMACOKINETICS. Atropine is an ester of tropic acid and a tertiary amine (tropine). Atropine and scopolamine are well absorbed from the gut and are distributed to the central nervous system. After systemic administration, they are excreted in the urine and have a fairly short half-life of about 2 hours. After topical ocular administration, they have longer-lasting effects because they bind to pigments in the iris, which slowly release the drugs over many days. People with darker irises bind more atropine and experience a more prolonged effect than do people with lighter irises. The ocular effects of atropine gradually subside over time but are still perceptible after several days.

PHARMACOLOGIC EFFECTS. The muscarinic receptor antagonists inhibit the effects of parasympathetic nerve stimulation and thereby relax smooth muscle, increase heart rate and cardiac conduction, and inhibit exocrine gland secretion. As shown in Figure 7–1, as the dose of atropine increases, the severity of its effects increases. The signs of atropine toxicity are expressed by the mnemonic "dry as a bone, blind as a bat, red as a beet, and mad as a hatter."

(1) OCULAR EFFECTS. Atropine and other muscarinic receptor blockers relax the iris sphincter muscle, and this leads to pupillary dilatation (mydriasis). Muscarinic blockers also relax the ciliary muscle, thereby increasing the tension on the suspensory ligaments attached to the lens and causing the lens to flatten so that it is focused on distant objects. This prevents the lens from increasing its refractive power to focus on near objects (accommodation), a condition that is called cycloplegia (paralysis of accommodation). Atropine also inhibits lacrimal gland secretion and can cause dry eyes.

(2) CARDIAC EFFECTS. Standard doses of atropine and related drugs increase the heart rate and atrioventricular conduction velocity by blocking the effects of the vagus nerve on the sinoatrial and atrioventricular nodes. When intravenous administration of atropine is begun, however, the low dose of the drug causes a paradoxical slowing of the heart rate. This effect probably results from stimulation of the vagal motor nucleus in the brain stem. After the full therapeutic dose has been administered, the increase in heart rate is observed.

(3) RESPIRATORY TRACT EFFECTS. In addition to producing bronchial smooth muscle relaxation and bronchodilation, atropine and other muscarinic receptor antagonists act as potent inhibitors of secretions in the upper and lower respiratory tract.

(4) GASTROINTESTINAL AND URINARY TRACT EFFECTS. Atropine reduces lower esophageal muscle tone and can cause gastroesophageal reflux. Muscarinic receptor blockers relax gastrointestinal muscle, except sphincters, and reduce intestinal motility, thereby increasing gastric emptying time and intestinal transit time. They also inhibit gastric acid secretion. Sufficient doses of these drugs can cause constipation. Atropine relaxes the detrusor muscle of the urinary bladder and can cause urinary retention.

(5) CENTRAL NERVOUS SYSTEM EFFECTS. Atropine, scopolamine, and other tertiary amines are distributed to the central nervous system, where they can block muscarinic receptors and produce either sedation or excitement. Scopolamine, which is more sedating than is atropine, has been used as an adjunct to anesthesia. Standard doses of atropine typically cause mild stimulation, followed by a slower and longer-lasting sedative effect. With higher doses of atropine, patients can experience an acute confusional state

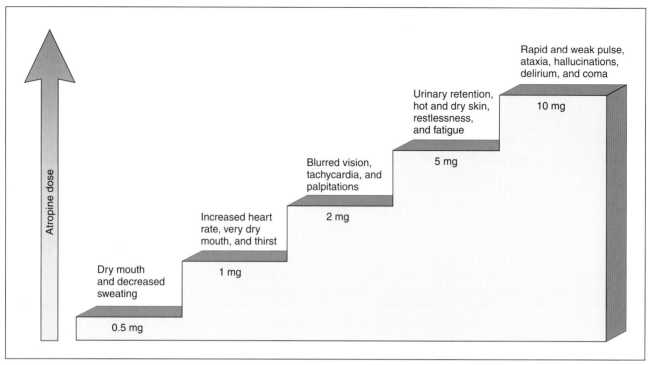

Figure 7-1. Dose-dependent effects of atropine. Low doses of atropine inhibit salivation and sweating, and the magnitude of these effects increases as the dosage increases. Higher doses produce tachycardia, urinary retention, and central nervous system effects.

known as delirium. Higher doses of muscarinic antagonists can also cause hallucinations.

(6) OTHER EFFECTS. The muscarinic receptor antagonists inhibit sweating, which can reduce heat loss and lead to hyperthermia, especially in children. The increased body temperature can cause cutaneous vasodilatation, and the skin can become hot, dry, and flushed.

INDICATIONS. (1) OCULAR INDICATIONS. To obtain a relatively localized effect on ocular tissues, muscarinic receptor blockers are administered via topical instillation of a solution or ointment. These drugs are typically used to produce mydriasis and facilitate ophthalmoscopic examination of the peripheral retina. They can also be used to produce cycloplegia and permit the accurate determination of refractive errors, especially in younger patients with a strong accommodation. Because muscarinic receptor blockers can reduce muscle spasm and pain caused by inflammation, they are useful in the treatment of iritis and cyclitis (inflammation of the iris and ciliary muscles) associated with infection, trauma, or surgery.

(2) CARDIAC INDICATIONS. Atropine can be used to treat sinus bradycardia in cases in which the slow sinus rhythm reduces the cardiac output and blood pressure and produces symptoms of hypotension or ischemia. This type of symptomatic bradycardia sometimes occurs after a myocardial infarction. Atropine is usually administered intravenously for this purpose, but it can be injected endotracheally if a vein is not accessible. In patients with symptomatic atrioventricular block, atropine or glycopyrrolate can be used to increase the atrioventricular conduction velocity.

(3) RESPIRATORY TRACT INDICATIONS. Because of its bronchodilating effects, atropine was once used to treat asthma and other obstructive lung diseases. It is no longer used for this purpose, however, because of its many adverse effects. For example, it impairs ciliary activity, thereby reducing the clearance of mucus from the lungs and causing accumulation of viscid material in the airways. As discussed later in this chapter (see "Ipratropium and Tiotropium"), ipratropium is now used instead of atropine to treat obstructive lung diseases. Atropine and other muscarinic receptor blockers are used to reduce salivary and respiratory secretions and thereby prevent airway obstruction in patients who are receiving general anesthetics. Glycopyrrolate is often used for this purpose today (see "Other Indications").

(4) GASTROINTESTINAL AND URINARY TRACT INDICATIONS. Atropine and related drugs are used to relieve **intestinal spasms and pain** associated with several gastrointestinal disorders, and they are also used to relieve urinary bladder spasms in persons with **overactive bladder.**

In the past, atropine was frequently used to reduce gastric acid secretion in patients with peptic ulcers. Large doses were required, however, and these doses often produced intolerable side effects, such as dry mouth, blurred vision, and urinary retention. For this reason, atropine and other nonselective muscarinic receptor blockers are seldom used to treat peptic ulcers today. As discussed later, a selective muscarinic M_1 receptor blocker, pirenzepine, is available in some countries to treat peptic ulcer disease.

(5) CENTRAL NERVOUS SYSTEM INDICATIONS. A transdermal formulation of scopolamine can be used to prevent motion sickness. The skin patch slowly releases scopolamine over a period of 3 days and is thought to work by blocking acetylcholine neurotransmission from the vestibular apparatus to the vomiting center in the brain stem. As discussed in Chapter 24, muscarinic receptor blockers are also used in the treatment of Parkinson's disease.

(6) OTHER INDICATIONS. Atropine and glycopyrrolate are used in two other clinical contexts. First, they are used to prevent muscarinic side effects when cholinesterase inhibitors are given to patients with myasthenia gravis. Second, as discussed in Chapter 6, they are used to reverse the muscarinic effects of cholinesterase inhibitor overdose. In this setting, supranormal doses may be required to counteract the large concentrations of acetylcholine that have accumulated at acetylcholine synapses, and the atropine dosage must be titrated to the patient's response. Atropine and glycopyrrolate will not counteract the effects of nicotinic receptor activation caused by cholinesterase inhibition. The muscle weakness resulting from nicotinic receptor stimulation can be attenuated by adding pralidoxime to the treatment regimen.

Hyoscyamine

Hyoscyamine, the levorotatory isomer of racemic atropine, is the natural form of the alkaloid that occurs in plants. It is primarily responsible for the pharmacologic effects of atropine. Formulations of hyoscyamine for oral or sublingual administration are used to treat **intestinal spasms** and other gastrointestinal symptoms.

Semisynthetic and Synthetic Muscarinic Receptor Antagonists

In the search for a more selective muscarinic receptor antagonist, investigators have developed a large number of semisynthetic and synthetic blocking agents. Although the pharmacologic effects of these agents are similar to those of atropine, their unique pharmacokinetic properties are advantageous in specific situations.

Ipratropium and Tiotropium

Ipratropium (ATROVENT) and tiotropium (SPIRIVA), quaternary amine derivatives of atropine, are administered by inhalation to patients with **obstructive lung diseases.** Because these drugs are not well absorbed from the lungs into the systemic circulation, they produce few adverse effects. For example, unlike atropine, they do not impair the ciliary clearance of secretions from the airways. This makes them particularly useful in treating patients with **asthma, emphysema** and **chronic bronchitis.** The respiratory effects and uses of these compounds are discussed more thoroughly in Chapter 27.

Dicyclomine, Oxybutynin, Solifenacin, Tolterodine, and Trospium

Dicyclomine is a synthetic tertiary amine used to relax intestinal smooth muscle and thereby relieve irritable bowel symptoms, such as intestinal cramping. Oxybutynin, tolterodine, darifenacin, solifenacin, and trospium are used to reduce the four major symptoms of **overactive bladder:** daytime urinary frequency, nocturia (frequent urination at night), urgency, and incontinence. Compared to other muscarinic receptor antagonists, darifenacin, solifenacin, tolterodine, and trospium appear to have a more selective action on the urinary bladder and cause fewer adverse effects such as dry mouth and blurred vision. These "uroselective" blockers are administered once or twice daily.

Glycopyrrolate

Glycopyrrolate blocks muscarinic receptors throughout the body. Low doses preferentially inhibit secretions, and the drug is administered preoperatively to inhibit excessive salivary and respiratory tract secretions. It is also used during anesthesia to inhibit the secretory and vagal effects of cholinesterase inhibitors (e.g., neostigmine) that are used to reverse nondepolarizing neuromuscular blockade induced by curariform drugs (e.g., vecuronium).

Tropicamide

Tropicamide is a tertiary amine that was developed for topical ocular administration as a mydriatic (pupillary dilator). It is given just before ophthalmoscopy to facilitate **examination of the peripheral retina.** It has a short duration of action (about 1 hour) and is often preferable to atropine and scopolamine for short-term mydriasis.

Pirenzepine

Pirenzepine, a muscarinic receptor antagonist that is selective for M_1 receptors, was developed to reduce vagally stimulated gastric acid secretion in patients with **peptic ulcers.** It blocks M_1 receptors on paracrine cells and inhibits the release of histamine, a potent gastric acid stimulant. Pirenzepine is available in Canada but not in the United States.

NICOTINIC RECEPTOR ANTAGONISTS

The acetylcholine nicotinic receptor antagonists include ganglionic blocking agents and neuromuscular blocking agents.

Ganglionic Blocking Agents

Drugs such as **trimethaphan** selectively block the ganglionic type of nicotinic receptors found on postjunctional neurons in sympathetic and parasympathetic ganglia. The effect of these drugs on a particular tissue depends on whether the sympathetic or parasympathetic system is dominant in that tissue. Blockade of sympathetic ganglia causes hypotension, whereas blockade of parasympathetic ganglia produces dry mouth, blurred vision, and urinary retention.

Ganglionic blockers were historically used to treat hypertension, but they are no longer used for this disorder because of the advent of more effective drugs with fewer adverse effects. Trimethaphan was formerly used in cases of a **hypertensive emergency**, when extremely high blood pressures must be reduced, but other drugs have replaced trimethaphan for this purpose.

Neuromuscular Blocking Agents

The neuromuscular blocking agents (also referred to as paralytics or muscle relaxants) bind to the muscle type of nicotinic acetylcholine receptor and inhibit neurotransmission at skeletal neuromuscular junctions, causing muscle weakness and paralysis. These agents can be divided into two groups, one consisting of **nondepolarizing blockers**, which

are competitive antagonists at the neuromuscular junction, and the other consisting of the **depolarizing blocker**, succinylcholine. The neuromuscular blocking agents are extremely dangerous compounds, since they can produce complete respiratory failure in a patient lacking external ventilatory support. The neuromuscular blockers are primarily responsible for the rare occurrence of awareness during surgery, since they can render a patient immobile without affecting mental status.

Nondepolarizing Neuromuscular Blocking Agents

General Properties

The nondepolarizing neuromuscular blocking agents, also known as **curariform drugs**, include **tubocurarine, atracurium, cisatracurium, pancuronium, rocuronium,** and **vecuronium.** Tubocurarine was originally extracted from plants used by native South Americans as arrow poisons for hunting wild game. The curariform drugs are not well absorbed from the gut and do not cross the blood-brain barrier. Hence, they do not cause poisoning when meat containing these substances is ingested. **Curare** is another name for the arrow poisons and their chemical derivatives.

CHEMISTRY AND PHARMACOKINETICS. The pharmacologic properties of curariform drugs are listed in Table 7–1. They are positively charged quaternary amines having an amino-steroid structure (pancuronium, rocuronium, and vecuronium) or a benzylisoquinoline structure (atracurium, cisatracurium, doxacurium, and tubocurarine). The nondepolarizing neuromuscular blocking agents are administered only via the intravenous route.

Whereas most nondepolarizing paralytic agents are eliminated by renal and biliary excretion of the unchanged compounds and hepatic metabolites, most of the isomers of racemic atracurium are hydrolyzed by plasma esterases. However, the specific isomer known as **cisatracurium** spontaneously decomposes by nonenzymatic Hoffman degradation. Hence, cisatracurium is the preferred paralytic agent for critically ill patients with impaired hepatic and renal function. In patients with normal renal and hepatic function, atracurium and cisatracurium have intermediate duration of action comparable to vecuronium and rocuronium.

MECHANISMS AND EFFECTS. The curariform drugs act as competitive antagonists of acetylcholine at nicotinic receptors in skeletal muscle, and this accounts for their muscle-relaxing effects. After a curariform drug is administered, it first paralyzes the small and rapidly moving muscles of the eyes and face and then paralyzes the larger muscles of the limbs and trunk. Finally, it paralyzes the intercostal muscles and diaphragm, causing respiration to cease. This sequence of paralysis is fortunate in that it enables relaxation of abdominal muscles for surgical procedures without producing apnea. Respiratory function should always be closely monitored in patients receiving a neuromuscular blocking agent, however.

Curariform drugs stimulate the release of histamine from mast cells, and they block autonomic ganglia and muscarinic receptors (see Table 7–1). These actions can cause bronchospasm, hypotension, and tachycardia. Newer drugs, such as doxacurium, cisatracurium, rocuronium, and vecuronium, tend to cause less histamine release and fewer autonomic side effects than do tubocurarine and pancuronium.

INTERACTIONS. The muscle-relaxing effects of curariform drugs are potentiated by volatile inhalational anesthetic agents (e.g., isoflurane) and by the aminoglycoside antibiotics, tetracycline antibiotics, and calcium channel blockers. The effects of paralytic agents are also more pronounced in patients who have neuromuscular disorders such as myasthenia gravis.

TABLE 7–1. Properties of Neuromuscular Blocking Agents

Drug	Depolarizing Agent	Histamine Release*	Ganglionic Blockade†	Effects Reversed by Cholinesterase Inhibitors	Duration of Action (Minutes)	Primary Mode(s) of Elimination
Succinylcholine	Yes	Minimal	None‡	No	Short (5–10)	Plasma (butyryl) cholinesterase
Atracurium	No	Varies‡‡	Low	Yes	Intermediate (30–60)	Plasma esterase
Cisatracurium	No	None	Low	Yes	Intermediate (30–60)	Spontaneous chemical degradation
Pancuronium	No	None	Medium	Yes	Long (60–120)	Renal excretion
Rocuronium	No	None	Low	Yes	Intermediate (30–60)	Biliary and renal excretion
Tubocurarine	No	High	High	Yes	Long (60-120)	Renal and biliary excretion
Vecuronium	No	None	Low	Yes	Intermediate (30–60)	Biliary and renal excretion and hepatic metabolism

*May cause bronchospasm, hypotension, and excessive salivary and bronchial secretions.
†May cause hypotension and tachycardia.
‡May cause bradycardia by stimulating parasympathetic (vagal) ganglia, or may cause tachycardia and hypertension by stimulating sympathetic ganglia.
‡‡At higher doses (e.g., for tracheal intubation), histamine release becomes clinically significant.

The muscle-relaxing effects of curariform drugs can be reversed by administering a cholinesterase inhibitor (e.g., neostigmine), which acts by increasing acetylcholine levels at the neuromuscular junction and counteracting the neuromuscular blockade. Neostigmine reversal should not be attempted until patients have demonstrated partial recovery of neuromuscular function as measured using a nerve stimulator.

A new drug called **sugammadex** is currently undergoing clinical testing for reversing steroidal neuromuscular blocking agents such as rocuronium. Sugammadex forms a tight water-soluble complex with rocuronium and thereby removes the drug from the neuromuscular junction and produces a fast recovery of neuromuscular function. In contrast to cholinesterase inhibitors, sugammadex is effective on subjects demonstrating complete paralysis when tested with a nerve stimulator. Sugammadex appears to be safe and well tolerated and may revolutionize the clinical use of neuromuscular blocking agents.

INDICATIONS. The neuromuscular blockers are primarily used to induce muscle relaxation during surgery and thereby facilitate surgical manipulations. These drugs are sometimes used as an adjunct to electroconvulsive therapy to prevent injuries that might be caused by involuntary muscle contractions. They have also been used to facilitate intubation of the respiratory tract so as to enable ventilation and endoscopic procedures (e.g., bronchoscopy). During the clinical use of neuromuscular blocking agents, the degree of neuromuscular blockade can be determined by monitoring the contraction of a small limb muscle in response to nerve stimulation.

Drug Selection

The selection of a nondepolarizing agent for a particular clinical application is usually based on the relative duration of action and the degree of drug-induced changes in blood pressure and heart rate. Atracurium, cisatracurium, rocuronium, and vecuronium provide an intermediate duration of action (30–60 minutes). With the exception of atracurium, which can cause histamine release at higher doses, the intermediate-acting drugs have minimal effects on cardiovascular and respiratory function. Doxacurium or pancuronium might be selected when a longer duration of action is required. Tubocurarine is no longer used because it is associated with a higher incidence of histamine release and adverse effects.

Depolarizing Neuromuscular Blocking Agents

Succinylcholine, the only depolarizing agent available for clinical use today, is composed of two covalently linked molecules of acetylcholine. Succinylcholine binds to nicotinic receptors in skeletal muscle and causes persistent depolarization of the motor end plate. When the drug is first administered, it produces transient muscle contractions called fasciculations. The fasciculations are quickly followed by a sustained muscle paralysis. Succinylcholine is not hydrolyzed as rapidly by cholinesterase as acetylcholine is, and this appears to partly account for the persistent depolarization and muscle paralysis.

Table 7–1 compares the properties of succinylcholine with those of the curariform drugs. Succinylcholine has a short duration of action (5–10 minutes) owing to its hydrolysis by plasma cholinesterase. The sequence of muscle paralysis produced by succinylcholine is similar to that produced by the curariform drugs. The effects of succinylcholine, however, are not reversed by cholinesterase inhibitors, and no pharmacologic antidote exists to reverse an overdose of succinylcholine.

Succinylcholine is used to produce muscle relaxation before and during surgery and to facilitate **intubation of the airway**. Because of its shorter duration of action, succinylcholine offers the best chance for resumption of spontaneous breathing if endotracheal intubation proves difficult; thus it is the preferred neuromuscular blocker for adults with emergency airway situations. Before the drug is administered in a nonemergent situation, patients should be interviewed to screen for personal or family history suggestive of atypical cholinesterase. Individuals with this inherited disorder cannot metabolize succinylcholine at normal rates and are susceptible to prolonged neuromuscular paralysis and apnea after receiving the usual doses of the drug.

When possible, a serum potassium level should be obtained before administering succinylcholine. Succinylcholine can cause hyperkalemia sufficient to cause cardiac arrest in persons with unhealed skeletal muscle injury such as follows third-degree burns, and it should not be used in these individuals until the injury heals. Many conditions involving muscle weakness, such as paralysis due to spinal cord injury, also present an increased risk of hyperkalemia due to up-regulation of acetylcholine receptors at the neuromuscular junction. Children are more susceptible to the consequences of hyperkalemia, and succinylcholine is therefore used less frequently in pediatric patients. Succinylcholine can also cause postoperative myalgia, particularly in the muscles of the neck, back, and abdomen. This effect probably results from the muscle fasciculations produced by the drug. Finally, succinylcholine has been associated with a rare complication known as malignant hyperthermia, which is also associated with volatile anesthetics (see Chapter 21).

SUMMARY OF IMPORTANT POINTS

- The muscarinic receptor antagonists relax smooth muscle, increase heart rate and cardiac conduction, and inhibit exocrine gland secretion. They include belladonna alkaloids (e.g., atropine and scopolamine) and semisynthetic and synthetic drugs (e.g., ipratropium).

- The muscarinic receptor blockers are used to treat bradycardia, obstructive lung diseases, intestinal spasms, and overactive urinary bladder. They are also used to reduce salivary and respiratory secretions and to produce mydriasis and cycloplegia.

- Atropine toxicity can cause dryness of the mouth and skin, blurred vision, tachycardia, palpitations, urinary retention, delirium, and hallucinations.

- The nicotinic receptor antagonists include ganglionic blocking agents (e.g., trimethaphan) and neuromuscular blocking agents (e.g., the curariform drugs, which are nondepolarizing, and succinylcholine, which is depolarizing).

■ Neuromuscular blockers such as cisatracurium are used primarily to produce muscle relaxation during anesthesia.

■ Curariform drugs competitively block nicotinic receptors in skeletal muscle. They do not cause muscle fasciculations, and their effects can be reversed by cholinesterase inhibitors.

■ Succinylcholine produces muscle fasciculations that are followed by muscle paralysis. The effects cannot be reversed by cholinesterase inhibitors.

Review Questions

1. Which drug produces transient muscle fasciculations followed by muscle paralysis that is not reversed by neostigmine?
   (A) rocuronium
   (B) hyoscyamine
   (C) ipratropium
   (D) succinylcholine
   (E) dicyclomine

2. Toxic doses of atropine typically cause all of the following effects EXCEPT
   (A) hallucinations
   (B) bronchospasm
   (C) hyperthermia
   (D) urinary retention
   (E) blurred vision

3. Topical ocular administration of tropicamide will cause
   (A) contraction of the ciliary muscle
   (B) vasoconstriction
   (C) miosis
   (D) relaxation of the iris sphincter muscle
   (E) lacrimation

4. The therapeutic use of darifenacin is based on its ability to
   (A) relax bronchial smooth muscle
   (B) relax urinary bladder smooth muscle
   (C) relax uterine smooth muscle
   (D) inhibit salivary secretions
   (E) relax ciliary muscle

Answers and Explanations

1. **The answer is D: succinylcholine.** Succinylcholine is a depolarizing neuromuscular blocking agent that produces persistent depolarization of the motor end plate, thereby causing transient muscle fasciculations followed by paralysis. Cholinesterase inhibitors, acting to increase acetylcholine levels, do not counteract the muscle paralysis produced by succinylcholine and can actually increase the degree of paralysis by prolonging muscle depolarization.

2. **The answer is B: bronchospasm.** Muscarinic receptor antagonists such as atropine cause relaxation of bronchial smooth muscle and bronchodilation. Atropine causes hyperthermia by inhibiting sweating, thereby leading to vasodilation and flushing. Atropine causes blurred vision by relaxing the ciliary muscle, thereby producing cycloplegia (paralysis of accommodation).

3. **The answer is D: relaxation of the iris sphincter muscle.** Tropicamide binds to muscarinic receptors and competitively blocks acetylcholine released by the parasympathetic oculomotor nerve. This action leads to relaxation of the iris sphincter muscle and dilation of the pupil (mydriasis), thereby facilitating ophthalmoscopic examination of the peripheral retina.

4. **The answer is B: relax urinary bladder smooth muscle.** Darifenacin is used to treat hyperactive bladder and relieve urgency, frequency, and incontinence. It is not used to relax uterine or bronchial smooth muscle. It can inhibit salivary secretions, causing dry mouth, and it can relax the ciliary muscle, causing blurred vision.

SELECTED READINGS

Chancellor, M.B., and F. de Migue. Treatment of overactive bladder: selective use of anticholinergic agents with low drug-drug interaction potential. Geriatrics 62:15–24, 2007.

Garely, A.D., V. Lucente, J. Vapnek, and N. Smith. Solifenacin for overactive bladder with incontinence. Ann Pharmacother 41:391-398, 2007.

Naguib, M. Sugammadex: another milestone in clinical neuromuscular pharmacology. Anesth Analg 104:575–581, 2007.

Adrenoceptor Agonists

CLASSIFICATION OF ADRENOCEPTOR AGONISTS

Direct-Acting Adrenoceptor Agonists
Catecholamines
- Dobutamine
- Dopamine
- Epinephrine
- Isoproterenol
- Norepinephrine

Noncatecholamines
- Albuterol (PROVENTIL, VENTOLIN)*
- Apraclonidine†
- Clonidine (CATAPRES)‡
- Midodrine (PROAMATINE)
- Oxymetazoline (AFRIN)
- Phenylephrine
- Ritodrine (YUTOPAR)

Indirect-Acting Adrenoceptor Agonists
- Amphetamine
- Cocaine

Mixed-Acting Adrenoceptor Agonists
- Ephedrine
- Pseudoephedrine

*Also fenoterol, formoterol, pirbuterol, salmeterol, and terbutaline.
†Also brimonidine.
‡Also dexmedetomidine.

OVERVIEW

The adrenoceptor agonists are a large group of drugs whose diverse pharmacologic effects make them valuable in the treatment of a wide spectrum of clinical conditions, ranging from cardiovascular emergencies to the common cold. Although some of the agonists exert their effects on multiple organ systems, others target a specific organ. The spectrum of effects produced by a particular adrenoceptor agonist depends on its affinity for different types of adrenoceptors.

Adrenoceptors

Adrenoceptors are classified as **α-adrenoceptors** and **β-adrenoceptors,** based on the relative potency of epinephrine, norepinephrine, and other adrenoceptor agonists in cardiac and smooth muscle. For example, epinephrine and norepinephrine are more potent than isoproterenol at α-adrenoceptors located in smooth muscle, whereas isoproterenol is more potent than epinephrine and norepinephrine at β-adrenoceptors located in cardiac muscle.

As shown in Table 8–1 and Figure 8–1, subtypes of α- and β-adrenoceptors have been identified on the basis of several criteria, including their molecular structure, differences in signal transduction and physiologic effects, and differences in agonist affinity for different receptors. The receptor subtypes have also been cloned, and their molecular structures have been determined.

α-Adrenoceptors

The α-adrenoceptors can be differentiated on the basis of their location and function. The **α₁-adrenoceptors** are primarily located in smooth muscle at sympathetic neuroeffector junctions, but these receptors are also found in exocrine glands and the central nervous system. Three subtypes of α_1-adrenoceptors have been identified (α_{1A}, α_{1B}, and α_{1D}), but the functional roles of these α_1-receptor subtypes have not been clearly established. The α_2-adrenoceptors are widely distributed in presynaptic neurons, various tissues, and blood platelets (see Fig. 8–1), and subtypes of these receptors have also been identified.

The α_1-adrenoceptors mediate contraction of vascular smooth muscle, the iris dilator muscle, and smooth muscle in the lower urinary tract (bladder, urethra, and prostate). The α_2-adrenoceptors located on sympathetic postganglionic neurons serve as **autoreceptors** whose activation leads

TABLE 8–1. Properties of Adrenergic, Dopamine, and Imidazoline Receptors

Type of Receptor	Mechanism of Signal Transduction	Effects
Adrenoceptors		
α_1	Phospholipase C activation, increased IP$_3$, release of calcium	Contraction of smooth muscles, exocrine gland secretion, neuronal excitation
α_2	Inhibition of adenylyl cyclase and decreased cAMP	Inhibition of norepinephrine release, decrease in secretion of aqueous humor, decrease in secretion of insulin, platelet aggregation, and central nervous system effects
β_1	Adenylyl cyclase activation, increased cAMP, protein kinase activation	Increase in secretion of renin and increase in heart rate, contractility, and conduction
β_2	Adenylyl cyclase activation, increased cAMP, protein kinase activation	Glycogenolysis, relaxation of smooth muscles, and uptake of potassium in skeletal muscles
β_3	Adenylyl cyclase activation, increased cAMP, protein kinase activation	Lipolysis
Dopamine Receptors		
D$_1$	Increased cAMP	Relaxation of vascular smooth muscles
D$_2$	Decreased cAMP, increased potassium currents, and decreased calcium influx	Modulation of neurotransmission in the sympathetic and central nervous systems
Imidazoline Receptors	Uncertain	Natriuresis and decrease of sympathetic outflow from the central nervous system

cAMP = cyclic adenosine monophosphate; IP$_3$ = inositol triphosphate.

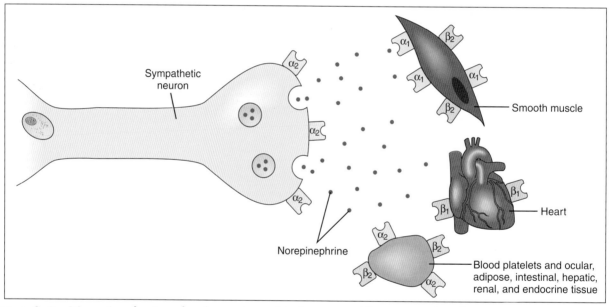

Figure 8–1. Primary tissue locations of α-adrenoceptors and β-adrenoceptors. Whereas α_1- and β_2-adrenoceptors are primarily located in smooth muscle, β_1-adrenoceptors are predominantly found in cardiac tissue. Some α_2-adrenoceptors are located on sympathetic neurons, where they produce feedback inhibition of neurotransmitter release. Other α_2- and β_2-adrenoceptors are located in blood platelets and a variety of organ tissues. The α- and β-adrenoceptors are also found in the central nervous system.

to feedback inhibition of norepinephrine release from nerve terminals. The α_2-receptors are also found in blood platelets and in ocular, adipose, intestinal, hepatic, renal, and endocrine tissue. In blood platelets, α_2-receptors mediate platelet aggregation. In the pancreas, α_2-receptors mediate the inhibition of insulin secretion that occurs when the sympathetic nervous system is activated.

β-Adrenoceptors

Table 8–1 summarizes the effects of three subtypes of β-adrenoceptors.

Activation of **β_1-adrenoceptors** produces cardiac stimulation, leading to a positive **chronotropic effect** (increased heart rate), a positive **inotropic effect** (increased contractility), and a positive **dromotropic effect** (increased cardiac impulse conduction velocity). Activation of β_1 receptors also increases **renin secretion** from renal juxtaglomerular cells.

The **β_2-adrenoceptors** mediate relaxation of bronchial, uterine, and vascular smooth muscle (see Fig. 11–3). In skeletal muscle, β_2-receptors mediate potassium uptake. In the liver, they mediate **glycogenolysis**, which increases the glucose concentration in the blood. Whereas epinephrine and norepinephrine are equally potent at β_1-receptors in cardiac tissue, epinephrine is more potent than norepinephrine at β_2-receptors in smooth muscle.

Activation of β_3-**adrenoceptors** produces **lipolysis**, a process in which the hydrolysis of triglycerides in adipose tissue leads to the release of fatty acids into the circulation. Investigators are currently searching for selective β_3-adrenoceptor agonists because they believe that the lipolytic effect of these agonists would be useful in the treatment of obesity.

Dopamine Receptors

Dopamine receptors are activated by dopamine but not by other adrenoceptor agonists. Several subtypes exist, including the D_1-**receptors**, which mediate muscle relaxation in vascular smooth muscle, and the D_2-**receptors**, which modulate neurotransmitter release.

Imidazoline Receptors

Imidazoline receptors are activated by adrenoceptor agonists and other substances that contain an imidazoline structure. One of the best-studied examples of these substances is clonidine. The imidazoline receptors are found in the central nervous system and a number of peripheral tissues. The antihypertensive effect of clonidine appears to result from activation of both α_2-adrenoceptors and imidazoline receptors in the central nervous system, leading to a reduced sympathetic outflow to the heart and vascular smooth muscle. The pharmacologic properties of antihypertensive imidazoline drugs are discussed in greater detail in Chapter 10.

Signal Transduction

The adrenergic, dopamine, and imidazoline receptors are guanine nucleotide protein–binding (G protein–binding) receptors that are located in cell membranes of target tissues.

Activation of α_1-adrenoceptors is coupled with activation of **phospholipase C**, which catalyzes the release of **inositol triphosphate (IP$_3$)** from membrane phospholipids. In smooth muscle, IP$_3$ stimulates the release of calcium from the sarcoplasmic reticulum, and this leads to muscle contraction. This is the mechanism by which α_1-adrenoceptor agonists cause vasoconstriction and increase blood pressure. In exocrine glands, formation of IP$_3$ leads to calcium release and gland secretion. Activation of α_2-adrenoceptors leads to inhibition of adenylyl cyclase and a decrease in the levels of cyclic adenosine monophosphate (cAMP) in sympathetic neurons and other tissues. This is the mechanism responsible for a decrease in aqueous humor secretion and for other effects of α_2-adrenoceptor agonists. Activation of D_2-receptors also reduces cAMP formation.

Activation of β-adrenoceptors and D_1-receptors leads to stimulation of adenylyl cyclase and an increase in the levels of cAMP in cardiac tissue and smooth muscle. Cyclic AMP activates **protein kinase A**, which phosphorylates other proteins and enzymes. The cellular response depends on the specific proteins that are phosphorylated in each tissue.

In cardiac tissue, calcium channels are phosphorylated, thereby augmenting calcium influx and cardiac contractility. In smooth muscle, cAMP produces muscle relaxation via effects on multiple targets, including potassium channels, calcium channels, and myosin light chain kinase (see Fig. 11–3).

Classification of Adrenoceptor Agonists

The adrenoceptor agonists mimic the effect of sympathetic nervous system stimulation and, therefore, are also called **sympathomimetic drugs**. These drugs can be divided into three groups on the basis of their mode of action. The **direct-acting agonists** bind to and activate adrenoceptors. As shown in Figure 8–2, the **indirect-acting agonists** increase the stimulation of adrenoceptors by increasing the concentration of norepinephrine at sympathetic neuroeffector junctions in one of two ways. Cocaine inhibits the **catecholamine transporter** located in the plasma membrane of the presynaptic sympathetic neuron and thereby decreases the neuronal reuptake of norepinephrine and increases its synaptic concentration. Amphetamine and related drugs are transported into the sympathetic nerve terminal by the catecholamine transporter. Once inside the sympathetic neuron, amphetamines inhibit the storage of norepinephrine by neuronal vesicles. This increases the cytoplasmic concentration of norepinephrine, leading to reverse norepinephrine transport into the synapse by the catecholamine transporter. The **mixed-acting agonists** (e.g., ephedrine) have both direct and indirect actions.

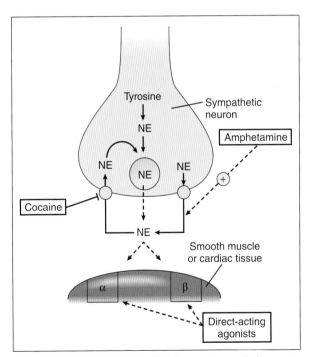

Figure 8–2. Mechanisms of indirect-acting and direct-acting adrenoceptor agonists. Cocaine blocks norepinephrine reuptake by the catecholamine transporter. Amphetamine inhibits the storage of norepinephrine by neuronal vesicles, leading to reverse transport of norepinephrine into the synapse by the catecholamine transporter. Direct-acting agonists bind to and activate adrenoceptors. α = α-adrenoceptor; β = β-adrenoceptor; NE = norepinephrine.

DIRECT-ACTING ADRENOCEPTOR AGONISTS

The direct-acting agonists can be subdivided into catecholamines and noncatecholamines.

Catecholamines

The naturally occurring catecholamines include **norepinephrine**, an endogenous sympathetic neurotransmitter; **epinephrine**, the principal hormone of the adrenal medulla; and **dopamine**, the precursor to norepinephrine and epinephrine. Synthetic catecholamines include **isoproterenol** and **dobutamine**.

General Properties

CHEMISTRY AND PHARMACOKINETICS. Each catecholamine consists of the catechol moiety and an ethylamine side chain (Fig. 8–3). The catecholamines are rapidly inactivated by **monoamine oxidase** (MAO) and **catechol-*O*-methyltransferase** (COMT), enzymes found in the gut, liver, and other tissues. The drugs have low oral bioavailabilities and short plasma half-lives. For these reasons, they must be administered parenterally when a systemic action is required (e.g., in the treatment of patients who are in anaphylactic shock).

MECHANISMS AND EFFECTS. As shown in Figure 8–3 and Table 8–2, the various catecholamines differ in their affinities and specificities for receptors. The size of the alkyl substitution on the amine nitrogen (R_2) determines the relative affinity for α- and β-adrenoceptors. Drugs with a large alkyl group (e.g., isoproterenol) have greater affinity for β-adrenoceptors than do drugs with a small alkyl group (e.g., epinephrine). Epinephrine is a potent agonist at all α- and β-adrenoceptors. Norepinephrine differs from epinephrine only in that it has greater affinity for β_1-adrenoceptors than for β_2-adrenoceptors. Because of this difference, norepinephrine constricts all blood vessels, whereas epinephrine constricts some blood vessels but dilates others. Isoproterenol is considered to be a selective β_1- and β_2-adrenoceptor agonist because it has little affinity for α-receptors. Dobutamine primarily stimulates β_1-receptors but has minor stimulatory effects on β_2- and α-receptors. Dopamine activates D_1-, β_1-, and α-receptors. Unlike the other catecholamines, dopamine also stimulates the release of norepinephrine from sympathetic neurons. For this reason, dopamine is both a direct-acting and an indirect-acting receptor agonist.

(1) CARDIOVASCULAR EFFECTS. Figure 8–4 compares the cardiovascular effects when norepinephrine, epinephrine, isoproterenol, and dopamine are given by intravenous infusion.

The cardiovascular effects of norepinephrine primarily result from activation of α_1-adrenoceptors. Activation produces vasoconstriction and increases peripheral resistance, which, in turn, increases the systolic and diastolic blood pressure. Norepinephrine can cause reflex bradycardia if blood pressure increases sufficiently to activate the baroreceptor reflex.

Epinephrine increases the systolic blood pressure but can increase or decrease the diastolic blood pressure. The

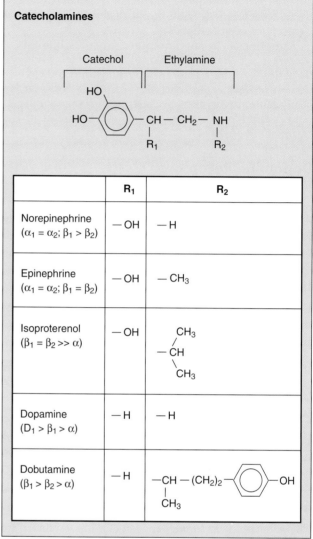

Figure 8–3. Structures of selected adrenoceptor agonists. Catecholamines contain the catechol moiety and an ethylamine side chain. The amine nitrogen substitution (R_2) determines the relative affinity for α- and β-adrenoceptors, with larger substitutions (e.g., in isoproterenol and dobutamine) decreasing the affinity for α-adrenoceptors and increasing the affinity for β-adrenoceptors. Note that dopamine has an even higher affinity for dopamine D_1 receptors than for adrenoceptors.

increased systolic pressure is partly due to an increased heart rate and cardiac output. The effect on diastolic pressure depends on the relative stimulation of α_1- and β_2-adrenoceptors, which mediate vasoconstriction and vasodilation, respectively. Lower doses of epinephrine produce greater stimulation of β_2-receptors than α_1-receptors, especially in the vascular beds of skeletal muscle, thereby causing vasodilation and decreasing diastolic blood pressure. Higher doses produce more vasoconstriction throughout the body and can increase both diastolic and systolic pressure.

Isoproterenol activates β_1- and β_2-adrenoceptors and produces vasodilation and cardiac stimulation. It usually lowers the diastolic and mean arterial pressure, but it can increase the systolic pressure by increasing the heart rate and contractility. Its potent chronotropic effect can cause tachycardia and cardiac arrhythmias. For this reason, an alternative

TABLE 8-2.	Pharmacologic Effects and Clinical Uses of Adrenoceptor Agonists	
Drug	**Pharmacologic Effect (and Receptor)**	**Clinical Use**
Direct-Acting Catecholamines		
Dobutamine	Cardiac stimulation (β_1) and vasodilation (β_2)	Cardiogenic shock, acute heart failure, and cardiac stimulation during heart surgery
Dopamine*	Renal vasodilation (D_1), cardiac stimulation (β_1), and increased blood pressure (β_1 and α_1)	Cardiogenic shock, septic shock, heart failure, and adjunct to fluid administration in hypovolemic shock
Epinephrine	Vasoconstriction and increased blood pressure (α_1), cardiac stimulation (β_1), and bronchodilation (β_2)	Anaphylactic shock, cardiac arrest, ventricular fibrillation, reduction in bleeding during surgery, and prolongation of the action of local anesthetics
Isoproterenol	Cardiac stimulation (β_1) and bronchodilation (β_2)	Asthma, atrioventricular block, and bradycardia
Norepinephrine	Vasoconstriction and increased blood pressure (α_1)	Hypotension and shock
Direct-Acting Noncatecholamines		
Albuterol	Bronchodilation (β_2)	Asthma
Apraclonidine	Decreased aqueous humor formation (α_2)	Short-term control of intraocular pressure
Clonidine	Decreased sympathetic outflow from central nervous system (α_2 and imidazoline)	Hypertension, opioid dependence
Dexmedetomidine	Sedation (α_2)	Adjunct to anesthesia
Midodrine	Vasoconstriction (α_1)	Orthostatic hypotension
Oxymetazoline	Vasoconstriction (α_1)	Nasal and ocular decongestion
Phenylephrine	Vasoconstriction, increased blood pressure, and mydriasis (α_1)	Nasal and ocular decongestion, mydriasis, maintenance of blood pressure and treatment of shock
Ritodrine	Uterine relaxation (β_2)	Premature labor
Terbutaline	Bronchodilation (β_2)	Asthma
Indirect-Acting Agents		
Amphetamine	Increase in norepinephrine release, central nervous system stimulation	Narcolepsy, attention-deficit disorder
Cocaine	Inhibition of norepinephrine uptake	Local anesthesia
Mixed-Acting Agents		
Ephedrine	Vasoconstriction (α_1)	Nasal decongestion
Pseudoephedrine	Vasoconstriction (α_1)	Nasal decongestion

*Dopamine is a catecholamine with mixed action.

drug (e.g., dobutamine) is usually administered to increase cardiac output in cases of heart failure.

Dobutamine selectively increases myocardial contractility and stroke volume while producing a smaller increase in heart rate. These actions can increase cardiac output in persons with acute heart failure. Dobutamine also reduces vascular resistance by activating β_2-adrenoceptors, thereby reducing the impedance to ventricular ejection. In patients with heart failure, this effect contributes to an increased stroke volume and cardiac output (see Chapter 12).

When given in low doses, dopamine selectively activates D_1-receptors in renal and other vascular beds, thereby causing vasodilation and an increase in renal blood flow. At slightly higher doses, dopamine activates β_1-adrenoceptors in the heart, thereby stimulating cardiac contractility and increasing cardiac output and tissue perfusion. At even higher doses, dopamine activates α_1-adrenoceptors and causes vasoconstriction. Hence, dopamine tends to increase vascular resistance, whereas dobutamine usually decreases vascular resistance.

(2) RESPIRATORY TRACT EFFECTS. Epinephrine and isoproterenol are potent bronchodilators. Although they have been used in the treatment of asthma, more selective β_2-adrenoceptor agonists are usually used for this purpose today.

(3) ADVERSE EFFECTS. Catecholamines can cause excessive vasoconstriction, leading to tissue ischemia and necrosis. Localized tissue ischemia can result from extravasation of an intravenous drug infusion or from the accidental injection of epinephrine into a finger when a patient is trying to stop an allergic reaction by self-injecting epinephrine. The administration of excessive doses of catecholamines can reduce blood flow to vital organs, such as the kidneys, or cause excessive cardiac stimulation that leads tachycardia and other cardiac arrhythmias. The β-adrenoceptor agonists can cause hyperglycemia secondary to glycogenolysis, and this is usually undesirable in patients with diabetes.

Specific Drugs

Catecholamines are used to treat several types of **shock**. Shock is a condition in which the circulation to vital organs is profoundly reduced as a result of inadequate blood volume (**hypovolemic shock**), inadequate cardiac function (**cardiogenic shock**), or inadequate vasomotor tone (**neurogenic shock and septic shock**). Septic shock is associated with massive vasodilation secondary to the production of toxins by pathogenic microorganisms. It is sometimes called "warm shock" to distinguish it from hypovolemic and cardiogenic shock, in which the patient's extremities are usually cold because of inadequate blood flow. Some cases of septic shock, however, are also manifested by hypoperfusion and cold extremities. **Anaphylactic shock**, resulting from severe immediate hypersensitivity reactions, is usually manifested by hypotension and difficult breathing.

Catecholamine drugs that increase blood pressure (**vasopressors**) are used in treating shock when organ

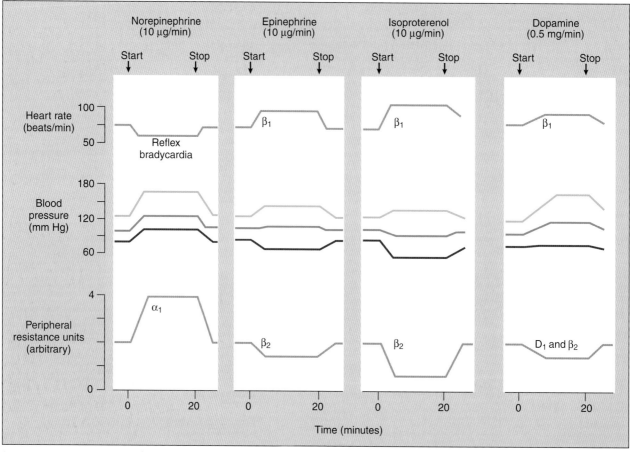

Figure 8–4. Comparison of the cardiovascular effects of four catecholamines when a low dose of each drug is given by intravenous infusion. Arrows indicate when the infusion was started and stopped. The blood pressure recordings show systolic, diastolic, and mean arterial pressure. Peripheral resistance is expressed on an arbitrary scale, ranging from 0 to 4 units. The reflex mechanism, adrenoceptors (α_1, β_1, and β_2), or dopamine (D_1) receptors responsible for changes in the heart rate and peripheral resistance are illustrated. Norepinephrine increases peripheral resistance and blood pressure, and this leads to reflex bradycardia. Epinephrine increases heart rate while reducing peripheral resistance, and the mean arterial blood pressure increases slightly. Isoproterenol increases heart rate but significantly lowers peripheral resistance, and the mean arterial pressure declines. Dopamine increases heart rate (and increases cardiac output) while lowering vascular resistance, and the mean arterial pressure increases.

function is impaired because mean arterial blood pressure is less than 60 mm Hg. **Hypovolemia** should be corrected by intravenous fluid administration before the use of vasopressors because vasopressors will not be effective if hypovolemia is present. In cases of cardiogenic shock, mechanical devices (e.g., the intra-aortic balloon pump) are usually superior to pharmacologic agents in their ability to improve coronary artery perfusion and cardiac performance while reducing myocardial ischemia and cardiac work. Such devices are often used in conjunction with vasopressor drugs in the treatment of this condition.

Dopamine is used to treat **septic or cardiogenic shock** when patients remain hypotensive despite adequate fluid administration. Dopamine is usually started at a dose of 2 mg/kg body weight per minute and then the dose is titrated to achieve the desired blood pressure. Although low doses of dopamine can increase urine output by augmenting renal blood flow in normal subjects, ample evidence indicates that low doses of dopamine are usually not effective in preventing and treating **acute renal failure**. The most effective means of protecting the kidneys in patients with shock appears to be the maintenance

of mean arterial pressure of greater than 60 mm Hg with intravenous fluids and adequate doses of a vasopressor agent.

Norepinephrine, which is a potent vasoconstrictor, is used to treat septic shock and is often given to persons with cardiogenic shock when the response to dopamine is inadequate or is accompanied by marked tachycardia. Norepinephrine is also used to treat hypotension caused by decreased peripheral resistance such as can occur in persons who have received excessive doses of a vasodilator drug. Phenylephrine is also used for this purpose, as described later in this chapter (see "Phenylephrine").

In cases of **anaphylaxis**, epinephrine is the treatment of choice (see Box 8–1). By producing bronchodilation and increasing blood pressure, epinephrine counteracts the effects of histamine and other mediators that are released from mast cells and basophils during immediate hypersensitivity reactions. Epinephrine is used as a vasoconstrictor to **reduce bleeding** during surgery and to **prolong the action of local anesthetics** by retarding their absorption into the general circulation. Epinephrine is also used as a cardiac stimulant in the treatment of

BOX 8-1. A CASE OF AIRWAY OBSTRUCTION

CASE PRESENTATION: A 6-year-old boy suffered a bee sting on the tongue. He developed edema of the face, lips, eyelids, tongue, and throat, and experienced breathing difficulties. Paramedics administered subcutaneous epinephrine and transported the patient to the hospital where he received intravenous dexamethasone (a corticosteroid). The child previously had a bee sting that did not require hospitalization. Because of his respiratory distress, he was intubated and mechanically ventilated for 24 hours. The edema subsided, and the boy was extubated and discharged in good condition.

CASE DISCUSSION: Insect stings are common and can result in immediate hypersensitivity reactions that range from localized pain and rash to more severe reactions involving laryngeal edema, bronchospasm, and hypotension. Stings in the oropharyngeal area have a greater potential to cause airway obstruction and may require intubation and more aggressive treatment than stings in other areas of the body. Hypersensitivity reactions are mediated by immunoglobulin E, which cross-links antigens on mast cells and basophils, leading to the release of histamine and other chemical mediators that cause edema and laryngospasm. The treatment of severe hypersensitivity reactions (anaphylaxis) typically includes epinephrine, antihistamine drugs, and corticosteroids. The corticosteroids counteract inflammation and edema. Hypotension and shock may occur in the most severe cases, and these reactions may require intravenous fluids, oxygen, and other medications.

cardiac arrest and **ventricular fibrillation**. Isoproterenol is used to treat refractory **bradycardia** and **atrioventricular block** when other measures have not been successful. Although it has been used to treat **asthma**, a selective β_2-adrenoceptor agonist is usually preferred for this indication because it does not increase the heart rate as much as isoproterenol.

Dobutamine is a cardiac stimulant (inotropic agent) that also produces vasodilation. It is used as a **cardiac stimulant during heart surgery** and in the short-term management of **acute heart failure** and **cardiogenic shock**. Dobutamine is not routinely used in treating septic shock, however, because its vasodilator effect can further reduce vascular resistance and blood pressure. Its utility in hypotensive patients is limited to situations in which hypotension is caused by bradycardia.

Noncatecholamines

These drugs do not contain a catechol moiety, and they are not substrates for COMT. Some of the noncatecholamines are also resistant to degradation by MAO. For this reason, noncatecholamines are effective after oral administration and have a longer duration of action than do the catecholamines.

Phenylephrine

PHARMACOKINETICS. Phenylephrine is adequately absorbed after oral or topical administration and can also be administered parenterally. The drug is partly metabolized by MAO in the intestine and liver.

MECHANISMS AND EFFECTS. Phenylephrine activates α_1-adrenoceptors and causes smooth muscle contraction. This produces vasoconstriction and increases vascular resistance and blood pressure. Ocular administration of phenylephrine leads to contraction of the iris dilator muscle and dilation of the pupil (mydriasis).

INDICATIONS. Phenylephrine is used as a **nasal decongestant** in patients with **viral rhinitis**, an infection that can be caused by more than a hundred serotypes of rhinovirus, as well as other viruses, and is referred to as the common cold. Phenylephrine is also used by patients with **allergic rhinitis**, an inflammation of the nasal mucosa that is caused by histamine released from mast cells during allergic reactions. The drug's vasoconstrictive effect on the nasal mucosa reduces vascular congestion and mucus secretion so as to open the nasal passages and facilitate breathing. Both topical and oral preparations are available for this purpose.

In patients with **allergic conjunctivitis**, an inflammation of the eyes associated with hay fever or other allergies, phenylephrine can be used as a topical **ocular decongestant**. The ocular preparation of phenylephrine is also used to induce **mydriasis** and thereby facilitate ophthalmoscopic examination of the retina. In contrast to the muscarinic receptor antagonists used for this purpose (e.g., tropicamide), phenylephrine does not relax the ciliary muscle so as to prevent accommodation for near vision.

Phenylephrine can be administered intravenously to treat forms of **hypotension** and **shock** caused by decreased peripheral vascular resistance. These include hypotension caused by excessive doses of vasodilator drugs, drug-induced shock, septic shock, and neurogenic shock such as resulting from spinal cord injury. Phenylephrine is also used to **maintain blood pressure during surgery** (e.g., when hypotension is induced by anesthetic agents).

Midodrine

Midodrine is used to treat postural (orthostatic) hypotension in persons who are considerably impaired by this condition (e.g., those with severe diabetic autonomic neuropathy). Midodrine has also been used to treat hypotension caused by infections in infants, hypotension induced by psychotropic agents, and hypotension in persons undergoing renal dialysis. The drug acts to increase both systolic and diastolic blood pressure of persons in the standing, sitting, and supine positions.

The primary adverse effect of the drug is hypertension, particularly when persons are supine. The drug, which is rapidly absorbed after oral administration, is extensively converted to an active metabolite in the liver and other tissues.

Albuterol, Ritodrine, Terbutaline, and Related Drugs

CHEMISTRY AND PHARMACOKINETICS. Albuterol, ritodrine, and terbutaline are selective β_2-adrenoceptor agonists that can be administered orally, parenterally, or by inhalation. Their oral bioavailability ranges from 30% to 50% because of their incomplete absorption and hepatic first-pass metabolism. They are partly metabolized to inactive compounds before undergoing renal excretion. About 50% of albuterol, for example, is converted to an inactive sulfate conjugate. To reduce their systemic absorption and adverse effects, albuterol and the related agonists are usually administered by inhalation in the treatment of asthma. The duration of action of these agonists is about 4 to 6 hours after inhalation or oral administration and is about 2 to 3 hours after intravenous administration.

MECHANISMS, EFFECTS, AND INDICATIONS. The β_2-adrenoceptor agonists act by causing smooth muscle relaxation. As discussed in greater detail in Chapter 27, these drugs are helpful in the treatment of **asthma** and other obstructive lung diseases because they produce bronchodilation. **Ritodrine** is specifically used in the treatment of **preterm labor**, which is defined as labor that begins before the 37th week of gestation and is believed to be caused by an imbalance in the hormonal regulation of uterine contractions. The administration of ritodrine will relax the uterus and maintain pregnancy for 24 to 48 hours in more than 80% of women with preterm labor. Although the effects of ritodrine are of limited duration in this setting, the treatment may delay delivery long enough to enable the administration of corticosteroids and thereby reduce the risk of neonatal respiratory distress syndrome and other problems associated with preterm delivery.

The adverse effects of albuterol and other selective β_2-adrenoceptor agonists include tachycardia, muscle tremor, and nervousness caused by activation of β_2-adrenoceptors in the heart, skeletal muscle, and central nervous system.

Several other β_2-adrenoceptor agonists have been introduced to treat asthma, including fenoterol, formoterol, pirbuterol, and salmeterol. The distinguishing properties and clinical use of these drugs are described in Chapter 27.

Imidazolines

CHEMISTRY AND PHARMACOKINETICS. The imidazoline compounds activate α-adrenergic and imidazoline receptors. Some imidazolines are administered by topical ocular or nasal administration, whereas others are administered by systemic routes. After systemic administration, the imidazolines have a duration of action of several hours and are partly metabolized and excreted in the urine.

MECHANISMS, EFFECTS, AND INDICATIONS. Based on their clinical use, the imidazolines can be divided into three groups. The first group consists of **oxymetazoline** and similar drugs that

activate α_1-adrenoceptors to produce vasoconstriction. These drugs are used as topical **nasal and ocular decongestants**. Oxymetazoline is available as a nasal spray without prescription. Because it may increase blood pressure, it should not be used by persons with hypertension or heart disease without consulting a health care provider. Topical nasal decongestants should never be used for more than 3 to 5 days in order to avoid rebound congestion that results from excessive vasoconstriction and tissue ischemia. Oxymetazoline and similar decongestants can also cause central nervous system and cardiovascular depression if they are absorbed into the systemic circulation and distributed to the brain. For this reason, these drugs should be used with caution in children under 6 years of age and in the elderly.

The second group of imidazoline compounds includes **apraclonidine** and **brimonidine**. Following topical ocular administration, these agents activate ocular α_2-adrenoceptors in the ciliary body and thereby reduce the level of aqueous humor secretion (see Box 6–1). Apraclonidine and brimonidine are primarily used to prevent short-term elevations of intraocular pressure after cataract surgery and other types of **ocular surgery**. The ability of these drugs to lower intraocular pressure is of limited duration, usually less than 3 months, and there is a high rate of tachyphylaxis (rapid development of tolerance). For this reason, the use of apraclonidine and brimonidine in treating chronic open-angle glaucoma is limited.

The third group consists of **clonidine** and **dexmedetomidine**, which activate α_2-adrenoceptors and imidazoline receptors in the central nervous system. Activation of these receptors leads to a reduction in sympathetic outflow from the vasomotor center in the medulla. For this reason, clonidine is used to treat **hypertension** (see Chapter 10). Clonidine is also used to facilitate abstinence from opioids in persons being treated for **drug dependence** (see Chapter 25). The activation of α_2-adrenoceptors in the central nervous system is also responsible for the sedative and analgesic effects of clonidine and dexmedetomidine. Dexmedetomidine is indicated for sedation of intubated and mechanically ventilated patients during treatment in an intensive care setting. It has also been used as an adjunct to anesthesia during surgical procedures because of its ability to facilitate sedation and analgesia and to prevent shivering.

INDIRECT-ACTING ADRENOCEPTOR AGONISTS

Amphetamine and Tyramine

Amphetamine and related compounds have high lipid solubility and indirectly increase synaptic concentrations of norepinephrine in the central and peripheral nervous systems by mechanisms previously described. Amphetamine produces vasoconstriction, cardiac stimulation, increased blood pressure, and central nervous system stimulation. The various **central nervous system effects** are discussed in greater detail in Chapters 22 and 25.

Tyramine is a naturally occurring amine found in a number of foods, including bananas. Under normal conditions, tyramine is rapidly degraded by MAO in the gut and liver. In patients receiving MAO inhibitors, however, tyramine can be absorbed from foods in a quantity that is high enough to exert a sympathomimetic effect and increase blood pressure. The interaction between foods containing tyramine and MAO inhibitors is discussed in greater detail in Chapter 22. Tyramine is not used as a therapeutic agent.

Cocaine

Cocaine, a naturally occurring alkaloid, acts as a local anesthetic and also stimulates the sympathetic nervous system by blocking the neuronal reuptake of norepinephrine at both peripheral and central synapses. The sympathomimetic effects of cocaine are similar to those of amphetamine. Cocaine produces both vasoconstriction and cardiac stimulation and thereby elevates blood pressure. When the drug is used as a local anesthetic, its vasoconstrictive effect serves to retard its absorption into the systemic circulation, and this prolongs its duration of action. The vasoconstrictive effect, however, can also cause ischemia and necrosis of the nasal mucosa in people who abuse cocaine. The sympathomimetic effects of cocaine also appear to be responsible for the severe hypertension and cardiac damage that may occur in people who abuse cocaine. The **local anesthetic** and **central nervous system effects** of cocaine are discussed further in Chapters 21 and 25.

MIXED-ACTING ADRENOCEPTOR AGONISTS

Among the drugs that activate adrenoceptors by both direct and indirect mechanisms are dopamine (see above), ephedrine, and pseudoephedrine. These agents indirectly increase synaptic concentrations of norepinephrine in a manner similar to that of amphetamine.

Ephedrine and Pseudoephedrine

PHARMACOKINETICS. Ephedrine is a naturally occurring compound obtained from plants of the genus *Ephedra*, which is also called *Ma Huang*. Ephedrine is well absorbed from the gut and has sufficient lipid solubility to enter the central nervous system. Relatively resistant to metabolism by MAO and COMT, ephedrine's duration of action is several hours. **Pseudoephedrine**, an isomer of ephedrine, has been used as a nasal decongestant in the treatment of colds and allergies.

MECHANISM, EFFECTS, AND INDICATIONS. Ephedrine and related drugs activate both α- and β-adrenoceptors by direct and indirect mechanisms. Via the activation of α_1-adrenoceptors, these drugs produce vasoconstriction. This makes them useful as **nasal decongestants** in the treatment of **viral and allergic rhinitis**. Via the action of β-adrenoceptors, the drugs produce bronchodilation. However, a selective β_2-adrenoceptor agonist such as albuterol is now preferred for this indication.

The adverse effects of ephedrine and pseudoephedrine include tachycardia caused by β_1-receptor stimulation, increased blood pressure, and urinary retention. Urinary retention is caused by stimulation of the sphincter muscle of the bladder. These drugs also cause central nervous system stimulation and can produce insomnia. Dietary supplements containing *Ephedra* have been widely used as appetite suppressants as an aid to losing weight. The U.S. Food and Drug Administration has banned the sale of such products because fatalities caused by hypertension and excessive cardiovascular stimulation have occurred following the use of these preparations.

Because of the risks of toxicity and limited evidence of effectiveness, the U.S. Food and Drug Administration recently recommended that **cough and cold medications** should not be used in children under 6 years of age. These products typically contain combinations of antihistamines, cough suppressants, and decongestants, such as phenylephrine and pseudoephedrine.

SUMMARY OF IMPORTANT POINTS

■ Activation of α_1-adrenoceptors mediates smooth muscle contraction, leading to vasoconstriction, dilation of the pupils, and contraction of the bladder sphincter muscle.

■ Activation of α_2-adrenoceptors inhibits the release of norepinephrine from sympathetic neurons, decreases the secretion of aqueous humor, and decreases the secretion of insulin.

■ Activation of β_1-adrenoceptors produces cardiac stimulation and increases the secretion of renin, whereas activation of β_2-adrenoceptors mediates smooth muscle relaxation.

■ The catecholamines include norepinephrine, epinephrine, isoproterenol, dopamine, and dobutamine. These drugs are rapidly metabolized, must be administered parenterally, and are used primarily to treat cardiac disorders and various types of shock.

■ In addition to activating adrenoceptors, dopamine activates D_1-receptors and thereby increases renal blood flow.

■ Noncatecholamines (e.g., phenylephrine and albuterol) are resistant to degradation by COMT. Phenylephrine activates α-adrenoceptors and causes vasoconstriction. Albuterol activates β_2-adrenoceptors and produces bronchodilation.

■ Imidazoline compounds are agents that activate both α-adrenoceptors and imidazoline receptors. Examples include oxymetazoline, a topical decongestant; clonidine, an antihypertensive agent; and apraclonidine, an agent used to treat glaucoma.

■ The indirect-acting adrenoceptor agonists increase the synaptic concentration of norepinephrine. Amphetamine causes reverse transport of norepinephrine by the catecholamine transporter, whereas cocaine blocks the reuptake of norepinephrine by the catecholamine transporter.

■ Mixed-acting agonists, such as pseudoephedrine, have both direct and indirect actions. Pseudoephedrine is used as a nasal decongestant.

Review Questions

1. A man with diabetic autonomic neuropathy complains of dizziness and fainting when arising from bed in the morning. Which drug would be most beneficial to this patient?
   (A) dobutamine
   (B) albuterol
   (C) midodrine
   (D) clonidine
   (E) isoproterenol

2. A woman requires a drug to lower intraocular pressure after cataract surgery. Which mechanism would most likely lead to the desired effect?
   (A) inhibition of adenylyl cyclase
   (B) stimulation of adenylyl cyclase
   (C) activation of phospholipase C
   (D) inhibition of phospholipase C
   (E) release of calcium from the sarcoplasmic reticulum

3. A child with asthma is being treated with an adrenoceptor agonist to prevent bronchospasm. Which side effect is typically associated with this drug?
   (A) sedation
   (B) rapid heart rate
   (C) muscle weakness
   (D) high blood pressure
   (E) blurred vision

4. After being stung by a bee, a woman experiences urticaria, laryngeal edema, difficult breathing and hypotension. She receives oxygen and administration of an adrenoceptor agonist. Which action would lead to bronchodilation?
   (A) increased cAMP levels
   (B) increased cyclic guanosine monophosphate (cGMP) levels
   (C) increased IP3 levels
   (D) calcium influx
   (E) sequestration of calcium

Answers and Explanations

1. **The answer is C: midodrine.** Midodrine is a selective α_1-adrenoceptor agonist that is used to treat postural (orthostatic) hypotension. None of the other options increases systemic vascular resistance or counteracts postural hypotension.

2. **The answer is A: inhibition of adenylyl cyclase.** α_2-Adrenoceptor agonists such as apraclonidine are used for short-term control of intraocular pressure after cataract surgery. Activation of α_2-adrenoceptors is coupled with inhibition of adenylyl cyclase and decreased cAMP levels.

3. **The answer is B: rapid heart rate.** β_2-Adrenoceptor agonists such as albuterol are used to relax bronchial smooth muscle and prevent bronchospasm in persons with asthma. These drugs also activate β-adrenoceptors in the heart and increase heart rate.

4. **The answer is A: increased cAMP levels.** The preferred treatment for severe hypersensitivity reactions (anaphylaxis) is epinephrine. The drug causes bronchodilation by activation of β_2-adrenoceptors in bronchial smooth muscle, leading to increased cAMP levels and smooth muscle relaxation. Although cGMP (Option B) also mediates smooth muscle relaxation, levels of this substance are not significantly increased by β_2-adrenoceptor activation. Increased IP3 levels (Option C) causes smooth muscle contraction, as does calcium influx (Option D). Sequestration of calcium (Option E) causes muscle relaxation, but this action is not invoked by β_2-receptor stimulation.

SELECTED READINGS

Centers for Disease Control and Prevention. Infant deaths associated with cough and cold medications—two states, 2005. Morb Mortal Wkly Rep 56:1–4, 2007.

Hieble, J.P. Subclassification and nomenclature of alpha- and beta-adrenoceptors. Curr Top Med Chem 7:129–134, 2007.

Kemp, S.F. Office approach to anaphylaxis: sooner better than later. Amer J Med 120:664–668, 2007.

Simhan, H.N., and Caritis. S.N. Prevention of preterm labor. N Engl J Med 357:477–487, 2007.

CHAPTER 9

Adrenoceptor Antagonists

OVERVIEW

Excessive sympathetic nervous system activity contributes to a number of diseases, including common cardiovascular disorders such as hypertension, angina pectoris, and cardiac arrhythmias. Drugs that reduce sympathetic stimulation, **sympatholytic drugs**, are used in the management of cardiovascular diseases and other diseases such as glaucoma, migraine headache, and urinary obstruction. The most important group of sympatholytic drugs consists of the adrenoceptor antagonists. Other drugs that have a sympatholytic effect include the ganglionic-blocking agents (discussed in Chapter 7) and the sympathetic neuronal blocking agents (discussed in Chapter 5).

Adrenoceptor antagonists can block α-adrenoceptors, β-adrenoceptors, or both. The **therapeutic effects** of the antagonists are caused primarily by blockade of α$_1$- or β$_1$-adrenoceptors, whereas the **adverse effects** tend to be related to blockade of α$_2$- or β$_2$-adrenoceptors. Drugs that selectively block either α$_1$- or β$_1$-adrenoceptors have been developed in an effort to avoid the adverse effects caused by α$_2$- or β$_2$-adrenoceptor blockade. Blockade of α$_1$-adrenoceptors relaxes vascular and other smooth muscles in tissues innervated by the sympathetic nervous system, whereas blockade of β$_1$-adrenoceptors reduces sympathetic stimulation of the heart.

α-ADRENOCEPTOR ANTAGONISTS

The α-adrenoceptor antagonists, or **α-blockers**, can be distinguished on the basis of their selectivity for adrenoceptor subtypes and by their noncompetitive or competitive blockade of these receptors.

Nonselective α-Blockers

Agents that block both α$_1$- and α$_2$-adrenoceptors are called nonselective α-blockers. Phenoxybenzamine and phentolamine are examples. Phenoxybenzamine is a noncompetitive antagonist, whereas phentolamine is a competitive adrenoceptor antagonist.

Phenoxybenzamine

MECHANISM OF ACTION. Phenoxybenzamine has a chemical structure and mechanism of action that are similar to the nitrogen mustard alkylating agents used in cancer chemotherapy. As with the alkylating agents, phenoxybenzamine undergoes spontaneous chemical transformation in the body to an active metabolite that forms a stable covalent bond with the α-adrenoceptor, resulting in a noncompetitive antagonism of epinephrine and other adrenoceptor agonists (Fig. 9–1).

PHARMACOKINETICS. When phenoxybenzamine is administered orally, it exhibits a gradual onset of action. This is because time is needed to form the active intermediate and bond covalently with α-adrenoceptors. The drug has a duration of action of 3 to 4 days because of its stable covalent bonding with α-adrenoceptors.

EFFECTS AND INDICATIONS. Phenoxybenzamine decreases vascular resistance and lowers both the supine and the standing blood pressure.

As shown in Table 9–1, phenoxybenzamine is used to treat **hypertensive episodes** in patients with **pheochromocytoma**. Because this tumor of the adrenal medulla secretes huge amounts of catecholamines, patients have extremely high blood pressure. Phenoxybenzamine has been used to control hypertension until surgery can be performed to remove the tumor (Box 9–1).

Phentolamine

CHEMISTRY AND PHARMACOKINETICS. Phentolamine is an imidazoline compound that is structurally related to oxymetazoline and other agents in the imidazoline class of adrenoceptor agonists. After intravenous administration of phentolamine, the onset of action is immediate, and the duration of action is 10 to 15 minutes. After intramuscular or subcutaneous administration, the onset of action is 15 to 20 minutes, and the duration is 3 to 4 hours. The drug is metabolized chiefly in the liver before excretion in the urine.

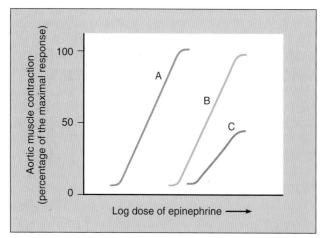

Figure 9–1. Competitive and noncompetitive blockade of epinephrine-induced aortic smooth muscle contraction by phentolamine and phenoxybenzamine. Three dose-response curves are compared. A is the curve of epinephrine alone. B is the curve of epinephrine in the presence of phentolamine. Because phentolamine is a competitive α-adrenoceptor antagonist, epinephrine can surmount its effect. C is the curve of epinephrine in the presence of phenoxybenzamine. Because phenoxybenzamine is a noncompetitive antagonist, it reduces the maximal effect of epinephrine.

MECHANISMS, EFFECTS, AND INDICATIONS. Phentolamine is a competitive adrenoceptor antagonist (see Fig. 9–1) that produces vasodilation, decreases peripheral vascular resistance, and decreases blood pressure. It is used in the treatment of **hypertensive episodes** caused by **α-adrenoceptor agonists.** In addition, it is used to treat **dermal necrosis and ischemia** caused by extravasation or accidental injection of epinephrine or other vasopressor amines. For example, if a patient who carries an epinephrine auto-injector for use in treating acute allergic reactions were to accidentally inject his or her finger and thereby cause ischemia, the patient could be treated by injecting phentolamine into the same site where epinephrine was injected. The phentolamine would competitively block the α-adrenoceptor stimulation and vasoconstriction produced by the epinephrine.

Phentolamine and other nonselective α-blockers are not useful in treating hypertension, partly because they evoke reflex tachycardia and cause dizziness, headache, and nasal congestion.

Selective α₁-Antagonists

Agents that selectively antagonize α₁-adrenoceptors include **alfuzosin, doxazosin, prazosin, tamsulosin,** and **terazosin.** Prazosin, the original drug in this class, was developed to treat hypertension. These drugs have also been used to treat urinary symptoms in men with benign prostatic hyperplasia.

General Properties

PHARMACOKINETICS. The selective α₁-adrenoceptor antagonists are administered orally and undergo varying amounts of first-pass and systemic metabolism. The drugs are highly bound to plasma proteins and they are excreted in the bile, urine, and feces.

MECHANISMS, EFFECTS, AND INDICATIONS. The selective α₁-blockers relax vascular and other smooth muscles, including those of the urinary bladder, urethra, and prostate. Because they produce vasodilation and decrease blood pressure, they are used to treat essential (primary) hypertension. The cardiovascular effects of α- and β-blockers in patients with hypertension are depicted in Figure 9–2.

The selective α₁-blockers do not cause as much reflex tachycardia as do phentolamine and other agents that nonselectively block both α₁- and α₂-adrenoceptors. This is because blockade of α₂-adrenoceptors on sympathetic neurons prevents feedback inhibition of norepinephrine release and thereby leads to increased activation of cardiac β₁-adrenoceptors and tachycardia (Fig. 9–3). The use of prazosin and other selective α₁-blockers to treat hypertension is discussed in greater detail in Chapter 10.

The selective α₁-blockers are quite useful in treating **lower urinary tract symptoms** associated with **benign prostatic hyperplasia** and other conditions. Men with these conditions complain of urinary frequency, urgency, and nocturia (need to urinate more frequently at night). Prostatic enlargement may contribute to urinary outflow obstruction in these men and the beneficial effects of α₁-blockers have been assumed to be due to relaxation of prostatic and urethral smooth muscle (Fig. 9–4). However, the weak correlation between lower urinary tract symptoms and prostatic

TABLE 9–1. Mechanisms, Pharmacologic Effects, and Clinical Uses of Selected Adrenoceptor Antagonists

Drug	Mechanism of Action	Pharmacologic Effects	Clinical Use
α-Blockers			
Doxazosin, Prazosin, Terazosin	Competitive α_1-blocker	Cause vasodilation and decrease blood pressure; relax bladder, urethral, and prostate smooth muscle	Hypertension; urinary symptoms due to benign prostatic hyperplasia
Alfuzosin, Tamsulosin	Competitive α_1-blocker	Relax bladder, urethral, and prostate smooth muscle	Urinary symptoms due to benign prostatic hyperplasia
Phenoxybenzamine	Noncompetitive α_1- and α_2-blocker	Causes vasodilation; decreases blood pressure	Hypertension in pheochromocytoma
Phentolamine	Competitive α_1- and α_2-blocker	Causes vasodilation; decreases vascular resistance and blood pressure	Hypertension in pheochromocytoma; treat necrosis and ischemia after injection of an α-adrenoceptor agonist
β-Blockers			
Acebutolol	β_1-Blocker with ISA and MSA	Decreases cardiac rate, output, AV node conduction, and O_2 demand; decreases blood pressure	Hypertension; cardiac arrhythmias
Atenolol	β_1-Blocker	Same as acebutolol	Hypertension; angina pectoris; acute myocardial infarction
Esmolol	β_1-Blocker	Same as acebutolol	Acute supraventricular tachycardia and hypertension
Metoprolol	β_1-Blocker with MSA	Same as acebutolol	Hypertension; angina pectoris; acute myocardial infarction
Nadolol	β_1- and β_2-Blocker	Same as acebutolol	Hypertension; angina pectoris; migraine headache
Pindolol	β_1- and β_2-Blocker with ISA and MSA	Same as acebutolol	Hypertension
Propranolol	β_1- and β_2-Blocker with MSA	Same as acebutolol	Hypertension; angina pectoris; cardiac arrhythmias; hypertrophic subaortic stenosis; essential tremor; migraine headache; acute thyrotoxicosis; acute myocardial infarction; pheochromocytoma
Timolol	β_1- and β_2-Blocker	Decreases cardiac rate, output, AV node conduction, and O_2 demand; decreases blood pressure; decreases intraocular pressure	Hypertension; acute myocardial infarction; migraine headache; glaucoma
α- and β-Blockers			
Carvedilol	β_1- and β_2-Blocker; α_1-blocker	Causes vasodilation; decreases heart rate and blood pressure in patients with hypertension; increases cardiac output in patients with heart failure	Hypertension; heart failure
Labetalol	β_1- and β_2-Blocker with MSA; α_1-blocker	Causes vasodilation; decreases heart rate and blood pressure	Hypertension

AV = atrioventricular; ISA = intrinsic sympathomimetic activity (partial agonist activity); MSA = membrane-stabilizing activity (local anesthetic activity).

enlargement has shifted the focus to the role of α_1-adrenoceptors in the bladder, urethra, and the nervous system in causing lower urinary tract symptoms. Blockade of α_1-receptors in these tissues is believed to contribute to the therapeutic effects of α_1-adrenoceptor antagonists in the relief of lower urinary tract symptoms.

The most common adverse effects of α_1-blockers include hypotension, dizziness, and sedation, and these effects have been attributed to excessive vasodilation as well as to the central nervous system effects of these drugs. Doxazosin and terazosin appear to be associated with a higher incidence of these adverse effects than tamsulosin and alfuzosin. A small percentage of men experience abnormal ejaculation when taking α_1-blockers.

Specific Drugs

Prazosin, whose half-life is shorter than the half-lives of other α_1-antagonists, has a duration of action of about 6 hours. It undergoes considerable first-pass and systemic metabolism before renal and biliary excretion.

Doxazosin and terazosin are longer acting α_1-blockers that are usually administered once a day to treat hypertension or to relieve lower urinary tract symptoms. Their duration of action ranges from about 20 hours (terazosin) to about 30 hours (doxazosin).

Alfuzosin and tamsulosin are more uroselective α_1-blockers that relieve lower urinary tract symptoms without causing as much hypotension, dizziness, and sedation as other

BOX 9–1. A CASE OF HEADACHE, ANXIETY, AND A RACING HEART

CASE PRESENTATION: A 38-year-old man complains of the recent onset of episodes of headache, nervousness, sweating, a racing heart, and rapid breathing. The episodes last from a few minutes to over an hour and occur several times a day. On physical examination his pulse is 86 beats/min, his respiration rate is 24/min, and his blood pressure is 210/110 mm Hg. The patient has no history of hypertension and is taking no medications. He is given oxygen and intravenous labetalol to gradually reduce heart rate and blood pressure. His 24-hour urinary vanillylmandelic acid concentration is 10.8 mg (normal <7 mg/24 h), his epinephrine is elevated at 186 μg (normal <22 μg/24 h), and norepinephrine is 135 μg (normal 12–85 μg/24 h). A computed tomography image shows a 1.7 × 2.1 cm soft tissue density in the left suprarenal area but no other abnormalities, and he is placed on metoprolol and phenoxybenzamine to control high blood pressure until surgery. His blood pressure is gradually reduced to 118/65 mm Hg, and he is started on a high-salt diet to maintain plasma volume. A week later he undergoes laparoscopic left adrenalectomy and his medications are gradually withdrawn. His blood pressure stabilizes at 120/70 mm Hg, and he is discharged after an uneventful recovery on no medication.

CASE DISCUSSION: Pheochromocytoma is a rare tumor of the adrenal medulla that secretes huge quantities of epinephrine and norepinephrine. The peak age of onset is 40 years. Symptoms may be intermittent or continuous and include headache, anxiety, sweating, rapid breathing, and tachycardia. The diagnosis is established by abdominal imaging and measurement of urinary catecholamines and vanillylmandelic acid. If the tumor has not metastasized, it can be surgically removed with no sequelae. Blood pressure should be controlled until surgery with adrenoceptor antagonists, and phenoxybenzamine is often used for this purpose along with a β-blocker to reduce cardiac stimulation and prevent arrhythmias and cardiac ischemia. Patients are usually given a high-sodium diet (>5000 mg daily) to counteract catecholamine-induced volume contraction and the orthostatic hypotension caused by α-receptor blockade. If the tumor is unilateral, replacement of corticosteroids is not necessary after adrenalectomy.

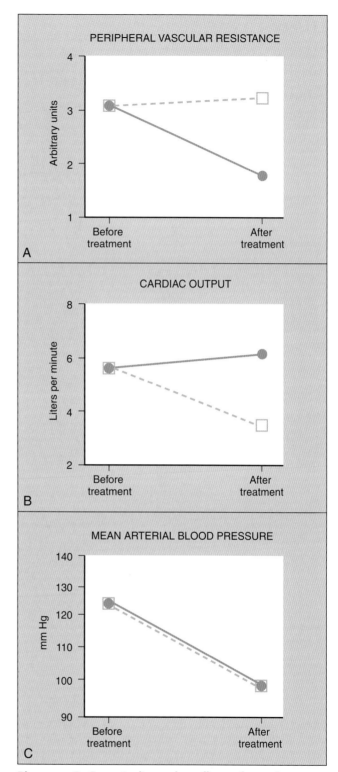

Figure 9-2. Cardiovascular effects of α_1-adrenoceptor antagonists (solid line) and β_1-adrenoceptor antagonists (dotted line) in patients with hypertension. (A) The α_1-blockers reduce peripheral vascular resistance. The α_1-blockers can cause a slight increase in peripheral vascular resistance, owing to reflex mechanisms. (B) The β_1-blockers reduce cardiac output. The β_1-blockers can increase cardiac output by decreasing cardiac afterload and aortic impedance to ventricular ejection of blood. (C) Both α_1-blockers and β_1-blockers reduce mean arterial blood pressure.

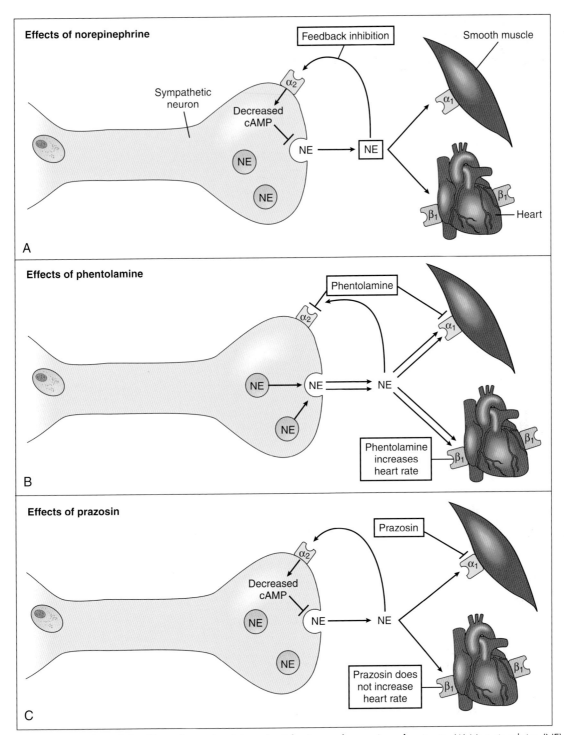

Figure 9-3. A comparison of the effects of norepinephrine, phentolamine, and prazosin on heart rate. (A) Norepinephrine (NE) activates presynaptic α_2-adrenoceptors (2), and this inhibits the formation of cyclic adenosine monophosphate (cAMP) and decreases the release of NE. (B) Phentolamine blocks α_2-adrenoceptor–mediated inhibition of NE release. This increases the stimulation of cardiac β_1-adrenoceptors (1) and results in tachycardia. (C) Prazosin, a selective α_1-blocker, does not block α_2-adrenoceptor–mediated inhibition of norepinephrine release. Therefore, prazosin causes less tachycardia than does phentolamine. $\alpha_1 = \alpha_1$-adrenoceptors.

α_1-blockers. In fact, their side effect profiles are similar to those of placebo. These drugs are only indicated for treating symptoms of urinary outflow obstruction in men with prostatic hyperplasia and are not used to treat hypertension.

β-ADRENOCEPTOR ANTAGONISTS

The β-adrenoceptor antagonists, or **β-blockers**, can be categorized as nonselective or selective.

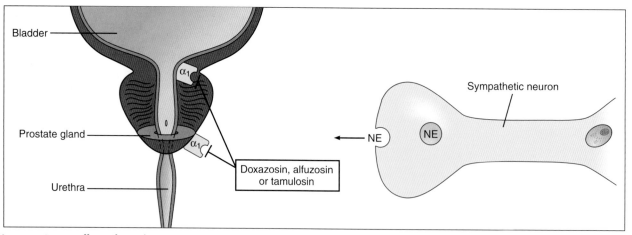

Figure 9–4. **Effects of α_1-adrenoceptor antagonists on the urinary bladder.** Prostatic hyperplasia leads to obstruction of urine outflow from the bladder through the urethra. An α_1-blocker (e.g., doxazosin, alfuzosin, or tamsulosin) will relax smooth muscle in the bladder, urethra, and prostate and thereby facilitate micturition in patients with prostatic hyperplasia. $\alpha_1 = \alpha_1$-adrenoceptors; NE = norepinephrine.

Nonselective β-Blockers

The nonselective β-blockers were the first β-blockers to be developed for clinical use. In addition to blocking β_1-adrenoceptors in heart tissue, they block β_2-adrenoceptors in smooth muscle, liver, and other tissues. Examples include **nadolol**, **pindolol**, **propranolol**, and **timolol**.

General Properties

CHEMISTRY AND PHARMACOKINETICS. The β-adrenoceptor antagonists are structural analogues of β-adrenoceptor agonists (see Fig. 3–2). Table 9–2 outlines the pharmacologic properties of various β-blockers. All of the nonselective β-blockers can be administered orally, and propranolol can also be administered parenterally.

MECHANISMS AND EFFECTS. The nonselective β-blockers competitively block the effects of norepinephrine and other adrenoceptor agonists at β_1- and β_2-adrenoceptors. In addition, some of them exhibit intrinsic sympathomimetic activity and membrane-stabilizing (local anesthetic) activity, as outlined in Table 9–2 and defined below.

Blockade of β_1-adrenoceptors reduces sympathetic stimulation of the heart and thereby produces a negative chronotropic, inotropic, and dromotropic effect. Because the β-blockers reduce cardiac output and blood pressure (see Fig. 9–2), they can be used to treat arterial hypertension. In the kidneys, β_1-adrenoceptor blockade reduces the secretion of renin from the juxtaglomerular cells. In the eye, adrenoceptor blockade reduces aqueous humor secretion and intraocular pressure.

Blockade of β_2-adrenoceptors produces several effects that can lead to adverse reactions in some patients receiving β-blockers, such as patients with asthma or diabetes. In the lungs, antagonism of β_2-adrenoceptors can cause bronchoconstriction in patients with asthma. These persons depend on endogenous epinephrine to prevent bronchospasm, so agents that block β_2-adrenoceptors should be avoided or used with great caution. If a β-blocker is required to treat an asthmatic patient, a selective β_1-blocker should be used. In the liver, β_2-adrenoceptor blockade inhibits epinephrine-stimulated glycogenolysis and can thereby slow the recovery of blood glucose after a hypoglycemic episode in a patient with diabetes. The β-blockers can also mask some of the early signs of hypoglycemia (e.g., tachycardia and sweating), which would otherwise alert the diabetic patient to this problem. For these reasons, β-blockers should be used cautiously in patients with diabetes and particularly in those who have insulin-dependent diabetes and are susceptible to hypoglycemic episodes associated with excessive insulin administration.

Specific Properties

Tables 9–1 and 9–2 compare the effects, uses, and properties of four nonselective β-blockers: nadolol, pindolol, propranolol, and timolol.

Of these four drugs, only pindolol has **intrinsic sympathomimetic activity**, or **partial agonist activity**, which enables it to exert a weak agonist effect on β-adrenoceptors. This effect is observed when the patient is resting and sympathetic tone is low, and it can result in a smaller reduction in heart rate than that caused by β-blockers without intrinsic sympathomimetic activity. When sympathetic tone is high, pindolol acts as a competitive receptor antagonist to inhibit sympathetic stimulation of the heart in the same manner as other β-blockers.

Although pindolol and propranolol exhibit **membrane-stabilizing activity**, or **local anesthetic activity**, nadolol and timolol do not. Drugs with local anesthetic activity can block sodium channels in nerves and heart tissue and thereby slow conduction velocity.

Pindolol is used only to treat **hypertension**. In contrast, propranolol has many clinical applications. Propranolol is used, for example, to treat patients with **hypertension, angina pectoris,** or **cardiac arrhythmias** (conditions discussed in detail in the chapters of Section III); patients with **hypertrophic subaortic stenosis** (a form of hypertrophic cardiomyopathy, a condition that impedes the ejection of blood from the ventricles and reduces cardiac output); and patients with **essential tremor** (a benign condition characterized by involuntary trembling of the hands). Propranolol is

TABLE 9–2. Pharmacokinetic Properties of Drugs That Cause β-Adrenoceptor Blockade

Drug	Lipid Solubility	Oral Bioavailability	Elimination Half-Life	Intrinsic Sympathomimetic Activity	Membrane-Stabilizing Activity
Nonselective β-Blockers					
Nadolol	Low	35%	15–20 hours	None	None
Pindolol	Medium	75%	3–4 hours	Medium	Low
Propranolol	High	25%	4–6 hours	None	High
Timolol	Medium	50%	4–6 hours	None	None
Selective β₁-Blockers					
Acebutolol	Medium	40%	10–12 hours*	Low	Medium
Atenolol	Low	50%	6–7 hours	None	None
Esmolol	Low	—	10 minutes	None	None
Metoprolol	Medium	40%	3–4 hours	None	Low
α- and β-Blockers					
Carvedilol	Not known	30%	6–8 hours	None	None
Labetalol	Medium	20%	6–8 hours	None	Low

*Includes half-life of active metabolite.

also used to prevent **migraine headache** and as adjunctive therapy in the treatment of **acute thyrotoxicosis, acute myocardial infarction**, and **pheochromocytoma**. Patients with thyrotoxicosis often experience tachycardia and palpitations because thyroid hormones increase the effects of sympathetic stimulation on the heart. Propranolol is used to reduce these symptoms until the underlying thyroid disorder can be treated. Propranolol and other β-blockers are frequently administered to patients with acute myocardial infarction because clinical trials have shown that β-blockers reduce the incidence of sudden death and mortality in these patients. In patients with pheochromocytoma, propranolol is used to reduce cardiac stimulation caused by circulating catecholamines released from this adrenal medullary tumor.

Propranolol, the first β-blocker approved for clinical use, is distinguished by its high lipid solubility and central nervous system penetration, which can cause a higher incidence of central nervous system side effects in some patients. Propranolol has a greater local anesthetic effect than do other β-blockers, but the clinical significance of this activity is uncertain.

Nadolol is a long-acting drug that is largely excreted unchanged in the urine. It is primarily used to treat **hypertension** and **angina pectoris** and to prevent **migraine headache**.

Timolol is administered orally to treat **hypertension**, to reduce the risk of death in patients with **acute myocardial infarction**, and to prevent **migraine headache**. Timolol was the first β-blocker to be used to treat **glaucoma** and is available as an ophthalmic solution for topical ocular administration. The drug is absorbed through the cornea and penetrates to the ciliary body. In glaucoma, which is discussed in greater detail in Chapter 6, β-blockers reduce aqueous humor secretion and intraocular pressure. Timolol was selected for ophthalmic use partly because it does not have membrane-stabilizing activity and, therefore, does not anesthetize the cornea when instilled into the eye.

Selective β₁-Blockers

General Properties

Examples of selective β₁-blockers include **acebutolol, atenolol, esmolol**, and **metoprolol**. These drugs have a greater affinity for β₁- than for β₂-adrenoceptors. Because β₁-adrenoceptors are primarily located in cardiac tissue, the β₁-blockers are also known as **cardioselective β-blockers**.

In comparison with the nonselective β-blockers, the selective β₁-blockers produce less bronchoconstriction and, other β₂-adrenoceptor–mediated effects. Their selectivity for β₁-adrenoceptors, however, is not absolute, and β₂-receptor blockade increases with dosage. For this reason, selective β₁-blockers should be used with caution in patients who have asthma.

Specific Properties

Tables 9–1 and 9–2 compare the effects, uses, and properties of four selective β₁-blockers.

Acebutolol is a cardioselective β-blocker with a low degree of intrinsic sympathomimetic activity. It is converted to an active metabolite, *N*-acetyl acebutolol, which has a longer half-life than the parent compound and accounts for the drug's relatively long duration of action. Acebutolol is administered orally to treat **hypertension** and **cardiac arrhythmias** (e.g., ventricular premature beats).

Atenolol shows less variability in its oral absorption than do other β-blockers and is excreted largely unchanged in the urine. It also has lower lipid solubility and has been associated with a lower incidence of central nervous system side effects (e.g., vivid dreams, tiredness, and depression). Atenolol is administered orally or parenterally and is primarily used to treat **hypertension, angina pectoris**, and **acute myocardial infarction**.

Esmolol has a much shorter half-life than other β-blockers and is administered intravenously to treat hypertension and **acute supraventricular tachycardia** when these occur during surgery. Esmolol is rapidly metabolized to inactive compounds by plasma esterase enzymes.

Metoprolol is used to treat **hypertension, angina pectoris,** and **acute myocardial infarction**. It can be administered orally or parenterally, and it is extensively metabolized by cytochrome P450 enzymes before undergoing renal excretion.

Other selective β_1-selective antagonists include bisoprolol and betaxolol. Both of these drugs are administered orally to treat hypertension, and betaxolol is also used to treat chronic open-angle glaucoma. Topical ocular administration of betaxolol reduces aqueous humor secretion while producing negligible blockade of systemic β-adrenoceptors.

α-AND β-ADRENOCEPTOR ANTAGONISTS

Carvedilol and **labetalol** are agents that block both α- and β-adrenoceptors. Their effects, uses, and properties are shown in Tables 9–1 and 9–2. Carvedilol blocks β_1-, β_2-, and α_1-adrenoceptors, and possesses antioxidant activity. Each of these actions contributes to its cardioprotective effects in persons with myocardial infarction. The antioxidant effects of carvedilol include (1) inhibition of lipid peroxidation in myocardial membranes, (2) scavenging of free radicals, and (3) inhibition of neutrophil release of O_2. In addition, carvedilol has antiapoptotic properties that can prevent myocyte death and reduce infarct size in persons suffering from myocardial ischemia. For these reasons, carvedilol has been called a "third-generation β-blocker and neurohumoral antagonist," and its value in treating myocardial infarction has been established in clinical trials.

Carvedilol decreases blood pressure and has been used in the treatment of hypertension. As discussed further in Chapter 12, it also decreases cardiac afterload, increases cardiac output, and reduces mortality in patients with heart failure.

Labetalol is a nonselective β-blocker and a selective α_1-blocker that is primarily used in the treatment of hypertension. It is 5 to 10 times more potent as a β-blocker than as an α-blocker, but both actions are believed to contribute to its antihypertensive effect. Labetalol decreases heart rate and cardiac output as a result of β_1-adrenoceptor blockade, and it decreases peripheral vascular resistance as a result of α_1-adrenoceptor blockade.

SUMMARY OF IMPORTANT POINTS

■ The α-adrenoceptor antagonists relax smooth muscle and decrease vascular resistance, whereas the β-adrenoceptor antagonists reduce heart rate and cardiac output. Both α- and β-blockers reduce blood pressure.

■ The nonselective α-blockers include phenoxybenzamine (a noncompetitive blocker) and phentolamine (a competitive blocker). These drugs block both α_1- and α_2-adrenoceptors and are primarily used to treat hypertensive episodes caused by pheochromocytoma.

■ The selective α_1-blockers include alfuzosin, doxazosin, prazosin, tamsulosin, and terazosin. These drugs are used to treat chronic essential (primary) hypertension or to treat urinary obstruction caused by benign prostatic hyperplasia and other conditions.

■ The nonselective β-blockers, which antagonize both β_1- and β_2-adrenoceptors, include nadolol, pindolol, propranolol, and timolol. In comparison with other β-blockers, pindolol has a higher degree of intrinsic sympathomimetic activity (partial agonist activity), and propranolol has a higher degree of membrane-stabilizing activity (local anesthetic activity).

■ The selective β_1-blockers include acebutolol, atenolol, esmolol, and metoprolol. These drugs cause less bronchoconstriction than do nonselective β-blockers.

■ The β-blockers have a variety of clinical applications, including the prevention of migraine headache and the treatment of hypertension, angina pectoris, cardiac arrhythmias, and glaucoma.

■ Carvedilol blocks α- and β-adrenoceptors and exerts other cardioprotective effects that make it useful in the treatment of myocardial infarction and heart failure.

Review Questions

Questions 1 to 4. For each patient described, select the most appropriate drug therapy from the lettered choices.
  (A) alfuzosin
  (B) carvedilol
  (C) metoprolol
  (D) phenoxybenzamine
  (E) phentolamine
  (F) timolol

1. A woman experiences pain and ischemia in her finger after accidentally injecting it with an auto-injector that she carries for emergency treatment of allergic reactions.

2. A man complains of urinary urgency, frequency, and nocturia and is found to have benign enlargement of the prostate gland.

3. A woman with essential hypertension requires a drug that reduces both cardiac output and peripheral resistance.

4. A man with episodic severe hypertension is found to have markedly elevated levels of epinephrine and norepinephrine metabolites in his urine and requires a long-acting drug to lower blood pressure before surgery.

Question 5. Choose the single best answer from the lettered choices.

5. Which drug is least likely to slow recovery from hypoglycemia in a diabetic patient who has taken an excessive dose of insulin?
  (A) metoprolol
  (B) labetalol

(C) nadolol
(D) propranolol
(E) timolol

Answers and Explanations

1. **The answer is E: phentolamine.** Epinephrine and other adrenoceptor agonists can cause excessive vasoconstriction and ischemia when injected into fingers, toes, or other tissues because of stimulation of α_1-adrenoceptors in vascular smooth muscle. Phentolamine is a nonselective α–adrenoceptor antagonist that can be injected directly into affected tissues to counteract the vasoconstrictive effects of adrenoceptor agonists.

2. **The answer is A: alfuzosin.** Alfuzosin is a selective α_1-adrenoceptor blocker that acts to relax smooth muscle in the bladder outflow tract and thereby relieve urinary obstruction caused by prostatic hyperplasia. The drug is sometimes used in combination with finasteride or other drugs that inhibit the 5α-reductase enzyme that converts testosterone to dihydrotestosterone and thereby contributes to stimulation of prostatic growth.

3. **The answer is B: carvedilol.** Carvedilol is a nonselective β-adrenoceptor antagonist and a selective α_1-receptor antagonist that is used to treat hypertension. It acts to reduce cardiac output by blocking cardiac β_1-adrenoceptors and to reduce peripheral resistance by blocking α_1-receptors in vascular smooth muscle.

4. **The answer is D: phenoxybenzamine.** The patient most likely has a tumor of the adrenal medulla called pheochromocytoma. This tumor secretes massive quantities of epinephrine and norepinephrine, thereby causing severe hypertension. Phenoxybenzamine is a noncompetitive, long-acting α-adrenoceptor antagonist that is sometimes used to reduce blood pressure in patients with this condition.

5. **The answer is A: metoprolol.** Selective β_1-blockers such as metoprolol are less likely to inhibit β_2-receptor–mediated glycogenolysis and thereby slow recovery from hypoglycemia. Drugs that block both β_1- and β_2-adrenoceptors (labetalol, nadolol, propranolol, and timolol) are more likely to prolong hypoglycemia after excessive insulin administration. Labetalol also blocks α_1-adrenoceptors.

SELECTED READINGS

Agabiti, R.E., and D. Rizzoni. Metabolic profile of nebivolol, a beta-adrenoceptor antagonist with unique characteristics. Drugs 67: 1097–1107, 2007.

Andersson, K.E., and C. Gratzke. Pharmacology of alpha$_1$-adrenoceptor antagonists in the lower urinary tract and central nervous system. Nat Clin Pract Urol 4:368–378, 2007.

Dandona, P., H. Ghanim, and D.P. Brooks. Antioxidant activity of carvedilol in cardiovascular disease. J Hypertens 25:731–741, 2007.

III

CARDIOVASCULAR, RENAL, AND HEMATOLOGIC PHARMACOLOGY

CHAPTER 10

Antihypertensive Drugs

CLASSIFICATION OF ANTIHYPERTENSIVE DRUGS

Diuretics
Thiazide and related diuretics
- Hydrochlorothiazide[a]

Potassium-sparing diuretics
- Amiloride[b]

Sympatholytics
Adrenoceptor antagonists
- Atenolol (TENORMIN)[c]
- Doxazosin (CARDURA)[d]
- Labetalol (NORMODYNE, TRANDATE)
- Carvedilol (COREG)
- Nebivolol (BYSTOLIC)

Centrally acting drugs
- Clonidine (CATAPRES)[e]

Angiotensin Inhibitors
Angiotensin-converting enzyme (ACE) inhibitors
- Enalapril (VASOTEC)[f]

Angiotensin receptor antagonists
- Losartan (COZAAR)[g]

Direct renin inhibitor
- Aliskiren (TEKTURNA)

Vasodilators
Calcium channel blockers (CCBs)
- Amlodipine (NORVASC)[h]

Other vasodilators
- Hydralazine[i]

Dopamine agonist
- Fenoldopam (CORLOPAM)

[a]Also indapamide and metolazone.
[b]Also spironolactone, eplerenone, and triamterene.
[c]Also betaxolol, bisoprolol, metoprolol, nadolol, pindolol, propranolol, and timolol.
[d]Also prazosin and terazosin.
[e]Also guanfacine and methyldopa.
[f]Also benazepril, captopril, fosinopril, lisinopril, moexipril, perindopril, quinapril, ramipril, and trandolapril.
[g]Also candesartan, eprosartan, irbesartan, telmisartan, and valsartan.
[h]Also diltiazem, felodipine, isradipine, nicardipine, nifedipine, nisoldipine, and verapamil.
[i]Also minoxidil and nitroprusside.

OVERVIEW

An estimated 50 million people in the United States have high blood pressure (hypertension), commonly defined as a sustained systolic blood pressure of 140 mm Hg or higher or a sustained diastolic blood pressure of 90 mm Hg or higher. Numerous studies have shown that untreated high blood pressure damages blood vessels, accelerates **atherosclerosis**, and produces **left ventricular hypertrophy.** The rate at which these changes occur is proportional to the severity of hypertension. Eventually, these abnormalities contribute to the development of **ischemic heart disease, stroke, heart failure**, and **renal failure**, which are the most common causes of death in patients who are hypertensive.

Hypertension

Over the past several decades, health professionals and public officials have increased their efforts to educate the public about the hazards of untreated hypertension, and this has led to a significant increase in the number of hypertensive individuals who are aware of their condition and treat it effectively via lifestyle modifications and pharmacologic agents. The effective treatment of high blood pressure appears to be one of the factors that has contributed to a nearly 60% reduction in the incidence of stroke and at least a 50% reduction in the mortality rate from coronary artery disease since 1970.

About 95% of the cases of hypertension are considered to be **primary hypertension** that cannot be attributed to a specific cause. The other 5% of cases are classified as **secondary hypertension**, which results from an identifiable cause such as chronic kidney disease, pheochromocytoma (a tumor of the adrenal medulla), or hyperaldosteronism. In some cases, secondary hypertension can be corrected by medication or surgery.

Although the cause of primary hypertension in any specific patient is usually unknown, numerous genetic and lifestyle factors are associated with it. These include obesity, lack of exercise, the so-called metabolic syndrome (abdominal obesity, hyperlipidemia, and insulin resistance), dietary sodium intake by individuals with salt sensitivity, and excessive consumption of alcohol.

In recent years, the role of vascular **endothelial cell dysfunction** in the genesis and maintenance of hypertension has received increased attention. The endothelium is an important regulator of vascular smooth muscle tone via the synthesis and release of several relaxing factors, including **nitric oxide** and **prostacyclin**, as well as vasoconstricting factors such as endothelin-1 and angiotensin II. In addition to its vasoconstrictive effect, angiotensin II produces vascular injury via activation of growth factors that cause vascular smooth muscle proliferation and hypertrophy as well as fibrotic changes in the vascular wall. Oxidative stress and other pathologic stimuli appear to alter the ratio of endothelial relaxing factors and vasoconstrictive factors, thereby contributing to the development of hypertension. Several antihypertensive drugs, including carvedilol and the angiotensin inhibitors, appear to counteract endothelial cell dysfunction and thereby reduce some of the adverse consequences of hypertensive disease.

Classification of Blood Pressure

The classification of blood pressure shown in Table 10–1 was presented in the Seventh Report of the Joint National Committee on the Prevention, Detection, Evaluation, and Treatment of High Blood Pressure (JNC 7; Chobanian et al., 2003). This classification includes the term *prehypertension* for those with blood pressures ranging from 120 to 139 mm

Hg systolic, 80 to 89 mm Hg diastolic blood pressure, or both. This designation is intended to identify persons in whom early adoption of **lifestyle changes** that decrease blood pressure could prevent the progression of blood pressure to hypertensive levels (see below). These persons are not candidates for drug therapy unless they have **diabetes** and a trial of lifestyle changes fails to reduce their blood pressure to the desired level of 130/80 mm Hg or less for diabetics.

The classification includes two stages of hypertension that confer differences in follow-up recommendations and management. In addition to providing information about lifestyle modifications, stage 1 hypertension should be confirmed within 2 months and then treated appropriately. Stage 2 hypertension should be treated immediately if blood pressure is greater than 180/110 mm Hg. For lower blood pressures, stage 2 hypertension should be evaluated and treated within 1 month.

Regulation of Blood Pressure

From a systemic hemodynamic perspective, blood pressure is regulated primarily by the **sympathetic nervous system** and the **kidneys** through their influence on cardiac output and peripheral vascular resistance. There is increasing awareness that vasoactive and other substances produced within the blood vessel wall may have a substantial role in the regulation of blood pressure and in the pathophysiology of hypertension.

Cardiac output, which is the product of stroke volume and heart rate, is increased by sympathetic stimulation via activation of β_1-adrenoceptors in the heart. Cardiac output is also influenced by the kidneys via their regulation of blood volume, which is one of the factors determining the cardiac filling pressure and stroke volume.

Peripheral vascular resistance (PVR) is chiefly determined by the resistance to blood flow through the arterioles, whose cross-sectional area depends on arteriolar smooth muscle tone in the various vascular beds. Via activation of α_1-adrenoceptors, the sympathetic nervous system stimulates arteriolar smooth muscle contraction, and this leads to vasoconstriction. Several blood-borne substances, including vasopressin and angiotensin II, produce vasoconstriction. In addition, adenosine, serotonin, endothelin, prostaglandins, and a number of other substances produced locally in various tissues have an effect on arteriolar smooth muscle tone. These substances serve to regulate blood flow through the tissues, and they can also affect systemic arterial pressure.

The sympathetic nervous system provides **short-term regulation** of blood pressure through the **baroreceptor reflex**. This reflex modulates sympathetic stimulation of cardiac output and PVR and adjusts blood pressure in response to postural changes and altered physical activity. The kidneys are primarily responsible for the **long-term control** of blood pressure, via regulation of plasma volume and the renin-angiotensin-aldosterone axis. By these mechanisms, the sympathetic system and kidneys maintain arterial blood pressure within a fairly narrow range when a person is at rest, and they adjust blood pressure appropriately in response to postural changes and physical activity.

TABLE 10–1. Classification of Blood Pressure for Adults and Follow-up Recommendations

Blood Pressure Classification	SBP mm Hg	DBP mm Hg	Follow-up Recommendations
Normal	<120	and <80	Check again in 2 years
Prehypertension	120–139	or 80–90	Check again in 1 year
Stage 1 hypertension	140–159	or 90–99	Confirm within 2 months
Stage 2 hypertension	>160	or >100	Evaluate within 1 week to 1 month*

From Chobanian A.V., G.L. Bakris, H.R. Black, W.C. Cushman, L.A. Green, et al. The seventh report of the Joint National Committee (JNC) on Prevention, Detection, Evaluation, and Treatment of High Blood Pressure. Hypertension 42:1206–1252, 2003.

*Based on blood pressure level and clinical situation.

DBP = diastolic blood pressure; SBP = systolic blood pressure.

In normotensive individuals, an increase in blood pressure leads to a proportional increase in sodium and water excretion by the kidneys, so that blood volume is reduced and blood pressure returns to its normal "set point." In hypertensive patients, the set point at which blood pressure is controlled is higher than normal; the regulation of blood pressure is defective; and an increase in blood pressure is not followed by a proportional increase in sodium and water excretion by the kidneys. Although studies have shown that PVR is elevated in most hypertensive patients, it is not clear whether this is the cause or the result of hypertension.

Sites and Effects of Antihypertensive Drug Action

The four major categories of antihypertensive drugs are the diuretics, sympatholytics, angiotensin inhibitors, and vasodilators. Subcategories and examples are listed at the beginning of the chapter. The various antihypertensive drugs lower blood pressure through actions exerted on one or more of the following sites: kidneys, sympathetic nervous system, renin-angiotensin-aldosterone axis, or vascular smooth muscle (Fig. 10–1).

Antihypertensive drugs can be characterized in terms of their cardiovascular effects (Table 10–2) and their pharmacologic effects on serum potassium and cholesterol measurements, which are important **cardiovascular risk factors** (Table 10–3). They can also be characterized in terms of the

compensatory mechanisms invoked by their hypotensive effect. The compensatory mechanisms tend to return blood pressure to the pretreatment level and include reflex tachycardia, fluid retention by the kidneys, and activation of the renin-angiotensin-aldosterone axis. Drugs that cause vasodilation tend to invoke compensatory mechanisms to a greater extent than do drugs that suppress cardiac output, cause diuresis, or inhibit angiotensin. For this reason, vasodilators are often combined with other types of drugs (e.g., diuretics) that prevent compensatory responses.

Whereas most antihypertensive drugs are taken orally on a long-term basis, some are administered parenterally for the management of **hypertensive emergencies**. The treatment of this condition is discussed at the end of the chapter.

DIURETICS

Chapter 13 provides detailed information about the various classes of diuretics and their uses, mechanisms of action, and pharmacologic properties. The discussion here focuses on the diuretics most commonly used to treat hypertension: the thiazide and related diuretics, and the potassium-sparing diuretics.

All diuretics cause an increase in renal sodium excretion. This **natriuretic effect**, or **natriuresis**, appears to be responsible for some of their antihypertensive activity. The thiazide

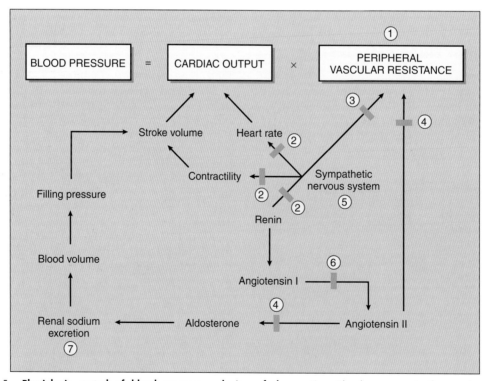

Figure 10–1. Physiologic control of blood pressure and sites of drug action. Blood pressure is the product of cardiac output and PVR. These parameters are regulated on a systemic level by the sympathetic nervous system and the kidneys. Antihypertensive drugs act to suppress excessive sympathetic activity and modify renal function to counteract the mechanisms responsible for hypertension. Sites of action of the following drugs are shown: (1) vasodilators, (2) β-adrenoceptor antagonists (β-blockers), (3) α-adrenoceptor antagonists (α-blockers), (4) angiotensin receptor antagonists, (5) centrally acting sympatholytics, (6) ACE inhibitors, and (7) diuretics. The vasodilators, sympatholytic drugs, and angiotensin inhibitors reduce PVR; β-adrenoceptor blockers reduce cardiac output; and diuretics promote sodium excretion and reduce blood volume. ACE = angiotensin-converting enzyme; PVR = peripheral vascular resistance.

TABLE 10–2.   Cardiovascular Effects of Antihypertensive Drugs

Drug Classification	Peripheral Vascular Resistance	Cardiac Output	Blood Volume	Plasma Renin Activity	Left Ventricular Hypertrophy
Diuretics					
Thiazide and loop diuretics	Decrease	Decrease	Decrease	Increase	No change or decrease
Potassium-sparing diuretics	Decrease	Decrease	Decrease	Increase	No change or decrease
Sympatholytic Drugs					
α-Adrenoceptor antagonists	Decrease	No change or increase	No change or increase	No change or decrease	Decrease
β-Adrenoceptor antagonists	No change or decrease	Decrease	No change or decrease	Decrease	Decrease
Centrally acting drugs	Decrease	No change or decrease	Increase*	Decrease	Decrease
Angiotensin Inhibitors**					
Angiotensin-converting enzyme inhibitors	Decrease	No change or increase	No change	Increase	Decrease
Angiotensin receptor antagonists	Decrease	No change or increase	No change or increase	Increase	Decrease
Vasodilators					
Calcium channel blockers	Decrease	No change or increase†	No change	No change or increase	Decrease
Other vasodilators					
Hydralazine	Decrease	Increase	Increase	Increase	Increase
Minoxidil	Decrease	Increase	Increase	Increase	Increase
Nitroprusside	Decrease	Increase	Increase	Increase	No change or increase
Fenoldopam	Decrease	Increase	No change	Increase	No change

*Two exceptions are guanabenz and guanfacine, which either cause no change in blood volume or decrease it slightly.
**Includes aliskiren, a direct renin inhibitor.
†An exception is verapamil, which may increase or decrease cardiac output.

TABLE 10–3.   Pharmacologic Effects of Antihypertensive Drugs on Serum Potassium and Cholesterol Measurements

Drug Classification	Serum Potassium	Total Cholesterol	Low-Density Lipoproteins	High-Density Lipoproteins	Triglycerides
Diuretics					
Thiazide and loop diuretics	Decrease	Increase	Increase	No change or decrease	Increase
Potassium-sparing diuretics	Increase	Unknown	Unknown	Unknown	Unknown
Sympatholytic Drugs					
α-Adrenoceptor antagonists	No change	Decrease	Decrease	Increase	Decrease
β-Adrenoceptor antagonists	Slight increase	No change or increase	No change or increase	Variable	No change or increase
Centrally acting drugs	No change	No change	No change	No change	No change
Angiotensin Inhibitors**					
Angiotensin-converting enzyme inhibitors	Increase	No change	No change	No change	No change
Angiotensin receptor antagonists	Increase	No change	No change	No change	No change
Vasodilators					
Calcium channel blockers	No change	No change	No change	No change	No change
Other vasodilators					
Hydralazine	No change	No change	No change	No change	No change
Minoxidil	No change	No change	No change	No change	No change
Nitroprusside	No change	Not applicable*	Not applicable*	Not applicable*	Not applicable*
Fencidopam	Decrease	No change	No change	No change	No change

*Nitroprusside is used only for short-term management of hypertension.
**Includes aliskiren, a direct renin inhibitor.

diuretics have a moderate natriuretic effect and are the diuretics used most frequently in the treatment of hypertension. The loop diuretics have the greatest natriuretic effect of all classes of diuretics, but are usually less effective in treating hypertension than are thiazide diuretics. Loop diuretics can be used to treat hypertension when a thiazide diuretic is not effective or is contraindicated. The potassium-sparing diuretics have a relatively low natriuretic effect and are primarily used in combination with a thiazide or loop diuretic to reduce potassium excretion and prevent hypokalemia.

Thiazide and Related Diuretics

Thiazide and related diuretics reduce blood pressure by two mechanisms, both stemming from their ability to increase sodium and water excretion. When they are first administered to a patient, the drugs decrease blood volume and thereby decrease cardiac output (Fig. 10–2 and Table 10–2). With continued administration over weeks and months, they also decrease PVR, and this appears to account for much of their long-term antihypertensive effect. The decreased PVR may result from a reduction in the sodium content of arteriolar smooth muscle cells, which decreases muscle contraction in response to vasopressor agents such as norepinephrine and angiotensin. This relationship is supported by the finding that the effect of a thiazide on PVR is reduced if patients ingest enough dietary sodium to counteract the natriuretic effect of the drug.

Use of a thiazide typically reduces the blood pressure by 10 to 15 mm Hg. **Hydrochlorothiazide** is the thiazide diuretic most often used to treat hypertension. **Indapamide, metolazone**, and other thiazide-like diuretics have equivalent efficacy in the treatment of hypertension and differ primarily in their pharmacokinetic properties. Indapamide can also cause vasodilation via calcium channel blockade.

The JNC 7 report recommends a thiazide diuretic for initial therapy of most patients with high blood pressure. Thiazide diuretics can be used alone or in combination with another type of antihypertensive agent (e.g., a sympatholytic, an angiotensin inhibitor, or a vasodilator). The two drugs usually have an additive effect on blood pressure, and the diuretic prevents the compensatory fluid retention that otherwise can be evoked by the other agent. The JNC 7 report indicates that more than two thirds of patients with hypertension cannot have their condition controlled with a single drug.

The common adverse effects and interactions of thiazide diuretics and other antihypertensive agents are summarized in Table 10–4. The primary disadvantage of thiazide diuretics is their tendency to cause hypokalemia, which can lead to cardiac arrhythmias. Using a low dosage of a thiazide diuretic (e.g., 25–50 mg/day of hydrochlorothiazide) usually produces a maximal antihypertensive effect with minimal hypokalemia. Using a higher dosage causes more hypokalemia but does not have a greater effect on blood pressure. Thiazides elevate plasma levels of glucose, uric acid, and lipids in some patients. Less commonly, they cause hematologic toxicity and aggravate hepatic disease. They can also evoke a compensatory increase in renin secretion, and this reduces their effectiveness in some patients.

An advantage of taking thiazide diuretics is that they appear to offer protection against **osteoporosis**, a condition in which bone demineralization and loss of bone mass make patients more susceptible to fractures. Thiazides are probably beneficial in this condition because they decrease the urinary excretion of calcium.

Loop Diuretics

Despite the greater natriuretic effect of loop diuretics, they are usually less effective than thiazide diuretics in the treatment of hypertensive patients with normal renal function. For this reason, loop diuretics are usually reserved for use in hypertensive patients who have poor renal function and a serum creatinine level greater than 2.3 mg/dL.

Potassium-Sparing Diuretics

Examples of potassium-sparing diuretics are **amiloride, spironolactone**, and **triamterene**. These agents exert a mild natriuretic and antihypertensive effect. They also reduce renal potassium excretion and thereby prevent hypokalemia, a common problem caused by other diuretics.

Several drug products that contain both a thiazide diuretic and amiloride or triamterene are available. Potassium chloride tablets can also be used to prevent and treat hypokalemia.

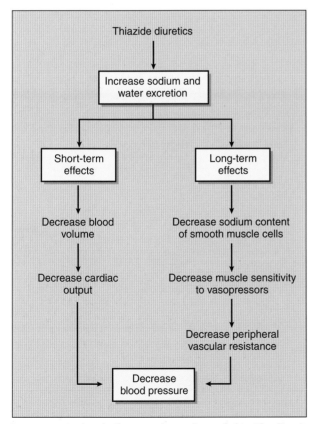

Figure 10–2. Antihypertensive actions of thiazide diuretics. Initially, thiazide diuretics decrease blood volume and thereby decrease cardiac output. Over time, the drugs decrease PVR, an action that may be secondary to a reduction in the sodium content of smooth muscle cells. PVR = peripheral vascular resistance.

TABLE 10-4. Adverse Effects, Contraindications, and Drug Interactions of Antihypertensive Agents

Drug Classification	Common Adverse Effects	Common Drug Interactions
Diuretics		
Thiazide and loop diuretics	Blood cell deficiencies, hyperlipidemia, hyperuricemia, hypokalemia, and other electrolyte changes. Aggravation of diabetes.	Increase serum levels of lithium. Hypotensive effect decreased by NSAIDs and augmented by ACE inhibitors.
Potassium-sparing diuretics	Hyperkalemia.	Hyperkalemic effect increased by ACE inhibitors and potassium supplements.
Sympatholytic Drugs		
α-Adrenoceptor antagonists	Dizziness, first-dose syncope, fluid retention, and orthostatic hypotension.	Hypotensive effect increased by β-adrenoceptor antagonists and diuretics.
β-Adrenoceptor antagonists	Bradycardia, bronchoconstriction, depression, fatigue, impaired glycogenolysis, and vivid dreams.	Cardiac depression increased by diltiazem and verapamil. Hypotensive effect decreased by NSAIDs.
Centrally acting drugs		
Clonidine	Dry mouth, fatigue, rebound hypertension, and sedation.	Hypotensive effect decreased by tricyclic antidepressants. Sedative effect increased by CNS depressants.
Guanabenz	Same as clonidine.	Same as clonidine.
Guanfacine	Same as clonidine but milder.	Same as clonidine.
Methyldopa	Autoimmune hemolytic anemia, hepatitis, and lupuslike syndrome. Other adverse effects same as those of clonidine.	Hypotensive effect increased by levodopa. Other interactions same as those of clonidine.
Angiotensin Inhibitors		
ACE inhibitors	Acute renal failure, angioedema, cough, hyperkalemia, loss of taste, neutropenia, and rash.	Increase serum levels of lithium. Hyperkalemic effect increased by potassium-sparing diuretics and potassium supplements. Hypotensive effect decreased by NSAIDs.
Angiotensin receptor antagonists	Hyperkalemia.	Serum levels of drug increased by cimetidine and decreased by phenobarbital.
Aliskiren	Hyperkalemia	Aliskiren reduces serum levels of furosemide. Cyclosporine increases levels of aliskiren.
Vasodilators		
Calcium channel blockers		
Dihydropyridine drugs*	Dizziness, edema, gingival hyperplasia, headache, and tachycardia.	Serum levels of drug increased by azole antifungal agents, cimetidine, and grapefruit juice.
Diltiazem	Atrioventricular block, bradycardia, constipation, dizziness, edema, gingival hyperplasia, headache, and heart failure.	Increases serum levels of carbamazepine, digoxin, and theophylline. Decreases serum levels of lithium.
Verapamil	Same as diltiazem.	Same as diltiazem.
Other vasodilators		
Hydralazine	Angina, dizziness, fluid retention, headache, lupuslike syndrome, and tachycardia.	Hypotensive effect decreased by NSAIDs.
Minoxidil	Angina, dizziness, fluid retention, headache, hypertrichosis, pericardial effusion, and tachycardia.	Hypotensive effect decreased by NSAIDs.
Nitroprusside	Dizziness, headache, increased intracranial pressure, methemoglobinemia, and thiocyanate/cyanide toxicity.	None.
Fenoldopam	Headache and Navsea.	None identified.

*The dihydropyridine drugs include amlodipine, felodipine, isradipine, nicardipine, and nifedipine.
ACE = angiotensin-converting enzyme; CNS = central nervous system; NSAIDs = nonsteroidal anti-inflammatory drugs.

Eplerenone is similar to spironolactone but has fewer endocrine side effects. Eplerenone has been found to cause regression of left ventricular hypertrophy in hypertensive patients and regression of microalbuminuria in patients with type 2 diabetes. These findings open the possibility of increased use of this drug in persons with these conditions.

SYMPATHOLYTIC DRUGS

The sympatholytic drugs used in the treatment of hypertension include adrenoceptor antagonists and the centrally acting α_2-adrenoceptor agonists. The pharmacologic effects of these drugs are summarized in Tables 10–2 and 10–3 and their common adverse effects and drug interactions are listed in Table 10–4.

Adrenoceptor Antagonists

α-Adrenoceptor Antagonists

Selective α_1-blockers, such as **doxazosin, prazosin**, and **terazosin**, are used in the treatment of hypertension. Although they effectively inhibit sympathetic stimulation of arteriolar contraction, leading to vasodilation and decreased vascular resistance, these drugs have several disadvantages. The α_1-blockers may evoke reflex activation of the sympathetic

nervous system and can increase the heart rate, contractile force, and circulating norepinephrine level. These drugs do not protect the heart against ventricular arrhythmias, and they are usually not employed in patients with ischemic heart disease because they often increase myocardial oxygen requirements. Because they also activate the renin-angiotensin-aldosterone system and can cause fluid retention, they frequently must be given in combination with a diuretic. The α_1-blockers can also cause orthostatic hypotension. For these reasons, α_1-blockers are not preferred drugs for the initial treatment of most patients with high blood pressure.

Selective α_1-blockers produce less reflex tachycardia than do nonselective α_1- and α_2-blockers (e.g., phentolamine and phenoxybenzamine), which are not used in the management of primary hypertension. **Phentolamine and phenoxybenzamine** have been used for short-term management of patients with hypertensive episodes caused by pheochromocytoma (see Chapter 9).

The administration of a selective α_1-blocker and a diuretic may cause first-dose syncope in some patients, but this can be prevented by beginning treatment with a low dose of the blocker at bedtime and withholding the diuretic for 1 day. The pharmacokinetic properties of α-blockers are covered in Chapter 9.

β-Adrenoceptor Antagonists

The β-blockers lower blood pressure by blocking β_1-adrenoceptors in the heart and other tissues. Blockade of cardiac β_1-receptors reduces cardiac output by decreasing the heart rate and contractility. Blockade of β_1-receptors in renal juxtaglomerular cells inhibits renin secretion which, in turn, reduces the formation of angiotensin II and the subsequent release of aldosterone. The drugs also appear to reduce sympathetic outflow from the central nervous system. Hence, β-blockers have multiple actions affecting blood pressure.

Numerous clinical trials have shown that β-blockers lower blood pressure in most patients with hypertension. The β-blockers also benefit persons with other cardiovascular conditions. In persons with **coronary heart disease**, β-blockers reduce myocardial ischemia and lower the risk of myocardial infarction (see Chapter 11). The β-blockers are cardioprotective and prevent sudden death in persons who have had a **myocardial infarction**. In persons with **heart failure**, β-blockers improve symptoms and survival (see Chapter 12). Hence, the benefits of using β-blockers to treat hypertension in patients with preexisting heart disease are substantial.

The role of β-blockers in treating hypertension in persons without preexisting cardiovascular disease is controversial. Recent meta-analyses of clinical trial data suggest that β-blockers such as atenolol are less likely to prevent stroke, myocardial infarction, and death in patients without coronary heart disease in comparison with the calcium-channel blockers, renin-angiotensin system inhibitors, and diuretics. Hence, some experts have suggested that β-blockers should not be used alone for the initial treatment of most hypertensive patients. In 2006, the U.K. National Institute for Health and Clinical Excellence published a clinical guideline in which β-blockers are no longer preferred as the initial therapy for hypertension and instead recommended a diuretic, angiotensin system inhibitor, or calcium channel blocker (CCB) for the initial treatment of most hypertensive patients. Many

patients with hypertension require more than one drug to control blood pressure without causing adverse effects, and the β-blockers can be combined with other drugs to achieve greater reductions in blood pressure. These drugs only rarely cause orthostatic hypotension or produce hepatic, renal, or hematopoietic toxicity. Analysis of pooled data from clinical trials suggests that β-blockers are only slightly more likely than a placebo to cause fatigue, sleep disturbances, and sexual dysfunction in persons receiving the drugs for hypertension.

Nonselective β-blockers are contraindicated in persons with asthma or chronic obstructive pulmonary disease because these drugs may cause bronchospasm due to β_2-blockade. Selective β_1-blockers may be used cautiously in these patients if a β-blocker is required. Beta blockers may improve cardiovascular outcomes in diabetic patients, but this comes at the price of slightly impaired glycemic control due to decreased insulin sensitivity. Not all β-blockers are alike in this regard, and third-generation β-blockers such as carvedilol may actually improve insulin sensitivity. Nonselective β-blockers may delay recovery from hypoglycemia by blocking β_2-receptor mediated glycogenolysis and hepatic glucose production. Hence, selective β_1-blockers are usually preferred for treating hypertension in diabetic patients.

Chapter 9 compares the pharmacologic properties of selective β_1-blockers (e.g., **atenolol, bisoprolol,** and **metoprolol**) with those of nonselective β-blockers (e.g., **nadolol, propranolol,** and **timolol**) and drugs that block both α and β receptors (**carvedilol** and **labetalol**). Atenolol is less lipophilic than other β-blockers and may cause fewer central nervous system side effects than more lipophilic drugs such as propranolol. **Labetalol** is used to treat both chronic hypertension and hypertensive emergencies. Because of its α-adrenoceptor-blocking activity, it can cause orthostatic hypotension. **Esmolol** is an intravenously administered, ultrashort-acting β_1-blocker that is used to treat hypertension in surgical patients and in persons with hypertensive emergencies. **Carvedilol** is a third-generation α- and β-blocker with antioxidant properties that can protect the vascular wall from free radicals that damage blood vessels and thereby contribute to the progression of cardiovascular disease. **Nebivolol** is a new third-generation drug undergoing clinical trials. This selective β_1-blocker with antioxidant properties also increases the release of endothelial **nitric oxide** and thereby exerts a vasodilating effect that contributes to the blood pressure-lowering effect of this drug. Nebivolol provides another option for treating hypertension in patients with heart failure, diabetes, and cardiac arrhythmias.

Centrally Acting Drugs

The centrally acting sympatholytic drugs include **clonidine, guanabenz, guanfacine,** and **methyldopa**. These drugs cause more side effects than many other antihypertensive drugs and are not recommended for the initial treatment of most patients with high blood pressure. They are primarily used when other drugs are ineffective or for the treatment of hypertensive emergencies. The centrally acting drugs are α_2-adrenoceptor agonists that reduce sympathetic outflow from the brain stem to the heart, blood vessels, and other tissues. These drugs also activate a class of receptors in the ventrolateral medulla known as **imidazoline receptors**, which appear to be partly responsible

for their antihypertensive action. They lower the blood pressure primarily by causing a reduction in PVR while the heart rate and cardiac output are either reduced or remain unchanged. Because tricyclic antidepressant drugs can block the effects of centrally acting sympatholytic drugs, the two classes of drugs should not be used concurrently.

Sedation, dry mouth, and other central nervous system side effects of centrally acting sympatholytics can be problematic in hypertensive patients whose work requires mental alertness, as well as in those who are elderly or have neurologic diseases. Because severe **rebound hypertension** can occur if clonidine and related drugs are discontinued abruptly, the dosage should be tapered gradually over 1 to 2 weeks if treatment is to be stopped.

Methyldopa is similar to clonidine in its actions and effects. Unlike clonidine and other centrally acting drugs, however, methyldopa is accumulated by central noradrenergic neurons and is converted to an active metabolite, methyl-norepinephrine. Methyldopa is well known for its ability to cause immunologic effects, including a Coombs-positive **hemolytic anemia** (reported in up to 2% of patients), autoimmune hepatitis, and other organ dysfunction. Methyldopa has been used to treat hypertension in pregnant women, because extensive experience has shown that it does not harm the fetus.

ANGIOTENSIN INHIBITORS

The angiotensin system inhibitors include the angiotensin-converting enzyme (ACE) inhibitors, the angiotensin receptor blockers (ARBs), and a direct renin inhibitor called aliskiren. The ACE inhibitors and ARBs are effective and well tolerated and are among the drugs indicated for the initial treatment of high blood pressure in most hypertensive patients. ACE inhibitors and ARBs have been shown to reduce the risk of stroke, and they are particularly useful in persons with diabetes or heart failure. The pharmacologic properties of these drugs are summarized in Tables 10–2

and 10–3, and their adverse effects and drug interactions are listed in Table 10–4.

Angiotensin-Converting Enzyme Inhibitors

Drug Properties

CHEMISTRY AND PHARMACOKINETICS. Molecular techniques were used to model the active site of ACE and design drugs that inhibit ACE by binding the zinc atom at the active site. The various ACE inhibitors have essentially identical mechanisms of action and pharmacologic effects, but they differ in their pharmacokinetic properties (Table 10–5). They undergo varying degrees of first-pass hepatic inactivation after oral administration, and several of the ACE inhibitors have active metabolites. Except for captopril, the duration of action of most ACE inhibitors is about 24 hours, and the drugs are administered once or twice daily to treat hypertension and other disorders.

MECHANISMS AND PHARMACOLOGIC EFFECTS. The actions of ACE inhibitors and other drugs affecting the renin-angiotensin-aldosterone axis are shown in Figure 10–3. Three primary stimuli to renin secretion exist: (1) a reduction in arterial pressure in renal afferent arterioles, (2) a fall in sodium chloride concentration in the distal renal tubule, and (3) sympathetic nervous system activation of β_1-adrenoceptors on renal juxtaglomerular cells.

When blood pressure falls and renin is released, this initiates a cascade of events that normally return blood pressure to the preexisting level. In the circulation, renin acts as a protease that converts circulating angiotensinogen to angiotensin I. ACE, a protease primarily located in the pulmonary vasculature, then converts the physiologically inactive angiotensin I to the active angiotensin II. Angiotensin II activates two types of **angiotensin receptors**, called AT_1 and AT_2. The AT_1 receptors are coupled with enzymes that increase the formation of inositol triphosphate and various arachidonic acid

TABLE 10-5. Pharmacokinetic Properties of Selected Angiotensin Inhibitors				
Drug	**Oral Bioavailability**	**Absorption Reduced by Food**	**Active Metabolite**	**Duration of Action (Hours)**
Angiotensin-Converting Enzyme Inhibitors				
Benazepril	37%	No	Benazeprilat	24
Captopril	75%	30%–40%	None	6–12
Enalapril	60%	No	Enalaprilat*	24
Fosinopril	36%	No	Fosinoprilat	24
Lisinopril	25%	No	None	24
Quinapril	60%	25%–30%	Quinaprilat	24
Ramipril	55%	No	Ramiprilat	24
Angiotensin Receptor Antagonists				
Condesartan	15%	No	None	24
Losartan	33%	10%	Carboxylic acid metabolite	24
Valsartan	25%	40%	None	24
Direct Renin Inhibitor				
Aliskiren	2.5%	Yes (high fat)	None	24

*Enalaprilat is available as a separate drug for intravenous administration.

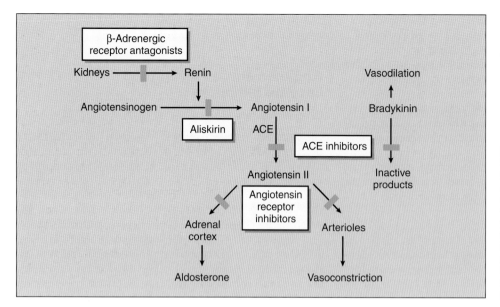

Figure 10-3. Actions of antihypertensive drugs on the renin-angiotensin-aldosterone axis. β-Adrenoceptor antagonists inhibit sympathetic stimulation of renin secretion. ACE inhibitors block the formation of angiotensin II and inhibit the breakdown of bradykinin, a vasodilator. Angiotensin receptor antagonists (e.g., losartan) block AT₁ receptors in smooth muscle and adrenal cortex. ACE = angiotensin-converting enzyme.

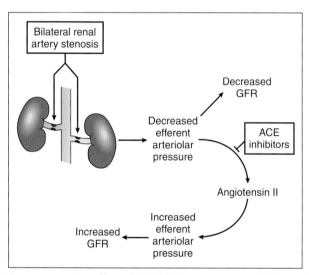

Figure 10-4. Effects of ACE inhibitors in patients with bilateral renal artery stenosis. Renal blood flow is reduced in the presence of bilateral renal artery stenosis. In affected patients, glomerular filtration is maintained by elevating efferent arteriolar pressure via vasoconstriction produced by angiotensin II. By blocking the formation of angiotensin II, ACE inhibitors can severely impair glomerular filtration and lead to renal failure. ACE = angiotensin-converting enzyme; GFR = glomerular filtration rate.

metabolites and decrease the formation of cyclic adenosine monophosphate. The effects resulting from activation of AT₁ receptors include (1) contraction of vascular smooth muscle leading to generalized vasoconstriction, (2) secretion of aldosterone from the adrenal cortex, (3) increased reabsorption of sodium from the proximal tubule, (4) increased release of norepinephrine from sympathetic nerves, and (5) stimulation of cell growth in the arteries and heart. The functional significance of AT₂ receptors has not been fully elucidated.

In the normal chain of events, ACE converts angiotensin I to angiotensin II and also catalyzes the inactivation of **bradykinin**, an endogenous vasodilator peptide. Drugs that inhibit ACE therefore exert hypotensive effects by blocking the

formation of a vasoconstrictor (angiotensin II) and the degradation of a vasodilator (bradykinin). Increased renal prostaglandin synthesis may also contribute to the hypotensive effects of these drugs. Some studies have found that angiotensin II levels can return toward pretreatment levels during long-term ACE inhibitor therapy, even though the blood pressure remains under control. This suggests that the effects on bradykinin and prostaglandins may be an important component of the antihypertensive action of these drugs.

The antihypertensive action of ACE inhibitors is primarily caused by a reduction in PVR, with little or no change in cardiac output or blood volume (see Table 10-2). ACE inhibitors decrease both arterial pressure and venous pressure, and this in turn reduces cardiac afterload and cardiac preload, respectively. By reducing angiotensin-stimulated aldosterone secretion, ACE inhibitors prevent the compensatory increase in sodium retention and plasma volume that can occur with some other antihypertensive drugs. In patients treated with ACE inhibitors, renal sodium retention is decreased, renal potassium retention is increased, and serum potassium levels typically increase by about 0.5 mEq/L.

ADVERSE EFFECTS. ACE inhibitors can cause fetal and neonatal injury and death when administered to pregnant women, especially during the second and third trimesters. Therefore, use of these drugs should be discontinued when pregnancy is detected. ACE inhibitors can also cause renal failure in patients who have a rare condition known as **bilateral renal artery stenosis**, because these persons depend on angiotensin II to maintain renal blood flow and glomerular filtration, as illustrated in Figure 10-4.

The ACE inhibitors are usually well tolerated and do not adversely affect the lifestyle of most hypertensive patients. The most common side effect is a **dry cough** that is probably caused by increased bradykinin levels. Less commonly, bradykinin accumulation may contribute to the development of **angioedema**, manifested as painful swelling of the lips, face, and throat. Rash and an **abnormal taste sensation** occur mostly in persons receiving captopril, which has a sulfhydryl group as the zinc-binding moiety. The presence of sulfhydryl groups in other drugs has been associated with these side effects.

INTERACTIONS. The antihypertensive action of ACE inhibitors is augmented by diuretics, and several combination products containing an ACE inhibitor and a thiazide diuretic are available. ACE inhibitors can interact with potassium-sparing diuretics and potassium supplements to increase serum potassium levels and cause hyperkalemia. They can also increase serum lithium levels and provoke lithium toxicity in patients receiving lithium compounds for the treatment of bipolar disorder. Nonsteroidal anti-inflammatory drugs, such as ibuprofen, can impede the effects of ACE inhibitors and other antihypertensive agents.

INDICATIONS. Because they have excellent antihypertensive action and few bothersome side effects, ACE inhibitors are used in the management of mild to severe hypertension in patients with a wide variety of traits and concomitant diseases, as outlined in Table 10–6. The drugs are of particular value in treating hypertensive patients with coexisting heart failure, myocardial infarction, chronic kidney disease, or diabetes mellitus.

Studies have shown that ACE inhibitors increase cardiac output and survival in patients with **heart** failure

TABLE 10–6. Selection of Antihypertensive Drugs for Patients with Specific Traits or Concurrent Diseases

Patient Characteristic	Most Preferred Drugs	Least Preferred Drugs
Age over 65 years	Diuretic, ACEI, CCB	Centrally acting α₂-agonist
African heritage	Diuretic (± ACEI, ARB), CCB	β-Blocker
Pregnant	Methyldopa, labetalol	ACEI, ARB, aliskiren
Angina pectoris	β-Blocker, CCB	Hydralazine, minoxidil
Myocardial infarction	β-Blocker, ACEI, ARB, aldosterone antagonist	
Congestive heart failure	ACEI, ARB, β-blocker, diuretic	
Stroke prevention	Diuretic + ACEI or ARB	
Kidney disease	ACEI or ARB (± verapamil or diltiazem)	
Diabetes	ACEI or ARB (± β-blocker, diuretic, or CCB)	
Asthma	CCB, ACEI, or ARB	β-Blocker
Benign prostatic hyperplasia	α-Blocker	
Migraine headache	β-Blocker, CCB	
Osteoporosis	Diuretic	

α-Blocker = α-adrenoceptor blocker; ACEI = angiotensin converting enzyme inhibitor; ARB = angiotensin receptor blocker; β-Blocker = β-adrenoceptor blocker; CCB = calcium channel blocker; diuretic = thiazide diuretic.

(see Chapter 12). These agents also reduce the incidence of overt heart failure and increase survival in persons with a myocardial infarction and significant left ventricular dysfunction (a cardiac ejection fraction of less than 40%). The ejection fraction is the percentage of blood that is ejected from the left ventricle during each systole.

In **diabetic patients** who exhibit early signs of renal impairment (e.g., albuminuria and increased serum creatinine levels), ACE inhibitors exert a renoprotective effect. Studies indicate that the ACE inhibitor **enalapril** reduces the progression of these harbingers of renal failure and the subsequent need for renal dialysis in these patients. Moreover, if enalapril is withdrawn from treatment, the progression of nephropathy resumes quickly. Based on these findings, experts now recommend that ACE inhibitor therapy be considered for diabetic patients with albuminuria or increased serum creatinine levels, regardless of whether they have hypertension.

Blood pressure is the most important determinant of the risk of **stroke**, and ACE inhibitors are among the agents that reduce the incidence of both primary and secondary stroke. The renin-angiotensin system appears to be involved in the development and progression of cerebrovascular disease, and some clinical trials suggest that ACE inhibitors and ARBs have a cerebroprotective effect beyond their blood pressure lowering ability.

Specific Drugs

Three classes of ACE inhibitors have been developed. In each class, a different chemical group binds the zinc ion in ACE. The only sulfhydryl compound is **captopril**; the phosphoryl agents include **fosinopril**; and the carboxyl derivatives include **benazepril, enalapril, lisinopril, quinapril**, and **ramipril**. All of these drugs, except captopril and lisinopril, are enzymatically transformed to active metabolites. **Enalaprilat**, the active metabolite of enalapril, is available for intravenous administration; the other ACE inhibitors are administered orally.

The orally administered ACE inhibitors undergo considerable first-pass inactivation, and their oral bioavailability ranges from 25% to 75% (see Table 10–5). In comparison with other ACE inhibitors, which are administered one or two times a day, captopril has a shorter half-life and must be administered two or three times a day.

Angiotensin Receptor Blockers

A more recent approach to angiotensin inhibition has been the development of ARBs. These drugs selectively block AT_1 receptors in various tissues and thereby reduce vasoconstriction, aldosterone secretion, sodium reabsorption by the proximal tubule, and norepinephrine release from sympathetic nerve terminals. ARBs are often effective when used alone, and they can be combined with a diuretic or other antihypertensive agent when greater blood pressure reduction is needed. Some studies show a benefit of combining an ACE inhibitor with an ARB in high-risk patients with diabetic nephropathy and other conditions.

Many orally effective ARBs are now available, including **candesartan, irbesartan, losartan, valsartan**, and others. In the treatment of hypertension, these drugs are as effective as the ACE inhibitors but only rarely cause the dry cough that occurs with ACE inhibitors. Recent clinical trials have found that the ARBs can reduce the risk of the cardiovascular consequences of hypertension. In these studies, losartan produced a greater reduction of **left ventricular hypertrophy** and the risk of **stroke** and new-onset **diabetes** than did atenolol, despite having similar blood pressure lowering effects. With regard to diabetes, ARBs such as **telmisartan** have been shown to increase insulin sensitivity by activating the peroxisome proliferator-activated receptor-gamma (see Chapter 35).

The ARBs do not increase serum glucose, uric acid, or cholesterol levels, but may cause **hyperkalemia**, neutropenia, and elevated serum levels of hepatic aminotransferase enzymes. As with the ACE inhibitors, the ARBs can cause **fetal injury and death** and should not be used during pregnancy.

Direct Renin Inhibitor

Aliskiren is the first orally effective direct renin inhibitor to be approved for treatment of hypertension. It binds to the active site of renin, preventing cleavage of angiotensinogen and formation of angiotensin I. Thus, aliskiren lowers **plasma renin activity** and levels of angiotensin I and angiotensin II. It has equal or superior blood pressure-lowering ability compared to other drugs and a placebo-like side effect profile. While the role of aliskiren in treating high blood pressure is still being defined, it may become a valuable adjunct to other drugs and thereby help patients achieve their blood pressure goals.

VASODILATORS

The vasodilators include the CCBs and other agents such as hydralazine, minoxidil, and nitroprusside. The pharmacologic effects, adverse effects, and drug interactions of these agents are summarized in Tables 10–2, 10–3, and 10–4.

Calcium Channel Blockers

CCBs are used to treat hypertension, angina pectoris, peripheral vascular disorders, and cardiac arrhythmias. Chapter 11 discusses the pharmacologic properties of these drugs in detail, while this chapter focuses on their antihypertensive actions.

By blocking calcium ion channels in the plasma membranes of smooth muscle, the CCBs relax vascular smooth muscle and cause vasodilation. CCBs have a greater effect on arteriolar smooth muscle than on venous smooth muscle, and their effect on blood pressure is primarily caused by a reduction in PVR, with relatively little impact on venous capacitance, cardiac filling pressure, and cardiac output. Some studies indicate that CCBs have a natriuretic effect that may contribute to their ability to lower blood pressure.

Whereas all of the CCBs relax vascular smooth muscle, **diltiazem** and **verapamil** also have significant effects on cardiac tissue and can reduce the heart rate and cardiac output. Most CCBs, including **amlodipine, felodipine, isradipine, nicardipine**, and **nifedipine**, belong to the dihydropyridine class. The dihydropyridines have little direct effect on cardiac tissue at usual therapeutic levels; however, they can evoke reflex tachycardia.

The CCBs are among the most widely recommended drugs for the initial treatment of high blood pressure, and they are often combined with diuretics or angiotensin system inhibitors. CCBs protect against stroke, coronary heart disease, and kidney disease. In fact, verapamil and diltiazem reduce protein excretion in patients with kidney disease and may be used with an ACE inhibitor or ARB for this purpose. The CCBs are relatively free of adverse effects and do not alter levels of serum glucose, lipids, uric acid, or electrolytes. They are particularly useful in treating hypertensive patients who have asthma or are of African heritage (see Table 10–6). Because of the need to obtain 24-hour blood pressure control in hypertensive patients, a long-acting CCB such as amlodipine or a sustained-release formulation such as the nifedipine gastrointestinal system should be employed.

Other Vasodilators

Hydralazine and Minoxidil

Hydralazine and minoxidil are orally effective vasodilators primarily used in combination with other antihypertensive drugs to treat moderate to very severe hypertension. When used alone, they often evoke reflex tachycardia and cause fluid retention, and they can precipitate angina in susceptible patients. To prevent these problems, hydralazine or minoxidil is usually given in combination with two other drugs: a diuretic plus either a β-adrenoceptor antagonist or another sympatholytic agent. Hydralazine has been associated with a **lupus-like syndrome**, whereas minoxidil can cause hypertrichosis (excessive hair growth), particularly in women. In fact, minoxidil has been marketed as a topical formulation for the treatment of several forms of **alopecia** (baldness) in men and women.

Nitroprusside

Sodium nitroprusside is one of several drugs used in the management of hypertensive emergencies. The drug is administered by intravenous infusion and has a short half-life. Nitroprusside is rapidly metabolized to cyanide in erythrocytes and other tissues. Cyanide is then converted to thiocyanate in the presence of a sulfur donor. Both thiocyanate and cyanide gradually accumulate during nitroprusside infusion. For this reason, the duration of therapy with this drug is usually limited to a few days. During drug administration, the patient's blood pressure should be monitored frequently, and thiocyanate levels should be checked every 72 hours to detect potential toxicity.

Fenoldopam

Fenoldopam represents a novel class of antihypertensive drugs. It is an agonist at dopamine D_1-like receptors, with moderate affinity for α_2-adrenoceptors. Fenoldopam is a rapid acting, intravenously administered drug used to treat hypertensive emergencies (see below). It causes arteriolar vasodilation in systemic vascular beds, including coronary, renal, and mesenteric vessels. In the kidney, fenoldopam dilates both afferent and efferent arterioles, thereby increasing renal blood flow. The drug is rapidly converted to inactive glucuronide and other conjugates and has a short half-life of about 5 minutes. Fenoldopam can reduce serum potassium levels, which should be monitored at 6-hour intervals during drug infusion.

THE MANAGEMENT OF HYPERTENSION

Lifestyle Modifications

Patients with hypertension should be encouraged to pursue lifestyle changes that will improve their general health and can substantially lower their blood pressure. Effective strategies include exercise and weight loss, reduction of alcohol intake, and institution of a diet that is low in sodium and provides an adequate intake of potassium, calcium, and magnesium. Patients should be encouraged to consume a diet rich in fruits and vegetables and low in saturated and total fat. Unless hypertension is severe, patients should be encouraged to try lifestyle modifications for several months before instituting drug therapy.

Single- and Multiple-Drug Therapy

Recent guidelines for the treatment of high blood pressure recommend using a **thiazide diuretic** for the initial therapy of most patients without comorbid diseases (Box 10–1). This recommendation is based on the ability of thiazide diuretics to prevent complications of hypertension, including stroke and coronary artery disease, as well as the synergistic effect of diuretics with other antihypertensive medications. Numerous clinical trials have shown that thiazide diuretics are effective and relatively safe when serum potassium, glucose, uric acid, and lipid levels are monitored appropriately. In addition, thiazides are among the least expensive agents available for treating hypertension.

Other drug classes that can be considered for the initial treatment of hypertension include (1) **angiotensin converting enzyme inhibitors**, (2) **ARBs**, and (3) **CCBs.** Selection of one of these drugs is recommended for initial therapy when a thiazide diuretic cannot be used or when a **comorbid condition** is present that requires the use of a specific drug, such as kidney or cerebrovascular disease (see Table 10–6). β-**Blockers** should be reserved for the initial treatment of patients with coronary heart disease (angina and myocardial infarction), heart failure, and certain cardiac arrhythmias.

Most patients with high blood pressure will require more than one drug to achieve target blood pressure levels. A number of **combination drug products** are now available to treat hypertension, most of which can be taken once or twice daily. These products are usually less expensive and more convenient to use than two single drug products, and they enhance patient compliance with the treatment regimen. Studies have found that the initiation of therapy with more than one drug increases the likelihood of achieving a desired blood pressure in a timely manner. Moreover, drug combinations often achieve blood pressure reduction with lower doses of the component drugs, thereby causing fewer adverse effects. Unless intolerable side effects occur or hypertension is severe, drugs should be given a trial of several weeks before evaluating their effectiveness or changing medications.

BOX 10–1 A CASE OF INCREASING BLOOD PRESSURE AND PROTEINURIA

CASE PRESENTATION: An overweight 56-year-old African American woman with an 8-year history of type 2 diabetes and a 5-year history of hypertension has been seen regularly by her health care providers. Her diabetes has been treated with dietary restrictions and metformin, though her target glycosylated hemoglobin A1c level (<7%) has not been achieved. Her blood pressure was initially controlled with a thiazide diuretic. Over the past 2 years, her blood pressure readings have increased and now average 138/86 mm Hg. Her latest test results showed microalbuminuria (proteinuria) of 50 µg/min over 24 hours. Lisinopril and glipizide were added to her treatment regimen, and she was scheduled to see a dietitian and exercise counselor.

CASE DISCUSSION: The prevalence of both type 2 diabetes and hypertension is higher in blacks than in other populations, and both diseases increase the risk of proteinuria and chronic kidney disease. A greater proportion of black hypertensive patients exhibit microalbuminuria (>30 µg/min) compared to white patients. For these reasons, it is important that patients achieve target A1c and blood pressure levels (<130/80 mm Hg) in order to slow the progression of kidney disease. Several types of drugs can be combined with metformin to help the woman control blood glucose and A1c levels, including glipizide and pioglitazone (see Chapter 35). The addition of lisinopril to her treatment regimen is aimed at achieving the target blood pressure level and at slowing progression of nephropathy. Although diuretics and CCBs are often preferred for the initial treatment of black hypertensive patients, angiotensin system inhibitors such as lisinopril are effective in black patients when combined with a diuretic. Lifestyle changes can help the patient achieve target A1c and blood pressure levels while controlling body weight.

Patients with Specific Traits or Diseases

Table 10–6 summarizes the most preferred and least preferred drugs for hypertensive patients with specific traits or concurrent diseases. These recommendations are only guidelines and individual patient characteristics should always been considered when selecting drug therapy.

In hypertensive patients over 65 years of age, the use of a thiazide diuretic, an ACE inhibitor, or a dihydropyridine

CCB may be preferred for initial therapy. In some patients over 70 years of age, β-blockers may reduce cardiac output too much. The cardioprotective effect of β-blockers, however, may still justify their use in this population if they are tolerated. In elderly black patients, β-blockers are often less effective than diuretics, so a diuretic or CCB should be used, with or without an angiotensin inhibitor.

Most patients with **ischemic heart disease**, including those with **angina pectoris** or **myocardial infarction**, should be treated with a β-blocker as well as an ACE inhibitor or ARB unless they are contraindicated. The β-blockers protect against sudden death in these patients.

For patients with **diabetes mellitus**, the JNC 7 report recommends that blood pressure be controlled to the level of 130/80 mm Hg or lower (see Box 10–1). This is because rigorous control of blood pressure is essential for reducing the progression of **diabetic nephropathy** to end-stage renal disease. Clinical trials show that ACE inhibitors, ARBs, β-blockers, and calcium antagonists have demonstrated benefits in both type 1 and type 2 diabetics. Thiazide diuretics are also beneficial in diabetics. The Antihypertensive and Lipid-Lowering Treatment to Prevent Heart Attack Trial found that thiazides reduced the incidence of fatal coronary artery disease and myocardial infarction to the same extent as an ACE inhibitor or calcium antagonist. Although diuretics can aggravate hyperglycemia, the effect is slight and easily managed in most patients.

The ACE inhibitors and ARBs are important components of antihypertensive regimens for diabetic patients because of their ability to reduce the progression of diabetic nephropathy. β-Adrenoceptor blockers are also beneficial in diabetic patients as part of multidrug therapy, particularly in patients who also have coronary heart disease. Although β-blockers can mask symptoms of hypoglycemia and slow recovery from hypoglycemia by blocking glycogenolysis, these problems are usually managed easily and are not absolute contraindications for β-blocker use in patients with diabetes.

In patients with **asthma**, treatment with β-blockers should be avoided, because these agents can cause bronchoconstriction. Use of a CCB or ACE inhibitor is usually preferred. CCBs can relax bronchial smooth muscle and thereby reduce bronchoconstriction in patients with asthma.

Hypertensive Emergencies and Urgencies

Hypertensive emergencies are characterized by severe elevations in blood pressure (>180/120 mm Hg) complicated by target organ dysfunction (e.g., encephalopathy or intracranial hemorrhage). These situations require immediate reduction in blood pressure to limit target organ damage. **Hypertensive urgencies** are situations with severe elevations of blood pressure without target organ dysfunction, such as with persons who have upper levels of stage 2 hypertension associated with severe headache, shortness of breath, or severe anxiety.

The initial goal of treatment of hypertensive emergencies is to reduce blood pressure by no more than 25% within minutes to 1 hour, and then to 160/100 mm Hg within the next 2 to 6 hours. If this level of blood pressure is well tolerated, gradual reductions to normal blood pressure can be implemented in the next 24 to 48 hours. Excessive reductions in blood pressure can precipitate renal, cerebral, or coronary ischemia and should be avoided. For this reason, short-acting nifedipine is no longer an acceptable treatment for hypertensive emergencies or urgencies.

A number of drugs can be used to treat hypertensive emergencies and urgencies. Parenterally administered drugs are usually used, although oral **clonidine** can be used for less severe hypertensive urgencies because it slowly reduces blood pressure to a safe level. The drugs most often used in treating most types of hypertensive emergencies include **fenoldopam, nicardipine, labetalol,** and **sodium nitroprusside. Hydralazine** has been used for hypertension associated with **eclampsia** of pregnancy. **Nitroglycerin** is used for hypertensive emergencies in persons with **acute coronary ischemia**, and **enalaprilat** may be of value in patients with acute **left ventricular failure** (but not acute myocardial infarction). **Esmolol** is useful in persons with **aortic dissection** and **perioperative hypertension**.

SUMMARY OF IMPORTANT POINTS

■ The four major classes of antihypertensive drugs are the diuretics, sympatholytic drugs, angiotensin inhibitors, and vasodilators.

■ Thiazide diuretics initially reduce blood volume and cardiac output, but their long-term effect on blood pressure is primarily caused by decreased PVR.

■ Sympatholytic drugs used in the treatment of hypertension include α-adrenoceptor antagonists, β-adrenoceptor antagonists, and centrally acting drugs. Except for the β-blockers, which reduce cardiac output, the sympatholytics reduce blood pressure primarily by decreasing PVR.

■ The two types of angiotensin inhibitors are the ACE inhibitors (e.g., lisinopril) and the ARBs (e.g., losartan). These drugs reduce PVR and aldosterone levels, with little effect on blood volume or cardiac output in patients who do not have heart failure.

■ The vasodilators include the CCBs, hydralazine, minoxidil, and nitroprusside. These drugs reduce PVR, and some of them provoke reflex tachycardia and fluid retention.

■ The management of high blood pressure begins with lifestyle modifications and then proceeds to the use of a diuretic, angiotensin system inhibitor, or CCB for patients without comorbid conditions. Patients with heart disease often benefit from use of a β-blocker and an angiotensin system inhibitor. Angiotensin system inhibitors are particularly useful in preventing kidney disease. ARBs appear to protect against stroke more than other drugs.

Review Questions

1. A man complains of tender and swollen gums during an appointment with his dentist. He has a history of poor dental hygiene and his exam shows extensive dental plaque. Which drug is most likely the cause of his distress?
   (A) irbesartan
   (B) metoprolol
   (C) nifedipine
   (D) hydrochlorothiazide
   (E) doxazosin

2. While away on a business trip, a salesman ingested his medication with grapefruit juice and then promptly fainted upon arising from the breakfast table. Which medication was he most likely taking?
   (A) clonidine
   (B) atenolol
   (C) enalapril
   (D) hydrochlorothiazide
   (E) felodipine

3. A man with a history of poor compliance with prescribed diuretic therapy suffers a mild stroke and is evaluated for follow-up therapy. He does not have diabetes, coronary heart disease, lung disease, or kidney disease. Which antihypertensive agent has the greatest ability to decrease the risk of another stroke in this patient?
   (A) atenolol
   (B) irbesartan
   (C) doxazosin
   (D) verapamil
   (E) hydralazine

4. A man is diagnosed with type 2 diabetes, coronary heart disease and hypertension. Which drug may increase insulin sensitivity and also reduce the risk of myocardial infarction and death in this patient?
   (A) carvedilol
   (B) amlodipine
   (C) propranolol
   (D) hydrochlorothiazide
   (E) doxazosin

Answers and Explanations

1. **The answer is C: nifedipine.** CCBs, particularly nifedipine, have been associated with gingival overgrowth or hyperplasia, which occurs in about 10% to 20% of persons taking these drugs. Poor dental hygiene is a strong risk factor for this condition in persons taking CCBs, and good hygiene can often relieve the condition in these patients. Other drugs associated with this condition include cyclosporine and phenytoin. None of the other options are typically responsible for gingival overgrowth.

2. **The answer is E: felodipine.** Felodipine and other dihydropyridine CCBs are metabolized to inactive compounds by cytochrome P450 3A4 in the gut and liver. Inhibitors of this enzyme, including compounds in grapefruit juice, may elevate the serum level and hypotensive effects of these drugs, leading to postural hypotension and syncope. None of the other options are significantly inactivated by cytochrome P450 3A4.

3. **The answer is B: irbesartan.** The most important factor in stroke prevention is to control blood pressure to target levels, and all commonly used antihypertensive agents lower the incidence of stroke. However, ARBs such as irbesartan have been shown to reduce the risk of cerebrovascular disease beyond their blood pressure lowering effect, and appear to be the best agents to prevent stroke at this time. ACE inhibitors may also reduce the risk of stroke beyond their ability to lower blood pressure, but the evidence is less compelling than for ARBs.

4. **The answer is A: carvedilol.** Carvedilol is a third-generation β-blocker. Unlike nonselective β-blockers such as propranolol (Option C), carvedilol does not decrease insulin sensitivity and may actually improve it. Thiazide diuretics such as hydrochlorothiazide (Option D) also cause a small decrease in insulin sensitivity. Amlodipine and doxazosin (Options B and E) do not usually affect insulin sensitivity.

SELECTED READINGS

Chobanian, A.V., G.L. Bakris, H.R. Black, W.C. Cushman, L.A. Green, et al. The seventh report of the Joint National Committee (JNC) on Prevention, Detection, Evaluation, and Treatment of High Blood Pressure. Hypertension 42:1206–1252, 2003.

Dahlöf, B. Prevention of stroke in patients with hypertension. Am J Cardiol 100:17J–24J, 2007.

Epstein, B.J., K. Vogel, and B.F. Palmer. Dihydropyridine calcium channel antagonists in the management of hypertension. Drugs 67:1309–1327, 2007.

Oh, B.H. Aliskiren, the first in a new class of direct renin inhibitors for hypertension: present and future perspectives. Expert Opin Pharmacother 8:2839–2849, 2007.

Tocci, G., S. Sciarretta, C. Facciolo, and M. Volepe. Antihypertensive strategy based on angiotensin II receptor blockers: a new gateway to reduce risk in hypertension. Expert Rev Cardiovascular Ther 5:767–776, 2007.

CHAPTER 11

Antianginal Drugs

CLASSIFICATION OF ANTIANGINAL DRUGS

Vasodilators
Organic nitrites and nitrates
- Amyl Nitrite
- Isosorbide Dinitrate
- Isosorbide Mononitrate
- Nitroglycerin

Calcium channel blockers
- Amlodipine (NORVASC)*
- Nifedipine (PROCARDIA)
- Bepridil (VASCOR)
- Diltiazem (CARDIZEM)
- Verapamil (CALAN)

β-Adrenoceptor antagonists
- Atenolol (TENORMIN)
- Metoprolol (LOPRESSOR)
- Nadolol (CORGARD)
- Propranolol (INDERAL)

Metabolic Modifier
- Ranolazine (RANEXA)

*Also felodipine (PLENDIL) and nicardipine (CARDENE).

OVERVIEW

Coronary Heart Disease

The spectrum of coronary heart disease (CHD) includes **chronic angina pectoris** (stable angina) and a group of acute coronary syndromes consisting of **unstable angina** and **myocardial infarction** (MI; Fig. 11–1). Two forms of MI can be distinguished by the presence or lack of ST-segment elevation on the electrocardiogram, as described more fully in Chapter 16. All of these conditions are caused by coronary artery ischemia (inadequate blood flow) resulting from atherosclerosis, formation of thrombi (blood clots), or coronary vasospasm.

Typical angina results from formation of atherosclerotic plaques in vessel walls that limit coronary blood flow and the supply of oxygen to the myocardium. The symptoms of angina, often described as resembling a heavy weight or pressure on the chest, occur when the oxygen supply is insufficient to meet the demand imposed by increased physical exertion. The condition is called **stable angina** if angina attacks have similar characteristics and occur in similar circumstances each time. It is known as **unstable angina** if the frequency and severity of attacks increase over time. Unstable angina, which may be caused by occlusion of a coronary vessel by small platelet thrombi and ruptured atheromatous plaque, is often the forerunner of MI. Variant

angina (**Prinzmetal's angina**) is caused by acute coronary vasospasm and may occur at rest or during sleep.

Table 11–1 lists five classes of drugs and compares their efficacy in treating different forms of CHD. This chapter focuses on the anti-ischemic agents: **organic nitrites and nitrates**, **calcium channel blockers** (CCBs), and **β-adrenoceptor antagonists** (β-blockers), which are the primary agents used to treat angina symptoms. Chapter 15 discusses drugs for hyperlipidemia, and Chapter 16 covers antithrombotic drugs (e.g., aspirin). These two groups of drugs have been shown to reduce the risk of MI and death in persons with CHD.

Mechanisms and Effects of Antianginal Drugs

The anti-ischemic agents used in treating angina serve to prevent or counteract myocardial ischemia and thereby increase exercise tolerance and reduce the frequency of anginal attacks. This is accomplished by restoring the balance between myocardial oxygen supply and demand, either by increasing oxygen supply or decreasing oxygen demand. The factors that determine supply and demand are illustrated in Figure 11–2.

Myocardial oxygen supply is primarily determined by **coronary blood flow** and **regional flow distribution** but is

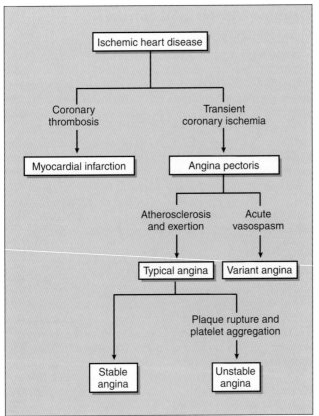

Figure 11-1. Classification and pathophysiology of ischemic heart disease. Variant angina, also called Prinzmetal's angina, is considered a form of unstable angina if the angina attacks occur with increasing severity or frequency.

TABLE 11-1.   Efficacy of Drugs Used in the Treatment of Coronary Heart Disease*

| Drug Class | TYPICAL ANGINA PECTORIS | | Variant Angina Pectoris | Myocardial Infarction |
	Stable Angina	Unstable Angina		
Anti-ischemic Agents				
Organic nitrites and nitrates	++	++	++	+
Calcium channel blockers	++	0 to ++	+++	0
β-adrenoceptor antagonists	++	++	0	+++
Preventive Agents				
Antithrombotic drugs (e.g., aspirin)†	+++	+++	0	++++
Cholesterol-lowering agents	+++	+++	0	+++

*Ratings range from 0 (not efficacious) to +++ (highly efficacious).
†Includes antiplatelet, anticoagulant, and fibronolytic drugs.

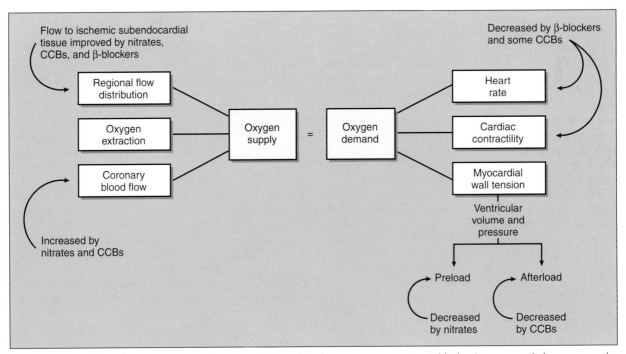

Figure 11-2. Effects of organic nitrites and nitrates, CCBs, and β-adrenoceptor antagonists (β-blockers) on myocardial oxygen supply and demand.

also influenced by **oxygen extraction.** In patients with coronary artery disease, the subendocardial tissue is more likely to suffer from ischemia because it is not as well perfused as the subepicardial tissue. The use of nitrates or CCBs (vasodilator drugs) can reduce ischemia by increasing both the total coronary flow and the distribution of coronary flow to ischemic subendocardial tissue. The drugs increase the distribution of blood flow to subendocardial tissue by dilating collateral vessels and by decreasing intraventricular pressure and the resistance to perfusion of this tissue. The use of β-blockers may improve the distribution of coronary flow by reducing intraventricular pressure. Cardiac tissue extracts a higher percentage of oxygen from blood than does any other tissue, and this factor is not affected by existing drugs.

Myocardial oxygen demand is largely determined by the amount of energy required to support the work of the heart. The factors that influence cardiac work include the **heart rate, cardiac contractility**, and **myocardial wall tension.** Contractility is directly related to the amount of cytosolic calcium that is available to stimulate the shortening of myocardial fibers. As contractility increases, the velocity of fiber shortening and the peak systolic muscle tension also increase. Myocardial wall tension is equal to the product of ventricular volume (radius) and pressure, divided by wall thickness. Ventricular wall tension is primarily determined by arterial and venous blood pressure.

Antianginal drugs act by several mechanisms to reduce myocardial oxygen demand. The β-blockers decrease heart rate and contractility, whereas the organic nitrates and CCBs reduce wall tension via their effects on ventricular volume and pressure. Dilation of veins decreases venous pressure, cardiac filling pressure, and ventricular diastolic pressure (preload). Dilation of arteries decreases arterial and aortic pressure and thereby reduces ventricular systolic pressure (afterload) and impedance to ventricular ejection of blood. The organic nitrates act primarily on venous tissue and predominantly affect preload, whereas the CCBs act mostly on arteriolar muscle to reduce afterload.

In **typical angina**, which is caused by increased oxygen demand in the face of a limited oxygen supply, vasodilators and β-blockers act primarily by decreasing oxygen demand through the mechanisms described above. They can also increase the perfusion of ischemic subendocardial tissue. In **variant angina**, chest pain usually occurs at rest (when oxygen demand is relatively low), and ischemia results in a reduction in oxygen supply secondary to coronary artery spasm. Under these conditions, vasodilators increase oxygen supply by relaxing coronary smooth muscle and restoring normal coronary flow. The β-blockers are not effective in the treatment of variant angina, because they cannot counteract vasospasm and increase coronary blood flow. The β-blockers may actually reduce coronary blood flow by blocking the vasodilative effect of epinephrine, an effect that is mediated by β_2-adrenoceptors in coronary smooth muscle.

VASODILATORS

Two classes of vasodilators are used in the management of angina pectoris. The first consists of organic nitrites and nitrates and the second consists of CCBs.

Organic Nitrites and Nitrates

The organic nitrites and nitrates are polyol esters of nitrous acid and nitric acid, respectively. Amyl nitrite, the only nitrite compound used to treat angina, is administered by inhalation. Nitroglycerin (glyceryl trinitrate), isosorbide dinitrate, and isosorbide mononitrate are compounds with sufficient solubility in water and lipids to enable rapid dissolution and absorption following sublingual, oral, or transdermal administration. The onset and duration of action of these drugs varies with their physical properties, route of administration, and rate of biotransformation. Amyl nitrite has the most rapid onset and the shortest duration of action, whereas isosorbide compounds have the slowest onset and the longest duration. Nitroglycerin has an intermediate onset and duration. All of these compounds are extensively metabolized in the liver.

Amyl Nitrite

Amyl nitrite is a volatile liquid that can be inhaled and absorbed through the lungs. Its action is rapid in onset (within 30 seconds) and brief in duration (3–5 minutes). Amyl nitrite is effective in the **treatment of acute angina attacks**, as well as in the **initial management of cyanide poisoning.** In patients with cyanide poisoning, amyl nitrite is used until intravenous sodium nitrite and sodium thiosulfate can be administered. The nitrites oxidize hemoglobin to methemoglobin. In comparison with hemoglobin, methemoglobin has a greater affinity for cyanide, and this allows it to trap the compound in the form of cyanmethemoglobin. Thiosulfate is then administered to convert cyanide to inactive thiocyanate.

Nitroglycerin, Isosorbide Dinitrate, and Isosorbide Mononitrate

PHARMACOKINETICS. Nitroglycerin and the isosorbide preparations are nitrate compounds used to **prevent and treat angina attacks.**

Nitroglycerin is available in formulations for sublingual, transdermal, topical, oral, and intravenous administration. The drug's solubility in water and lipids permits its rapid dissolution and absorption after sublingual or buccal administration for the treatment of acute angina attacks. Its high lipid solubility and low dosage have enabled the formulation of skin patches for transdermal administration. The patches slowly release the drug for absorption through the skin into the circulation and are used in the prevention of angina attacks. In ointment form, nitroglycerin is absorbed through the skin over a period of several hours. The ointment is primarily used in hospitalized patients with **angina** or **MI.** Nitroglycerin is administered orally in the form of sustained-release capsules that are used to prevent angina attacks. The drug is well absorbed from the gut but undergoes considerable first-pass inactivation, thereby necessitating the use of larger doses when administered orally. Nitroglycerin is also available as an intravenous solution that is used chiefly to reduce preload but also to reduce afterload in patients who have **acute heart failure** associated with MI and other conditions.

Isosorbide dinitrate can be administered sublingually or orally and is used for both the prevention and the treatment of angina attacks. Isosorbide dinitrate produces the same

pharmacologic effects as nitroglycerin, but it has a slightly slower onset of action and a greater duration of action. It is converted to an active compound, isosorbide mononitrate, which is now available as a drug preparation itself.

MECHANISMS AND PHARMACOLOGIC EFFECTS. The organic nitrates are believed to act by releasing **nitric oxide** in vascular smooth muscle cells (Fig. 11–3). The precise mechanisms by which nitroglycerin and other organic nitrates release nitric oxide are still under investigation. Some evidence suggests the involvement of thiol (−SH) compounds in this process. Recent evidence supports the involvement of **aldehyde dehydrogenase** in the release of nitric oxide as well as in the development of nitrate tolerance (see "TOLERANCE").

Nitric oxide is a gas that activates guanylyl cyclase, forming **cyclic guanosine monophosphate** (cGMP). Cyclic GMP activates cGMP-dependent kinases that appear to cause relaxation of vascular smooth muscle by phosphorylating proteins that decrease intracellular calcium mobilization and decrease phosphorylation of myosin light chains by increasing activity of myosin light-chain phosphatase (an enzyme that removes phosphate; Fig. 11–3).

The organic nitrates preferentially relax venous smooth muscle and have a relatively smaller effect on arteriolar smooth muscle. This leads to venous pooling of blood, a decrease in venous blood return to the heart, and a decrease in ventricular volume, pressure, and wall tension. By these mechanisms, the nitrates reduce cardiac work and oxygen demand and thereby relieve or prevent angina pectoris. By reducing cardiac preload, the nitrates also reduce cardiac output and thereby contribute to a reduction in blood pressure. If blood pressure falls sufficiently, reflex tachycardia can be invoked. The nitrates do not have any direct effects on myocardial tissue.

TOLERANCE. Continuous administration of nitroglycerin and other organic nitrates often leads to pharmacodynamic tolerance to their vasodilative effects. It has been demonstrated to occur with intravenous, transdermal, and oral administration of the nitrates, including sustained-release preparations of them. To prevent nitrate tolerance and loss of therapeutic effect, skin patches should be removed for at least 10 hours each day, and long-acting oral medications should be administered only once or twice a day.

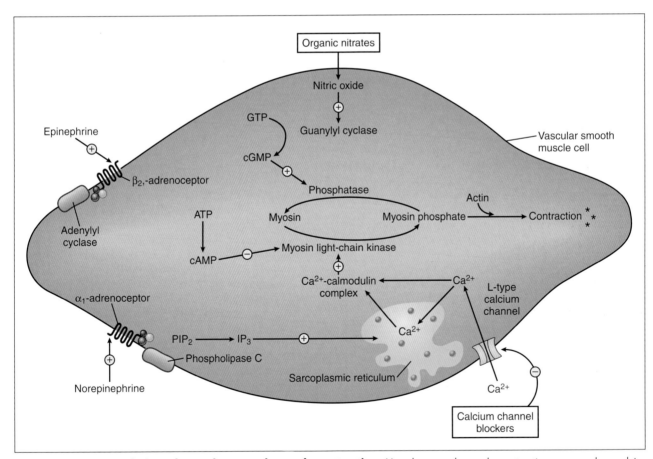

Figure 11–3. Regulation of vascular smooth muscle contraction. Vascular smooth muscle contraction occurs when calcium (Ca^{2+}) enters smooth muscle via L-type calcium channels, binds to calmodulin, and activates myosin light-chain kinase. This leads to formation of myosin phosphate, which interacts with actin to cause muscle contraction. Calcium influx is inhibited by CCBs, leading to muscle relaxation. Organic nitrates release nitric oxide, which activates guanylyl cyclase and increases formation of cGMP. Investigators believe that cGMP causes smooth muscle relaxation by activating kinases that increase myosin phosphatase activity and decrease myosin phosphate levels. α_1-adrenoceptor agonists activate phospholipase C (PLC), which increases formation of inositol triphosphate (IP$_3$) from phosphatidylinositol bisphosphate (PIP$_2$), leading to increased release of calcium from the sarcoplasmic reticulum. β_2-adrenoceptor agonists increase formation of cAMP, which activates kinases that inhibit myosin light-chain kinase.

Several mechanisms have been proposed to explain nitrate tolerance but none has been proved conclusively. Recent studies have suggested that anion free radicals (O_2^-) are formed during the release of nitric oxide from organic nitrates by mitochondrial **aldehyde dehydrogenase** and that these radicals then inactivate aldehyde dehydrogenase and thereby lead to tolerance.

ADVERSE EFFECTS AND INTERACTIONS. The most common adverse effects of organic nitrates, which are caused by excessive vasodilation, include headache, hypotension, dizziness, and reflex tachycardia. Tachycardia increases oxygen demand and can counteract the beneficial effects of nitrates, so patients should be cautioned to avoid excessive doses of these drugs. To prevent reflex tachycardia, a β-blocker can be used together with an organic nitrate or other type of vasodilator.

Calcium Channel Blockers

Calcium channel blockers belong to numerous chemical classes. **Amlodipine, felodipine, isradipine, nicardipine, nifedipine**, and **nimodipine** belong to the dihydropyridine class and have similar pharmacologic properties. **Bepridil, diltiazem**, and **verapamil** are unique members of other chemical classes.

All of the CCBs, except bepridil and nimodipine, are indicated for the treatment of **hypertension** (see Chapter 10). Diltiazem and verapamil are also used to treat certain types of **cardiac arrhythmias** (see Chapter 14). Nimodipine is indicated for the treatment of **subarachnoid hemorrhage**, which is one of the causes of stroke. In this setting, the drug is believed to dilate small cerebral vessels and thereby increase collateral circulation. Nimodipine can also reduce neuronal damage caused by an excessive release of calcium invoked by cerebral ischemia.

The discussion below focuses on the CCBs used in the management of **angina pectoris**. These antianginal CCBs include several dihydropyridines (amlodipine, felodipine, nicardipine, and nifedipine), bepridil, diltiazem, and verapamil.

TABLE 11–2. Pharmacokinetic Properties of Calcium Channel Blockers Used in the Treatment of Coronary Heart Disease*

Drug	Oral Bioavailability	Excreted Unchanged in Urine	Elimination Half-Life (Hours)
Dihydropyridines			
Amlodipine	75%	10%	40
Felodipine	20%	1%	14
Nicardipine	35%	1%	3
Nifedipine	60%	1%	3
Other Calcium Channel Blockers			
Bepridil	60%	5%	25
Diltiazem	55%	3%	5
Verapamil	25%	3%	5

*Values shown are the mean of values reported in the literature.

Drug Properties

PHARMACOKINETICS. The pharmacokinetic properties of the seven antianginal CCBs are summarized in Table 11–2. These CCBs are well absorbed after oral administration, but most of them undergo significant first-pass metabolism. Diltiazem, nicardipine, nifedipine, and verapamil have relatively short half-lives and are available in sustained-release preparations that are administered once or twice daily. Amlodipine, felodipine, and bepridil have longer half-lives, and their immediate-release formulations are administered once or twice a day.

MECHANISMS AND PHARMACOLOGIC EFFECTS. The **calcium ion channels** are located in the plasma membrane of smooth muscle and cardiac tissues. The influx of calcium through these channels leads to membrane depolarization and initiates or strengthens muscle contraction. CCBs bind to these channels and alter their conformation in a way that prevents the entry of calcium into cells (see Fig. 11–3). By this mechanism, CCBs produce smooth muscle relaxation and suppress cardiac activity.

Calcium channels are classified on the basis of their electrophysiologic properties. The two main types of voltage-activated calcium channels are the L (long) type and the T (transient) type. **L-type calcium channels** are high-voltage channels that are slowly inactivated, and their calcium influx has a relatively long duration. **T-type calcium channels** are low-voltage channels that are rapidly inactivated, and their calcium influx is more transient. Both L-type and T-type channels are found in vascular smooth muscle and in the sinoatrial (SA) and atrioventricular (AV) nodes. Only L-type channels, however, are found in the muscle cells of the heart. CCBs differ in their affinity for the different types of calcium channels. All of the currently available CCBs selectively bind to L-type channels.

Whereas all CCBs cause vascular smooth muscle to relax, they differ markedly in their effects on cardiac tissue (Table 11–3). The dihydropyridine drugs, which are potent vasodilators, can reduce blood pressure sufficiently to evoke reflex tachycardia. At therapeutic doses, the dihydropyridines do not suppress cardiac function as much as the other CCBs do. Diltiazem and verapamil decrease SA node automaticity, cardiac contractility, and AV node conduction velocity to a greater degree than the other CCBs do and can significantly reduce cardiac output in patients with heart failure.

ADVERSE EFFECTS. The most common side effects of CCBs are fatigue, headache, dizziness, flushing, **peripheral edema**, and other manifestations of vasodilation and hypotension. In retrospective case-control studies, investigators found a higher incidence of MI, congestive heart failure, and deaths from CHD in the group of patients who took immediate-release forms of nifedipine and other short-acting CCBs than in the control group. Authorities now recommend that a long-acting CCB or a sustained release formulation of a shorter-acting CCB, such as the nifedipine gastrointestinal system, be used for treating chronic cardiovascular disorders. The CCBs occasionally cause **gingival hyperplasia** (gingival overgrowth). Unlike diltiazem and verapamil, dihydropyridine CCBs do not affect digoxin serum levels significantly.

TABLE 11–3. Cardiovascular Effects of Calcium Channel Blockers Used in the Treatment of Coronary Heart Disease

Drug	Coronary Blood Flow	Sinoatrial Node Automaticity*	Cardiac Contractility*	Atrioventricular Node Conduction Velocity*
Dihydropyridine Drugs				
Amlodipine	Increases	None	None	None
Nicardipine	Increases	None	None	None
Nifedipine	Increases	None	None	None
Felodipine	Increases	None	None	None
Other Calcium Channel Blockers				
Bepridil	Increases	Decreases slightly	Decreases slightly	Decreases slightly
Diltiazem	Increases	Decreases	Decreases slightly	Decreases
Verapamil	Increases	Decreases	Decreases	Decreases

*Direct effects may be counteracted by reflex activity.

Amlodipine and Related Drugs

Amlodipine, felodipine nicardipine, and nifedipine are the dihydropyridine CCBs approved for the treatment of angina. Amlodipine has a long elimination half-life and is administered once a day. Felodipine and nifedipine are available in sustained-release formulations given once daily.

Bepridil

Unlike the other CCBs, bepridil is a multiple ion-channel blocker in cardiac tissue. For example, it blocks the sodium-calcium transporter (exchanger) as well as L-type calcium channels. Bepridil slows the heart rate slightly and reduces AV node conduction while increasing the AV node refractory period. Bepridil also prolongs the QT interval of the electrocardiogram, and may cause ventricular tachycardia (torsades de pointes). Hence, it is indicated for patients that fail to respond to or are intolerant of other antianginal medications. It may be combined with nitrates or beta blockers.

Diltiazem and Verapamil

Diltiazem or verapamil are effective treatments for typical and variant angina. Because these drugs can suppress cardiac contractility, caution should be exercised when administering them to patients with heart failure, especially verapamil. In patients who have typical angina without heart failure, the drugs have the advantage of reducing the heart rate and contractility in addition to their effects on myocardial wall tension.

Verapamil and other CCBs can cause constipation, probably because of relaxation of gastrointestinal smooth muscle and reduced peristalsis. Both verapamil and diltiazem reduce the clearance of digoxin and can thereby increase serum digoxin levels and precipitate digoxin toxicity. Digoxin doses should be reduced in patients receiving these drugs.

β-ADRENOCEPTOR ANTAGONISTS

The pharmacologic properties of β-adrenoceptor antagonists, or β-blockers, are discussed in Chapter 9, and their use in the treatment of hypertension and arrhythmias is discussed in Chapters 10 and 14, respectively.

Among the β-blockers used in the management of angina are **atenolol, metoprolol, nadolol,** and **propranolol.** These β-blockers are often used in **typical angina pectoris** and **acute MI,** but they are not used in the management of vasospastic angina or acute anginal attacks. In typical angina, they prevent ischemic episodes because of their ability to prevent exercise-induced tachycardia and increased myocardial oxygen demand. They can also prevent reflex tachycardia induced by either organic nitrates or dihydropyridine CCBs. In the post-MI setting, β-blockers decrease the risk of a recurrence and improve survival.

The β-blockers have a negative inotropic effect that can be hazardous to patients with heart failure if large doses are given. Because the combination of verapamil and a β-blocker may significantly reduce cardiac output, it should usually be avoided. The combination of a β-blocker and diltiazem is less hazardous.

DRUGS THAT MODIFY MYOCARDIAL METABOLISM

A newer group of antianginal drugs act by modifying myocardial metabolism. Trimetazidine is available in Europe and ranolazine has been approved in the United States. These agents improve exercise capacity and reduce angina episodes without causing significant hemodynamic changes (alteration of arterial or venous pressure).

The heart uses glucose, fatty acids, and lactate as sources of energy. Although fatty acids are the major fuel for the heart, glucose is metabolized more efficiently and generates about 15% more energy per oxygen utilized. **Trimetazidine** inhibits fatty acid oxidation, leading to increased glucose metabolism and efficiency of oxygen utilization by the heart. **Ranolazine** improves cardiac diastolic function, apparently by limiting sodium influx and the congruent calcium overload that can have detrimental effects on cardiac performance. Clinically, ranolazine reduces the frequency of angina attacks in persons with stable angina, and thereby decreases the need for nitroglycerin in these patients. Ranolazine appears to be a useful alternative or adjunct to conventional antianginal agents.

MANAGEMENT OF ANGINA PECTORIS

In patients with a history of angina pectoris, the primary objectives of drug therapy are to relieve acute symptoms, to prevent ischemic attacks, improve the quality of life, and to reduce the risks of MI and other potential cardiovascular problems, as illustrated in Box 11–1. Treatment of concurrent hypertension, hyperlipidemia, diabetes, and obesity can slow coronary artery disease progression, whereas antithrombotic agents (e.g., aspirin) reduce the risk of coronary thrombosis and MI. In fact, aspirin has been shown to prolong the life of persons with stable angina.

If a patient has only an occasional angina episode, sublingual nitroglycerin can be used as needed to relieve acute symptoms. If episodes occur predictably with exertion, sublingual nitroglycerin or isosorbide dinitrate can be taken as a prophylactic measure just before exertion. If the severity of angina requires regular use of sublingual nitroglycerin, however, prophylactic therapy should be considered. In some cases, angiography should be performed to determine if percutaneous coronary intervention (angioplasty) or coronary artery bypass grafting is appropriate.

For patients who have stable angina and require long-term treatment, either a β-blocker, a long-acting nitrate, or a CCB can be chosen for initial therapy, with other drugs added or substituted depending on the response. Some studies show that β-blockers lower the risk of MI and possibly improve survival in patients with stable angina, and a meta-analysis of 90 clinical studies found that β-blockers reduced anginal episodes more than did CCBs. However, rates of cardiac death and MI were similar in patients receiving β-blockers and CCBs.

Patients with unstable angina have a high risk of MI and should also receive aspirin or other antithrombotic drugs to prevent platelet aggregation and thrombus formation. CCBs are less suitable than β-blockers for patients with unstable angina or a recent MI, because the dihydropyridine CCBs have the potential to cause reflex tachycardia and because verapamil and diltiazem have the potential to suppress cardiac contractility and can increase the frequency of heart failure in persons with ventricular systolic dysfunction.

The β-blockers are ineffective in treating variant angina, which is caused by coronary vasospasm. This condition is usually treated with a CCB.

In patients who have angina and concomitant asthma, a CCB is usually preferred because of its potential ability to relax bronchial smooth muscle. The β-blockers should usually be avoided in persons with asthma because of their tendency to cause bronchoconstriction. In patients with diabetes, a CCB is often used; however, a β_1-adrenoceptor blocker or a third-generation β-blocker such as carvedilol may be advantageous in some patients. In patients with heart failure, a long-acting nitrate may be preferred for angina prophylaxis, because the low doses of β-blockers typically used in persons with heart failure may not adequately control angina (see Chapter 12).

BOX 11–1   A CASE OF CHEST PAIN UPON EXERTION

CASE PRESENTATION: A 57-year-old construction foreman who is a heavy smoker complained to his physician of a pressurelike discomfort in the retrosternal area. The problem began about a month ago and occurs two or three times a week. The discomfort occurs only when he is working, disappears when he rests, and never lasts for more than 15 minutes. Except for a blood pressure of 150/100 mm Hg, his physical examination and electrocardiogram were normal. Blood samples were obtained for chemical analysis, including a complete lipid profile.

After ruling out other causes of the patient's chest discomfort, the physician made a provisional diagnosis of typical angina pectoris and prescribed sublingual nitroglycerin for relief of acute chest discomfort. The patient was started on a thiazide diuretic and amlodipine, and a low dose of aspirin. He was also encouraged to monitor his blood pressure regularly and to enroll in a smoking cessation program. He was scheduled to see his physician again in 3 weeks.

CASE DISCUSSION: The risk factors for CHD include hypertension and smoking. While β-blockers have often been preferred for treating hypertension in persons with CHD, recent clinical trials have indicated that long-acting CCBs are as effective as β-blockers for the prevention of death and MI in angina patients. Moreover, CCBs may be more effective than β-blockers for the prevention of stroke. Amlodipine is a long-acting dihydropyridine CCB that is suitable for control of blood pressure and prevention of angina symptoms. Studies have shown that amlodipine reduces hospitalization and the need for revascularization in angina patients. Combining amlodipine with a diuretic will enable the patient to achieve normal blood pressure in a shorter amount of time using lower doses of each drug.

Aspirin can prevent formation of platelet thrombi and reduce the risk of MI and death in persons with angina. Patients with CHD should be evaluated for hyperlipidemia and treated appropriately with dietary restrictions and drug therapy to retard the progression of atherosclerosis. These patients should also be considered for angiographic evaluation of their coronary arteries to determine whether angioplasty or coronary artery bypass grafting would be beneficial.

SUMMARY OF IMPORTANT POINTS

■ Lifestyle changes and drugs that lower cholesterol levels (e.g., statins) may slow the progression of atherosclerosis. Aspirin and statins decrease coronary events and mortality in persons with CHD.

■ In patients with typical angina, the antianginal drugs act by decreasing myocardial oxygen demand. The organic nitrites and nitrates and the CCBs decrease myocardial wall tension, whereas the β-adrenoceptor antagonists (β-blockers) and some CCBs decrease the heart rate and contractility.

■ Nitrates and dihydropyridine CCBs have the potential to cause reflex tachycardia, but this effect can be prevented by concurrent administration of a β-blocker.

■ Continuous exposure to nitrates leads to tolerance. Nitrate tolerance is caused by inactivation of aldehyde dehydrogenase and decreased release of nitric oxide.

■ All CCBs have similar vasodilating activity. Verapamil and diltiazem also produce significant cardiac depression, and verapamil has a greater effect than diltiazem on cardiac contractility. Verapamil and diltiazem can increase serum digoxin levels and cause digitalis toxicity.

■ In patients with a history of MI, the β-blockers have been found to reduce the incidence of ventricular arrhythmias that cause sudden death.

■ Calcium channel blockers and organic nitrates are effective in the treatment of vasospastic angina, whereas the β-blockers are not.

■ Ranolazine is a novel agent that reduces ischemic symptoms in angina patients by preventing myocardial sodium and calcium overload.

Review Questions

1. A woman taking an antianginal drug complains of chronic constipation despite appropriate dietary intake. The smooth muscle relaxation produced by her medication most likely results from which signal transduction event?
   (A) increased levels of cGMP
   (B) decreased binding of calcium to calmodulin
   (C) decreased formation of IP3
   (D) decreased myosin light-chain kinase activity
   (E) increased metabolic efficiency

2. A man is placed on atenolol and diltiazem for prevention of angina. Which effect is caused by both of these drugs?
   (A) decreased cyclic AMP levels
   (B) increased cGMP levels
   (C) decreased heart rate
   (D) relaxation of arterial smooth muscle
   (E) inhibition of sodium influx

3. A woman is taking an antianginal medication that increases cGMP levels in vascular smooth muscle. Which drug action is responsible for this effect?
   (A) inhibition of phosphodiesterase

   (B) inactivation of aldehyde dehydrogenase
   (C) blockade of β-adrenoceptors
   (D) release of nitric oxide
   (E) blockade of calcium channels

4. A man with obstructive pulmonary disease requires therapy to prevent anginal attacks. Which drug should be avoided in this patient?
   (A) verapamil
   (B) felodipine
   (C) isosorbide mononitrate
   (D) diltiazem
   (E) propranolol

Answers and Explanations

1. **The answer is B: decreased binding of calcium to calmodulin.** The CCBs such as nifedipine are the only anti-ischemic drugs that typically cause constipation, most likely because they relax gastrointestinal smooth muscle. These drugs reduce calcium influx, thereby reducing formation of the calcium-calmodulin complex that increases myosin light-chain kinase activity. None of the other options are associated with CCBs.

2. **The answer is C: decreased heart rate.** Atenolol, a β₁-adrenoceptor blocker, and diltiazem, a nondihydropyridine CCB, decrease heart rate and contractility. Option A (decreased cyclic adenosine monophosphate [cAMP] levels) is only caused by atenolol. Option B (increased cGMP levels) is caused by neither atenolol nor diltiazem. Option D (relaxation of arterial smooth muscle) is caused only by diltiazem, whereas neither drug inhibits sodium influx (Option E).

3. **The answer is D: release of nitric oxide.** Organic nitrates release nitric oxide, which activates guanylyl cyclase and increases cGMP levels. Option A (inhibition of phosphodiesterase) is the mechanism by which sildenafil relaxes vascular smooth muscle. Option B (inactivation of aldehyde dehydrogenase) may lead to decreased release of nitric oxide and nitrate tolerance. Options C (blockade of β-adrenoceptors) and E (blockade of calcium channels) are not caused by organic nitrates.

4. **The answer is E: propranolol.** Nonselective β-blockers such as propranolol may cause bronchoconstriction by blocking β₂-adrenoceptors. Calcium channel blockers (Options A, B, and D) appear to relax bronchial smooth muscle and are preferred for treating angina in persons with obstructive lung disease. Organic nitrates (Option C) do not significantly affect bronchial smooth muscle and can also be used in obstructive lung disease patients.

SELECTED READINGS

Bassand, J.-P., C. Hamm, D. Ardissino, E. Boersma, A. Budaj, et al. Guidelines for the diagnosis and treatment of non-ST-segment elevation acute coronary syndromes. Eur Heart J 28:1598–1660, 2007.

Ben-Dor, I., and A. Battler. Treatment of stable angina. Heart 93:868–874, 2007.

Scirica, B.M. Ranolazine in patients with coronary artery disease. Expert Opin Pharmacother 8:2149–2157, 2007.

CHAPTER 12

Drugs for Heart Failure

CLASSIFICATION OF DRUGS FOR HEART FAILURE

Positively Inotropic Drugs
Digitalis glycoside
- Digoxin

Adrenoceptor agonist
- Dobutamine

Phosphodiesterase inhibitor
- Milrinone (PRIMACOR)

Vasodilators
Angiotensin inhibitors
- Enalapril (VASOTEC)[a]
- Valsartan (DIOVAN)[b]

Other vasodilators
- Hydralazine
- Isosorbide Dinitrate
- Nesiritide (NATRECOR)

Aldosterone Antagonists
- Spironolactone (ALDACTONE)
- Eplerenone (INSPRA)

β-Adrenoceptor Blocker
- Carvedilol (COREG)[c]

Diuretic
- Furosemide (LASIX)[d]

[a]Also lisinopril, ramipril, and others.
[b]Also candesartan and others.
[c]Also bisoprolol and metoprolol.
[d]Also bumetanide and torsemide.

OVERVIEW

In the United States, **heart failure** affects nearly 5 million individuals, is the primary cause of more than 40,000 deaths per year, and is a contributing factor in an additional 220,000 deaths. The overall mortality rate in patients with heart failure is about eight times as high as that in the normal population, and the 5-year mortality rate for patients with heart failure approaches 50%.

Pathophysiology of Heart Failure

Heart failure is the end-stage of a number of cardiovascular disorders that ultimately impair the ability of the ventricle to fill with blood or to eject blood into the circulation. **Ischemic heart disease** is the most common cause of heart failure. Other important causes of heart failure include hypertension, valvular disorders, arrhythmias, viral and congenital cardiomyopathy, and constrictive pericarditis. Less commonly, heart failure results from severe anemia, thiamine deficiency, or the use of certain anticancer drugs, such as doxorubicin (see Chapter 45). Over time, these disorders produce molecular and cellular changes in cardiac myocytes

and connective tissue that lead to a series of structural and functional alternations in the ventricular wall. This process, known as **cardiac** or **ventricular remodeling**, is characterized by cardiac dilatation, ventricular wall thinning, interstitial fibrosis, and wall stiffness. These changes impair the ability of the heart to relax or contract.

Cardiac remodeling is believed to result primarily from the activation of neurohumoral systems in response to myocardial ischemia, excessive stretch of muscle fibers, or other pathologic stimuli. The neurohumoral systems implicated in this process include the renin-angiotensin-aldosterone axis, sympathetic nervous system, various inflammatory cytokines, and local mediators such as endothelin. These mediators activate biochemical pathways that induce myocyte hypertrophy, apoptosis, collagen production, fibrosis, and other effects that lead to cardiac remodeling and loss of ventricular function. For example, angiotensin II, which is formed locally in the myocardium in response to mechanical stretch and other stimuli, can induce collagen production and proliferation of fibroblasts. Chronic sympathetic nervous system stimulation of the injured myocardium produces myocyte hypertrophy, increases production of myocardial cytokines (e.g., tumor necrosis factor-α), and ultimately leads to myocyte death via activation of apoptotic pathways.

The hallmark of heart failure is a **reduction in stroke volume and cardiac output** at any given diastolic muscle fiber length, as determined by measuring the ventricular end-diastolic pressure (preload). The reduced stroke volume can be caused by **diastolic dysfunction** or **systolic dysfunction** and is manifested as an inability of the ventricles either to fill properly or to empty properly, respectively. Systolic dysfunction can result from decreased cardiac contractility secondary to a dilated or ischemic myocardium. Diastolic dysfunction can result from decreased compliance (increased stiffness) of ventricular tissue secondary to left ventricular hypertrophy or fibrosis. Hence, both systolic and diastolic heart failure can be caused or exacerbated by the process of cardiac remodeling.

In cases of **left ventricular failure** (**left-sided heart failure**), the left ventricle does not adequately pump blood forward, so the pressure in the pulmonary circulation increases. When the increased pressure forces fluid into the lung interstitium, this causes **congestion** and **edema** (Fig. 12–1). **Pulmonary edema** reduces the diffusion of oxygen and carbon dioxide between alveoli and the pulmonary capillaries. This causes **hypoxemia** (deficient oxygenation of the blood) and can lead to **dyspnea** (difficulty in breathing), including **exertional dyspnea** (dyspnea provoked by exercise), **orthopnea** (intensified dyspnea when lying flat), and **paroxysmal nocturnal dyspnea** (edema-induced bronchoconstriction when sleeping).

The combination of edema-related hypoxemia and the heart's failure to pump sufficient blood to adequately perfuse the tissues can lead to generalized tissue hypoxia and organ dysfunction. For this reason, patients with heart failure often experience symptoms of weakness and fatigue and have reduced exercise capacity.

In cases of **right ventricular failure** (**right-sided heart failure**), congestion in the peripheral veins leads to **ankle edema** in the ambulatory patient and to **sacral edema** in the bedridden patient. It also leads to **hepatojugular reflux**, characterized by an increase in jugular vein distention when pressure is applied over the liver. Ultimately, right-sided

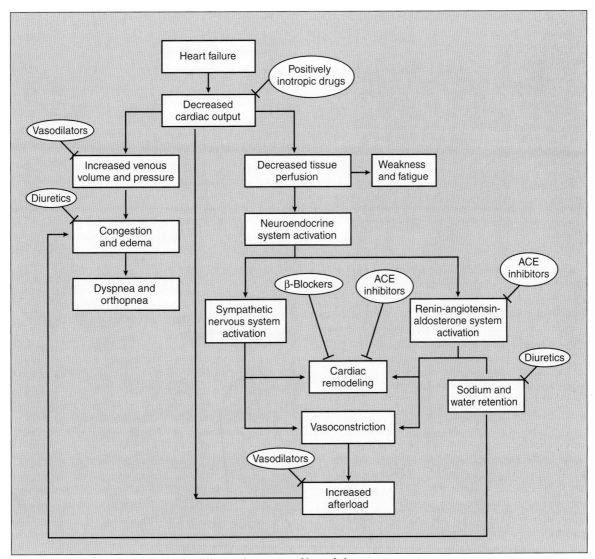

Figure 12–1. Pathophysiology and treatment of heart failure. ACE = angiotensin-converting enzyme.

TABLE 12-1. **Cardiovascular Effects of Drugs Used in the Treatment of Heart Failure***

Drug	Cardiac Contractility	Heart Rate	Preload Reduction	Afterload Reduction	Risk of Arrhythmia	Other Effects
Positively Inotropic Drugs						
Digitalis Glycoside						
Digoxin	+	–	++	0 to +	++	Increases parasympathetic tone and decreases sympathetic tone
β-Adrenoceptor Agonist						
Dobutamine	++	+ to +	0 to +	+ to ++	+ to ++	
Phosphodiesterase Inhibitor						
Milrinone	+	0 to ++	++	++		
Vasodilators						
Angiotensin-Converting Enzyme Inhibitors						
Captopril	0	0	++	++	0	
Enalapril	0	0	++	++	0	
Lisinopril	0	0	++	++	0	
Other Vasodilators						
Hydralazine	0	+ (R)	0	++	+	Reduces blood pressure
Isosorbide dinitrate	0	+ (R)	++	+	0	Reduces pulmonary congestion
Loop-Acting Diuretics						
Bumetanide	0	0	+	0	0	Reduces edema and congestion
Furosemide	0	0	+	0	0	Reduces edema and congestion
Torsemide	0	0	+	0	0	Reduces edema and congestion
β-Adrenoceptor Antagonist						
Carvedilol	0	0 to –	0	+	0	Blocks α- and β-adrenoceptors

*Effects are indicated as follows: decrease (–); no change or variable (0); increase ranging from small (+) to large (++); and reflex (R).

failure can lead to left-sided failure as the left ventricle is forced to work harder in an attempt to maintain cardiac output.

The reduction in cardiac output that occurs in heart failure triggers a cascade of **compensatory neurohumoral responses**. Although these responses attempt to restore cardiac output via the Frank-Starling mechanism (see Fig. 12–1), they are often maladaptive and counterproductive. The reduction in tissue perfusion activates both the sympathetic nervous system and the renin-angiotensin-aldosterone system, both of which in turn stimulate vasoconstriction. Arterial vasoconstriction increases aortic impedance to left ventricular ejection and thereby decreases cardiac output, especially in patients with a weak, dilated heart. When angiotensin II stimulates the secretion of aldosterone and antidiuretic hormone, this increases the amount of sodium and water retention, the plasma volume, and the venous pressure. In addition, angiotensin II and sympathetic activation lead to cardiac remodeling and ventricular wall thinning or fibrosis, which often reduce systolic and diastolic function. Hence, the net result of the neurohumoral responses is often a further reduction in cardiac output and an increase in circulatory congestion.

Mechanisms and Effects of Drugs for Heart Failure

The primary goals of drug therapy for heart failure are to improve symptoms, slow or reverse deterioration in myocardial function, and prolong survival. Drugs can also be used to treat underlying conditions, control arrhythmias, prevent thrombosis, and treat anemia.

The pharmacologic agents used to treat heart failure include drugs that (1) increase cardiac output, (2) reduce pulmonary and systemic congestion, and (3) slow or reverse cardiac remodeling. Cardiac output can be increased by positively inotropic drugs that increase cardiac contractility and by vasodilators that reduce cardiac afterload and the impedance to left ventricular ejection. Vasodilators also reduce venous pressure, circulatory congestion, and edema. Diuretics are used to mobilize edematous fluid and reduce plasma volume, thereby decreasing circulatory congestion.

TABLE 12-2. Pharmacokinetic Properties of Positively Inotropic Drugs*

Drug	Oral Bioavailability	Onset of Action	Duration of Action	Elimination Half-Life	Excreted Unchanged in Urine	Therapeutic Serum Level
Digitalis Glycoside						
Digoxin	75%	1 hour	24 hours	36 hours	60%	0.5–2 ng/mL
β-Adrenoceptor Agonist						
Dobutamine	NA	1 minute	<10 minutes	2 minutes	0%	NA
Phosphodiesterase Inhibitors						
Inamrinone and milrinone	NA	3 minutes	Variable	4 hours	60%	NA

*Values shown are the mean of values reported in the literature.
NA = not applicable (not administered orally).

Angiotensin and sympathetic inhibitors have been shown to favorably influence cardiac remodeling and increase survival in persons with heart failure.

Table 12–1 compares the cardiovascular effects of drugs discussed in this chapter. Each of these drugs partly counteracts the loss of myocardial function and the maladaptive responses that occur during heart failure; however, none of the current therapies, either alone or in combination, has been completely satisfactory. Because heart failure has such a high incidence and poor prognosis, a much greater effort has been expended in the search for better means to treat it. The most significant development in recent decades has been the use of angiotensin inhibitors, β-adrenoceptor blockers, and other agents that attenuate cardiac remodeling and reduce the mortality rate in patients with heart failure. Ultimately, however, the successful treatment of patients with heart failure may require the development of novel drugs that activate genes capable of repairing or replacing myocardial tissue.

POSITIVELY INOTROPIC DRUGS

Derived from the Greek words for fiber (*inos*) and changing (*tropikos*), the term *inotropic* refers to a change in muscle contractility. Drugs that increase cardiac contractility are said to have a positive inotropic effect, whereas drugs that decrease contractility have a negative inotropic effect. Drugs with a positive effect include members of three groups: digitalis glycosides, β-adrenoceptor agonists, and phosphodiesterase inhibitors. The calcium-sensitizing agents represent a new class of inotropic drugs that are currently under investigation for the treatment of heart failure. These include levosimendan.

All of the currently available inotropic agents increase calcium influx into cardiac muscle cells, thereby increasing cardiac contractility. The β-receptor agonists and phosphodiesterase inhibitors increase calcium influx by increasing intracellular cyclic adenosine monophosphate (cAMP) levels. β-Agonists increase cAMP formation by activating adenylyl cyclase, whereas milrinone inhibits cAMP degradation. The mechanism by which digitalis glycosides increase calcium influx is described next.

Digitalis Glycosides

Despite the fact that the digitalis glycosides have been used to treat heart failure for more than 200 years, their effectiveness and place in therapy have been difficult to determine. Recent clinical trials indicate that digoxin provides a definite, yet limited, benefit to patients with heart failure caused by systolic dysfunction.

Drug Properties

Many digitalis glycosides have been isolated from plant and animal sources, including the leaves of *Digitalis* (foxglove) plants and the skin secretions of certain toads. Digoxin is the only digitalis glycoside that is extensively used today, having replaced digitoxin and crude digitalis leaf preparations in the treatment of heart failure and other cardiac disorders.

CHEMISTRY AND PHARMACOKINETICS. The digitalis glycosides are composed of a steroid nucleus, a lactone ring, and three sugar residues linked by glycosidic bonds. The stereochemical configuration of the steroid nucleus of digitalis glycosides is different than that of human steroids, and the digitalis glycosides lack most of the effects produced by gonadal or adrenal steroids.

As shown in Table 12–2, digoxin is adequately absorbed from the gut and has a long half-life of about 36 hours. It is primarily eliminated by renal excretion of the parent compound. Because digoxin has a low therapeutic index, serum concentrations are useful in assessing the adequacy of the dosage and evaluating potential toxicity and should be in the range of 0.5 to 2 ng/mL.

MECHANISMS AND PHARMACOLOGIC EFFECTS. The direct and indirect actions of digoxin produce a unique constellation of effects on the cardiovascular system. It has a positive inotropic effect (an increase in the force of contraction), a negative chronotropic effect (a decrease in the heart rate), and a negative dromotropic effect (a decrease in conduction velocity). Among the various types of positively inotropic drugs, digoxin is unique in its ability to strengthen cardiac contraction while decreasing heart rate. Moreover, digoxin indirectly increases parasympathetic tone while reducing sympathetic tone. This contributes to its effects on heart rate and conduction velocity and may partly account for its important role in the treatment of heart failure and other cardiac disorders.

(1) POSITIVE INOTROPIC EFFECT. Digoxin produces a modest positive inotropic effect that is caused by an increase in intracellular calcium and is secondary to inhibition of the sodium pump (Na+,K+-ATPase) in the plasma membrane (sarcolemma). When the sodium pump is inhibited, the concentration of intracellular sodium is increased, thereby increasing the activity of the sodium-calcium exchanger and causing more calcium to enter the cardiac myocyte (Fig. 12–2). The increase in cytoplasmic calcium stimulates the release of additional calcium from the sarcoplasmic reticulum and leads to greater myofibril shortening (contraction).

The positive inotropic effect of digoxin increases the velocity of cardiac muscle contraction and the peak systolic muscle tension. These actions increase stroke volume and cardiac output at any given diastolic fiber length (preload), as shown in Figure 12–3. The stroke volume is the amount of blood pumped by the ventricle during each systole, and the cardiac output is the amount of blood ejected from either ventricle of the heart per minute.

(2) ELECTROPHYSIOLOGIC AND ELECTROCARDIO-GRAPHIC EFFECTS. Digoxin has several indirect effects on cardiac electrophysiology. It causes an increase in parasympathetic (vagal) tone, and this decreases the heart rate and atrioventricular (AV) node conduction velocity while increasing the AV node refractory period (Fig. 12–4). At the same time, it causes a decrease in sympathetic tone. In patients with heart failure, the reduction in sympathetic tone is caused partly by the withdrawal of reflex sympathetic stimulation secondary to the improved cardiac output produced by digoxin. The drug also appears to directly inhibit sympathetic nerve activity. The reduction in sympathetic tone augments the effect of vagal activation on the sinoatrial and AV nodes, and it also decreases sympathetic vasoconstriction and thereby counteracts the direct vasoconstrictive effect of digoxin. The effects of digoxin on the AV node account for its ability to slow the ventricular rate in patients with atrial fibrillation (see below).

Digoxin also has direct effects on cardiac electrophysiology. Of particular importance is the drug's ability to increase abnormal impulse formation by evoking spontaneous **afterdepolarizations** (see Fig. 12–4). These abnormal depolarizations occur during or immediately after normal cardiac repolarization and lead to **extrasystoles** (premature or coupled beats) and **tachycardia** (rapid beating of the heart). The afterdepolarizations appear to be caused by excessive calcium influx into cardiac cells, and they are more likely to occur after higher doses of digoxin are given.

Digoxin has several electrocardiographic effects (see Fig. 12–4). It shortens the ventricular action potential duration by accelerating repolarization, and this decreases the QT interval. It reduces the AV node conduction velocity and thereby increases the PR interval. Finally, it causes ST segment depression, which gives rise to the so-called hockey stick configuration of the ST segment.

ADVERSE EFFECTS. The most common adverse effects of digoxin are gastrointestinal, cardiac, and neurologic reactions. Frequently, the earliest signs of toxicity are anorexia, nausea, and vomiting. These reactions are often associated with elevated serum concentrations and may forewarn of more serious toxicity.

Arrhythmias, usually the most serious manifestation of digoxin toxicity, can include AV block and various tachyarrhythmias. Atrial tachycardia with 2:1 or 3:1 AV block is one of the most common types of digitalis-induced arrhythmia, but digoxin can also cause ventricular arrhythmias. Hypokalemia can precipitate arrhythmias in patients receiving digoxin, and the serum potassium level should be determined immediately if arrhythmias occur in these patients.

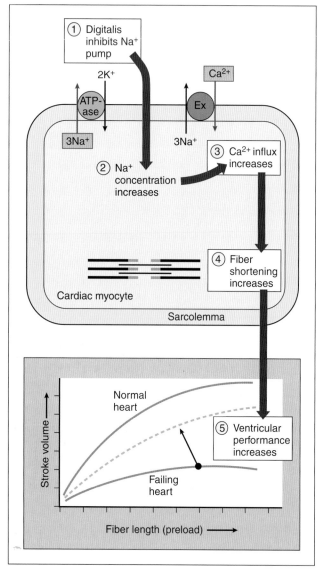

Figure 12–2. **Mechanisms by which digoxin exerts its positive inotropic effect on the heart.** Digoxin inhibits the sodium pump (ATPase) in the sarcolemma and increases the concentration of intracellular sodium. The high sodium concentration increases the activity of the sodium-calcium exchanger (Ex), thereby causing more calcium to enter the cardiac myocyte. Calcium activates muscle fiber shortening and increases cardiac contractility, which, in turn, increases stroke volume at any given fiber length (preload).

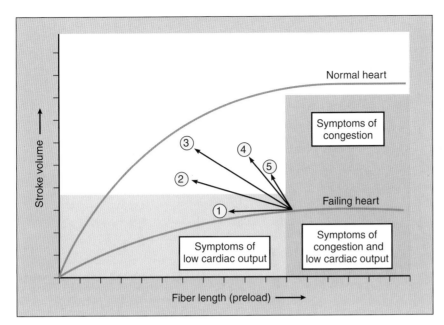

Figure 12–3. **Effect of drug treatment on ventricular performance.** Effects of the following drugs or drug combinations are shown: (1) a diuretic or a nitrate; (2) nitroprusside or an ACE inhibitor; (3) a positively inotropic drug plus a vasodilator; (4) dobutamine; and (5) digoxin. The positively inotropic drugs increase stroke volume at any given fiber length and thereby decrease venous pressure and preload. Some vasodilators (e.g., ACE inhibitors) decrease afterload and thereby increase stroke volume. Vasodilators can also decrease preload.

The neurologic effects of digoxin include blurred vision and yellow, green, or blue chromatopsia (a condition in which objects appear unnaturally colored). Severe digoxin toxicity can precipitate seizures.

Because digoxin has some estrogenic activity, it occasionally causes gynecomastia (excessive growth of male mammary glands).

INTERACTIONS. Several drugs can interact with digoxin and thereby affect its efficacy and toxicity (Table 12–3). Because antacids and cholestyramine can reduce the absorption of digoxin and decrease its therapeutic effects, their administration should be separated from the administration of digoxin by at least 2 hours. Diltiazem, quinidine, and verapamil reduce digoxin clearance and increase serum digoxin levels, which can cause digitalis toxicity. When digoxin is used concurrently with these drugs, only 50% of the usual dose of digoxin should be given, and serum digoxin levels should be monitored. Diuretics should be used cautiously with digoxin. Diuretic-induced hypokalemia can precipitate digitalis toxicity because the reduced serum potassium concentration increases digitalis binding to the sodium pump. Hypokalemia can also contribute directly to arrhythmias.

INDICATIONS. Digitalis glycosides have been used to treat **heart failure** for centuries, but their benefits have been uncertain, whereas their toxicity has been substantial. The improvement produced by digoxin in patients with systolic heart failure probably results from a combination of a modest positive inotropic effect and attenuation of the neurohumoral consequences of heart failure. As previously discussed, digoxin augments parasympathetic tone while reducing sympathetic tone, and these actions reduce heart rate, sympathetic vasoconstriction, and cardiac afterload. Digoxin is generally not used to treat diastolic heart failure because contractility is not impaired in this disorder.

In patients with heart failure, clinical trials have shown that although digoxin treatment does not prolong survival, it reduces symptoms and the need for hospitalization, and thereby improves the quality of life of persons with heart failure. Moreover, patients who have been withdrawn from digoxin exhibit worsening of heart failure. Hence, digitalis will probably continue to have a role in treating heart failure in combination with angiotensin inhibitors, diuretics, β-adrenoceptor antagonists, and other drugs.

The most certain indication for digoxin, however, appears to be the treatment of patients with **both heart failure and atrial fibrillation.** In these patients, the ventricular rate is often rapid and irregular, thereby causing palpitations and reducing cardiac output. By slowing the AV node conduction velocity and increasing the AV node refractory period, digoxin reduces the number of ectopic impulses that are transmitted from the atria to the ventricles and thereby slows the ventricular rate.

Digoxin Immune Fab

An antidote for serious digoxin toxicity is available in the form of **digoxin immune Fab.** This antibody preparation is administered intravenously and can rapidly reverse severe digoxin toxicity.

β-Adrenoceptor Agonists

Dobutamine is the β-adrenoceptor agonist most frequently used in patients with heart failure. This agent must be administered by continuous intravenous infusion, and this usually restricts its use to the short-term management of **acute heart failure** and **cardiogenic shock.** Symptomatic improvement has been documented in patients with heart failure receiving a continuous infusion of dobutamine for 3 to 5 days, and some patients may benefit from dobutamine administration for up to 30 days. No evidence indicates that such treatments improve survival and intermittent high-dose dobutamine can increase mortality. Hence, some

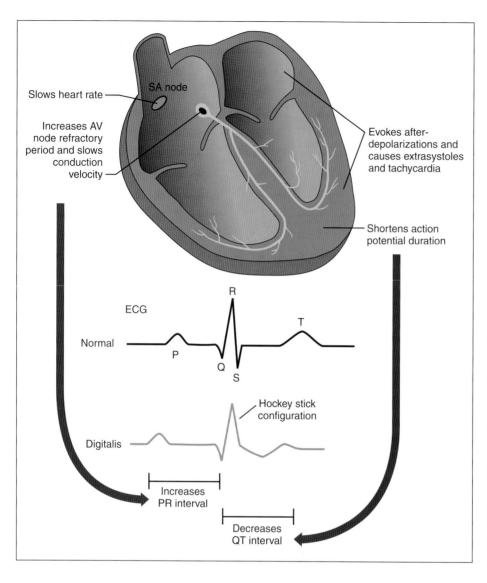

Figure 12-4. **Electrophysiologic and electrocardiographic effects of digoxin.** Digoxin causes an increase in parasympathetic (vagal) tone and a decrease in sympathetic tone. These actions slow the heart rate by decreasing sinoatrial (SA) node automaticity. The increased vagal tone and decreased sympathetic tone also slow the AV node conduction velocity while increasing the AV node refractory period. The reduced AV conduction velocity increases the PR interval on the electrocardiogram. In ventricular tissue, digoxin shortens the action potential duration, and this decreases the QT interval. Toxic concentrations of digoxin may evoke afterdepolarizations throughout the heart and thereby cause extra systoles and tachycardia. Digoxin also causes ST segment depression, which gives rise to the so-called hockey stick configuration on the electrocardiogram.

authorities believe dobutamine and other intravenous inotropes should be limited to the short-term management of patients with severe decompensated heart failure.

Dobutamine selectively stimulates cardiac contractility and usually causes less tachycardia than do other β-adrenoceptor agonists, such as isoproterenol. Dobutamine also activates β$_2$-adrenoceptors in vascular smooth muscle and thereby decreases vascular resistance and cardiac afterload.

The properties and effects of dobutamine are summarized in Tables 12–1, 12–2, and 12–3 and are described in greater detail in Chapter 8.

Milrinone

Milrinone is a unique inotropic agent with a bi-pyridine structure. It is occasionally used in treating acute heart failure and other conditions requiring myocardial stimulation. Milrinone acts by inhibiting **type 3 phosphodiesterase**, an enzyme that converts cAMP to inactive 5′-AMP. By increasing the concentration of cAMP in myocytes, milrinone stimulates cardiac contractility. It also increases cAMP in vascular smooth muscle and produces vasodilation (see Fig. 11–3).

Milrinone is used for the short-term management of heart failure in patients who are not responsive to other drugs. It has also been used for inotropic support of infants and children awaiting cardiac transplantation and for other conditions requiring myocardial stimulation. Intravenous administration of milrinone can provide both hemodynamic and symptomatic improvement in persons with advanced heart failure. However, long-term use can cause thrombocytopenia and ventricular arrhythmias and is associated with increased mortality in patients with severe heart failure (Table 12–4). Despite these limitations, infants awaiting cardiac transplantation have received the drug for up to 6 months without serious adverse effects.

VASODILATORS

The vasodilators used in treating heart failure include the angiotensin inhibitors and the combination of hydralazine and isosorbide dinitrate. The angiotensin inhibitors include the angiotensin-converting enzyme (ACE) inhibitors and the angiotensin receptor antagonists. Vasodilators are useful

TABLE 12-3. Adverse Effects, Contraindications, and Drug Interactions of Positively Inotropic Drugs

Drug	Common Adverse Effects	Common Drug Interactions
Digitalis Glycoside		
Digoxin	Anorexia, nausea, and vomiting; arrhythmias; blurred vision; chromatopsia; gynecomastia; and seizures.	Digitalis absorption inhibited by antacids and cholestyramine. Digitalis clearance reduced by diltiazem, quinidine, and verapamil. Diuretic-induced hypokalemia precipitates digitalis toxicity.
β-Adrenoceptor Agonist		
Dobutamine	Excessive vaso-constriction and tachyarrhythmias.	Activity affected by other agonists and antagonists.
Phosphodiesterase Inhibitor		
Milrinone	Arrhythmias; hypotension; and thrombocytopenia.	Unknown.

in the treatment of heart failure because of their ability to reduce venous and arterial pressure. The reduction in venous pressure decreases edema, while the dilation of arteries reduces cardiac afterload and increases cardiac output. In addition, the angiotensin inhibitors slow or reverse **cardiac remodeling**, which is probably responsible for their beneficial effect on the survival of patients with heart failure.

Angiotensin-Converting Enzyme Inhibitors

The ACE inhibitors reduce the formation of angiotensin II and are used in the treatment of **diabetic nephropathy, hypertension,** and **heart failure**. The general pharmacologic properties of these drugs are described in Chapter 10.

Angiotensin II has several actions that contribute to the pathogenesis of heart failure, including vasoconstriction and increased secretion of aldosterone and antidiuretic hormone. **Ramipril, enalapril, lisinopril,** and other ACE inhibitors act by producing venous and arterial dilation and decreasing the secretion of these two hormones. These actions in turn reduce the plasma volume, venous pressure, and level of edema, and they can increase cardiac output by reducing arterial pressure and cardiac afterload. In addition, ACE inhibitors can counteract the adverse effects of angiotensin that contribute to cardiac (ventricular) remodeling in patients with heart failure.

As described in Table 12–4, enalapril and other vasodilators have been shown to decrease the mortality rate in patients with heart failure. The Cooperative North Scandinavian Enalapril Survival Study (CONSENSUS) trial found that enalapril reduced the mortality rate by 40% in patients with **severe heart failure**. The Vasodilator Heart Failure Trial (V-HeFT-II) trial showed that treatment with enalapril reduced the mortality rate more than did treatment with the combination of a nitrate and hydralazine in patients with **chronic heart failure**. The Survival and Ventricular Enlargement (SAVE) and Studies of Left Ventricular Dysfunction (SOLVD) studies showed that treatment with captopril or enalapril can prevent the transition from asymptomatic to overt heart failure, thereby supporting the early use of an ACE inhibitor in patients with **asymptomatic heart failure**.

In patients with **acute myocardial infarction**, treatment with an ACE inhibitor has been found to improve the survival rate when it is administered within 24 hours of the onset of symptoms. Investigators believe that this benefit is partly caused by the inhibition of angiotensin II–induced cardiac remodeling, which would otherwise lead to cardiac dilatation, wall thinning, and expansion of the infarct zone in these patients.

Angiotensin Receptor Blockers

Angiotensin II receptor blockers (ARBs), such as valsartan and candesartan, selectively reduce the binding of angiotensin II to AT_1 receptors and have pharmacologic and clinical effects that are similar to those of the ACE inhibitors. Unlike ACE inhibitors, ARBs do not inhibit bradykinin degradation, an effect that may be responsible for some of the beneficial as well as adverse effects of ACE inhibitors (see Chapter 10). For example, ARBs do not induce chronic cough, an effect that occurs in 3% to 20% of persons treated with ACE inhibitors.

Clinical trials have found that valsartan and candesartan reduce mortality and hospitalization in persons with heart failure. The ARBs appear to be as effective as, or possibly slightly less effective than, ACE inhibitors in treating heart failure, and most authorities recommend that ARBs not be used in preference to an ACE inhibitor to treat heart failure. The ARBs are particularly indicated in patients with heart failure who cannot tolerate an ACE inhibitor, and valsartan is approved by the U.S. Food and Drug Administration for this indication. In addition, the Assessment of Reduction in Mortality and Morbidity (CHARM-Added) trial showed that patients receiving an ACE inhibitor benefited from the addition of an ARB, and some authorities recommend adding an ARB to heart failure therapy in patients who are stable on ACE inhibitors and β-blockers.

Hydralazine and Nitrates

Isosorbide dinitrate primarily relaxes venous smooth muscle, whereas hydralazine preferentially relaxes arterial smooth muscle. The combined use of these two drugs reduces cardiac preload and afterload, leading to reduced venous pressure and edema and to increased cardiac output, respectively. Hence, the effects of isosorbide dinitrate plus hydralazine are similar to those produced by the angiotensin inhibitors. The V-HeFT trials (see Table 12–4) found that this drug combination decreased mortality more than placebo but less than enalapril. For this reason, the hydralazine–isosorbide dinitrate combination is sometimes used

TABLE 12-4. **Findings in Clinical Studies of Drugs Used in the Treatment of Heart Failure**

Drug	Study	Findings
Positively Inotropic Drugs		
Amrinone (an early phosphodiesterase inhibitor)	Packer et al.[1]	Amrinone increased mortality rate in patients with severe heart failure.
Digoxin versus milrinone	BiBianco et al.[2]	Digoxin was superior to milrinone; milrinone caused arrhythmia in more patients.
Digoxin versus placebo	DIG[3]	Digoxin did not decrease mortality rate but decreased rate of hospitalization admissions for heart failure and other causes.
Digoxin withdrawal	PROVED[4] RADLANCE[5]	Clinical worsening of heart failure occurred with digoxin withdrawal. Clinical worsening of heart failure occurred with digoxin withdrawal.
Milrinone	PROMISE[6]	Milrinone increased mortality rate in patients with severe heart failure.
Vasodilators		
Captopril	SAVE[7]	Captopril decreased risk of congestive heart failure by 37% in post–myocardial infarction patients with left ventricular dysfunction.
Enalapril	CONSENSUS[8]	Enalapril decreased mortality rate by 40% at 6 months in patients with severe heart failure.
Enalapril	SOLVD[9]	Enalapril decreased mortality rate by 18% in patients with mild to moderate heart failure; also decreased risk of congestive heart failure by 37% in patients with asymptomatic left ventricular dysfunction.
Enalapril versus combination of nitrate plus hydralazine versus placebo	V-HeFT-II[10]	Enalapril decreased risk of sudden death by 36% in patients with chronic heart failure; nitrate plus hydralazine decreased mortality rate more than placebo did but less than enalapril did.
Other Drugs		
Carvedilol	AUZ-NZ[11]	Carvedilol decreased mortality rate and improved ejection fractions but did not change exercise tolerance or global assessment in patients with congestive heart failure.
Carvedilol	PRECISE[12]	Carvedilol increased exercise tolerance and improved ejection fractions in patients with congestive heart failure.
Carvedilol	US mild CHF[13]	Carvedilol decreased mortality rate, decreased rate of hospital admissions, increased exercise tolerance, and improved global assessment in patients with mild congestive heart failure.
Carvedilol versus metoprolol	COMET[14]	Carvedilol reduced mortality more than did metoprolol.
Candesartan plus ACE inhibitor	CHARM-Added[15]	Addition of candesartan reduced mortality.
Spironolactone	RALES[16]	Spironolactone decreased mortality 30% at 24 months.

ACE = angiotensin-converting enzyme.

[1]Packer, M., et al. Circulation 70:1038–1047, 1984.

[2]BiBianco, R., et al. N Engl J Med 320:677–683, 1989.

[3]Digitalis Investigational Group. N Engl J Med 336:525–533, 1997.

[4]Uretsky, B.F., et al. J Am Coll Cardiol 22:955–962, 1993.

[5]Packer, M., et al. N Engl J Med 329:1–7, 1993.

[6]Packer, M., et al. N Engl J Med 325:1468–1475, 1991.

[7]Pfeffer, M.A., et al. N Engl J Med 327:669–677, 1992.

[8]CONSENSUS Trial Study Group. N Engl J Med 316:1429–1435, 1987.

[9]SOLVD Investigators. N Engl J Med 325:293–302, 1991.

[10]Cohn, J.N., et al. N Engl J Med 325:293–302, 1991.

[11]Australia–New Zealand Heart Failure Research Collaborative Group. Lancet 349:375–380, 1997.

[12]Packer, M., et al. Circulation 94:2793–2799, 1996.

[13]Packer, M., et al. N Engl J Med 334:1349–1355, 1996.

[14]Poole-Wilson, P.A., et al. Lancet 362:7–13, 2003.

[15]McMurray, J.J., et al. Lancet 362:767–771, 2003.

[16]Pitt, B., et al. N Engl J Med 341:709–717, 1999.

to treat patients with heart failure who cannot tolerate an angiotensin inhibitor.

In the V-HeFT trials, black patients had a lesser benefit from ACE inhibitors than did whites, whereas the effect of hydralazine plus isosorbide dinitrate was greater in black patients. The recently completed African-American Heart Failure Trial provided further evidence of the beneficial effects of the combination of hydralazine and isosorbide dinitrate on the survival of black patients with heart failure.

Nesiritide

Nesiritide (NATRECOR) is a form of **human B–type natriuretic peptide** obtained from *Escherichia coli* using recombinant DNA technology. It is approved for the treatment of patients with acutely decompensated heart failure who have shortness of breath (dyspnea) at rest or with minimal activity.

Nesiritide binds to a guanylate cyclase receptor in vascular smooth muscle and endothelial cells, leading to increased intracellular concentrations of cyclic guanosine monophosphate (cGMP). Cyclic GMP acts as a second messenger to dilate venous and arterial smooth muscle, thereby leading to reductions in venous and arterial pressure in patients with heart failure. Clinical trials show that nesiritide reduced pulmonary capillary wedge pressure, a clinical measure of venous pressure and cardiac preload, and thereby decreased vascular congestion and dyspnea in decompensated patients with heart failure. The most common adverse effect of nesiritide is hypotension, although most cases were not symptomatic. Because nesiritide is a peptide drug, it must be given intravenously, and it is primarily eliminated by intracellular proteolysis. The drug can be used alone or with other standard therapies for heart failure.

β-ADRENOCEPTOR ANTAGONISTS

Once contraindicated in heart failure because of their negative inotropic effect, the β-adrenoceptor antagonists (β-blockers) have emerged as one of the newer treatments for this cardiac condition. This paradigm shift resulted from advances in the understanding of the role of the sympathetic nervous system in cardiac remodeling and the progression of heart failure.

Excessive sympathetic nervous system activity contributes to cardiac remodeling in several ways. Sympathetic activation of cardiac β-receptors produces tachycardia and increased oxygen demand, thereby increasing infarct size and the propensity for cardiac remodeling in persons with myocardial infarction. Sympathetic activation also increases activation of the renin-angiotensin-aldosterone system, whose role in cardiac remodeling is described above. In addition, chronic stimulation of cardiac β-receptors leads to both myocyte hypertrophy and apoptosis in a manner that contributes to cardiac dilatation and ventricular wall thinning. Finally, activation of the sympathetic system increases production of cardiac cytokines, including tumor necrosis factor-α and interleukins. These cytokines also induce myocyte hypertrophy and apoptosis and produce alterations in the intracellular matrix that contribute to fibrosis and ventricular wall stiffness.

The benefits of therapy with β-blockers are caused by the ability of these drugs to reduce excessive sympathetic stimulation of the heart and circulation in patients with heart failure. Several clinical trials have shown that some β-blockers, particularly carvedilol, metoprolol, and bisoprolol, benefit patients with mild to moderate heart failure caused by left ventricular systolic dysfunction.

Much of the attention concerning β-blocker therapy in heart failure has been focused on carvedilol. Carvedilol is a third-generation β- and β$_2$-blocker that also produces vasodilation via α$_1$-receptor blockade. In addition, carvedilol and its metabolites have antioxidant properties (described in Chapter 9), and it also exhibits anti-inflammatory and anti-apoptotic properties that can contribute to its beneficial effects in heart failure. For these reasons, carvedilol has been called a **multiple-action neurohumoral antagonist**.

In several clinical trials, carvedilol has been found to increase left ventricular ejection fraction, improve symptoms, and slow disease progression. These studies show that carvedilol reduces both hospitalization and mortality in persons with heart failure when it is added to a standard treatment regimen. Carvedilol is currently recommended for all patients with symptomatic heart failure who do not have significant hypotension, pulmonary congestion, or atrioventricular block. Patients should be monitored for the adverse effects of carvedilol, which include bradycardia, worsening heart failure, and dizziness or light-headedness caused by vasodilation and decreased blood pressure.

Metoprolol and bisoprolol have also been shown to produce beneficial effects in patients with heart failure. Some studies, however, suggest that these drugs are not as beneficial as carvedilol in some patients with heart failure. In the COMET study of patients with heart failure, carvedilol reduced mortality more than did metoprolol. This study has been criticized with respect to whether the doses of the β-blockers used in the study produced the same degree of β-blockade. Further clinical trials may help decide whether carvedilol is superior to other β-blockers.

The initiation of β-blocker therapy in patients with heart failure requires careful attention to dosage titration. Because the beneficial effects of β-blockers in heart failure have a delayed onset of action, whereas potential adverse cardiac effects can occur immediately, patients are started on low doses of a β-blocker and the dose is then gradually titrated upward every 2 to 3 weeks until the target dose is achieved over a period of several months. Patients should be monitored regularly during the titration period and informed that β-blockers can lead to increased symptoms for 4 to 10 weeks before any improvement is noted.

ALDOSTERONE ANTAGONISTS

Spironolactone (ALDACTONE) and eplerenone (INSPRA) are aldosterone antagonists that compete with aldosterone for the mineralocorticoid receptor in renal tubules and other tissues. These drugs act on the kidneys to increase sodium excretion, decrease potassium excretion, and exert a moderate diuretic effect. For this reason, spironolactone has been classified as a potassium-sparing diuretic; its pharmacologic properties and use are described in Chapter 13.

The Randomized ALDACTONE Evaluation Study (RALES) clinical trial found that spironolactone reduced mortality in persons with severe heart failure. This benefit has been attributed to the prevention of the adverse effects of excessive aldosterone levels on the heart and to an elevation of the serum potassium level. The survival benefits of these drugs were in addition to those provided by angiotensin inhibitors and β-blockers. Current guidelines recommend using an aldosterone antagonist only for the treatment of severe heart failure. Following the RALES study, many physicians began using aldosterone antagonists in patients with mild to moderate heart failure. The increased use of these drugs in elderly patients who may have renal insufficiency has been associated with about a 100% increase in the incidence of hospitalization and death caused by hyperkalemia. This illustrates one of the differences between clinical trials, in which patients are carefully selected and monitored, and typical medical care practices.

Aldosterone produces endocrine side effects resulting from its binding to androgen and progesterone receptors and leading to gynecomastia and impotence in some male patients. Eplerenone produces fewer endocrine side effects than spironolactone (1% vs. 10% in clinical trials). Eplerenone is much more expensive, however, and it seems reasonable to begin with spironolactone and switch to eplerenone if endocrine side effects develop.

DIURETICS

In patients with heart failure, diuretics are used to reduce plasma volume and edema and thereby relieve the symptoms of circulatory congestion such as shortness of breath (dyspnea).

Loop diuretics (e.g., **bumetanide, furosemide**, and **torsemide**) have more natriuretic activity than other types of diuretics and are the preferred diuretics for reducing plasma volume to control symptoms of circulatory congestion in most cases of heart failure. Loop diuretics must be used carefully to avoid excessive diuresis, dehydration, and electrolyte imbalances. Hypokalemia predisposes patients to digoxin toxicity, and patients with heart failure should be closely monitored for this condition. Thiazide diuretics can be used when a lesser degree of diuresis is required in the treatment of heart failure.

The pharmacologic properties of diuretics are described in Chapter 13.

MANAGEMENT OF HEART FAILURE

In patients with heart failure, the goals are to (1) relieve the symptoms of disease, (2) prevent disease progression, and (3) prolong survival. Acute heart failure may require hospitalization and the administration of intravenous vasodilators, positively inotropic drugs, diuretics, and oxygen. Once stabilized, patients with heart failure are usually managed with oral medications, dietary restrictions, and exercise guidelines (Box 12–1). Although bed rest may relieve symptoms of heart failure during the early course of therapy, many patients benefit from an incremental exercise program after their condition has been stabilized by medication.

The selection of medication for chronic heart failure depends on the severity of the condition and the particular signs and symptoms exhibited by the patient. The standard drug therapy for chronic heart failure caused by systolic dysfunction consists of the following types of medications: (1) an ACE inhibitor in combination with a β-adrenoceptor blocker to slow progression of heart failure and improve survival, (2) spironolactone or eplerenone (if spironolactone is not tolerated) to improve survival in persons with severe heart failure or with left ventricular dysfunction after an acute myocardial infarction, (3) a loop diuretic to reduce plasma volume and thereby control edema and shortness of breath, and (4) digoxin to improve symptoms of weakness and fatigue caused by low cardiac output and to reduce the need for hospitalization.

Angiotensin receptor blockers can be used in persons who cannot tolerate an ACE inhibitor, and some patients taking ACE inhibitors benefit from the addition of an ARB to the drug regimen. Several other classes of drugs are currently under investigation, and the treatment of heart failure will continue to evolve as new drugs with unique mechanisms of action are developed.

BOX 12–1 A CASE OF DYSPNEA UPON EXERTION

CASE PRESENTATION: A 70-year-old woman complains to her physician of shortness of breath and fatigue while climbing stairs. She has a history of hypertension and coronary artery disease treated with diltiazem. She smoked cigarettes for many years but quit 5 years ago. On physical exam, her pulse is 85 beats per minute and regular, her respiration rate is 25 breaths per minute, and her blood pressure is 138 over 84 mm Hg. Her chest radiograph shows mild cardiomegaly and pulmonary edema, and echocardiography reveals left ventricular dilatation with an ejection fraction of 40%. Her serum electrolytes are normal, but her total and LDL (low-density lipoprotein) cholesterol levels are elevated. She is hospitalized and treated with oxygen and intravenous administration of furosemide and enalaprilat, and her symptoms gradually improve. Long-term management will include lisinopril, gradually increasing doses of carvedilol, and simvastatin. She will be referred to a dietitian for guidance in planning a diet low in sodium, saturated fat, and cholesterol, and she is enrolled in a structured exercise program.

CASE DISCUSSION: Heart failure is the most frequent cause of hospitalization in U.S. patients older than 65 years, and the disease is responsible for over 250,000 deaths per year. Despite recent advances in the treatment of heart failure, morbidity and mortality remain high. In systolic heart failure, the heart is dilated and the ejection fraction is less than 50%. Diuretics reduce pulmonary edema and are the only treatment that acutely produces symptomatic benefits and improves exercise capacity. ACE inhibitors should be used by all patients with heart failure because they improve survival and quality of life. β-Blockers improve clinical outcomes over time and decrease mortality and should be used in heart failure patients who are stable on ACE inhibitors. Exercise programs improve physical and psychological well-being and can increase maximal oxygen consumption (VO_2) in medically stable heart failure patients.

SUMMARY OF IMPORTANT POINTS

■ Heart failure is a common manifestation of coronary heart disease, chronic hypertension, valvular disorders, and other cardiovascular conditions.

■ Angiotensin inhibitors and β-adrenoceptor blockers attenuate cardiac remodeling and disease progression while increasing cardiac output and survival in persons with heart failure.

■ In patients with heart failure, digoxin increases cardiac contractility and cardiac output and reduces symptoms of weakness and fatigue and the need for hospitalization.

■ Digoxin augments parasympathetic tone and thereby slows the AV node conduction velocity and increases the AV node refractory period. These actions slow the ventricular rate in patients with atrial fibrillation.

■ Digoxin is primarily eliminated by renal excretion and has a relatively long half-life.

■ The adverse gastrointestinal, cardiac, and neurologic effects of digoxin include anorexia, nausea, vomiting, arrhythmias, blurred vision, chromatopsia, and seizures.

■ Digoxin immune Fab can be used to treat life-threatening digoxin toxicity.

■ Loop-acting diuretics are used to mobilize edematous fluid in patients with heart failure.

■ Positively inotropic drugs (e.g., dobutamine) and vasodilators (e.g., nesiritide, a recombinant human B–type natriuretic peptide) are used in the treatment of acute decompensated heart failure.

Review Questions

1. Which process is most directly involved in cardiac remodeling in heart failure?
   (A) decompensation
   (B) myocyte apoptosis
   (C) venous congestion
   (D) sodium and water retention
   (E) increased afterload

2. A man is brought to the emergency department complaining of nausea and vomiting, blurred and abnormally-colored vision, and palpitations. Which drug is most likely responsible for these effects?
   (A) dobutamine
   (B) lisinopril
   (C) digoxin
   (D) milrinone
   (E) furosemide

3. Which drug has been demonstrated to increase survival in persons with heart failure?
   (A) furosemide
   (B) carvedilol
   (C) milrinone
   (D) digoxin
   (E) hydralazine-isosorbide dinitrate

4. A woman is given a recombinant form of a human natriuretic peptide. Which mechanism is responsible for the cardiovascular effects of this drug?
   (A) inhibition of adenylyl cyclase
   (B) stimulation of adenylyl cyclase
   (C) inhibition of guanylyl cyclase
   (D) stimulation of guanylyl cyclase
   (E) inhibition of phosphodiesterase, type III

Answers and Explanations

1. **The correct answer is B: myocyte apoptosis.** Cardiac remodeling in heart failure is characterized by ventricular wall thinning, collagen production, fibrosis, and cardiac dilatation. Myocyte apoptosis (programmed cell death) contributes to wall thinning and impaired systolic function. The other options (A,C,D, and E) are partly the result of cardiac remodeling.

2. **The correct answer is C: digoxin.** Excessive doses of digitalis glycosides cause nausea and vomiting, visual disturbances, and cardiac arrhythmias. Dobutamine and milrinone (Options A and D) may also cause cardiac arrhythmias but do not typically caused blurred vision, nausea, and vomiting. Lisinopril and furosemide (Options B and E) do not usually cause any of these adverse effects.

3. **The correct answer is B: carvedilol.** Carvedilol, a third generation β-blocker, has been shown to improve cardiac performance, reduce symptoms, slow disease progression and increase survival in heart failure. Angiotensin inhibitors also increase cardiac output and reduce mortality. Inotropic agents (Options C and D), diuretics (Option A), and hydralazine-isosorbide dinitrate (Option E) improve symptoms but have not been shown to increase survival.

4. **The correct answer is D: stimulation of guanylyl cyclase.** The woman was most likely given nesiritide, a recombinant form of type B human natriuretic peptide. This drug activates guanylyl cyclase in vascular smooth muscle and endothelial cells, leading to increased cyclic GMP and vasodilation. Nesiritide is used to treat acutely decompensated heart failure (heart failure in which the stroke volume is no longer proportional to the diastolic fiber length). Vasodilation reduces congestion and dyspnea in these patients.

SELECTED READINGS

Hasselblad, V., W. Gattis Stough, M.R. Shah, Y. Lokhnygina, C.M. O'Connor, et al. Relation between dose of loop diuretics and outcomes in a heart failure population: results of the ESCAPE trial. Eur J Heart Fail 9:1064–1069, 2007.

McMahon, C.J., H. Murchan, T. Prendiville, and M. Burch. Long-term support with milrinone prior to cardiac transplantation in a neonate with left ventricular noncompaction cardiomyopathy. Pediatr Cardiol 28:317–318, 2007.

Parissis, J.T., D. Farmakis, and M. Nieminen. Classical inotropes and new cardiac enhancers. Heart Fail Rev 12:149–156, 2007.

Sica, D.A., T.W. Gehr, and W.H. Frishman. Use of diuretics in the treatment of heart failure in the elderly. Heart Fail Clin 3:455–464, 2007.

CHAPTER 13

Diuretics

CLASSIFICATION OF DIURETICS

Thiazide and Related Diuretics
- Hydrochlorothiazide
- Indapamide (LOZOL)
- Metolazone

Loop Diuretics
- Ethacrynic Acid (EDECRIN)
- Furosemide (LASIX)*

Potassium-Sparing Diuretics
- Amiloride (MIDAMOR)
- Spironolactone (ALDACTONE)
- Triamterene (DYRENIUM)

Osmotic Diuretics
- Glycerol
- Mannitol

Carbonic Anhydrase Inhibitors
- Acetazolamide (DIAMOX)
- Dorzolamide (TRUSOPT)

Antidiuretic Hormone Antagonist
- Conivaptan (VAPRISOL)

*Also bumetanide (BUMEX) and torsemide (DEMADEX).

OVERVIEW

Diuretics are used in the management of edema associated with cardiovascular, renal, and endocrine abnormalities, as well as in the treatment of hypertension, glaucoma, and several other clinical disorders (Table 13–1). The drugs act at various sites in the nephron to cause **diuresis** (an increase in urine production). Most diuretics inhibit the reabsorption of sodium from the nephron into the circulation and thereby cause an increase in **natriuresis** (the excretion of sodium in the urine). Several types of diuretics also cause an increase in **kaliuresis** (the excretion of potassium in the urine). Diuretics also affect the excretion of magnesium, calcium, chloride, and bicarbonate ions.

NEPHRON FUNCTION AND SITES OF DRUG ACTION

Sodium and other electrolytes are reabsorbed into the circulation at various sites throughout the nephron by active and passive processes that involve **ion channels, transport proteins**, and the **sodium pump** (Na^+,K^+-ATPase). Ion channels are unique membrane proteins through which a specific ion moves across the cell membrane in the direction that is determined by the electrochemical gradient for the ion. The transport proteins include **symporters**, which transport two or more ions in the same direction, and **antiporters**, which transport ions in opposite directions across cell membranes. Most diuretics act by blocking a specific ion channel or transporter in the tubular epithelial cells. The effects of diuretics on ion reabsorption and secretion in the nephron are illustrated in Box 13–1.

Glomerular Filtration

Urine formation begins with glomerular filtration, a process in which an ultrafiltrate of blood is forced out of the glomerular capillaries and into the nephron lumen by the hydrostatic pressure in these capillaries. In healthy individuals, this filtrate is essentially free of blood cells and plasma proteins. **Digitalis glycosides** and other cardiac stimulants can indirectly cause diuresis by increasing cardiac output, renal blood flow, and the glomerular filtration rate. The renal actions of these drugs are described in greater detail in Chapter 12. The diuretic drugs described in this chapter do not increase the glomerular filtration rate, and some of them may indirectly reduce it by decreasing plasma volume and renal blood flow.

Proximal Tubule

The proximal tubule is an important site of tubular reabsorption and secretion. Essentially all of the filtered glucose, amino acids, and other organic solutes are reabsorbed in the early portion of the proximal tubule. About 85% of filtered sodium bicarbonate is reabsorbed in the proximal tubule, and this reabsorption is inhibited by a class of diuretics known as **carbonic anhydrase inhibitors**. For reasons described later in this chapter, these drugs are relatively weak diuretics and are seldom used for this purpose, although their actions are useful in the treatment of glaucoma and other conditions.

About 40% of filtered sodium chloride is reabsorbed in the proximal tubule. This is a relatively unimportant site of diuretic action, however, because inhibition of sodium chloride reabsorption in the proximal tubule almost invariably leads to increased sodium chloride reabsorption in more distal segments of the nephron.

The proximal tubule is the major site of the active tubular secretion of organic acids and bases into the nephron lumen, including natural compounds (e.g., uric acid) and drugs (e.g., penicillins). The **loop diuretics** and **thiazide diuretics** are also secreted by proximal tubular cells, and then these drugs are carried in the tubular fluid to their site of action in the loop of Henle and the distal tubule, respectively.

Loop of Henle

The loop of Henle is responsible for the reabsorption of about 35% of the filtered sodium chloride. This segment also participates in the formation of a concentrated urine by transporting sodium chloride into the surrounding interstitium, where

---

TABLE 13-1. **Usefulness of Diuretics in the Management of Various Clinical Disorders***

Disorder	Thiazide and Related Diuretics	Loop Diuretics	Potassium-Sparing Diuretics	Osmotic Diuretics	Carbonic Anhydrase Inhibitors
Cerebral edema	0	0	0	+	0
Cirrhosis	+	++	+	0	0
Congestive heart failure	+	++	+	0	0
Diabetes insipidus	++	0	0	0	0
Epilepsy	0	0	0	0	+
Glaucoma	0	0	0	+	++
High-altitude sickness	0	0	0	0	++
Hyperaldosteronism	0	0	+	0	0
Hypercalcemia	0	++	0	0	0
Hypertension	++	+	+	0	0
Hypokalemia	0	0	++	0	0
Nephrolithiasis	++	0	0	0	0
Nephrotic syndrome	+	++	+	0	0
Pulmonary edema	+	++	+	0	0
Renal impairment	+	++	0	+	0

*Ratings range from 0 (not useful) to ++ (highly useful).

BOX 13-1   SITES AND MECHANISMS OF ACTION OF DIURETICS

In the proximal tubule (**A**), carbonic anhydrase catalyzes the reversible conversion of hydrogen ion and bicarbonate to carbon dioxide and water, thereby enabling the reabsorption of sodium bicarbonate. This process is inhibited by **carbonic anhydrase inhibitors**, such as **acetazolamide**.

In the thick ascending limb of the loop of Henle (**B**), the $Na^+,K^+,2Cl^-$ symporter transports sodium, potassium, and chloride ions into the tubular cells, and then sodium is transferred to the interstitial fluid by the sodium pump. Potassium back-diffuses into the lumen and contributes to the positive transepithelial potential that drives paracellular calcium and magnesium reabsorption. By inhibiting the symporter, the **loop diuretics** reduce the back-diffusion of potassium and increase the excretion of calcium and magnesium.

In the distal tubule (**C**), sodium is transported into tubular epithelial cells by the Na^+,Cl^- symporter and then is transferred to interstitial fluid by the sodium pump. The Na^+,Cl^- symporter is inhibited by **thiazide and related diuretics**.

In the collecting duct (**D**), sodium enters the principal cells through sodium channels. Sodium is then transferred into the interstitial fluid by the sodium pump, while potassium is pumped in the opposite direction and then moves through potassium channels into the tubular fluid. Aldosterone stimulates these processes by increasing the synthesis of messenger RNA that encodes for sodium channel and sodium pump proteins. The **potassium-sparing diuretics** exert their effects via two mechanisms: **amiloride** and **triamterene** inhibit the entrance of sodium into the principal cells, whereas **spironolactone** blocks the mineralocorticoid receptor and thereby inhibits sodium reabsorption and potassium secretion.

A = antiporter; ALDO = aldosterone; CA = carbonic anhydrase; MR = mineralocorticoid receptor; mRNA = messenger RNA; S = symporter.

(Continued)

BOX 13-1   SITES AND MECHANISMS OF ACTION OF DIURETICS—cont'd

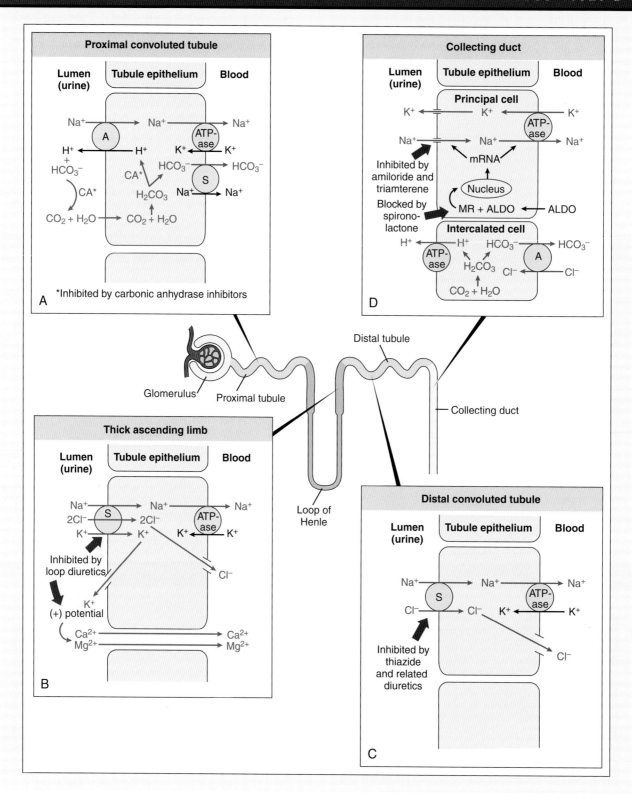

a hypertonic interstitial fluid is formed. This fluid attracts water from the collecting duct under the influence of antidiuretic hormone. The reabsorption of sodium from the thick ascending limb is inhibited by **loop diuretics**, which produce a greater diuretic effect than any other class of diuretics.

Distal Tubule

The early distal tubule is responsible for the reabsorption of 5% to 10% of the filtered sodium chloride, and this reabsorption is inhibited by **thiazide and related diuretics**. Because a relatively small percentage of sodium reabsorption can be inhibited by these drugs, they have a more modest diuretic action than the loop diuretics.

Collecting Duct

The collecting duct serves to adjust the final composition and volume of urine to regulate extracellular fluid composition and pH and thereby maintain physiologic homeostasis. The collecting duct is the site of action of **aldosterone** and **antidiuretic hormone**. Aldosterone is a mineralocorticoid that increases sodium reabsorption, thereby promoting sodium retention by the body. Antidiuretic hormone increases the reabsorption of water from the collecting duct, which conserves body water and concentrates the urine. The actions of these hormones are partly responsible for maintaining plasma volume and osmolality in the normal range.

The collecting duct is responsible for the reabsorption of about 3% of the filtered sodium chloride. This reabsorption is coupled with potassium and hydrogen excretion. The **potassium-sparing diuretics** inhibit these processes and are used to reduce potassium excretion and prevent hypokalemia.

DIURETIC AGENTS

Thiazide and Related Diuretics

The thiazides and related diuretics are the most commonly used diuretics. They are orally efficacious, have a moderate natriuretic effect, and have few adverse effects in most patients.

Drug Properties

CHEMISTRY AND PHARMACOKINETICS. Thiazides are sulfonamide compounds that contain a benzothiadiazide (thiazide) moiety. They exhibit good oral bioavailability and were the first orally administered diuretics to be widely used for the treatment of hypertension and edema. Thiazides are actively secreted into the nephron by proximal tubular cells, and they travel through the nephron lumen to reach their site of action in the distal tubule. Some of the thiazides are partially metabolized before excretion in the urine (Table 13–2).

TABLE 13-2. Pharmacokinetic Properties of Diuretics*

Drug	Oral Bioavailability	Elimination Half-Life (Hours)	Route of Elimination	Duration of Action (Hours)
Thiazide and Related Diuretics				
Hydrochlorothiazide	70%	5	60% R and 40% M	12 for oral
Indapamide	90%	16	70% R and 30% M	30 for oral
Metolazone	65%	8	80% R and 20% M	18 for oral
Loop Diuretics				
Bumetanide	85%	1.25	65% R and 35% M	5 for oral 1 for IV
Ethacrynic acid	100%	1	65% R and 35% M	7 for oral 2 for IV
Furosemide	60%	2	60% R and 40% M	7 for oral 2 for IV
Torsemide	80%	3.5	30% R and 70% M	7 for oral 7 for IV
Potassium-Sparing Diuretics				
Amiloride	20%	8	R	24 for oral
Spironolactone	65%	1.5	M	60 for oral
Triamterene	50%	4	M	14 for oral
Osmotic Diuretics				
Glycerol	95%	0.07	M	1 for oral
Mannitol	NA	1	R	7 for IV
Carbonic anhydrase inhibitors				
Acetazolamide	70%	7.5	R	10 for oral
Dorzolamide	NA	Biphasic†	R and M	8 for topical

*Values shown are the mean of values reported in the literature.
†Dorzolamide is eliminated in a biphasic manner, with a rapid decline in serum levels followed by a much slower release from erythrocytes, and has a half-life of 4 months.
IV = intravenous; M = metabolism; NA = not applicable (not administered orally); R = renal; U = unknown.

MECHANISMS AND PHARMACOLOGIC EFFECTS. Thiazide diuretics act primarily on the early portion of the distal tubule to inhibit the Na^+,Cl^- symporter that participates in the reabsorption of sodium and chloride from this segment of the nephron (see Box 13–1). This action leads to the delivery of a greater volume of sodium chloride-enriched tubular fluid to the late distal tubule and collecting duct, which in turn stimulates the exchange of sodium and potassium at these sites. In the process, a small amount of sodium is reabsorbed as potassium is secreted into urine in the tubules. By this mechanism, thiazides have a kaliuretic effect that leads to hypokalemia in some patients.

As shown in Table 13–3, thiazides increase magnesium excretion, but (unlike many diuretics) they decrease calcium excretion in the urine. The hypocalciuria induced by thiazides appears to result from decreased expression of calcium transport proteins, including the epithelial calcium channel, calbindin, and the sodium-calcium exchanger protein, in renal tubules. The ability of thiazides to reduce calcium excretion is the basis for their use in the treatment of kidney stones caused by excessive calcium in the urine.

ADVERSE EFFECTS AND INTERACTIONS. Table 13–4 lists the common adverse effects and interactions of thiazides and other diuretics.

Thiazide diuretics sometimes cause hypokalemia, particularly in patients whose dietary potassium intake is inadequate. Hypokalemia can eventually lead to hypokalemic metabolic alkalosis (Fig. 13–1). In this disorder, hydrogen ions enter body cells as potassium leaves these cells in an attempt to correct the plasma potassium deficiency. As the plasma potassium level falls, more hydrogen ions are secreted into urine in the tubules in exchange for sodium, and this further contributes to the development of metabolic alkalosis. In cases of hypokalemic metabolic alkalosis, potassium chloride is administered intravenously and orally. Correction of the serum potassium level then leads to correction of the acid-base disturbance as potassium displaces hydrogen ions from body cells and fewer hydrogen ions are secreted by the collecting duct.

In addition to causing electrolyte and acid-base disturbances, the thiazides can cause several metabolic abnormalities, including elevated blood glucose, uric acid, and lipid levels. An increase in blood glucose levels can be caused, in part, by diuretic-induced potassium deficiency, because hypokalemia reduces the secretion of insulin by pancreatic β-cells and thereby increases plasma glucose concentrations. Hyperuricemia, which is caused by inhibition of uric acid secretion from the proximal tubule, can lead to the development of gout. The effects of thiazide diuretics on serum lipid levels are discussed in greater detail in Chapter 10.

INDICATIONS. Thiazide diuretics are widely used in the management of cardiovascular and renal diseases (see Table 13–1). They are often prescribed for **hypertension** and can be used to treat **edema** associated with **heart failure, cirrhosis, corticosteroid and estrogen therapy,** and **renal disorders** such as **nephrotic syndrome.** Because thiazides reduce calcium excretion and decrease urinary calcium levels, they are helpful in treating patients with **nephrolithiasis** (kidney stones) associated with **hypercalciuria.**

Thiazides are also used to treat nephrogenic **diabetes insipidus.** In this disorder, the kidneys are not responsive to circulating antidiuretic hormone, and patients may excrete from 10 to 20 L of urine per day. Thiazides exert a paradoxical antidiuretic effect in these patients and reduce the excessive urine volume dramatically. In cases of diabetes insipidus, the effectiveness of thiazides is believed to stem from a reduction in plasma volume caused by these drugs. The reduced plasma volume serves to increase sodium and water reabsorption from the proximal tubule, so that less water is delivered to the diluting segments of the nephron. As a result, the urine output falls.

Hydrochlorothiazide

The several thiazide compounds that are available have almost identical actions but differ in their potency and pharmacokinetic properties. Hydrochlorothiazide is the most frequently prescribed thiazide diuretic.

Thiazide-like Diuretics

Several thiazide-like diuretics exist whose structures are slightly different from those of the thiazide compounds but whose actions and uses are generally similar. One of them is **indapamide,** an agent primarily used to treat **hypertension** and **heart failure.** Another is **metolazone,** a diuretic that may be more effective than thiazide compounds in the treatment of patients with **impaired renal function.** Metolazone is sometimes combined with a loop diuretic to treat patients with **diuretic resistance.** Patients with diuretic resistance do not adequately respond to any single diuretic agent, but they may respond to the combination of a thiazide-like diuretic and a loop diuretic. The combined use of these diuretics produces **sequential nephron blockade,** in which the drugs inhibit the reabsorption of sodium in the ascending limb and the early distal tubule.

TABLE 13–3. Effects of Diuretics on Plasma pH and Urinary Excretion of Electrolytes*

Drug	Plasma pH	ELECTROLYTES EXCRETED				
		Ca^{2+}	HCO_3^-	K^+	Mg^{2+}	Na^+
Thiazide and related diuretics	0 or +	–	0 or +	++	++	++
Loop diuretics	0 or +	++	0	++	++	+++
Potassium-sparing diuretics	0 or –	–	0	–	–	+
Osmotic diuretics	0	+	+	+	++	+++
Carbonic anhydrase inhibitors	–	0 or +	+++	+	–	+

*Acute effects are shown and are indicated as follows: decrease (–); no change or variable (0); and increase ranging from small (+) to large (+++).

TABLE 13-4. Adverse Effects and Drug Interactions of Diuretics

Drug	Common Adverse Effects	Common Drug Interactions
Thiazide and Related Diuretics		
Hydrochlorothiazide	Blood cell deficiencies; electrolyte imbalances; and increased blood cholesterol, glucose, or uric acid levels.	Potentiates the diuretic effect of loop diuretics.
Indapamide	Electrolyte imbalances and increased blood cholesterol, glucose, or uric acid levels.	Same as hydrochlorothiazide.
Metolazone	Blood cell deficiencies; electrolyte imbalances; and increased blood cholesterol or glucose levels.	Same as hydrochlorothiazide.
Loop Diuretics		
Bumetanide	Blood cell deficiencies; electrolyte imbalances; hearing impairment; and hypersensitivity reactions.	Diuretic effect decreased by NSAIDs. Administration with ACE inhibitors may cause excessive hypotension.
Ethacrynic acid	Blood cell deficiencies; electrolyte imbalances; hearing impairment; and rash.	Diuretic effect decreased by NSAIDs.
Furosemide	Blood cell deficiencies; electrolyte imbalances; hearing impairment; hypersensitivity reactions; increased blood cholesterol, glucose, or uric acid levels; and photosensitivity.	Same as bumetanide.
Torsemide	Electrolyte imbalances and increased blood cholesterol, glucose, or uric acid levels.	Same as bumetanide.
Potassium-Sparing Diuretics		
Amiloride	Blood cell deficiencies; gastrointestinal distress; and hyperkalemia.	Administration with ACE inhibitors or potassium supplements may cause hyperkalemia. Administration with NSAIDs may cause renal failure.
Spironolactone	Gynecomastia; hyperkalemia; and impotence.	Administration with ACE inhibitors or potassium supplements may cause hyperkalemia.
Triamterene	Same as amiloride.	Same as amiloride.
Osmotic Diuretics		
Glycerol	Heart failure; nausea and vomiting; and pulmonary congestion and edema.	Potentiates effects of other diuretics.
Mannitol	Same as glycerol.	Same as glycerol.
Carbonic Anhydrase Inhibitors		
Acetazolamide	Blood cell deficiencies; drowsiness; hepatic insufficiency; hyperglycemia; hypokalemia; metabolic acidosis; paresthesia, and uremia.	Serum levels of weak bases, such as amphetamine, ephedrine, and quinidine, are increased by CA inhibitors. Serum levels of CA inhibitors are increased by salicylates.
Dorzolamide	Bitter taste; blurred vision; ocular discomfort and allergic reactions.	Unknown.

ACE = angiotensin-converting enzyme; CA = carbonic anhydrase; NSAIDs = nonsteroidal anti-inflammatory drugs.

Loop Diuretics

Drug Properties

CHEMISTRY AND PHARMACOKINETICS. With the exception of ethacrynic acid, loop-acting diuretics contain a sulfonamide moiety but lack the thiadiazide structure found in thiazide diuretics. The pharmacokinetic properties of loop diuretics are summarized in Table 13–2.

MECHANISMS AND PHARMACOLOGIC EFFECTS. Loop diuretics inhibit the $Na^+,K^+,2Cl^-$ symporter in the ascending limb of the loop of Henle and thereby exert a powerful natriuretic effect. In comparison with other diuretics, loop diuretics can inhibit the reabsorption of a greater percentage of filtered sodium. Loop diuretics are sometimes called **high-ceiling diuretics** because they produce a dose-dependent diuresis throughout their clinical dosage range. This property can be contrasted with the rather flat dose-response curve and limited diuretic efficacy of thiazides and other diuretic drugs (Fig. 13–2).

In addition to their natriuretic effect, the loop diuretics produce kaliuresis by increasing the exchange of sodium and potassium in the late distal tubule and collecting duct via the same mechanisms as those described for the thiazide diuretics. Loop diuretics also increase magnesium and calcium excretion by reducing the reabsorption of these ions in the ascending limb (see Box 13–1). This action results from inhibition of the $Na^+,K^+,2Cl^-$ symporter, which reduces the back-diffusion of potassium into the nephron lumen. The reduction of potassium back-diffusion decreases the transepithelial electrical potential that normally drives the paracellular reabsorption of magnesium and calcium. Inhibition of this process thereby increases magnesium and calcium excretion.

ADVERSE EFFECTS AND INTERACTIONS. Loop diuretics can produce a variety of electrolyte abnormalities, including hypokalemia, hypocalcemia, hypomagnesemia, and metabolic alkalosis. These diuretics can also increase blood glucose and uric acid levels in the same manner as the thiazide diuretics. In some

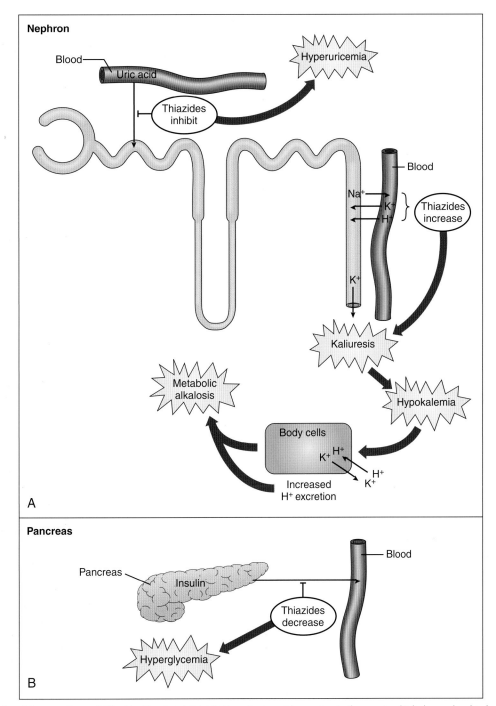

Figure 13-1. Adverse effects of thiazide diuretics. (A) Inhibition of uric acid secretion in the proximal tubule can lead to hyperuricemia and gout. Increased potassium secretion in the collecting duct can cause hypokalemia. Hypokalemia can lead to metabolic alkalosis by promoting the exchange of intracellular potassium for hydrogen ions and by increasing the excretion of hydrogen ions. The increased excretion is caused by lack of availability of potassium for exchange with sodium in the collecting duct. (B) In the presence of hypokalemia, the amount of insulin secreted by the pancreas can be reduced, thereby leading to hyperglycemia. Other mechanisms can also be involved in the development of hyperglycemia.

patients, use of loop diuretics causes ototoxicity with manifestations such as tinnitus, ear pain, vertigo, and hearing deficits. In most cases, the hearing loss is reversible. Other adverse effects and drug interactions are listed in Table 13–4.

INDICATIONS. Loop diuretics are used when intensive diuresis is required and cannot be achieved with other diuretics. Loop

diuretics are highly effective in the treatment of pulmonary edema, partly because of the vasodilation that occurs when they are administered intravenously. They are the preferred diuretics in the treatment of persons with renal impairment, because (unlike thiazide and other diuretics) they are effective in patients whose creatinine clearance drops below 30 mL/min. Loop diuretics are often the drugs of choice for patients with

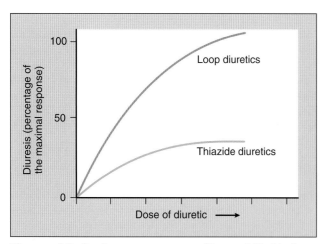

Figure 13-2. Dose-response curves of loop and thiazide diuretics. Loop diuretics produce dose-dependent diuresis throughout their therapeutic dosage range, whereas thiazide diuretics have a relatively flat dose-response curve and a limited maximal response.

edema caused by heart failure, cirrhosis, and other disorders. Although they are prescribed for patients with hypertension, the thiazide diuretics are usually preferred for this condition. Loop diuretics can be used to treat hypercalcemia, whereas the thiazide diuretics can increase serum calcium levels slightly.

Bumetanide, Furosemide, and Torsemide

Bumetanide, furosemide, and torsemide are sulfonamide derivatives with similar pharmacologic actions and effects. These drugs can be administered orally or intravenously. In comparison with other loop diuretics, torsemide has a somewhat longer half-life and a significantly longer duration of action after intravenous administration (see Table 13–2). All three of the drugs are partly metabolized before they are excreted in the urine.

Ethacrynic Acid

Ethacrynic acid is the only loop diuretic that is not a sulfonamide derivative. It is available for use when patients are hypersensitive to other drugs in this class. Otherwise, it is seldom used because it produces more ototoxicity than do the other loop diuretics.

Potassium-Sparing Diuretics

Two types of potassium-sparing diuretics exist: the epithelial sodium channel blockers and the aldosterone receptor antagonists.

Amiloride and Triamterene

Amiloride and triamterene are epithelial sodium channel antagonists. By blocking the entry of sodium into the principal tubular cells of the late distal tubule and collecting duct (see Box 13–1), these drugs prevent sodium reabsorption at this site and indirectly reduce the secretion of potassium into the tubular filtrate and urine. Through these actions,

the potassium-sparing diuretics produce a modest amount of natriuresis while decreasing kaliuresis, and they are primarily used to prevent and treat **hypokalemia** induced by thiazide and loop diuretics. The properties, effects, and uses of amiloride, triamterene, and other potassium-sparing diuretics are outlined in Tables 13–1 to 13–4.

The most characteristic adverse effect of the potassium-sparing diuretics is hyperkalemia, but this is unlikely to occur unless the patient also ingests potassium supplements or other drugs that increase serum potassium levels (e.g., angiotensin antagonists) or unless the patient has a renal disorder that predisposes to hyperkalemia.

Spironolactone

Spironolactone, a steroid congener of aldosterone, competitively blocks the binding of aldosterone to the mineralocorticoid receptor in tubular epithelial cells of the late distal convoluted tubule and collecting duct. Normally, the mineralocorticoid receptor is activated by aldosterone and then interacts with nuclear DNA to promote the transcription of genes that encode proteins of the epithelial sodium channels, sodium pump, and related compounds involved in the reabsorption of sodium and secretion of potassium in these tubular segments. By blocking these actions, spironolactone reduces sodium reabsorption and the coupled secretion of potassium.

Spironolactone is adequately absorbed from the gut and has a long duration of action, despite its short elimination half-life, indicating that its cellular actions persist longer than its circulating drug levels (see Table 13–2). Spironolactone is used to prevent hypokalemia in the same manner as amiloride and triamterene, and it has a special role in the treatment of primary hyperaldosteronism. Clinical trials have shown that spironolactone reduces mortality in persons with heart failure, as described in Chapter 12. Its use in this condition, however, has been associated with an increased incidence of hyperkalemia. Because of its antiandrogenic effect, spironolactone is also used in the treatment of polycystic ovary disease and hirsutism in women.

The adverse effects of spironolactone include gynecomastia and impotence in men (caused by the drug's antiandrogenic effects) and hyperkalemia. Eplerenone is a new aldosterone antagonist that produces less endocrine side effects than does spironolactone. Eplerenone is used to counteract the effects of excessive aldosterone in persons with heart failure (see Chapter 12).

Osmotic Diuretics

Glycerol and **mannitol** are examples of osmotic diuretics. These diuretics increase the osmotic pressure of the plasma and thereby attract water from interstitial and transcellular fluids. Because of this action, mannitol is used to treat **cerebral edema** and reduce intracranial pressure. Glycerol and mannitol are both used in the treatment of **acute glaucoma**. By attracting water from ocular fluids into the circulation, the drugs reduce intraocular volume and pressure. Glycerol is administered orally for this purpose, whereas mannitol is administered intravenously.

Mannitol is also used as a diuretic. Following intravenous administration, it is filtered at the glomerulus but is not

reabsorbed from the renal tubules. It osmotically attracts and retains water as it moves through the nephron and into the urine. This action reduces the tubular sodium concentration and the concentration gradient between the tubular fluid and cells and thereby retards the reabsorption of sodium. Hence, mannitol has both direct and indirect actions that promote diuresis. The diuretic effect of mannitol has been used to improve renal function in the oliguric phase of **acute renal failure**. Evidence for a renoprotective effect of mannitol has been obtained in studies of persons having renal transplantation.

Mannitol has also been administered along with intravenous fluids to maintain renal function and reduce the renal toxicity of antineoplastic platinum compounds (e.g., cisplatin), and mannitol is used to promote the renal excretion of toxic substances in cases of drug overdose or poisoning.

The primary adverse effect of mannitol is excessive plasma volume expansion, which is most likely to occur if the drug is administered too rapidly or with too large a volume of intravenous fluid. Excessive plasma volume can lead to heart failure and pulmonary congestion and edema in susceptible patients.

Carbonic Anhydrase Inhibitors

Drug Properties

The carbonic anhydrase (CA) inhibitors were the first sulfonamide derivatives to be used as diuretics, and their discovery eventually led to the development of the thiazide and loop diuretics. **Acetazolamide, dorzolamide**, and other CA inhibitors are relatively weak diuretics and are seldom used for this purpose today. Instead, their ability to inhibit CA has led to their use in the treatment of disorders such as high-altitude sickness and glaucoma.

Specific Drugs

PHARMACOKINETICS. Acetazolamide is one of several orally administered CA inhibitors, whereas dorzolamide is used as an ophthalmic solution to treat glaucoma. Dorzolamide is partly absorbed from the eye into the circulation and undergoes some metabolic transformation before it is excreted in the urine. The drug is eliminated in a biphasic manner, with a rapid decline in serum levels followed by a much slower release from erythrocytes, and it has a half-life of 4 months. The pharmacokinetic properties of acetazolamide and dorzolamide are outlined in Table 13–2.

MECHANISMS, PHARMACOLOGIC EFFECTS, AND INDICATIONS. Acetazolamide and other drugs in this class inhibit CA throughout the body. This enzyme catalyzes the conversion of carbon dioxide and water to carbonic acid, which spontaneously decomposes to bicarbonate and hydrogen ions.

$$CO_2 + H_2O \rightleftharpoons H_2CO_3 \longrightarrow HCO_3^- + H^+$$

When the ciliary process forms aqueous humor, CA participates by catalyzing the formation of bicarbonate, which is secreted into the posterior chamber of the eye, along with water and other substances that make up the aqueous humor. In patients with **glaucoma**, inhibition of CA reduces

aqueous humor secretion and intraocular pressure. The CA inhibitors are used in the treatment of both the acute and the chronic form of glaucoma, although they must be combined with other drugs to treat the acute form. Traditionally, the CA inhibitors have been administered orally to patients with glaucoma. Now some of these drugs, including dorzolamide, are available for topical ocular administration. Dorzolamide is administered every 8 hours in the treatment of **chronic ocular hypertension** and **open-angle glaucoma**.

Carbonic anhydrase is also required for the reabsorption of sodium bicarbonate from the proximal tubule and for the secretion of hydrogen ion in the collecting duct. In the reabsorption of sodium bicarbonate, bicarbonate must be converted to carbon dioxide and water by CA, because the apical cell membrane of the tubular epithelial cells is impermeable to bicarbonate. The carbon dioxide and water can diffuse into the tubular cells, where CA converts them back to bicarbonate, which is then transported into the interstitial fluid for diffusion into the circulation (see Box 13–1). Inhibition of this process by acetazolamide and other CA inhibitors causes a marked reduction in the reabsorption of sodium bicarbonate and a corresponding increase in its renal excretion. This leads to alkalinization of the urine and produces a mild form of hyperchloremic metabolic acidosis. The hyperchloremia results from the increased reabsorption of chloride as a compensation for reduced bicarbonate reabsorption.

Carbonic anhydrase inhibitors are seldom used as **diuretics**, although they are used occasionally to **alkalinize the urine**. They are effective in the prevention and treatment of **high-altitude sickness (mountain sickness)**, in part because the metabolic acidosis produced by the drugs counteracts the respiratory alkalosis that can result from hyperventilation in this condition. By counteracting respiratory alkalosis, the drugs enhance ventilation acclimatization and maintain oxygenation during sleep at a high altitude. The drugs also counteract fluid retention and cause a decrease in cerebral spinal fluid (CSF) pressure, which can be elevated with acute high-altitude sickness. At the same time, CA inhibitors prevent the fall in CSF pH that occurs in this disorder.

Inhibition of CA in the central nervous system elevates the seizure threshold. For this reason, CA inhibitors have been used occasionally for the treatment of **epilepsy**.

ADVERSE EFFECTS AND INTERACTIONS. Acetazolamide and other orally administered CA inhibitors can cause drowsiness, paresthesia, and other central nervous system effects as well as hypokalemia and hyperglycemia. Less commonly, they are associated with various hypersensitivity reactions and blood cell deficiencies. By increasing the pH of the renal tubular fluid and alkalinizing the urine, the CA inhibitors decrease the excretion of weak bases, such as amphetamine, pseudoephedrine, and quinidine, and thereby increase their serum levels and cause drug toxicity.

MANAGEMENT OF EDEMA

Edema is a condition in which fluid accumulates in the interstitial space and body cavities, either because of increased hydrostatic pressure in the capillary beds or because

of inadequate colloid osmotic pressure in the plasma. The plasma osmotic pressure is primarily influenced by the osmotic attraction of water by sodium and plasma proteins. Conditions that cause edema as a result of increased hydrostatic pressure include heart failure and certain renal diseases, all of which cause sodium and water retention. Conditions that cause edema as a result of inadequate colloid osmotic pressure include severe dietary protein deficiency and hepatic diseases (e.g., cirrhosis). In conditions such as cirrhosis, the liver is unable to synthesize adequate albumin and other plasma proteins to maintain plasma osmotic pressure. Hepatic cirrhosis can lead to ascites (accumulation of fluid within the peritoneal cavity) and portal hypertension. This disorder can be managed with dietary salt restriction and the use of diuretics (e.g., spironolactone and furosemide).

Nephrotic syndrome, a renal disease that leads to excessive protein excretion in the urine (proteinuria), can cause edema by this mechanism. Infection, neoplasms, and thromboembolism can also cause edema by various mechanisms that include inflammation, increased capillary fluid permeability, and increased hydrostatic pressure caused by obstruction of blood vessels.

The primary treatment of edema is to **correct the underlying disorder** and restore plasma osmotic pressure and hydrostatic pressure to normal values. In acute life-threatening situations (e.g., cerebral edema and pulmonary edema) **diuretics** and other drugs must be administered immediately to prevent tissue hypoxia, injury, and death. In milder forms of edema, diuretics can be used as short-term adjunct treatments that serve to mobilize edematous fluid while an attempt is made to correct the underlying cause. Most cases of mild peripheral edema, however, can be managed without pharmacologic therapy by correcting the underlying disorder or discontinuing a causative drug.

ANTIDIURETIC HORMONE ANTAGONIST

Conivaptan is a nonpeptide antagonist of antidiuretic hormone (arginine vasopressin) V_{IA} and V_2 receptors. V_2 receptors are coupled with insertion of aquaporin channels in the apical membranes of the renal collecting ducts, leading to reabsorption of water (antidiuretic effect). By activating these receptors, antidiuretic hormone helps maintain plasma osmolality in the normal range. Antagonism of V_2 receptors by conivaptan causes **free water excretion** or aquaresis, and the drug has been called an **aquaretic**.

Conivaptan is approved for treating **euvolemic and hypervolemic hyponatremia** (low serum sodium concentration) in hospitalized patients. However, it is contraindicated in patients with hypovolemic hyponatremia. The drug is given as an intravenous infusion, usually for 4 days, and typically increases free water clearance by 3800 mL and serum sodium concentration by 6.5 mEq/L. Almost 70% of patients achieve a normal serum sodium concentration of 135 mEq/L after 4 days of conivaptan therapy.

Conivaptan is extensively metabolized by CYP3A4, and is a potent inhibitor of this enzyme. Hence, conivaptan increases serum levels of midazolam, simvastatin, and other drugs metabolized by CYP3A4. The coadministration of conivaptan with potent CYP3A4 inhibitors is contraindicated. The most common adverse reactions reported with conivaptan are infusion site reactions.

SUMMARY OF IMPORTANT POINTS

■ Diuretics are drugs that increase urine production. Most diuretics inhibit the reabsorption of sodium from various sites in the nephron.

■ Thiazide diuretics inhibit sodium chloride reabsorption from the distal tubule. They cause natriuresis and kaliuresis, but they decrease calcium excretion. They are primarily used to treat hypertension, edema, hypercalciuria, and nephrogenic diabetes insipidus.

■ Loop diuretics inhibit the $Na^+,K^+,2Cl^-$ symporter in the ascending limb and thereby increase sodium, potassium, calcium, and magnesium excretion. They are chiefly used to treat heart failure, renal failure, pulmonary edema, and hypercalcemia.

■ Thiazide and loop diuretics can cause hypokalemia and other electrolyte disturbances, as well as hyperglycemia and hyperuricemia.

■ Potassium-sparing diuretics, which inhibit potassium secretion in the collecting duct, are primarily used to prevent hypokalemia, which can be caused by thiazide and loop diuretics. Spironolactone is used to treat severe heart failure and hyperaldosteronism.

■ Osmotic diuretics increase the osmotic pressure of plasma and retain water in the nephron. They are used to treat cerebral edema, glaucoma, and the oliguria of acute renal failure.

■ Carbonic anhydrase inhibitors, which are weak diuretics that inhibit sodium bicarbonate reabsorption from the proximal tubule, can cause a mild form of metabolic acidosis. They reduce aqueous humor secretion and are primarily used to treat glaucoma.

■ Conivaptan is an antidiuretic hormone receptor antagonist that increases free water excretion and is used to treat euvolemic or hypervolemic hyponatremia.

SELECTED READINGS

Carter, B.L., and D.A. Sica. Strategies to improve the cardiovascular risk profile of thiazide-type diuretics as used in the management of hypertension. Expert Opin Drug Saf 6:583–594, 2007.

Ivengar, S., and W.T. Abraham. Diuretics for the treatment of acute decompensated heart failure. Heart Fail Rev 12:125–130, 2007.

Patel, J., M. Smith, and J.T. Heywood. Optimal use of diuretics in patients with heart failure. Curr Treat Options Cardiovas Med 9:332–342, 2007.

Wermers, R.A., A.E. Kearns, G.D. Jenkins, and L.J. Melton, 3rd. Incidence and clinical spectrum of thiazide-associated hypercalcemia. Am J Med 120:911. e9–e15, 2007.

CHAPTER 14

Antiarrhythmic Drugs

CLASSIFICATION OF ANTIARRHYTHMIC DRUGS

Sodium Channel Blockers
Class IA drugs
- Disopyramide (NORPACE)
- Procainamide (PRONESTYL)
- Quinidine

Class IB drugs
- Lidocaine (XYLOCAINE)
- Mexiletine (MEXITIL)ᵃ

Class IC drugs
- Flecainide (TAMBOCOR)
- Propafenone (RYTHMOL)

Class II drugs
- Esmolol (BREVIBLOC)
- Metoprolol (LOPRESSOR)
- Propranolol (INDERAL)

Class III drugs
- Amiodarone (CORDARONE)
- Ibutilide (CORVERT)
- Dofetilide (TIKOSYN)
- Sotalol (BETAPACE)

Class IV drugs
- Diltiazem (CARDIZEM)
- Verapamil (CALAN, ISOPTIN)

Miscellaneous Drugs
- Adenosine (ADENOCARD)
- Digoxin (LANOXIN)
- Magnesium Sulfate

ᵃAlso tocainide (TONOCARD).

OVERVIEW

In a healthy adult with a normal heart, each heartbeat originates in the sinoatrial (SA) node, the rhythm of heartbeats is regular, and the heart rate is about 70 beats per minute at rest. If the origin, rhythm, or rate of heartbeats is abnormal, the condition is called an arrhythmia (dysrhythmia). Arrhythmias occur primarily because of disturbances in cardiac impulse formation or conduction, and they can originate in any part of the heart. Those arising in the atria or atrioventricular (AV) node are called supraventricular arrhythmias, whereas those arising in the ventricles are called ventricular arrhythmias. Those in which the heart rate is too rapid are called tachyarrhythmias, and those in which the heart rate is too slow are called bradyarrhythmias.

Some arrhythmias are benign and do not necessarily require treatment. Others require treatment because they reduce cardiac output and blood pressure significantly or because they can precipitate more serious and even lethal rhythm disturbances. Both pharmacologic and electrophysiologic methods are used to terminate and prevent arrhythmias. This chapter describes the pathophysiology of arrhythmias and the mechanisms by which antiarrhythmic drugs work.

Cardiac Action Potentials and Electrocardiographic Findings

Figure 14–1 depicts the relationships between ion currents, cardiac action potentials in phases 0 through 4, and findings on the surface electrocardiogram (EGG).

The SA node, located in the right atrium, is the site of origin of the normal heartbeat. The SA node spontaneously depolarizes to form an impulse that is conducted through the atrium to the AV node and then through the bundle of His, bundle branches, and Purkinje fibers to the ventricular muscle.

The spontaneous depolarization of the SA node is caused by the influx of sodium and calcium as the efflux of potassium subsides. When the threshold potential (TP) is reached at about −40 mV, the SA node is more rapidly depolarized by sodium and calcium influx to generate an impulse that can be conducted to the rest of the heart. As the impulse is conducted to atrial and ventricular muscle cells, these cells are rapidly depolarized by the influx of sodium through the fast sodium channel. As the cells depolarize to about −40 mV, the slow calcium channels open. The influx of calcium through these channels during phase 2 serves to

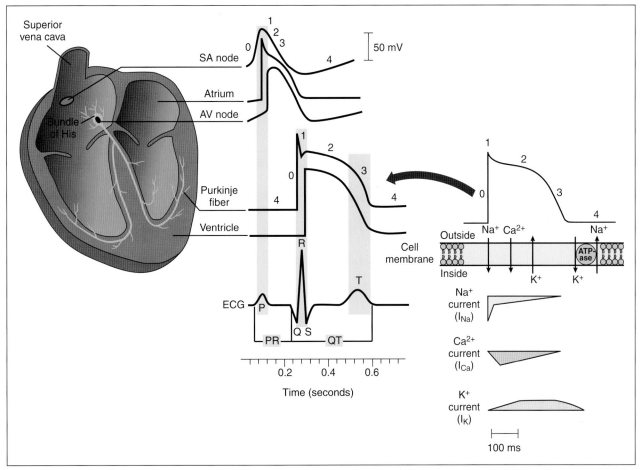

Figure 14-1. Relationships between ion currents, cardiac action potentials, and the findings on surface ECG. The normal heartbeat originates in the SA node. The impulse is conducted through internodal fibers to the AV node and then through the bundle of His, bundle branches, and Purkinje fibers to the ventricular muscle. On the ECG, the P wave represents atrial depolarization, the QRS complex represents ventricular depolarization, and the T wave represents ventricular repolarization. The PR interval is primarily related to the conduction time through the AV node, and the QT interval represents the time between ventricular depolarization and repolarization. In phase 0, ventricular depolarization is caused by sodium influx through the fast sodium channel. In phase 1, the membrane is transiently repolarized as a result of potassium efflux. In phase 2, the membrane potential is relatively stable because of the concurrent influx of calcium and efflux of potassium. In phase 3, repolarization is caused by continued potassium efflux as calcium influx declines. In phase 4, the ion balance is returned to normal by the action of the sodium pump (Na$^+$,K$^+$-adenosine triphosphatase [ATPase]). Calcium is removed from the cell by the sodium-calcium exchanger and the calcium ATPase (not shown).

activate muscle contraction. Cardiac tissues become repolarized during phase 3 as a result of the efflux of potassium through several types of rectifier potassium channels, an efflux that occurs when the influx of calcium declines.

As shown in Figure 14–1, the surface ECG is a summation of action potentials generated by the heart during the cardiac cycle. The **P wave** represents atrial depolarization, whereas the **PR interval** corresponds to the time required to conduct the action potential through both the atria and the AV node. The **QRS complex** and the **T wave** represent ventricular depolarization and ventricular repolarization, respectively. Hence, the **QT interval** represents the duration of the ventricular action potential.

Pathophysiology of Arrhythmias

Arrhythmias can be caused by coronary ischemia and tissue hypoxia, electrolyte disturbances, overstimulation of the sympathetic nervous system, general anesthetics, and

other conditions or drugs that perturb cardiac transmembrane potentials and lead to abnormal impulse formation or abnormal impulse conduction.

Abnormal Impulse Formation

Abnormal impulse formation can generate extrasystoles and result in tachycardia. The two mechanisms that are primarily responsible for abnormal impulse formation are increased automaticity and the occurrence of afterdepolarizations. These are depicted in Box 14–1.

INCREASED AUTOMATICITY. Spontaneous phase 4 depolarization generates an action potential that can be propagated to other parts of the heart. The SA node is the usual site of spontaneous impulse initiation (automaticity), but other cardiac tissues, including the AV node and the His-Purkinje system tissues, are also capable of spontaneous depolarization. Pathologic conditions or drugs can cause these tissues to depolarize more rapidly and thereby generate abnormal

BOX 14–1 THE ELECTROPHYSIOLOGIC BASIS OF ARRHYTHMIAS

Abnormal Impulse Formation

The two mechanisms primarily responsible for abnormal impulse formation are increased automaticity and afterdepolarizations.

Increased automaticity can be caused by any change that decreases the time required for depolarization from the maximal diastolic potential (MDP) to the TP. Increased automaticity occurs if the rate of diastolic depolarization (the slope of phase 4) in the SA node or in latent pacemakers is increased. It also occurs if a shift of the TP occurs to a more negative value or if a shift occurs of the MDP to a more positive value.

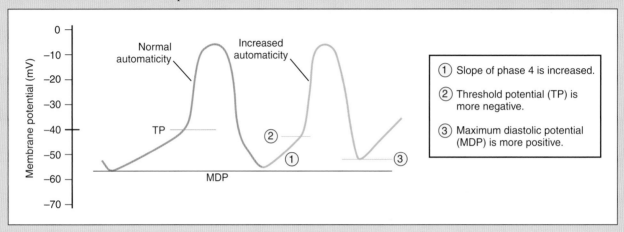

1. Slope of phase 4 is increased.
2. Threshold potential (TP) is more negative.
3. Maximum diastolic potential (MDP) is more positive.

Afterdepolarizations are believed to result from abnormal calcium influx into cardiac cells during or immediately after phase 3 of the ventricular action potential. Afterdepolarizations can lead to extrasystoles and tachycardia.

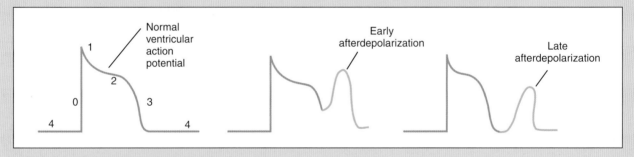

Abnormal Impulse Conduction

Reentry is characterized by the retrograde conduction of an impulse into previously depolarized tissue. It is usually caused by the presence of a unidirectional conduction block in a bifurcating conduction pathway. For reentry to occur, the conduction time through the retrograde pathway must exceed the refractory period of the reentered tissue.

In **ventricular tissue**, the unidirectional block is often caused by decremental conduction of the impulse in the anterograde direction, with normal conduction of the impulse in the retrograde direction.

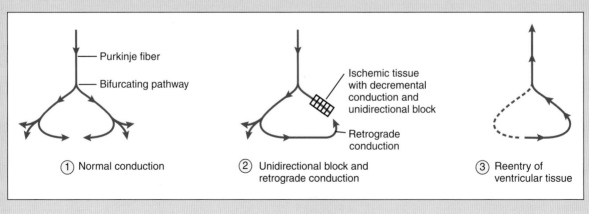

(Continued)

BOX 14-1 THE ELECTROPHYSIOLOGIC BASIS OF ARRHYTHMIAS—cont'd

Reentry in the **AV node** is the most common electrophysiologic mechanism responsible for PSVT. Reentry occurs when a premature atrial depolarization arrives at the AV node and finds that one pathway (β) is still refractory from the previous depolarization. The other pathway (α), however, is able to conduct the impulse to the ventricle. Retrograde conduction of the impulse through pathway β leads to reentry of the atrium and results in tachycardia. In the AV node, the unidirectional block results from the β pathway's longer refractory period, which blocks anterograde conduction but permits retrograde conduction after it has recovered its excitability.

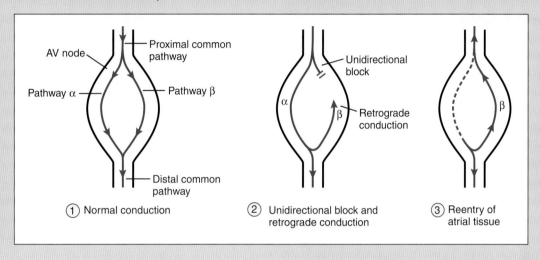

impulses. For example, overstimulation of the sympathetic nervous system or use of sympathomimetic drugs increases automaticity and can cause tachyarrhythmia.

The rate at which action potentials are generated in the SA node and elsewhere in the heart depends on the time required to depolarize the tissue from the maximal diastolic potential (MDP) to the TP. Automaticity is increased if MDP becomes more positive or if the TP becomes more negative. Serum electrolyte abnormalities, hypoxia, and other pathologic changes can affect the MDP or TP in this manner and lead to arrhythmias.

AFTERDEPOLARIZATIONS. Afterdepolarizations are abnormal impulses resulting from the spontaneous generation of action potentials during or immediately after phase 3 repolarization. Depending on the time they occur, the abnormal impulses are designated as early afterdepolarizations or late afterdepolarizations. Afterdepolarizations are believed to be triggered by abnormal calcium influx and can be provoked by digitalis glycosides and by other drugs or pathologic events that prolong cardiac repolarization and the QT interval.

Abnormal Impulse Conduction

Abnormal impulse conduction is the basis for the formation of arrhythmias by the process of **reentry**, a process that involves reexcitation of a particular zone of cardiac tissue by the same impulse. Reentry is believed to be the most common mechanism responsible for the genesis of arrhythmias. It is usually caused by the presence of a **unidirectional conduction block** in a bifurcating conduction pathway (see Box 14–1).

REENTRY IN VENTRICULAR TISSUE. In ventricular tissue, ischemia and tissue hypoxia can cause a reduction in the resting membrane potential and a decrease in membrane responsiveness. Under these conditions, the cells do not depolarize as rapidly or completely during phase 0, and this reduces the rate at which the impulse is conducted to surrounding ventricular tissue. When a cardiac impulse is conducted through ischemic or infarcted tissue, the conduction velocity gradually slows until conduction ceases. This phenomenon, called **decremental conduction**, is the most common cause of a unidirectional block in ventricular tissue. If the unidirectional block occurs in one arm of a bifurcating pathway, the impulse can continue through the other arm in the normal (anterograde) direction and then reenter the ventricular tissue by retrograde conduction.

The reason that the impulse is blocked in the anterograde direction but is conducted in the retrograde direction is related to the characteristics of decremental conduction. In this type of conduction, the impulse encounters increasing resistance as it moves in the anterograde direction, and its velocity slows until the impulse is finally extinguished. The retrograde impulse has full velocity as it encounters the area of greatest resistance, and this enables it to jump across the ischemic area without being extinguished.

REENTRY IN THE ATRIOVENTRICULAR NODE. Reentry in the AV node is the most common electrophysiologic mechanism responsible for paroxysmal supraventricular tachycardia (PSVT). Of the several forms of PSVT, the form that occurs in patients with Wolff-Parkinson-White syndrome involves an accessory AV node conduction pathway through the bundle of Kent. In patients with the most common form of PSVT, however, the reentrant circuit is located entirely within the AV node. In the common form of PSVT, a premature atrial impulse is blocked in one pathway, is conducted through the AV node via the other pathway, and reenters the atrium by retrograde conduction. In AV node reentry, the unidirectional block does not result from decremental conduction but, instead, is caused by the difference in the refractory periods of the two pathways.

Drug-Induced Arrhythmias

Drugs can induce arrhythmias by several mechanisms.

Sympathomimetic drugs can increase the automaticity of the SA node, AV node, or His-Purkinje fibers and thereby produce tachyarrhythmias.

Digitalis glycosides sometimes evoke afterdepolarizations by increasing calcium influx into cardiac cells, and they can also impair AV node conduction and cause AV block.

Other drugs cause arrhythmias via their effects on ventricular conduction and repolarization. Drugs that slow ventricular repolarization and cause QT prolongation can evoke a form of polymorphic ventricular tachycardia called **torsades de pointes** (based on a French term meaning "fringe of pointed tips"). In this disorder, each QRS complex has a configuration that differs from the preceding one, and QT prolongation probably predisposes the ventricular tissue to afterdepolarizations that produce extrasystoles and tachycardia. Types of drugs that have been reported to induce torsades de pointes include **antiarrhythmic drugs** (e.g., quinidine and sotalol), **histamine antagonists** (e.g., astemizole and terfenadine), **psychotropic drugs** (e.g., phenothiazines), and other agents (e.g., cisapride).

Mechanisms and Classification of Antiarrhythmic Drugs

Antiarrhythmic drugs act primarily by suppressing or preventing abnormal impulse formation or conduction. Drugs that block sodium or calcium channels can reduce abnormal automaticity and slow conduction of the cardiac impulse. Drugs that block potassium channels can prolong repolarization and the action potential duration and thereby increase the refractory period of cardiac tissue. Drugs that block β-adrenoceptors reduce the sympathetic stimulation of cardiac automaticity and conduction velocity and thereby prevent the overstimulation that contributes to some arrhythmias.

BOX 14–2   ELECTROPHYSIOLOGIC PROPERTIES OF SODIUM CHANNEL BLOCKERS

During phase 0 of the ventricular action potential, the sodium channels open to depolarize the cell. The channels are then inactivated and no longer permit sodium entry during phases 1, 2, and 3. The channels must return to the resting state (phase 4) before they can open again during the next action potential.

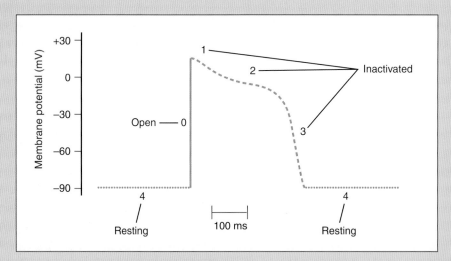

Drugs dissociate from the sodium channels at different rates (recovery). Drugs with a slow recovery have a greater effect on cardiac conduction velocity.

Drug Class	Example	Sodium Channel Affinity	Rate of Dissociation
Class IA	Quinidine	Open > inactivated	Slow
Class IB	Lidocaine	Inactivated > open	Rapid
Class IC	Flecainide	Open > inactivated	Very slow

On the basis of these mechanisms, Vaughan-Williams has divided the antiarrhythmic drugs into four main classes, with **Class I** consisting of sodium channel blockers, **Class II** consisting of β-adrenoceptor antagonists (β-blockers), **Class III** consisting of potassium channel blockers and other drugs that prolong the action potential duration, and **Class IV** consisting of calcium channel blockers. Although this classification system is helpful, a few drugs (e.g, adenosine) do not fit into any of these categories, and some drugs (e.g., amiodarone) could be included in more than one category.

SODIUM CHANNEL BLOCKERS

Class I, the largest group of antiarrhythmic drugs, consists of sodium channel blockers. These drugs bind to sodium channels when the channels are in the open and inactivated states, and they dissociate from the channels during the resting state (Box 14–2). The sodium channel blockers have the most pronounced effect on cardiac tissue that is firing rapidly, because sodium channels in this tissue spend more time in the open and inactivated states than in the resting state. This is called **use-dependent blockade**. Because of use-dependent blockade, sodium channel blockers suppress cardiac conduction more in a person with tachycardia than in a person with a normal heart rate.

The drugs in Class I have been subdivided into three groups (IA, IB, and IC), based on whether they have greater affinity for the open state or the inactivated state and based on their rate of dissociation from sodium channels (rate of recovery). As shown in Box 14–2, **Class IA drugs** have greater affinity for the open state and have a slow recovery; **Class IB drugs** have greater affinity for the inactivated state and have a rapid recovery; and **Class IC drugs** have greater affinity for the open state and a very slow recovery.

Class IA Drugs

Disopyramide, procainamide, and quinidine are Class IA drugs. These drugs have similar electrophysiologic effects and clinical indications, but they differ in their pharmacokinetic properties and adverse effects.

Drug Properties

The Class IA drugs block the fast sodium channel and also block potassium channels. Therefore, they slow phase 0 depolarization and phase 3 repolarization in ventricular tissue (Fig. 14–2). These actions decrease the ventricular conduction velocity and prolong the ventricular action potential duration and refractory period (Table 14–1). On the ECG, this increases the QRS duration and prolongs the QT interval. Class IA drugs suppress abnormal (ectopic) automaticity, but they usually do not significantly affect SA node automaticity and the heart rate.

All of the Class IA drugs have some degree of antimuscarinic (atropine-like) activity and may inhibit parasympathetic (vagal) effects on the SA and AV nodes. Disopyramide has the greatest antimuscarinic effect, procainamide has the least, and quinidine has an intermediate effect.

Quinidine

Quinidine is an isomer of quinine, an alkaloid obtained from the bark of the cinchona tree that is used to treat fever and malaria. The pharmacokinetic properties of quinidine and other antiarrhythmic drugs are summarized in Table 14–2. Quinidine is usually administered orally. It undergoes hepatic biotransformation and is excreted in the urine as the parent compound and metabolites. Because it has a moderately short half-life, quinidine is often given as a sustained-release preparation. The most common adverse effect of quinidine is diarrhea, which occurs in up to 30% of patients taking the drug and is often responsible for their discontinuation of its use. Less commonly, quinidine causes excessive prolongation of the QT interval and torsade de pointes, which can cause syncope secondary to a reduction in cardiac output. Thrombocytopenia has also been reported with quinidine use. Higher doses of quinidine can cause cinchonism, characterized by a constellation of neurologic symptoms that include tinnitus, dizziness, and blurred vision. Although its use has declined, quinidine is occasionally used to suppress supraventricular and ventricular arrhythmias.

Procainamide

Procainamide is the amide derivative of the local anesthetic procaine. It is well absorbed from the gut and is converted to an active metabolite, N-acetylprocainamide. Long-term use of procainamide often causes a syndrome that resembles lupus erythematous, presents with arthralgia and a butterfly rash on the face, and is reversible. This syndrome can be distinguished from idiopathic lupus on the basis of serologic tests for anti-DNA antibodies. It is often responsible for discontinuation of the drug. The clinical use of procainamide has declined in recent years. Although not a first-line drug for any arrhythmia, procainamide is occasionally used to terminate acute ventricular arrhythmias, and it may be given orally for long-term suppression.

Disopyramide

Disopyramide is administered orally to prevent **ventricular arrhythmias**. Because it has greater negative inotropic and antimuscarinic effects than do other Class IA drugs, it should be used with caution in patients with heart failure and in elderly patients.

Class IB Drugs

Lidocaine, mexiletine, and tocainide are Class IB drugs. Class IB drugs have a greater affinity for inactivated sodium channels than for open channels.

Drug Properties

CHEMISTRY AND PHARMACOKINETICS. Lidocaine is a local anesthetic that also has antiarrhythmic activity. It undergoes extensive first-pass hepatic inactivation after oral administration and is not suitable for administration by this route. Mexiletine and tocainide are lidocaine congeners that are not susceptible to first-pass inactivation and are intended for oral administration. Lidocaine is rapidly inactivated

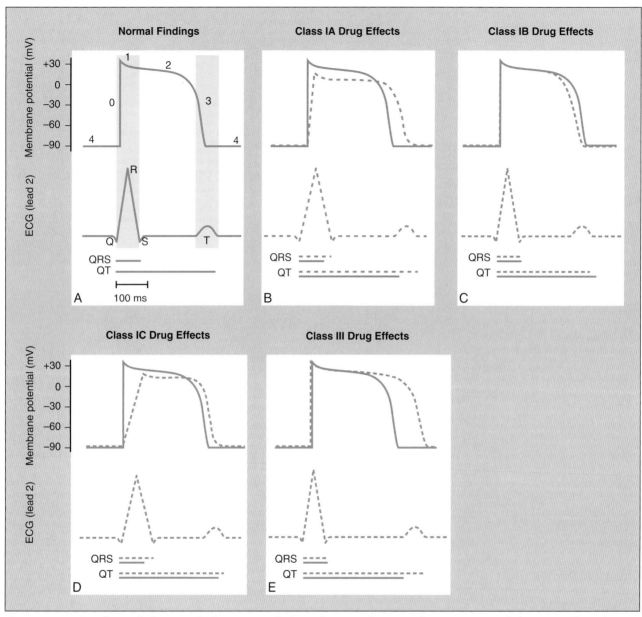

Figure 14–2. Effects of Class I and Class III antiarrhythmic drugs on the ventricular action potential duration and on the ECG. In each panel, the membrane potential scale is in millivolts (mV), and the time scale is in milliseconds (ms). Blue tracings and blue lines for the time scale depict normal findings; dashed lines and tracings depict the effects of drug administration. (A) Lightly shaded vertical bars show the relationship between the ventricular action potential duration and the findings on ECG in the normally functioning heart. (B) Class IA drugs slow phase 0 depolarization and phase 3 repolarization, thereby increasing the QRS duration and the QT interval. (C) Class IB drugs have little effect on normal cardiac tissue, but they can accelerate phase 3 repolarization and decrease the QT interval slightly. (D) Class IC drugs have the greatest effect on phase 0 depolarization and increase the QRS duration markedly, but they have little effect on phase 3 and the QT interval. (E) Class III drugs have no effect on phase 0, but they markedly prolong phase 3 and increase the QT interval.

by hepatic enzymes, whereas mexiletine and tocainide are more slowly metabolized and have much longer half-lives (see Table 14–2).

MECHANISMS AND EFFECTS. Lidocaine has a more pronounced effect on ischemic tissue than on nonischemic tissue. In ischemic tissue, cells are partly depolarized because they lack sufficient adenosine triphosphate to operate the sodium pump. As a result, sodium channels in ischemic tissue spend more time in the inactivated state than do channels in

nonischemic tissue. Because lidocaine has a greater affinity for inactivated channels, it suppresses conduction more in ischemic tissue than in normal tissue.

Lidocaine has little effect on normal cardiac tissue and electrocardiographic findings at therapeutic levels. Hence, it is not very effective in the treatment of supraventricular arrhythmias because these arrhythmias usually arise in nonischemic tissue. However, mexiletine and tocainide have a greater effect on normal cardiac tissue than does lidocaine.

TABLE 14–1. Electrophysiologic Properties of Antiarrhythmic Drugs*

Drug	ATRIOVENTRICULAR (AV) NODE			HIS-PURKINJE SYSTEM AND VENTRICLE			ELECTROCARDIOGRAM		
	Ectopic Automaticity	Conduction Velocity	Refractory Period	Conduction Velocity	Refractory Period	Heart Rate	PR Interval	QRS Duration	QT Interval
Class I Drugs									
IA drugs	D	±	O/I	D	I	±	±	I	I
IB drugs	D	O	O	O/D†	±	O	O	O	O/D
IC drugs	D	D	O/I	D	I	O	I	I	O/I
Class II Drugs	D	D	I	O	O	D	I	O	O/D
Class III Drugs									
Amiodarone	D	D	I	D	I	D	I	I	I
Dofetilide	O	O/D	I	O	I	O/D	O	O	I
Ibutilide	U	O/D	I	O	I	O/D	O/I	O	I
Sotalol	D	D	I	O	I	D	I	O	I
Class IV Drugs	D	D	I	O	O	D	I	O	O
Other Drugs									
Adenosine	D	D	I	O	O	I	I	O	O
Digoxin	I	D	I	O	D	D	I	O	D
Magnesium sulfate	D	O	O	O	O	O	O	O	O

*Effects are indicated as follows: decrease (D); increase (I); variable increase or decrease (±); no change (O); and unknown (U).
†Slow conduction in ischemic tissue.

TABLE 14-2. **Pharmacokinetic Properties of Antiarrhythmic Drugs***

Drug	Oral Bioavailability	Onset of Action	Duration of Action	Elimination Half-Life	Excreted Unchanged in Urine	Therapeutic Serum Concentration
Class IA Drugs						
Disopyramide	90%	1 hour	6 hours	7 hours	50%	2–7 µg/mL
Procainamide	85%	1 hour	5 hours	3.5 hours	55%	4–8 µg/mL
Quinidine	75%	1 hour	7 hours	6 hours	30%	2–5 µg/mL
Class IB Drugs						
Lidocaine	NA	See text	See text	1.5 hours	1%	1.5–6 µg/mL
Mexiletine	90%	1 hour	10 hours	11 hours	10%	0.5–2 µg/mL
Tocainide	92%	1 hour	12 hours	12 hours	40%	4–10 µg/mL
Class IC Drugs						
Flecainide	75%	3 hours	21 hours	14 hours	30%	0.2–1 µg/mL
Propafenone	10%	3 hours	10 hours	6 hours	<1%	0.06–0.1 µg/mL
Class II Drugs						
Esmolol	NA	<5 minutes	20–30 minutes	0.15 hour	<2%	0.5–1 µg/mL
Metoprolol	35%	1 hour	15 hours	3.5 hours	7%	15–25 µg/mL
Propranolol	35%	0.5 hour	4 hours	4 hours	<0.5%	0.2–1 µg/mL
Class III Drugs						
Amiodarone	45%	2 weeks	4 weeks	40 days	0%	0.5–2.5 µg/mL
Dofetilide	90%	1 hour	12 hours	10 hours	80%	NA
Ibutilide	NA	5 minutes	N/A	6 hours	<10%	NA
Sotalol	90%	2 hours	15 hours	12 hours	90%	1–4 µg/mL
Class IV Drugs						
Diltiazem	55%	2 hours	8 hours	5 hours	3%	0.1–0.2 µg/mL
Verapamil	25%	2 hours	9 hours	5 hours	3%	0.1–0.3 µg/mL
Miscellaneous Drugs						
Adenosine	NA	30 seconds	1.5 minutes	<10 seconds	0%	NA
Digoxin	75%	1 hour	24 hours	35 hours	60%	0.5–2 ng/mL
Magnesium sulfate	NA	<5 minutes	NA	NA	100%	NA

NA = not applicable (not administered orally).
*Values shown are the mean of values reported in the literature.

ADVERSE EFFECTS. A high serum concentration of lidocaine can cause central nervous system side effects such as nervousness, tremor, and paresthesia. Higher or toxic doses also slow the conduction velocity in normal cardiac tissue and may cause cardiac arrest. Because lidocaine is extensively metabolized, concurrent use of a drug that inhibits cytochrome P450 enzymes (e.g., cimetidine) can increase the serum concentration of lidocaine and precipitate lidocaine toxicity.

Because use of tocainide can lead to agranulocytosis and other blood cell deficiencies, patients receiving this drug should have blood counts performed periodically. Mexiletine is less frequently associated with these adverse effects.

INDICATIONS. Lidocaine has been administered intravenously as a loading dose (bolus) followed by a continuous intravenous infusion in the treatment of **ventricular tachycardia** and **other acute ventricular arrhythmias**. Recent guidelines of the American College of Cardiology and American Heart Association, however, do not recommend lidocaine for treatment of recurrent sustained ventricular tachycardia or ventricular fibrillation (see below).

Mexiletine and tocainide are administered orally on a long-term basis for the suppression of **ventricular arrhythmias**.

Class IC Drugs

Flecainide and propafenone, which are Class IC drugs, are administered orally. Their properties are outlined in Tables 14–1 and 14–2.

Class IC drugs block both fast sodium channels and the rate of rise of the action potential during phase 0 to a greater extent than do other Class I drugs. By this mechanism, the Class IC drugs slow conduction throughout the heart and especially in the His-Purkinje system. Flecainide and propafenone usually have less effect on the potassium rectifier current and do not prolong the QT interval as much as do Class IA drugs, such as quinidine.

Flecainide

Flecainide is indicated for the treatment of **supraventricular arrhythmias** and **documented life-threatening ventricular arrhythmias**. In the past, it was also routinely used to suppress ventricular arrhythmias in patients with cardiac disorders. This practice has changed, however, since a clinical study called the **Cardiac Arrhythmia Suppression Trial (CAST)** showed that flecainide actually increased the mortality rate in patients who were recovering from myocardial infarction.

Although flecainide does not cause afterdepolarizations and torsades de pointes, it is capable of increasing the ventricular rate and causing reentrant ventricular tachycardia. Other adverse effects of flecainide include bronchospasm, leukopenia, thrombocytopenia, and seizures.

Propafenone

The effect of propafenone on fast sodium channels and cardiac conduction is similar to that of flecainide. As with flecainide, propafenone prolongs the PR interval and QRS duration. Propafenone can also cause some degree of QT prolongation.

Propafenone is administered orally on a long-term basis to suppress supraventricular tachycardia and atrial fibrillation. The drug is also used to treat life-threatening forms of ventricular arrhythmia, such as sustained ventricular tachycardia.

Propafenone has the potential to cause ventricular arrhythmias and several hematologic abnormalities, including agranulocytosis, anemia, and thrombocytopenia.

OTHER ANTIARRHYTHMIC DRUGS

Tables 14–1 and 14–2 compare the electrophysiologic and pharmacokinetic properties of the various groups and subgroups of antiarrhythmic drugs.

Class II Drugs

Drug Properties

The Class II antiarrhythmics are β-adrenoceptor antagonists (β-blockers), including esmolol, metoprolol, and propranolol. These drugs are used to prevent and treat supraventricular arrhythmias and to reduce ventricular ectopic depolarizations and sudden death in patients with myocardial infarction.

The β-blockers have antiarrhythmic effects because of their ability to inhibit sympathetic activation of cardiac automaticity and conduction. β-blockers slow the heart rate, decrease the AV node conduction velocity, and increase the AV node refractory period (Fig. 14–3). They have little effect on ventricular conduction and repolarization. The general pharmacologic properties of β-blockers are discussed in Chapter 9.

Esmolol

Esmolol, a β-blocker given intravenously, is rapidly metabolized by plasma esterase and has an extremely short half-life. Its pharmacologic properties make it ideally suited for the treatment of **acute supraventricular tachycardia** or **hypertension** during or immediately after surgery, where its short duration of action enables continuous control of the patient's heart rate and blood pressure.

Metoprolol and Propranolol

Metoprolol and propranolol can be administered orally or intravenously to treat and suppress **supraventricular and ventricular arrhythmias**. In patients with **myocardial infarction**, metoprolol is often administered intravenously during the early phase of treatment, followed by oral maintenance therapy that can continue for several months. The β-blockers have been demonstrated to protect the heart against the damage caused by ischemia and free radicals that may be formed during reperfusion of the coronary arteries when fibrinolytic drugs are used.

Class III Drugs

Amiodarone, dofetilide, ibutilide, and sotalol are Class III antiarrhythmics. The most common attribute of this heterogeneous group of drugs is the prolongation of the ventricular action potential duration and refractory period. Class III drugs act mostly by blocking potassium rectifier

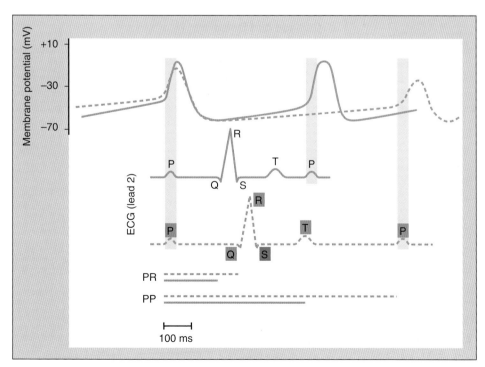

Figure 14–3. Effects of Class II and Class IV antiarrhythmic drugs on the SA node action potential duration and on the ECG. The membrane potential scale is in millivolts (mV), and the time scale is in milliseconds (ms). Solid tracings and dashed lines for the time scale depict normal findings; dashed lines and tracings depict the effects of drug administration. Vertical bars show the relationship between the action potential and the findings on ECG. Class II drugs (β-adrenoceptor antagonists) and Class IV drugs (calcium channel blockers) slow phase 4 depolarization in the SA node and increase the PP interval. They also slow the AV node conduction velocity and increase the PR interval.

currents that repolarize the heart during phase 3 of the action potential. Except for amiodarone, these drugs do not slow the ventricular conduction velocity or increase the QRS duration significantly.

Amiodarone

CHEMISTRY AND PHARMACOKINETICS. Amiodarone is an organic iodine compound that is structurally related to thyroid hormones (Fig. 14–4). It can be administered orally or intravenously, and has unusual pharmacokinetic properties. After oral administration, amiodarone is slowly and variably absorbed and is primarily eliminated by biliary excretion. As shown in Table 14–2, the drug's action may not begin for about 2 weeks if loading doses are not given. In most cases, oral or intravenous administration of loading doses is used to accelerate the drug's onset of action. The half-life of amiodarone is extremely long (about 40 days with a range of 26 to 107 days).

MECHANISMS AND PHARMACOLOGIC EFFECTS. Although amiodarone has Class III antiarrhythmic activity, it also blocks sodium channels, calcium channels, and β-adrenoceptors. Hence, it is difficult to assign its antiarrhythmic activity to a specific mechanism.

As shown in Table 14–1, amiodarone decreases SA node automaticity, decreases AV node conduction velocity, and prolongs AV node and ventricular refractory periods. It increases the PR interval and the QT interval and causes a slight prolongation of the QRS duration. Amiodarone is a powerful inhibitor of ectopic pacemaker automaticity, and it prolongs repolarization and refractory periods throughout the heart. These actions probably account for much of its antiarrhythmic effects.

ADVERSE EFFECTS AND INTERACTIONS. Amiodarone may cause a number of adverse effects, most of which are reversible and can be managed by dosage reduction or discontinuation. The reversible cardiac effects of amiodarone include bradycardia, impaired AV conduction, and QT interval prolongation leading to torsades de pointes. Amiodarone causes corneal micro-deposits in over 90% of patients, but these are usually benign and do not require intervention. Amiodarone causes photosensitivity to ultraviolet light and patients should avoid sun exposure and use sunscreen.

The drug also causes a **blue-gray skin discoloration** that may require dosage reduction or discontinuation. The more serious adverse effects include **hypothyroidism** (6% of patients) or hyperthyroidism (0.9%–2% of patients). Hypothyroidism may be managed with levothyroxine replacement therapy, whereas hyperthyroidism usually requires discontinuation of amiodarone. Tremor, ataxia, and optic or peripheral **neuropathy** may also occur. Hepatic dysfunction should be monitored by determining serum levels of hepatic enzymes such as alanine transaminase every 6 months during amiodarone treatment.

Pulmonary fibrosis is an uncommon but potentially fatal reaction to amiodarone and patients should have pulmonary function tests and a chest radiograph before starting treatment, with a yearly radiograph thereafter. The drug must be discontinued immediately if any sign of pulmonary toxicity occurs.

Amiodarone inhibits the metabolism of a number of pharmacologic agents and significantly elevates the plasma concentrations of drugs such as digoxin, flecainide, phenytoin, procainamide, and warfarin. The dosage of these drugs should be decreased in patients receiving concurrent amiodarone therapy. Amiodarone also interacts with inhalational anesthetics and other central nervous system depressants to cause an increased incidence of adverse cardiovascular effects such as bradycardia.

INDICATIONS. Amiodarone is given orally on a long-term basis to suppress both supraventricular and ventricular arrhythmias, including atrial fibrillation, atrial flutter, supraventricular tachycardia, and ventricular tachycardia. Amiodarone is used intravenously to terminate ventricular fibrillation or sustained ventricular tachycardia. In this setting, the drug can be given as a loading infusion followed by a maintenance infusion. Amiodarone also appears to be an effective adjunct to implantable cardioverter-defibrillators to reduce the number of shocks required to maintain sinus rhythm.

Ibutilide and Dofetilide

Ibutilide and dofetilide selectively block several types of outward potassium channels. These channels are called delayed rectifier channels because they are responsible for repolarizing myocardial tissue during phase 3 of the action potential. By inhibiting these currents, dofetilide and

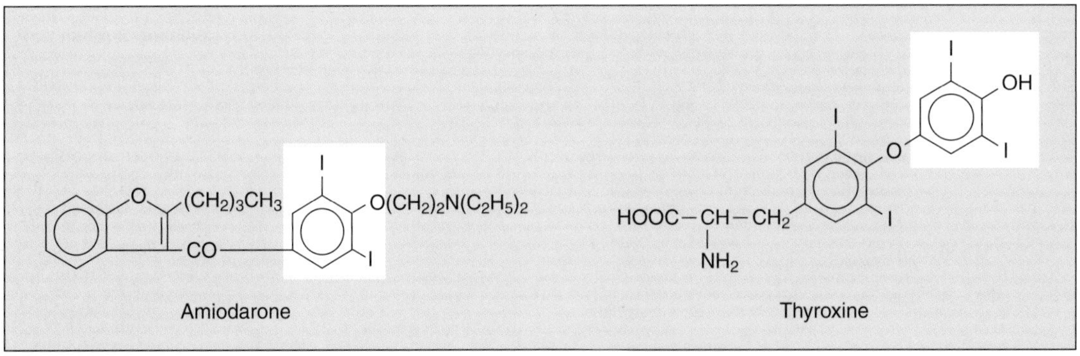

Figure 14–4. Structures of amiodarone and thyroxine. The structure of amiodarone, which contains two iodine atoms, has some similarity to the structure of thyroid hormones such as thyroxine. Amiodarone can cause hypothyroidism and, less commonly, hyperthyroidism in some persons. The similar parts of the structures of amiodarone and thyroxine are unshaded.

ibutilide prolong ventricular repolarization and increase the QT interval of the ECG. Ibutilide also prolongs the action potential duration by promoting the influx of sodium through slow inward sodium channels. The sodium influx counteracts the outward potassium current and thereby prolongs repolarization.

Ibutilide is administered by intravenous infusion. It is rapidly metabolized in the liver, and its metabolites are eliminated in the urine and feces, with an average half-life of 6 hours. The drug is indicated for the rapid conversion of **atrial fibrillation or flutter** to normal sinus rhythm. It does not significantly affect the heart rate, blood pressure, QRS duration, or PR interval. It can induce torsades de pointes, and continuous ECG monitoring is required during administration of the drug. Ibutilide should be avoided in patients with a prolonged QT interval (QTc > 440 msec) and those with a history of polymorphic ventricular tachycardia.

Dofetilide selectively blocks the rapidly activating delayed rectifier channel. The drug is administered orally to convert **atrial fibrillation** and for long-term suppression of the arrhythmia. Because of its potent ability to prolong the QT interval and induce torsades de pointes, the ECG must be closely monitored during dosage titration. When therapy is initiated, dosage adjustments are based on the degree of QT prolongation. The drug is primarily eliminated by renal excretion, and doses must be reduced in persons with renal insufficiency.

Sotalol

Sotalol is a nonselective β-adrenoceptor antagonist that prolongs the cardiac action potential duration and QT interval by blocking the delayed potassium rectifier current during phase 3 of the ventricular action potential (see Fig. 14–2). The drug also decreases automaticity, slows the AV node conduction velocity, and increases the AV node refractory period without affecting the ventricular conduction and QRS duration.

Sotalol is approved for the treatment of **ventricular arrhythmias** and is also effective in the management of **atrial arrhythmias**, including **atrial fibrillation**. It produces a dose-dependent incidence of torsades de pointes, most likely because of QT prolongation. Some of its adverse effects (e.g., bronchospasm) are caused by β-adrenoceptor blockade.

Class IV Drugs

Diltiazem and **verapamil** are calcium channel blockers that have significant effects on cardiac tissue. They primarily act to decrease the AV node conduction velocity and increase the AV node refractory period, and they have a smaller effect on the SA node and heart rate. As shown in Table 14–1, they have little effect on the ventricular conduction velocity and refractory period.

Diltiazem and verapamil can be administered intravenously to terminate **acute supraventricular tachycardia**. They are also used to reduce the ventricular rate in patients who have **atrial fibrillation** with a rapid ventricular response. These drugs can exacerbate ventricular tachycardia, so it is important that arrhythmias be correctly diagnosed before beginning treatment with diltiazem or verapamil. Other calcium channel blockers (including dihydropyridine

drugs such as amlodipine) have less effect on cardiac tissue and no role in the treatment of arrhythmias.

Miscellaneous Drugs

Adenosine

Adenosine is a naturally occurring nucleoside composed of adenine and ribose. When administered as a rapid intravenous bolus, it has an extremely short half-life of 10 seconds or less. In the body, adenosine is derived from adenosine triphosphate and activates specific G protein–coupled adenosine receptors. Stimulation of these receptors leads to activation of acetylcholine-sensitive potassium channels and blockade of calcium influx in the SA node, atrium, and AV node. It thereby causes cell hyperpolarization, slows the AV node conduction velocity, and increases the AV node refractory period. In fact, AV node conduction can be completely blocked for a few seconds, resulting in a brief period of asystole. These actions serve to terminate supraventricular tachycardia by preventing the retrograde conduction of reentrant impulses through the AV node. Because of its brief duration of action, adenosine has been termed a pharmacologic counterpart to electrical cardioversion.

Adenosine is primarily used to terminate **acute PSVT**, including the type associated with Wolff-Parkinson-White syndrome. It is not indicated for the treatment of atrial fibrillation or flutter. Dipyridamole, a vasodilator used to facilitate angiographic studies, inhibits the cellular uptake of adenosine and markedly increases its cardiac effects. Doses of adenosine, therefore, should be reduced in persons who have recently received dipyridamole. Adenosine can cause bronchospasm and should be used cautiously in persons with obstructive lung disease.

Digoxin

Digoxin, a digitalis glycoside discussed in Chapter 12, acts indirectly to increase vagal tone and thereby slow the AV node conduction velocity and increase the AV node refractory period. Digoxin has been used to slow the ventricular rate in patients with **atrial fibrillation**, although β-blockers and calcium channel blockers are usually preferred for this purpose because of their more rapid onset of action and greater degree of AV nodal blockade. Digoxin is sometimes used for this indication because it does not cause as much bradycardia as β-blockers and it does not reduce cardiac contractility as much as calcium channel blockers such as verapamil. In fact, digoxin has a positive inotropic effect and is also used to treat **heart failure** (see Chapter 12).

Magnesium Sulfate

The magnesium ion, the second most common intracellular cation, has a number of roles in normal cardiac function. Magnesium deficiency can be caused by use of drugs such as loop diuretics or by pathologic states, and this deficiency can contribute to the development of arrhythmias and congestive heart failure, as well as to gastrointestinal and renal disorders.

Magnesium sulfate is administered intravenously to suppress drug-induced torsades de pointes, to treat digitalis-induced ventricular arrhythmias, and to treat supraventricular arrhythmias associated with magnesium deficiency.

MANAGEMENT OF SUPRAVENTRICULAR ARRHYTHMIAS

Atrial Fibrillation and Flutter

Atrial fibrillation is thought to be caused by a disorganized form of reentry in atrial tissue, a form in which atrial cells are continuously reexcited by reentrant wavelets as soon as they have repolarized. Under these conditions, the AV node is continuously bombarded with atrial impulses, some of which are conducted to the ventricles, so that the ventricular rate is often rapid and usually irregular.

The first objective of treatment is to control ventricular rate. This is accomplished by administering drugs that slow the conduction velocity and increase the refractory period of the AV node, so that fewer atrial impulses are transmitted to the ventricles. Drugs used for this purpose include β-blockers, calcium channel blockers, and digoxin. Although these drugs may slow the ventricular rate, they usually do not affect the underlying atrial fibrillation (Box 14–3).

After controlling the ventricular rate, atrial fibrillation can be converted to normal sinus rhythm by the use of direct current cardioversion (provided the arrhythmia is of less than 48 hours duration) or by administration of ibutilide or dofetilide. Many patients whose condition is successfully converted will relapse, however. Long-term suppression of atrial fibrillation with Class I or Class III drugs may be effective in some patients after conversion to normal sinus rhythm. For example, amiodarone may be beneficial in patients with heart failure and atrial fibrillation. However, drugs used to suppress atrial fibrillation are not always effective and have numerous adverse effects. For this reason, many patients with atrial fibrillation are treated with a drug to control the ventricular rate and with an anticoagulant to prevent thromboembolism and stroke (see Chapter 16). Surgical ablation of arrhythmogenic tissue is a treatment option in some patients.

Patients who have Wolff-Parkinson-White syndrome and develop atrial fibrillation should not be treated with digoxin or verapamil, because these drugs can decrease accessory pathway refractoriness and lead to ventricular tachycardia.

BOX 14–3   A CASE OF SHORTNESS OF BREATH AND PALPITATIONS

CASE PRESENTATION: A 76-year-old man presents to the emergency department complaining of shortness of breath and chest palpitations for a duration of 3 hours while at rest. He has a history of hypertension controlled with hydrochlorothiazide and type 2 diabetes controlled with diet and metformin. His ECG shows atrial fibrillation with a rapid and irregular ventricular rate averaging 120 beats per minute. He receives diltiazem intravenously, and his ventricular rate becomes more regular with a rate of 85 breaths per minute, and his symptoms subside. Over the next 24 hours, his ECG continues to show atrial fibrillation with a ventricular rate of 75 beats per minute. His serum electrolytes, thyroid function tests, and blood chemistries are within normal limits, and he is placed on heparin and warfarin anticoagulants to prevent thromboembolism and stroke. After discussing treatment options with his physician, he undergoes pharmacologic cardioversion to sinus rhythm with intravenous dofetilide with continuous ECG monitoring, and he is discharged on metformin and lisinopril. He is instructed to call his physician if symptoms of atrial fibrillation resume, and he is scheduled for follow-up evaluations and electrophysiologic studies to determine the most appropriate long-term therapy.

CASE DISCUSSION: Atrial fibrillation is the most common arrhythmia requiring medical care. Its prevalence increases with age such that 8% of persons over 80 years of age have atrial fibrillation. The arrhythmia typically causes dyspnea and palpitations and may lead to clot formation on fibrillating atrial leaflets. Hence, most patients receive anticoagulants to prevent thromboembolism and stroke. Atrial fibrillation may also cause heart failure because it impairs ventricular filling and emptying. There are two approaches to the long-term management of atrial fibrillation: rate control and rhythm control. In the rate control method, a β-blocker or calcium antagonist is administered to control ventricular rate by slowing AV conduction and increasing AV refractory period, without affecting the underlying atrial fibrillation. In the rhythm control method, electrical or pharmacologic cardioversion is used to restore sinus rhythm, which is then maintained with a Class I or Class III antiarrhythmic drug such as flecainide or amiodarone. However, most patients will have a recurrence of atrial fibrillation despite treatment, and drugs used for long-term suppression of atrial fibrillation have the potential to cause serious ventricular arrhythmias. Angiotensin inhibitors appear to lower the relapse rate after cardioversion. A number of new therapies are under development that may overcome some of the limitations of currently available drugs. Some patients benefit from catheter ablation surgery to remove the arrhythmogenic tissue causing atrial fibrillation.

Atrial flutter is usually treated in the same manner as atrial fibrillation. Surgical ablation of the arrhythmogenic tissue can be effective in some patients with atrial flutter.

Supraventricular Tachycardia

PSVT is caused most frequently by a reentrant circuit in the AV node. Acute PSVT is often treated with intravenous adenosine, which causes AV block and interrupts the reentrant pathway. Alternatively, AV block can be produced by a calcium channel blocker (e.g., verapamil) or by a β-blocker (e.g., esmolol). Esmolol is a short-acting drug whose use is often preferred in perioperative patients. Long-term suppression is usually accomplished by use of a calcium channel blocker, β-blocker, or digitalis glycoside. Surgical ablation of the arrhythmogenic tissue can also be effective.

Patients with Wolff-Parkinson-White syndrome exhibit an atypical form of PSVT caused by reentry through an accessory bypass conduction pathway between the atria and ventricles. This form of PSVT can also be terminated with drugs that cause AV block. Long-term treatment may consist of surgical ablation of arrhythmogenic tissue or use of a sodium or potassium channel blocker to suppress the arrhythmia.

MANAGEMENT OF VENTRICULAR ARRHYTHMIAS

Ventricular Tachycardia

Ventricular tachycardia is an arrhythmia that usually presents with a monomorphic, regular, wide QRS complex with a rate greater than 100 to 120 beats per minute. It is often associated with myocardial infarction and is thought to be caused by decremental conduction and reentry in ventricular tissue, phenomena that are described earlier in this chapter.

Sustained ventricular tachycardia should be treated immediately because of its deleterious effect on cardiac output and myocardial ischemia, and because it can lead to ventricular fibrillation (see "Ventricular Fibrillation").

If the patient with ventricular tachycardia does not have a pulse or is hemodynamically unstable, electric (direct current) cardioversion should be used to terminate the arrhythmia. If such persons do not respond to three shocks, they should be treated as if they have ventricular fibrillation (see below) and given epinephrine and amiodarone with continued attempts at cardioversion.

Persons with recurrent episodes of sustained ventricular tachycardia not resulting from a reversible cause (e.g., hypokalemia) are usually treated with intravenous **amiodarone** administered as a series of bolus doses or as an intravenous infusion. Intravenous **procainamide** is an alternative to amiodarone. These treatments are given to prevent further episodes of ventricular tachycardia and reduce the need for cardioversion. An **implantable cardioverter-defibrillator** is usually inserted in patients with hemodynamically significant sustained ventricular tachycardia that occurs more than 2 days after a myocardial infarction.

Clinical trials have shown that amiodarone is not as effective as an implantable cardioverter-defibrillator for the long-term suppression of ventricular arrhythmias in patients with a history of syncope or aborted sudden cardiac death. Amiodarone, however, is sometimes used in conjunction with an implantable cardioverter-defibrillator to reduce the number of shocks required to maintain normal sinus rhythm. Amiodarone or sotalol can also be used to control benign symptomatic arrhythmias, such as nonsustained ventricular tachycardia and frequent premature ventricular beats.

The choice of drug therapy for long-term prophylaxis of ventricular arrhythmias is controversial. Clinical trials have found that amiodarone reduced arrhythmic deaths and arrhythmias requiring resuscitation in patients after myocardial infarction with frequent ventricular premature beats or a low ventricular ejection fraction, but amiodarone did not reduce total or cardiac mortality. The combination of **β-blockers** and **amiodarone**, however, significantly reduced both nonarrhythmic and arrhythmic death. In addition, β-blockers are the only drugs currently recommended to prevent sudden death in persons who have had a myocardial infarction and do not have recurrent ventricular arrhythmias.

Patients who have taken an overdose of a **tricyclic antidepressant drug** (e.g., imipramine) can develop a wide QRS complex tachycardia that is believed to result from the blockade of cardiac sodium channels by the antidepressant. The treatment for this particular form of ventricular tachycardia includes the intravenous administration of sodium bicarbonate, which increases dissociation of the antidepressant from sodium channels. Magnesium sulfate and β-blockers have also been used in successfully treated cases.

Torsades de Pointes

Torsades de pointes is a polymorphic ventricular tachycardia that can be induced by drugs (such as tricyclic antidepressants and phenothiazine antipsychotic agents) or electrolyte abnormalities that prolong the QT interval and predispose cardiac cells to afterdepolarizations. This arrhythmia can also result from a congenital, prolonged QT syndrome. Patients with a drug-induced arrhythmia can be treated by withdrawal of the causative agent, correction of any electrolyte abnormalities such as hypokalemia, intravenous administration of **magnesium sulfate**, cardiac overdrive pacing, or intravenous administration of isoproterenol (a β-adrenoceptor agonist). These treatments act in part by shortening the QT interval.

Ventricular Fibrillation

Ventricular fibrillation is the most common cause of sudden cardiac death in persons with ischemic heart disease. In ventricular fibrillation, the ECG shows rapid (300–400/min), irregular, shapeless depolarizations of variable amplitude and shape. Ventricular fibrillation is thought to be caused by a disorganized reentry circuit in the ventricles. Electrical defibrillation is the treatment of choice for patients with this disorder. If ventricular fibrillation persists after three rapid shocks, intravenous **epinephrine** (or vasopressin) and **amiodarone** are administered followed by continued attempts at defibrillation. **Lidocaine** is no longer used routinely for this purpose, but some authorities suggest trying it if other measures fail.

Long-term therapy to prevent sudden cardiac death in patients who developed sustained ventricular tachycardia or ventricular fibrillation 24 to 48 hours after a myocardial infarction usually consists of an implantable cardioverter-defibrillator and a β-blocker.

SUMMARY OF IMPORTANT POINTS

■ Antiarrhythmic drugs suppress the abnormal impulse formation or conduction that causes arrhythmias.

■ Antiarrhythmic drugs are divided into four main classes, with Class I consisting of sodium channel blockers, Class II consisting of β-adrenoceptor antagonists (β-blockers), Class III consisting of potassium channel blockers and other drugs that prolong the action potential duration, and Class IV consisting of calcium channel blockers.

■ Class IA drugs (e.g., quinidine) slow conduction and prolong refractory periods, thereby increasing the QRS duration and the QT interval. They are primarily used for the long-term suppression of arrhythmias.

■ Class IB drugs have little effect on normal cardiac tissue and electrocardiographic findings, but they can decrease the QT interval slightly. Lidocaine has been administered intravenously for the treatment of acute ventricular arrhythmias. Mexiletine and tocainide, oral congeners of lidocaine, have been used for long-term prophylaxis.

■ Class IC drugs have a greater effect than other sodium channel blockers on cardiac conduction but have little effect on the action potential duration. Flecainide and propafenone are used to treat supraventricular arrhythmias and life-threatening ventricular arrhythmias.

■ Class II drugs (β-blockers), which slow the AV node conduction velocity and prolong the AV node refractory period, are used to treat supraventricular arrhythmias. They also reduce the incidence of fatal ventricular arrhythmias in patients with myocardial infarction.

■ Class III drugs (e.g., amiodarone, dofetilide, ibutilide, and sotalol) prolong the action potential duration, refractory periods, and QT interval.

■ Amiodarone is given intravenously in the treatment of ventricular tachycardia and fibrillation, and can be given orally for chronic prophylaxis. Ibutilide and dofetilide are used for acute termination and chronic prophylaxis of atrial fibrillation. Sotalol is used for both acute and chronic treatment of supraventricular and ventricular arrhythmias.

■ Class IV drugs (calcium channel blockers) slow the AV node conduction velocity, prolong the AV node refractory period, and thereby terminate the AV node reentry that is responsible for supraventricular tachycardia.

■ Adenosine is administered as a rapid intravenous bolus to terminate acute supraventricular tachycardia.

Review Questions

1. After beginning drug therapy to suppress ventricular tachycardia, a man complains of cold intolerance and of being tired all the time. His thyroid-stimulating hormone level is found to be elevated. Which drug is most likely responsible for this adverse reaction?
   (A) procainamide
   (B) sotalol
   (C) dofetilide
   (D) verapamil
   (E) amiodarone

2. A woman is placed on an antiarrhythmic drug that dissociates very slowly from ventricular sodium channels. Which electrocardiographic finding results from this property?
   (A) prolonged PR interval
   (B) shortened PR interval
   (C) prolonged QRS duration
   (D) prolonged QT interval
   (E) sinus bradycardia

3. A man is taking a drug that selectively blocks the rapidly activating delayed rectifier channels. Which electrocardiographic change should guide dosage adjustments with this drug?
   (A) QT prolongation
   (B) QRS widening
   (C) PR prolongation
   (D) T wave inversion
   (E) premature ventricular depolarizations

4. A woman complains of a racing heart that began while playing softball 2 hours ago. Her ECG shows a rapid and regular heart beat, and she is given an intravenous bolus of a drug that activates G protein–coupled receptors. Which drug mechanism may lead to termination of the arrhythmia?
   (A) increased chloride influx
   (B) increased cyclic guanosine monophosphate
   (C) increased calcium influx
   (D) increased potassium efflux
   (E) decreased sodium influx

5. Which drug should be avoided in persons with asthma?
   (A) sotalol
   (B) diltiazem
   (C) flecainide
   (D) quinidine
   (E) lidocaine

Answers and Explanations

1. **The answer is E: amiodarone.** Amiodarone is a thyroxine analogue that can cause hypothyroidism and, less commonly, hyperthyroidism. None of the other options is associated with this adverse effect.

2. **The answer is C: prolonged QRS duration.** The woman was most likely taking a Class IC antiarrhythmic agent such as flecainide. These drugs dissociate very slowly from sodium channels and thereby slow ventricular depolarization and increase QRS duration. A prolonged or shortened PR interval (Options A and B) result from slower or faster impulse conduction, respectively, in the AV node. A prolonged QT interval (Option D) results from delayed ventricular repolarization. Sinus bradycardia (Option E) results from decreased a decreased rate of depolarization of the SA node pacemaker.

3. **The answer is A: QT prolongation.** The man is most likely taking dofetilide, which blocks the delayed rectifying potassium channels that repolarize ventricular tissue. Because of its tendency to prolong the QT interval, the ECG must be monitored during dosage titration of this drug. Potassium channel blockade is not associated with changes in the PR interval, QRS duration, or heart rate.

4. **The answer is D: increased potassium efflux.** The woman most likely had supraventricular tachycardia, which may be precipitated by a premature atrial depolarization. She was treated with adenosine, which activates G protein–coupled adenosine receptors and leads to increased potassium efflux and hyperpolarization of supraventricular tissue.

5. **The answer is A: sotalol.** In addition to having Class III antiarrhythmic activity, sotalol is a β-adrenoceptor antagonist. It may cause bronchospasm in sensitive persons by blocking β_2-adrenoceptors in bronchial smooth muscle. Hence, the drug should be avoided in persons with asthma and chronic obstructive lung disease.

SELECTED READINGS

Gupta, A., A.T. Lawrence, and K. Krishnan, and C.J. Kavinsky, R.G. Trohman. Current concepts in the mechanisms and management of drug-induced QT prolongation and torsades de pointes. Am Heart J 153:891–899, 2007.

Kistler, P.M., and M.N. Obeyesekere. Pharmacologic management of tachycardia. Aust Fam Physician 36:500–505, 2007.

Lip, G.Y., and H.F. Tse. Management of atrial fibrillation. Lancet 370:604–618, 2007.

Reiffel, J.A. Adjunctive therapy for recurrent ventricular tachycardia in patients with implantable cardioverter defibrillators. Curr Cardiol Rep 9:381–386, 2007.

Vassallo, P., and R.G. Trohman. Prescribing amiodarone: an evidence-based review of clinical indications. JAMA 298:1312–1322, 2007.

CHAPTER 15

Drugs for Hyperlipidemia

CLASSIFICATION OF DRUGS FOR HYPERLIPIDEMIA

HMG-CoA Reductase Inhibitors
- Atorvastatin (LIPITOR)
- Fluvastatin (LESCOL)
- Lovastatin (MEVACOR)
- Pravastatin (PRAVACHOL)
- Rosuvastatin (CRESTOR)
- Simvastatin (ZOCOR)

Bile Acid–binding Resins
- Cholestyramine (QUESTRAN)
- Colestipol (COLESTID)
- Colesevelam (WELCHOL)

Cholesterol Absorption Inhibitor
- Ezetimibe (ZETIA)

Fibric Acid Derivatives
- Fenofibrate (TRICOR)
- Gemfibrozil (LOPID)

Other Drugs
- Niacin (NICOTINIC ACID)

OVERVIEW

Lipids are necessary molecules for human life. **Cholesterol,** which is an essential component of cell membranes, is the precursor to the sterol and steroid compounds that are synthesized in the body. **Triglycerides,** composed of three **fatty acids** and glycerol, are the main storage form of fuel used to generate high-energy compounds, such as adenosine triphosphate, that provide the energy for muscle contraction and metabolic reactions. Despite the vital functions of these and other lipids, elevated concentrations of cholesterol and triglycerides play an important role in the development of atherosclerotic heart disease and other disorders.

Whereas **hyperlipidemia** and **hyperlipoproteinemia** are general terms for elevated concentrations of lipids and lipoproteins in the blood, **hypercholesterolemia** and **hypertriglyceridemia** refer specifically to high concentrations of cholesterol and triglycerides, respectively. Hypercholesterolemia contributes to the pathogenesis of **atherosclerosis** and has been causally associated with **coronary artery disease** and other atherosclerotic vascular diseases (Fig. 15–1). Hypertriglyceridemia is a risk factor for **pancreatitis** and is believed to have a role in the development of atherosclerosis and heart disease in some patients, although its role in cardiovascular disorders appears to be less significant than that of hypercholesterolemia.

Because **coronary heart disease** (CHD) is the main cause of premature death in industrialized countries, it is important to detect and eliminate **modifiable risk factors** associated with it. In addition to hyperlipidemia, these risk factors include hypertension, cigarette smoking, and a low high-density lipoprotein (HDL) cholesterol level (<40 mg/dL). Unmodifiable risk factors include male gender, family history of premature CHD (CHD in first-degree male relative under 55 years of age or first-degree female under 65 years of age), and advanced age (men over 45 years, women over 55 years). Diabetes mellitus and clinical manifestations of noncoronary forms of atherosclerotic disease (e.g., aortic aneurysm and carotid artery disease) are considered CHD risk equivalents when health care professionals are determining goals for treatment of hyperlipidemia. This means that persons with these conditions are considered to have the same risk for future occurrences of CHD as persons who already have some form of CHD (e.g., angina pectoris, myocardial infarction, or other types of clinically significant myocardial ischemia).

Women have a lower risk of heart disease until after menopause, and this lower risk may be partly owing to the favorable effect of estrogens on serum lipoprotein levels. Estrogens may also have beneficial effects on the microcirculation and energy metabolism.

After discussing lipoproteins, lipid transport, and the causes and types of hyperlipoproteinemia, this chapter

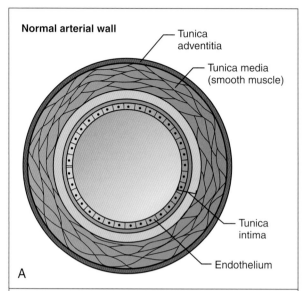

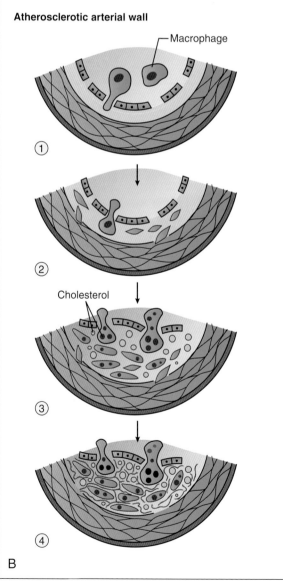

describes how dietary restrictions, alone or in combination with drug treatment, can reduce serum lipoprotein levels and thereby reduce the risk of CHD.

Lipoproteins and Lipid Transport

Because lipids are insoluble in plasma, they must be transported in the circulation in the form of lipoproteins. There are numerous **types of lipoproteins,** including chylomicrons, very low-density lipoproteins (VLDLs), low-density lipoproteins (LDLs), intermediate-density lipoproteins, HDLs, and lipoprotein(a). The various types are distinguished in terms of their buoyant density, lipid and protein composition, and role in lipid transport. Moreover, each type is associated with a unique group of **apoproteins.** Some of the apoproteins are exchanged between different types of lipoproteins as they transport lipids to various tissues. The composition and metabolism of lipoproteins is depicted in Box 15–1.

Chylomicrons

Chylomicrons are involved primarily in the transport of dietary lipids from the gut to the adipose tissue and liver. When cholesterol and triglycerides are ingested, they are emulsified in the intestines by the bile acids and other bile secretions, and the emulsified lipids are combined with proteins to form chylomicrons in the gut wall. After chylomicrons are secreted into the circulation, they deliver triglycerides to adipose tissue via the action of a **lipoprotein lipase** located in the vascular endothelial cells. By this process, chylomicrons are converted to a cholesterol-rich chylomicron remnant, which transports cholesterol to the liver.

Very Low-Density and Low-Density Lipoproteins

Golgi bodies in the liver form VLDLs from triglycerides, cholesterol, and protein and then secrete the VLDLs into the circulation. The VLDLs deliver triglycerides to adipose tissue in the same manner as do the chylomicrons. During the process, the VLDLs are transformed into intermediate-density lipoproteins and LDLs that contain a high percentage of cholesterol.

The LDLs transport cholesterol to peripheral tissues for incorporation into cell membranes and steroids. In this process, the LDLs bind to specific LDL receptors that are located in the plasma membrane of cells and recognize apoprotein B-100 on the surface of LDL molecules. After binding to their receptors, the LDLs undergo endocytosis and are incorporated into lysosomes for further processing of cholesterol and protein.

The LDLs can also deliver cholesterol to nascent atheromas and thereby contribute to the development of atherosclerosis (see Fig. 15–1). In atheromas, cholesterol is

Figure 15–1. Comparison of normal (A) and atherosclerotic (B) arterial walls. Steps in the pathogenesis of atherosclerosis are as follows: (1) Damage to the endothelium is followed by invasion of macrophages. (2) Endothelial and macrophage growth factors stimulate smooth muscle cells to migrate into the tunica intima and to proliferate. (3) Oxidized cholesterol accumulates in and around macrophages (foam cells) and muscle cells. (4) Collagen and elastic fibers form a connective tissue matrix that results in a fibrous plaque.

BOX 15–1   LIPOPROTEIN METABOLISM AND ATHEROSCLEROSIS

The liver is the central processing site for lipoprotein metabolism. Cholesterol is derived from three sources: (1) biosynthesis from acetyl-CoA, (2) delivery of dietary cholesterol by chylomicron remnants, and (3) endocytosis of LDL cholesterol by LDL receptors.

Triglycerides are formed in the liver from fatty acids, which are derived from lipolysis of triglycerides in adipose tissue. Triglycerides, cholesterol, and protein are packaged by Golgi bodies in the liver to form VLDLs, which are secreted into the circulation. The VLDLs accept apoproteins C and E from HDLs and then return these apoproteins to HDL as they deliver triglycerides (as fatty acids) to adipose and other tissues via the action of lipoprotein lipase located in the capillary endothelium.

COMPOSITION OF LIPOPROTEINS

Lipoprotein	Core Lipids*	Apoproteins*
Chylomicron	Dietary triglycerides and cholesteryl esters	B-48, C, E, and A
VLDL	Endogenous triglycerides and cholesteryl esters	C, B-100, and E
LDL	Cholesteryl esters	B-100
HDL	Cholesteryl esters and phospholipids	A-I, A-II, C, E, and D

*Listed in order of quantitative importance.

With the removal of apoproteins and triglycerides, VLDLs are transformed into LDLs and intermediate-density lipoproteins. The LDLs deliver cholesterol to various sites in the body, including peripheral tissues and the liver via endocytosis by LDL receptors. LDL cholesterol is also incorporated into atherosclerotic plaques.

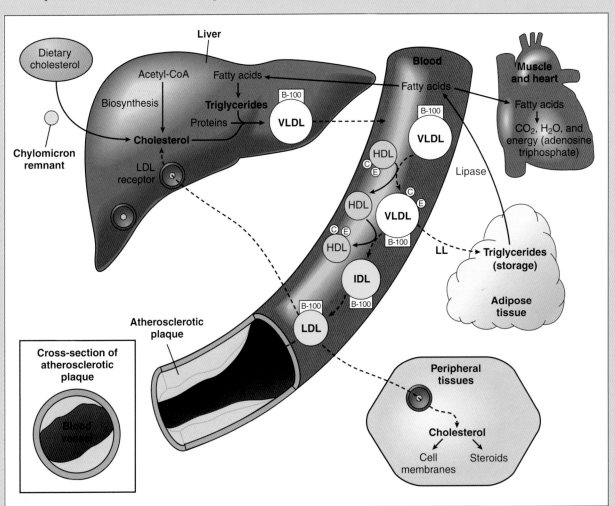

phagocytosed by macrophages, which are transformed into foam cells as they become filled with oxidized cholesterol.

High-Density Lipoproteins

The HDLs are small lipoproteins whose high density is caused by their high ratio of protein to lipid. Nascent pre-β-HDL particles are formed in the liver and intestines from apoprotein A-I and a small quantity of cholesterol and phospholipid. The cholesterol is then esterified by **lecithin-cholesterol acyltransferase** so as to convert pre-β-HDL into mature α-HDL particles. As HDL circulates in the blood, it exchanges apoproteins C and E with VLDL, so as to enable delivery of VLDL triglycerides to adipose tissue via lipoprotein lipase.

HDL transports cholesterol from atheromas and peripheral tissues to the liver. During this process of **reverse cholesterol transport**, the α-HDLs acquire additional cholesterol from macrophages in blood vessel walls (via adenosine triphosphate–binding cassette transporters) and esterify the cholesterol via lecithin-cholesterol acyltransferase. The cholesteryl esters are either transported by HDL directly to the liver or are transferred to LDL for transport to the liver (indirect pathway). The contribution of reverse cholesterol transport to CHD has been supported by epidemiologic studies that show an inverse correlation between HDL levels and the risk of this disease.

Lipoprotein(a)

Lipoprotein(a) is a unique lipoprotein whose physiologic function is unknown and whose occurrence is genetically determined. It is found in atherosclerotic plaques of some individuals, and plasma levels of lipoprotein(a) are highly correlated with angiographically demonstrable coronary artery disease.

Causes and Types of Hyperlipoproteinemia

Hyperlipoproteinemia occurs as a result of genetic or environmental factors that increase the formation of lipoproteins or reduce the clearance of lipoproteins from the circulation. These factors include biochemical defects in lipoprotein metabolism, excessive dietary intake of lipids, endocrine abnormalities, and use of drugs that perturb lipoprotein formation or catabolism. Table 15–1 provides information about the characteristics and types of hyperlipoproteinemia.

Primary hyperlipoproteinemias are relatively rare disorders, each of which is caused by a **monogenic defect** (a specific defect at a single gene). In some disorders, LDL cholesterol (LDL-C) levels are severely elevated because of a deficiency of LDL receptors or a defect in the structure of apoprotein B. In the latter case, LDL receptors do not recognize LDL, so LDL removal from the circulation is markedly impaired. In another disorder, VLDL and triglyceride levels are severely elevated because of a lipoprotein lipase deficiency that prevents delivery of triglycerides to adipose tissue.

Most cases of hyperlipoproteinemia do not result from a single gene defect but instead result from the influence of several genes that predispose the patient to milder forms of hyperlipoproteinemia, particularly in the presence of excessive dietary intake of lipids. These milder forms, called **polygenic-environmental hyperlipoproteinemias**, which are much more common than primary hyperlipoproteinemias, are responsible for most cases of accelerated atherosclerosis.

Secondary hyperlipoproteinemias are commonly caused by the presence of alcoholism, diabetes mellitus, or uremia or by the use of drugs such as β-adrenoceptor antagonists, isotretinoin, oral contraceptives, or thiazide diuretics. They are less commonly caused by hypothyroidism, nephrotic syndrome, or obstructive liver disease.

Guidelines for Management of Hypercholesterolemia

The Adult Treatment Panel III of the **National Cholesterol Education Program** (NCEP) issued evidence-based guidelines for the management of high blood cholesterol and related disorders in 2001. These recommendations were updated in 2004 based on evidence from five clinical trials

TABLE 15–1. Types and Characteristics of Hyperlipoproteinemia			
Types	**Incidence**	**Total Cholesterol Concentration (mg/dL)**	**Triglyceride Concentration (mg/dL)**
Primary (Monogenic) Types			
Hypercholesterolemia	Rare	>300	<250
Hypertriglyceridemia	Rare	<250	>300
Mixed hyperlipidemia	Rare	>250	>300
Polygenic-Environmental Types			
Hypercholesterolemia	Common	200–270	<250
Mixed hyperlipidemia	Less common	>200	>300
Secondary Types			
Hyperlipoproteinemia due to alcoholism, diabetes mellitus, uremia, or use of β-adrenoceptor antagonists,[†] isotretinoin, oral contraceptives, or thiazide diuretics	Common	Usually normal*	Increased
Hyperlipoproteinemia due to hypothyroidism, nephrotic syndrome, or obstructive liver disease	Less common	Increased	Normal or slightly increased

*Use of thiazide diuretics may increase the total cholesterol concentration.
[†]Use of β-adrenoceptor antagonist may decrease the high-density lipoprotein (HDL) cholesterol concentration.

published since the Adult Treatment Panel III guidelines were issued. These trials confirmed the benefits of cholesterol-lowering therapy in high-risk patients and encourage more aggressive reductions in LDL-C in very high-risk patients.

The NCEP guidelines (Table 15–2) establish LDL-C goals and levels for initiating **therapeutic lifestyle changes** (TLCs) and drug therapy for persons in different risk categories. For **high-risk** patients (who already have CHD or have CHD risk equivalents), the basic goal is to achieve a LDL-C of less than 100 mg/dL, and TLC and drug therapy should be initiated if the patient's LDL-C is higher than 100 mg/dL. The updated guidelines suggest an optional LDL-C goal for high-risk patients of less than 70 mg/dL, particularly for those whose LDL-C is less than 100 mg/dL at baseline. This optional goal is based on clinical trials that show that high-risk patients benefit from LDL-C reduction regardless of their baseline level.

For **moderately high-risk** patients (persons with two or more CHD risk factors and a 10% to 20% risk of developing CHD in 10 years), the original guidelines suggest a LDL-C goal of less than 130 mg/dL, with TLC and drug therapy initiated if levels are higher than 130 mg/dL. The updated guidelines recommend considering drug therapy for patients with LDL-C levels between 100 and 129 mg/dL. The 10-year risk of developing CHD can be estimated using calculators such as the one provided by the National Heart, Lung, and Blood Institute (see Table 15–2).

Patients with a **moderate risk** of CHD (two or more risk factors and <10% risk of developing CHD in 10 years) have the same LDL-C goal and TLC initiation level as moderately high-risk patients, but drug therapy is recommended only at the start of therapy if LDL-C levels are above 160 mg/dL. If TLCs do not achieve the target level in 6 to 12 months, drug therapy should be considered for persons with a moderate risk of CHD.

For persons with a **lower risk** of CHD (zero to one risk factor), the target LDL-C level is less than 160 mg/dL. For this reason, TLC should be initiated in persons exceeding this level. The original guidelines recommended drug therapy only at the start of treatment if LDL-C levels exceed 190 mg/dL, but the updated recommendations suggest considering drug therapy if levels are between 160 and 189 mg/dL.

The updated guidelines also suggest that high-risk patients with high triglycerides or a low HDL-cholesterol (HDL-C) level receive niacin or a fibrate drug in combination with a LDL-C lowering drug to raise HDL-C levels and lower triglyceride levels. This is because epidemiologic studies show a correlation between CHD and high levels of plasma triglycerides or low levels of HDL.

Secondary causes of hyperlipidemia should be excluded before treatment is considered, because abnormal levels of cholesterol or triglycerides can often be corrected by proper management of the underlying condition or by replacing the offending drug with an alternative.

Therapeutic Lifestyle Changes

TLCs are an essential modality in the management of high cholesterol and triglyceride levels and may be effective by themselves in patients with mildly elevated cholesterol or triglyceride levels. The TLC modality includes recommendations for diet, weight management, and physical activity. The diet of patients with hypercholesterolemia should be low in cholesterol, saturated fat, and calories. **Saturated fat** and **cholesterol** are restricted because each independently increases LDL-C, and **calories** are restricted to help the patient achieve or maintain an ideal body weight. The Adult Treatment Panel III guidelines recommend the **American Heart Association step II diet** as the initial diet for lowering cholesterol and triglyceride levels and suggest adding **plant stanol or sterol esters**, also called **phytosterols** (2 g/day), and soluble fiber (10 to 25 g/day) to enhance LDL-C reduction.

The American Health Association step II diet mandates that cholesterol intake should be under 200 mg/day, and total calories from fat should be limited to 25% to 35% of total calories, with saturated fat limited to less than 7% of total calories. Foods containing partially hydrogenated plant oils should be avoided because hydrogenation produces the **trans isomers of fatty acids** that acts to increase

TABLE 15–2. **National Cholesterol Education Program Guidelines for Management of High Blood Cholesterol Levels for Persons in Different Risk Categories***

Risk Category	LDL-C goal	Initiate TLC*	Consider Drug Therapy*
High risk: CHD or CHD equivalents[†] (10-year risk[‡] of CHD >20%)	<100 mg/dL (optional: <70 mg/dL)	≥100 mg/dL	≥100 mg/dL (optional goal: <100 mg/dL)
Moderately high risk: 2+ risk factors[§] (10-year risk of CHD 10%–20%)	<130 mg/dL (optional: <100 mg/dL)	≥130 mg/dL	≥130 mg/dL (optional: 100–129 mg/dL)
Moderate risk: 2+ risk factors (10-year risk of CHD <10%)	<130 mg/dL	≥130 mg/dL	≥160 mg/dL
Lower risk: 0–1 risk factor	<160 mg/dL	≥160 mg/dL	≥190 mg/dL (optional: 160–190 mg/dL)

From Adult Treatment Panel III Guidelines, issued in 2001 and updated in 2004 (see Grundy et al). [J Am Coll Cardiol 2001;44:720–732.]
*LDL-C levels at which TLC or drug therapy initiated.
[†]Includes myocardial infarction, angina, myocardial ischemia, noncoronary forms of atherosclerosis, and diabetes mellitus.
[‡]Electronic 10-year risk calculators available at www.nhlbi.nih.gov/guidelines/cholesterol.
[§]Risk factors include cigarette smoking, hypertension, low HDL-C, family history of premature CHD, and age (see chapter text for details).
CHD = coronary heart disease; HDL-C = high-density lipoprotein cholesterol; LDL-C = low-density lipoprotein cholesterol; TLC = therapeutic lifestyle change.

LDL-C levels, decrease HDL-C levels, increase systemic inflammation, and reduce the availability of fatty acid precursors to anticoagulant prostaglandins.

Dietary modulations are particularly useful in persons with multiple risk factors or angiographic evidence of coronary artery disease. Studies have shown that diets low in saturated and trans fatty acids and high in linoleic acid and **omega-3 fatty acids** (linolenic acid and those in **fish oils**) improve the LDL-C to HDL-C ratio. These diets may also reverse the angiographic evidence of coronary atherosclerosis and reduce mortality rate in patients with CHD. In patients with hypertriglyceridemia, supplementing the diet with fish oils that contain **omega-3 fatty acids** often lowers triglyceride levels. The omega-3 fatty acids contain a double bond between the third and fourth carbon from the end of the molecule.

DRUGS FOR HYPERCHOLESTEROLEMIA

The 3-hydroxy-3-methylglutaryl–coenzyme A (HMG-CoA) reductase inhibitors (statins), the bile acid–binding resins, and ezetimibe are used primarily to treat hypercholesterolemia, whereas the fibric acid derivatives and niacin are used to reduce elevated triglyceride levels and to raise HDL levels. Table 15–3, Table 15–4, and Table 15–5 outline the effects and pharmacokinetic properties of the drugs used to treat hypercholesterolemia and compare them with the effects and properties of other drugs discussed in this chapter.

HMG-CoA Reductase Inhibitors (Statins)

Among the HMG-CoA reductase inhibitors are **atorvastatin, fluvastatin, lovastatin, pravastatin, rosuvastatin,** and **simvastatin.** The statins are the most effective drugs for lowering blood cholesterol levels, and clinical trials have shown that they prevent coronary artery disease and reduce mortality. The statins have a good safety record, and their once-daily dosage regimen is highly convenient and fosters patient adherence.

CHEMISTRY AND PHARMACOKINETICS. The statins are structurally related to HMG-CoA, which is the substrate for HMG-CoA reductase (see Fig. 15–3). The drugs have a relatively low bioavailability, owing largely to extensive first-pass metabolism. Lovastatin and simvastatin are inactive prodrugs that must be converted to active metabolites in the liver, whereas the other statins are active compounds. All of the drugs, except atorvastatin, have relatively short half-lives (see Table 15–4). Some of the reductase inhibitors are metabolized by cytochrome P450 (CYP) enzymes (see below).

Statins with shorter half-lives are taken in the evening or at bedtime to ensure inhibition of nocturnal cholesterol biosynthesis. Atorvastatin and rosuvastatin have longer half-lives and can be taken at any time of day. Lovastatin should be taken with the evening meal to facilitate its absorption, whereas the other drugs can be taken without regard to food. Lovastatin and simvastatin cross the blood-brain barrier and can cause sleep disturbances in some patients.

MECHANISMS AND PHARMACOLOGIC EFFECTS. HMG-CoA reductase converts HMG-CoA to mevalonic acid and is the rate-limiting enzyme in cholesterol biosynthesis (Fig. 15–2 and Fig. 15–3). By competitively inhibiting this enzyme, statins reduce hepatic cholesterol biosynthesis and the amount of cholesterol available for incorporation into VLDL. This leads to a compensatory increase in the number of hepatic LDL receptors, which increases hepatic uptake of LDL-C. Together, these actions cause a substantial reduction in LDL-C. In patients with hypercholesterolemia, statins typically decrease LDL-C levels by 20% to 50%, whereas HDL-C levels are increased by 10% (see Table 15–3). The statins also reduce serum triglycerides but are usually not a sufficient treatment for hypertriglyceridemia by themselves.

INDICATIONS. The statins are used to reduce blood cholesterol levels in persons with **hypercholesterolemia** to achieve the LDL-C goals recommended by the NCEP. The NCEP guidelines recommend using a statin dose that can achieve a 30% to 40% reduction in LDL-C levels. The statins do not have equal potency with respect to reducing LDL-C levels. Rosuvastatin is the most potent statin currently available,

TABLE 15–3. Effects of Diet and Drug Therapy on Serum Lipid Concentrations

Therapy	LDL Cholesterol Concentration	HDL Cholesterol Concentration	Total Triglyceride Concentration	Other Effects
Dietary modifications alone	↓ 10%–15%	↑ (variable)	↓ 10%–20%	Reduction of weight and decrease in blood pressure
Drug Therapy				
HMG-CoA reductase inhibitors	↓ 20%–50%	↑ 10%	↓ 10%–40%	Increase in hepatic LDL receptors
Bile acid–binding resins	↓ 10%–20%	↑ 0%–4%	↓ 0%–5%	Increase in hepatic LDL receptors
Fibric acid derivatives	↓ 10%*	↑ 10%–20%	↓ 40%–50%	Activation of lipoprotein lipase
Other Drugs				
Ezetimibe	↓ 18%–22%	↑ 1%–3%	↓ 8%–12%	—
Niacin	↓ 10%–20%	↑ 10%–25%	↓ 20%–80%	Decrease in lipolysis and lipoprotein(a) levels

*Fenofibrate has a greater effect than gemfibrozil on the LDL cholesterol concentration.
HDL = high-density lipoprotein; HMG-CoA = 3-hydroxy-3-methylglutaryl–coenzyme A; LDL = low-density lipoprotein.

TABLE 15–4. **Pharmacokinetic Properties of Drugs for Hyperlipidemia**

Drug	Oral Bioavailability	Elimination Half-Life (Hours)	Major Routes of Elimination	Other Properties
HMG-CoA Reductase Inhibitors				
Atorvastatin	12%	14	M and F	Does not cross the blood-brain barrier
Fluvastatin	25%	<1	M and F	Does not cross the blood-brain barrier
Lovastatin	5%	3.5	M and F	Is a prodrug; crosses the blood-brain barrier
Pravastatin	17%	1.8	M and F	Does not cross the blood-brain barrier
Rosuvastatin	20%	19	M and F	—
Simvastatin	<5%	3	M and F	Is a prodrug; crosses the blood-brain barrier
Bile Acid–binding Resins				
Cholestyramine	0%	NA	F	Is a high-molecular-weight polymer
Colestipol	0%	NA	F	Is a high-molecular-weight polymer
Fibric acid derivatives				
Fenofibrate	100%	23	M	Is a prodrug
Gemfibrozil	100%	2	M (98%)	Undergoes enterohepatic cycling
Other Drugs				
Ezetimibe	Variable	22	M and F	Localizes in small intestine
Niacin	100%	0.5	M and R	—

F = fecal; HMG-CoA = 3-hydroxy-3-methylglutaryl–coenzyme A; M = metabolism; NA = not applicable; R = renal.

TABLE 15–5. **Adverse Effects and Interactions of Drugs for Hyperlipidemia**

Drug	Common Adverse Effects	Common Drug Interactions
HMG-CoA reductase inhibitors	Elevated serum levels of hepatic enzymes; hepatitis; and myalgia, rhabdomyolysis, and other myopathies.	Cause slight increase in serum levels of warfarin. Increase risk of myopathies when taken with erythromycin, gemfibrozil, or niacin.*
Bile acid–binding resins	Constipation; fecal impaction; and rash.	Decrease absorption of digoxin, thyroxin, warfarin, and other drugs.
Fibric acid derivatives	Allergic reactions; blood cell deficiencies; and myalgia, rhabdomyolysis, and other myopathies.	Increase risk of myopathy when taken with HMG-CoA reductase inhibitors or niacin.
Other Drugs		
Ezetimibe	Headache, myalgia.	Absorption decreased by cholestyramine.
Niacin	Gastric irritation; glucose intolerance; myalgia, rhabdomyolysis, and other myopathies; and vasodilation, flushing, and pruritus.	Increases risk of myopathy when taken with gemfibrozil or HMG-CoA reductase inhibitors.*

*If niacin must be used in combination with an HMG-CoA reductase inhibitor, the safest combination is niacin plus fluvastatin and the combination that poses the greatest risk is niacin plus lovastatin.
HMG-CoA = 3-hydroxy-3-methylglutaryl–coenzyme A.

followed by atorvastatin. Atorvastatin and rosuvastatin also have the greatest effect on triglyceride levels and can be useful in treating patients with **mixed hyperlipidemia.** Statins also lower levels of lipoprotein(a).

Clinical trials of reductase inhibitors have demonstrated that these drugs slow the progression of atherosclerosis, reduce the risk of CHD and other atherosclerotic vascular diseases, and reduce the cardiac mortality rate. A large prospective study of 4444 patients with CHD found that patients treated with simvastatin had a lower rate of **death, myocardial infarction, stroke, and revascularization procedures.** Some of the benefits produced by statins may result from their ability to improve vascular endothelial function and reduce inflammation. Clinical trials also indicate that statins may also protect against **osteoporosis** and certain forms of **cancer.**

ADVERSE EFFECTS. The statins are generally well tolerated but may cause serious adverse effects in a small percentage of persons. The most frequent adverse effects are gastrointestinal problems, including abdominal cramps, constipation,

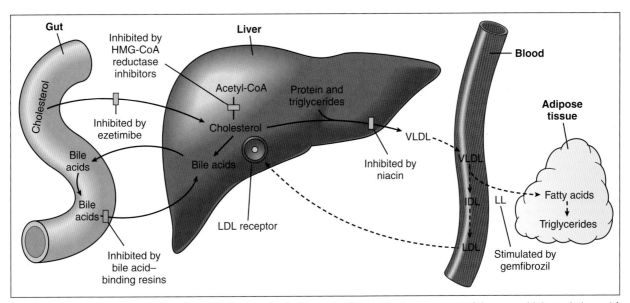

Figure 15-2. Sites and mechanisms of drugs for hyperlipidemia. Ezetimibe inhibits the absorption of dietary and biliary cholesterol from the intestines. The HMG-CoA reductase inhibitors block the rate-limiting step in cholesterol biosynthesis. The bile acid–binding resins inhibit the reabsorption of bile acids from the gut. Niacin inhibits the secretion of VLDLs from the liver, while fibrates such as gemfibrozil stimulate lipoprotein lipase to increase the hydrolysis of VLDL triglycerides and the delivery of fatty acids to adipose and other tissues. IDL = intermediate-density lipoprotein.

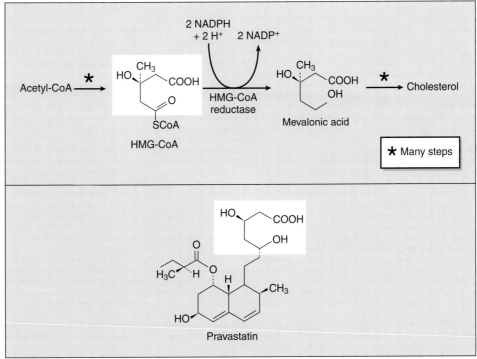

Figure 15-3. Inhibition of cholesterol biosynthesis by HMG-CoA reductase inhibitors. HMG-CoA reductase catalyzes the conversion of HMG-CoA to mevalonic acid, the rate-limiting enzyme in cholesterol biosynthesis. The reductase inhibitors contain a structure that is similar to the structure of HMG-CoA (the unshaded portions of pravastatin and HMG-CoA), and they compete with the substrate for the catalytic site of the enzyme.

diarrhea, and heartburn. Less frequently, statins cause hepatitis and elevate serum levels of hepatic enzymes (see Table 15–5). The most serious adverse effect of statins is rhabdomyolysis, which is a potentially fatal form of skeletal muscle toxicity (myopathy). Only about 0.2% of patients receiving statins develop myopathy, and only a few of these cases progress to rhabdomyolysis.

The precise mechanisms by which statins cause **myopathy** are still being elucidated. By inhibiting cholesterol synthesis, statins can alter cell membrane composition and electrical properties, but exactly how this is related to myopathy remains uncertain. The earliest stage of statin-induced myopathy is **myalgia**, which consists of muscle ache or weakness without elevated creatine kinase levels. This stage is reversible on statin withdrawal and resolves in 2 to 3 weeks. Myalgia can be followed by **myositis** or muscle inflammation accompanied by muscle pain, leakage of muscle creatine kinase into the plasma, and elevated creatine kinase levels. Myositis can eventually lead to **rhabdomyolysis** in which muscle cells disintegrate, thereby releasing myoglobin into the circulation. Myoglobin then accumulates in the kidneys and causes acute renal failure. Creatine kinase levels in rhabdomyolysis are often greater than 10 times the upper limit of normal, and persons with this affliction have dark urine resulting from **myoglobinuria.**

Patients taking a statin should be asked to report any sign of unusual, diffuse, or persistent muscle tenderness, pain, or weakness, especially if it is accompanied by malaise, fever, or dark urine. Factors that increase the risk of statin-induced myopathy include increasing age, female gender, renal or hepatic disease, hypothyroidism, and the use of drugs that inhibit statin metabolism. Use of the statin must be discontinued if myopathy is diagnosed or if levels of creatine kinase are found to be significantly elevated. No specific treatment exists for rhabdomyolysis except drug withdrawal and fluid administration to maintain renal function.

INTERACTIONS. Atorvastatin, lovastatin, and simvastatin are metabolized by CYP3A4, and their plasma concentrations are greatly increased by strong inhibitors of this isozyme, such as erythromycin, itraconazole, and ritonavir. Pravastatin and rosuvastatin are mostly excreted unchanged, and their plasma concentrations are not significantly increased by CYP3A4 inhibitors. Fluvastatin is metabolized by CYP2C9, and its plasma levels may be increased by inhibitors of this CYP, including some nonsteroidal anti-inflammatory drugs.

Statins inhibit the metabolism of certain other drugs by CYP enzymes. For example, they increase warfarin levels slightly by inhibiting warfarin metabolism. Because both statins and fibric acid derivatives may cause myopathies, the combined use of drugs should be avoided or used with great caution.

Bile Acid–binding Resins

Drug Properties

Bile acid–binding resins are moderately effective drugs for hypercholesterolemia and have an excellent safety record. They are especially valuable for patients who cannot tolerate other drugs and for patients who are young and therefore may need to take drug therapy for a long time.

CHEMISTRY AND PHARMACOKINETICS. The bile acid–binding resins are large-molecular-weight polymers containing a chloride ion that can be exchanged for bile acids in the gut. The resins are not absorbed from the gut and are excreted in the feces.

MECHANISMS AND PHARMACOLOGIC EFFECTS. After the resins bind to bile acids, the bile acid–resin complex is excreted. This action prevents the enterohepatic cycling of bile acids and obligates the liver to synthesize replacement bile acids from cholesterol. To obtain more cholesterol for this purpose, the liver increases the number of LDL receptors. Then the levels of LDL-C in the serum are reduced as more cholesterol is delivered to the liver. As shown in Table 15–3, the resins have relatively little effect on levels of HDL-C and triglycerides, which are usually increased slightly.

ADVERSE EFFECTS AND INTERACTIONS. The bile acid–binding resins have few adverse effects. They can cause constipation, fecal impaction, and other gastrointestinal side effects, some of which can be prevented by taking the drugs with a full glass of water. Occasionally, they cause irritation of the perianal area and a skin rash. In the gut, cholestyramine and colestipol can bind to digoxin, thyroxin, warfarin, and other drugs. For this reason, it is best to take these resins 2 hours before or after taking other medications. A newer resin, colesevelam, does not affect the oral bioavailability of digoxin, warfarin, or lovastatin, and, therefore, can be co-administered with most drugs, including HMG-CoA reductase inhibitors.

INDICATIONS. The resins are indicated for the treatment of **hypercholesterolemia** and are particularly useful in patients who cannot tolerate other drugs. Although the resins are less effective than the statins, they do not cause hepatitis or myopathy, and they can be given in combination with other drugs to produce an additive effect on serum cholesterol levels. The resins have also been used to treat **diarrhea** and **pruritus** (itching) caused by excessive levels of bile acids.

Cholestyramine, Colestipol, and Colesevelam

Cholestyramine and colestipol are bile acid–binding resins that are available in powder (granular) form for mixing with water or juice just before administration. To obtain the maximal effect on serum cholesterol levels, these drugs must be taken before each meal and at bedtime. **Colesevelam** is a newer resin that is available as solid tablets that are usually taken twice daily with meals. It decreases LDL-C to a similar degree as do the other resins and is more convenient and palatable.

Ezetimibe

Ezetimibe is a unique drug that inhibits the absorption of dietary cholesterol. After oral administration, ezetimibe is absorbed from the intestines and then is mostly converted to pharmacologically active ezetimibe-glucuronide. This metabolite is distributed by the circulation to the small intestines where it localizes in the brush border and inhibits the absorption of both biliary and dietary cholesterol. Studies suggest that ezetimibe acts by disrupting a complex of two proteins, annexin 2 and caveolin 1, which mediate cholesterol transport in intestinal brush border cells. The half-lives of ezetimibe and ezetimibe-glucuronide are both 22 hours. The drugs are eliminated in the urine and feces.

Because of its unique mechanism of action, ezetimibe can be used alone or in combination with a statin to treat hypercholesterolemia. A fixed-dose combination of ezetimibe and simvastatin (VYTORIN) is available for this purpose. When administered alone, ezetimibe lowers LDL-C 19% to

23%. An incremental reduction of LDL-C of about 22% was obtained when ezetimibe was added to statin therapy in one study. Hence, the co-administration of ezetimibe and a statin can achieve reductions in LDL-C similar to that obtained with the highest statin doses. This may permit the use of lower doses of statins to obtain desired LDL-C levels with correspondingly less risk of statin toxicity (Box 15–2). This combination has been found to be effective in treating persons with homozygous familial hypercholesterolemia.

Ezetimibe has been well tolerated in clinical trials, although some persons complained of headache and myalgia.

OTHER DRUGS FOR HYPERLIPIDEMIA

Niacin and the fibric acid derivatives are used to treat hypertriglyceridemia and to increase HDL-C levels in persons with abnormally low levels of this lipoprotein. The effects and properties of these drugs are shown in Tables 15–3, 15–4, and 15–5.

Niacin (Nicotinic Acid)

Pharmacologic doses of niacin have profound effects on serum lipid levels, and niacin has a valuable role in the treatment of patients with dyslipidemia.

CHEMISTRY AND PHARMACOKINETICS. Niacin is also known as vitamin B_3. The small amount of niacin that is ingested in food is converted in the body to enzyme cofactors required for oxidative reactions in intermediary metabolism. These cofactors are nicotinamide adenine dinucleotide and its phosphate derivative. Niacin is well absorbed from the gut and is extensively metabolized before undergoing renal excretion.

MECHANISMS AND PHARMACOLOGIC EFFECTS. The quantity of niacin ingested in food does not have any measurable effect on serum lipid levels. The action of niacin on lipids is a pharmacologic effect that requires the administration of several grams of the compound each day. Pharmacologic doses of niacin lower LDL-C and triglyceride levels while raising HDL-C levels.

Niacin acts primarily by inhibiting the formation and secretion of hepatic VLDL, the major carrier of plasma triglycerides and the precursor to LDL (see Fig. 15–3). The effect on VLDL secretion is caused partly by **inhibition of lipolysis** in adipose tissue. This action reduces the supply of circulating free fatty acids that the liver uses to synthesize triglycerides for incorporation into VLDL. The inhibition of lipolysis has been attributed to the binding of niacin to a **G protein–coupled receptor** in adipose tissue. Niacin decreases LDL-C levels and particularly the levels of small, dense LDL particles associated with atherosclerosis. At the same time, niacin increases HDL-C levels (see Table 15–3), including the levels of the beneficial HDL_2 component of HDL.

INDICATIONS. Because of its favorable effects on VLDL, LDL, and HDL levels, niacin is an effective treatment for hypercholesterolemia, hypertriglyceridemia, and **mixed hyperlipidemia,**

BOX 15–2 A CASE OF WEIGHT GAIN AND DYSLIPIDEMIA

CASE PRESENTATION: A 56-year-old man with a family history of CHD came to his physician to review recent lab work. He has battled weight gain over the past several years and now weighs 215 pounds. His waist circumference is 41 inches and his body mass index is 28. He has had hypertension for 4 years that has been treated with lisinopril, and his recent blood pressure readings have averaged 136 over 84 mm Hg. The patient's lab work shows an LDL-C level of 175 mg/dL, an HDL-C level of 40 mg/dL, and a triglyceride level of 180 mg/dL. His other lab values are within normal limits. The patient expresses a desire to lose weight and agrees to begin an American Heart Association step II diet and a structured exercise program. He is placed on atorvastatin to reduce LDL-C levels and is referred to a dietitian and exercise physiologist.

Two month later, the patient returns to his physician for follow-up. He has lost 8 pounds, and his lipid profile now includes a LDL-C of 150 mg/dL, a HDL-C of 44 mg/dL, and a triglyceride level of 150 mg/dL. To further reduce his LDL-C level, ezetimibe is added to the patient's treatment regimen, and he is scheduled to see his physician again in 2 months.

CASE DISCUSSION: An estimated 13 million Americans have CHD, which is the leading cause of mortality in the United States. The death rate for CHD has been decreasing steadily for several decades, partly due to lifestyle changes and improved medical care, but CHD still causes nearly 1 in 5 deaths. The patient in this case has several risk factors for CHD, including advanced age, male gender, hypertension, and an atherogenic dyslipidemia. He also meets several criteria for the so-called metabolic syndrome. Hence, it is important to address his modifiable risk factors and prevent progression to symptomatic CHD. The patient has shown adherence to lifestyle modifications that may enable him to achieve a normal body weight and triglyceride level. Because of his multiple risk factors for CHD, his LDL-C goal is less than 100 mg/dL, with an optional goal of less than 70 mg/dL. Statins have been shown to reduce LDL-C and prevent cardiovascular death, while ezetimibe may enable the patient to achieve his LDL-C goal more easily and with less risk of toxicity. The patient will benefit from working with a health care team that may include a physician's assistant, nurse, pharmacist, dietician, and exercise counselor.

and it can be used to treat **HDL deficiency**. In the Coronary Drug Project trial, niacin reduced the risk of myocardial infarction among men with hypercholesterolemia and atherosclerosis, and it decreased total mortality. Niacin may be combined with a statin to treat patients with mixed lipidemia (see below).

ADVERSE EFFECTS AND INTERACTIONS. The large doses of niacin required to lower serum lipids typically cause vasodilation and flushing of the skin, accompanied by pruritus and a feeling of warmth and tingling. This effect can be reduced by pretreatment with aspirin, and some tolerance to this effect develops with continued drug administration. These effects are also reduced with the use of a sustained-release niacin preparation. In a small percentage of patients, niacin can elevate serum transaminase levels and cause hepatitis. It can also cause gastric distress and may activate a peptic ulcer. Although niacin can cause glucose intolerance and aggravate diabetes, clinical trials show it can be used in persons whose diabetes is well controlled with little effect on glucose levels.

Fibric Acid Derivatives

Drug Properties

High triglyceride levels (>1000–1500 mg/dL) are associated with pancreatitis and are usually treated with fibrates to reduce the risk of this disorder. The benefit of treating mild-to-moderate elevations in triglyceride levels is less clear. While hypertriglyceridemia appears to be a risk factor for premature CHD, the utility of fibrate drugs in preventing CHD is uncertain because clinical trials have generally shown that fibrates reduce the onset of CHD but do not significantly lower the rates of fatal myocardial infarction or total mortality. In a trial of fenofibrate in patients with type 2 diabetes and dyslipidemia, fenofibrate did not reduce the rates of either fatal or nonfatal myocardial infarction. For this reason, some authorities suggest using niacin, rather than a fibrate, to control dyslipidemia in these patients (see below).

CHEMISTRY AND PHARMACOKINETICS. These drugs are derivatives of a branched-chain carboxylic acid known as fibric acid or **fibrate**. The first drug in this class, clofibrate, is largely obsolete because of its high incidence of adverse effects. **Gemfibrozil** and **fenofibrate** are currently available in the United States.

MECHANISMS AND PHARMACOLOGIC EFFECTS. The fibrates reduce plasma levels of VLDL triglycerides and LDL-C, while raising levels of HDL-C. The fibrates produce these effects primarily by activating a receptor in cell nuclei that regulates gene transcription and is called the **peroxisome proliferator-activated receptor-α** (PPAR-α). In the liver and elsewhere, PPAR-α increases the transcription of specific genes while inhibiting the transcription of other genes.

The effect of fibrates on plasma triglyceride levels can be partly attributed to PPAR-α–mediated expression of **lipoprotein lipase.** This enzyme is located in the vascular endothelium and catalyzes the hydrolysis and removal of triglycerides from VLDL, thereby lowering plasma triglyceride levels (see Fig. 15–2). PPAR-α activation also reduces expression of an inhibitor of lipoprotein lipase, **apolipoprotein C-III.** Other effects of PPAR-α activation include expression of enzymes that oxidize fatty acids. The effects of fibrates on HDL-C are primarily caused by PPAR-α–mediated expression of apoproteins A-I and A-II, which are important components of HDL. PPAR-α also increases expression of cholesterol transport proteins (adenosine triphosphate–binding cassette transporters A1 and G1) involved in reverse cholesterol transport (see "High-Density Lipoproteins").

Fenofibrate reduces plasma LDL-C levels, in part, by increasing expression of hepatic LDL receptors via activation of PPAR-α. PPAR-α activation also results in changes in the triglyceride and cholesterol content of LDL that increase LDL affinity for the LDL receptor. Together, these actions increase the uptake of LDL-C by the liver and reduce plasma LDL-C levels. Fenofibrate causes a greater reduction in LDL-C than does gemfibrozil.

ADVERSE EFFECTS AND INTERACTIONS. The fibrates often cause gastrointestinal side effects and, less commonly, blood cell deficiencies and other hypersensitivity reactions. As with the statin drugs, the fibrates can cause myopathy and rhabdomyolysis (see Table 15–5). For this reason, the combined administration of statins and fibrates should be avoided or used with great caution. Fibrates can be given with cholestyramine and colestipol, but the doses must be separated by more than 2 hours, because the resins reduce fibrate absorption.

Gemfibrozil

Gemfibrozil is indicated primarily for the treatment of **hypertriglyceridemia.** It is also useful in patients with combined hypertriglyceridemia and hypercholesterolemia and can be administered to increase HDL-C in patients with an isolated **HDL deficiency.**

The Helsinki Heart Study, which involved 2000 men with hypercholesterolemia, found that gemfibrozil increased HDL-C levels and decreased LDL-C and triglyceride levels. It also reduced the CHD-related mortality rate, but the overall mortality rate was not affected.

Fenofibrate

Fenofibrate is indicated for the treatment of elevated triglyceride levels and mixed hyperlipidemia with elevated triglyceride and cholesterol levels.

DRUG COMBINATIONS

Drugs can be used in combination to treat high blood cholesterol in patients who do not respond to a single drug. The most useful combinations are those consisting of ezetimibe or a bile acid–binding resin in combination with a statin drug. Ezetimibe and simvastatin are available in a combination product (VYTORIN), which enables the use of a lower dose of the statin to achieve target LDL-C levels and reduce the risk of myopathy. Colesevelam is a newer resin that can be co-administered with statins.

For patients with elevated levels of both cholesterol and triglycerides, a statin can be combined with niacin or a fibrate drug. Niacin is often preferred for this purpose for several reasons: (1) niacin has a greater effect on cholesterol levels than do fibrates and may enable the use of lower doses of a statin to control hypercholesterolemia; (2) clinical trials show that niacin lowers cardiovascular and overall mortality; and (3) niacin is less likely than fibrates to cause myopathy and rhabdomyolysis when used in combination with a statin.

SUMMARY OF IMPORTANT POINTS

■ Cholesterol and triglycerides are secreted by the liver in the form of VLDL. After delivering triglycerides to adipose tissue, VLDL becomes LDL. LDL delivers cholesterol to peripheral tissues, the liver, and atheromas. HDL transports cholesterol from tissues and atheromas to the liver.

■ Hypercholesterolemia is a risk factor for atherosclerosis and coronary artery disease. Hypertriglyceridemia, which is associated with pancreatitis, also has a role in the development of heart disease.

■ Patients with high blood cholesterol levels should be managed with TLC and drug therapy based on the guidelines of the NCEP.

■ Ezetimibe inhibits the absorption of dietary and biliary cholesterol from the intestines, thereby causing a reduction in LDL-cholesterol levels.

■ Atorvastatin and other HMG-CoA reductase inhibitors block the rate-limiting enzyme in cholesterol biosynthesis and lead to a secondary increase in hepatic LDL receptors and cholesterol uptake, thereby causing a reduction in LDL-C levels.

■ Cholestyramine, colestipol, and colesevelam are bile acid–binding resins that prevent the enterohepatic cycling of bile acids and increase hepatic cholesterol conversion to replacement bile acids, thereby leading to a reduction in LDL-C levels.

■ Niacin and the fibric acid derivatives (gemfibrozil and fenofibrate) reduce triglyceride levels and increase HDL-C levels. Niacin inhibits VLDL secretion and reduces triglyceride and LDL-C levels. Fibrates increase VLDL clearance by increasing lipoprotein lipase activity via activation of the PPAR-α.

Review Questions

1. An otherwise healthy 58-year-old man is found to have an LDL-C level of 170 mg/dL, an HDL-C level of 50 mg/dL, and a triglyceride level of 105 mg/dL. He has no other risk factors for CHD. In addition to TLC, which drug treatment is most appropriate for this patient?
   (A) cholestyramine
   (B) simvastatin
   (C) niacin
   (D) ezetimibe
   (E) gemfibrozil

2. A man with hyperlipidemia is treated with an agent that increases expression of lipoprotein lipase. Which of the following effects would be expected to result from this action?
   (A) increased LDL-C levels
   (B) decreased HDL-C levels
   (C) increased plasma triglyceride levels
   (D) decreased plasma triglyceride levels
   (E) decreased LDL-C levels

3. A woman experiences flushing and pruritus over her upper body after starting a drug for hyperlipidemia. Which mechanism is responsible for the effect of this drug on hepatic triglyceride synthesis?
   (A) activation of the PPAR-α
   (B) increased lipolysis
   (C) binding to a G protein–coupled receptor
   (D) inhibition of HMG-CoA reductase
   (E) binding to deoxycholic acid

4. A man is placed on a drug that disrupts annexin and caveolin. Which effect results from this action?
   (A) decreased cholesterol synthesis
   (B) decreased triglyceride synthesis
   (C) decreased cholesterol absorption
   (D) decreased triglyceride absorption
   (E) increased bile acid excretion

Answers and Explanations

1. **The answer is B: simvastatin.** The man has two risk factors for CHD (male gender and advanced age) and a moderate risk of CHD. Because his LDL-C level is greater than 160 mg/dL, drug therapy should be considered. Statins such as simvastatin have been shown to reduce the incidence of heart disease in persons with elevated cholesterol levels and would be the most appropriate drug therapy for this patient.

2. **The answer is D: decreased plasma triglyceride levels.** The man was treated with a fibrate drug that activates the PPAR-α and thereby increases expression of lipoprotein lipase. This enzyme catalyzes the removal of triglycerides from VLDL and thereby decreases plasma triglyceride levels.

3. **The answer is C: binding to a G protein–coupled receptor.** Flushing and pruritus are most likely caused by niacin, which inhibits lipolysis by binding to a G protein–coupled receptor. Fibrates such as gemfibrozil activate the PPAR-α (Option A), whereas ezetimibe disrupts the annexin-caveolin complex (Option B). Statins such as fluvastatin inhibit HMG-CoA reductase and cholesterol synthesis (Option D), and resins such as cholestyramine bind to bile acids such as deoxycholic acid (Option E).

4. The answer is C: decreased cholesterol absorption. Ezetimibe disrupts the annexin-caveolin complex in intestinal brush border cells and thereby inhibits absorption of dietary cholesterol. Ezetimibe has no effect on cholesterol or triglyceride synthesis (Options A and B), triglyceride absorption (Option D), or bile acid excretion (Option E).

SELECTED READINGS

Benatar, J.R. and R.A. Stewart. Is it time to stop treating dyslipidemia with fibrates? N Z Med J 120:U2706, 2007.

Bouknight, P., L. Mackler and M. Heffington. FPIN's clinical inquiries. Best alternatives to statins for treating hyperlipidemia. Am Fam Physician 76:1027–1029, 2007.

Brunzell, J.D. Clinical practice. Hypertriglyceridemia. N Engl J Med 357: 1009–1017, 2007.

Cahoon, W.D. Jr., M.A. Crouch. Preprocedural statin therapy in percutaneous coronary intervention. Ann Pharmacother 41:1687–1693, 2007.

Singh, I.M., M.H. Shishehbor and J.A. Benjamin. High-density lipoprotein as a therapeutic target. JAMA 298:786–798, 2007.

CHAPTER 16

Anticoagulant, Antiplatelet, and Fibrinolytic Drugs

OVERVIEW

Excessive platelet aggregation and blood coagulation play a central role in a number of important diseases, including coronary artery disease, cerebrovascular disease, and venous thromboembolism. This chapter focuses on drugs that prevent the formation of pathologic thrombi or which cause lysis of thrombi. These agents are frequently used in the prevention and treatment of heart attacks, stroke, and other disorders.

BLOOD COAGULATION

Normal Hemostasis

When a small blood vessel is injured, hemorrhage is prevented by **vasospasm**, the formation of a **platelet plug** and a **fibrin clot** (Fig. 16–1). After the vessel is repaired, the clot is removed via the process of **fibrinolysis**.

Vasospasm reduces bleeding and blood flow and thereby facilitates platelet adhesion and coagulation.

Exposure of the blood to extravascular collagen causes adherence of platelets to the injured vessel wall and initiates the sequential activation of numerous **coagulation factors**, or **blood clotting factors**. These factors and their synonyms are listed in Table 16–1, and the **coagulation pathways** are illustrated in Figure 16–2. The **intrinsic pathway** may be activated by surface contact with a foreign body or extravascular tissue, whereas the **extrinsic pathway** is activated by a complex tissue factor. The pathways converge with the activation of **factor X**, which is the major rate-limiting step in the coagulation cascade. The activation of factor X leads to the formation of **thrombin**, and thrombin, in turn, catalyzes the conversion of **fibrinogen** to **fibrin**. The fibrin meshwork traps erythrocytes and platelets to complete the formation of a hemostatic thrombus (clot).

Pathologic Thrombus Formation

The processes leading to **thrombosis** and **embolism** are complex and not completely understood.

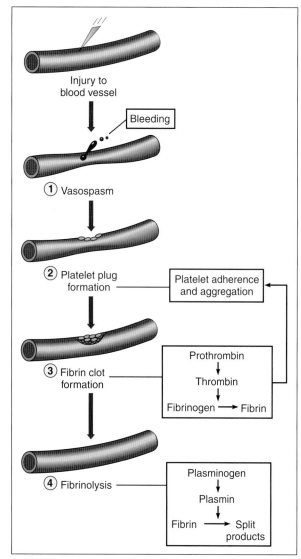

Figure 16-1. Normal hemostasis. (1) When a small blood vessel is injured, vasospasm reduces blood flow and facilitates platelet aggregation and coagulation. (2) The platelets, which adhere to extravascular collagen, are activated to release mediators that cause platelet aggregation and the formation of a platelet plug to arrest bleeding. (3) Exposure of the blood to tissue factors also activates coagulation and leads to the formation of a fibrin clot, which arrests bleeding until the vessel is repaired. (4) After the vessel is repaired, the clot is removed by the process of fibrinolysis.

Atherosclerosis and other abnormalities affecting the vascular endothelium can serve as a stimulus for platelet aggregation and blood coagulation in arteries. Venous pooling, sluggish blood flow, and inflammation of veins may permit inappropriate platelet adhesion and coagulation in vessels. Platelet aggregation appears to have a larger role in the formation of **arterial thrombi (white thrombi)**, whereas coagulation predominates in the formation of **venous thrombi (red thrombi)**. Platelet aggregation followed by coagulation, however, occurs both in arteries and in veins, and the processes differ only in the degree of contribution by platelets or coagulation to the thrombus.

TABLE 16-1. Coagulation Factors

Factor*	Common Synonym	Dependent on Vitamin K†
I	Fibrinogen	No
II	Prothrombin	Yes
III	Tissue thromboplastin	No
IV	Calcium	No
V	Proaccelerin	No
VII	Proconvertin	Yes
VIII	Antihemophilic factor	No
IX	Plasma thromboplastin component	Yes
X	Stuart factor	Yes
XI	Plasma thromboplastin antecedent	No
XII	Hageman factor	No
XIII	Fibrin stabilizing factor	No

*Factor VI is no longer considered to be a coagulation factor.
†Proteins C and S, which are endogenous anticoagulants that inactivate factors Va and VIIIa and promote fibrinolysis, are also dependent on vitamin K.

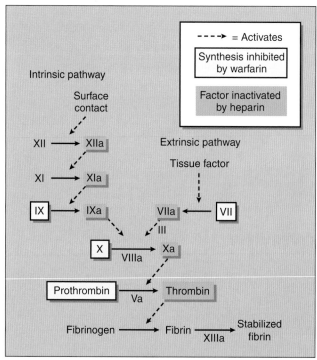

Figure 16-2. Blood coagulation and sites of drug action. Blood coagulation involves the sequential activation of proteolytic clotting factors. The intrinsic pathway can be activated by surface contact with a foreign body, whereas the extrinsic pathway is activated by tissue factor. The pathways converge with the activation of factor X, which leads to the formation of thrombin and fibrin. Warfarin and other oral anticoagulants inhibit the synthesis of the vitamin K–dependent clotting factors. Heparin inactivates various clotting factors.

An arterial or venous thrombus can become dislodged from the vessel wall and form an **embolus** that travels through the circulation and eventually occludes a smaller vessel in the lungs or brain, thereby causing pulmonary embolism or a cerebrovascular accident (stroke), respectively.

ANTICOAGULANT DRUGS

Oral Anticoagulants

Anticoagulants are drugs that retard coagulation and thereby prevent the occurrence or enlargement of a thrombus. Table 16–2 compares the properties of oral anticoagulants (e.g., warfarin) with those of parenteral anticoagulants (e.g., heparin).

Drug Properties

CHEMISTRY AND MECHANISMS. Coumarin compounds were originally discovered in spoiled clover hay and identified as substances that caused hemorrhage in cattle. Coumarin derivatives (e.g., warfarin and dicumarol) were subsequently developed as anticoagulants.

Warfarin and other coumarin derivatives are structurally related to vitamin K. These drugs work by inhibiting the synthesis of clotting factors II (prothrombin), VII, IX, and X, whose carboxylation is dependent on a reduced form of vitamin K. As shown in Figure 16–3, warfarin blocks the reduction of oxidized vitamin K and thereby prevents the post-translational carboxylation of these four factors. Oral anticoagulants also inhibit the synthesis of proteins C and S, which are endogenous anticoagulants that inactivate factors V and VIII and promote fibrinolysis. It is possible that the inhibition of proteins C and S contributes to a transient procoagulant effect of the oral anticoagulants when they are first administered.

PHARMACOKINETIC AND PHARMACOLOGIC EFFECTS. Coumarin anticoagulants, which are absorbed from the gut, are extensively metabolized before being excreted in the urine. Unlike heparin and related anticoagulants, the coumarins cross the placenta and can cause fetal hemorrhage and malformations.

The vitamin K antagonists have a delayed onset of action, owing to the time required to deplete the pool of circulating clotting factors after synthesis of new factors is inhibited. The half-life of circulating factors II, VII, IX, and X ranges from 6 hours (factor VII) to 50 hours (factor II). Therefore, the maximal effect of oral anticoagulants is not observed until 3 to 5 days after starting therapy with these drugs. Patients with acute thromboembolism are usually treated with a low-molecular-weight heparin (LMWH) and warfarin, and the LMWH is then withdrawn after warfarin becomes effective. A period of several days is also required for coagulation factor levels to return to normal after coumarin anticoagulants are discontinued. The recovery of clotting factors can be accelerated by administration of phytonadione (vitamin K_1), as described later.

ADVERSE EFFECTS AND INTERACTIONS. The most common adverse effect of coumarin anticoagulants is bleeding (Table 16–3), which can range in severity from mild nosebleed to life-threatening hemorrhage. Patients should be instructed to report any signs of bleeding, including hematuria and bleeding into the skin (ecchymoses).

The coumarin anticoagulants are contraindicated in pregnancy because of their potential to cause fetal hemorrhage and various structural malformations referred to as the fetal warfarin syndrome. These malformations are caused partly by antagonism of vitamin K–dependent maturation of bone proteins during a process in which certain proteins undergo carboxylation in the same manner as the nascent clotting factors. Warfarin and other oral anticoagulants block the process and can cause bone deformities and various birth defects that are listed in Table 4–6.

Most drug interactions with warfarin and other coumarin anticoagulants are caused by induction or inhibition of cytochrome P450 (CYP) enzymes, but a few are caused by the antagonism or potentiation of the anticoagulant effect. The most serious interactions are with drugs that increase the anticoagulant effect and place the patient at risk for hemorrhage. Because the number of drugs that interact with warfarin is large, patients who are taking this drug should be instructed to consult their physician before starting or discontinuing any other medication.

Treatment with high doses of salicylates or with some third-generation cephalosporins has a direct hypoprothrombinemic effect and thereby increases the anticoagulant effect of warfarin and related drugs. In contrast, treatment

TABLE 16-2. Comparison of the Pharmacologic Properties of Warfarin and Heparin Anticoagulants		
Property	**Warfarin Anticoagulants**	**Heparin Anticoagulants**
Active in vitro	No	Yes
Routes of administration	Oral	Parenteral
Onset of action	Delayed	Immediate
Mechanism of action	Inhibit synthesis of clotting factors	Inactivate clotting factors
Safe to take during pregnancy	No	Yes
Antidote	Phytonadione (vitamin K_1)	Protamine sulfate

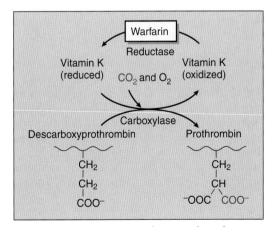

Figure 16-3. **Mechanisms of action of warfarin.** Warfarin blocks the reduction of oxidized vitamin K (vitamin K epoxide) and thereby prevents vitamin K–dependent carboxylation of clotting factors.

TABLE 16-3. Adverse Effects and Drug Interactions of Anticoagulant, Antiplatelet, and Fibrinolytic Drugs

Drug	Common Adverse Effects	Common Drug Interactions
Oral Anticoagulants		
Warfarin	Birth defects and bleeding	Serum levels altered by drugs that induce or inhibit cytochrome P450, by drugs that inhibit gut absorption, and by drugs that directly increase or decrease the anticoagulant effect (see text)
Parenteral Anticoagulants		
Dalteparin	Bleeding and thrombocytopenia	Risk of bleeding increased by salicylates
Enoxaparin heparin	Same as dalteparin	Same as dalteparin
	Bleeding, hyperkalemia, and thrombocytopenia	Same as dalteparin
Hirudin and related drugs	Bleeding	Same as dalteparin
Antiplatelet Drugs		
Abciximab	Bleeding, bradycardia, hypotension, and thrombocytopenia	Unknown
Aspirin	Gastrointestinal irritation and bleeding, hypersensitivity reactions, and tinnitus	Increases hypoglycemic effect of sulfonylureas. Increases risk of gastrointestinal bleeding and ulceration associated with methotrexate, valproate, and other drugs. Inhibits uricosuric effect of probenecid
Dipyridamole	Gastrointestinal distress, headache, mild and transient dizziness, and rash	Decreases metabolism of adenosine. Increases risk of bradycardia associated with β-adrenergic receptor antagonists
Clopidogrel	Bleeding, diarrhea, gastrointestinal pain, increased cholesterol and triglyceride levels, nausea, and neutropenia	Increases levels of drugs metabolized by liver microsomal enzymes
Fibrinolytic Drugs	Bleeding, hypersensitivity reactions, and reperfusion arrhythmias	Increases risk of bleeding associated with anticoagulant and antiplatelet drugs

with rifampin or barbiturates induces CYP enzymes and thereby decreases the anticoagulant effect of warfarin. Cholestyramine inhibits the absorption of warfarin from the gut. Amiodarone, cimetidine, erythromycin, fluconazole, gemfibrozil, isoniazid, metronidazole, sulfinpyrazone, and other drugs inhibit the metabolism of warfarin and increase the risk of bleeding. The **prothrombin time (PT)** should be monitored when adding or deleting drugs with persons taking coumarin anticoagulants.

Phytonadione directly antagonizes the effect of coumarin anticoagulants on clotting factor synthesis and is used to treat hemorrhage caused by anticoagulant activity.

INDICATIONS. Warfarin and related anticoagulants are primarily used in the long-term treatment of patients who have a thromboembolic disorder such as **deep vein thrombosis** or **atrial fibrillation** and patients who have an **artificial heart valve** (Table 16-4). They are also used in conjunction with a heparin-type anticoagulant for the treatment of **myocardial infarction**. The goal of anticoagulant use is to inhibit embolization and thereby prevent the serious and potentially fatal sequelae of thrombosis. Anticoagulants can keep an established thrombus from extending, but they cannot dissolve one.

The dosage of oral anticoagulants to be given is based on the patient's PT. This measurement is determined by drawing a blood sample, adding a tissue thromboplastin preparation to initiate coagulation in it, and comparing the in

TABLE 16-4. Clinical Uses of Antithrombotic Agents

Clinical Use	Primary Drugs
Venous Thromboembolism	
Acute	LMWH
Surgical prophylaxis	LMWH or fondaparinux
Long-term prophylaxis	Warfarin or LMWH
Pulmonary embolism	Heparin, fibrinolytic drug
Acute Coronary Syndromes	
Unstable angina and non-STE ACS	Aspirin ± clopidogrel; eptifibatide or tirofiban; LMWH
STEMI	Fibrinolytic drug and aspirin ± heparin
Percutaneous coronary interventions*	Aspirin ± clopidogrel; abciximab or eptifibatide (alternative: bivalirudin)
Stroke, thrombotic	
Acute	Fibrinolytic drug or aspirin
Prophylaxis, including transient ischemic attacks	Aspirin and dipyridamole combined; clopidogrel or prasugrel
Atrial fibrillation	Heparin followed by warfarin
Artificial heart valve	Warfarin, aspirin

*Coronary angioplasty and stent placement.
LMWH = low-molecular-weight heparin; non-STE ACS = non–ST segment elevation acute coronary syndrome; STEMI = ST segment elevation myocardial infarction.

vitro clotting time in the sample with that in a standardized control preparation. As a general rule, the dosage of warfarin to be given should prolong the PT of the patient so that it is 1.3 to 1.5 times the PT of the control.

When the international reference thromboplastin preparation is used as the standardized control preparation, the ratio is expressed as the **international normalized ratio** (INR) and is calculated as follows:

$$INR = (PT_{observed}/PT_{control})^{ISI}$$

where the $PT_{observed}$ and $PT_{control}$ are the prothrombin times of the patient and control, respectively, and the ISI is the international sensitivity index of the thromboplastin reagent being used. For most indications, an INR of 2 to 3 is recommended. For patients with mechanical prosthetic heart valves and for those with recurrent systemic embolization, an INR of 3 to 4.5 is recommended.

The patient's PT should be monitored daily during the initiation of warfarin therapy and whenever another drug is added to or withdrawn from the treatment regimen. Concurrent heparin therapy can cause an increase of 10% to 20% in the patient's PT, so the target PT and INR levels should be increased by the same amount. Once the patient's PT has stabilized, it should be monitored every 4 to 6 weeks.

TREATMENT OF BLEEDING. If bleeding occurs, the coumarin anticoagulant should be withheld until the bleeding can be evaluated and the patient's PT can be determined. The treatment of bleeding can include a reduction in drug dosage and the administration of phytonadione (vitamin K_1). If bleeding is serious or if the INR is markedly elevated (>20), fresh frozen plasma or factor IX concentrate can be warmed and administered to rapidly replace clotting factors.

Specific Drugs

Warfarin is the most widely used orally administered anticoagulant. It is completely absorbed after oral administration. About 99% of the drug is bound to plasma proteins, and it is almost completely metabolized by CYP enzymes. Warfarin is primarily metabolized by CYP2C9, with smaller contributions from CYP1A2, CYP2C19, and CYP3A4. Drug interactions caused by induction or inhibition of these enzymes are described above. Other oral anticoagulants either have less favorable pharmacologic and pharmacokinetic properties or are more toxic and should be used only in cases in which the patient is intolerant of warfarin.

Dicumarol is a coumarin derivative that is incompletely absorbed from the gut and can cause considerable gastrointestinal distress. For these reasons, it is rarely used.

Parenteral Anticoagulants

The parenteral anticoagulants include heparin, hirudin, and related compounds.

Heparin and Related Drugs

The heparin family of anticoagulants includes unfractionated heparin, low molecular weight heparins, a heparinoid drug, and fondaparinux. In its natural form, **heparin** contains fractions with high molecular weights ranging from 5000 to 30,000 and fractions with low molecular weights ranging from 2000 to 9000. Low-molecular-weight fractions have been developed for specific clinical uses, including **enoxaparin, dalteparin,** and **tinzaparin**. Danaparoid, a so-called heparinoid anticoagulant, is a sulfated polysaccharide that is structurally distinct from heparin. Fondaparinux is a synthetic pentasaccharide whose mechanism and effects are similar to those of other heparin-like drugs.

CHEMISTRY AND MECHANISMS. Heparin is a naturally occurring mixture of sulfated mucopolysaccharides found in mast cells, basophils, and the vascular endothelium. For pharmaceutical use, it is obtained from porcine intestine or bovine lung.

As shown in Figure 16–2, heparin inactivates clotting factors. Heparin accomplishes this by potentiating the activity of an endogenous anticoagulant called **antithrombin III** (AT-III), which is the most powerful endogenous inhibitor of thrombin (active factor II) and active factor X (Stuart factor). The activation of AT-III by a heparin-containing pentasaccharide is depicted in Figure 16–4.

In contrast to unfractionated heparin, LMWHs, such as enoxaparin and dalteparin, primarily inactivate active factor X because the LMWH–AT-III complex has less affinity for thrombin than does the heparin–AT-III complex. Fondaparinux is an even more selective active factor X inhibitor (see Fig. 16–4).

PHARMACOKINETIC AND PHARMACOLOGIC EFFECTS. Heparin and related anticoagulants are not absorbed from the gut and must be given parenterally. Heparin is usually administered by continuous intravenous infusion. It is removed from the circulation by the reticuloendothelial system, is eliminated from the body by renal and hepatic mechanisms, and has a half-life of about 90 minutes. The dosage of heparin is generally determined by monitoring the **activated partial thromboplastin time** (aPTT). The dosage is considered adequate when the aPTT is 1.5 to 2 times normal.

Enoxaparin, dalteparin, tinzaparin, and danaparoid are administered subcutaneously, and their maximal effect occurs from 3 to 5 hours after injection. When they are used, the aPTT usually does not need to be monitored because the anticoagulant activity of LMWHs and danaparoid is more predictable than is the activity of unfractionated heparin.

ADVERSE EFFECTS AND INTERACTIONS. Adverse effects and drug interactions are listed in Table 16–3. The most common serious adverse effect of fractionated and unfractionated heparin is bleeding caused by excessive anticoagulation.

Heparin can also cause two types of **heparin-induced thrombocytopenia** (HIT). Type 1 HIT, which occurs in about 25% of patients treated with heparin, is caused by a direct interaction between heparin and platelets, leading to platelet aggregation. Type 1 HIT is usually mild and is reversible within 4 days despite continued heparin treatment. Type 2 HIT is a much less common but more serious condition caused by immunoglobulin-mediated platelet inactivation, and has a high risk of thrombotic complications and mortality. Heparin must be discontinued if type 2 HIT occurs.

Heparin occasionally causes **hyperkalemia** because of the suppression of aldosterone secretion.

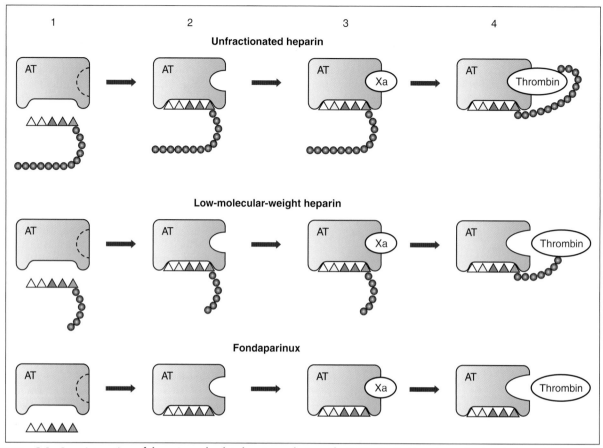

Figure 16–4. **Interaction of heparin and related anticoagulants with AT-III.** (1–2) Heparin and related drugs bind to the pentasaccharide-binding site on AT-III. (3) Anticoagulant–AT-III complexes inactivate factor Xa (active Stuart factor). (4) Unfractionated heparin–AT-III also inactivates thrombin, whereas low-molecular-weight heparin–AT-III and fondaparinux–AT-III produce little or no inactivation of thrombin, respectively.

INDICATIONS. Heparin is indicated for the treatment of **acute thromboembolic disorders**, including peripheral and pulmonary embolism, venous thrombosis, and coagulopathies such as disseminated intravascular coagulation. It is used prophylactically to prevent clotting in **arterial and heart surgery**, during **blood transfusions**, and in **renal dialysis** and **blood sample collection**. Heparin is also used to prevent embolization of thrombi that might cause a cerebrovascular event in patients with **acute atrial fibrillation**. Low doses of heparin can be administered subcutaneously to prevent **deep vein thrombosis** and **pulmonary embolism** in high-risk patients.

Low molecular weight heparins (e.g., enoxaparin and dalteparin) are used to prevent **venous thromboembolism** associated with abdominal surgery and knee or hip replacement surgery. For this purpose, the drugs are administered once before surgery and for 5 to 10 days after surgery. Enoxaparin and dalteparin are also approved to prevent ischemic complications of **unstable angina** or non–ST segment elevation (non–Q wave) myocardial infarction. Enoxaparin is approved for the treatment of deep vein thrombosis and to prevent thromboembolism caused by severely restricted mobility during acute illness.

Fondaparinux is administered subcutaneously for the prophylaxis of deep vein thrombosis in patients having hip fracture or hip replacement surgery or knee replacement surgery.

TREATMENT OF BLEEDING. The treatment of bleeding caused by unfractionated or LMWHs consists of administering protamine sulfate, which is a positively charged basic protein that physically combines with negatively charged heparin and thereby inactivates it. Protamine is administered intravenously for this purpose, and the dosage is based on the estimated amount of residual heparin in the body. Measurement of the aPTT 2 to 4 hours after protamine administration is used to guide the need for further protamine treatment. Severe bleeding may require the administration of fresh frozen plasma.

Hirudin Analogues

Hirudin is a mixture of homologous polypeptides produced by the salivary gland of *Hirudo medicinalis*, the medicinal leech. Hirudin and its analogues are direct thrombin inhibitors that do not require AT-III as a cofactor and have a more predictable anticoagulant effect than does heparin. **Lepirudin** is a recombinant hirudin obtained from yeast cells, whereas **bivalirudin** is a synthetic derivative of hirudin. The hirudin compounds do not cause thrombocytopenia and lepirudin is indicated for management of thromboembolic disorders in persons who have experienced **HIT**. Both lepirudin and bivalirudin have been used to prevent thrombosis in patients with **unstable angina** and **acute myocardial infarction**, including those having coronary

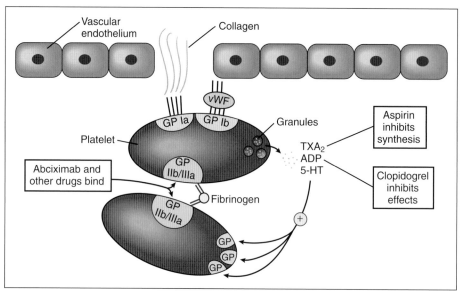

Figure 16–5. **Platelet aggregation and sites of drug action.** Platelets adhere to damaged endothelium via linkage of GP Ia receptors with exposed collagen and via linkage of GP Ib receptors with von Willebrand's factor. This activates the platelets and leads to the synthesis and release (degranulation) of various mediators of platelet aggregation, including TXA_2, ADP, and 5-hydroxytryptamine (or serotonin). These mediators increase the expression of GP receptors and promote platelet aggregation via the binding of fibrinogen to GP IIb/IIIa receptors.

angioplasty and stent insertion. Several clinical trials have established the efficacy and safety of these drugs in these settings.

The hirudin drugs are administered intravenously and their subcutaneous use is being studied. The most serious adverse effect of these drugs is bleeding. Orally administered direct thrombin inhibitors are currently being developed.

ANTIPLATELET DRUGS

The mechanisms of platelet aggregation and the sites of antiplatelet drug action are depicted in Figure 16–5.

Platelets adhere to the damaged vascular endothelium via linkage of glycoprotein (GP) Ia receptors with exposed collagen and via linkage of Ib receptors with von Willebrand's factor, a circulating factor that is similar to clotting factor VIII. The adherence of platelets to vascular endothelium activates the platelets and leads to the synthesis and release (degranulation) of various mediators of platelet aggregation, including thromboxane A_2 (TXA_2), adenosine diphosphate (ADP), and 5-hydroxytryptamine (or serotonin). These mediators increase the expression of GP IIb/IIIa receptors that bind to fibrinogen and thereby cause platelet aggregation. Aspirin and clopidogrel inhibit the synthesis or activity of specific mediators of platelet aggregation, whereas abciximab, tirofiban, and eptifibatide block GP IIb/IIIa receptors.

Aspirin

Aspirin is a nonsteroidal anti-inflammatory drug (NSAID) that has analgesic, antipyretic, and anti-inflammatory effects. It also inhibits platelet aggregation and is used to prevent and treat arterial thromboembolic disorders.

MECHANISMS AND PHARMACOLOGIC EFFECTS. Aspirin and most other NSAIDs inhibit the synthesis of prostaglandins from arachidonic acid, as described in greater detail in Chapter 30. The most important prostaglandins affecting platelet aggregation are prostacyclin (also called prostaglandin I_2, or PGI_2) and TXA_2. Prostacyclin is synthesized by vascular endothelial cells and inhibits platelet aggregation, whereas TXA_2 is synthesized by platelets and promotes platelet aggregation. Under normal conditions, prostacyclin serves to prevent platelet aggregation and thrombosis, whereas TXA_2 becomes predominant during thrombus formation.

Low doses of aspirin have been found to selectively inhibit the synthesis of TXA_2 without having as much effect on prostacyclin, whereas higher doses inhibit the synthesis of both prostaglandins. Hence, the dosage of aspirin used to inhibit platelet aggregation is sometimes lower than that used to produce other pharmacologic effects. Unlike other NSAIDs, aspirin irreversibly inhibits cyclooxygenase, the enzyme that catalyzes an early step in TXA_2 synthesis. For this reason, aspirin inhibits platelet aggregation for the life of the platelet and effectively reduces platelet aggregation when administered once a day or every other day.

INDICATIONS. Aspirin is primarily used to prevent arterial thrombosis in patients with ischemic heart disease and stroke, but it has many other indications as well. In patients with unstable angina, it is used to prevent myocardial infarction. In patients with recent myocardial infarction (Box 16–1), it is used to prevent enlargement of a coronary thrombus and potentially reduce the severity of cardiac damage. In patients with transient ischemic attacks, it can be used to prevent an initial or subsequent stroke. In patients who have artificial heart valves or are having percutaneous transluminal coronary angioplasty, it is used to prevent thrombosis. Aspirin is also used to treat persons

CASE PRESENTATION: A 61-year-old male presented to the emergency department with crushing chest pain at rest, which began an hour ago. He had a history of hypertension treated with hydrochlorothiazide. His vital signs included a blood pressure of 142 over 92 mm Hg and a heart rate of 88 beats per minute. The electrocardiogram showed a 2-mm ST segment elevation in the anterior leads. The man was promptly treated with aspirin and three sublingual doses nitroglycerin at 5-minute intervals followed by a continuous nitroglycerin intravenous infusion, and metoprolol and morphine by intravenous injection. Because the ST segment elevation and chest pain continued, the patient received clopidogrel and enoxaparin, and then fibrinolysis was accomplished with tenecteplase. He was placed on metoprolol, lisinopril, and clopidogrel, and was subsequently transferred to another hospital for angiography and further treatment.

CASE DISCUSSION: There are an estimated 500,000 ST segment elevation myocardial infarction (STEMI) events in the United States annually. The immediate treatment of STEMI includes aspirin to slow progression of coronary thrombosis and nitroglycerin to reduce myocardial oxygen demand, ischemia, and infarct size. The most important objective is restoration of coronary blood flow as soon as possible, and patients with STEMI typically receive fibrinolytic therapy or undergo percutaneous coronary intervention (angioplasty ± stent insertion). For patients that present to hospitals without facilities for percutaneous coronary intervention, fibrinolysis with a drug such as tenecteplase is the most viable option. Studies show that clopidogrel and enoxaparin reduce cardiovascular mortality in persons undergoing fibrinolysis or angioplasty. Angiotensin inhibitors may improve left ventricular function in STEMI patients, and β-adrenoceptor antagonists reduce secondary cardiovascular events and mortality.

with peripheral arterial occlusive disease and chronic limb ischemia.

ADVERSE EFFECTS AND INTERACTIONS. Aspirin can cause bleeding, especially in the gastrointestinal tract, where it inhibits the synthesis of prostaglandins that promote secretion of bicarbonate and mucus. These substances protect the gastric mucosa from the potentially damaging effects of stomach acid and pepsin. High doses of aspirin and other salicylates

may cause hypoprothrombinemia and thereby increase the likelihood of bleeding. Other adverse effects of aspirin are discussed in Chapter 30, and interactions are listed in Table 16–3.

Dipyridamole

Dipyridamole is a coronary vasodilator and a relatively weak antiplatelet drug.

As a vasodilator, dipyridamole is used during **myocardial perfusion imaging (thallium imaging)** to dilate and evaluate the arteries of patients with coronary artery disease.

As an antiplatelet drug, dipyridamole acts primarily by inhibiting platelet adhesion to the vessel wall. It can also inhibit platelet aggregation by increasing the formation of cyclic adenosine monophosphate and lowering the level of platelet calcium. Dipyridamole is used in combination with aspirin to prevent **ischemic (thrombotic) stroke** in persons who have previously had an atherothrombotic stroke and in persons experiencing transient ischemic attacks. Some authorities believe the combination of aspirin and dipyridamole is superior to aspirin alone, and to clopidogrel, for stroke prevention. A combination product containing aspirin and extended release dipyridamole is marketed as **Aggrenox**.

Adenosine Diphosphate Inhibitors

Clopidogrel, prasugrel, and ticlopidine are oral antiplatelet drugs unrelated to aspirin and dipyridamole. These drugs produce irreversible blockade of the ADP P2Y receptor, and thereby inhibit expression of GP IIb/IIIa receptors and prevent ADP-induced platelet aggregation (see Fig. 16–5). As with aspirin, the ADP inhibitors prolong bleeding time and inhibit platelet function for the life of the platelet.

ADP inhibitors are well absorbed following oral administration. Clopidogrel and prasugrel are prodrugs that are metabolized to active antiplatelet metabolites. **Prasugrel** is a newer drug that has a higher potency and a more rapid onset of action because of the more efficient generation of its active metabolite. Prasugrel produces a higher and more consistent level of platelet inhibition than clopidogrel, which translates into less response variability and a decreased prevalence of nonresponsiveness compared to clopidogrel.

Because it can cause mild to severe neutropenia, patients who are treated with **ticlopidine** must have a complete blood count with white cell differential every 2 weeks from the second week to the third month of treatment. After 3 months, a complete blood count is required only when patients exhibit signs or symptoms of an infection. Clopidogrel and prasugrel cause significantly less neutropenia than ticlopidine and white blood cell counts are not required in persons taking these drugs. For this reason, clopidogrel and prasugrel have replaced ticlopidine for most purposes.

In patients who are intolerant of or unresponsive to aspirin, clopidogrel and prasugrel are used to prevent **thrombotic stroke**, and they are used with aspirin to treat acute coronary syndromes. Clinical trials (CLARITY-TIMI 28 and COMMIT) have shown that clopidogrel should be included in coronary reperfusion regimens (thrombolysis and angioplasty) in persons with ST segment elevation myocardial infarction. Clopidogrel is also used in patients with

TABLE 16–5. **Characteristics of Selected Fibrinolytic Drugs**

	Streptokinase	Alteplase	Reteplase	Tenecteplase
Administration	Infusion	Infusion	Bolus	Bolus
Allergic reactions	Yes	No	No	No
Systemic fibrinogen depletion	Marked	Mild	Moderate	Minimal
Fibrin specificity	–	++	+	+++
TIMI coronary flow grade 2 out of 3*	55%	75%	83%	83%

*Percentage of patients in TIMI trial with a 2 out of 3 coronary blood flow grade after fibrinolysis.
TIMI = thrombolysis in myocardial infarction.

intermittent claudication of blood vessels, chronic arterial occlusion, atrioventricular shunts or fistulas, open heart surgery, and sickle cell anemia.

Glycoprotein IIb/IIIa Antagonists

The final common pathway in platelet aggregation is the cross-linking of platelets by fibrinogen, which binds to an activated GP IIb/IIIa complex on the platelet surface (see Fig. 16–5). The GP IIb/IIIa complex is a type of **integrin**. Integrins are cell surface transmembrane glycoproteins that function as adhesion receptors to structurally link the cell surface to the cytoskeleton.

Abciximab

Abciximab was the first platelet integrin GP IIb/IIIa inhibitor approved by the U.S. Food and Drug Administration. It consists of the Fab fragment of a chimeric human-murine monoclonal antibody. The drug prevents platelet aggregation by binding to platelet GP IIb/IIIa receptors to prevent fibrinogen binding and cross-linking of platelets.

Abciximab is used to prevent platelet aggregation and thrombosis in patients having **percutaneous coronary interventions**, including coronary angioplasty and stent placement. In this setting, it is administered in combination with aspirin and heparin or LMWH. Abciximab has been shown to significantly prevent vessel restenosis, reinfarction, and death. It has also been used as an adjunct to thrombolysis with alteplase and similar drugs (see "Fibrinolytic Drugs").

The most common adverse effect of abciximab is bleeding. Other adverse reactions include thrombocytopenia, hypotension, and bradycardia.

Tirofiban and Eptifibatide

Tirofiban and eptifibatide also prevent platelet aggregation by preventing fibrinogen cross-linking of platelets. Unlike abciximab, tirofiban and eptifibatide are competitive, reversible inhibitors of fibrinogen binding to GP IIb/IIIa receptors. Eptifibatide is a cyclic heptapeptide from rattlesnake venom, whereas tirofiban is a tyrosine derivative. Both of these agents have short half-lives and are given as an intravenous loading dose followed by a maintenance infusion.

Tirofiban and eptifibatide are primarily used in persons with **acute coronary syndromes** (unstable angina and myocardial infarction). Eptifibatide is used in two ways: (1) to prevent coronary thrombosis in persons with unstable angina or non–ST segment elevation (non–Q wave) acute

coronary syndrome, and (2) to prevent thrombosis in persons having coronary angioplasty or stent placement for ST segment elevation myocardial infarction.

Bleeding is the major adverse effect of tirofiban and eptifibatide. The incidence of intracranial bleeding and gastrointestinal or genitourinary bleeding caused by tirofiban in one study was 0.1% and 0.2%, respectively.

FIBRINOLYTIC DRUGS

The fibrinolytic drugs, or **thrombolytic drugs**, include **alteplase**, **reteplase**, **and tenecteplase**, which are recombinant forms of human tissue plasminogen activator (t-PA); **urokinase**, an enzyme obtained from human urine; **streptokinase**, a protein obtained from streptococci; and **anistreplase**, a complex of streptokinase and plasminogen. Unlike the anticoagulant and antiplatelet drugs, these drugs are administered intravenously to degrade an existing thrombus in patients having **myocardial infarction, thrombotic stroke**, or **pulmonary embolism**. Their use in patients with acute ischemic (thrombotic) stroke reduces the incidence of the neurologic sequelae of stroke. For patients with ST segment elevation myocardial infarction, fibrinolytic drugs are the primary means of restoring coronary blood flow in hospitals without facilities for angioplasty (see Box 16–1). The characteristics of selected fibrinolytic agents are listed in Table 16–5.

CHEMISTRY AND PHARMACOLOGIC EFFECTS. The fibrinolytic drugs are enzymes that convert plasminogen to plasmin. Plasmin degrades fibrin and fibrinogen and thereby causes clot dissolution (Fig. 16–6). Streptokinase must first combine with plasminogen to form an activator complex that converts inactive plasminogen to plasmin. In anistreplase, streptokinase and plasminogen are already formed into a complex (the anisoylated plasminogen streptokinase activator complex).

ADVERSE EFFECTS AND INTERACTIONS. Table 16–3 lists adverse effects and drug interactions. The most common adverse effect is hemorrhage. Fibrinolytic drugs create a general lytic state that can lyse both normal and pathologic thrombi. Because t-PA selectively activates plasminogen that is bound to fibrin, the recombinant forms of t-PA can cause less bleeding than does streptokinase. Arrhythmias (e.g., bradycardia and tachycardia), which have been reported in patients

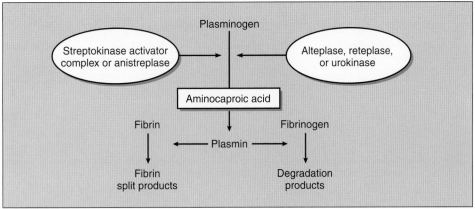

Figure 16–6. **Fibrinolysis and sites of drug action.** Alteplase, reteplase, and tenecteplase catalyze the conversion of plasminogen to plasmin. Streptokinase combines with plasminogen to form an active catalyst (activator complex) that converts inactive plasminogen to plasmin. In anistreplase, streptokinase and plasminogen are already formed into a complex. Plasmin is a protease that breaks down fibrinogen and fibrin to degradation (split) products. Aminocaproic acid inhibits the conversion of plasminogen to plasmin.

treated with fibrinolytic drugs, are believed to be caused by free radicals that are generated during the reperfusion of the coronary artery after fibrinolysis. The administration of streptokinase can cause various types of hypersensitivity reactions, including fatal anaphylactic shock. For this reason, it should not be used repeatedly in the same patient.

TREATMENT OF BLEEDING. By competitively blocking plasminogen activation, aminocaproic acid inhibits fibrinolysis. This drug is used to stop the bleeding caused by fibrinolytic drugs. It is also used to prevent bleeding in patients who have hemophilia, patients who are recovering from gastrointestinal or prostate surgery, or patients who have cancer and are undergoing radiation therapy or chemotherapy. Aminocaproic acid can be administered orally or intravenously and is excreted by the kidneys. Its adverse effects include thrombosis, hypotension, and arrhythmias.

SUMMARY OF IMPORTANT POINTS

■ When a small blood vessel is injured, hemorrhage is prevented by the processes involved in normal hemostasis: vasospasm, platelet plug formation, and fibrin clot formation. After the vessel is repaired, the clot is removed via the process of fibrinolysis.

■ Orally administered coumarin anticoagulants (e.g., warfarin) inhibit vitamin K–dependent synthesis of clotting factors II, VII, IX, and X.

■ Parenteral anticoagulants, including heparin and hirudin derivatives, inactivate clotting factors. Unfractionated heparin primarily inactivates thrombin by activating AT-III, whereas low molecular-weight heparins and fondaparinux primarily inactivate factor Xa. These drugs are used to prevent and treat venous thromboembolism.

■ Bivalirudin is a direct thrombin inhibitor used in persons having coronary angioplasty, whereas lepirudin is indicated for treating thromboembolic disease in persons with HIT.

■ Oral antiplatelet drugs act by interfering with the synthesis or activity of mediators of platelet aggregation. Aspirin inhibits TXA_2 synthesis, and clopidogrel inhibits ADP activity. Abciximab, tirofiban, and eptifibatide are parenteral antiplatelet drugs that prevent the binding of fibrinogen to GP IIb/IIIa receptors and are primarily used in persons with acute coronary syndromes.

■ Fibrinolytic drugs (e.g., alteplase, reteplase, and tenecteplase) convert plasminogen to plasmin and thereby stimulate fibrin degradation. These drugs are used to lyse clots in patients having myocardial infarction, thrombotic stroke, or pulmonary embolism.

■ Any of the anticoagulant, antiplatelet, or fibrinolytic drugs can cause bleeding. Phytonadione (vitamin K_1) is used to counteract bleeding caused by oral anticoagulants. Protamine sulfate is used to neutralize heparins, and aminocaproic acid is used to inhibit fibrinolysis.

SELECTED READINGS

Cattaneo, M. Platelet P2 receptors: old and new targets for antithrombotic drugs. Expert Rev Cardiovasc Ther 5:45–55, 2007.

Eikelboom, J.W., and J. Hirsh. Combined antiplatelet and anticoagulant therapy: benefits and risks. J Thromb Haemost 5:255–263, 2007.

Gumina, R.J. New trials and therapies for acute myocardial infarction. Med Clin N Amer 91:729–749, 2007.

Hammwohner, M., A. D'Alessandro, O. Wolfram, and A. Goette. New pharmacologic approaches to prevent thromboembolism in patients with atrial fibrillation. Curr Vasc Pharmacol 5:211–219, 2007.

Jakubowski, J.A., C.D. Payne, G.J. Weerakkody, J.T. Brandt, N.A. Farid, et al. Dose-dependent inhibition of human platelet aggregation by prasugrel and its interaction with aspirin in healthy subjects. J Cardiovasc Pharmacol 49:167–173, 2007.

CHAPTER 17

Hematopoietic Drugs

CLASSIFICATION OF HEMATOPOIETIC DRUGS

Minerals
- Ferrous sulfate[a]
- Iron Dextran

Vitamins
- Folic Acid
- Vitamin B_{12} (CYANOCOBALAMIN AND HYDROXOCOBALAMIN)

Hematopoietic Growth Factors
- Epoetin-α (EPOGEN, PROCRIT)[b]
- Filgrastim (NEUPOGEN)[c]
- Sargramostim (LEUKINE)

[a]Also ferrous fumarate and ferrous gluconate.
[b]Also epoetin-β (NEORECORMON) and darbepoetin-α (ARANESP).
[c]Also pegfilgrastim (NEULASTA).

OVERVIEW

Mature blood cells are continuously formed in the bone marrow and are removed from the circulation by reticuloendothelial cells in the liver and spleen. The process by which blood cells are replaced is called **hematopoiesis**. This process requires minerals and vitamins and is regulated by hematopoietic growth factors that promote the differentiation and maturation of marrow stem cells to form leukocytes, erythrocytes, and platelets.

Anemia, a subnormal concentration of erythrocytes or hemoglobin in the blood, can result from inadequate erythropoiesis, blood loss, or accelerated hemolysis. Erythropoiesis can be impaired by the lack of essential nutrients or by the myelosuppressive effects of certain drugs or irradiation. Infection, cancer, endocrine deficiencies, and chronic inflammation can also cause anemia. **Iron, folic acid, and vitamin B_{12} deficiencies** are the most common causes of **nutritional anemia**.

This chapter describes the pharmacologic properties and uses of minerals, vitamins, and hematopoietic growth factors in the treatment of anemia and other blood cell deficiencies.

DRUGS

Minerals

Iron, an essential dietary mineral, serves as an important component of hemoglobin, myoglobin, and a number of enzymes. The average dietary intake of iron is 18 to 20 mg/day, but people with normal iron stores absorb only about 10% of this amount. Absorption is enhanced twofold or threefold when stored iron is depleted or when erythropoiesis occurs at an accelerated rate. The absorption of iron is regulated by the amount of iron that is stored in the intestinal mucosa.

Iron is absorbed from the intestines into the circulation, where it is bound to **transferrin** and transported to various tissues, including the bone marrow and liver. In these tissues, iron is stored as **ferritin** (Fig. 17–1). In the marrow, iron is incorporated into heme and packaged in new erythrocytes. The erythrocytes circulate in the blood for about 120 days and then are taken up and degraded by reticuloendothelial cells. These cells later return most of the iron to the plasma so that it can be used again in erythropoiesis. Iron is highly conserved by the body, and only small amounts of it are excreted via the intestinal tract.

The dietary iron requirement per kilogram of body weight is highest in infants and pregnant women, somewhat lower in children and nonpregnant women, and lowest in men. Pregnant women have the greatest need for routine **iron supplementation** because their dietary iron often cannot meet the requirements for maternal and fetal erythropoiesis. Most multivitamin supplements contain iron, and many processed foods, including bread, are supplemented with iron.

If dietary iron intake is inadequate to support sufficient erythropoiesis and maintain a normal hemoglobin concentration in the blood, the body will utilize stored iron to maintain erythropoiesis until the stores are depleted. When iron stores are significantly depleted, the plasma iron level begins to fall and erythropoiesis is reduced. Over time, these

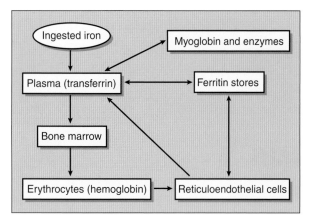

Figure 17–1. Iron metabolism. Ingested iron is absorbed from the intestinal mucosa into the circulation, where it is bound to transferrin. Iron is distributed to tissues for incorporation into hemoglobin, myoglobin, and enzymes, or it is stored as ferritin. After about 120 days, erythrocytes are degraded by reticuloendothelial cells, and the iron is returned to the plasma or stored.

changes lead to **hypochromic microcytic anemia**, a form of anemia in which the mean corpuscular hemoglobin concentration and the mean corpuscular volume are decreased. The iron preparations described in the following paragraphs are used to prevent and treat **iron deficiency anemia** in affected individuals.

Ferrous Sulfate and Related Compounds

Iron is administered orally in the form of **ferrous salts**, including **ferrous sulfate, ferrous gluconate,** and **ferrous fumarate**. Iron contained in these preparations is absorbed in the same manner as is dietary iron. In patients with iron deficiency, the amount of iron absorbed increases progressively with larger doses, but the percentage absorbed decreases as the dosage increases. Food can retard iron absorption by 40% to 60%, but the gastric distress caused by iron often necessitates administering iron preparations with food. The percentage of iron absorbed from sustained-release preparations is lower than that absorbed from immediate-release preparations. This is because iron is primarily absorbed from the duodenum, and some of the sustained-release iron is transported to the lower intestinal tract before it is released for absorption.

In iron deficiency states, oral iron preparations are usually administered three times a day in doses that provide a total of 100 to 200 mg of elemental iron daily. The various iron salts contain different percentages of elemental iron. Ferrous sulfate contains about 20%, so that a 300-mg tablet contains approximately 60 mg of elemental iron. The duration of iron therapy depends on the cause and severity of the iron deficiency. In general, about 4 to 6 months of oral iron therapy is required to reverse uncomplicated iron deficiency anemia.

At therapeutic doses, iron salts have few adverse effects, but they sometimes cause epigastric pain, nausea, vomiting, diarrhea or constipation, and black stools. Liquid iron preparations can also stain the teeth. Bile acid–binding resins

(e.g., cholestyramine) reduce the absorption of iron, whereas ascorbic acid increases iron absorption by maintaining iron in the reduced ferrous state. Ferrous iron is better absorbed than is ferric iron. Iron can reduce the absorption of tetracyclines, fluoroquinolones, levothyroxine, and vitamin E. The administration of these drugs should be separated from iron administration by at least 2 hours. The ingestion of large quantities of iron can cause serious and potentially lethal toxicity. Hence, iron preparations should be kept out of the reach of children.

Iron Dextran

Iron dextran is a mixture of ferric hydroxide and dextran. It is intended for intramuscular or intravenous treatment of iron deficiency anemia in patients who cannot tolerate oral iron preparations or fail to respond to oral iron therapy. The dosage of iron dextran required for each patient is calculated on the basis of the observed hemoglobin concentration and body weight.

Following administration, the iron dextran complex is removed from the circulation by the reticuloendothelial system, and the iron is transferred to the plasma for distribution to the bone marrow and other tissues.

Because treatment with iron dextran has been associated with fatal anaphylactic reactions, it should be limited to the indications described. Intramuscular administration of iron dextran can cause several adverse reactions at the injection site, including pain, inflammation, sterile abscesses, and brown discoloration of skin. For this reason, the iron preparation must be given by deep intramuscular injection into the outer quadrant of the buttock. A Z-track technique, in which the skin is displaced laterally before injection, is used to avoid leakage into the subcutaneous tissue. Intravenous administration can cause peripheral flushing and hypotensive reactions.

Vitamins

Although many vitamins participate in the formation and function of erythrocytes, **folic acid** and **vitamin B$_{12}$** have a critical role in erythropoiesis, and a deficiency of either of them may cause **megaloblastic anemia**. The two vitamins serve as cofactors in biochemical reactions involving the addition of single-carbon units to various substrates, and the administration of one of the vitamins can partially compensate for a deficiency of the other. Therefore, it is critical that the specific vitamin deficiency be correctly identified before therapy is started.

Folic Acid

The structure of folic acid is shown in Figure 17–2A. Active forms of this vitamin serve as enzyme cofactors that donate single-carbon atoms in the biosynthesis of amino acids and the purine and pyrimidine bases contained in DNA (Fig. 17–3A). Hence, folic acid plays a critical role in cell proliferation and erythropoiesis.

The requirement for folic acid increases markedly during pregnancy, and inadequate dietary intake of this vitamin can cause **neural tube birth defects**, such as **spina bifida**, and **megaloblastic anemia**. For this reason, folic acid supplementation is especially important before and during

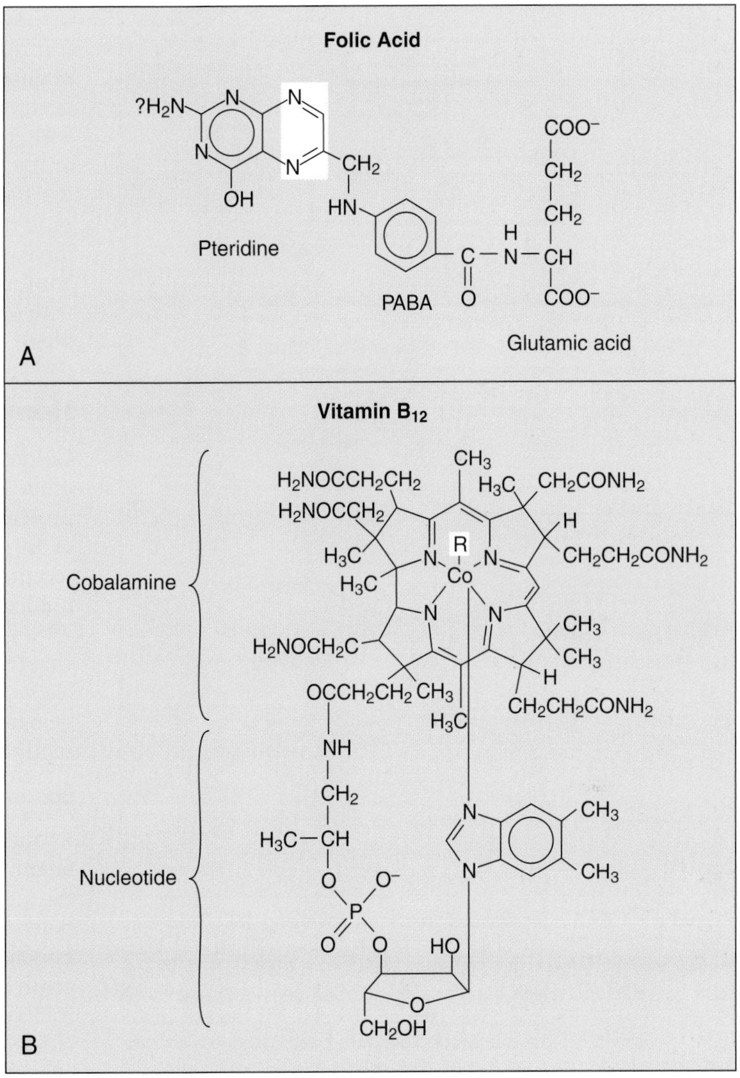

Figure 17-2. Structures of folic acid and vitamin B₁₂. (A) Folic acid consists of pteridine, PABA, and glutamic acid. The unshaded areas represent the bonds that are reduced by folate reductase to form tetrahydrofolic acid. (B) Vitamin B₁₂ consists of a porphyrin-like ring with a central cobalt (Co) atom attached to a nucleotide. PABA = p-aminobenzoic acid; R = CN⁻ (cyanocobalamin) or OH⁻ (hydroxocobalamin).

pregnancy. The standard U.S. diet provides 50 to 500 μg of absorbable folic acid daily. Women of childbearing age should take an additional 400 μg/day of folic acid, the amount contained in most multivitamin preparations. Since 1998, the U.S. Food and Drug Administration has required fortification of all enriched cereal grains sold in the United States with 140 μg of folic acid per 100 g of grain. The incidence of neural tube defects in the United States, which had been declining for decades, has fallen an additional 25% since fortification of cereals began.

Folic acid is well absorbed from the jejunum, and oral supplementation is effective both in preventing and in treating megaloblastic anemia associated with **folic acid deficiency**. This disorder often results from insufficient folic acid intake in the diet, but it can also result from impaired folic acid absorption, such as that seen in patients with alcoholism and certain malabsorption syndromes. In patients with megaloblastic anemia, vitamin B₁₂ deficiency must be ruled out before treatment with folic acid is begun. This is because treatment with folic acid may partly correct

the anemia caused by a vitamin B₁₂ deficiency but will not correct other problems associated with it. Irreversible neurologic damage can occur if a B₁₂ deficiency is incorrectly treated with folic acid.

Several drugs can contribute to folate deficiency. These include chemotherapeutic **folate reductase inhibitors,** such as trimethoprim, pyrimethamine, and methotrexate (see Chapters 40, 44, and 45). Other drugs inhibit folate absorption, including cholestyramine and certain anticonvulsant drugs (e.g., phenytoin).

Vitamin B₁₂

Vitamin B₁₂ consists of a porphyrin-like ring with a central cobalt atom attached to a nucleotide (see Fig. 17–2B). Two synthetic forms of vitamin B₁₂, **cyanocobalamin** and **hydroxocobalamin**, are available for the treatment of B₁₂ deficiency. In the body, these forms of the vitamin are converted to methylcobalamin or deoxyadenosylcobalamin, which are cofactors for biochemical reactions. Vitamin B₁₂ serves as a cofactor for methylation reactions, including the

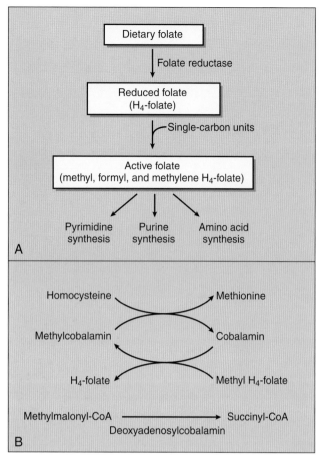

Figure 17–3. Biochemical reactions involving folic acid and vitamin B$_{12}$. (A) Dietary folate is reduced by folate reductase to tetrahydrofolate (H$_4$-folate). Single-carbon units are added to H$_4$-folate to form active folate, which donates single-carbon units in the synthesis of pyrimidine and purine bases and amino acids. (B) The two active forms of vitamin B$_{12}$ are methylcobalamin and deoxyadenosylcobalamin. These forms are cofactors for methylation reactions, including the conversion of homocysteine to methionine and the conversion of methylmalonyl-CoA to succinyl-CoA. Methyl H$_4$-folate donates a methyl group to cobalamin to form methylcobalamin.

conversion of homocysteine to methionine and the conversion of methylmalonyl coenzyme A (CoA) to succinyl CoA (see Fig. 17–3B).

Vitamin B$_{12}$ is essential for growth, cell replication, hematopoiesis, and myelin synthesis. It is obtained from dietary meats, dairy products, and eggs, and it is absorbed from the gut in the presence of **intrinsic factor** (a glycoprotein secreted by gastric parietal cells) and calcium. An inadequate secretion of intrinsic factor leads to **vitamin B$_{12}$ deficiency** and eventually results in **pernicious anemia**. Vitamin B$_{12}$ deficiency is also seen in patients who have malabsorption disorders, in individuals who have had gastrectomy, and in strict vegetarians who have a low dietary intake of the vitamin.

Because vitamin B$_{12}$ is not absorbed from the gut in the absence of intrinsic factor, the vitamin must be administered intramuscularly in the treatment of pernicious anemia, and treatment must be continued for life. At the start of therapy, injections are given daily for 5 to 10 days. Thereafter,

maintenance doses are given once a month. A nasal spray formulation of cyanocobalamin (**CALOMIST**) is available for maintenance therapy after normalization of serum B$_{12}$ concentrations with intramuscular B$_{12}$ injections. In patients with a dietary deficiency of vitamin B$_{12}$, treatment is given orally.

Hydroxocobalamin is also utilized for out-of-hospital empiric treatment of **cyanide poisoning** resulting from smoke inhalation. In this setting, hydroxocobalamin (**CYANOKIT**) is administered intravenously, and then it rapidly combines with cyanide to form harmless cyanocobalamin in the blood.

Hematopoietic Growth Factors

Colony-stimulating factors (CSFs), **erythropoietin**, and other hematopoietic growth factors are endogenous glycoproteins that stimulate the differentiation and maturation of bone marrow progenitor cells. The growth factors bind to receptors on specific myeloid progenitor cells and thereby induce their differentiation and proliferation.

Some growth factors, including those discussed in this chapter, have been manufactured by recombinant DNA technology, and these are administered parenterally to treat hematopoietic deficiencies. Other growth factors are currently undergoing development.

Epoetin and Darbepoetin

Endogenous **erythropoietin** stimulates erythroid cell differentiation and proliferation and is secreted primarily by the kidney. Epoetin-α was the first form of human erythropoietin to be produced by recombinant DNA technology. Epoetin-β and darbepoetin-α have been marketed more recently, and a pegylated form of epoetin-β is in Phase III clinical trials. Recombinant human erythropoietin (r-HuEPO) is used to treat anemia caused by **chronic renal failure, cancer chemotherapy**, and **zidovudine therapy** for human immunodeficiency virus. It is also used to treat anemia in patients with **hematologic malignancies** (e.g., lymphoma) and to treat anemia in patients with **heart failure** and other chronic diseases.

In persons with cancer-related anemia, administration of r-HuEPO has been found to cause reticulocytosis, increase hemoglobin levels, reduce the need for blood transfusions, and improve quality of life. The standard treatment has been to administer r-HuEPO intravenously or subcutaneously three times a week, but studies show that once weekly epoetin-β or darbepoetin-α is as effective as a three times weekly regimen. This is partly because darbepoetin-α has a threefold longer half-life than epoetin-α because of its increased sialic acid content. The dosage and duration of therapy are determined by the hematocrit response to epoetin treatment. Clinical trials have shown that using larger doses of r-HuEPO to achieve hemoglobin levels above 12 g/dL is associated with increased **risk of hypertension, stroke, myocardial infarction, heart failure,** and **death** in comparison with doses used to achieve hemoglobin levels of below 12 g/dL. Hence, caution should be exercised in dosing erythropoietin because of the increased risk of thrombotic and other complications.

Recombinant erythropoietin is a safe and effective treatment for anemia in patients with chronic renal failure, but higher doses pose the same risks as described in the previous paragraph. The drug is usually well tolerated, and most of the adverse reactions that occur during therapy are attributable to the underlying disease state. The utilization of iron stores, however, is increased in patients treated with r-HuEPO. Therefore, patients should be given iron supplements to maintain transferrin saturation levels that will support epoetin-stimulated erythropoiesis.

Filgrastim, Pegfilgrastim, and Sargramostim

Filgrastim is recombinant human **granulocyte CSF** (G-CSF), and sargramostim is recombinant human **granulocyte-macrophage CSF** (GM-CSF). The endogenous forms of these growth factors are produced by various leukocytes, fibroblasts, and endothelial cells. Because filgrastim is produced in *Escherichia coli* by recombinant DNA technology, it is not glycosylated and differs in this manner from G-CSF isolated from human cells.

The addition of a **polyethylene glycol** moiety to filgrastim has resulted in the development of pegfilgrastim. Pegylation of filgrastim increases its molecular size so that it is too large for renal clearance, thereby increasing the half-life from about 3.5 hours for filgrastim to 42 hours for pegfilgrastim. Pegfilgrastim is eliminated primarily by neutrophil uptake and metabolism. The longer half-life of pegfilgrastim has enabled less frequent administration for treating cancer chemotherapy-induced neutropenia.

Filgrastim, pegfilgrastim, and sargramostim are used primarily to treat **neutropenia associated with cancer chemotherapy and bone marrow transplantation.**

Filgrastim accelerates granulocyte recovery after myelosuppressive chemotherapy and thereby reduces the incidence of infections and shortens the period of hospitalization. Filgrastim is also used to mobilize hematopoietic progenitor cells into the peripheral blood when blood is being collected for leukapheresis. Studies indicate that filgrastim may be beneficial in the treatment of aplastic anemia, hairy cell leukemia, myelodysplasia, drug-induced and congenital agranulocytosis, and other forms of congenital or acquired neutropenia.

Sargramostim is used to accelerate myeloid cell recovery in patients who have **lymphoma,** acute lymphoblastic **leukemia,** or **Hodgkin's disease** and are having autologous **bone marrow transplantation** or chemotherapy. It has also been used to reduce the incidence of fever and infections in patients with severe chronic neutropenia. Although endogenous GM-CSF stimulates the production of several types of cells, sargramostim has little effect on erythrocytes or platelets in deficiency states and serves primarily to accelerate the development of neutrophils.

Filgrastim and sargramostim are administered subcutaneously or intravenously once a day for 2 weeks or until the absolute neutrophil count has reached 10,000/μL. Because of its longer half-life, pegfilgrastim requires administration only once during each cycle of cancer chemotherapy in order to manage chemotherapy-induced neutropenia.

SUMMARY OF IMPORTANT POINTS

■ Iron deficiency causes hypochromic microcytic anemia, whereas folic acid or vitamin B_{12} deficiency causes megaloblastic anemia.

■ Ferrous sulfate and other ferrous salts are administered orally for several months in the treatment of iron deficiency anemia.

■ Folic acid supplementation is used during pregnancy to prevent anemia and birth defects.

■ Folic acid treatment can partly mask the hematologic effect of vitamin B_{12} deficiency but does not prevent irreversible neurologic damage.

■ Pernicious anemia is caused by inadequate secretion of intrinsic factor and reduced vitamin B_{12} absorption. It is treated with intramuscular injections of cyanocobalamin or hydroxocobalamin.

■ Epoetin-α, epoetin-β, and darbepoetin-α are recombinant forms of human erythropoietin used to treat anemia caused by chronic renal failure, cancer-related anemia, and anemia caused by other conditions.

■ Filgrastim, pegfilgrastim, and sargramostim are recombinant forms of G-CSF or GM-CSF. They are used to treat neutropenia associated with cancer chemotherapy, bone marrow transplantation, and various disease states.

Review Questions

For each numbered patient, select the most appropriate drug therapy from the lettered choices provided.

1. A 19-year-old woman who complains of lethargy and fatigue is found to have a blood hemoglobin concentration of 9.8 g/dL (normal range 12–16 g/dL), a low mean corpuscular volume, and a low mean corpuscular hemoglobin concentration.

2. A 47-year-old woman exhibits severe neutropenia following a course of chemotherapy for breast cancer.

3. A 66-year-old man with progressive fatigability and anorexia is found to have a low blood hemoglobin concentration, an elevated mean corpuscular volume, and an elevated serum concentration of methylmalonic acid.

4. A 68-year-old man with diabetic nephropathy and end-stage renal disease exhibits peripheral reticulocytopenia and anemia.
   (A) cyanocobalamin
   (B) epoetin
   (C) ferrous gluconate
   (D) filgrastim
   (E) folic acid

Answers and Explanations

1. **The answer is C: ferrous gluconate.** Iron deficiency anemia is a hypochromic (low mean corpuscular hemoglobin concentration), microcytic (low mean corpuscular volume) anemia. Several months of treatment with oral ferrous sulfate or another ferrous salt may be required to correct the iron deficiency and restore hemoglobin concentrations to normal. Patients should also consume a diet containing adequate amounts of folic acid and vitamin B_{12} to ensure adequate erythropoiesis.

2. **The answer is D: filgrastim.** Filgrastim is a recombinant G-CSF that is used to treat cancer chemotherapy–induced neutropenia in patients with neoplasms, such as breast cancer. Sargramostim has similar indications. Folic acid and vitamin B_{12} are required for normal leucopoiesis, but these vitamins will not by themselves accelerate leucopoiesis caused by drug-induced myelosuppression.

3. **The answer is A: cyanocobalamin.** Pernicious anemia usually results from inadequate vitamin B_{12} absorption because of decreased production of intrinsic factor by gastric parietal cells. Vitamin B_{12} deficiency causes a megaloblastic anemia characterized by an abnormally high mean corpuscular volume. Persons with pernicious anemia will also have a low serum level of vitamin B_{12} and a high serum concentration of methylmalonic acid, because B_{12} is required to convert methylmalonyl CoA to succinyl CoA.

4. **The answer is B: epoetin.** Epoetin is a recombinant form of erythropoietin. Patients with end-stage renal disease often require epoetin treatment to prevent anemia because their kidneys are unable to produce sufficient erythropoietin to maintain adequate erythrocyte production.

SELECTED READINGS

Ciurea, S.O., and R. Hoffman. Cytokines for the treatment of thrombocytopenia. Semin Hematol 44:166–182, 2007.

Hurter, B., and N.J. Bush. Cancer-related anemia: clinical review and management update. Clin J Oncol Nurs 11:349–359, 2007.

Huston, A., and G.H. Lyman. Agents under investigation for the treatment and prevention of neutropenia. Expert Opin Investig Drugs 16:1831–1840, 2007.

Panchapakesan, U., S. Sumual, and C. Pollock. Nanomedicines in the treatment of anemia in renal disease: focus on CERE (Continuous Erythropoietin Receptor Activator). Int J Nanomedicine 2:33–38, 2007.

CENTRAL NERVOUS SYSTEM PHARMACOLOGY

CHAPTER 18

Introduction to Central Nervous System Pharmacology

OVERVIEW

The central nervous system (CNS) consists of the brain and spinal cord. Sensory information arrives to the CNS from the special senses and peripheral nerves and is integrated with memories and internal drive states to generate cognitive, emotional, and motor (behavioral) responses. This processing occurs because of the complex interplay of **neurotransmitters** and **neuromodulators** acting on their **receptors** to excite or inhibit CNS neurons. In persons with **brain disorders**, structural or functional disturbances of CNS processing produce aberrant cognitive, emotional, or motor responses. Brain disorders are seen in association with a variety of disease processes, including degenerative, ischemic, and psychological disturbances.

Most CNS drugs correct an **imbalance in neurotransmitters or their receptors**. Drugs are used to relieve the symptoms of brain dysfunction, but they usually do not correct the underlying disorder. Although short-term drug treatment may be effective in relieving acute symptoms such as pain and insomnia, drug therapy for many brain disorders is a life-long process.

After reviewing pertinent concepts of CNS function and neurotransmission, this chapter explains the general mechanisms by which drugs alter CNS activities and processes.

NEUROTRANSMISSION IN THE CENTRAL NERVOUS SYSTEM

Principles of Neurotransmission

In the past century, great debates raged about the nature of neuronal communication in the CNS. The early physiologists believed that neurons communicated by electrical signals directly passing from neuron to neuron in a **hardwired** fashion much like wires in a telegraph relay. The early pharmacologists argued for chemical transmission, with substances released into the **synapse** between communicating neurons. Modern research shows that both were right to some degree because most neuronal communication occurs by chemical **neurotransmitters** serving as messengers that

enable neurons to communicate with one another. However there is also evidence of direct voltage signaling between neurons at **electrotonic** or **gap junctions**.

The details of chemical neurotransmission undergo constant refinement as new mechanisms and neurotransmitters as discovered. An early statement by Sir Henry Dale, known as **Dale's principle**, suggested that each neuron contained only one type of neurotransmitter. This principle was revised with the finding that neurons may release more than one neurotransmitter, as is the case with co-transmitters (see below). It was also thought that neurotransmitter action was limited to the single synapse where released. The neuroanatomical demonstration of diffuse neuronal systems with fine, widespread projections throughout the CNS, such as norepinephrine and serotonergic fibers arising from brain stem nuclei, led to the concept of the **chemical "soup"** or **chemical milieu** model of neurotransmission. Newer methods using in vitro brain slice preparations and other techniques show that neurotransmitters can diffuse far from the synapse and affect other neurons at other synapses. Identification of neuroactive substances both intrinsic and extrinsic to the CNS that exert generalized effects on neurons strengthened the concept of action at a distance. A **neuromodulator** is a general term for any substance that exerts an effect on neurotransmission among a set of neurons in the brain.

The action of drugs on the CNS is similar to the chemical milieu model of neurotransmission, because drug molecules are widely distributed throughout the brain and can simultaneously interact with receptors on neurons in several different neuronal tracts. This lack of specificity can lead to therapeutic effects and adverse effects at the same time. For this reason, the development of agents that are more selective for specific receptor types and subtypes is a useful approach to improving the therapeutic index of CNS drugs.

Neurotransmitter Synthesis and Metabolism

Neurotransmitters are synthesized in neuronal cell bodies or terminals, and they are stored in neuronal **vesicles** until they are released into a synapse (Fig. 18–1). The release of neurotransmitters is activated by membrane depolarization and calcium influx into the cell. Calcium evokes the

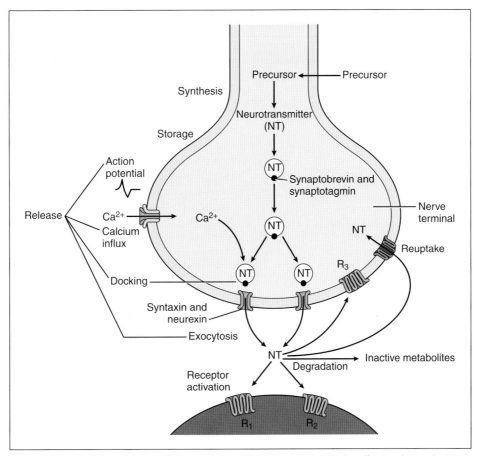

Figure 18-1. CNS neurotransmission and sites of drug action. CNS drugs act primarily by affecting the synthesis, storage, release, reuptake, or degradation of neurotransmitters (NTs) or by activating receptors. NTs are synthesized from precursors accumulated or synthesized in the neurons. The NTs are stored in vesicles whose membranes contain proteins involved in NT release (synaptobrevin and synaptotagmin). The NTs are released when an action potential–mediated calcium influx initiates interaction of synaptobrevin and synaptotagmin with neuronal membrane–docking proteins (syntaxin and neurexin). This leads to docking and exocytosis. Synaptic NTs can activate presynaptic (R_3) or postsynaptic receptors (R_1, R_2). The action of NTs is terminated by reuptake into the presynaptic neuron or by enzymatic degradation.

interaction of storage vesicle proteins (synaptobrevin and synaptotagmin) and membrane-docking proteins (syntaxin and neurexin) and leads to **vesicle fusion** with the membrane and **exocytosis** of the neurotransmitter.

Following exocytosis, the neurotransmitter may activate presynaptic and postsynaptic receptors. A neurotransmitter's action is then terminated either by its reuptake into the presynaptic neuron or by its degradation to inactive compounds, with degradation catalyzed by enzymes located on presynaptic and postsynaptic neuronal membranes or within the cytoplasm.

Neurotransmitters can also diffuse from the synapse of their origin to affect neurons in the surrounding vicinity. In this way, different neurotransmitters released from different types of neurons form a **chemical milieu**, as described previously. The net influence of the chemical milieu on neurotransmission depends on the concentrations of the excitatory and inhibitory neurotransmitters acting at a particular synapse.

Excitatory and Inhibitory Neurotransmission

CNS neurotransmitters can evoke either an excitatory or an inhibitory synaptic membrane potential and trigger effects at presynaptic and postsynaptic sites on target neurons. If an **excitatory postsynaptic membrane potential** reaches firing threshold, an action potential is conducted along the dendritic and axonal membrane and evokes the release of a neurotransmitter from the nerve terminal. An **inhibitory postsynaptic membrane potential** hyperpolarizes the neuronal membrane and inhibits the firing of action potentials. Depending on whether a **presynaptic membrane potential** is excitatory or inhibitory, it will increase or decrease the release of a neurotransmitter from the neuron. Presynaptic receptors, also called **autoreceptors**, can also be coupled with **cyclic adenosine monophosphate (cAMP)** or other **second messengers** that modulate neurotransmitter release.

As shown in Box 18–1, the interaction of multiple neurotransmitters at a particular site in a neuronal tract enables the complex interplay of various neuronal systems and contributes to the wide range of functional expression exhibited in the CNS. For example, inhibition of the release of an inhibitory neurotransmitter will actually increase neurotransmission in the target neuron. Similarly, drugs can act in complex ways to affect neurotransmission. **Ethanol** (ethyl alcohol), for instance, can diminish the inhibitory influence of the cerebral cortex on certain human behaviors and thereby increase drug-induced behaviors, a phenomenon called **behavioral**

BOX 18–1. PATTERNS OF NEUROTRANSMISSION IN THE CENTRAL NERVOUS SYSTEM

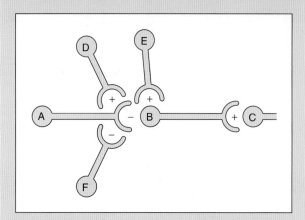

A, B, C, D, E, and F are neurons in a tract that projects from left to right. Neurons B, D, and E release excitatory neurotransmitters (+). Neurons A and F release inhibitory neurotransmitters (−). The net effect of neuronal interactions on neurotransmission from B to C is shown in the table below. Each interaction presupposes that the other neurons are quiescent at that time. Other, more complex interactions are possible.

Interaction	Effect on Neurotransmission (B → C)
A → B	Decreased
D → A → B	Greatly decreased
F → A → B	Increased
E → B	Increased

disinhibition. Ethanol and other CNS depressants, initially or at low doses, exert their effects on the smaller and more numerous inhibitory neurons, creating disinhibition via excitation due to removal of inhibitory neurotransmitters. At higher doses, larger excitatory neurons are inhibited and profound depression of CNS activity can occur.

Fast versus Slow Signals

Neurotransmitters in the CNS can be characterized as slow or fast, depending on the receptors that are activated and the persistence of signal transduction pathways. The best examples of **fast neurotransmitters** are γ-aminobutyric acid (GABA) and glutamate acting at **ligand-gated ion channels.** Binding of these amino acid neurotransmitters directly to subunits of the ion channel protein directly initiates ion flow with a signal that lasts for only a few milliseconds. Examples of **slow neurotransmitters** are norepinephrine and serotonin acting at **G protein–coupled receptors.** These activated G protein–coupled receptor proteins initiate a slower, multistep process with alterations in second messengers and membrane effects that can last from many milliseconds to as long as a second. A slow (long-acting) signal can influence the overall tone of a neuron because it can modulate the signals of several other fast neurotransmitters acting on the same neuron. For this reason, slow neurotransmitters can also be called **neuromodulators**.

Neurotransmitters and Receptors

Important neurotransmitters in the CNS include acetylcholine and several amino acids, biogenic amines, and neuropeptides. Table 18–1 lists the names, receptors, mechanisms of signal transduction, and functions of the major neurotransmitters.

The receptors can be divided into two basic groups: **ionotropic receptors**, also called **ligand-gated ion channels**, which are directly associated with ion channels, and **metabotropic receptors**, which are typical **G protein–coupled receptors** (see Chapter 3). Although this terminology is most frequently applied to receptors for amino acid neurotransmitters (e.g., GABA and glutamate), it is equally appropriate for other classes of neurotransmitter receptors.

The **mechanisms of signal transduction** for neurotransmitters in the CNS are similar to those for neurotransmitters in the autonomic nervous system. The activation of ionotropic receptors alters chloride, sodium, potassium, or calcium influx and thereby evokes excitatory or inhibitory membrane potentials. The linkage of metabotropic receptors with G proteins leads to activation or inhibition of adenylyl cyclase and alteration in the levels of intracellular cAMP, or activation of phospholipase C and the formation of inositol triphosphate and diacylglycerol. Metabotropic receptor activity can also modulate ion channel activity via **second messengers** (most notably calcium) that activate protein kinases responsible for the phosphorylation of ion channels. Signal transduction for other receptors in the CNS is discussed in Chapter 3.

Acetylcholine

Acetylcholine, synthesized from acetyl coenzyme A and choline, is degraded to acetate and choline by the enzyme acetylcholinesterase (Fig. 18–2). **Acetylcholine receptors** (also known as **cholinergic receptors**) consist of two main types: **muscarinic receptors** and **nicotinic receptors**. The properties and mechanisms of these receptors are compared in Table 6–1.

Drugs can affect acetylcholine neurotransmission by activating or blocking acetylcholine receptors or by inhibiting cholinesterase. The general pharmacologic properties of acetylcholine receptor agonists and antagonists are described in Chapters 6 and 7, respectively.

In the CNS, acetylcholine acts as an excitatory or inhibitory neurotransmitter in a number of neuronal tracts, including those that innervate the hippocampus, cerebral cortex, and basal ganglia. These tracts participate in memory, sensory processing, and motor coordination, respectively.

Amino Acids

Several amino acids are important neurotransmitters in the brain and spinal cord. Some of them, most notably, **GABA** and **glycine**, are inhibitory. Others, such as **glutamate** and **aspartate**, are excitatory.

γ-AMINOBUTYRIC ACID. GABA, which is synthesized from glutamic acid, is the most ubiquitous inhibitory

TABLE 18–1. Major Neurotransmitters and Their Receptors in the CNS

Neurotransmitter	Receptors	Signal Transduction	Function
Acetylcholine	Muscarinic		
	M_1, M_3, M_5	$\uparrow IP_3$, $\uparrow DAG$, $\uparrow iCa^{2+}$	Excitatory; role in arousal and consciousness, memory consolidation
	M_2, M_4	$\downarrow cAMP$, $\uparrow gK^+$, $\downarrow gCa^{2+}$	Inhibitory; autoreceptor and heteroreceptor, decreases NT release
	Nicotinic	$\uparrow gNa^+$, $\uparrow gCa^{2+}$	Excitatory; increases NT release, role in nicotine dependence
Amino Acids			
GABA	$GABA_A$	$\uparrow gCl^-$	Inhibitory (major); ligand-gated ion channel site of action of sedative-hypnotics, alcohol, general anesthetics
	$GABA_B$	$\downarrow cAMP$, $\uparrow gK^+$, $\downarrow gCa^{2+}$	Inhibitory; modulates motor neuron excitability
Glutamate	NMDA, AMPA, KA	$\uparrow gNa^+$, $\uparrow gCa^{2+}$	Excitatory (major); roles in LTP (memory), excitotoxicity of neurons
	$mGlu_1$, $mGlu_5$	$\uparrow IP_3$, $\uparrow DAG$, $\uparrow iCa^{2+}$	Excitatory; memory consolidation, neuronal excitation
	$mGlu_2$-$mGlu_4$, $mGlu_6$-$mGlu_8$	$\downarrow cAMP$, $\uparrow gK^+$, $\downarrow gCa^{2+}$	Inhibitory; role in thalamic sensory processing
Glycine	Strychnine-sensitive	$\uparrow gCl^-$	Inhibitory; highest levels in spinal cord
	Strychnine-insensitive	Co-agonist at NMDA receptor	Excitatory; obligate co-agonist for function of NMDA receptor
Biogenic Amines			
Dopamine	D_1, D_5	$\uparrow cAMP$, $\uparrow PKA$	Excitatory; basal ganglia function, memory and performance
	D_2, D_3, D_4	$\downarrow cAMP$, $\uparrow gK^+$, $\downarrow gCa^{2+}$	Inhibitory; decreases dopamine release, reduces firing of neurons
Norepinephrine	α_1	$\uparrow IP_3$, $\uparrow DAG$, $\uparrow iCa^{2+}$	Excitatory; autonomic nuclei in brain stem
	α_2	$\downarrow cAMP$, $\uparrow gK^+$, $\downarrow gCa^{2+}$	Inhibitory; sympathetic outflow from CNS; decreases pain transmission
	β_1, β_2	$\uparrow cAMP$, $\uparrow PKA$	Excitatory; cortex, limbic system, nucleus accumbens
Serotonin (5-HT)*	$5\text{-}HT_1$	$\downarrow cAMP$, $\uparrow gK^+$, $\downarrow gCa^{2+}$	Inhibitory; role in anxiety and depression
	$5\text{-}HT_2$	$\uparrow IP_3$, $\uparrow DAG$, $\uparrow iCa^{2+}$	Excitatory; widespread distribution, role in antipsychotic action
	$5\text{-}HT_3$	$\uparrow gNa^+$, $\uparrow gCa^{2+}$	Excitatory; mediate fast neuronal transmission in neocortex; presynaptic modulation of NT release
	$5\text{-}HT_4$	$\uparrow cAMP$, $\uparrow PKA$	Excitatory; role in cognitive processes, anxiety
Histamine	H_1	$\uparrow IP_3$, $\uparrow DAG$, $\uparrow iCa^{2+}$	Excitatory; increases NT release, role in arousal, anxiety
	H_2	$\uparrow cAMP$, $\uparrow PKA$	Excitatory; located in hippocampus, amygdala and basal ganglia
	H_3	$\downarrow cAMP$, $\uparrow gK^+$, $\downarrow gCa^{2+}$	Inhibitory; autoreceptor and heteroreceptor, decreases NT release
Neuropeptides			
Opioid peptides	*Mu, delta, kappa*	$\downarrow cAMP$, $\uparrow gK^+$, $\downarrow gCa^{2+}$	Inhibitory; analgesic role in sensory processing, role in drug dependence for opioids and other substances
Tachykinins	NK_1, NK_2, NK_3	$\uparrow IP_3$, $\uparrow DAG$, $\uparrow iCa^{2+}$	Excitatory; role in pain processing, autonomic regulation

*Over a dozen types of serotonin receptors are cloned; the four given here are the main types.
AMPA = α-amino-3-hydroxy-5-methyl-4-isoxazole propionate; cAMP = cyclic adenosine monophosphate; CNS = central nervous system; DAG = diacylglycerol; 5-HT = 5-hydroxytryptamine (serotonin); g = ion channel conductance; GABA = γ-aminobutyric acid; i = intracellular; IP_3 = inositol triphosphate; KA = kainate; LTP = long-term potentiation; NK = neurokinin; NMDA = N-methyl-D-aspartate; NT = neurotransmitter; PKA = cAMP-dependent protein kinase.

neurotransmitter in the brain and spinal cord. Its receptors are the **ionotropic $GABA_A$ receptors** and the **metabotropic $GABA_B$ receptors**. Most drugs affecting GABA neurotransmission primarily activate or inhibit the **$GABA_A$-chloride ion channel** complex. This ion channel complex contains receptors for several types of drugs, including the **benzodiazepines** and **barbiturates** (see Chapter 19), **general anesthetics** (Chapter 21), and **alcohol** (Chapter 25). Drugs acting at the **$GABA_B$ receptor** are used to control spasticity (Chapter 24).

The functions of GABA include regulation of neuronal excitability throughout the CNS and motor coordination.

GLYCINE AND TAURINE. Glycine is a major inhibitory transmitter in the spinal cord. Its **strychnine-sensitive receptors** are coupled with the chloride ion channel, and activation of these receptors leads to membrane hyperpolarization. The inhibitory actions of glycine are potently antagonized by the alkaloid **strychnine**, a convulsant poison used as a

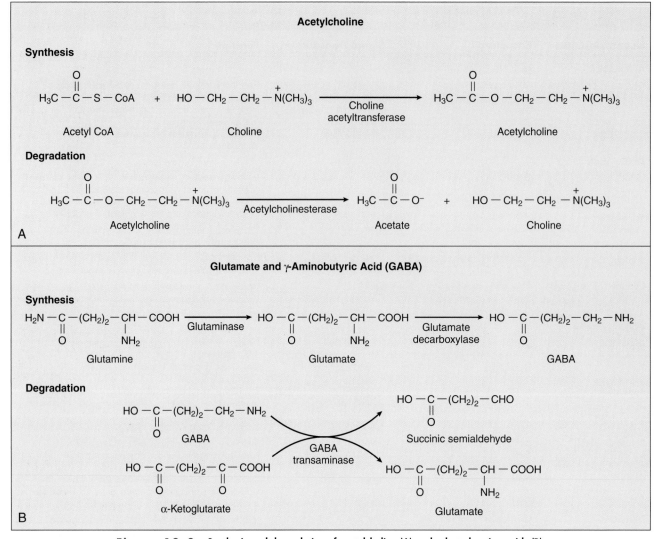

Figure 18-2. Synthesis and degradation of acetylcholine (A) and selected amino acids (B).

rodenticide. Strychnine poisoning causes disinhibition of motoneurons, leading to convulsions and death through respiratory failure. Glycine also acts as a **co-agonist** to the excitatory amino acid, glutamate, at **NMDA receptors**, by binding to an allosteric **strychnine-insensitive** site.

Taurine is a sulfur-containing amino acid that is postulated to act as a neurotransmitter or neuromodulator in the CNS. Taurine is believed to activate both strychnine-sensitive and strychnine-insensitive types of **glycine-binding sites**.

GLUTAMATE AND ASPARTATE. Glutamate and aspartate are acidic amino acids that function as excitatory neurotransmitters throughout the CNS. Their ionotropic receptors consist of three types that differ in their subunit composition and are named for drugs that show the most selectivity for each type: **NMDA** (*N*-methyl-*D*-aspartate), **AMPA** (α-amino-3-hydroxy-5-methyl-4-isoxazole propionate), and **kainate** receptors. These receptors are excitatory because their associated ion channels allow the flow of sodium or calcium ions into neurons causing depolarization. Metabotropic

glutamate receptors consist of two main classes that are either coupled to phospholipase C and intracellular calcium signaling or are negatively coupled to adenylyl cyclase. Glutamate and aspartate participate in the long-term potentiation needed for learning and memory and have a role in neuronal toxicity and apoptosis (cell death) evoked by trauma and ischemia. Antagonists of these excitatory amino acid receptors are used in the treatment of **seizures** (Chapter 20) and may find use in blocking the overexcitation of neurons that occurs following stroke and other disorders.

Biogenic Amines

The biogenic amines or monoamines that function as CNS neurotransmitters are the catecholamines, dopamine and norepinephrine; and serotonin (5-hydroxytryptamine); and histamine. These neurotransmitters, which are formed by decarboxylation of amino acids, are catabolized in part by the enzyme, monoamine oxidase.

DOPAMINE. Dopamine is a major CNS neurotransmitter that binds to five types of dopamine receptors. The D_1 and D_5

receptors activate adenylyl cyclase and thereby increase cAMP levels. In contrast, the D_2, D_3, and D_4 receptors inhibit adenylyl cyclase and decrease cAMP levels. As shown in Table 18–2, levodopa, clozapine, and other drugs have effects on various steps in the synthesis and metabolism of dopamine. Dopamine is found in several neuronal tracts originating from the ventral tegmental area, plays a significant role in behavioral and drug reinforcement, and regulates emesis (vomiting), prolactin release, mood states, motor coordination, and olfaction. Its degradation by monoamine oxidase results in the formation of homovanillic acid, a metabolite that is subsequently excreted in the urine (Fig. 18–3). Inhibitors of monoamine oxidase increase dopamine levels in the brain and are used for the treatment of Parkinsonism.

NOREPINEPHRINE. Norepinephrine, which is formed from dopamine, is degraded by **monoamine oxidase** and **catechol-O-methyltransferase** to a number of metabolites. The major metabolite excreted in the urine is **3-methoxy-4-hydroxy-mandelic acid**, or **vanillylmandelic acid**. The receptors for norepinephrine are **α-adrenoceptors** and **β-adrenoceptors** (also known as α- and β-adrenergic receptors), and their classification and properties are described in detail in Chapter 8. Norepinephrine is associated with several neuronal tracts projecting from the **locus ceruleus** in the medulla (brainstem) to the thalamus, cerebral cortex, cerebellum, and spinal cord, and it is found in tracts projecting from the midbrain to the hypothalamus. This ubiquitous neurotransmitter participates in the regulation of anxiety, cerebellar function, learning, memory, mood, sensory processing (including pain), and sleep. Drugs can alter norepinephrine neurotransmission by activating or blocking its receptors or by inhibiting its presynaptic neuronal uptake.

SEROTONIN. Serotonin, or 5-hydroxytryptamine (5-HT), is synthesized from tryptophan, is degraded to **5-hydroxy-indoleacetic acid**, and functions as both an excitatory and inhibitory neurotransmitter. Serotonin is found in neuronal tracts projecting from the **raphe nuclei** in the medulla to many other parts of the brain. These tracts are involved in emotional processing and pain processing and have an effect on appetite, mood, sleep, and hallucina-

tions. Serotonin (5-HT) acts on more than a dozen types of receptors; all of them are metabotropic receptors, except for the **5-HT₃ receptor** which is a ligand-gated ion channel protein. The main types and effector mechanisms of 5-HT receptors are outlined in Table 18–1. In most areas of the brain, serotonin has an inhibitory effect mediated by the 5-HT$_{1A}$ receptor, decreasing cAMP levels and increasing potassium conductance causing membrane hyperpolarization. Drugs can affect serotonergic function by stimulating or blocking 5-HT receptors or by blocking serotonin reuptake.

HISTAMINE. Histamine is a neurotransmitter found in **hypothalamic neurons** that project to all the major parts of the brain, including the cerebral cortex. It is involved in the regulation of the sleep-wake cycle, cardiovascular control, regulation of the hypothalamic-pituitary-adrenal axis, learning, and memory. Histamine acts on two types of receptors in the brain, **H₁ and H₃**, with action on a third type, **H₂**, in the periphery. All histamine receptors are metabotropic, with H₁ receptors coupled to the phospholipase C pathway and H₃ receptors negatively coupled to adenylate cyclase. H₃ receptors were originally discovered as autoreceptors on histaminergic neurons but are now known to also inhibit the release of other neurotransmitters. CNS histamine receptors are not currently considered a major site of therapeutic drug action, but antagonism of H₁ receptors is partly responsible for the drowsiness and sedation caused by some **antihistamines**.

Neuropeptides

A number of peptides function as slow neurotransmitters or neuromodulators in the CNS. Unlike other neurotransmitters, **neuropeptides** are synthesized in neuronal cell bodies and are then transported to nerve terminals for release. Once released, they are metabolized by various peptidases, but they do not undergo presynaptic reuptake. Some of the neuropeptides are released as **co-transmitters** with other, nonpeptide neurotransmitters. The co-transmitter neuropeptides usually serve to amplify or prolong the effects of these other neurotransmitters.

A growing number of neuropeptides are known to function as neuromodulators in the CNS. One of the first classes

TABLE 18–2. Sites of CNS Drug Action

Process	Mechanism	Drug Example	Major Use
NT synthesis	Increase synthesis of NT by precursor loading	Levodopa	Parkinsonism
NT storage	Block transport of NT into vesicles	Reserpine	Hypertension
NT release	Increase NT release	Methylphenidate	Attention deficit-hyperactivity disorder
NT reuptake	Block reuptake of NT	Fluoxetine	Depression
NT degradation	Block NT degradation enzyme	Donepezil	Alzheimer's disease
Receptor activation	Agonist activity at receptor	Morphine	Pain states
Receptor blockade	Antagonist activity at receptor	Clozapine	Schizophrenia
Signal transduction	Block formation of second messengers	Lithium	Bipolar disorder
Neuronal conduction	Block axonal action potentials	Lidocaine	Local anesthesia

CNS = central nervous system; NT = neurotransmitter.

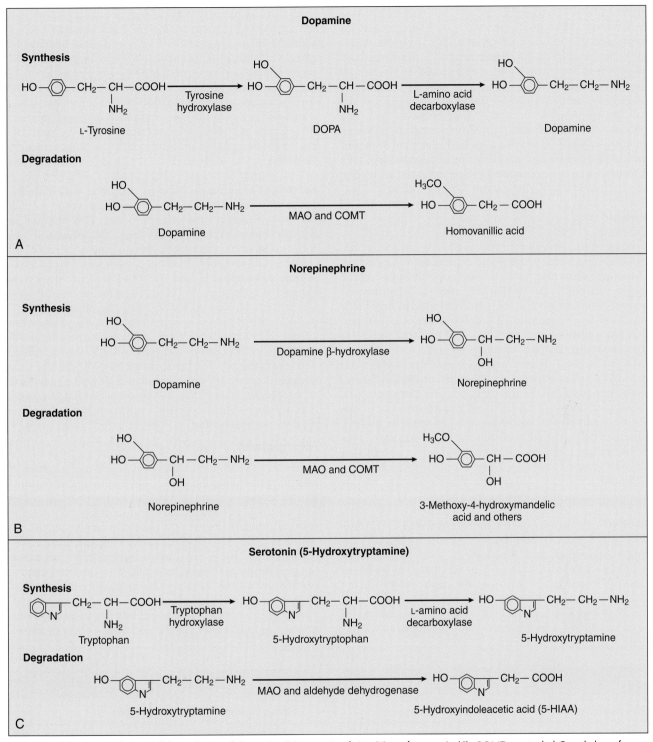

Figure 18-3. Synthesis and degradation of dopamine (A), norepinephrine (B), and serotonin (C). COMT = catechol-*O*-methyltransferase; DOPA = dihydroxyphenylalanine; MAO = monoamine oxidase.

of neuropeptides discovered are the **endogenous opioid peptides (endorphins)** and includes **Met-enkephalin, dynorphin, and β-endorphin**. The opioid peptides inhibit pain transmission in the spinal cord and midbrain, among other CNS effects. A second important group consists of **tachykinins** and includes **neurokinins A and B,** and **substance P.** Neurokinins modulate cardiovascular and behavioral responses to stress, and substance P participates in pain processing, emesis, and anxiety.

Other peptides that were originally isolated from peripheral tissues are thought to function as neuromodulators in the CNS. These neuropeptides include **cholecystokinin, gastrin, somatostatin,** and **vasoactive intestinal polypeptide.**

Other Neurotransmitters

Several additional substances, including the gases **nitric oxide** and **carbon monoxide**, appetite-regulating peptides, and purines, may also serve as neurotransmitters or neuromodulators in the CNS.

Nitric oxide is a gas formed from arginine by calcium-calmodulin–stimulated nitric oxide synthase in CNS neurons. Evidence suggests that nitric oxide acts as a **retrograde neurotransmitter** in that it is released by the postsynaptic neuron and diffuses to the presynaptic terminal, where it facilitates future neurotransmitter release by elevating levels of cyclic guanosine monophosphate. This action may contribute to long-term potentiation, which is a key process to establish memory. A similar function is also postulated for **carbon monoxide** in the CNS.

Several recently discovered **appetite-regulating peptides** may function as neuromodulators in the CNS. These include **ghrelin**, a peptide synthesized in the stomach and hypothalamus, and **neuropeptide Y** and **orexin**, contained in neurons in the lateral hypothalamus. All three peptides stimulate food intake and increase body weight in animal models. Conversely, **leptin** is a peptide hormone secreted from fat cells and acts on the brain to reduce food intake and increase peripheral energy expenditure. As expected, the pharmaceutical industry has intense interest in developing drug therapies for the treatment of obesity based on these discoveries.

Purines that can serve as neurotransmitters include **adenosine** and **adenosine triphosphate (ATP)**. Adenosine activates specific receptors identified as A_1, A_2, and A_3 **receptors.** Activation of A_1 and A_3 receptors increases cAMP formation, whereas activation of A_2 receptors inhibits cAMP formation. The role of adenosine as a central neurotransmitter is not clearly established, but inhibition of A_2 receptors by methylxanthines (e.g., caffeine) causes CNS stimulation. ATP acts on both ionotropic receptors, called **P2X receptors**, and metabotropic **P2Y receptors**. Similarly, the role of ATP in neurotransmission is unclear, but some evidence indicates that ATP is a co-transmitter that is released with other neurotransmitters in the brain and serves to augment the effects of these neurotransmitters.

MECHANISMS OF DRUG ACTION

Table 18–2 lists the many processes by which drugs affect the CNS and provides examples of agents acting via each process.

Drugs that alter CNS neurotransmitter function generally do so by altering the **synthesis**, **storage**, or **release** of a neurotransmitter; blocking the **reuptake** of a neurotransmitter; inhibiting the **degradation** of a neurotransmitter; or **activating** or **blocking** neurotransmitter receptors. A few CNS drugs act by directly blocking membrane ion channels or by altering the physiochemical properties of neuronal membranes to inhibit neurotransmission. Although bypassing the membrane receptor and directly modulating second-messenger or signal transduction pathways is an attractive target for novel pharmacologic agents; **lithium** is currently the only CNS drug shown to act by this mechanism.

Neurotransmitter Synthesis, Storage, and Release

Neurotransmitter synthesis can be increased by administering a precursor to a neurotransmitter, such as levodopa. **Levodopa** is taken up by dopamine neurons and is converted to dopamine, thereby increasing the amount of dopamine available for neurotransmission. The vesicular storage of norepinephrine is blocked by **reserpine**, a plant alkaloid first used to treat hypertension. The side effect of severe depression in patients treated with reserpine provided an early clue that neurotransmitter levels may be inadequate in persons with this type of affective disorder (see Chapter 22). Drugs can cause non-exocytotic release of neurotransmitter by interacting with the presynaptic neurotransmitter transporter. For example, **amphetamine** increases the release of norepinephrine by this mechanism, and **amantadine** is used therapeutically to increase the release of dopamine in patients with parkinsonism.

Neurotransmitter Reuptake and Degradation

Presynaptic reuptake and enzymatic degradation are the two primary mechanisms for terminating the action of most CNS neurotransmitters, and drugs inhibit both of these processes. **Cocaine** and many of the antidepressant drugs act by blocking the reuptake of dopamine, norepinephrine, or serotonin. **Donepezil** and **selegiline** are examples of agents that inhibit the degradation of acetylcholine or dopamine and thereby elevate the synaptic concentration of these neurotransmitters.

Receptor Activation or Blockade

Postsynaptic receptors are activated or blocked by several types of CNS drugs. For example, **bromocriptine**, a drug used in the treatment of parkinsonism, acts as an agonist at dopamine receptors, whereas antipsychotic drugs act as antagonists at dopamine and serotonin receptors.

Presynaptic receptors are involved in feedback inhibition of neurotransmitter release. They are called **autoreceptors** when they are activated by the same neurotransmitter that is released by the neuron and **heteroreceptors** when they are activated by a different neurotransmitter. Activation of presynaptic receptors decreases the concentration of the released neurotransmitter found in synapses, whereas blockade of these receptors increases the concentration. For example, activation of 5-HT_{1D} autoreceptors inhibits the release of serotonin and decreases its concentration in synapses.

Receptor Alterations Caused by CNS Drug Treatment

As detailed in Chapter 3, receptor proteins not only regulate cell processes but are themselves regulated. Receptors undergo **dynamic alteration** in response to changes in synaptic neurotransmitter concentrations or in response to long-term drug administration. These alterations can affect the efficiency of receptor coupling to signal transduction

pathways (**desensitization** or **sensitization**) or affect the number of receptor proteins expressed by the neuron (**down-regulation** or **up-regulation**). CNS drugs that act on metabotropic or G protein–coupled receptors are particularly noted for their alteration of receptor numbers. Receptor down-regulation may follow a sustained increase in neurotransmitter release, a sustained blockade of neurotransmitter reuptake, or long-term receptor activation by a drug. For example, long-term administration of **morphine** in a patient with chronic pain can cause

down-regulation of opioid receptors in the brain and spinal cord (Fig. 18–4). Receptor down-regulation is one of the primary mechanisms of pharmacodynamic drug tolerance. Receptor **up-regulation** is a compensatory reaction to a sustained decrease in neurotransmission, a condition that can be caused either by a **reduction** in neurotransmitter release or by long-term **receptor antagonism**. For example, daily administration of **haloperidol**, a dopamine receptor antagonist, in a schizophrenic patient can lead to up-regulation of D_2 receptors.

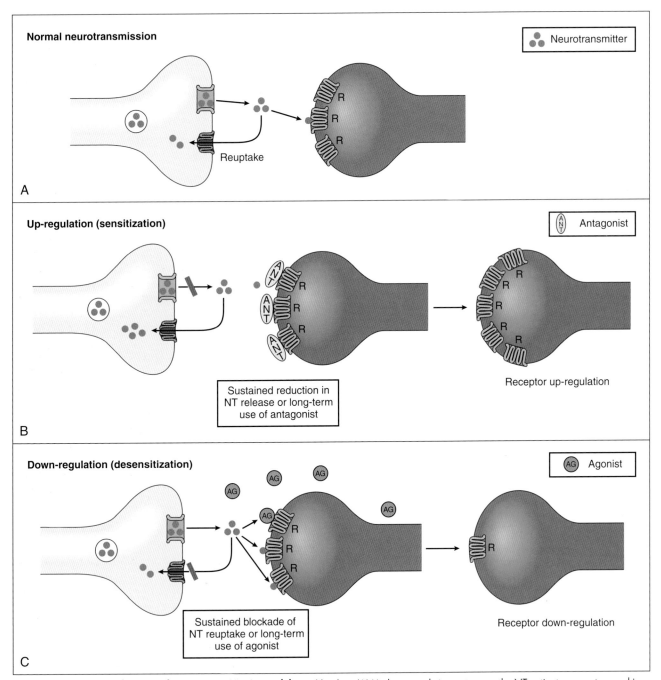

Figure 18–4. Mechanisms of receptor sensitization and desensitization. (A) Under normal circumstances, the NT activates receptors and is removed from the synapse by neuronal reuptake. (B) The number of receptors can be increased (up-regulated) by a sustained reduction in NT release or by the long-term administration of a receptor ANT. (C) The number of receptors can be decreased (down-regulated) by a sustained blockade of NT reuptake or by the long-term administration of a receptor AG. ANT = antagonist; AG = agonist; NT = neurotransmitter.

NEURONAL SYSTEMS IN THE CENTRAL NERVOUS SYSTEM

Many CNS diseases and drug treatments affect cognitive processing, memory, motor coordination, and other complex brain functions. It is difficult to attribute these complex functions to specific neuronal tracts, because many of the functions are accomplished through the interaction of tracts that communicate with several brain regions and utilize various neurotransmitters. These six broad areas of functional processing, however, provide an introduction to the neuroanatomy and neuropharmacology of CNS agents.

Cognitive Processing

Cognitive processing occurs in **prefrontal cortical structures**, where sensory information is integrated with past experience and interpreted in a manner that can result in thoughts and behavioral action. The neuronal systems involved in cognitive processing include **association fibers** that arise from areas throughout the brain and converge on the anteromedial frontal, orbital frontal, and cingulate areas of the prefrontal cortex.

Cognitive processing utilizes memory and is influenced by emotions. At the same time, emotions are largely derived from past experience and cognition. Cognitive processing also encompasses abstract reasoning and forethought, which are processes that do not necessarily result in motor expression but can influence emotional processing and future acts.

Delirium is a general term that refers to disorders of cognitive processing, and one of the manifestations of **schizophrenia** is impaired cognitive processing.

Drugs that affect cognitive processing include **antipsychotics, CNS stimulants, hallucinogens,** and **sedative-hypnotics.**

Memory

Memory is the ability to recall events and integrate them into cognitive processing, emotional processing, and ongoing motor activities. One form of memory, called **procedural memory**, is used to recall a set of practiced motor actions (e.g., riding a bicycle or typing on a keyboard) and it involves the interaction of **limbic structures**, the **cerebellum**, and the **basal ganglia**. Another form of memory, called **declarative memory**, involves thoughts and associations that may be used to determine future actions. For example, remembering that touching a hot stove is painful may keep a child from playing near the stove in the future, and remembering that a family member's birthday is approaching may trigger activities such as planning a dinner party. Declarative memory involves neuronal tracts in the **hippocampus, amygdala, thalamus,** and **neocortex**.

Dementia is a term used to describe a number of memory disorders, including **Alzheimer's disease**. The involvement of the basal ganglia in procedural memory may explain why some patients with **Parkinson's disease** have difficulties with practiced motor actions.

Drugs that affect memory include the **cholinesterase inhibitors** and CNS depressants such as the **benzodiazepines**.

Emotional Processing

Emotional processing is responsible for the generation of emotions such as anger, anxiety, fear, happiness, love, and sadness. These emotions represent the conscious perception of neuronal activity originating in the **limbic system**, including the hypothalamus, amygdala, septum, hippocampus, and mammillary bodies, as well as the cingulate and entorhinal portions of the frontal lobe cortex. Emotions contribute to a state of mental preparedness for anticipated future activities. For example, anxiety contributes to a state of heightened vigilance, which may amplify the response to a future stimulus or event.

Disorders in which emotional processing is defective include **anxiety states, mood disorders,** and **schizophrenia**.

Drugs that affect emotional processing in the limbic system include **anxiolytic (antianxiety) drugs, antidepressants, antipsychotics, CNS stimulants, opioids,** and **all drugs that produce drug dependence**. Hence, most CNS drugs have some effect on emotional processing.

Sensory Processing

Sensory processing involves neuronal tracts that perceive external stimuli and transmit that information to the brain. These include the sensory systems responsible for vision, hearing, olfaction, touch, and pain.

The spinothalamic tracts relay touch and pain sensations to the **thalamus**, which projects this information to the **cortex**. The brainstem region known as the **reticular formation** plays a significant role in filtering sensory information before it is relayed to the thalamus and hypothalamus and eventually to the cortex. The reticular formation includes the **locus ceruleus** and **raphe nuclei**, whose neurons release norepinephrine and serotonin, respectively, and play an important role in determining the level of consciousness, sleep, and wakefulness. The cortex of the parietal and occipital lobes and part of the temporal lobe is involved in the recognition and integration of sensory perceptions.

Disorders in which sensory processing is defective include **sleep disorders, chronic pain syndromes,** and **disorders of the special senses** such as blindness, deafness, and taste and olfactory dysfunction.

Among the drugs that affect sensory processing are **antidepressants, hallucinogens, local and general anesthetics, opioid analgesics,** and **sedative-hypnotics**.

Motor Processing

Motor processing refers to the neuronal activity that enables body movement. The structures involved in motor processing include the **cerebellum**, the motor strip of the **frontal lobe cortex**, the **basal ganglia**, and the suprasegmental nuclei that are found in the **brainstem** and are involved in the control of posture (e.g., the vestibular nuclei).

Disturbances in motor processing occur in **Parkinson's disease, Huntington's disease,** and a variety of degenerative and demyelinating neuron disorders.

Drugs that affect motor processing include **antiparkinsonian drugs, antispasmodics, CNS stimulants, muscle relaxants,** and **sedative-hypnotics**.

Autonomic Processing

Autonomic processing involves areas of the brain that integrate the activities of the **peripheral autonomic nervous system** (see Chapter 5). These areas include the **hypothalamus** and portions of the **brainstem**, such as the vasomotor center and the cranial nuclei of parasympathetic nerves.

Disorders of autonomic processing include **orthostatic hypotension** and **postural tachycardia syndrome**.

Some CNS drugs alter autonomic processing by affecting the actions of hypothalamic and brain stem nuclei, and others have a direct effect on peripheral autonomic neurotransmission. The drugs that affect autonomic processing include **antidepressants**, **antiparkinsonian drugs**, **antipsychotics**, and **drugs used to treat Alzheimer's disease**.

SUMMARY OF IMPORTANT POINTS

■ CNS drugs act primarily by affecting the synthesis, storage, release, reuptake, or degradation of neurotransmitters or by activating or blocking receptors.

■ Long-term administration of drugs sometimes causes up-regulation or down-regulation of receptors. Up-regulation is evoked by receptor antagonists, whereas down-regulation is evoked by receptor agonists or reuptake inhibitors.

■ Major CNS neurotransmitters include acetylcholine; amino acids (aspartate, GABA, glutamate, and glycine); biogenic amines (dopamine, histamine, norepinephrine, and serotonin); and neuropeptides such as the endogenous opioid peptides and the tachykinins.

■ Some CNS neurotransmitters (e.g., aspartate, glutamate, histamine, and tachykinins) are excitatory; others (e.g., dopamine, GABA, glycine, and opioid peptides) are inhibitory; and still others (e.g., acetylcholine, norepinephrine, and serotonin) are both excitatory and inhibitory, with these actions exerted via different receptors.

■ Neurotransmitters can be classified as fast or slow, depending on the type of receptor they activate and on the duration of the neuronal signal that they evoke. GABA and glutamate are fast, whereas norepinephrine, neuropeptides, and serotonin are slow.

■ Receptors for CNS neurotransmitters can be classified as ionotropic (directly coupled with ion channels) or metabotropic (coupled with G proteins and second messengers).

■ Many diseases of the CNS and the corresponding drugs used to treat these diseases have an effect on one or more of the following complex brain functions: cognitive processing, emotional processing, memory, motor processing, sensory processing, and autonomic processing.

Review Questions

1. Which of the following terms best describes a receptor located on a neuronal terminal that binds a neurotransmitter released from another neuron and decreases release of neurotransmitter from the neuronal terminal?
   (A) presynaptic receptor
   (B) heteroreceptor
   (C) postsynaptic receptor
   (D) autoreceptor
   (E) ionotropic receptor

2. Neurotransmitters are made in neurons and released when vesicles fuse with the neuronal membrane. What name is given to this process?
   (A) apoptosis
   (B) phagocytosis
   (C) endocytosis
   (D) pinocytosis
   (E) exocytosis

3. Which one of the following statements best describes the differences between classical neurotransmitters and neuropeptides?
   (A) neuropeptides are synthesized in the cell body
   (B) classical neurotransmitters have a longer duration of action
   (C) neuropeptides undergo rapid reuptake into the presynaptic terminal
   (D) classical neurotransmitters are packaged into vesicles
   (E) neuropeptides are degraded by acetylcholinesterase in the synapse

4. A patient with metastatic lung cancer is treated for chronic pain with daily doses of a long-acting morphine formulation and oxycodone for breakthrough pain. He complains that the medicines are no longer working. Which one of the following mechanisms may explain the lack of effect of his medicines?
   (A) the metabolism of morphine is up-regulated
   (B) pain intensity has greatly increased
   (C) the efficiency of G protein coupling is decreased
   (D) opioid receptors are down-regulated
   (E) the patient is a "drug seeker" and addicted to opioid medications

5. Which one of the following drugs acts by inhibiting neurotransmitter re-uptake?
   (A) lithium
   (B) morphine
   (C) fluoxetine
   (D) levodopa
   (E) donepezil

Answers and Explanations

1. **The correct answer is B: heteroreceptor.** A heteroreceptor is a type of presynaptic receptor that is also located on the neuronal terminal but binds a different neurotransmitter than the one being released from the terminal.

The signaling through this type of receptor usually causes decreased release of the neurotransmitter. Answer (A), presynaptic receptor, is a general term for any type of receptor located on the neuronal terminal. Answer (C), postsynaptic receptor, is incorrect because this receptor is located on the postsynaptic membrane. Answer (D), autoreceptor, is a type of presynaptic receptor in which the binding of the same neurotransmitter released from the neuronal terminal decreases further release of that neurotransmitter. Answer (E), ionotropic receptor, is the term for a receptor associated with an ion channel and could be located on either the presynaptic or postsynaptic membrane.

2. **The correct answer is E: exocytosis.** Fusion of the neurotransmitter vesicle is triggered with an influx of Ca^{+2} into the presynaptic terminal. This process is called exocytosis. Answer (A), apoptosis, is incorrect as this means programmed cell death. Answer (B), phagocytosis, means the engulfing of cellular debris or bacteria by another cell, usually a macrophage. Answer (C), endocytosis, is the process whereby receptors and other membrane proteins are recycled back into the neuron. Answer (D), pinocytosis, refers to is a form of endocytosis in which small particles of liquids are brought into the cell within small vesicles formed from the membrane.

3. **The best answer is A: neuropeptides are synthesized in the cell body.** Unlike classical neurotransmitters that are synthesized in vesicles en route or at the neuronal terminal from precursor substances, neuropeptides arise from the transcription of a neuropeptide gene, processing of the neuropeptide messenger RNA (mRNA), and translation of the mRNA into a neuropeptide product in the endoplasmic reticulum in the cell body of a neuron. Answer (B), classical neurotransmitters have a longer duration of action, is not true in general, and many studies show that neuropeptides act more as neuromodulators with longer duration of action than classical neurotransmitters. Answer (C), neuropeptides undergo rapid reuptake into the presynaptic terminal, is incorrect as there are no known transport proteins in presynaptic membranes to facilitate the reuptake of neuropeptides back into the terminal. Answer (D), classical neurotransmitters are packaged into vesicles, is true but does not differentiate between the two types of substances because neuropeptides are also packaged into vesicles for release, albeit into different types called dense-core vesicles. Answer (E), neuropeptides are degraded by acetylcholinesterase in the synapse, is incorrect because other enzymes called peptidases are responsible for the degradation of neuropeptides after release into the synapse.

4. **The best answer is D: opioid receptors are downregulated.** Chronic administration of an agonist, such as the opioid agonists morphine and oxycodone, will cause a decrease in the number of receptor proteins expressed by the neuron in an attempt to decrease the signaling through that pathway and establish homeostasis. Answer (A), the metabolism of morphine is up-regulated, could be true because the metabolism of some CNS agents, most notably the barbiturates, self-induce metabolic enzymes, but this mechanism is not known to occur with opioid analgesics. Answer (B), pain intensity has greatly increased, could also be true but there is no information given in the question to assume that this might be the case. Answer (C), the efficiency of G protein coupling is decreased, is a mechanism more noted for acute changes after agonist administration, whereas down-regulation is more likely with long-term or chronic administration of an agonist. Answer (E), the patient is a "drug seeker" and addicted to opioid medications, is very unlikely because metastatic lung cancer can be a very painful condition and less than 4% of patients treated with opioid analgesics develop substance abuse disorders.

5. **The best answer is C: fluoxetine.** Fluoxetine, with the trade name of Prozac, is one of the classes of antidepressants called selective serotonin reuptake inhibitors, or SSRIs. Answer (A), lithium, is incorrect as this agent to treat bipolar disorder acts at the level of signal transduction. Answer (B), morphine, is incorrect as this opioid agonist acts by receptor activation. Answer (D), levodopa, is an antiparkinsonian agent that acts by a strategy known as "precursor loading," which feeds the biosynthetic pathway for the synthesis of dopamine. Answer (E), donepezil, is incorrect as this drug to treat Alzheimer's disease acts by inhibiting the breakdown of acetylcholine, the neurotransmitter that is reduced in Alzheimer's disease.

SELECTED READINGS

Dorostkar, M.M., and S. Boehm. Presynaptic ionotropic receptors. Handb Exp Pharmacol 184:479–527, 2008.

Harvey, J. Leptin regulation of neuronal excitability and cognitive function. Curr Opin Pharmacol 7:643–647, 2007.

McKay, B.E., A.N. Placzek, and J.A. Dani. Regulation of synaptic transmission and plasticity by neuronal nicotinic acetylcholine receptors. Biochem Pharmacol 74:1120–1133, 2007.

Rostène, W., P. Kitabgi, and S.M. Parsadaniantz. Chemokines: a new class of neuromodulator? Nat Rev Neurosci 8:895–903, 2007.

Upton, R.N. Cerebral uptake of drugs in humans. Clin Exp Pharmacol Physiol 34:695–701, 2007.

CHAPTER 19

Sedative-Hypnotic and Anxiolytic Drugs

CLASSIFICATION OF SEDATIVE-HYPNOTIC AND ANXIOLYTIC DRUGS

Benzodiazepines
- Alprazolam (XANAX)
- Chlordiazepoxide (LIBRIUM)
- Clonazepam (KLONOPIN)
- Diazepam (VALIUM)
- Lorazepam (ATIVAN)
- Midazolam (VERSED)
- Triazolam (HALCION)[a]
- Flumazenil (ROMAZICON)[b]

Barbiturates
- Amobarbital (AMYTAL)
- Pentobarbital (NEMBUTAL)
- Phenobarbital (LUMINAL)
- Thiopental (PENTOTHAL)

Antihistamines
- Diphenhydramine (BENADRYL)
- Hydroxyzine (ATARAX)

Other Sedative-Hypnotic Drugs
- Zolpidem (AMBIEN)
- Zaleplon (SONATA)
- Eszopiclone (LUNESTA)
- Ramelteon (ROZEREM)

Nonsedating Anxiolytic Drugs
- Buspirone (BUSPAR)
- Propranolol (INDERAL)

[a]Also estazolam (PROSOM), flurazepam (DALMANE), oxazepam (SERAX), temazepam (RESTORIL), and others.
[b]Benzodiazepine antagonist.

OVERVIEW

Sedative-hypnotic drugs are among the most widely used pharmaceutical agents in the world. The **sedative** part of their name refers to the ability of these agents to calm or reduce anxiety, known as an **anxiolytic** effect. The **hypnotic** part of their name describes the ability of these agents to induce drowsiness and promote sleep. This latter action is caused by a greater depression of central nervous system (CNS) activity and most sedative-hypnotic drugs will first cause sedation, then at higher doses, produce hypnosis, the medical term for sleep. A few agents, however, exert anxiolytic effects without causing sedation or hypnosis.

This chapter describes the pharmacologic properties of benzodiazepines, barbiturates, and other sedative-hypnotic and anxiolytic drugs that are used in the treatment of anxiety and sleep disorders. Because of their greater safety, less adverse effects, and the availability of an antagonist, the benzodiazepines have largely replaced the older barbiturates for these indications. Although ethanol (alcohol) has sedative-hypnotic effects, it is not used therapeutically for these purposes; its pharmacologic effects are described in Chapter 25.

ANXIETY DISORDERS

Anxiety is normally an **adaptive response** that prepares a person to react to the challenges of life. Anxiety is characterized by changes in mood (apprehension and fear), sympathetic nervous system arousal, and hypervigilance. When anxiety becomes chronic, it can impair a person's ability to perform the activities of daily living. Moreover, chronic anxiety often leads to visceral organ dysfunction and unpleasant symptoms. For example, patients with chronic anxiety may develop gastrointestinal, cardiovascular, and neurologic problems, including diarrhea, tachycardia, sweating, tremors, and dizziness. Ultimately, anxiety can contribute to heart disease and other disorders, including self-medication which may lead to substance abuse.

Neurologic Basis of Anxiety

The neuronal pathways involved in anxiety disorders include the **sensory, cognitive, behavioral, motor,** and **autonomic pathways.** Sensory systems, cortical processing, and memory are involved in interpreting a stimulus to be dangerous and creating a state of heightened arousal. Motor systems and autonomic processing participate in the exaggerated responses to an anxiety state.

Growing evidence indicates that the **amygdala,** an almond-shaped structure in the temporal lobe, plays a central role in mediating most of the manifestations of anxiety, including the **conditioned avoidance reaction** (conditioned fear reaction) that underlies anxiety states. In experimental protocols, this reaction can be induced in animals by teaching them that a cue (e.g., a flashing light) will be followed by a noxious stimulus (e.g., a shock to the foot). During the anticipatory period, the animals conditioned in this manner will exhibit signs of anxiety, such as autonomic and behavioral arousal. Electrical stimulation of the amygdala induces signs of anxiety, whereas lesioning the amygdala or the administration of anxiolytic drugs prevents the behavioral and physiologic manifestations of anxiety during the anticipatory period. It is believed that **long-term potentiation** in amygdala neurons establishes the memory of adverse events underlying anticipatory anxiety.

Classification and Treatment of Anxiety Disorders

The appropriate management of anxiety disorders requires an accurate diagnosis, and treatment may involve the use of pharmacologic agents, psychotherapy, or both.

Acute Anxiety

Acute anxiety may develop in response to various factors, such as illness, separation from loved ones, or the anticipation of stressful events. Acute anxiety is often self-limiting and may resolve in a few weeks to a few months without drug treatment. A **benzodiazepine** might provide short-term relief from more severe acute anxiety conditions.

Panic Disorder

Panic disorder is characterized by acute episodes of severe anxiety with marked psychologic and physiologic symptoms. During a panic attack, an individual may feel an impending sense of doom that is often accompanied by sweating, tachycardia, tremor, and other visceral symptoms. Patients with panic disorder often respond to drug therapy with a **benzodiazepine** or an **antidepressant drug,** such as a **selective serotonin reuptake inhibitor** (**SSRI;** see Chapter 22). Benzodiazepines may provide immediate relief from panic attacks during the early phase of therapy, and **alprazolam** and **clonazepam** are benzodiazepines that have been particularly useful in this regard. For long-term treatment, an SSRI antidepressant, such as **sertraline,** is often prescribed.

Phobic Disorders

Phobic disorders can be grouped into specific phobia, social anxiety disorder (social phobia), or agoraphobia. Phobias are conditions in which an individual is overly fearful about a particular situation or condition, such as a fear of spiders or traveling in an airplane. Panic disorder can coexist with **agoraphobia,** an intense fear of being in a public place from which it might be difficult or embarrassing to cope with a panic attack. Patients with panic disorder and agoraphobia often show the best outcomes when treated with a combination of psychotherapy and drug therapy. As with panic disorder, phobic disorders are treated with a **benzodiazepine** or an **antidepressant drug.** Benzodiazepines provide acute relief of symptoms and enable patients to more easily benefit from psychotherapy, whereas antidepressants are usually the most effective long-term drug therapy for agoraphobia and social phobia. **Propranolol** is useful in the prevention of **stage fright,** or **acute situational** or **performance anxiety.**

Obsessive-Compulsive Disorder

Obsessive-compulsive disorder is characterized by **obsessions,** which are recurring or persistent thoughts and impulses, and **compulsions,** defined as repetitive behaviors in response to obsessions. Obsessive-compulsive disorder can be treated effectively with an **antidepressant drug** (see Chapter 22) and psychotherapy.

Generalized Anxiety Disorder

Generalized anxiety disorder is characterized by chronic worry and apprehension concerning future events. Short-term therapy with a **benzodiazepine** may relieve acute symptoms and provide a useful bridge to psychotherapy. The severity of the disorder often fluctuates over time, and benzodiazepines may be effectively used on an intermittent basis to help patients deal with exacerbations of the disorder. **Buspirone,** a **nonsedating anxiolytic,** provides a useful alternative to benzodiazepines for the treatment of chronic anxiety states, because it produces little sedation and is not associated with tolerance or dependence. It must be taken for 3 or 4 weeks, however, before its anxiolytic effects are felt. SSRIs, such as **paroxetine,** and the norepinephrine and serotonin reuptake inhibitors, **venlafaxine** and **duloxetine,** are also used in the treatment of this condition.

Posttraumatic Stress Disorder

Posttraumatic stress disorder may develop after exposure to a traumatic event, such as sexual assault or military combat. SSRIs are used in the treatment of posttraumatic stress disorder. Other medications, such as benzodiazepines, may also be used to treat associated symptoms, such as an exaggerated **startle response** and **flashbacks.**

SLEEP DISORDERS

Sleep is a reversible state of reduced consciousness that is accompanied by characteristic changes in the EEG. Five distinct patterns of brainwave activity occur during sleep, grouped into the four stages of **non–rapid eye movement sleep (NREM),** and a pattern characterized by paralysis of voluntary muscles and quick, saccadic movement of the eye called **rapid eye movement sleep (REM).**

As an individual falls asleep, the high-frequency and low-amplitude activity of the alert state gradually diminishes during stages 1 and 2 and is replaced by the low-frequency and high-amplitude activity of **slow-wave sleep** (stages 3 and 4). Over time, the individual returns to stage 1 and eventually to the REM stage. REM sleep is also known as **paradoxical sleep** because the EEG pattern is similar to the awake state. A normal adult cycles through the sleep stages about every 90 minutes (Box 19–1).

BOX 19-1. EFFECT OF SEDATIVE-HYPNOTIC DRUGS ON SLEEP ARCHITECTURE TERMINOLOGY

Patterns on the EEG vary with the stage of sleep. When a person falls asleep, the high-frequency and low-amplitude pattern of the **awake state** is gradually replaced by the progressively lower-frequency and higher-amplitude patterns of stages 1 through 4, which collectively are called **non–rapid eye movement sleep (NREM sleep)**. Stages 3 and 4 are called **slow-wave sleep**. Another stage, called **rapid eye movement sleep (REM sleep)**, is characterized by rapid, jerky eye movements. REM sleep is also called **paradoxical sleep** because it is during this stage that the pattern on EEG returns to the pattern seen during the awake state.

Normal and Abnormal Sleep Patterns

The normal sleep pattern in adults consists of about five cycles, each of which lasts approximately 90 minutes. During each cycle, an individual progresses from stage 1 to stage 4 and then returns to stage 1, followed by a period of REM sleep. As the cycles progress through the night, they become shorter, and the amount of slow-wave sleep decreases.

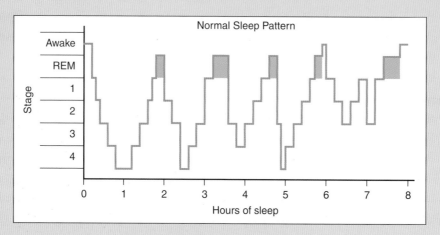

Effects of Drugs on Sleep Architecture

The sleep patterns of patients with insomnia vary widely but are often characterized by reduced amounts of slow-wave sleep and by one or more awakenings during the night. The time required to fall asleep (sleep latency) is usually prolonged, and the total sleep time is decreased in most patients with insomnia. Elderly adults often have a similar sleep pattern.

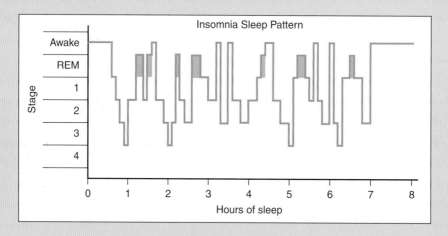

Benzodiazepines and most other hypnotics suppress the stages of 3, slow-wave sleep, and REM sleep. In contrast, zolpidem, zaleplon, eszopiclone, and ramelteon (new agents) have little effect on sleep architecture. Therefore, use of these new agents may better restore the sleep pattern to normal.

(Continued)

BOX 19–1. EFFECT OF SEDATIVE-HYPNOTIC DRUGS ON SLEEP ARCHITECTURE TERMINOLOG—cont'd

State	Rapid Eye Movements	Pattern on EEG	Effect of Benzodiazepines	Effect of New Agent
Awake	No	High-frequency, low-amplitude pattern	Induce sleep	Induces sleep
Stages 1 and 2 sleep	No	Lower-frequency, higher-amplitude pattern than awake state	Increase length of stages	Little change
Stages 3 and 4 sleep	No	Lower-frequency, higher-amplitude pattern than stages 1 and 2	Decrease length of stages	Little change
REM sleep	Yes	High-frequency, low-amplitude pattern	Decrease length of stage	Little change

Sleep patterns change with age and are altered by sedative-hypnotic and other CNS drugs.

Neurologic Basis of Sleep

The neuronal systems involved in sleep include the **basal forebrain nuclei** and the **reticular formation**. Projecting from the basal forebrain to the cortex are cholinergic fibers that are believed to be involved in the induction of sleep. The basal forebrain is the only region of the brain that is active during slow-wave sleep and quiescent at other stages. The reticular formation facilitates the flow of sensory information from the thalamus to the cortex. When reticular nuclei are quiescent, the thalamus does not transfer information to the cortex, and this facilitates the onset of sleep.

Classification and Treatment of Sleep Disorders

Insomnia

Some patients with insomnia find it difficult to go to sleep or to stay asleep during the night, whereas others awaken too early in the morning. In general, the management of insomnia depends on whether the sleep disorder is caused by physiologic, psychologic, or medical conditions. As shown in Box 19–1, the patterns of sleep stages in patients with insomnia are irregular and include longer latency to fall asleep and frequent awakenings.

Occasional sleeplessness caused by acute stress or a minor illness is usually self-limiting and may not require treatment. More severe insomnia caused by medical conditions whose symptoms interfere with sleep is effectively treated with **benzodiazepines** or other **sedative-hypnotic drugs**, such as **zolpidem** and **zaleplon**, whereas insomnia related to psychologic and psychiatric disturbances is best managed with a combination of psychotherapy and sedative-hypnotic drugs. Benzodiazepines and most other hypnotic drugs **decrease sleep latency** (the time required to go to sleep) and **increase sleep duration**. The newest agents, zolpidem, zaleplon, eszopiclone, and ramelteon, have the advantages of not significantly affecting sleep architecture and not causing as much tolerance and dependence as do the older drugs. For these reasons, **zolpidem, zaleplon, eszopiclone**, and

ramelteon have become the drugs of choice to treat most types of insomnia.

Other Sleep Disorders

Other sleep disorders include **hypersomnia** (difficulty in awakening), **narcolepsy** (sleep attacks), **enuresis** (bedwetting during sleep), **somnambulism** (sleepwalking), **sleep apnea** (episodes of hypoventilation during sleep), and **nightmares** and **night terrors**. Most of these disorders are managed with a combination of psychotherapy and **antidepressant drugs** or **CNS stimulants**. **Sodium oxybate** (XYREM), a form of the abused drug γ-hydroxybutyrate, was recently approved for the treatment of cataplexy associated with **narcoleptic attacks**. CNS stimulants used to treat narcolepsy and other sleep disorders are discussed in Chapter 22.

SEDATIVE-HYPNOTIC DRUGS

The sedative-hypnotic drugs include **benzodiazepines, barbiturates**, some **antihistamines**, and a few nonbenzodiazepine agents, such as **zolpidem, zaleplon, eszopiclone**, and **ramelteon**. The properties of these drugs are summarized in Table 19–1, and their adverse effects, and drug interactions are listed in Table 19–2.

Because the benzodiazepines have fewer adverse reactions and drug interactions and are safer in cases of overdose, they have largely replaced the barbiturates and other older drugs. Nevertheless, barbiturates are still used when benzodiazepines are ineffective or contraindicated. The sedating antihistamines are occasionally used to treat mild insomnia and anxiety and have less potential for abuse than do benzodiazepines and barbiturates. Many over-the-counter (nonprescription) sleep aids contain antihistamines as their effective ingredient.

Benzodiazepines

The benzodiazepines are a large group of drugs that have similar pharmacologic effects. They are so named because they share the common chemical structure of a benzene ring (*benzo*) joined to a seven-member ring containing two nitrogen molecules (*diazepine*). The particular use of specific drugs is largely determined by their pharmacokinetic properties and route of administration. Some benzodiazepines were developed and

TABLE 19–1. **Pharmacokinetic Properties and Clinical Uses of Sedative-Hypnotic and Anxiolytic Drugs**

Drug	Onset of Action*	Duration of Action*	Active Metabolites	Major Clinical Uses
Benzodiazepines				
Alprazolam	Fast	Medium	Yes	Anxiety, including panic disorder
Chlordiazepoxide	Fast; very fast (IV)	Long	Yes	Alcohol detoxification; anxiety
Clonazepam	Fast	Medium	No	Anxiety, including panic disorder; seizure disorders
Diazepam	Fast; very fast (IV)	Long	Yes	Alcohol detoxification; anxiety; muscle spasm; seizure disorders; spasticity
Estazolam	Fast	Medium	Yes	Insomnia
Flurazepam	Fast	Long	Yes	Insomnia
Lorazepam	Fast; very fast (IV)	Medium	No	Anxiety; seizure disorders
Midazolam	Very fast (IV)	Short (IV)	Yes	Anesthesia
Oxazepam	Fast	Short	No	Anxiety
Temazepam	Fast	Medium	No	Insomnia
Triazolam	Fast	Short	Yes	Insomnia
Barbiturates				
Amobarbital	Fast	Medium	No	Insomnia
Pentobarbital	Fast	Short	No	Insomnia
Phenobarbital	Slow	Long	No	Seizure disorders
Thiopental	Very fast (IV)	Short (IV)	No	Induction of anesthesia
Antihistamines				
Diphenhydramine	Fast	Medium	No	Insomnia
Hydroxyzine	Fast	Long	No	Anxiety; sedation
Other sedative-hypnotic drugs				
Zolpidem	Fast	Short	No	Insomnia
Zaleplon	Fast	Very short	No	Insomnia; mid-sleep awakenings
Eszopiclone	Fast	Short	No	Insomnia
Ramelteon	Slow	Short	Yes	Sleep-onset insomnia
Nonsedating Anxiolytic Drugs				
Buspirone	Very slow	Long	No	Chronic anxiety
Propranolol	Fast	Medium	Yes	Situational or performance anxiety

*Unless onset and duration of action are specifically indicated for intravenous (IV) administration, they are for oral administration. Very fast = <15 minutes; fast = 15–59 minutes; slow = 1–4 hours; very slow = 3–4 weeks; short = 1–6 hours; medium = 7–12 hours; and long = >12 hours.

approved to treat anxiety, whereas others are approved for the management of insomnia or for other purposes.

Drug Properties

PHARMACOKINETICS. The pharmacokinetic properties of various benzodiazepines are compared in Table 19–1. The benzodiazepines are absorbed from the gut and distributed to the brain at rates that are proportional to their **lipid solubility**, which varies 50-fold among individual drugs in the class. As the plasma concentration of a benzodiazepine declines, the drug is redistributed from the brain to the blood, and this mechanism contributes significantly to the termination of its effects on the CNS.

All benzodiazepines are **extensively metabolized** in the liver. Most benzodiazepines are converted to **active metabolites** in phase I oxidative reactions catalyzed by cytochrome

P450 enzymes. The active metabolites of chlordiazepoxide, diazepam, and flurazepam are long acting and contribute to the long duration of action of these agents. The active metabolites of alprazolam, estazolam, midazolam, and triazolam are shorter acting. Each of these active metabolites is eventually conjugated with glucuronate to form an inactive polar metabolite that is excreted in the urine. Other drugs, namely **oxazepam, temazepam,** and **lorazepam,** bypass phase I oxidation and are metabolized only by phase II conjugation (Fig. 19–1). These three drugs may be safer for use by elderly patients, because the capacity to conjugate drugs does not decline with age as much as the capacity for oxidative biotransformation does. Hence, these three drugs are less likely to accumulate to toxic levels in elderly patients.

Benzodiazepines also undergo some degree of **enterohepatic cycling** that prolongs their duration of action. In fact, some patients who are taking a drug such as diazepam may

TABLE 19-2. **Adverse Effects and Drug Interactions of Sedative-Hypnotic and Anxiolytic Drugs**

Drug	Common Adverse Effects	Common Drug Interactions
Benzodiazepines		
Alprazolam	Arrhythmia, CNS depression, drug dependence, hypotension, and mild respiratory depression	Alcohol and other CNS depressants potentiate effects. Fluoxetine and fluvoxamine increase serum levels and effects
Chlordiazepoxide	Same as alprazolam	Alcohol and other CNS depressants potentiate effects. Cimetidine increases and rifampin decreases serum levels
Clonazepam	Same as alprazolam	Same as chlordiazepoxide
Diazepam	Same as alprazolam	Same as chlordiazepoxide
Estazolam	Same as alprazolam	Same as chlordiazepoxide
Flurazepam	Same as alprazolam	Same as chlordiazepoxide
Lorazepam	Same as alprazolam	Alcohol and other CNS depressants potentiate effects. Rifampin decreases serum levels
Midazolam	Same as alprazolam	Alcohol and other CNS depressants potentiate effects. Calcium channel blockers, erythromycin, and ketoconazole increase serum levels
Oxazepam	Same as alprazolam	Same as lorazepam
Temazepam	Same as alprazolam	Same as chlordiazepoxide
Triazolam	Amnesia, confusion, and delirium. Other adverse effects same as alprazolam	Alcohol and other CNS depressants potentiate effects. Cimetidine, erythromycin, ketoconazole, and oral contraceptives increase serum levels
Barbiturates		
Amobarbital	CNS depression, drug dependence, and respiratory depression	Induces cytochrome P450 enzymes and increases metabolism of many drugs. Potentiates effects of other CNS depressants
Pentobarbital	Same as amobarbital	Same as amobarbital
Phenobarbital	Same as amobarbital	Same as amobarbital
Thiopental	Same as amobarbital	Same as amobarbital
Antihistamines		
Diphenhydramine	Anticholinergic effects, such as blurred vision, dry mouth, and urinary retention; dizziness; and drowsiness	Alcohol, barbiturates, and other CNS depressants potentiate CNS effects
Hydroxyzine	Same as diphenhydramine	Same as diphenhydramine
Other sedative-hypnotic drugs		
Zolpidem	Dizziness, drowsiness, and headache	Potentiation by alcohol and other CNS depressants
Zaleplon	Same as zolpidem	Same as zolpidem
Eszopiclone	Drowsiness, dizziness, difficulty with coordination	Potentiation by alcohol and other CNS depressants
Ramelteon	Dizziness; drowsiness; alteration of reproductive hormone levels	Potentiation by alcohol and other CNS depressants. Fluvoxamine increases plasma ramelteon levels
Nonsedating Anxiolytic Drugs		
Buspirone	Dizziness, headache, and nervousness	None
Propranolol	Bradycardia, bronchoconstriction, depression, fatigue, hypersensitivity, hypotension, impaired glycogenolysis, and vivid dreams	Cardiac depression increased by calcium channel blockers

CNS = central nervous system.

notice an increased sedative effect after eating a high-fat meal. The fatty meal causes the gallbladder to empty and thereby delivers bile containing diazepam to the intestines for reabsorption into the circulation.

MECHANISM OF ACTION. The **benzodiazepines** and **barbiturates** are believed to exert their effects on consciousness and sleep by facilitating the activity of **γ-aminobutyric acid (GABA)** at various sites in the neuraxis. GABA, the most ubiquitous

inhibitory neurotransmitter in the CNS, regulates the excitability of neurons in almost every neuronal tract. As shown in Figure 19–2, the **GABA$_A$ receptor–chloride ion channel** has binding sites for benzodiazepines and barbiturates, as well as alcohols, steroids, and inhalational anesthetics. This receptor–ion channel complex is made up of five subunits with the major form of the complex containing α, β, and γ subunits. However, there are at least 16 types of these protein subunits (e.g., α_1, α_2, β_1, β_2, etc.), and it is not entirely clear which types

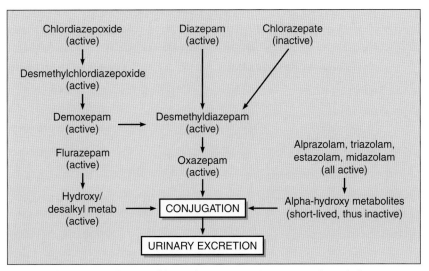

Figure 19–1. Major biotransformation pathways of benzodiazepines. Chlordiazepoxide and diazepam are converted to long-acting active metabolites. Alprazolam, midazolam, and triazolam are converted to a short-acting active metabolite. All benzodiazepines, including those with no active metabolites, are eventually converted to glucuronide compounds that are pharmacologically inactive and are excreted in the urine. The benzodiazepines that have no active metabolites include oxazepam, temazepam, and lorazepam ("out the liver"), and these may be the safest benzodiazepines to use in treating elderly patients.

BOX 19–2. THE CASE OF THE GROGGY GRANDMOTHER

CASE PRESENTATION: A 68-year-old female was prescribed 5 mg diazepam for anxiety by her primary care physician after her husband died. She was told to take one in the morning, along with her breakfast, and was advised to increase her activities to "take her mind off her worries." After following the prescribed regimen for a week, she finds that she has problems going to sleep and without consulting her physician, takes another diazepam pill at night. She continues taking one diazepam pill in the morning and one pill at night for the next few days. Her friends note that she is not coming out of her room at the assisted living center as much as she used to, and they knock on her door to check up on her. They find her still in her nightgown and disorientated. They convince her to call her doctor who tells her to stop taking the second pill of diazepam at night; the doctor prescribes zolpidem, at a dose of 5 mg, to be taken at night to help her sleep. Over the next few days, the patient is more alert during the day and resumes her activities.

CASE DISCUSSION: The use of benzodiazepines for anxiety disorders has largely replaced any other type of sedative-hypnotic agent, such as barbiturates, for this indication because of their increased safety and effectiveness. However, benzodiazepines are metabolized into many active metabolites, some that have longer durations of actions than their parent drug. Phase 1 or oxidative drug biotransformation (metabolism) in the elderly is reduced and this patient population is especially sensitive to the buildup of active metabolites of many benzodiazepines, including diazepam. Three agents are better suited in elderly patients; oxazepam, temazepam, and lorazepam do not undergo Phase 1 metabolism but are directly conjugated to inactive metabolites. Phase 2 metabolic reactions, such as conjugation, are less affected with aging. The use of zolpidem, a nonbenzodiazepine drug used for insomnia, has a short elimination half-life and leads to little hangover effect the next day, allowing for resumption of normal daytime activities for the elderly patient.

---

of subunits make up the $GABA_A$ receptors that mediate the clinical and adverse effects of drugs that bind to them.

The **benzodiazepine binding site** is located at the interface between α and γ subunits at a site different than the binding site of GABA. Benzodiazepines bind to this site and increase the affinity of GABA for its binding site on the $GABA_A$ receptor–chloride ion channel complex. This is an example of an **allosteric binding site**. Benzodiazepines bind

to receptors made up of both α_1 and α_2 subunits, whereas the newer nonbenzodiazepine agents (see below) are selective for receptors containing α_1 subunits.

Benzodiazepines increase the **frequency** with which the channel opens, whereas barbiturates increase the **length of time** that the channel remains open. By increasing chloride conductance, these drugs cause neuronal membrane **hyperpolarization** and this, in turn, counteracts the depolarizing

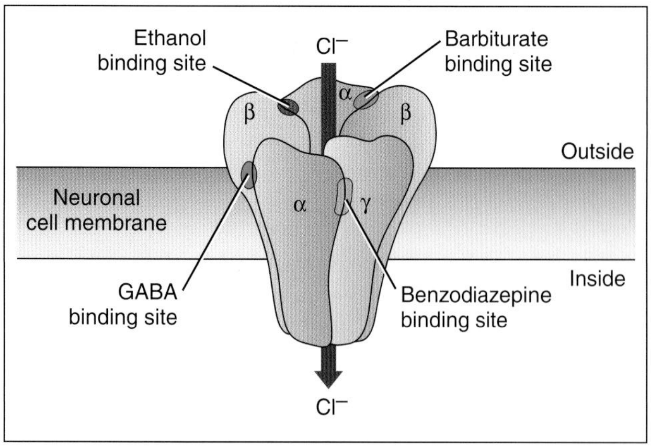

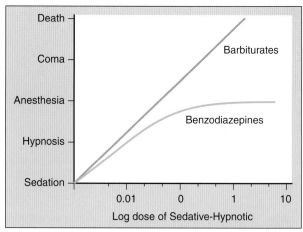

Figure 19-2. Receptor sites for GABA, benzodiazepines, barbiturates, and ethanol on the GABA$_A$ chloride ion channel. The GABA$_A$ chloride ion channel is a protein complex pentameric form that has varying combinations of α, β, and γ subunits. GABA binds to a site near the junction of α and β subunits, and this causes conformational changes that open the chloride ion channel and lead to neuronal membrane hyperpolarization. Benzodiazepines bind to an allosteric site formed by the cleft between α and γ subunits, and this facilitates GABA binding and increases the frequency of chloride channel opening. Barbiturates bind adjacent to α and β subunits and increase the duration of chloride channel opening, both in the presence and in the absence of GABA. Ethanol (ethyl alcohol) binds to a distinct site on the ionophore and enhances chloride influx. The ionophore also contains binding sites for steroids and inhalational anesthetics.

Figure 19-3. Dose-response curves of barbiturates and benzodiazepines. The barbiturates exhibit a linear dose-response effect, which progresses from sedation to respiratory depression, coma, and death. Benzodiazepines exhibit a ceiling effect, which precludes severe CNS depression following oral administration of these drugs. Intravenous administration of benzodiazepines can produce anesthesia and mild respiratory depression.

effect of excitatory neurotransmitters. Barbiturates increase chloride conductance **independent** of the presence of GABA, which is why they are capable of causing greater CNS depression and toxicity than the benzodiazepines.

In addition to their effects on GABA, benzodiazepines also inhibit the neuronal reuptake of **adenosine**. This action increases the inhibitory effect of adenosine on neurons that release acetylcholine from the pedunculopontine nucleus of the reticular formation, which is a brain structure mediating arousal. The effect of benzodiazepines on adenosine may also explain why these drugs dilate coronary arteries and decrease total peripheral resistance.

PHARMACOLOGIC EFFECTS. The benzodiazepines produce a dose-dependent but limited depression of the CNS. Lower doses have a sedative and anxiolytic effect, whereas higher doses produce hypnosis (sleep) and anesthesia (Fig. 19–3). Benzodiazepines can relieve anxiety at doses that produce relatively little sedation. In contrast to the barbiturates, the orally administered benzodiazepines do not produce significant respiratory depression, coma, or death unless they are administered with another CNS depressant (e.g., alcohol). Because benzodiazepines only work in the presence of GABA released by neurons, the depth of CNS depression is limited. Barbiturates do not exhibit this **ceiling effect** and can produce severe respiratory depression and death after administration of an excessive amount.

In addition to producing sedative-hypnotic and anxiolytic effects, benzodiazepines can produce **anterograde amnesia**, which means that an individual will not remember what happens from the time that the drug is administered to the time that the drug effects dissipate. This is in contrast to

retrograde amnesia, in which a person cannot remember what happened before a certain point in time. The benzodiazepines produce anterograde amnesia because they interfere with the formation of new memory; they do not affect the ability to recall past events. The amnesic property of benzodiazepines is often useful when patients are undergoing stressful procedures, such as endoscopy or outpatient surgery. When these drugs are used on a long-term basis, such as in treating anxiety, the amnesic properties can have an adverse effect on the patient's ability to function. **Triazolam**, a widely used hypnotic, has been associated with problems caused by its amnesic effect.

The benzodiazepines have anticonvulsant effects and are used in the treatment of seizure disorders (see Chapter 20). Although benzodiazepines cause muscle relaxation only at doses that produce considerable sedation, they are occasionally used to treat muscle spasm and spasticity. The muscle-relaxing effects of benzodiazepines are probably caused by the fact that these drugs potentiate the effects of GABA on interneurons in the spinal cord.

ADVERSE EFFECTS. The adverse effects of benzodiazepines are largely caused by CNS depression. The drugs frequently cause motor incoordination, dizziness, and excessive drowsiness. They impair cognitive processing and can affect concentration, judgment, and planning. They can also interfere with **driving** and other **psychomotor skills**. When longer-acting benzodiazepines (e.g., flurazepam) are used to treat insomnia, they can cause drowsiness and a drug hangover the next day. If this occurs, a shorter-acting drug (e.g., estazolam or zolpidem) should be substituted for the longer-acting drug.

Intravenous administration of benzodiazepines produces greater CNS depression than does oral administration, and intravenous administration can cause respiratory depression. Specific warnings of respiratory depression were issued by the U.S. Food and Drug Administration (FDA) for

midazolam, an agent indicated solely for intravenous administration. The greater effect produced by intravenous administration probably results from the more rapid uptake of the drug by brain tissue, which results in a greater potentiation of GABA before the self-limiting effect on GABA release has had time to develop.

The benzodiazepines have a mild euphoric effect and can reduce behavioral inhibitions in a manner similar to the **disinhibitory** effect of alcohol. The behavioral reinforcement produced by these drugs may contribute to their recreational abuse by polydrug abusers and to their inappropriate long-term use by patients. It appears that the reinforcing effects of benzodiazepines are less than the reinforcing effects of barbiturates but greater than the reinforcing effects of sedating antihistamines and possibly **zolpidem, zaleplon,** and **eszopiclone**. The newest agent, **ramelteon** is the only unscheduled, prescription sedative-hypnotic agent, which is thought to have fewer reinforcing effects as it is an agonist at **melatonin receptors**.

Long-term use of the benzodiazepines can produce **physical dependence**, the severity of which is proportional to the dosage and duration of administration. After several months of continued use, most patients develop some degree of physical dependence. If their medication is abruptly discontinued, they will experience a withdrawal syndrome, characterized by rebound anxiety, insomnia, headache, irritability, and muscle twitches. The withdrawal syndrome is usually mild and not life-threatening. Abrupt withdrawal from **alprazolam** has been associated with seizures. Therefore, to prevent its occurrence, the dosage of benzodiazepines should be gradually tapered over a period of several weeks. Because the various drugs in the benzodiazepine class exhibit cross-tolerance, any of them can be substituted for another one to prevent or counteract the withdrawal reaction.

Pharmacodynamic tolerance also occurs during long-term use of benzodiazepines. Unlike barbiturates, however, the benzodiazepines do not induce their own metabolism or cause pharmacokinetic tolerance.

Although the overall safety of the benzodiazepines is high, their use has been associated with hypotension, arrhythmia (tachycardia or bradycardia), and a number of other, less common effects. Rarely, a massive overdose of a benzodiazepine has been fatal, but it is less likely than in the case of barbiturates because of the availability of the selective benzodiazepine antagonist, **flumazenil**.

The incidence of fetal malformations in the offspring of women who take benzodiazepines during pregnancy is very low. Nevertheless, chronic use of benzodiazepines during pregnancy is not recommended, and benzodiazepines are included in pregnancy category D by the FDA. **Zolpidem** and **zaleplon** appear to be safer in pregnancy and are listed as pregnancy category B.

INTERACTIONS AND TREATMENT OF ADVERSE EFFECTS. Several drugs, including flumazenil and β-carboline derivatives, interact with benzodiazepine receptors.

Flumazenil is a competitive **benzodiazepine receptor antagonist**. In addition to blocking the effects of agonists, such as diazepam, it also blocks the effects of inverse agonists (see later text) at the benzodiazepine receptor.

Flumazenil can be used to counteract the adverse effects of benzodiazepines, such as respiratory depression resulting from intravenous administration of these drugs or in the case of accidental or intentional overdose. Flumazenil is given intravenously and has a rapid onset and a short duration of action. Its potential adverse effects include seizures, arrhythmias, blurred vision, emotional lability, and dizziness.

The **β-carboline derivatives** act as **inverse agonists**. An inverse agonist is a drug that decreases the response of an effector system below the basal level (see Chapter 3). The β-carboline drugs act to decrease chloride conductance by the $GABA_A$ receptor–chloride ion channel, and this can cause anxiety and seizures. Some experimental inverse agonists enhance cognitive function and are being studied for the treatment of Alzheimer's disease.

Table 19–2 lists the individual benzodiazepines and outlines their interactions with various other drugs.

INDICATIONS. The benzodiazepines are effective in the treatment of anxiety disorders, insomnia, muscle spasm, seizure disorders, and spasticity. They are also used for the treatment of alcohol withdrawal. When possible, the use of benzodiazepines should be limited to the short-term treatment of these conditions. If long-term use is medically justified, the physician should carefully monitor drug usage to prevent dosage escalation.

Specific Agents

Alprazolam is converted to a short-acting α-hydroxyl metabolite before undergoing glucuronide formation. Alprazolam has a medium duration of action and is used primarily in the management of **anxiety**. Although it has special utility in the treatment of **panic disorder**, the larger doses usually required for controlling panic attacks can cause considerable sedation and contribute to drug dependence. Therefore, for many patients, the panic disorder can be treated instead with antidepressants and behavioral therapy. Alprazolam is useful as a short-term measure to relieve acute symptoms while other therapies are instituted.

Chlordiazepoxide and **diazepam** are converted to long-acting metabolites, including desmethyldiazepam (also called nordiazepam). Desmethyldiazepam is converted to **oxazepam**, which is excreted as a polar glucuronate conjugate (see Fig. 19–1). Chlordiazepoxide and diazepam are effective in the treatment of **anxiety**. In patients undergoing **alcohol detoxification**, these drugs can be used to prevent seizures and other acute withdrawal reactions. The drug dosage is gradually tapered over several weeks.

Diazepam is also used to terminate **acute recurrent seizures** (see Chapter 20), to treat **severe muscle spasm** and to treat **spasticity** associated with degenerative and demyelinating neurologic disorders.

Lorazepam, oxazepam, and temazepam do not form long-acting metabolites, so they have a short or medium duration of action. They are biotransformed to inactive glucuronide compounds. As mentioned, they may be preferable in the treatment of elderly patients because glucuronide conjugation does not decline significantly with aging. Lorazepam can be administered orally or intravenously and is used to treat **anxiety** and to control **seizures**. Oxazepam is a

short-acting drug that is administered to patients with **anxiety**. Temazepam is used primarily to treat **insomnia**.

Estazolam, flurazepam, and triazolam have active metabolites with varying durations of action. Estazolam has a medium duration of action, whereas flurazepam has a longer one and triazolam has a shorter one. All three drugs are used to treat **insomnia**. A short- or medium-acting drug may be preferred for patients whose primary problem is getting to sleep, whereas a medium- or long-acting drug may be preferred for patients who complain of waking up too early. The short-acting triazolam is more likely to cause rebound insomnia when it is discontinued. The long-acting flurazepam is less likely to cause rebound insomnia but is more likely to cause daytime drowsiness. Triazolam has been associated with a higher incidence of amnesia, confusion, and delirium, especially in elderly patients. The dosage of triazolam in formulations marketed in the United States has been reduced by the FDA, and triazolam was banned in the United Kingdom.

Recently, label revisions for all of the previously mentioned sedative-hypnotic agents indicated for sleep disorders were made to include warnings for the risk of **hypersensitivity reactions,** including anaphylaxis (severe allergic reaction) and angioedema (severe facial swelling), which can occur as early as the first time the sedative-hypnotic agents is taken. Additionally, warnings were included for the risk of **complex sleep-related behaviors,** which may include driving, making phone calls, having sex, and preparing and eating food, all while still asleep and with no memory of the behaviors occurring.

Other Benzodiazepines

Clonazepam is used for the treatment of **panic disorder** and **other anxiety disorders**, as well as for the treatment of **seizure disorders** (see Chapter 20).

Midazolam is used intravenously as an **anesthetic** for patients undergoing endoscopy, other diagnostic procedures, or minor surgery.

Barbiturates

The barbiturates include **amobarbital, pentobarbital, phenobarbital,** and **thiopental**. The properties, adverse effects, and interactions of these drugs are outlined in Tables 19–1 and 19–2.

Drug Properties

PHARMACOKINETICS. The onset and duration of action of barbiturates are determined by their lipid solubility and rate of metabolic inactivation. Highly lipid-soluble drugs (e.g., **amobarbital, pentobarbital,** and **thiopental**) are well absorbed from the gut, rapidly redistributed from the brain to peripheral tissues as plasma concentrations fall, and extensively metabolized to inactive compounds before they are excreted in the urine. Phenobarbital, a more polar drug, is slowly absorbed from the gut and more slowly redistributed from the brain, and this contributes to its longer duration of action. **Phenobarbital** is partly converted to inactive metabolites, but a significant fraction of the parent compound is excreted unchanged in the urine.

MECHANISM OF ACTION. Barbiturates bind to an **allosteric site** on the GABA$_A$ receptor–chloride ion channel that is distinct from the allosteric site to which benzodiazepines bind (see Fig. 19–2). The barbiturates increase the affinity of the receptor for GABA and the duration of time that the chloride channel remains open. In contrast to the benzodiazepines, the barbiturates also act to directly increase chloride influx in the absence of GABA. For this reason, barbiturates do not exhibit a ceiling effect. As shown in Figure 19–3, they have a linear dose-response curve. Higher doses of barbiturates increasingly depress the neuronal activity of the CNS, causing respiratory depression, coma, and death. This accounts for the fact that barbiturates exhibit greater toxicity and a smaller therapeutic index than benzodiazepines.

PHARMACOLOGIC EFFECTS. Unlike the anxiolytic effect of benzodiazepines, that of barbiturates is associated with considerable sedation. When used to treat insomnia, the barbiturates can cause hangover and daytime sedation. As with the benzodiazepines, the barbiturates suppress slow-wave and REM sleep. Barbiturates can also cause tolerance and physical dependence during continuous use, and a withdrawal syndrome occurs if the drugs are abruptly discontinued. Short-acting barbiturates (e.g., **pentobarbital**) have been extensively abused.

INTERACTIONS. The barbiturates induce cytochrome P450 enzymes in the liver and thereby accelerate their own metabolism as well as that of other drugs metabolized by these enzymes. Maximal enzyme induction is obtained by the daily administration of phenobarbital, a long-acting agent. Barbiturates also induce the rate-limiting enzyme in porphyrin biosynthesis, α-aminolevulinate synthase, and may thereby exacerbate **porphyria,** a condition in which a hereditary defect causes excessive porphyrin synthesis and excretion, with attendant neurologic and cutaneous manifestations.

INDICATIONS. The barbiturates were extensively used to treat anxiety disorders and insomnia before the development of benzodiazepines, but they are seldom used for these purposes today. Unlike the benzodiazepines, the barbiturates do not produce significant muscle relaxation and are not used in treating muscle spasm or spasticity disorders. They are indicated for the treatment of seizure disorders (see Chapter 20) and for the induction of general anesthesia.

Specific Agents

Amobarbital and **pentobarbital** have been used primarily to treat **insomnia. Phenobarbital** is used occasionally to treat **seizure disorders**, and **thiopental** is administered intravenously to induce **anesthesia**. Thiopental has a high degree of lipid solubility and a very fast onset of action. It is also rapidly redistributed from the brain to other tissues (muscle and fat), which accounts for its short duration of action.

Antihistamines

Some of the **histamine antagonists** (antihistamines) cross the blood-brain barrier and produce varying degrees of sedation, and these drugs have been used to treat **mild insomnia** and **anxiety disorders**. For example, **diphenhydramine** is the active ingredient in several nonprescription sleep preparations, and **hydroxyzine** has been used in the treatment of mild anxiety and is sometimes used as a **sedative** before surgery. The sedative action of these drugs is caused by their ability to bind to H_1 heteroreceptors and reduce acetylcholine released by neurons in the reticular activating system.

Drugs that block acetylcholine release, including the **antihistamines**, induce drowsiness and sleep via their effects on the cholinergic projections of the reticular nuclei. In contrast, **caffeine** and related **methylxanthines** can increase arousal by blocking presynaptic adenosine receptors and thereby increasing cholinergic activity in the reticular nuclei.

Some tolerance can occur during the long-term use of antihistamines, but these drugs are not associated with physical dependence or significant drug abuse. The pharmacologic properties of antihistamines are discussed in detail in Chapter 26.

Other Sedative-Hypnotic Drugs

Zolpidem, Zaleplon, and Eszopiclone

The newer agents, zolpidem (AMBIEN), zaleplon (SONATA), and eszopiclone (LUNESTA), have largely replaced older benzodiazepines for the treatment of insomnia. The popularity of these agents is due to less adverse effects compared to the older benzodiazepine agents, such as relative lack of effect on REM or slow-wave sleep, and less potential for tolerance and dependence. Their shorter duration of action usually precludes daytime sedation and hangover effects. There is evidence that this is due to greater selectivity at targeting only $GABA_A$ receptors that are composed of particular subunit combinations, in particular those receptors composed of $alpha_1$ subunits. (This site of action was previously classified as $omega_1$ sites). The older benzodiazepines are less selective and bind to a more widespread distribution of receptor, producing a greater degree of adverse effects on sleep, cognitive performance, and memory. Additionally, the elimination half-life of these newer agents is shorter than that of the older benzodiazepine agents, which accounts for a weaker hangover effect. **Zaleplon** has the advantage that its elimination half-life is the shortest at about 1 hour and can be taken in patients that awaken in the middle of the night and have difficulty going back to sleep.

Melatonin and Ramelteon

Melatonin is a neuroendocrine hormone synthesized in the pineal gland. The hormone interacts with specific receptors in the CNS and elsewhere, and it is believed to be the principal mediator of the biologic clock that determines circadian, seasonal, and reproductive rhythms in animal species. In humans, melatonin is released before the onset of sleep and produces drowsiness that facilitates sleep. Studies show that melatonin produces drowsiness even if administered during the daytime.

Melatonin is available without prescription and may be effective in the treatment of **jet lag** in individuals who have rapidly traveled across several time zones and in the treatment of **insomnia in shift-change workers**. If melatonin is taken at bedtime for a few nights, it may accelerate the resetting of the biologic clock in these persons. Melatonin may also be effective in treating **insomnia in elderly patients** who do not secrete adequate melatonin, and it appears to be effective in treating **delayed sleep-phase syndrome** and **non–24-hour sleep-wake disorder**. It should be noted that melatonin is not an FDA-approved drug.

Ramelteon (ROZEREM) is a new drug that acts at selective **melatonin receptors** and is approved to treat **sleep-onset insomnia**. Ramelteon dose not appear to produce dependence and shows little potential for abuse. As compared to benzodiazepine drugs, there is no evidence for **rebound insomnia** after cessation of ramelteon. It is currently the only nonscheduled prescription drug for the treatment of insomnia available. It should not be used with fluvoxamine (LUVOX) as this antidepressant is a strong CYP1A2 inhibitor and concurrent use with ramelteon increases the peak plasma concentration of ramelteon 70-fold.

Chloral Hydrate

Chloral hydrate is an older hypnotic that is largely obsolete today. It is a prodrug that is converted to its active metabolite, trichloroethanol, by liver enzymes. Its effects are potentiated by alcohol, and the combination of alcohol and chloral hydrate gained fame under the monikers of "Mickey Finn" and "knock-out drops." Chloral hydrate is occasionally used for **preanesthetic sedation** in pediatric patients.

NONSEDATING ANXIOLYTIC DRUGS

Buspirone

Buspirone is a unique anxiolytic agent that does not share structural similarity with the other agents. The drug is used in the treatment of **chronic anxiety** and produces an anxiolytic effect without causing marked sedation, amnesia, tolerance, dependence, or muscle relaxation. In some patients, it can cause headache, dizziness, and nervousness, but these side effects are usually mild and temporary.

Buspirone is a **partial agonist** at serotonin 5-HT_{1A} receptors and may exert its anxiolytic effect by activating feedback inhibition of serotonin release. By this action, it can cause up-regulation of postsynaptic serotonin receptors. This effect takes time to develop and is consistent with the 3- to 4-week delay in the onset of the anxiolytic effect of buspirone. Buspirone and other drugs affecting serotonin are discussed further in Chapter 26.

Propranolol

Propranolol, a β-adrenoceptor antagonist (β-blocker), is sometimes used to prevent the physiologic manifestations of **stage fright**, or **acute situational or performance anxiety**. When taken an hour before the anticipated anxiety-provoking event, propranolol prevents tachycardia and other signs and symptoms of acute anxiety caused by sympathetic stimulation. The mechanisms and properties of β-blockers are discussed in detail in Chapter 9.

SUMMARY OF IMPORTANT POINTS

■ Benzodiazepines, the most widely used sedative-hypnotic drugs, are indicated for the treatment of anxiety disorders, insomnia, muscle spasm, seizure disorders, and spasticity.

■ Benzodiazepines bind to an allosteric receptor site on the $GABA_A$ receptor–chloride ion channel and thereby facilitate the binding of GABA and increase the frequency with which the chloride channel opens. Benzodiazepines also decrease the release of GABA, which limits the magnitude of CNS depression produced by these drugs.

■ Some benzodiazepines (e.g., chlordiazepoxide and diazepam) have long-acting active metabolites. Others (e.g., alprazolam, midazolam, and triazolam) have shorter-acting active metabolites. All benzodiazepines, including those with no active metabolites, are eventually converted to inactive glucuronide compounds. The benzodiazepines that have no active metabolites (e.g., oxazepam, temazepam, and lorazepam) may be the safest ones to use in the treatment of elderly patients.

■ Benzodiazepines and other hypnotic drugs reduce the time required to fall asleep (sleep latency), reduce early awakenings, and increase total sleep time. Benzodiazepines and barbiturates reduce slow-wave sleep and REM sleep.

■ Pentobarbital, phenobarbital, and other barbiturates bind to the $GABA_A$ receptor–chloride ion channel but do not exhibit a ceiling effect and can cause respiratory depression, coma, and death.

■ Unlike benzodiazepines, barbiturates induce their own metabolism as well as that of many other drugs metabolized by cytochrome P450 enzymes.

■ Long-term administration of benzodiazepines and barbiturates can lead to tolerance and physical dependence, and abrupt discontinuation of their use will cause symptoms of withdrawal.

■ Zolpidem, zaleplon, and eszopiclone are effective, short-acting sedative-hypnotic agents that have little effect on normal sleep architecture and produce few adverse effects. Ramelteon is the first prescription drug to treat insomnia that acts on melatonin receptors.

■ Sedating antihistamines (e.g., diphenhydramine and hydroxyzine) have been used to treat mild insomnia and anxiety. Older hypnotics (e.g., chloral hydrate) are largely obsolete but are occasionally used for preanesthetic sedation.

■ Propranolol and other β-adrenoceptor antagonists can be used to prevent the physiologic manifestations of situational or performance anxiety, including tachycardia.

■ Flumazenil is a benzodiazepine receptor antagonist that can be used to counteract respiratory depression and other reactions that are usually caused by excessive doses of intravenously administered benzodiazepines.

Review Questions

1. Which of the following molecular processes best describes the mechanism of action of benzodiazepines?
   (A) potentiating the effect of GABA at chloride ion channels
   (B) blocking glutamate excitation
   (C) blocking the inactivation of sodium ion channels
   (D) binding to opioid receptors to produce sedation
   (E) potentiating the action of the inhibitory amino acid, glycine

2. Benzodiazepines are noted for altering which one of the following aspects of sleep?
   (A) increasing the time to sleep onset
   (B) decreasing stage 2 NREM sleep
   (C) increasing slow-wave sleep
   (D) decreasing the REM stage of sleep
   (E) increasing sleep awakenings

3. Which one of the following statement best describes flumazenil?
   (A) does not produce withdrawal seizures
   (B) has the longest elimination half-life
   (C) is not metabolized into an active agent
   (D) is also used for the treatment of epilepsy
   (E) is a selective benzodiazepine antagonist

4. Zaleplon differs from zolpidem in which one of the following ways?
   (A) produces withdrawal seizures
   (B) has a shorter elimination half-life
   (C) has a different chemical structure than benzodiazepines
   (D) shows less tolerance to sedative effects
   (E) produces greater morning sedation

5. Which one of the following anxiolytic drugs is noted for its lack of sedation?
   (A) hydroxyzine
   (B) diazepam
   (C) oxazepam
   (D) alprazolam
   (E) buspirone

Answers and Explanations

1. **The correct answer is A: potentiating the effect of GABA at chloride ion channels.** Benzodiazepines bind to an allosteric site on the $GABA_A$ receptor–ion channel complex to increase the affinity of GABA. GABA action increases the conductance of chloride ion into the neuron, thereby hyperpolarizing the membrane and making it harder to reach depolarization threshold and fire action potentials. Answer (B), blocking glutamate excitation, is the mechanism of action of N-methyl-D-aspartate receptor antagonists. Answer (C), blocking the inactivation of sodium ion channels, is the mechanism of action of certain antiepileptic agents. Answer (D), binding to opioid receptors to produce sedation, is the site

of opioid analgesic action. Answer (E), potentiating the action of the inhibitory amino acid, glycine, is incorrect because benzodiazepines do not have significant binding affinity for the glycine receptor.

2. **The correct choice is D: decreasing the REM stage of sleep.** Benzodiazepines are noted for decreasing the time spent in REM sleep, an effect that is unmasked by REM rebound after the administration of the benzodiazepine is stopped. Answer (A), increasing the time to sleep onset, is the opposite effect of sedative-hypnotics, which decrease the latency to sleep. Answer (B), decreasing stage 2 NREM sleep, is not correct, because studies do not show a consistent effect of benzodiazepines on stage 2 NREM sleep. Answer (C), increasing slow-wave sleep, may be beneficial to a restful sleep, but no evidence suggests that benzodiazepines produce this effect. Choice (E), increasing sleep awakenings, occurs in patients with insomnia, a symptom that benzodiazepines and other sedative-hypnotic agents aim to treat.

3. **The correct choice is E: is a selective benzodiazepine antagonist.** Flumazenil is a competitive antagonist of the benzodiazepine receptor. The availability of flumazenil to reverse benzodiazepine action is useful in cases of drug overdose or in outpatient procedures to bring patients back to normal wakefulness. Answer (A), does not produce withdrawal seizures, is certainly true; however, it is not the best statement describing flumazenil. Answer (B), has the longest elimination half-life, is not true because often flumazenil must be given in repeated administrations to reverse the effects of a longer-lasting benzodiazepine such as diazepam. Answer (C), is not metabolized into an active agent, is also true but is not the best choice. Answer (D), is also used for the treatment of epilepsy, is incorrect regarding the indicated uses of flumazenil.

4. **The correct answer is B: has a shorter elimination half-life.** Zaleplon, as with zolpidem, has a more selective action than benzodiazepines. It has the advantage that it has a shorter half-life and therefore is approved for those patients who awaken in the middle of the night and cannot return to sleep. Answer (A), produces withdrawal seizures, does not appear to be true for both agents, but is noted upon cessation from chronic doses of alprazolam. Answer (C), has a different chemical structure than benzodiazepines, and answer (D), shows less tolerance to sedative effects, are also true for both agents. Answer (E), produces greater morning sedation, is not true, and neither agent produces much sedation after its initial hypnotic effect.

5. **The correct answer is E: buspirone.** Buspirone is a unique, nonsedating anxiolytic agent mediating its effects by way of the 5-HT receptor. No sedative effects are associated with its action, although it differs in that it may take from 2 to 4 weeks of daily administration for clinical effectiveness. Answers (A) through (D) are all sedating drugs, including the antihistamine, hydroxyzine, and the benzodiazepines, diazepam, oxazepam, and alprazolam.

SELECTED READINGS

Bateson, A.N. The benzodiazepine site of the $GABA_A$ receptor: an old target with new potential? Sleep Med 5(Suppl 1):S9–S15, 2004.

Tariq, S., and S. Pulisetty. Pharmacotherapy for insomnia. Clin Geriatric Med 24:93–105, 2008.

Verster, J.C., D.S. Veldhuijzen, and E.R. Volkerts. Residual effects of sleep medication on driving ability. Sleep Med Rev 8:309–325, 2004.

Yaksh, T.L., and J.W. Allen. The use of intrathecal midazolam in humans: a case study of process. Anesth Analg 98:1536–1545, 2004.

Zhdanova, I.V. Advances in the management of insomnia. Expert Opin Pharmacother 5:1573–1579, 2004.

CHAPTER 20

Antiepileptic Drugs

CLASSIFICATION OF ANTIEPILEPTIC DRUGS*

Drugs for Partial Seizures and Generalized Tonic-Clonic Seizures
- Carbamazepine (TEGRETOL)
- Oxcarbazepine (TRILEPTAL)
- Phenytoin (DILANTIN)
- Phenobarbital (LUMINAL)
- Primidone (MYSOLINE)
- Valproic acid (DEPAKENE)

Adjunct Drugs for Partial Seizures
- Clorazepate (TRANXENE)
- Felbamate (FELBATOL)
- Gabapentin (NEURONTIN)
- Lamotrigine (LAMICTAL)
- Topiramate (TOPAMAX)[a]

Drugs for Generalized Absence, Myoclonic, or Atonic Seizures
- Clonazepam (KLONOPIN)
- Ethosuximide (ZARONTIN)
- Lamotrigine (LAMICTAL)
- Valproate (Valproic acid, DEPAKENE)

Drugs for Status Epilepticus
- Diazepam (VALIUM)
- Lorazepam (ATIVAN)
- Phenobarbital (LUMINAL)
- Fosphenytoin (CEREBYX)

*Note that some drugs are listed more than once.
[a]Also tiagabine (GABITRIL), levetiracetam (KEPPRA), zonisamide (ZONEGRAN), pregabalin (LYRICA), and vigabatrin (SABRIL).

OVERVIEW

Seizures are episodes of abnormal electrical activity in the brain that cause involuntary movements, sensations, or thoughts. Seizures can result from head trauma, stroke, brain tumors, hypoxia, hypoglycemia, fever, chronic alcohol withdrawal, and other conditions that alter neuronal function. Recurrent seizures that cannot be attributed to any proximal cause are seen in patients with epilepsy. In some patients, epilepsy appears to have a genetic basis. Environmental perturbations (e.g., intrauterine or neonatal complications) have also been implicated in the development of epilepsy. In the United States, epilepsy affects 1% to 2% of the population and is the second most common neurological disease after stroke.

Classification of Seizures

The two main categories of seizures are partial (focal) seizures and generalized seizures (Table 20–1). A partial seizure originates in one cerebral hemisphere, and the patient does not lose consciousness during the seizure. A generalized seizure arises in both cerebral hemispheres and involves loss of consciousness. Seizures are accompanied by characteristic changes in the electroencephalogram (EEG), as shown in Figure 20–1. Most seizures are self-limited and last from about 10 seconds to 5 minutes. Some seizures are preceded by an aura, which is a sensation or mood that may help identify the anatomic location of the seizure focus.

About 60% of epileptic seizures are partial seizures. Electroencephalographic abnormalities are seen in one or more lobes of a cerebral hemisphere, and the patient may exhibit motor, sensory, and autonomic symptoms. In **simple partial seizures**, consciousness is not altered. In **complex partial seizures**, however, patients have an altered consciousness and exhibit repetitive behaviors (automatisms). Complex partial seizures often originate in the temporal lobe, in which case the disorder is called either **temporal lobe epilepsy** or **psychomotor epilepsy**. Some partial seizures progress along anatomical lines as the electrical discharges spread across the cortex. For example, a seizure may first involve the fingers, then the hand, and finally the entire arm. This is characteristic of **jacksonian epilepsy,** or **"jacksonian march."** Partial seizures can also evolve into generalized seizures.

The two main types of generalized seizures are tonic-clonic seizures and absence seizures. Generalized tonic-clonic seizures, which were formerly called *grand mal*

TABLE 20-1. **International Classification of Partial and Generalized Seizures**

Classification	Characterization
Partial (Focal) Seizures	Arise in one cerebral hemisphere
Simple partial seizure	No alteration of consciousness
Complex partial seizure	Altered consciousness, automatisms, and behavioral changes
Secondarily generalized seizure	Focal seizure becomes generalized and is accompanied by loss of consciousness
Generalized Seizures	Arise in both cerebral hemispheres and are accompanied by loss of consciousness
Tonic-clonic (grand mal) seizure	Increased muscle tone is followed by spasms of muscle contraction and relaxation
Tonic seizure	Increased muscle tone
Clonic seizure	Spasms of muscle contraction and relaxation
Myoclonic seizure	Rhythmic, jerking spasms
Atonic seizure	Sudden loss of all muscle tone
Absence (petit mal) seizure	Brief loss of consciousness, with minor muscle twitches and eye blinking

seizures, begin with a brief tonic phase that is followed by a clonic phase with muscle spasms lasting 3 to 5 minutes, and they conclude with a postictal period of drowsiness, confusion, and a glazed look in the eyes. **Status epilepticus** is a condition in which patients experience recurrent episodes of tonic-clonic seizures without regaining consciousness or normal muscle movement between episodes. Generalized **absence seizures,** or *petit mal* **seizures,** are characterized by abrupt loss of consciousness and decreased muscle tone, and they can include a mild clonic component, automatisms, and autonomic effects. On the EEG, generalized absence seizures exhibit a synchronous 3-Hz (three cycles per second) spike-and-dome pattern that usually lasts 10 to 15 seconds.

Less common types of generalized seizures include **myoclonic seizures** and **atonic seizures** (see Table 20–1).

Neurobiology of Seizures

Epileptic seizures are caused by synchronous neuronal discharges within a particular group of neurons, or **seizure focus,** which is often located in the cerebral cortex but can be found in other areas of the brain. Once initiated, the abnormal discharges spread to other parts of the brain and produce abnormal movements, sensations, or thoughts. The neuronal mechanisms that initiate a seizure are not fully understood, but growing evidence indicates the involvement of excessive excitatory neurotransmission mediated by **glutamate** (Fig. 20–2). Investigators believe that excessive activation by glutamate of N-methyl-D-aspartate (NMDA) receptors displaces Mg^{2+} ions from the **NMDA receptor–calcium ion channel** and thereby facilitates calcium entry into neurons. Calcium contributes to the long-term potentiation of excitatory glutamate neurotransmission by activating the synthesis of **nitric oxide.**

Nitric oxide is a gas that can diffuse backward to the presynaptic neuron, where it facilitates glutamate release via stimulation of a G protein that activates the synthesis of cyclic guanosine monophosphate. These actions further increase NMDA receptor activation and calcium influx, which are believed to contribute to the **depolarization shift** that is observed in seizure foci. The depolarization shift consists of abnormally prolonged action potentials (depolarizations) that have spikelets. The shift recruits and synchronizes

depolarizations by surrounding neurons and thereby initiates a seizure.

Several other mechanisms can be involved in seizures. One is the suppression of inhibitory neurotransmission of **γ-aminobutyric acid (GABA),** and another is an increase in calcium influx via T-type calcium channels in thalamic neurons.

Mechanisms of Antiepileptic Drugs

Antiepileptic drugs are believed to suppress the formation or spread of abnormal electrical discharges in the brain. As shown in Table 20–2, the currently available drugs accomplish these actions via three mechanisms: (1) inhibition of the sodium or calcium influx responsible for neuronal depolarization, (2) augmentation of inhibitory GABA neurotransmission, and (3) inhibition of excitatory glutamate neurotransmission.

Effects on Ion Channels

Under normal circumstances, **voltage-sensitive (voltage-gated) sodium channels** are rapidly opened when the neuronal membrane potential (voltage) reaches its threshold. This causes rapid depolarization of the membrane and the conduction of an action potential along the neuronal axon. When the action potential reaches the nerve terminal, it evokes the release of a neurotransmitter. After the neuronal membrane is depolarized, the sodium channel is inactivated by closure of the channel's inactivation gate. The inactivation gate must be opened before the next action potential can occur.

Many antiepileptic drugs, including **carbamazepine, lamotrigine, phenytoin,** and **topiramate,** prolong the time that the sodium channel's inactivation gate remains closed, and this delays the formation of the next action potential. These drugs bind to the channel when it is opened. Because rapidly firing neurons are opened a greater percentage of the time than are slowly firing neurons, the drugs exhibit **use-dependent blockade.** For this reason, the drugs suppress abnormal repetitive depolarizations in a seizure focus more than they suppress normal neuronal activity. By these actions, carbamazepine and other drugs prevent the spread of abnormal discharges in a seizure focus to other neurons.

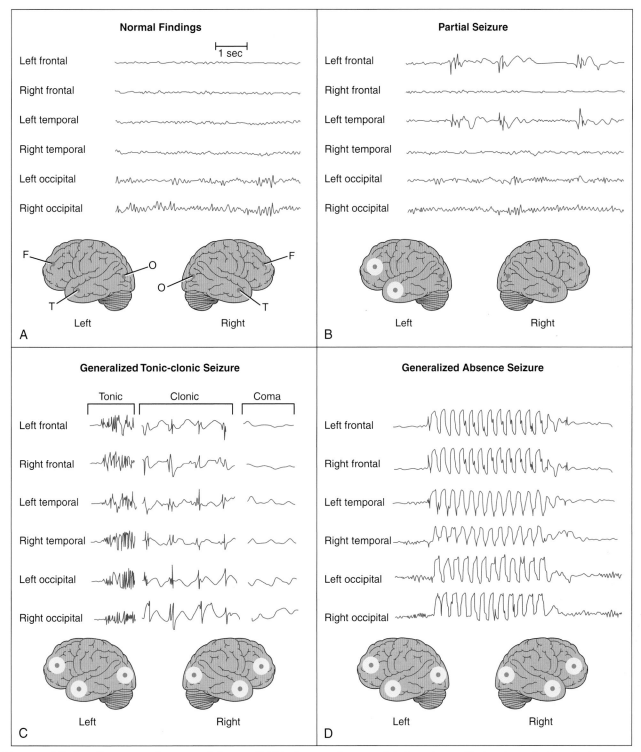

Figure 20-1. **Patterns on electroencephalogram (EEG) in the normal state and during seizures.** The locations of seizure foci are shown as shaded areas on the cerebral hemispheres. (A) In the normal state, the EEG shows asynchronous alpha (8–12 Hz) and beta (12–30 Hz) rhythms originating in the cortex of the frontal (F), temporal (T), and occipital (O) lobes. (B) During a partial seizure, synchronous discharges are observed in various areas of the brain. In this example, they are seen in the left frontal and left temporal lobes, but they are not seen in other lobes. (C) During a generalized tonic-clonic seizure, the tonic phase is characterized by low-frequency and high-amplitude waves, whereas the clonic phase shows synchronous oscillations. (D) During a generalized absence seizure, a synchronous 3-Hz spike-and-wave pattern is seen throughout the cortex.

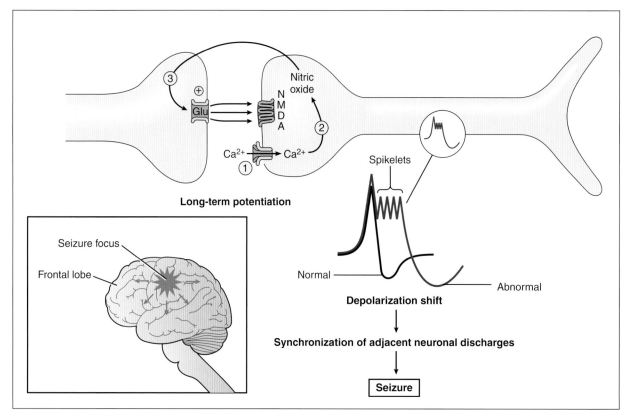

Figure 20–2. **Neuronal mechanisms underlying seizures.** In this example, a seizure is caused by the synchronous discharge of a group of neurons (focus) in the cortex. Activation of NMDA receptors increases calcium influx and nitric oxide synthesis. Nitric oxide then diffuses to the presynaptic neuron and increases the release of glutamate via formation of cyclic guanosine monophosphate. Increased excitatory glutamate neurotransmission leads to long-term potentiation. Long-term potentiation is believed to facilitate a depolarization shift, characterized by prolonged depolarizations with spikelets. The depolarization shift can cause adjacent neurons to discharge synchronously and thereby precipitate a seizure.

A few drugs, such as **ethosuximide** and **valproate**, block **T-type (low-threshold) calcium channels** that are located in thalamic neurons and participate in the initiation of generalized absence seizures.

Effects on GABAergic Systems

Antiepileptic drugs facilitate GABA neurotransmission by various means. Benzodiazepines, like clonazepam and barbiturates, such as phenobarbital, enhance GABA activation of the **GABA$_A$ receptor-chloride ion channel** (see Chapter 19). Topiramate also activates the GABA$_A$ receptor. **Gabapentin** increases GABA release, whereas **valproate** inhibits GABA degradation. Drugs that augment GABA may serve to counteract the excessive excitatory neurotransmission responsible for initiating and spreading abnormal electrical discharges.

Effects on Glutaminergic Systems

A few antiepileptic drugs, including **felbamate, topiramate**, and **valproate**, inhibit glutamate neurotransmission, and other drugs that work via this mechanism are under development. This is an attractive mechanism of action because it may affect the formation of a seizure focus and thereby terminate a seizure at an early stage of its development.

TREATMENT OF SEIZURE DISORDERS

As indicated in the drugs listed in the box at the beginning of this chapter, some are active against only one or two types of seizures. In contrast, valproate has a broad spectrum of activity and is active against most types of seizures. The newer agents, such as **lamotrigine, topiramate, tiagabine, levetiracetam, zonisamide,** and **pregabalin**, are considered adjunct agents and primarily used in combination with older drugs for the treatment of partial seizures. These newer agents are particularly useful because complex partial seizures are more resistant to treatment than are other types of seizures.

The pharmacologic properties of antiepileptic drugs are described below, whereas the mechanisms of action, adverse effects, contraindications, and drug interactions are given in Tables 20–2, 20–3, and 20–4.

Drugs for Partial and Generalized Tonic-Clonic Seizures

The first-line drugs for partial seizures and generalized tonic-clonic seizures are carbamazepine, phenytoin, and valproate. Carbamazepine and phenytoin have a similar

TABLE 20–2. Mechanisms of Antiepileptic Drugs

Drug	Effects on Ion Flux	Effects on GABA	Effects on Glutamate
Carbamazepine	Blocks voltage-sensitive sodium channels	—	—
Clonazepam	—	Enhances GABA-mediated chloride flux	—
Clorazepate	—	Enhances GABA-mediated chloride flux	—
Diazepam	—	Enhances GABA-mediated chloride flux	—
Ethosuximide	Blocks T-type calcium channels	—	—
Felbamate	—	—	Blocks glycine activation of NMDA receptors
Gabapentin	—	Increases GABA release	—
Lamotrigine	Blocks voltage-sensitive sodium channels	—	—
Lorazepam	—	Enhances GABA-mediated chloride flux	—
Phenobarbital	—	Enhances GABA-mediated chloride flux	—
Phenytoin	Blocks voltage-sensitive sodium channels	—	—
Primidone	Possibly blocks voltage-sensitive sodium channels	Enhances GABA-mediated chloride flux	—
Topiramate	Blocks voltage-sensitive sodium channels	Increases GABA activation of GABA$_A$ receptors	Blocks kainate and AMPA receptors
Valproate	Possibly blocks voltage-sensitive sodium channels and T-type calcium channels	Increases GABA synthesis and inhibits GABA degradation	Possibly decreases glutamate synthesis

AMPA = α-amino-3-hydroxy-5-methyl-4-isoxazole propionic acid; GABA = γ-aminobutyric acid; NMDA = N-methyl-D-aspartate.

mechanism of action and clinical effectiveness, and both drugs induce cytochrome P450 enzymes and increase drug metabolism. Valproate acts by a different mechanism and inhibits cytochrome P450 enzymes. Two other drugs that are effective against partial seizures as well as generalized tonic-clonic seizures are phenobarbital and primidone.

Carbamazepine

PHARMACOKINETICS. Carbamazepine is adequately absorbed after oral administration, and it is biotransformed to an active metabolite, **carbamazepine epoxide**. Almost all the drug is excreted as metabolites in the urine and feces.

MECHANISMS AND EFFECTS. Carbamazepine blocks voltage-sensitive sodium channels in neuronal cell membranes. As described, blockade of these channels inhibits the spread of abnormal electrical discharges from the seizure focus to other neurons by preventing the release of excitatory neurotransmitters from nerve terminals. Carbamazepine has additional mechanisms of action, but their contributions to its antiepileptic effects are unknown. For example, carbamazepine blocks adenosine receptors in a way that leads to up-regulation of these receptors, and it blocks norepinephrine reuptake in the same way that tricyclic antidepressants block it. The latter action is probably responsible for the mood-elevating effect of carbamazepine.

Carbamazepine can cause drowsiness, ataxia, and other symptoms of central nervous system (CNS) depression, as well as gastrointestinal reactions. Rarely, its use has been associated with **aplastic anemia**. In general, carbamazepine usually produces fewer adverse effects than does phenytoin.

INTERACTIONS. Carbamazepine is a **potent inducer** of cytochrome P450 enzymes that metabolize a wide range of drugs. Carbamazepine accelerates its own metabolism as well as that of many other drugs, including lamotrigine, phenytoin,

topiramate, and valproate. For this reason, it decreases the serum level and effects of these drugs. Carbamazepine can also increase lithium toxicity.

INDICATIONS. In addition to its use in treating **partial seizures** and generalized tonic-clonic seizures, carbamazepine is the drug of choice for **trigeminal neuralgia** *(tic douloureux)*, a condition that can cause chronic and intense pain on one or both sides of the face. Carbamazepine is also effective as an alternative to lithium in the treatment of **bipolar disease**, a mood disorder discussed in Chapter 22.

Phenytoin and Fosphenytoin

PHARMACOKINETICS. Phenytoin is a hydantoin derivative formerly called diphenylhydantoin. It is poorly soluble in water, and different pharmaceutical formulations of it may have different bioavailability. Hence, it is prudent to avoid switching from one formulation to another. If a switch must be made, serum drug levels should be monitored. A new formulation, called **fosphenytoin**, has become available for parenteral administration. Fosphenytoin is more soluble in water, and this prevents precipitation of the drug after intramuscular or intravenous administration.

Phenytoin is converted to an inactive hydroxylated metabolite by cytochrome P450 enzymes. The drug exhibits **dose-dependent kinetics**, whereby lower concentrations are eliminated by a **first-order** process, but higher concentrations saturate biotransformation enzymes and exhibit **zero-order** kinetics. Phenytoin hydroxylation also exhibits genetic **polymorphism**. These factors are responsible for the considerable patient variation in the plasma drug concentrations produced by a given dose. Because of this variation, serum drug levels should be monitored at the start of therapy and whenever toxicity or therapeutic failure occurs.

TABLE 20-3. **Adverse Effects, Contraindications, and Pregnancy Risk Data for Antiepileptic Drugs**

Drug	Major Adverse Effects	Contraindications	Risk Category and Effects of Use During Pregnancy*
Carbamazepine	Aplastic anemia (rare); ataxia, drowsiness, and other symptoms of central nervous system (CNS) depression; gastrointestinal reactions; and nausea	Hypersensitivity	Category C; increased risk of birth defects; abnormal facial features; neural tube defects, such as spina bifida; reduced head size; and other anomalies
Clonazepam	Arrhythmia; CNS depression; drug dependence; hypotension; and mild respiratory depression	Acute angle-closure glaucoma; hypersensitivity; and severe liver disease	Category C; apnea in newborns; increased risk of birth defects
Clorazepate	Confusion; drowsiness; drug tolerance; and lethargy	Hypersensitivity	Category D; increased risk of birth defects
Diazepam	Same as clonazepam	Same as clonazepam	Category D; increased risk of birth defects
Ethosuximide	Dizziness; drowsiness; gastric distress; lethargy; and nausea	Hypersensitivity	Category C
Felbamate	Aplastic anemia; fatigue; gastrointestinal reactions; headache; hepatic toxicity; and insomnia	Bone marrow depression; hepatic disease; and hypersensitivity	Category C
Gabapentin	Ataxia; dizziness; drowsiness; nystagmus; and tremor	Hypersensitivity	Category C
Lamotrigine	Ataxia; diplopia; dizziness; drowsiness; headache; nausea; rash; and Stevens-Johnson syndrome	Hypersensitivity. Use cautiously in patients who are taking valproate or have hepatic or renal disease	Category C; may reduce folate levels
Levetiracetam	Somnolence; asthenia (weakness); infection; and dizziness	Hypersensitivity	Category C; levetiracetam produced evidence of developmental toxicity at doses similar to or greater than human therapeutic doses
Lorazepam	Same as clonazepam	Same as clonazepam	Category D; increased risk of birth defects
Phenobarbital	Ataxia; cognitive impairment; dizziness; drowsiness; drug dependence; rash; and respiratory depression	Hypersensitivity; porphyria; respiratory depression; and severe liver disease	Category D; bleeding at birth; minor congenital defects
Phenytoin	Cerebellar symptoms; gastrointestinal disturbances; gingival hyperplasia; hirsutism; megaloblastic anemia and other blood cell deficiencies; osteomalacia; and psychiatric changes	Bradycardia; hypersensitivity; and severe atrioventricular block or sinoatrial dysfunction	Category D; may reduce folate levels; 2–3 times increased risk of birth defects; fetal hydantoin syndrome
Primidone	Same as phenobarbital	Hypersensitivity	Category D
Tiagabine	Dizziness, somnolence, nausea, nervousness, abdominal pain, and difficulty with concentration or attention	Hypersensitivity	Category C; adverse effects on embryo-fetal development, including teratogenic effects at doses greater than the human therapeutic dose
Topiramate	Ataxia; dizziness; drowsiness; nystagmus; paresthesia; and psychomotor impairment	Hypersensitivity. Use cautiously during pregnancy, during lactation, or in the presence of hepatic or renal disease	Category C
Valproate	Drowsiness; gastrointestinal disturbances; hepatic toxicity (rare); nausea; and weight gain	Hepatic disease and hypersensitivity	Category D; may reduce folate levels; teratogenic during the first trimester; neural tube defects, such as spina bifida
Vigabatrin	Amnesia; blurred vision; blue-yellow color blindness; decreased vision or other vision changes; eye pains; increase in seizures (rare)	Hypersensitivity	Category C; studies in rabbits have shown that vigabatrin causes birth defects
Zonisamide	Somnolence, anorexia, dizziness, headache, nausea, and agitation/irritability	Hypersensitivity	Category C; teratogenic in mice, rats, and dogs and embryolethal in monkeys when administered during the period of organogenesis at zonisamide dosage and maternal plasma levels similar to or lower than therapeutic levels in humans

*Pregnancy risk categories are defined by the FDA as follows: A = controlled studies show no risk; B = no evidence of risk in humans; C = risk cannot be ruled out; D = positive evidence of risk; and X = contraindicated in pregnancy.

TABLE 20-4. Interactions of Antiepileptic Drugs

Antiepileptic Drug	Interacting Drugs That Increase Serum Levels*	Interacting Drugs That Decrease Serum Levels†	Interactions That Cause Other Effects
Carbamazepine	Cimetidine, diltiazem, erythromycin, fluoxetine, isoniazid, and propoxyphene	Carbamazepine	Decreases serum levels of calcium channel blockers, clozapine, haloperidol, steroids, theophylline, thyroid, and warfarin
Clonazepam	Cimetidine and disulfiram	Rifampin	Increases lithium toxicity. Increases CNS depression if alcohol is ingested
Clorazepate	Cimetidine and disulfiram	Rifampin	Increases CNS depression if alcohol is ingested.
Diazepam	Cimetidine	Rifampin	Increases CNS depression if alcohol is ingested
Ethosuximide	Valproate	—	May alter seizure pattern if taken in combination with haloperidol
Felbamate	—	Carbamazepine and phenytoin	Increases CNS depression if alcohol is ingested
Gabapentin	—	Antacids	—
Lamotrigine	Valproate	Carbamazepine, phenobarbital, and phenytoin	Decreases serum levels of valproate
Lorazepam	—	Rifampin	Increases CNS depression if alcohol is ingested
Phenobarbital	Valproate	Phenobarbital	Decreases serum levels of many drugs. Increases meperidine toxicity
Phenytoin	Chloramphenicol, cimetidine, isoniazid, and sulfonamides	Carbamazepine	Decreases serum levels of amiodarone, digoxin, quinidines, steroids, theophylline, vitamin K, and other agents
Primidone	Valproate	Phenobarbital	—
Topiramate	—	Carbamazepine and phenytoin	Decreases serum levels of oral contraceptives
Valproate	Salicylates	Carbamazepine, lamotrigine, and phenytoin	May increase or decrease serum levels of carbamazepine and phenytoin

*These drugs inhibit metabolism.
†Except for antacids (which reduce the absorption of gabapentin), these drugs induce metabolism.

MECHANISMS AND EFFECTS. As with carbamazepine, phenytoin **blocks voltage-sensitive sodium channels** by prolonging the inactivation state of these channels. This enables phenytoin to inhibit the repetitive firing of neurons in a seizure focus.

Phenytoin can cause a number of adverse effects. The drug interferes with **folate metabolism**, and this can lead to **megaloblastic anemia**. Folate antagonism can also contribute to birth defects such as those seen in **fetal hydantoin syndrome**. This syndrome is characterized by cardiac defects; malformation of ears, lips, palate, mouth, and nasal bridge; mental retardation; and microcephaly. By impairing cerebellar function, phenytoin can cause ataxia, diplopia, nystagmus, and slurred speech. By interfering with vitamin D metabolism and decreasing calcium absorption from the gut, phenytoin sometimes causes osteomalacia. Phenytoin adversely affects collagen metabolism and thereby contributes to **gingival hyperplasia**, a condition in which the gums can extend down over the teeth if good dental hygiene is not practiced. It can also cause excessive hair growth, known as **hirsutism**. Because of these adverse effects, phenytoin use in children should generally be avoided.

INTERACTIONS. Phenytoin induces the **CYP3A4** isozyme and **accelerates the metabolism** of other antiepileptic agents, including felbamate, lamotrigine, topiramate, and valproate.

It can also reduce levels of digoxin, steroids, vitamin K, and other drugs. In patients who are being treated with phenytoin, vitamin K supplements are given to prevent hypoprothrombinemia and bleeding. Carbamazepine induces the metabolism of phenytoin and decreases its serum levels, whereas cimetidine and other drugs inhibit the metabolism of phenytoin and increase its serum levels.

INDICATIONS. Despite its many adverse effects and drug interactions, phenytoin is widely used in the treatment of **partial seizures** and **generalized tonic-clonic seizures**. As with carbamazepine, it can worsen absence seizures and should not be used in patients with this type of seizures.

Phenobarbital and Primidone

Phenobarbital and primidone are both second-line drugs for **partial seizures** and **generalized tonic-clonic seizures**. Phenobarbital, a barbiturate, is the oldest of the currently used antiepileptic drugs. Its pharmacologic properties are discussed in Chapter 19. Primidone has two active metabolites, phenobarbital and phenylethylmalonamide (PEMA), and the parent drug and its active metabolites probably all contribute to its antiepileptic effects.

Phenobarbital enhances the GABA-mediated chloride flux that causes membrane hyperpolarization. Primidone

probably acts primarily by blocking sodium channels and preventing membrane depolarization. It can also **potentiate GABA** via formation of phenobarbital. Both primidone and phenobarbital are well absorbed from the gut, but primidone has a shorter half-life and therefore reaches steady-state levels more rapidly. Both drugs can cause ataxia, dizziness, drowsiness, and cognitive impairment. In excessive doses, they can depress respiration. **Hypersensitivity** to these drugs develops in a few patients and most frequently presents as a rash.

Valproate

PHARMACOKINETICS. Several valproate formulations are available, including the free acid form (**valproic acid**), the sodium salt of valproic acid (**valproate sodium**), and a 1:1 mixture of valproic acid and valproate sodium (**divalproex sodium**). Divalproex sodium is absorbed more slowly than the other formulations, and it usually causes fewer adverse gastrointestinal and CNS side effects. Valproate is well absorbed from the gut and is metabolized to active metabolites and inactive conjugates before it is excreted.

MECHANISMS AND EFFECTS. Valproate has **several mechanisms of action** that probably contribute to its broad spectrum of antiepileptic effects. It inhibits voltage-sensitive sodium channels and T-type calcium channels; it increases GABA synthesis and decreases GABA degradation; and it may decrease glutamate synthesis. By these actions, valproate inhibits the repetitive firing of neurons and the spread of epileptic seizures.

Valproate produces relatively little sedation or drowsiness, but it occasionally causes nausea, gastrointestinal complaints, and weight gain. Mild hepatic toxicity sometimes occurs and is usually reversible. Rarely, the drug has been associated with **fatal hepatic toxicity**. To prevent liver damage, the hepatic function of patients should be monitored when they begin therapy with valproate. Patients under 2 years of age are at the greatest risk of liver failure.

Valproate has been associated with an increased incidence of **spina bifida** and other birth defects in the offspring of women treated with the drug during pregnancy.

INTERACTIONS. Valproate inhibits the metabolism of other drugs and can increase the serum levels of lamotrigine, phenobarbital, and primidone. It can either increase or decrease the levels of carbamazepine and phenytoin, whereas these drugs decrease the levels of valproate. Because of these interactions, serum levels should always be monitored when another drug is added to or removed from the treatment regimen of a patient with seizure disorders. Patients should be warned that salicylates can increase the serum levels of valproate.

INDICATIONS. Of the various antiepileptic drugs, valproate has the **broadest spectrum of activity**. It is effective in the treatment of partial seizures and all forms of generalized seizures, and it can be given in combination with other drugs when a single drug does not adequately control seizures (see below). Valproate is also used as an alternative to lithium to treat bipolar disorder (see Chapter 22).

Adjunct Drugs for Partial Seizures

The most difficult seizures to control with drug therapy are partial seizures and, especially, complex partial seizures. Efforts, therefore, have focused on developing new drugs for these seizures. Unlike clorazepate, the other drugs discussed below were recently introduced.

Clorazepate

Clorazepate is a prodrug that is converted to diazepam in the body. Although it primarily has been used to treat patients with **anxiety disorders**, it also has been found useful as an adjunct drug for the treatment of **partial seizures**. It can cause drowsiness and lethargy, and tolerance can occur during long-term use of the drug.

Felbamate

Felbamate was a promising new drug for the treatment of partial seizures and other types of seizures until cases of **fatal aplastic anemia** and **acute hepatic failure** were reported. Since 1994, felbamate has been limited to the treatment of **partial seizures that are refractory** to other drugs. Felbamate has a unique mechanism of action in that it **blocks glycine co-activation of NMDA receptors** and thereby can inhibit processes responsible for the initiation of seizures. Efforts are under way to develop other drugs that act via this mechanism but exhibit less toxicity than felbamate.

Gabapentin

Gabapentin is a GABA analogue that appears to act by **increasing the release of GABA** from central neurons. It has no direct effect on GABA receptors itself. The absorption of gabapentin from the gut is inversely related to the dose. Because the drug has a relatively short half-life, it must be given several times a day. Gabapentin is effective when used in combination with other drugs to treat **all forms of partial seizures**, and studies indicate that for many patients it is also effective when used alone. Its adverse effects are minimal at usual therapeutic doses, but it can cause ataxia, dizziness, drowsiness, nystagmus, and tremor.

Lamotrigine

Lamotrigine blocks voltage-sensitive sodium channels and thereby interferes with neuronal membrane conduction and the release of excitatory neurotransmitters such as glutamate. It appears to be one of the more effective adjunct drugs for treating **partial seizures** in adults and children. It also appears to be useful in the treatment of **generalized tonic-clonic, atonic, and absence seizures** and in the treatment of **Lennox-Gastaut syndrome**, a syndrome characterized by multiple types of seizures in patients with mental retardation and other neurologic abnormalities.

Lamotrigine has excellent oral bioavailability. It is mostly conjugated with glucuronate in the liver and excreted by the kidneys. Serum levels of lamotrigine are decreased by carbamazepine and phenytoin and are increased by valproate. Serum levels of valproate are decreased by lamotrigine.

The primary side effects of lamotrigine include cerebellar dysfunction, drowsiness, and rash. Patients should be

advised to report early signs of skin changes, because the rash can progress to **Stevens-Johnson syndrome**. This potentially fatal syndrome, a severe form of erythema multiforme, is characterized by mucocutaneous and systemic lesions, including ocular, gastrointestinal, cardiac, renal, and pulmonary inflammation and hemorrhage. The syndrome is more common in patients who are being treated with the **combination** of lamotrigine and valproate, possibly because valproate increases the serum level of lamotrigine. If children are treated with both drugs, the dosage of lamotrigine should be lower than that used in other patients. Dosage guidelines are provided in the prescription inserts.

Topiramate

Topiramate is a monosaccharide derivative that has several **mechanisms of action**, including blockade of voltage-sensitive sodium channels; **augmentation** of GABA activation of $GABA_A$ receptors; and **blockade** of two types of glutamate receptors, namely, **kainate receptors** and α-amino-3-hydroxy-5-methyl-4-isoxazole propionic acid **(AMPA) receptors**.

Clinical studies indicate that about half of patients who have intractable partial seizures experience a 50% reduction in seizure frequency when topiramate is added to their treatment regimen. Therefore, topiramate is approved for adjunct use in the treatment of **partial seizures**. Because it has also demonstrated effectiveness as single-drug therapy (monotherapy) for partial seizures and as an adjunct in the treatment of generalized seizures, it may receive approval for these indications in the future.

Topiramate is adequately absorbed from the gut, is partly metabolized before excretion in the urine, and has a half-life of about 21 hours. Carbamazepine and phenytoin may induce the metabolism of topiramate and decrease its serum level. Topiramate may reduce the serum level of oral contraceptives. The side effects of topiramate include ataxia, dizziness, drowsiness, and other CNS effects listed in Table 20–3.

Tiagabine

Tiagabine binds to recognition sites associated with the GABA reuptake transport protein. By this action, tiagabine **blocks GABA reuptake** into presynaptic neurons, permitting greater levels of GABA in the synapse.

Levetiracetam

The mechanism of action for **levetiracetam** is not clearly delineated. *In vitro* and *in vivo* recordings of epileptiform activity from the hippocampus have shown that levetiracetam inhibits burst firing without affecting normal neuronal excitability, suggesting that levetiracetam selectively prevents hypersynchronization of burst firing and propagation of seizure activity. It does not appear to directly facilitate GABAergic neurotransmission, but has been shown to oppose the activity of negative modulators of GABA- and glycine-gated currents in neuronal cell culture. A saturable and stereoselective neuronal binding site in rat brain tissue has been described for levetiracetam; however, the identification and function of this binding site is currently unknown. It has shown exceptional promise as an adjunct drug in treating **partial seizures** in children.

Zonisamide

Zonisamide acts at **sodium channels** and voltage-dependent, transient inward currents of **calcium channels** (low-threshold, T-type Ca^{2+} currents). Zonisamide blocks Na^+ channels in the inactivated state and reduces the ion flow in Ca^{2+} channel proteins.

Pregabalin

The most recently approved drug for seizure disorders in the United States, **pregabalin** binds to the alpha$_2$-delta site on an auxiliary subunit of voltage-gated calcium channels and **reduces the calcium current**. This action may be responsible for its antiseizure effects, as well as analgesic effects, as it is also indicated for **neuropathic pain** associated with diabetes, **postherpetic neuralgia**, and the first drug approved specifically for **fibromyalgia**.

Vigabatrin

Vigabatrin is an **irreversible inhibitor** of γ-aminobutyric acid transaminase (GABA-T), the enzyme responsible for the breakdown of GABA in the brain. The inhibition of the GABA-T enzyme leads to increased levels of the inhibitory neurotransmitter, GABA. It is not yet available in the United States, but prescribed in Canada and Europe.

Drugs for Generalized Absence, Myoclonic, or Atonic Seizures

Ethosuximide

PHARMACOKINETICS. Ethosuximide is the most effective and least toxic of the several succinimide derivatives that have been used to treat epilepsy over the past 50 years. It is well absorbed from the gut, widely distributed to tissues, and metabolized to inactive compounds before it is excreted in the urine. Ethosuximide has a **long half-life** of about 30 hours in children and 55 hours in adults.

MECHANISMS AND EFFECTS. Ethosuximide **inhibits T-type calcium channels** in thalamic neurons. These low-threshold channels are believed to be responsible for the pacemaker current that generates the synchronous 3-Hz (three cycles per second) spike-and-dome depolarizations observed in the EEG during absence seizures (see Fig. 20–1). Ethosuximide produces little toxicity, but it can cause dizziness, drowsiness, gastric distress, and nausea, which can usually be minimized by starting treatment with lower doses and then gradually increasing doses to the desired level.

INTERACTIONS. Valproate inhibits the metabolism of ethosuximide and increases its serum levels. **Haloperidol**, a high-potency antipsychotic drug, can alter the seizure pattern in patients treated with ethosuximide. No other important interactions have been identified.

INDICATIONS. Ethosuximide is safe and highly effective in the treatment of generalized absence seizures in children and is the drug of choice for this particular group of patients. Ethosuximide is not very effective, however, in the

treatment of adults with absence seizures or of patients with other types of seizures, so valproate (discussed above) is often used instead.

Clonazepam and Other Drugs

Clonazepam is a benzodiazepine that is used to treat **absence, myoclonic, and atonic seizures**. It often produces more sedation than other antiepileptic drugs when used at doses that suppress seizures.

Because the efficacy of valproate is equal to or greater than that of clonazepam, it is frequently used instead to treat patients with absence, myoclonic, and atonic seizures.

Lamotrigine is sometimes used as an adjunct for the treatment of absence and atonic seizures.

The pharmacologic properties of valproate and lamotrigine are discussed earlier in this chapter, and those of clonazepam are discussed in Chapter 19.

Drugs for Status Epilepticus

Status epilepticus is a life-threatening emergency. Patients with this condition have recurrent episodes of tonic-clonic seizures without regaining consciousness or normal muscle movement between episodes. If their seizures are not controlled, prolonged hypoxia can lead to **severe brain damage**. Immediate attention must be given to cardiopulmonary support and to the administration of drugs that rapidly terminate the seizures. In fact, published reports indicate that seizures must be controlled within 60 minutes of the onset of an episode in order to have a favorable prognosis.

The drug of choice for status epilepticus is **diazepam** or **lorazepam**. Either drug is administered as a slow intravenous injection given every 10 to 15 minutes until seizures are controlled or a maximal dosage has been administered. The pharmacologic properties of these drugs are described in Chapter 19.

After diazepam or lorazepam is administered, **phenytoin** (or the newer form, **fosphenytoin**) is often administered intravenously to provide a longer duration of seizure control than is provided by a benzodiazepine. Large doses of **phenobarbital** may be effective if a benzodiazepine or phenytoin fails to control the seizures. In highly resistant cases, general anesthesia can be used to control the seizures.

THE MANAGEMENT OF SEIZURE DISORDERS

The effective management of patients with epilepsy requires an accurate diagnosis of the type of seizures that occur and also requires the rational selection and use of drugs.

First-Line Drugs

For **partial seizures** and **generalized tonic-clonic seizures**, carbamazepine, phenytoin, and valproate are first-line drugs, and phenobarbital and primidone are second-line drugs. Carbamazepine generally causes fewer adverse effects than phenytoin, although phenytoin can be slightly less sedating than carbamazepine at equally effective doses. Of the

several drugs that have been recently developed as adjunct medications for partial seizures, lamotrigine and topiramate appear particularly attractive at this time. The relative safety and efficacy of these drugs are still being evaluated.

For **generalized absence seizures**, ethosuximide is clearly the first choice in treating children with this condition, which usually has its onset during childhood and often remits during adolescence. Valproate is generally more effective in treating adults with absence seizures and in treating patients with multiple types of seizures.

For **generalized myoclonic and atonic seizures**, valproate is the drug of choice.

For **status epilepticus**, intravenous treatment with diazepam or lorazepam can be followed by intravenous treatment with fosphenytoin or phenobarbital.

Principles of Drug Use

In most cases, an attempt should be made to control seizures with single-drug therapy (monotherapy) because this will minimize side effects, reduce costs, and increase patient compliance.

Unless the patient is experiencing frequent seizures, it is usually best to start with a single drug and give it in a low dose (one fourth to one third of the therapeutic dose). The dose can be gradually increased until effective serum concentrations are achieved or intolerable adverse effects occur. Starting with a low dose enables the patient to develop tolerance to the CNS side effects of antiepileptic drugs and improves compliance.

If a single drug has significantly reduced the occurrence of seizures but has not eliminated them, it is usually prudent to add another drug to the regimen, rather than to switch to a new drug. Two drugs acting by different mechanisms may control seizures when a single drug is not adequate. The second drug should be given initially in a low dose, and the dosage should be gradually increased until therapeutic concentrations are reached or adverse effects occur. Because of the many interactions between antiepileptic drugs (see Table 20–4), the doses that are both safe and effective for combination therapy may differ from the doses that are safe and effective for monotherapy. For example, lamotrigine causes a much higher incidence of serious **dermatologic toxicity in children** who are concurrently taking valproate, and lamotrigine should be started at much lower doses in these patients.

Once a satisfactory drug regimen is achieved, the patient should be monitored periodically for drug toxicity and efficacy. Serum drug levels should be determined if there is evidence or suspicion of adverse effects, therapeutic failure, or patient noncompliance.

The appropriate duration of antiepileptic drug therapy is a topic of considerable controversy. If a patient who is undergoing drug therapy has not had a seizure for several years, it seems prudent to consider slowly withdrawing the medication, because this will minimize long-term side effects and offer life-style benefits and cost savings. About 25% of patients who withdraw from medication will relapse within 1 year, however. Factors that increase the likelihood of relapse include onset of seizures during adolescence, occurrence of complex partial seizures or generalized seizures, and abnormal interictal findings on EEGs. If antiepileptic

medication is to be discontinued, the dosage should be tapered slowly over several weeks, because abrupt withdrawal from medication is associated with a higher incidence of rebound seizures.

CASE PRESENTATION: Suzy B., a 7-year-old girl of good health with normal development and intelligence, is having problems keeping up with her classroom activities at school. Her parents are called to the school to meet her teacher and are told that Suzy is not paying attention and at times seems to be "spacing out" with a blank stare and is unresponsive to the teacher's questions. The teacher says that at times Suzy "blanks out" from 10 to 15 seconds at a time, sometimes with repetitive blinking. She states that after these episodes, Suzy seems fine and behaves as if nothing happened and reports that on some days, Suzy may have five or more of these episodes. The concerned parents take Suzy to a neurologist who obtains an EEG trace while Suzy is having one of these episodes. He notes a characteristic 3-Hz spike-and-dome pattern and tells the parents that Suzy has absence seizures. He starts Suzy on a course of ethosuximide at 250 mg twice a day. Suzy returns to school, and her teacher calls the concerned parents in a few days to report that Suzy is no longer having any more episodes.

CASE DISCUSSION: Absence seizures (also called *petit mal* seizures) usually less than 10 seconds, but they can last as long as 20 seconds. The seizures begin and end suddenly, and during the seizure, awareness and responsiveness are impaired. Children who have a seizure are not usually aware that they have had one and are completely alert immediately afterward. Simple absence seizures are just "stares." Many absence seizures are complex absence seizures, meaning that muscle activity, such as blinking, occurs. Absence seizures usually begin between ages 4 and 12 and occur in children with normal development and intelligence. The most effective medications for absence seizures include ethosuximide, valproic acid, and lamotrigine. Most children take the medicine for 2 years and then, if no episodes have occurred, can usually discontinue antiseizure medications with a good prognosis. In about 75% of cases, absence seizures stop by the age of 18. Children who develop absence seizures before age 9 have a better prognosis for spontaneous remission than children whose absence seizures start after age 10.

A number of the antiseizure agents are currently in clinical trials for various other indications including bipolar disorder, trigeminal neuralgia, fibromyalgia, and neuropathic pain states, and others. They are also being used "off-label" for these disorders and others. Significantly, in 2008 the FDA issued a **warning letter** of increased risk of suicidal thoughts and behaviors (**suicidality**) in patients who take these drugs, which may limit expansion of these agents for wider indications.

SUMMARY OF IMPORTANT POINTS

■ Seizures are caused by episodic, synchronous neuronal discharges in the cerebral cortex or elsewhere in the brain. They are classified as partial or generalized seizures on the basis of their clinical characteristics and electroencephalographic pattern.

■ Some antiepileptic drugs work by blocking voltage sensitive sodium channels or T-type calcium channels. Others augment inhibitory GABA neurotransmission or block excitatory glutamate neurotransmission.

■ Carbamazepine, phenytoin, and valproate are the first-line drugs for partial seizures and generalized tonic-clonic seizures.

■ Ethosuximide is the drug of choice for generalized absence seizures in children. Valproate and clonazepam are effective in absence, myoclonic, and atonic seizures.

■ Gabapentin, lamotrigine, topiramate, and several other new drugs are used as adjuncts in the treatment of partial seizures, and some of these agents have activity against other types of seizures.

■ Status epilepticus is a medical emergency that requires intravenous administration of diazepam or lorazepam, sometimes followed by intravenous use of phenytoin (fosphenytoin) or phenobarbital.

■ Many antiepileptic drugs interact with other medications. Carbamazepine and phenytoin induce cytochrome P450 enzymes and decrease serum levels of the drugs with which they interact, whereas valproate inhibits the metabolism of the drugs with which it interacts.

■ Antiepileptic drugs frequently produce CNS and gastrointestinal side effects, and some drugs cause infrequent but severe hematologic or hepatic toxicity. Valproate and phenytoin are known to cause birth defects, and both of these drugs can reduce folate levels.

■ Except in urgent situations, antiepileptic therapy should begin with a low dose of a single drug, and the dosage should be increased until the desired serum concentration or full dosage is achieved. If a single drug is not effective, another drug can be added to the regimen or substituted. Drug use should be discontinued slowly. Serum levels should be monitored to verify adequate dosage and whenever toxicity, therapeutic failure, or noncompliance occurs or is suspected.

Review Questions

1. The molecular mechanism underlying the antiepileptic effects of carbamazepine and phenytoin is best described by which one of the following statements?
   (A) inhibiting low threshold Ca^{2+} ion channels
   (B) prolonging the inactivation of the Na^+ ion channel
   (C) potentiating the release of GABA by inhibiting GABA reuptake
   (D) increasing the release of GABA by vesicular fusion
   (E) blocking glutamate receptor excitation

2. Which antiepileptic agent gained wider therapeutic use also to treat trigeminal neuralgia and the manic phase of bipolar disorder?
   (A) ethosuximide
   (B) zonisamide
   (C) levetiracetam
   (D) carbamazepine
   (E) phenytoin

3. Which one of the following agents is considered the drug of choice for initial treatment of generalized absence seizure (petit mal) in children?
   (A) ethosuximide
   (B) zonisamide
   (C) levetiracetam
   (D) carbamazepine
   (E) phenytoin

4. Topiramate has which set of three mechanisms of action?
   (A) increases Na^+ channel inactivation, increases GABA, blocks glutamate
   (B) decreases Na^+ channel inactivation, decreases GABA, blocks glutamate
   (C) increases Ca^{2+} channel inactivation, increases GABA, blocks glutamate
   (D) decreases Ca^{2+} channel inactivation, increases GABA, blocks glutamate
   (E) decreases Ca^{2+} channel flow, increases GABA, blocks glutamate

5. Gabapentin has which mechanism of action?
   (A) inhibits monoamine oxidase
   (B) agonist effect at dopamine receptors
   (C) increases Na^+ channel inactivation
   (D) blocks reuptake of neurotransmitters
   (E) increases release of neurotransmitter

Answers and Explanations

1. **The correct answer is B: prolonging the inactivation of the Na^+ ion channel.** Both these agents bind to the Na^+ channel protein and prolong the state of inactivation. This leads to a decrease of repetitively firing neurons. Answer (A), inhibiting low threshold Ca^{2+} ion channels, is the mechanism of action of ethosuximide and valproic acid, particularly useful in controlling absence seizures. Answer (C), potentiating the release of GABA by inhibiting GABA reuptake, is the mechanism of action of tiagabine. Answer (D), increasing the release of GABA by vesicular fusion, is the action of gabapentin, although the precise mechanisms are unknown. Answer (E), blocking glutamate receptor excitation, is part of the mechanism of action of topiramate.

2. **The correct choice is D: carbamazepine.** This agent has also gained approval for the use as an antimanic agent or mood stabilizer, for treatment of bipolar disorder and for trigeminal neuralgia. Answer (A), ethosuximide, is the drug of choice for treating absence seizures in children. Answers (B), zonisamide, and (C), levetiracetam, are approved only for adjunct treatment of partial seizures. Answer (E), phenytoin, has gained some acclaim as a mood stabilizer but has not been mentioned for use in trigeminal neuralgia.

3. **The correct answer is A: ethosuximide.** Ethosuximide acts by inhibiting the low-threshold Ca^{2+} channels thought to be active during absence seizures. Answers (B), zonisamide, and (C), levetiracetam, are newer agents for the treatment of partial seizures. Answers (D), carbamazepine, and (E), phenytoin, are classic drugs used to treat partial seizures and generalized tonic-clonic seizures.

4. **The correct answer is A: increases Na^+ channel inactivation, increases GABA, blocks glutamate.** Topiramate is a newer agent with three known mechanisms of action. The other answers (B) through (E) contain at least one mechanism of action that would produce greater excitation of neurons, or is not a mechanism of topiramate.

5. **The correct choice is E: increases release of neurotransmitter.** Gabapentin is an analogue of GABA and is known to cause greater release of GABA from neurons but the precise mechanism is unknown. Answer (A), inhibits monoamine oxidase, is an action of certain types of antidepressant drugs. Answer (B), agonist effect at dopamine receptors, is an action of some antiparkinsonism agents. Answer (C), increases Na^+ channel inactivation, and answer (D), blocks reuptake of neurotransmitters, describes the action of the newer antiepileptic agent, tiagabine.

SELECTED READINGS

Johannessen-Landmark, C. Antiepileptic drugs in non-epilepsy disorders: relations between mechanisms of action and clinical efficacy. CNS Drugs 22:27–47, 2008.

Karceski, S.C. Seizure medications and their side effects. Neurology 69:E27–29, 2007.

McCorry, D., D. Chadwick, and A. Marson. Current drug treatment of epilepsy in adults. Lancet Neurol 3:729–735, 2004.

Vezzani, A. The promise of gene therapy for the treatment of epilepsy. Expert Rev Neurother 7:1685–1692, 2007.

Yogeeswari, P., J.V. Ragavendran, R. Thirumurugan, A. Saxena, D. Sriram. Ion channels as important targets for antiepileptic drug design. Curr Drug Targets 5:589–602, 2004.

Local and General Anesthetics

CLASSIFICATION OF LOCAL AND GENERAL ANESTHETICS

Local Anesthetics
Ester-Type Drugs
- Cocaine
- Procaine (NOVOCAIN)
- Benzocaine (AMERICAINE)
- Chloroprocaine (NESACAINE)[a]

Amide-Type Drugs
- Lidocaine (XYLOCAINE)
- Bupivacaine (MARCAINE)
- Etidocaine (DURANEST)
- Prilocaine (CITANEST)
- Ropivacaine (NAROPIN)[b]

General Anesthetics
Inhalational Anesthetics
- Nitrous oxide
- Halothane (FLUOTHANE)
- Desflurane (SUPRANE)
- Isoflurane (FORANE)

- Sevoflurane (ULTANE)[c]
- Dantrolene (DANTRIUM)*

Parenteral Anesthetics
- Thiopental (PENTOTHAL)
- Methohexital (BREVITAL)
- Midazolam (VERSED)
- Ketamine (KETALAR)
- Propofol (DIPRIVAN)
- Etomidate (AMIDATE)
- Fentanyl (SUBLIMAZE)[d]

*Dantrolene is not an anesthetic, but used to treat malignant hyperthermia.
[a]Also tetracaine (PONTOCAINE), proparacaine (OPHTHAINE), and dibucaine (NUPERCAINAL).
[b]Also levobupivacaine (CHIROCAINE) and mepivacaine (CARBOCAINE).
[c]Also enflurane (ETHRANE).
[d]Also sufentanil (SUFENTA), alfentanil (ALFENTA), and remifentanil (ULTIVA).

OVERVIEW

Anesthesia is the loss of all sensation, whereas analgesia is the selective loss of pain sensation. Local anesthetics block the conduction of nerve impulses in the peripheral nerves or spinal cord. General anesthetics block cortical neuronal activity underlying consciousness and all sensation.

Local anesthetics, which are used to anesthetize a particular part or region of the body, are given to patients undergoing surgery on the skin and subcutaneous tissues, ears, eyes, joints, or pelvis. They are also used for anesthesia during labor and delivery and for diagnostic procedures such as gastrointestinal endoscopy. Occasionally, local anesthetics are used to relieve pain associated with pathologic conditions.

General anesthetics are used to prevent consciousness during major surgical procedures. Unlike local anesthetics, general anesthetics produce loss of consciousness and amnesia and thereby prevent the anesthetized patient from recalling the surgical procedure.

LOCAL ANESTHETICS

Drug Properties

Chemistry and Pharmacokinetics

Based on their chemical structure, local anesthetics can be divided into **ester-type** drugs and **amide-type** drugs. Each local anesthetic has a lipophilic (hydrophobic) portion and a hydrophilic portion (Fig. 21–1). The hydrophilic portion, an amine that is a weak base, exists in both ionized and non-ionized forms. The ionized, protonated form predominates at lower pH levels, and the non-ionized, unprotonated form predominates at higher pH levels. Only the non-ionized form can **penetrate neuronal membranes** to reach binding sites on the internal surface of sodium channels. Inflammation and acidosis decrease the pH of tissues, thereby increasing the ionization of local anesthetics. For this reason, local anesthetics are less effective in the presence of these conditions, requiring larger doses.

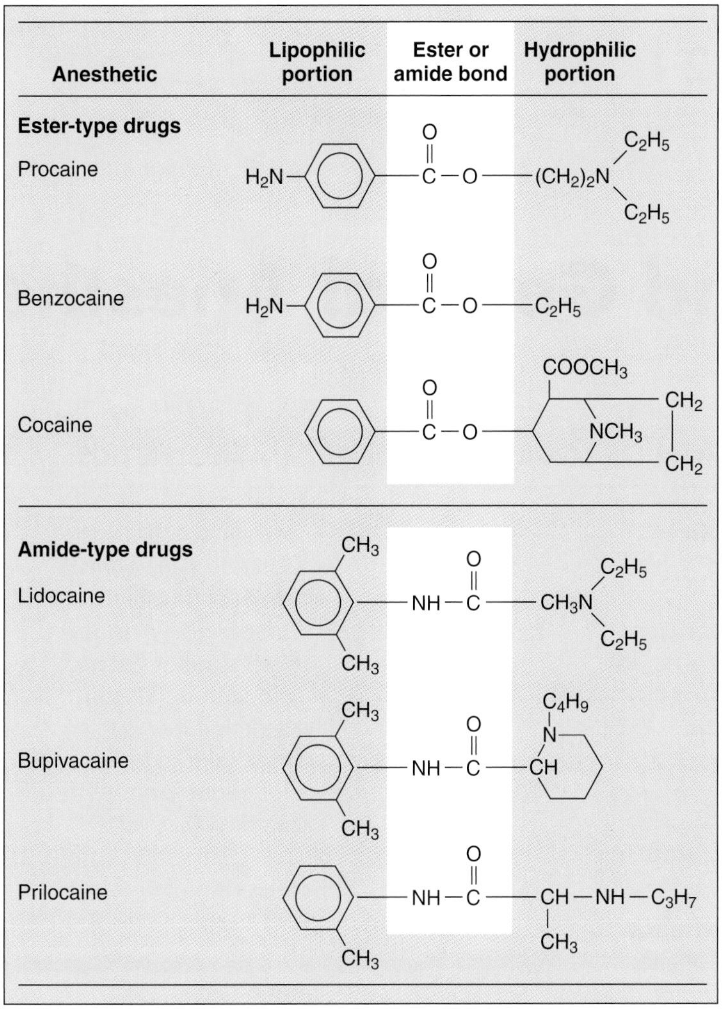

Figure 21–1. Structures of selected local anesthetics.

Local anesthetics are formulated as hydrochloride salts with a pH less than 7, as the ionized molecule is more soluble and stable than the free base. Once injected, the local anesthetic solution is quickly buffered to the pH of the tissue.

The duration of action of local anesthetics can be **short, medium, or long** (Table 21–1). Because local anesthetics act directly at the site of administration, their duration of action is determined primarily by the rate of diffusion and absorption away from the site of administration. Diffusion and absorption, in turn, depend on the chemical properties of the anesthetics and on such factors as local pH and blood flow. In some formulations, **epinephrine** is added to prolong a local anesthetic's duration of action by producing vasoconstriction and slowing its rate of absorption. Because of the risk of ischemia and necrosis, however, local anesthetics with epinephrine are not used to anesthetize tissues with end arteries, such as tissues of the fingers, toes, ears, nose, and penis.

Following systemic absorption, **ester-type local anesthetics** are metabolized in the plasma by butyrylcholinesterases to *p*-aminobenzoic acid (PABA) derivatives. **Amide-type local anesthetics** undergo metabolism by hepatic P450 enzymes to yield polar metabolites. In both cases, the metabolites are excreted in the urine.

Mechanism of Action

Local anesthetics cause a reversible inhibition of action potential conduction by **binding to the sodium channel** and decreasing the nerve membrane permeability to sodium. The nonpolar, lipophilic form of the anesthetic molecule passes through the neuronal membrane and switches to the polar, hydrophilic form in the cytoplasm of the neuron. This cationic form of the anesthetic binds to the cytoplasmic side of the sodium channel protein and **prolongs the inactivation state** of the sodium channel (Fig. 21–2). With sodium channels blocked, action potentials cannot propagate along the neuronal fiber and sensory input is lost.

Pharmacologic Effects

Local anesthetics have a greater affinity for sodium channels that are in the depolarized (open) configuration than for channels that are closed. Nerve fibers that are firing, therefore, are more susceptible to sodium channel blockade. This **use-dependent blockade** causes a selective inhibition of nerve fibers that are stimulated by the surgical procedure, such as pain fibers during suturing. **Size-dependent blockade** refers to the finding that small diameter fibers are

TABLE 21–1. Properties of Selected Local Anesthetics

Drug	Potency	Duration of Action*	Parenteral Uses	Topical Uses
Ester-Type Drugs				
Procaine	Low	Short	Infiltration, nerve block, and spinal anesthesia	None
Benzocaine	Low	Medium	None	Dermal, laryngeal, and oral
Chloroprocaine	Low	Short	Epidural, infiltration, and nerve block anesthesia	None
Cocaine	Low	Medium	None	Laryngeal, nasal, and urogenital
Amide-Type Drugs				
Lidocaine	Intermediate	Short	Epidural, infiltration, nerve block, and spinal anesthesia	Dermal, laryngeal, and oral
Bupivacaine	High	Medium	Epidural, infiltration, nerve block, and spinal anesthesia	None
Etidocaine	Intermediate	Long	Infiltration and nerve block anesthesia	None
Mepivacaine	Intermediate	Short	Epidural, infiltration, nerve block, and spinal anesthesia	None
Prilocaine	Intermediate	Short	Infiltration anesthesia	Dermal
Ropivacaine	High	Long	Epidural, infiltration, and nerve block anesthesia	None

*The duration varies with the dose and route of administration. Short = 0.25–1.5 hours; medium = >1.5–5 hours; and long = >5 hours.

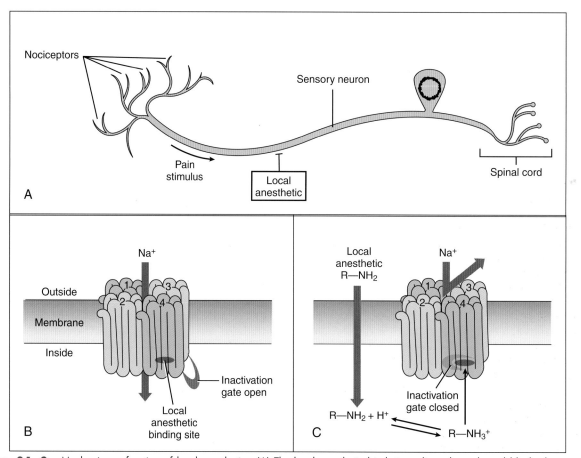

Figure 21–2. Mechanisms of action of local anesthetics. (A) The local anesthetic binds to sodium channels and blocks the generation and conduction of action potentials in peripheral neurons. (B) The sodium channel includes four large transmembrane domains, each with six transmembrane spanning regions. The inactivation gate is a short, intracellular loop between domains 3 and 4. The local anesthetic binds to amino acid residues located on domain 4. (C) The non-ionized form of the local anesthetic (R—NH$_2$) penetrates the axonal membrane and is then converted to the ionized form (R—NH$_3^+$). The ionized form binds to the sodium channel in the open state, and this prolongs the sodium channel inactivation state. Sodium entry is blocked during the inactivation state.

blocked more easily than are larger fibers. Small unmyelinated **C** and lightly myelinated **Aδ** pain fibers, therefore, are more easily anesthetized than are large myelinated touch fibers. Autonomic and sensory nerves are blocked more easily than are motor nerves. Nerves recover from blockade in the reverse order.

Adverse Effects and Interactions

The adverse effects of local anesthetics are primarily caused by their absorption into the systemic circulation and subsequent alteration of **central nervous system (CNS), cardiovascular**, and other organ system functions.

Local anesthetics often produce **CNS stimulation** (restlessness, tremor, and euphoria) followed by **inhibition** (drowsiness and sedation). Other symptoms of local anesthetic toxicity include headache, paresthesias, and nausea. Higher concentrations can cause seizures followed by coma. Death is usually caused by respiratory failure.

Adverse cardiovascular effects include **hypotension** and **cardiac depression**. Most local anesthetics are vasodilators, and they also block vasoconstriction induced by the sympathetic nervous system. Most local anesthetics have **antiarrhythmic activity**, but toxic levels of local anesthetics suppress cardiac conduction and can cause tachyarrhythmia characterized by a wide QRS complex.

Local anesthetic **blockade of autonomic ganglia** and **neuromuscular transmission** can lead to loss of visceral and skeletal muscle tone. For this reason, local anesthetics potentiate the effect of neuromuscular blocking drugs (e.g., tubocurarine) and must be used with great caution in patients with **myasthenia gravis**.

Allergic reactions to local anesthetics are fairly common. Patients who have repeated applications of topical anesthetics are particularly susceptible to sensitization. The ester-type anesthetics cause **hypersensitivity reactions** more frequently than do the amide-type anesthetics. This is because ester-type anesthetics (e.g., procaine) are metabolized to PABA. PABA causes allergic reactions in a small percentage of individuals. Patients who are allergic to an ester-type anesthetic will usually tolerate an amide-type anesthetic.

Indications

Local anesthetics are usually administered parenterally but are sometimes applied topically. The route of administration depends on factors such as the site of anesthesia.

TOPICAL ANESTHESIA. The topical application of local anesthetics is used to anesthetize the skin, mucous membranes, or cornea. A local anesthetic can be applied to the skin to treat **pruritus** (itching) caused by poison ivy, insect bites, eczema, or cutaneous manifestations of systemic diseases such as chickenpox (varicella). A eutectic mixture of local anesthetics (EMLA), consisting of two or more solid compounds that form a liquid when they are combined, is sometimes used to anesthetize the skin before venipuncture or minor surgery. The topical application of a local anesthetic to mucous membranes can **relieve pain** caused by oral, nasal, laryngeal, rectal disorders, or surgery. For example, an anesthetic ointment is used to relieve the discomfort of hemorrhoids. The topical ocular

administration of local anesthetics is used to anesthetize the cornea before diagnostic or surgical procedures (e.g., radial keratotomy), the removal of foreign bodies, and cataract surgery.

INFILTRATION ANESTHESIA. Infiltration is probably the most common route used to administer local anesthetics. The process involves injecting an anesthetic directly into **subcutaneous tissue** just under the skin. Infiltration is used primarily for minor surgical procedures (e.g., suturing a wound) or for the removal of foreign bodies. It is also frequently used for dental procedures. When a local anesthetic is to be administered by infiltration, epinephrine can be added to it to decrease its dosage and prolong its duration of action. As mentioned earlier, however, **epinephrine** should not be used to anesthetize fingers, toes, and other tissues with end arteries.

IONTOPHORESIS. Local anesthetics can also be administered by iontophoresis. This technique uses a small electric current to force molecules of the anesthetic into the tissue. Iontophoresis is used primarily in dentistry. It eliminates the need to inject the anesthetic and is used by some dentists for this reason. A new, **needle-free device** with the trade name of ZINGO delivers powdered **lidocaine** by rapid gas pressure to reduce the pain of subsequent peripheral injections or blood draws. It is approved for use in children.

NERVE BLOCK AND FIELD BLOCK ANESTHESIA. Nerve block and field block anesthesia are forms of regional anesthesia, the goal of which is to anesthetize an area of the body by blocking the conductivity of sensory nerves from that area. In nerve block anesthesia, a local anesthetic is injected into or **adjacent to a peripheral nerve or nerve plexus**. For example, a radial nerve block can be used to anesthetize the structures innervated by the radial nerve, including portions of the forearm and hand. **Intraorbital block** is often used for ocular surgery. Other examples of nerve block anesthesia are brachial plexus and cervical plexus blocks. In field block anesthesia, a local anesthetic is administered in a series of injections to form a wall of anesthesia encircling the operative field.

SPINAL INTRATHECAL ANESTHESIA. Spinal anesthesia is used to block somatic sensory and motor fibers during procedures such as surgery on the lower limb or pelvic structures. A local anesthetic is injected into the subarachnoid, intrathecal space below the level at which the spinal cord terminates. The spread of the anesthetic along the neuraxis is controlled by the horizontal tilt of the patient and by the **specific gravity** (baricity) of the local anesthetic solution. Hyperbaric solutions of local anesthetics are available for this purpose, and these spread along the neuraxis for about 15 minutes. By this time, they have mixed with cerebrospinal fluid to become isobaric and are said to be "fixed" at a certain level of the spinal cord. Spinal anesthesia can cause headaches associated with cerebrospinal fluid leakage from the **lumbar puncture**, and respiratory depression can occur if the anesthetic ascends too high up the spinal cord. Entry into the CNS by spinal injection also carries a small risk of infection or meningitis.

EPIDURAL ANESTHESIA. Epidural anesthesia is produced by injecting a local anesthetic into the lumbar or caudal epidural (extradural) space. A local anesthetic, such as bupivacaine, is often administered by this route to provide **anesthesia during labor and delivery**. After epidural administration, the local anesthetic is absorbed into the systemic circulation. Therefore, doses must be carefully monitored to prevent cardiac depression and neurotoxicity in the mother and neonate.

SPECIFIC AGENTS

Ester-Type Local Anesthetics

Cocaine, a naturally occurring plant alkaloid, was the first local anesthetic to be discovered. It has both local anesthetic and CNS stimulant properties, and it is the only local anesthetic that causes significant vasoconstriction as a result of its **sympathomimetic effect**. Because of its CNS effects and potential for abuse (see Chapter 25), cocaine is seldom used as a local anesthetic. It is occasionally used, however, to anesthetize the internal structures of the nose, where its vasoconstrictive action helps prevent bleeding after nasal surgery. A cocaine solution is applied to gauze and inserted into the nose for this purpose.

Procaine, the first synthetic local anesthetic drug to be prepared after the discovery of cocaine, became the standard of comparison for many years. Procaine and **chloroprocaine** have a low potency and a relatively short duration of action. They are not effective after topical administration and must be administered parenterally. Both drugs are metabolized to PABA. For this reason, they are more likely to cause **allergic reactions** than are the amide-type local anesthetics. Tetracaine is another ester-type local anesthetic with a longer duration of action than procaine. It is used for infiltration anesthesia. It is also available in a topical spray and gel formulation in combination with butamben (butyl aminobenzoate) and benzocaine in a preparation called CETACAINE.

Benzocaine, a frequently used topical anesthetic, is available in a number of nonprescription products for the treatment of **sunburn**, **pruritus**, and other skin conditions. In some patients, the drug causes hypersensitivity reactions, which can exacerbate preexisting dermatitis. Benzocaine is also used to **anesthetize mucous membranes** and is available in cough lozenges and sprays to relieve coughing.

Proparacaine is available in a 0.5% solution for instillation during eye surgery and other ophthalmic procedures. **Dibucaine** is formulated in an ointment used to relieve the pain and itching of hemorrhoids (piles) and other problems in the rectal area.

Amide-Type Local Anesthetics

Lidocaine produces local anesthesia after topical or parenteral administration. The most widely used local anesthetic, it is available in a number of formulations. These include topical solutions and ointments, oral sprays, viscous gels for oral and laryngeal application, and various parenteral formulations. A eutectic mixture of **lidocaine** and **prilocaine** is available as a cream to anesthetize intact skin to a depth of 5 mm. In pediatric patients, **EMLA cream** has been used for local anesthesia before venipuncture, intravenous cannulation, or circumcision. Lidocaine is also used for infiltration, nerve block, epidural, and spinal anesthesia.

Etidocaine has properties similar to those of lidocaine, but its duration of action is considerably longer. It is primarily used for infiltration and nerve block anesthesia.

Bupivacaine, mepivacaine, and **ropivacaine** have similar clinical uses but differ in their duration of action, as shown in Table 21–1. **Bupivacaine** has been the most widely used local anesthetic for obstetrical anesthesia, but it causes cardiac depression more frequently than do many other local anesthetics. **Ropivacaine** is a newer drug that may cause fewer cases of cardiac toxicity. **Levobupivacaine** is the isolated S(-)-stereoisomer of racemic bupivacaine, which is the active form of the chiral drug mixture. It is used in epidural anesthesia for labor and delivery.

Prilocaine is a congener of lidocaine. It is converted to O-toluidine, a **toxic metabolite** that can cause methemoglobinemia if it is allowed to accumulate. For this reason, prilocaine use is limited to topical and infiltration anesthesia.

GENERAL ANESTHETICS

The first demonstration of general anesthesia for surgery was performed by William Morton at Massachusetts General Hospital in 1846. The anesthetic that Morton used was **diethyl ether**, and his demonstration had a profound impact on the field of surgery. Before that time, surgery was limited to rapid procedures such as limb amputations. General anesthesia and the subsequent development of aseptic techniques permitted the evolution of surgical procedures to the sophisticated level achieved today.

Diethyl ether is no longer used in developed countries, because it has a slow rate of induction, causes considerable postoperative nausea and vomiting, and is highly flammable. Use of another anesthetic gas, cyclopropane, has also been abandoned, because of its explosive nature and its tendency to cause cardiac arrhythmias. A variety of anesthetics are currently available for inhalational use, however. These include **nitrous oxide** and a growing number of halogenated hydrocarbons. The pharmacologic properties and adverse effects of these drugs are listed in Tables 21–2 and 21–3, respectively.

INHALATIONAL ANESTHETICS

Drug Properties

Pharmacokinetics

The inhalational anesthetics are divided into **nonhalogenated** drugs and **halogenated** drugs. These anesthetics are either gases or volatile liquids whose gaseous phase can be inhaled.

The **potency** of inhalational anesthetics is expressed in terms of the inspired concentration of the anesthetic required to produce anesthesia in half of the subjects. This is called the **minimal alveolar concentration**. The minimal alveolar concentration value is used to compare potency among different inhalational agents similar to the median effective dose of other drugs.

TABLE 21-2. **Properties of Inhalation Anesthetics**

Drug	Minimum Alveolar Concentration (% Vol/Vol)*	Blood:Gas Partition Coefficient	Rate of Induction	Amount Metabolized	Amount of Skeletal Muscle Relaxation
Nonhalogenated Drugs					
Nitrous oxide	>100	0.47	Fast	0%	None
Halogenated Drugs					
Desflurane	6.0	0.42	Fast	<2%	Medium
Enflurane	1.7	1.9	Medium	5% (fluoride)	Medium
Halothane	0.75	2.3	Slow	20%	Low
Isoflurane	1.2	1.4	Medium	<2% (fluoride)	Medium
Sevoflurane	1.9	0.63	Fast	<2%	Medium

*The minimum alveolar concentration (MAC) is the concentration needed to produce anesthesia in half of the subjects.

TABLE 21-3. **Adverse Effects of Inhalational Anesthetics**

Drug	Airway Irritation	Respiratory Depression	Bronchodilation	Hypotensive Effect	Arrhythmia Potential*
Nonhalogenated Drugs					
Nitrous oxide	Low	None	None	None	None
Halogenated Drugs					
Desflurane	Moderate	Low	None	Reduced systemic vascular resistance	Low
Enflurane	Low	Moderate	Moderate	Reduced cardiac output	Low
Halothane	Moderate	Low	Moderate	Reduced cardiac output	Moderate
Isoflurane	Moderate	Moderate	Moderate	Reduced systemic vascular resistance	Low
Sevoflurane	Low	Low	None	Reduced systemic vascular resistance	Low

*Anesthetics that sensitize the heart to catecholamines have the potential to cause epinephrine-induced arrhythmias.

The pharmacokinetics of inhalational anesthetics differs from those of other drugs because the gaseous anesthetics are absorbed and eliminated through the same organ, the lungs. Moreover, as the activity of inhalational agents is caused by anesthetic molecules in the gas phase, molecules that enter the liquid phase and become soluble in the blood decrease the onset of anesthesia. The movement of anesthetic molecules between the lungs and other tissues is determined by the **partial pressure** of the anesthetic and, as the anesthetic's partial pressure in the blood increases, molecules of the anesthetic move across the blood-brain barrier into the brain and produce anesthesia.

The **induction rate** of anesthesia is determined by three primary factors: (1) the alveolar partial pressure of the anesthetic in the inspired air, (2) the ventilation rate, and (3) the rate at which the anesthetic's partial pressure in the blood increases as the anesthetic is administered. This third factor is largely dependent on the **blood:gas partition coefficient** (Box 21–1).

Because anesthetic molecules move from an area of higher partial pressure to an area of lower partial pressure,

both the rate of induction and the depth of anesthesia can be rapidly adjusted by increasing or decreasing the partial pressure of the anesthetic in the patient's inspired air. After the concentration in inspired air is increased or decreased, the concentration in the blood and brain will increase or decrease. The ability to control rapidly the depth of anesthesia increases the safety of the inhalational anesthetics.

Mechanism of Action

It was thought that the action of inhalational anesthetics resulted from a nonspecific interaction of anesthetic molecules within the lipid bilayer of neuronal membranes, causing a disruption of ion flow and inhibiting neuronal activity. This hypothesis was supported by the correlation of the anesthetic potency with its lipophilicity, known as the Meyer-Overton principle (see oil:gas partition coefficient, Box 21–2).

More recently, the molecular actions of inhalational anesthetics were elucidated. These agents bind to specific amino acid residues in the transmembrane portions of

BOX 21–1. PHARMACOKINETICS OF INHALATIONAL ANESTHETICS RATE OF INDUCTION OF ANESTHESIA

The rate of induction of anesthesia is determined by three primary factors: (1) the alveolar concentration, or alveolar partial pressure, of the anesthetic; (2) the ventilation rate; and (3) the rate at which the anesthetic's partial pressure in the blood increases as the anesthetic is administered. This third factor, in turn, is influenced by the blood:gas partition coefficient.

The blood:gas partition coefficient is a measure of the anesthetic's solubility in the blood. In the example shown here, the coefficient of nitrous oxide is 0.47, whereas that of halothane is 2.3.

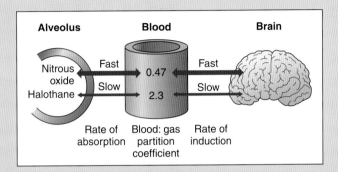

A high blood:gas partition coefficient corresponds with a high degree of solubility in the blood and with a low rate of rise in the anesthetic's partial pressure in the blood during induction. Anesthetics with a low coefficient (e.g., nitrous oxide) have a fast rate of induction because they saturate the blood quickly and their partial pressure rises quickly. Anesthetics with a higher coefficient (e.g., halothane) have a slow rate of induction because they dissolve slowly in the blood and it takes a long time for their partial pressure in the blood to rise.

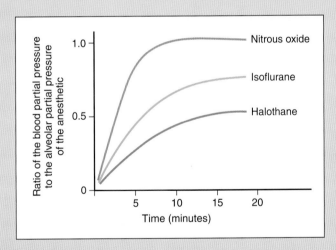

Adjusting the Rate or Depth of Anesthesia

The anesthetic's alveolar concentration and the ventilation rate can be altered by the anesthesiologist to accelerate or slow the rate of induction or recovery, to adjust the depth of anesthesia during surgery, or to maintain tissue oxygenation and eliminate carbon dioxide.

The anesthetic's alveolar concentration after induction is usually about half as high as during induction. In patients having mechanical ventilation, the rate of induction or depth of anesthesia can be adjusted by changing the respiratory rate or tidal volume.

γ-aminobutyric acid$_A$ (GABA$_A$) receptor–chloride ion channel. The inhalational anesthetics appear to increase chloride influx and potassium efflux from neurons. Both of these actions cause hyperpolarization of neuronal membranes and reduce membrane excitability. The effect of the anesthetics on chloride flux appears to be caused by potentiation of the action of GABA at the GABA$_A$ receptor–chloride ion channel. Inhalational anesthetics also reduce sodium and calcium influx, and this prevents nerve firing and the release of neurotransmitters.

Pharmacologic Effects

The induction by general anesthetics is characterized by four stages. In **stage I**, neurons in the spinal cord are prevented from firing, and **analgesia** and **conscious sedation** occurs. In **stage II**, inhibition of firing in small inhibitory

BOX 21–2. MECHANISMS OF ACTION OF INHALATIONAL ANESTHETICS

The potency of an inhalational anesthetic, expressed in terms of the minimal alveolar concentration, is highly correlated with the lipid solubility (oil:gas partition coefficient) of the anesthetic. This correlation suggests that anesthetics interact with a hydrophobic component of neuronal membranes.

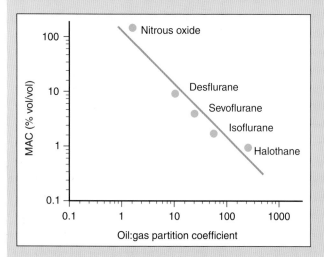

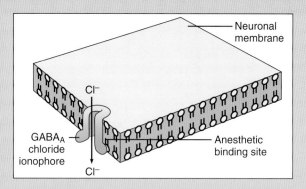

Because of their effects on neuronal membrane proteins, anesthetics disrupt neuronal firing and sensory processing in the thalamus and thereby cause loss of consciousness and analgesia. Anesthetics also inhibit neuronal output from layer V (the internal pyramidal layer) of the cortex, and this reduces motor activity.

Inhalational anesthetics are believed to bind stereoselectively to hydrophobic regions of neuronal membrane proteins that interface with membrane lipids. The anesthetics potentiate GABA activity at the GABA$_A$ chloride ionophore and thereby increase chloride flux through the ionophore. They may also inhibit sodium and calcium influx through membrane channels. These actions hyperpolarize the neuronal membrane and inhibit neuron firing and the release of neurotransmitters.

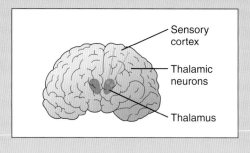

neurons can cause **paradoxical excitation**, although with modern balanced anesthesia, this stage is often not observed. **Stage III** is the goal of surgical anesthesia with **suppression** of the reticular-activating system, **loss of consciousness**, and **inhibition of spinal reflexes**. The latter effect contributes to the muscle relaxation needed for surgery; however, adjunct muscle relaxant agents (see Chapter 7) are commonly used. **Stage IV**, which is to be avoided because it can lead to **cardiovascular collapse**, is noted by depression of the respiratory and vasomotor nuclei in the brainstem.

Adverse Effects

Table 21–3 compares the adverse effects of nonhalogenated and halogenated anesthetics. Of particular importance with the administration of **halothane** is toxicity of the liver, called **halothane hepatitis**, which results from a reactive intermediate metabolite that acetylates liver proteins and produces an immune reaction that is fatal in about half of all cases.

Halothane and other halogenated anesthetics can also trigger **malignant hyperthermia**, a rare condition leading to muscle fiber breakdown, rhabdomyolysis (muscle proteins released into the blood), and renal failure. Prompt

discontinuation of the anesthetic and treatment with **dantrolene**, which prevents Ca^{+2} release from the sarcoplasmic reticulum, is necessary to prevent fatality. Dantrolene is also used in the management of **neuroleptic malignant syndrome** (see Chapter 22).

Because of a reactive fluoride group incorporated as one of the halogens in methoxyflurane, fluoride ion **nephrotoxicity** has occurred; as a result, **methoxyflurane was recently withdrawn** from the market.

SPECIFIC AGENTS

Nonhalogenated Drugs

Nitrous oxide is the only nonhalogenated anesthetic gas used today. It is the least potent of the inhalational anesthetics, and it does not reduce consciousness to the extent required for major surgical procedures. Nitrous oxide, however, produces more analgesia than do the other inhalational anesthetics, and it is often used for minor surgery and dental procedures that do not require loss of consciousness. Nitrous oxide is frequently used as a component of **balanced anesthesia** in combination with

CASE PRESENTATION: A 21-year-old male presents to a small-town hospital with nausea, a low-grade fever, and pain radiating from the lower right quadrant of his abdomen. A history reveals that he was backpacking in the country and was fed some wild berries by his girlfriend. Physical examination reveals tenderness and pain in the lower abdomen, which is worse after the physician presses down and quickly removes his hand. He is diagnosed with acute appendicitis and prepped for emergency surgery. He undergoes general anesthesia with halothane and the operation begins. During the surgery, he develops a fever, severe muscle rigidity and contractions, and tachycardia. The anesthesiologist recognizes a case of malignant hyperthermia, quickly stops the anesthetic, and administers dantrolene.

CASE DISCUSSION: Appendicitis is inflammation of the appendix, a small pocket off the large intestine that is commonly thought of as a vestigial organ but recently suggested to play a role as a reservoir for intestinal flora and as serving an immune function. When treated promptly by appendectomy, most patients with acute appendicitis recover without difficulty, but if treatment is delayed, the appendix can burst, causing infection and death. Many cases of appendicitis are linked to a blockage in the lumen of the organ and can occur by impacted feces or even a fruit pit. Malignant hyperthermia is associated with over 80 genetic defects and appears to be inherited with an autosomal dominant inheritance pattern. Most defects are related to mutations of the ryanodine receptor located on intracellular organelles, such as the sarcoplasmic reticulum, which mediate the release of Ca^{+2} from these intracellular stores. Dantrolene is given by the intravenous route, binds to the ryanodine receptor, and blocks the release of Ca^{+2} and the resultant sequelae that characterize malignant hyperthermia.

another anesthetic agent and other drugs (see below). The nitrous oxide in balanced anesthesia provides greater analgesia and enables the use of a lower concentration of the other anesthetic agent.

Because nitrous oxide has a low blood:gas partition coefficient, induction and recovery are rapid when it is used. The anesthetic produces virtually no cardiovascular or respiratory depression, and it is generally considered quite safe. It oxidizes the cobalt moiety of vitamin B_{12}, however, and

thereby inhibits methylation of nucleic acids and proteins. Although these effects are minimal during acute exposure, chronic exposure to nitrous oxide can cause **megaloblastic anemia.**

Nitrous oxide, which is also called **"laughing gas,"** often produces mild euphoria when it is administered. For this reason, some recreational use of the drug occurs.

Halogenated Anesthetics

In most areas of the world, the halogenated anesthetics replaced older volatile liquid anesthetics (e.g., **diethyl ether**) because of several advantages. The halogenated drugs have a more **rapid rate** of induction and recovery, cause a much lower incidence of postoperative nausea and vomiting, and are not flammable. However, they produce dose-dependent respiratory and cardiovascular depression. For this reason, respiratory and cardiovascular functions are monitored during the use of halogenated anesthetics, and artificial ventilation and circulatory support are often required. The halogenated anesthetics cause uterine relaxation, which usually limits their use in obstetrics to women having cesarean section. Because halogenated anesthetics produce relatively little analgesia or skeletal muscle relaxation, they are often given in combination with nitrous oxide, opioids, muscle relaxants, and other adjunct drugs in what is called **balanced anesthesia.**

Halothane is the prototypical halogenated anesthetic, and **desflurane, enflurane, isoflurane,** and **sevoflurane** are newer halogenated anesthetics.

Halothane is the most potent inhalational agent, but it has several disadvantages. Because of its relatively high blood:gas partition coefficient, its rate of induction and recovery is slower than that of other halogenated anesthetics. Because it sensitizes the heart to catecholamines more than other anesthetics do, it places patients at greater risk for **cardiac arrhythmias.** Hence, the utilization of epinephrine for hemostasis must be strictly limited in patients receiving halothane. Halothane undergoes appreciable hepatic metabolism and is converted to reactive intermediate metabolites that can produce a hypersensitivity reaction and hepatitis (see above). For this reason, a patient who is anesthetized with halothane should not be re-exposed to it for 6 to 12 months. It is no longer used in the USA.

Enflurane and **isoflurane** exhibit more rapid induction and recovery than halothane exhibits. They undergo less metabolic degradation and produce little cardiac arrhythmia. Enflurane and isoflurane produce more **muscle relaxation,** so this reduces the need for muscle relaxants during surgery. They cause more respiratory depression, however, than the other halogenated drugs cause. At high concentrations, enflurane can produce CNS excitation, leading to seizures.

Desflurane and **sevoflurane** have a more rapid rate of induction and recovery than other halogenated anesthetics do, but desflurane is irritating to the respiratory tract, so this limits the concentrations of this agent that can be administered during induction. Sevoflurane is close to an ideal anesthetic. It exhibits a rapid and smooth induction and recovery, and it causes little cardiovascular or other organ system toxicity.

TABLE 21–4. **Properties of Parenteral Anesthetics***

Drug	Duration of Action (Minutes)	Analgesia	Muscle Relaxation	Other Effects
Fentanyl	5–10 for IV 30–60 for IM	++++	0	Respiratory depression
Remifentanil	As long as infused	++++	0	Respiratory depression, corrected by stopping infusion
Ketamine	5–10 for IV 12–25 for IM	+++	0	Postanesthetic delirium and hallucinations
Midazolam	5–20 for IV 20–40 for IM	0	+++	Amnesia
Etomidate	5–10 for IV	0	0	Little effect on blood pressure
Propofol	5–10 for IV	0	0	Respiratory depression
Thiopental	5–10 for IV	0	0	Respiratory depression

*Values shown are the mean of values reported in the literature. Ratings range from range from none (0) to high (++++).
IM = intramuscular; IV = intravenous.

PARENTERAL ANESTHETICS

The parenteral anesthetics include barbiturates, benzodiazepines, opioids, and other compounds such as propofol. These drugs are used for a variety of purposes, including preanesthetic sedation, induction of anesthesia, perioperative analgesia, and anesthesia for minor surgical and diagnostic procedures. The properties of parenteral anesthetics are given in Table 21–4.

Thiopental is a thiobarbiturate, whereas **propofol** is a diisopropyl phenol compound. These drugs potentiate GABA activity at the GABA$_A$ receptor–chloride ion channel, and they are primarily used for induction of anesthesia. Their use is followed by the administration of an inhalational anesthetic to maintain anesthesia. Both drugs have a rapid onset of action, causing unconsciousness in about 20 seconds. Their duration of action is short (5–10 minutes) because they are redistributed from the brain to the peripheral tissues as their blood concentrations fall. Propofol has the advantages of being rapidly metabolized and eliminated from the body and causing little hangover. **Thiopental** is accumulated in fat and muscle. It is more slowly eliminated from the body, and some hangover can occur. Either drug can depress cardiovascular and respiratory function. **Methohexital** is also a barbiturate used for rapid induction of anesthesia and has similar properties to thiopental.

Etomidate is structurally distinct from the other parenteral anesthetics and commonly used in the emergency room for rapid induction to induce anesthesia or for conscious sedation. It has a rapid onset of action with low cardiovascular risks and is less likely to cause a significant drop in blood pressure than other induction agents.

Fentanyl is a strong opioid agonist used to treat moderate to severe pain (see Chapter 23). Because of its potent analgesic properties, it is also administered intravenously or epidurally in combination with other drugs for surgical or obstetric analgesia and anesthesia. For example, it is used to provide anesthesia during **cardiac surgery** (e.g., coronary artery bypass grafting), because it does not cause cardiovascular toxicity. Fentanyl does not produce amnesia or complete loss of consciousness, so it is often combined with a benzodiazepine (e.g., **diazepam**) to produce amnesia and increased sedation.

Fentanyl has been used in combination with **droperidol,** a member of the antipsychotic class of agents (previously called neuroleptics) that produces a condition called **neuroleptanesthesia** ("twilight sleep"). Droperidol is a butyrophenone compound whose properties are similar to those of haloperidol (see Chapter 22). The advantage of neuroleptanesthesia is that it provides adequate analgesia and sedation during surgery while maintaining a sufficient level of consciousness to permit the patient to respond to questions during the surgical procedure. The disadvantages of neuroleptanesthesia include **chest wall rigidity**, which is caused by the effects of fentanyl and droperidol on the basal ganglia. Fentanyl has a much shorter half-life than does droperidol, and supplemental doses of fentanyl may be needed during long surgical procedures.

Fentanyl and **sufentanil**, a closely related opioid, are also used with or without a local anesthetic for epidural administration or by the spinal intrathecal route during labor or to provide postoperative analgesia. Other shorter-acting opioids (e.g., **alfentanil** and **remifentanil**) are used intravenously for induction or for ambulatory surgery. **Remifentanil** is unique as it is metabolized extremely rapidly by esterases in the blood and tissues (see Chapter 23).

Ketamine is chemically and pharmacologically related to **phencyclidine (PCP)**, a street drug that is abused because of its pronounced effects on sensory perception (see Chapter 25). Both ketamine and PCP act by blocking the action of excitatory amino acids, primarily glutamate, at N-methyl-D-aspartate (NMDA) receptors. Ketamine produces less sensory distortion and euphoria than does PCP and, therefore, is more suitable for use as an anesthetic.

When administered intravenously, ketamine produces **dissociative anesthesia**, a mental state in which the individual appears to be dissociated from the environment without complete loss of consciousness. This type of anesthesia is characterized by analgesia, reduced sensory perception, immobility, and amnesia. Unlike many inhalational anesthetics, ketamine usually increases blood pressure, but it has little effect on respiration with typical doses. The main drawback of ketamine is its tendency to cause unpleasant effects during recovery, including delirium, hallucinations, and irrational behavior. Because children are less likely than adults to experience these adverse effects, ketamine is most often used in **pediatric patients** and is given in combination with a benzodiazepine for anesthesia during minor surgical or diagnostic procedures.

Midazolam is a short-acting benzodiazepine used for preoperative sedation as well as for endoscopy and other diagnostic procedures that do not require a high level of analgesia. Although its onset of action is slower than that of thiopental or propofol, it has the advantage of causing little cardiovascular or respiratory depression. If an overdose of midazolam occurs, the effects of the drug can be reversed by administration of flumazenil, a benzodiazepine antagonist.

SUMMARY OF IMPORTANT POINTS

■ Local anesthetics produce use-dependent blockade of nerve conduction and thereby prevent pain associated with surgical and diagnostic procedures. Autonomic and sensory nerves are blocked more easily than are nerves affecting proprioception, muscle tone, and somatic motor activity.

■ Local anesthetics are weak bases. The non-ionized form permeates neuronal membranes, and the ionized form binds to the internal surface of sodium channels.

■ Ester-type anesthetics (e.g., procaine and chloroprocaine) are converted to PABA and may elicit hypersensitivity reactions.

■ Amide-type anesthetics (e.g., lidocaine and mepivacaine) produce fewer allergic reactions than do ester-type anesthetics.

■ All local anesthetics can cause CNS and cardiac toxicity, including seizures and cardiac arrhythmias.

■ General anesthetics include inhalational agents (e.g., nitrous oxide and halothane) and parenteral agents (e.g., ketamine and propofol).

■ The potency of inhalational anesthetics is expressed as the minimal alveolar concentration required to produce anesthesia. The potency is proportional to the oil:gas partition coefficient.

■ The rate of induction of inhalational anesthetics is determined in part by the blood:gas partition coefficient. Nitrous oxide has a low coefficient and a rapid rate of induction. Halothane has a higher coefficient and a slower rate of induction.

■ All inhalational anesthetics, except nitrous oxide, suppress respiratory function and decrease blood pressure in a dose-dependent manner.

■ Parenteral anesthetics are used to induce anesthesia and to provide anesthesia during minor surgical and diagnostic procedures. They are also used in combination with other anesthetics during major surgical procedures.

Review Questions

1. Local anesthetics exert their effects by which one of the following mechanisms?
   (A) increasing K^+ conductance and hyperpolarizing nerves
   (B) blocking the Na^+ channels in nerves
   (C) inactivating the N^+-K^+ adenosine triphosphatase (ATPase) pump
   (D) blocking excitation at postsynaptic receptors
   (E) blocking by a direct action only at the synapse

2. Epinephrine is sometimes added to commercial local anesthetic solutions for which purpose?
   (A) decrease the rate of absorption of the local anesthetic
   (B) decrease the duration of action of the local anesthetic
   (C) block the metabolism of ester-type local anesthetics
   (D) enhance the distribution of the local anesthetic
   (E) act synergistically with the local anesthetic at the nerve ion channel

3. Which of the following characteristics is used to quantitate and compare the potency of gaseous general anesthetics?
   (A) blood:gas partition coefficient
   (B) minimal alveolar concentration
   (C) blood:brain partition coefficient
   (D) rate of uptake and elimination
   (E) relative analgesic potency

4. Which one of the following inhalational anesthetics can only provide anesthetic effectiveness under hyperbaric conditions?
   (A) enflurane
   (B) nitrous oxide
   (C) halothane
   (D) methoxyflurane
   (E) isoflurane

5. Muscle rigidity can be a side effect of which intravenous anesthetic?
   (A) fentanyl
   (B) midazolam
   (C) ketamine
   (D) propofol
   (E) thiopental

Answers and Explanations

1. **The correct choice is B: blocking the Na^+ channels in nerves.** Local anesthetics produce a block of voltage-gated sodium channels needed to conduct action potentials along nerve fibers. The unprotonated form of the local anesthetic molecule passes through the neuronal membrane and is changed to the protonated form in the cytoplasm. This form then binds to the inside of the sodium channel protein. Answer (A), increasing K^+ conductance and hyperpolarizing nerves, would cause inhibition of firing but not total blockade of action potentials because they are not dependent on potassium channels for nerve fiber

conduction. Answer (C), inactivating the Na^+-K^+ ATPase pump, is the action of some cardiovascular agents used for congestive heart failure. Answer (D), blocking excitation at postsynaptic receptors, is the action of a receptor antagonist. Answer (E), blocking by a direct action only at the synapse, again, is not the action of an local anesthetic, which can block all along the nerve fiber.

2. **The correct answer is A: decrease the rate of absorption of the local anesthetic.** Epinephrine causes vasoconstriction acting at α_1 receptors and thus decreases the amount of systemic absorption of the local anesthetic. Answer (B), decrease the duration of action of the local anesthetic, is wrong because epinephrine actually prolongs the duration of action by reducing absorption away from the nerve fiber. Answer (C), block the metabolism of ester-type local anesthetics, and (E), act synergistically with local anesthetic at the nerve ion channel, are wrong because no evidence exists for epinephrine having this effect. Answer (D), enhance the distribution of local anesthetic, is incorrect because epinephrine affects the pharmacokinetic property of absorption directly.

3. **The correct answer is B: minimal alveolar concentration.** The minimal alveolar concentration value, which is used for inhalational agents to determine potency, is defined as the percent concentration in the administered air that produces no response to surgical incision in 50% of the subjects. Answers (A), (C), and (D) are measures of the characteristics of anesthetics but do not give the potency. Answer (E), relative analgesic potency, is a term used when comparing analgesic agents.

4. **The correct answer is B: nitrous oxide.** Although nitrous oxide has the fastest rate of induction and is safe to use, the potency is such that would have to administer the gas under hyperbaric conditions to be the sole inhalational agent. It is often used in dental procedures for its analgesic effects and as an adjunct in other procedures.

5. **The correct choice is A: fentanyl.** Fentanyl is a potent opioid agonist given as part of balanced anesthesia. It can cause chest-wall (truncal) rigidity because of interactions in the striatum. This effect has not been noted for (B) midazolam, (C) ketamine, (D) propofol, or (E) thiopental.

SELECTED READINGS

Bischoff, P., G. Schneider, E. Kochs. Anesthetics drug pharmacodynamics. Handb Exp Pharmacol 182:379–408, 2008.

Lehr, V.T., Taddio A. Topical anesthesia in neonates: clinical practices and practical considerations. Semin Perinatol 31:323–329, 2007.

Miller, K.W. The nature of sites of general anaesthetic action. Br J Anaesth 89(1):17–31, 2002.

Phillips, J.F., A.B. Yates and R.D. Deshazo. Approach to patients with suspected hypersensitivity to local anesthetics. Am J Med Sci 334:190–196, 2007.

Sneyd, J.R. Recent advances in intravenous anaesthesia. Br J Anaesth 93(5):725–736, 2004.

CHAPTER 22

Psychotherapeutic Drugs

CLASSIFICATION OF PSYCHOTHERAPEUTIC DRUGS

Antipsychotic Drugs
Typical Antipsychotics
- Haloperidol (HALDOL)
- Chlorpromazine (THORAZINE)
- Fluphenazine (PROLIXIN)
- Thioridazine (MELLARIL)[a]

Atypical Antipsychotics
- Clozapine (CLOZARIL)
- Olanzapine (ZYPREXA)
- Molindone (MOBAN)
- Risperidone (RISPERDAL)[b]

Antidepressant Drugs
Tricyclic Antidepressants
- Amitriptyline (ELAVIL)
- Clomipramine (ANAFRANIL)[c]

Selective Serotonin Reuptake Inhibitors
- Fluoxetine (PROZAC)
- Fluvoxamine (LUVOX)
- Paroxetine (PAXIL)
- Sertraline (ZOLOFT)[d]

Monoamine Oxidase Inhibitors
- Phenelzine (NARDIL)
- Tranylcypromine (PARNATE)
- Selegiline (EMSAM)

Other Antidepressant Drugs
- Bupropion (WELLBUTRIN)
- Mirtazapine (REMERON)
- Trazodone (DESYREL)
- Venlafaxine (EFFEXOR)
- Duloxetine (CYMBALTA)

Mood-Stabilizing Drugs
- Lithium (LITHOTAB)
- Carbamazepine (TEGRETOL)
- Valproate (DEPAKOTE)

CNS Stimulants
- Amphetamines (ADDERALL)[e]
- Methylphenidate (RITALIN)
- Modafinil (PROVIGIL)
- Armodafinil (NUVIGIL)
- Atomoxetine (STRATTERA)
- Phentermine (ADIPEX-P)
- Sibutramine (MERIDIA)

[a] Also trifluoperazine (STELAZINE), thiothixene (NAVANE), and loxapine (LOXITANE).
[b] Also quetiapine (SEROQUEL), aripiprazole (ABILIFY), ziprasidone (GEODON), and paliperidone (INVEGA).
[c] Also desipramine (NORPRAMIN), imipramine (TOFRANIL), nortriptyline (PAMELOR).
[d] Also citalopram (CELEXA), escitalopram (LEXAPRO).
[e] Also dextroamphetamine (DEXEDRINE), methamphetamine (DESOXYN), lisdexamfetamine (VYVANSE).

OVERVIEW

The major psychiatric disorders include psychoses, such as schizophrenia, and affective disorders, such as depression. Psychoses are disorders in which patients exhibit gross disturbances in their comprehension of reality, as evidenced by false perceptions (hallucinations) and false beliefs (delusions). In contrast, affective disorders are emotional disturbances in which the mood is excessively low (depression) or high (mania). During the past 50 years, tremendous advances have been made in the treatment of these disorders. The newer antipsychotic drugs used to treat schizophrenia and the newer antidepressant and mood-stabilizing drugs used to treat affective disorders cause fewer adverse reactions and are more effective than the older psychotherapeutic agents. Treatment-resistant disorders still pose a significant problem to clinicians, but some progress has been made in the treatment of refractory disease. The chapter ends with central nervous system (CNS) stimulants used for attention-deficit/hyperactivity disorder, narcolepsy and other sleep disorders, and obesity.

SCHIZOPHRENIA

Clinical Findings

Schizophrenia, the most common form of psychosis, affects about 1% of the world's population. Its hallmarks are delusions, hallucinations, disorganized thinking, and emotional abnormalities. Several forms of the disease, including paranoid, disorganized, and catatonic forms, are differentiated on the basis of symptoms.

As shown in Table 22–1, the symptoms of schizophrenia can be divided into two groups. The **positive symptoms**, which include delusions and hallucinations, probably result from excessive neuronal activity in mesolimbic neuronal pathways. These symptoms are usually the primary manifestations of acute psychotic episodes. The **negative symptoms**, which include apathy, withdrawal, and lack of motivation and pleasure, probably result from insufficient activity in mesocortical neuronal pathways. The negative symptoms generally are more difficult to treat, often persist after positive symptoms resolve, and are associated with a poor prognosis.

Dopamine Hypothesis

Many hypotheses exist regarding the biologic basis of schizophrenia. According to the **dopamine hypothesis**, schizophrenia results from abnormalities in dopamine neurotransmission in mesolimbic and mesocortical neuronal pathways (Box 22–1). Much of the evidence supporting this hypothesis is based on the clinical effects of agents that alter dopaminergic transmission.

Several observations support the dopamine hypothesis. First, most antipsychotic drugs block **dopamine D_2 receptors**, and an excellent correlation exists between the clinical potency of these drugs and their in vitro binding affinity for these receptors. Second, drugs that act by increasing the neuronal release of dopamine (amantadine) or by blocking the reuptake of dopamine (drugs such as amphetamines and cocaine) can **induce psychotic behavior** that resembles the behavior of schizophrenic patients.

Dopamine turnover in the brain, which reflects the neuronal release of dopamine, can be studied by measuring the concentration of the principal metabolite of dopamine, homovanillic acid, in the cerebrospinal fluid. Although elevated levels of homovanillic acid are not found in patients with chronic schizophrenia, they are found in some schizophrenic patients having acute psychotic episodes. Evidence also exists for a dopamine receptor defect in schizophrenic

patients. Positive emission tomography scanning using D_2 receptor ligands has revealed that schizophrenic patients have **decreased D_2 receptor densities** in the prefrontal lobe cortex (but increased D_2 receptor densities in the caudate nucleus). These findings lend overall support to the dopamine hypothesis, although it is clear from the clinical effectiveness of atypical antipsychotics that 5-hydroxytryptamine ($5\text{-}HT_2$) and other types of dopamine receptors may be involved.

ANTIPSYCHOTIC DRUGS

Antipsychotic drugs are agents that reduce psychotic symptoms and improve the behavior of schizophrenic patients. Antipsychotic drugs were also called **neuroleptic drugs** because they suppress motor activity and emotional expression. The accidental discovery of the antipsychotic properties of chlorpromazine in the early 1950s began a new era in the treatment of schizophrenia and stimulated research concerning the neurobiology of mental illness and psychopharmacology. Nearly 40 years later, the introduction of **clozapine** had an equally important impact. Clozapine was the first agent to show greater activity against the **negative symptoms** of schizophrenia and to produce significantly **fewer extrapyramidal side effects** than the previous antipsychotic drugs. For this reason, the discovery of clozapine has stimulated the development of new antipsychotic drugs with improved pharmacologic properties.

Drug Properties

MECHANISM OF ACTION. The antipsychotic drugs interact with multiple neurotransmitter systems. Whereas the therapeutic effects of these drugs are believed to result from competitive blockade of **dopamine receptors** and **serotonin (5-HT) receptors**, the adverse effects are attributed to the blockade of a variety of receptors (Table 22–2).

Typical antipsychotic drugs have an equal or greater affinity for D_2 receptors than for $5\text{-}HT_2$ receptors. As shown in Figure 22–1, an excellent correlation exists between the clinical potency of these drugs and their in vitro affinity for D_2 receptors. Whereas antagonism of D_2 receptors in mesolimbic pathways is thought to repress the positive symptoms of schizophrenia, blockade of D_2 receptors in the basal ganglia is believed to be responsible for the parkinsonian and other extrapyramidal side effects that sometimes occur in patients taking antipsychotic drugs.

Atypical antipsychotic drugs (e.g., **clozapine**) have a greater affinity for 5-HT receptors than for D_2 receptors, and some atypical drugs have increased the affinity for D_3 or D_4 receptors.

PHARMACOLOGIC EFFECTS. The mechanisms by which the blockade of dopamine and serotonin receptors alleviates the symptoms of schizophrenia are not completely understood. Whereas these receptors are blocked immediately when antipsychotic drugs are first administered, the therapeutic effects of the drugs usually require several weeks to fully develop. This is because antipsychotic drugs produce three

TABLE 22–1.	Classification of Symptoms of Schizophrenia
Positive Symptoms	**Negative Symptoms**
Agitation	Apathy (avolition)
Delusions	Affective flattening
Disorganized speech	Lack of motivation
Disorganized thinking	Lack of pleasure (anhedonia)
Hallucinations	Poverty of speech (alogia)
Insomnia	Social isolation

BOX 22–1.   NEUROBIOLOGY OF SCHIZOPHRENIA AND SITES OF DRUG ACTION

Postulated Neuronal Dysfunction in Schizophrenia

As shown in the accompanying figure, numerous dopamine pathways are found in the brain.

(1) **Mesolimbic pathway.** Dopamine travels from the midbrain tegmental area to the nucleus accumbens. Increased activity in this pathway may cause delusions, hallucinations, and other so-called positive symptoms of schizophrenia.

(2) **Mesocortical pathways.** There are several mesocortical pathways. Decreased activity in the pathway that goes from the midbrain to the prefrontal lobe cortex can cause apathy, withdrawal, lack of motivation and pleasure, and other so-called negative symptoms of schizophrenia. Mesocortical dysfunction also disinhibits the mesolimbic pathway.

(3) **Nigrostriatal pathway.** The pathway from the substantia nigra to the striatum is involved in the coordination of body movements. Inhibition of this pathway causes the extrapyramidal side effects of antipsychotic drugs.

(4) **Tuberoinfundibular pathway.** The pathway from the hypothalamus to the pituitary inhibits the release of prolactin. Inhibition of this pathway leads to elevated serum prolactin levels.

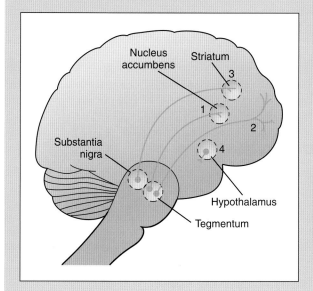

Sites of Drug Action

Some antipsychotic drugs (e.g., clozapine, olanzapine, and risperidone) block serotonin 5-HT$_2$ receptors in the mesocortical pathway to the prefrontal lobe cortex. This increases the release of dopamine (DA) and thereby alleviates the negative symptoms of schizophrenia. Most antipsychotic drugs (including those listed above) block dopamine D$_2$ receptors in the mesolimbic pathway to the nucleus accumbens, and this alleviates the positive symptoms of schizophrenia.

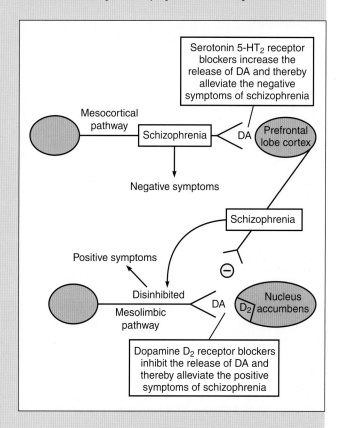

time-dependent **changes in dopamine neurotransmission**. When first administered, the drugs cause an increase in dopamine synthesis, release, and metabolism. This probably represents a compensatory response to the acute blockade of postsynaptic dopamine receptors produced by antipsychotic drugs. Over time, continued dopamine receptor blockade leads to inactivation of dopaminergic neurons and produces what has been called **depolarization blockade.** Depolarization blockade results in reduced dopamine release from mesolimbic and nigrostriatal neurons. This action is believed to alleviate the positive symptoms of schizophrenia while causing extrapyramidal side effects. Eventually, the reduction in dopamine release caused by depolarization blockade leads to dopamine receptor upregulation and supersensitivity to dopamine agonists. This supersensitivity may contribute to the development of a delayed type of extrapyramidal side effect called **tardive dyskinesia** (see below).

CASE PRESENTATION: A 24-year-old male employed as a policeman locks himself in an interrogation room, waving his handgun, and yelling incoherent statements like "They aren't going to take me alive" and "Get out of my head." His partner tells the police chief that he has been acting strangely, talking about a conspiracy against him by the other policemen, and arriving for work in dirty clothes and unshaven. He was overheard talking and arguing with himself in the locker room that morning, and the partner says they almost got into a fight just minutes ago because the partner wouldn't agree to shoot him when he insisted that he "wouldn't be hurt and was immortal." A medical emergency team arrives on the scene and at a moment when he is sitting in the corner cowering in fear, they forcibly enter the room, disarm him, and inject haloperidol into his thigh. He is transported to the locked ward of a psychiatric hospital and diagnosed with paranoid schizophrenia.

CASE DISCUSSION: Schizophrenia afflicts about 1 in 100 males and can be one of the most dangerous of all mental disorders as it causes its victims to lose touch with reality. They often show signs of confusion, inability to make decisions, auditory hallucinations, delusions, neglect of personal hygiene, strange statements or behavior, and changes in eating or sleeping habits, energy level, or weight. In the paranoid form of this disorder, schizophrenics develop delusions of persecution or personal grandeur. The first sign of paranoid schizophrenia usually surfaces between the ages of 15 and 30, and schizophrenia is much more common in males than females. There is no cure, but the disorder can be controlled with antipsychotic medications like haloperidol. Haloperidol is a good choice for acute psychotic episodes as it is rapidly absorbed and has a high bioavailability after intramuscular injection, with plasma levels reaching their maximum within 20 minutes after injection.

In mesocortical and nigrostriatal pathways, 5-HT$_2$ receptors mediate presynaptic inhibition of dopamine release. Blockade of these receptors by atypical antipsychotic drugs may increase dopamine release in these pathways. In the mesocortical pathway, this action may alleviate the negative symptoms of schizophrenia. In the nigrostriatal pathway, increased dopamine release counteracts the extrapyramidal side effects caused by D$_2$ receptor blockade.

ADVERSE EFFECTS. In the peripheral autonomic nervous system, antipsychotic drugs also block **muscarinic** receptors and α_1-**adrenoceptors,** thereby causing adverse effects described in Tables 22–2 and 22–3. Antagonism at α_1-adrenoceptors produces dizziness, orthostatic hypotension, and reflex tachycardia. Muscarinic receptor antagonism produces blurred vision, dry mouth, constipation, and urinary retention. Antagonism of brain H$_1$ receptors produces drowsiness and weight gain.

The most disturbing adverse effect is the development of **motor abnormalities** following the administration of high-potency, typical antipsychotics. These and other adverse effects specific to particular agents are discussed below.

Neuroleptic malignant syndrome is a severe form of drug toxicity that occurs in 0.5% to 1% of patients treated with antipsychotic drugs. It is a **life-threatening condition** characterized by muscle rigidity, elevated temperature (>38° C), altered consciousness, and autonomic dysfunction (tachycardia, diaphoresis, tachypnea, and urinary and fecal incontinence). The syndrome resembles malignant hyperthermia triggered by halogenated anesthetics in its rapid onset and mortality rate. Neuroleptic malignant syndrome is managed by immediately discontinuing treatment with the offending antipsychotic drug, administering **dantrolene** to prevent further muscle abnormality (see Chapter 21), and providing supportive care. If future antipsychotic therapy is required in patients who have experienced this syndrome, an atypical drug should be used because the atypical drugs are associated with a lower incidence of neuroleptic malignant syndrome.

INDICATIONS. Antipsychotic agents are primarily used to treat **schizophrenia** and other forms of psychosis, including drug-induced psychosis and psychosis associated with the manic phase of bipolar disorder. They are also used to treat severely agitated patients, including those with dementia and severe mental retardation. Because the phenothiazines have antiemetic activity, some of them are used in the management of nausea and vomiting (see Chapter 28).

Drug Classification

Antipsychotic drugs were traditionally classified on the basis of their chemical structure, but they are also classified according to whether they display **typical** or **atypical** pharmacologic properties. The **typical antipsychotic drugs** are also considered first-generation antipsychotic agents and the **atypical antipsychotic drugs,** second-generation antipsychotic agents.

Typical Antipsychotic Agents

Numerous typical antipsychotics are available for the treatment of schizophrenia and related conditions. The four representative examples discussed in detail here are **chlorpromazine, fluphenazine, thioridazine,** and **haloperidol.** These drugs have similar therapeutic effects but differ in their relative potency (Table 22–4) and in their side effect profiles (see Table 22–3).

PHARMACOKINETICS. The typical antipsychotics are adequately absorbed from the gut after oral administration. Several agents are also administered parenterally, including long-acting

TABLE 22–2. **Mechanisms Responsible for the Therapeutic and Adverse Effects of Antipsychotic Drugs**

Mechanism	Therapeutic Effects	Adverse Effects
Blockade of α_1-adrenoceptors	—	Dizziness, orthostatic hypotension, and reflex tachycardia
Blockade of dopamine D_2 receptors	Alleviation of positive symptoms of schizophrenia	Extrapyramidal effects (akathisia, dystonia, and pseudoparkinsonism) and elevated serum prolactin levels
Blockade of dopamine D_4 receptors	Alleviation of negative symptoms of schizophrenia and decrease in the incidence of extrapyramidal side effects	—
Blockade of histamine H_1 receptors	—(sedation)*	Drowsiness and increase in appetite and weight
Blockade of muscarinic receptors	—	Blurred vision, constipation, dry mouth, and urinary retention
Blockade of serotonin 5-HT_2 receptors	Alleviation of negative symptoms of schizophrenia and decrease in the incidence of extrapyramidal side effects	Anxiety and insomnia

*Sedation may be considered a therapeutic effect with a typical antipsychotic administered for acute psychosis.

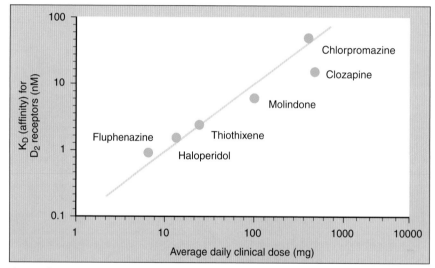

Figure 22–1. **Correlation of antipsychotic drug potency and dopamine D_2 receptor binding.** The clinical potency of the typical antipsychotic drugs is highly correlated with their in vitro affinity for D_2 (but not D_1) receptors.

depot preparations for intramuscular injection. These agents are extensively metabolized to a large number of active and inactive metabolites before they are excreted in the urine, and they have elimination half-lives ranging from 20 to 30 hours (see Table 22–4).

MECHANISMS AND PHARMACOLOGIC EFFECTS. The typical antipsychotic drugs exert their therapeutic effects primarily due to D_2 receptor antagonism. After therapy is initiated, the positive symptoms of schizophrenia usually subside in 1 to 3 weeks. Patients become **less agitated** and experience fewer **auditory hallucinations**. Grandiose or paranoid delusions subside and can disappear completely in some patients with continued treatment. At the same time, sleeping and eating patterns become normalized, and behavioral improvement occurs in the form of decreased hostility, combativeness, and aggression. Typical antipsychotic drugs can have some impact on negative symptoms, but it is usually less pronounced than the impact of atypical antipsychotic drugs.

Chlorpromazine and **thioridazine** are considered low-potency agents, **fluphenazine** has a slightly greater potency, and **haloperidol** is a high-potency antipsychotic agent.

ADVERSE EFFECTS. The most common adverse effects produced by typical antipsychotic drugs are summarized in Table 22–3.

Blockade of dopamine receptors in the striatum can cause several forms of extrapyramidal side effects, including **akathisia**, **pseudoparkinsonism**, and **dystonias**. Patients with **akathisia**, or "motor restlessness," feel compelled to pace, shuffle their feet, or shift positions and are unable to sit quietly. **Pseudoparkinsonism** resembles idiopathic Parkinson's disease and is characterized by rigidity, bradykinesia, and tremor. **Dystonia** is a state of abnormal muscle tension that often affects the neck and facial muscles, including the tongue, pharynx, larynx, and eyes. Patients with dystonia can experience severe reactions, such as oculogyric crisis (a condition in which the eyeballs become fixed in one position, usually upward), glossospasm, tongue protrusion, and torticollis (a contracted

TABLE 22-3. Adverse Effects of Selected Antipsychotic Drugs*

Drug	Extrapyramidal Effects	Sedation	Anticholinergic Effects	Orthostatic Hypotension	Other Adverse Effects
Typical Antipsychotics					
Chlorpromazine	+++	++++	+++	++++	Elevated serum prolactin levels and poikilothermy
Fluphenazine	+++++	++	++	++	Same as chlorpromazine
Thioridazine	++	++++	++++	++++	Cardiac arrhythmia, elevated serum prolactin levels, poikilothermy, and retinopathy
Trifluoperazine	++++	++	++	++	Same as chlorpromazine
Thiothixene	++++	++	++	++	Same as chlorpromazine
Haloperidol	+++++	+	+	+	Same as chlorpromazine
Loxapine	++++	+++	++	+++	Same as chlorpromazine
Atypical Antipsychotics					
Clozapine	+	+++++	+++++	++++	Agranulocytosis and cardiac arrhythmia
Olanzapine	+	++	+	+	Weight gain
Molindone	+++	+	++	++	Same as chlorpromazine
Risperidone	++	+	+	++	Cardiac arrhythmia and elevated serum prolactin levels

*Ratings range from extremely low (+) to extremely high (+++++).

state of the cervical muscles, producing twisting of the neck and an unnatural position of the head). Such reactions can be frightening and painful, and pharyngolaryngeal dystonias can be life threatening. Young males who are given large doses of high-potency drugs are at great risk of developing dystonias.

Although akathisia, pseudoparkinsonism, and dystonias are acute extrapyramidal side effects that often occur early in the course of treatment with antipsychotic drugs, **tardive dyskinesia** is a disorder that usually develops after months or years of treatment. The disorder is characterized by abnormal oral and facial movements (e.g., tongue protrusion and lip smacking). In later stages, abnormal limb and truncal movements may also be observed. Investigators believe that tardive dyskinesia results from supersensitivity to dopamine, which develops during **long-term dopamine receptor antagonism** (see Chapter 18). This hypothesis is supported by the fact that the symptoms of tardive dyskinesia temporarily subside if dopamine receptor blockade is increased by giving larger doses of an antipsychotic drug. This approach, however, eventually leads to further receptor supersensitivity and worsening of the manifestations of tardive dyskinesia.

Typical antipsychotic agents can increase serum **prolactin** levels by blocking dopamine receptors in the tuberoinfundibular pathway (see Box 22–1) and thereby cause **gynecomastia** in men and **menstrual irregularities** in women. Via their effects on the hypothalamus, antipsychotic drugs sometimes impair thermoregulation and cause **poikilothermy**, a condition in which the body temperature tends to approach the ambient temperature. This can lead to hyperthermia (including heat stroke) or hypothermia. In addition, high doses of **thioridazine** can cause **pigmentary retinopathy** and **cardiac toxicity**.

TREATMENT OF ADVERSE EFFECTS. Acute extrapyramidal effects (akathisia, pseudoparkinsonism, and dystonias) that are caused by typical antipsychotic drugs can be managed by lowering the drug dosage, changing to an atypical antipsychotic drug, or administering an additional drug to counteract the adverse effects. Drugs that counteract the effects include **benztropine,** an anticholinergic drug; **diphenhydramine,** an antihistamine with significant anticholinergic activity; and **amantadine,** an agent that increases dopamine release in the basal ganglia and can be used in conjunction with an anticholinergic drug.

Tardive dyskinesia is not easily managed and does not necessarily subside if a causative drug is discontinued. Hence, prevention is important. To prevent tardive dyskinesia, antipsychotic drugs should be used in the **lowest doses** for the shortest period of time required to control symptoms of schizophrenia. The drugs should be discontinued periodically to assess the need for continued treatment and possibly to reduce the development of **dopamine supersensitivity.** Patients should be evaluated regularly for early signs of tardive dyskinesia, which are sometimes reversible. Tardive dyskinesia often becomes irreversible if it is not detected early or is allowed to persist.

Once detected, tardive dyskinesia is best managed by reducing the dosage of antipsychotic medication. This results in significant improvement in many patients. No drugs are approved for the treatment of tardive dyskinesia, but some success has been reported with the use of **amantadine, dopamine receptor agonists**, and **clozapine.** Other drugs that may be effective include **physostigmine,** an indirect-acting cholinergic agonist, and the **benzodiazepines.**

INTERACTIONS. The major drug interactions of antipsychotic agents are listed in Table 22–4. The interactions include additive effects on CNS depression when used with other CNS drugs and pharmacokinetic interactions caused by antipsychotics and other drugs existing as substrates for the same cytochrome P450 isozymes.

TABLE 22-4. Pharmacologic Properties of Selected Antipsychotic Drugs*

Drug	Relative Potency†	Receptor Selectivity	Route of Administration	Elimination Half-Life and Route	Major Drug Interactions
Typical Antipsychotics					
Chlorpromazine	Low	$D_2 > 5\text{-}HT_2$	Oral, IM, and IV	30 hours (M)	Additive effects with antiadrenergic, anticholinergic, and CNS depressants. Decreases serum levels of lithium. Concurrent use of a β-adrenoceptor antagonist or an antidepressant may increase serum levels of both drugs.
Fluphenazine	High	$D_2 > 5\text{-}HT_2$	Oral and depot IM	20 hours (M)	Additive effects with anticholinergic and CNS depressants. Concurrent use of a β-adrenoceptor antagonist or an antidepressant may increase serum levels of both drugs.
Thioridazine	Low	$D_2 > 5\text{-}HT_2$	Oral	30 hours (M)	Same as chlorpromazine
Trifluoperazine	High	$D_2 > 5\text{-}HT_2$	Oral and IM	24 hours (M)	Same as chlorpromazine
Thiothixene	High	$D_2 > 5\text{-}HT_2$	Oral and IM	35 hours (M)	Additive effects with anticholinergic and CNS depressants. Concurrent use of a β-adrenoceptor antagonist may increase serum levels of both drugs.
Haloperidol	High	$D_2 > 5\text{-}HT_2$	Oral and depot IM	24 hours (M)	Barbiturates and carbamazepine decrease serum levels. Quinidine increases serum levels.
Loxapine	Medium	$D_2 > 5\text{-}HT_2$	Oral and IM	20 hours (M)	Concurrent use of an antidepressant may increase serum levels of both drugs.
Atypical Antipsychotics					
Clozapine	Low	$5\text{-}HT_2 = D_4$ and $> D_2$	Oral	24, hours (M)	Not established; possible interaction with drugs that induce or inhibit cytochrome P450 isozyme CYP1A2.
Olanzapine	High	$5\text{-}HT_2 > D_2$	Oral	30 hours (M)	Same as clozapine
Molindone	Medium	$D_2 > 5\text{-}HT_2$	Oral	2 hours (M)	Additive effects with anticholinergic and CNS depressants. Concurrent use of a β-adrenoceptor antagonist or an antidepressant may increase serum levels of both drugs.
Risperidone	High	$5\text{-}HT_2 > D_2$	Oral	24 hours (M)	Not established; possible interaction with drugs that induce or inhibit cytochrome P450 isozyme CYP2D6.

*Values shown are the mean of values reported in the literature.
†Low = 50–2000 mg/day; medium = 20–250 mg/day; and high = 1–100 mg/day.
CNS = central nervous system; D_2 = dopamine D_2 receptor; depot = long-acting form; $5\text{-}HT_2$ = serotonin $5\text{-}HT_2$ receptor; IM = intramuscular; IV = intravenous; M = metabolized.

Chlorpromazine and Thioridazine

Chlorpromazine and thioridazine are low-potency phenothiazines with similar properties. Of the two agents, thioridazine produces greater anticholinergic effects, and this probably accounts for its tendency to cause fewer extrapyramidal side effects.

Fluphenazine

Fluphenazine is a relatively high-potency typical antipsychotic agent that produces fewer autonomic side effects but more extrapyramidal side effects than do low-potency antipsychotics. Fluphenazine is available in a long-acting depot preparation that is intended for intramuscular injection every 1 to 3 weeks and is useful for treating patients who are not compliant with oral medication or are unable to take oral drugs.

Haloperidol

The first of the high-potency agents and one of the most widely used typical antipsychotics agents is **haloperidol.** Haloperidol has properties similar to those of fluphenazine and can cause significant extrapyramidal side effects (see Tables 22–3 and 22–4). As with fluphenazine, haloperidol is available in a long-acting depot preparation for intramuscular administration. Haloperidol is extensively metabolized in the liver, and its metabolites are excreted in the urine and bile.

In addition to its use in treating psychoses (e.g., **schizophrenia**), haloperidol is used in the treatment of **Tourette's syndrome** (Gilles de la Tourette's syndrome). This syndrome is characterized by facial and vocal tics, coprolalia (compulsive use of obscene words, particularly those related to feces), and echolalia (repetition of another person's words or phrases).

Atypical Antipsychotic Agents

Clozapine and olanzapine are atypical antipsychotics that produce fewer extrapyramidal side effects than do other antipsychotic drugs. Another member of this class, **quetiapine**, was recently approved for the treatment of schizophrenia and for acute manic episodes associated with bipolar disorder, as either monotherapy or adjunct therapy to lithium or valproate (see later text).

Clozapine

Clozapine has a unique profile of pharmacologic and clinical effects. It was the first of a new generation of **atypical antipsychotic** drugs that cause significantly fewer extrapyramidal side effects while exhibiting greater activity against the **negative symptoms** of schizophrenia.

Because clozapine is a potent antagonist of a large number of receptors, it has been difficult to attribute its effects to a particular mechanism of action. It seems likely that its therapeutic effects result from **blockade of D_4 receptors and $5\text{-}HT_2$ receptors**. Both of these actions may contribute to its greater efficacy against the negative symptoms of schizophrenia and to its **lower incidence of extrapyramidal side effects**. The use of clozapine is associated with significant sedation and autonomic side effects. These adverse reactions are caused by antagonism of histamine, muscarinic, and α_1-adrenoceptors. The use of clozapine is also associated with a 1.3% first-year incidence of potentially fatal **agranulocytosis**. For this reason, the U.S. Food and Drug Administration requires weekly monitoring of leukocyte counts during the first 6 months of therapy, the period during which the risk of agranulocytosis is greatest. After 6 months, biweekly monitoring of leukocyte counts is required.

Olanzapine

Olanzapine is a chemical analog of clozapine. Its pharmacologic properties are similar to those of clozapine, but olanzapine causes **fewer autonomic side effects** and has not been reported to cause agranulocytosis. As with clozapine, olanzapine causes few extrapyramidal side effects.

Olanzapine has about twice the affinity for $5\text{-}HT_2$ receptors as it does for D_2 receptors, and it can block dopamine D_3 and D_4 receptors. Although it also blocks histamine, muscarinic, and α_1-adrenoceptors, it does so to a lesser extent than does clozapine.

Clinical trials indicate that olanzapine is as effective as haloperidol in alleviating the **positive symptoms** of schizophrenia, is superior to haloperidol in alleviating the **negative symptoms**, and produces significantly fewer extrapyramidal side effects than does haloperidol. The most common adverse reactions to olanzapine are **sedation** and **weight gain**. At higher doses, olanzapine can cause akathisia, pseudoparkinsonism, and dystonias.

Risperidone

Risperidone is a newer atypical antipsychotic drug. Its pharmacologic properties are similar to those of olanzapine, but it appears to cause less sedation, more orthostatic hypotension, and a higher incidence of extrapyramidal side effects than does olanzapine. Its effects on treating both the positive and negative symptoms of schizophrenia are caused by antagonism at both D_2 and serotonin ($5\text{-}HT_{2A}$) receptors. In some patients, risperidone elevates levels of serum prolactin. It also **lengthens the QT interval** seen on the electrocardiogram and can predispose patients to cardiac arrhythmias, including *torsades de pointes*. Another agent sharing the pharmacologic profile of risperidone is **ziprasidone**. A newer agent, **aripiprazole**, differs slightly in that it is a **partial agonist** at dopamine receptors but a 5-HT receptor antagonist. **Paliperidone** is the major active metabolite of risperidone and shares its pharmacologic activity as an antagonist at both D_2 and $5\text{-}HT_{2A}$ receptors. Paliperidone is available in a once-a-day formulation using osmotic drug-release technology to deliver a controlled amount of drug throughout the 24-hour period.

Molindone

Molindone is an atypical antipsychotic with a unique spectrum of pharmacologic activities. It appears to cause a relatively low incidence of autonomic side effects and sedation. Although its incidence of extrapyramidal side effects also appears to be relatively low, it is probably higher than that of the newer atypical antipsychotic agents when they are given in equivalent doses. Molindone has a relatively short half-life but is metabolized to active and inactive compounds that have a longer half-life. Molindone is sometimes effective in patients who do not tolerate or respond to other drugs.

Treatment Considerations

All typical antipsychotic drugs appear to be equally effective when used in equipotent doses for the treatment of schizophrenia. The highly sedating drugs are no more effective than the less-sedating drugs in calming agitated patients, and the less-sedating drugs are no more effective than the highly sedating drugs in treating withdrawn patients. Hence, the choice of drug is primarily based on the need to minimize autonomic or extrapyramidal side effects. Several controlled trials indicate that low-dose regimens are as effective as high-dose regimens and produce fewer side effects.

The **atypical antipsychotic drugs** represent an appealing choice for the treatment of schizophrenia, and they may become the drugs of choice for treating most forms of psychosis. In comparison with the typical drugs, the atypical drugs produce a lower incidence of extrapyramidal side effects and appear to be more effective against the negative symptoms of schizophrenia. Data on the long-term effectiveness of atypical drugs in patients with chronic schizophrenia, however, have not yet been obtained.

During the first 2 weeks of treatment with an antipsychotic drug, many patients exhibit some alleviation of positive symptoms and an improvement in socialization, mood, and self-care habits. The maximal response to treatment, however, generally requires 6 weeks or longer, at which time it may be possible to reduce the dosage during maintenance therapy. Antipsychotic medication is usually continued for at least 12 months after the remission of acute psychotic symptoms. At that time, a low-dose regimen or gradual withdrawal of medication should be considered in order to reduce the probability of developing **tardive dyskinesia**. Antipsychotic drugs should be tapered slowly before discontinuation, because abrupt discontinuation can cause

withdrawal symptoms such as insomnia, nightmares, nausea, vomiting, diarrhea, restlessness, salivation, and sweating.

AFFECTIVE DISORDERS

Affective disorders are also called **mood disorders.** The two most common affective disorders are **major depressive disorder** and **bipolar disorder.** The primary drugs used in their treatment are antidepressant drugs and mood-stabilizing drugs.

Clinical Findings

Major Depressive Disorder

Major depressive disorder (unipolar depression) is characterized by depressed mood, loss of interest or pleasure in life, sleep disturbances, feelings of worthlessness, diminished ability to think or concentrate, and recurrent thoughts of suicide. Depressed patients can also be irritable or anxious.

Bipolar Disorder

Bipolar disorder (previously called **manic-depressive disorder**) is characterized by recurrent fluctuations in mood, energy, and behavior that encompass the extremes of human experience. This disorder differs from major depression in that periods of mania alternate or occur simultaneously with depressive symptoms. The clinical presentation varies widely. The manic phase is characterized by elevated mood, inflated self-esteem (grandiosity), increased talking (pressure of speech), racing thoughts (flight of ideas), increased social or work activity, and decreased need for sleep. Manic patients can become hostile and uncooperative. As the manic phase intensifies, some patients experience psychotic symptoms such as delusions.

Typically, the manic phase occurs just before or just after a depressive episode. In many patients, depressive and manic episodes last several weeks or months. In some patients, however, the episodes change within hours or days (rapid cycling bipolar disorder).

Biogenic Amine Hypothesis

According to the **biogenic amine hypothesis,** mood disorders result from abnormalities in serotonin, norepinephrine, or dopamine neurotransmission. Serotonergic fibers projecting from the raphe nuclei in the midbrain to limbic structures are important in regulating mood, among other functions. The serotonergic system is activated during behavioral arousal and increases cortical awareness of emotional reactions to environmental events. It is believed that impaired serotonin neurotransmission can decrease cortical responsiveness to emotional activation, leading to **affective dysfunction** and **depression.** Noradrenergic fibers that project from the locus ceruleus to the cerebral cortex can also play a role in depression, as can dopaminergic fibers innervating the nucleus accumbens.

Evidence also links depression with abnormal circadian rhythms and melatonin regulation. **Melatonin,** the principal mediator of biologic rhythms, is known to suppress the activity of serotonergic neurons. Investigators postulate that excess melatonin production contributes to the development of depression. This hypothesis is particularly relevant to **seasonal affective disorder,** which usually occurs during the winter months, when daylight is reduced and melatonin levels are increased. Abnormalities in melatonin and serotonin metabolism can also contribute to the sleep disturbances seen in patients with affective disorders.

The biogenic amine hypothesis is supported by the fact that all antidepressant drugs act to **increase serotonin, norepinephrine,** or **dopamine neurotransmission** in the brain. Most antidepressant drugs increase the synaptic concentration of serotonin, and this leads to down-regulation of presynaptic autoreceptors. Investigators believe that the down-regulation, in turn, increases the firing rate of serotonergic neurons and thereby produces the delayed therapeutic effect of antidepressant drugs. These mechanisms are depicted in Figure 22–2.

Recent data that antidepressant medications produce an increase in the rate of appearance of new neurons, called **neurogenesis,** in the brain of nonhuman mammals suggest a novel mechanism of antidepressant drug action. Studies have yet to show the correlation between increased appearance of brain neurons and the clinical effectiveness of antidepressants, but this interesting finding provides another view to the possible causes of depression and its treatment.

ANTIDEPRESSANT DRUGS

Depression can be treated with **tricyclic antidepressants (TCAs), selective serotonin reuptake inhibitors (SSRIs),** and a host of other antidepressants that have different structures and act by various mechanisms of action. If patients fail to respond to these drugs, **monoamine oxidase inhibitors (MAOIs)** can be used.

Because depressed patients might attempt suicide, the safety of an antidepressant in overdose is an important consideration when selecting a drug for a particular patient. Additionally, all antidepressant medications now contain **boxed warnings** highlighting the risk of increased **suicidal thoughts** and **behavior** in children, adolescents, and adults.

Indications

Antidepressants have been used to treat all forms of **depression** and to treat several other conditions. The antidepressants are also effective in the treatment of certain **anxiety disorders,** such as panic disorder, phobic disorders, and obsessive-compulsive disorder. **Clomipramine** is particularly effective in treating patients with obsessive-compulsive behavior. Some antidepressants are beneficial in the management of certain **sleep disorders,** including somnambulism, night terrors, and enuresis. Antidepressants repress excessive rapid eye movement (REM) sleep and dreaming, which are conditions that contribute to somnambulism and night terrors. In patients with enuresis, antidepressants appear to increase the awareness of the need to urinate and thereby facilitate waking up for this purpose. Other antidepressants also have a role in the treatment of **chronic pain syndromes** because of their mood-elevating effect and analgesic activity.

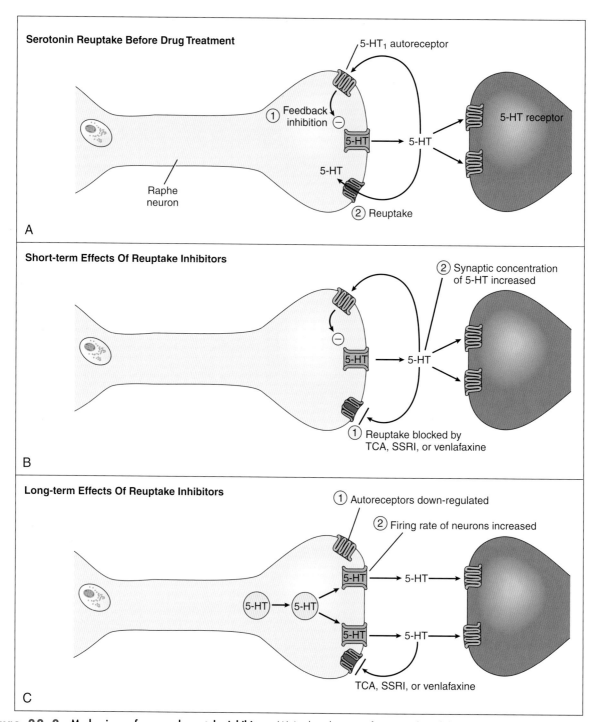

Figure 22-2. Mechanisms of neuronal reuptake inhibitors. (A) In the absence of a reuptake inhibitor, serotonin (5-hydroxytryptamine, or 5-HT) is released from raphe neurons that project to limbic structures. Serotonin activates postsynaptic and presynaptic 5-HT receptors and undergoes reuptake into the presynaptic neuron. (B) When a tricyclic antidepressant (TCA), a selective serotonin reuptake inhibitor (SSRI), or venlafaxine is initially given, the drug blocks the reuptake of 5-HT and increases its synaptic concentration. (C) With continued use of a TCA, an SSRI, or venlafaxine, increased synaptic concentrations of 5-HT cause the down-regulation of presynaptic autoreceptors and an increase in the firing rate of raphe neurons.

The SSRIs are used to treat **depression, eating disorders** (e.g., bulimia nervosa and anorexia nervosa), and **anxiety disorders** (e.g., panic disorder, phobic disorders, and obsessive-compulsive disorder). SSRIs may also be effective in the management of other conditions (e.g., **fibromyalgia, autism**, and **premenstrual dysphoric disorder**).

Tricyclic Antidepressants

The TCAs include **amitriptyline, clomipramine, desipramine, imipramine**, and **nortriptyline**. These agents are highly effective in the treatment of depression and several other disorders, but they are associated with a high incidence of adverse effects. They also cause severe toxicity when taken in excessive doses.

Drug Properties

PHARMACOKINETICS. The TCAs are incompletely absorbed after oral administration and are extensively metabolized to active and inactive metabolites in the liver. The **tertiary amine** TCAs are deaminated to pharmacologically active **secondary amine** TCAs, and several of these metabolites are available as drugs. For example, **amitriptyline** is converted to **nortriptyline**, and **imipramine** is metabolized to **desipramine**. The type of amine group determines the selectivity of the pharmacologic action. The TCAs and their active metabolites have relatively long half-lives, ranging from 18 to 70 hours.

MECHANISM OF ACTION. All TCAs block the neuronal reuptake of norepinephrine and serotonin, but they do so to differing degrees. The blockade occurs as soon as drug administration begins and causes an immediate increase in the synaptic concentration of serotonin and norepinephrine. The blockade is also believed to trigger a series of adaptive changes in norepinephrine and serotonin neurotransmission.

PHARMACOLOGIC EFFECTS. TCAs produce an antidepressant effect that becomes apparent about 2 to 4 weeks after drug therapy is started. Over time, the increased synaptic concentration of serotonin can cause down-regulation of presynaptic autoreceptors and thereby increase the firing rate of serotonergic neurons. The short-term and long-term effects of TCAs and other reuptake inhibitors on serotonin neurotransmission are illustrated in Figure 22–2.

ADVERSE EFFECTS. As with many of the antipsychotic drugs, the TCAs produce autonomic side effects by blocking **muscarinic** and α_1-adrenoceptors. Some of the TCAs also produce marked sedation (Table 22–5). In fact, TCAs are often administered at bedtime, when their sedative effects can have the added benefit of promoting sleep. The TCAs lower the seizure threshold and can induce seizures at therapeutic as well as toxic serum concentrations.

Taking an overdose of a TCA can cause life-threatening **cardiac arrhythmia**, which frequently presents as a wide QRS complex tachycardia; marked autonomic effects, including hypotension and sinus tachycardia; excessive sedation; and seizures.

TREATMENT OF ADVERSE EFFECTS. The type of arrhythmia that occurs with an overdose can be treated by the intravenous administration of **sodium bicarbonate**. Sodium bicarbonate increases the ratio of non-ionized TCA to ionized TCA and thereby decreases the binding of the TCA to the sodium channel in cardiac membranes.

Specific Drugs

Nortriptyline and **desipramine** are secondary amines formed by the demethylation of amitriptyline and imipramine, respectively. Secondary amines block norepinephrine uptake more than they block serotonin reuptake, and this is especially true of desipramine.

TABLE 22–5. Adverse Effects of Selected Antidepressant Drugs*				
Drug	Sedation	Anticholinergic Effects	Orthostatic Hypotension	Cardiac Conduction Disturbances
Tricyclic Antidepressants				
Amitriptyline	++++	++++	+++	+++
Clomipramine	++++	++++	++	+++
Desipramine	++	++	++	++
Imipramine	+++	+++	+++	+++
Nortriptyline	++	++	++	++
Selective Serotonin Reuptake Inhibitors				
Fluoxetine	0	0	0	0
Fluvoxamine	+	0	0	0
Paroxetine	+	+	0	0
Sertraline	0	0	0	0
Monoamine Oxidase Inhibitors				
Phenelzine	++	++	++	+
Tranylcypromine	+	++	++	+
Other Antidepressant Drugs				
Bupropion	+	+	0	+
Mirtazapine	+	+	++	+
Nefazodone	+++	0	+++	+
Trazodone	++++	0	+++	+
Venlafaxine	+	+	0	+

*Ratings range from none (0) to high (++++).

Amitriptyline, clomipramine, and **imipramine** are tertiary amines. They block serotonin reuptake to a greater extent than do secondary amines. They also produce more sedation and autonomic side effects than do secondary amines.

Studies have shown that all TCAs are equally effective in relieving depression, although some patients respond better to one drug than to another. The choice of a TCA is based primarily on the relative incidence of adverse effects produced by the different drugs. A drug that causes a higher degree of sedation may be chosen for highly agitated or anxious patients with depression, whereas a drug that causes a lower degree of sedation may be preferred for patients who are more apathetic or withdrawn.

Selective Serotonin Reuptake Inhibitors

The **SSRIs** are a newer class of antidepressants that include **fluoxetine, fluvoxamine, paroxetine, sertraline, citalopram**, and **escitalopram**. The SSRIs have become the most widely used drugs for the treatment of depression and certain anxiety disorders, such as panic disorder and obsessive-compulsive disorder. They are as effective as the TCAs but cause fewer autonomic side effects and less sedation. They are also much safer than the TCAs following an overdose, in that the SSRIs seldom cause cardiac arrhythmia and are less likely to induce seizures.

As opposed to older TCA agents that also block both serotonin and norepinephrine reuptake but also interact with many other receptor types to produce adverse effects, new drugs that are selective for both of the reuptake transporters, but not other receptors, are now available. Preclinical studies show that **duloxetine** (CYMBALTA) is a potent and selective inhibitor of **both** neuronal serotonin and norepinephrine reuptake. It is indicated for **major depressive disorder, diabetic peripheral neuropathic pain,** and **generalized anxiety disorder**. Duloxetine is the first approved agent for these disorders in the class of **selective serotonin norepinephrine reuptake inhibitors (SNSRI)**. **Venlafaxine** is also classified as an SNSRI and shares the properties and indications of duloxetine.

Drug Properties

PHARMACOKINETICS. The SSRIs are well absorbed from the gut after oral administration and are extensively metabolized by cytochrome P450 isozymes. **Fluoxetine**, which has a longer half-life than the other drugs in this class, is converted to an **active metabolite** that has an even longer half-life. The metabolites of other SSRIs have little or no pharmacologic activity.

MECHANISM OF ACTION AND PHARMACOLOGIC EFFECTS. The SSRIs selectively block the neuronal reuptake of serotonin and have much less effect on the reuptake of norepinephrine. Their efficacy in the treatment of depression supports the hypothesis that **serotonin dysfunction** plays a significant role in the pathophysiology of depression. The short-term and long-term effects of serotonin reuptake inhibition are illustrated in Figure 22–2.

ADVERSE EFFECTS. The SSRIs produce fewer sedative, autonomic, and cardiovascular side effects than do the TCAs. Unlike the TCAs, the SSRIs are usually administered in the morning, because they tend to increase alertness in patients. Their most common adverse effects are nervousness, dizziness, and insomnia. They occasionally cause **male sexual dysfunction** in the forms of priapism and impotence. Many of the side effects of SSRIs subside with continued use. The SSRIs should be used with caution in patients with seizure disorders, hepatic disorders, diabetes, or bipolar disorder.

Fluoxetine

Fluoxetine (PROZAC), is one of the most popular drugs for the treatment of depression, and the first drug approved for the treatment of **bulimia nervosa**; it is also effective in the management of **anorexia nervosa**. The drug is well absorbed orally and is converted to an active metabolite, **norfluoxetine**. The parent compound has a half-life of 2.5 days, but its active metabolite has a half-life of about 8 days. This long duration of action can be a disadvantage if severe adverse effects occur.

Fluoxetine causes more drug interactions than do other SSRIs. It can impair the regulation of blood glucose levels in diabetic patients. It can also cause a syndrome of **inappropriate antidiuretic hormone secretion**, characterized by persistent hyponatremia and elevated urine osmolality.

Fluvoxamine

Fluvoxamine is approved for the treatment of **obsessive-compulsive disorder** but has also been used to treat **depression** and **panic disorder**. Fluvoxamine has a half-life of about 15 hours and can be associated with sedative effects.

Paroxetine and Sertraline

Paroxetine and sertraline have half-lives of 21 and 26 hours, respectively. Paroxetine has a high bioavailability, whereas sertraline undergoes extensive first-pass elimination. Sertraline has relatively little effect on P450 isozymes and causes fewer drug interactions than does fluoxetine. Sertraline may be preferred in **elderly patients** because its elimination is not affected substantially by aging. Paroxetine is somewhat more sedating than either fluoxetine or sertraline.

Citalopram and Escitalopram

Citalopram has chemical structure unrelated to that of other SSRIs or of tricyclic, tetracyclic, or other available antidepressant agents. It is a racemic mixture (contains both R and S enantiomers of the drug molecule) and highly selective for serotonin reuptake transporters in preclinical models. **Escitalopram** is the pure S-enantiomer (single isomer) of the racemic citalopram drug. Escitalopram (the S-form) is at least 100 times more potent than the R-enantiomer with respect to inhibition of 5-HT reuptake.

Monoamine Oxidase Inhibitors

Because the **MAOIs** have many potentially serious interactions with other drugs and with food, they are not considered drugs of choice in the treatment of depression. They are generally used as alternative therapy when patients have failed to respond adequately to other drugs.

Drug Properties

PHARMACOKINETICS. The first-generation MAOIs, **phenelzine** and **tranylcypromine**, are adequately absorbed from the gut and have relatively short half-lives. They **irreversibly** bind to and inhibit monoamine oxidase, however, and their pharmacologic effects persist for many hours after their serum levels have declined. Phenelzine and tranylcypromine increase serotonin levels more than they do norepinephrine levels in the brain, and their antidepressant effects are probably caused by down-regulation of presynaptic autoreceptors and subsequent increased firing of serotonergic neurons. As with other antidepressants, the clinical effects of MAOIs are delayed for **several weeks** after therapy begins.

MECHANISM OF ACTION. The MAOIs bind **irreversibly** to an enzyme, **monoamine oxidase (MAO)**, responsible for the degradation of the biogenic amine neurotransmitters, norepinephrine, dopamine, and serotonin. The binding of MAOI prevents the substrate from reaching the active site on the enzyme.

The MAOIs are classified according to their selectivity for the two main types of MAO. MAO-A preferentially oxidizes serotonin but will also metabolize norepinephrine and dopamine. MAO-B preferentially metabolizes dopamine. The inhibition of MAO-A is believed to be responsible for the antidepressant effects of most of the MAOIs, except those with selectivity for MAO-B.

PHARMACOLOGIC EFFECTS. MAOIs increase the concentration of dopamine, norepinephrine and serotonin in storage sites throughout the nervous system and, in theory, this increased concentration of monoamines in the brain is the basis for its antidepressant activity.

ADVERSE EFFECTS. The major adverse effect reported with MAOIs is the occurrence of a **hypertensive crisis**, which is sometimes fatal. Such crises are characterized by some or all of the following symptoms: occipital headache which may radiate frontally, palpitation, neck stiffness or soreness, nausea or vomiting, sweating, and photophobia. Hypertensive crisis can occur with an MAOI alone or, more commonly, following the administration of sympathomimetic amines or eating food containing **tyramine** (see "Interactions").

Specific Agents

The first-generation MAOIs for treating depression include **phenelzine** and **tranylcypromine**, which are irreversible inhibitors of both MAO-A and MAO-B. The second-generation MAOIs include **moclobemide** and are reversible inhibitors of MAO-A (RIMA). This RIMA is used in many countries to treat depression but is not yet available in the United States. **Selegiline** represents a third type of MAOI, which selectively inhibits MAO-B and is also used in the treatment of Parkinson's disease (see Chapter 24). **Selegiline** was recently approved for the treatment of depression in a transdermal patch formulation called EMSAM.

Other Antidepressant Drugs

Several other drugs with diverse mechanisms of action are available for the treatment of depression.

Bupropion

The mechanism of action of bupropion is not well understood. It is a relatively weak inhibitor of the neuronal reuptake of dopamine, norepinephrine, and serotonin. Bupropion produces few anticholinergic side effects, causes very little sedation, and rarely produces cardiovascular effects or sexual dysfunction. It can cause agitation, insomnia, nausea, and weight loss. A formulation of bupropion was developed as adjunct therapy for patients who are attempting to quit smoking cigarettes (see Chapter 25).

Mirtazapine

Mirtazapine is structurally different from other antidepressants and has both **antidepressant** and **antianxiety** effects. Mirtazapine blocks presynaptic α_2-adrenergic **autoreceptors** and **heteroreceptors** and thereby increases the neuronal release of norepinephrine and serotonin, respectively. It increases central norepinephrine concentrations to a greater degree than do the TCAs, and it is also a potent antagonist of 5-HT$_2$ and 5-HT$_3$ receptors. Mirtazapine is better tolerated and causes fewer adverse reactions than do the TCAs. It can significantly elevate hepatic enzyme levels, however, and it has been associated with a few cases of **agranulocytosis**.

Trazodone

Trazodone selectively inhibits the neuronal reuptake of serotonin. It causes considerable sedation and orthostatic hypotension, but it does not produce anticholinergic side effects and has minimal effects on cardiac conduction.

Venlafaxine and Duloxetine

Venlafaxine and duloxetine are structurally unique antidepressants that strongly inhibit the reuptake of both norepinephrine and serotonin (see Fig. 22–2). Both have a side effect profile similar to that of the SSRIs. These agents do not antagonize muscarinic, adrenergic, or histamine receptors, and produce few autonomic, sedative, or cardiovascular side effects.

Hypericin

Extracts of the plant called St. John's wort (*Hypericum perforatum*) exhibit antidepressant activity, and products containing these extracts are available in health food stores. The extracts contain a substance called **hypericin** and several flavones. Some of these compounds inhibit MAO, whereas others appear to block the neuronal reuptake of serotonin. *Hypericum* extracts appear to cause fewer adverse effects than other antidepressants but are not as effective as prescription antidepressants.

Interactions

The serum levels of TCAs are elevated by concurrent administration of antipsychotic drugs, calcium channel blockers, cimetidine, and SSRI, which compete with TCA for metabolic enzymes in the liver. Barbiturates, carbamazepine, and phenytoin **decrease the serum levels** of TCAs because of up-regulation of hepatic metabolic enzymes. As with SSRIs (see below), TCAs should not be used with an MAOI.

Because of their ability to inhibit cytochrome P450 isozymes, the SSRIs have significant interactions with a variety of drugs. Among the SSRIs, **fluoxetine** has the greatest effect on the **CYP2D isozyme** and **sertraline** has the least effect. Inhibition of CYP2D can increase the serum levels of antipsychotic drugs, TCAs, and dextromethorphan. Inhibition by SSRIs of CYP2C and CYP3A can increase serum levels of alprazolam, diazepam, carbamazepine, phenytoin, and other drugs. SSRIs can also increase the **hypoprothrombinemic** effect of warfarin.

The SSRIs should not be used concurrently with MAOIs because both types of drugs increase the serotonin levels in the brain and their concurrent use can precipitate the **serotonin syndrome**. This syndrome is characterized by agitation, restlessness, confusion, insomnia, seizures, severe hypertension, and gastrointestinal symptoms. At least 2 weeks should elapse between the discontinuation of treatment with either an MAOI or an SSRI and the start of treatment with the other drug. The exception is that 5 weeks must elapse between the discontinuation of fluoxetine and the administration of an MAOI. Additionally, SSRIs should not be taken concurrently with **triptan** agents used to treat migraine (see Chapter 29). The Food and Drug Administration noted in 2006 that the concurrent use of these drugs increases the risk of triggering a **serotonin syndrome**.

MAOIs interact with SSRIs, TCAs, and other antidepressant drugs and have the potential to cause severe toxicity when administered with these drugs. Concurrent administration of MAOIs and TCAs or other antidepressants requires dosage reduction and careful monitoring.

MAOIs can cause severe hypertension when administered with sympathomimetic amines or with foods containing **tyramines**. These foods include many types of cheese (especially aged cheeses), beer, some wines (especially Chianti), some meats and fish (especially canned meat, liver, sardines, and herring), some fruits and vegetables (especially raisins, broad beans, avocados, and canned figs), and some products when consumed in large quantities (especially chocolate and coffee). The **selegiline patch** (EMSAM) at its lowest strength (6 mg) can be used without these dietary restrictions.

Treatment Considerations

Depression is one of the most common mental illnesses. Because it tends to be underdiagnosed, it often goes untreated. The primary treatment for patients with depression is drug therapy, but psychotherapy enhances the response to pharmacologic treatment and increases patient compliance with medication. **Electroconvulsive therapy** is sometimes used as an alternative when antidepressants have been ineffective or are not tolerated. More than 80% of patients respond to treatment with drugs, psychotherapy, electroconvulsive therapy, or a combination of these modalities.

The initial drug used in the treatment of depression is usually either a TCA or an SSRI, depending on clinician preference. A growing body of evidence indicates that SSRIs are better tolerated by patients, produce fewer adverse effects, and are safer in overdose than are TCAs. The

disadvantages of SSRIs include their higher cost and the increased tendency of some SSRIs to cause drug interactions. **Sertraline** causes fewer drug interactions than do other SSRIs and may be preferred in the treatment of patients who are taking other drugs that can interact with SSRIs.

If TCAs or SSRIs are not effective or well tolerated, the clinician has a growing choice of other antidepressants (e.g., mirtazapine, nefazodone, and venlafaxine). Mirtazapine and venlafaxine are attractive because of their **low incidence of sedation**, **autonomic side effects**, and **cardiac toxicity** (see Table 22–5). In comparison with other antidepressants, nefazodone has demonstrated a lower incidence of activating side effects, such as nervousness, agitation, and insomnia, and it does not cause sexual dysfunction.

It usually takes 2 to 4 weeks for antidepressants to elevate the mood of depressed patients, and some patients do not respond until after 6 weeks or longer. Some authorities believe that many cases of treatment-resistant depression are caused by inadequate drug dosage, inadequate duration of therapy, or patient noncompliance. Moreover, studies indicate that many patients who failed to respond to treatment in the past will respond to adequate doses of SSRIs or other new antidepressants.

To prevent relapse, antidepressants are usually continued for 4 to 9 months after remission of depressive symptoms.

MOOD-STABILIZING DRUGS

Indications

Mood-stabilizing drugs act to normalize the swings of affect in **bipolar disorder**. Although the element lithium is the standard agent in this class, a number of other agents are being tested and used for this indication. **Lithium** has been called a mood stabilizer because it reduces both manic and depressive symptoms and thereby tends to normalize the mood in patients with bipolar disorder. Lithium, as with other mood stabilizers, however, has greater activity against manic symptoms than it does against depression, and it is primarily used to treat or prevent the **manic phase of bipolar disorder**.

Lithium

Lithium, the lightest of the alkali metal elements, has a single valence electron which it readily loses to form a cation (Li^+). It was discovered to have a calming effect in patients during the early use of lithium solutions to dissolve urate crystal deposits in patients with gout.

Drug Properties

PHARMACOKINETICS. Lithium, which is administered orally in the form of lithium carbonate or lithium citrate, is available in immediate-release and sustained-release preparations. About 95% to 100% of the administered dose is absorbed from the gut. Lithium is widely distributed throughout the body, with the highest concentrations found in the thyroid gland, bone, and some areas of the brain. The drug is **not**

metabolized. It has a half-life of about 24 hours and is excreted in the urine. Lithium is extensively reabsorbed from the renal tubules, and the renal clearance of lithium is about 20% of the glomerular filtration rate. Lithium clearance increases during pregnancy. Sodium competes with lithium for renal tubular reabsorption and, thereby, can increase the excretion of lithium.

MECHANISM OF ACTION. The mechanisms by which lithium produces its mood-stabilizing effects are not well understood. The drug appears to act by suppressing the formation of second messengers involved in neurotransmitter signal transduction, but the relationship between this action and the drug's clinical effect is unclear. Lithium **reduces the formation of inositol triphosphate (IP$_3$)** by inhibiting myo-inositol-1-phosphatase, an enzyme in the inositol phosphate pathway. This enzyme participates in the regeneration of inositol and the inositol phosphate precursors to IP$_3$. By reducing IP$_3$ formation, lithium reduces the neuronal response to serotonin and norepinephrine, whose effects are partly mediated by IP$_3$ (see Table 18–1). Lithium also interferes with the formation of cyclic adenosine monophosphate.

PHARMACOLOGIC EFFECTS. Lithium produces a calming effect in manic patients, but the maximal response to lithium often requires several days or weeks of treatment. For this reason, other drugs may need to be used during the early phase of treatment while awaiting the full response to lithium (see below). The serum concentration of lithium should be **monitored** after initiating therapy and at periodic intervals thereafter. Although the concentration should be between 0.6 and 1.2 mEq/L, a concentration of 0.8 to 1.0 mEq/L is considered optimal for most patients. Monitoring the concentration serves to verify the adequacy of dosage and may warn of potential toxicity.

ADVERSE EFFECTS. Lithium has a relatively **low margin of safety** (therapeutic index). Elevated lithium levels can cause neurotoxicity and cardiac toxicity leading to arrhythmia. Nausea with vomiting can be one of the earliest signs of lithium overdose. It is important for the clinician and patient to distinguish the signs of lithium toxicity from the adverse effects of lithium that often occur with therapeutic serum levels.

Lithium is fairly well tolerated by most patients, but it produces a number of unpleasant side effects that decrease patient compliance. Common side effects include **drowsiness**, **weight gain**, a fine **hand tremor**, and **polyuria**. The hand tremor can usually be controlled by the administration of a β-adrenoceptor antagonist. Lithium causes polyuria because it interferes with the action of antidiuretic hormone and thereby inhibits the kidney's ability to concentrate the urine. In some patients, lithium causes **hypothyroidism** by blocking thyroid hormone synthesis and release.

INTERACTIONS. Nonsteroidal anti-inflammatory drugs and diuretics **decrease lithium clearance** by about 25% and increase lithium levels. Other drugs can increase lithium neurotoxicity.

Other Mood-Stabilizing Drugs

Although lithium is the primary drug used to treat and prevent manic symptoms in bipolar disorder, other drugs have been found to have equal or greater efficacy and may be better tolerated by some patients. These include **carbamazepine** and **valproate**, antiepileptic drugs whose pharmacologic properties are described in Chapter 20.

Treatment Considerations

Treatment of bipolar disorder must be individualized on the basis of symptoms, response to drug therapy and other treatment modalities, and the minimization of adverse effects. Drug treatment with **lithium** is often the cornerstone of therapy, because lithium can abort an acute manic episode, can prevent future manic episodes, and also appears to exert a mild antidepressive effect. Because of the dynamic nature of the disorder, however, therapy must be frequently reevaluated and modified.

Lithium usually controls an acute manic episode within 1 or 2 weeks after initiating therapy. Other drugs may be required to control acute symptoms while awaiting the full effect of lithium to develop. **Benzodiazepines** can relieve manic symptoms and promote sleep. An antipsychotic drug may be required to suppress delusions and other psychotic symptoms accompanying mania. **Risperidone** and **olanzapine** are effective in patients with bipolar disorder and cause fewer adverse effects than do typical antipsychotic drugs (e.g., haloperidol).

Lithium is usually continued for 9 to 12 months after the initial manic episode, and then its use can be slowly tapered, with continued monitoring of symptoms. Many patients experience **hypomanic symptoms** for several days or longer before developing a full manic episode, and lithium therapy can be reinstituted in these patients in an attempt to abort a full manic episode. Long-term prophylactic therapy can be given to patients who have had two or three episodes and to those whose symptoms develop rapidly. Long-term patient compliance with lithium, however, is often poor.

Depression that persists after lithium therapy is instituted may respond to **antidepressant drugs**. The use of antidepressants in patients who have bipolar disorder and are not taking lithium or another mood-stabilizing drug will evoke a manic response (switch phenomenon) in many patients.

A growing list of alternatives to lithium for bipolar disorder includes several antiepileptic drugs. **Carbamazepine** exhibits antimanic, antidepressant, and prophylactic effects that are equivalent to those of lithium, and it causes fewer adverse effects in many patients. Moreover, about 60% of manic patients who do not respond to lithium will respond to carbamazepine within the first several days of treatment. Evidence also suggests that lithium and carbamazepine can be synergistic in their antimanic activity in patients with refractory bipolar disorder. **Valproate** is another drug that is approved for the treatment of mania in bipolar disorder. It appears to be especially useful in patients with rapid cycling of manic and depressive episodes and in patients with coexisting substance abuse. Other antiepileptic drugs have demonstrated antimanic activity in clinical studies and may be approved for treating bipolar disorder in the future.

CENTRAL NERVOUS SYSTEM STIMULANTS

Amphetamine is the prototypical CNS stimulant, classified as an indirect-acting adrenergic agonist (see Chapter 8). It increases the release of norepinephrine and dopamine from nerve terminals; entering via the reuptake transporter, reversing the transport mechanism, and inhibiting further reuptake of catecholamines. It is available as a **mixture of amphetamine salts** in a formulation called ADDERALL. Other amphetamine derivatives include **dextroamphetamine** (DEXEDRINE), the active isomer of the racemic mixture of amphetamine; **methamphetamine** (DESOXYN), the same agent infamous for drug abuse and easy manufacture; and **lisdexamfetamine** (VYVANSE), a recently approved prodrug that is converted to dextroamphetamine after absorption.

Methylphenidate (RITALIN), **modafinil** (PROVIGIL), and **armodafinil** (NUVIGIL), the active isomer of modafinil, are also sympathomimetic agents and increase the levels of catecholamines in central and peripheral synapses like amphetamines but appear primarily to inhibit dopamine reuptake. These stimulants usually cause less irritability, anxiety, and anorexia than does amphetamine. **Atomoxetine** (STRATTERA) is a nonamphetamine drug that has some selectivity as a norepinephrine reuptake inhibitor.

Once-a-day formulations are available for the amphetamine mixture (ADDERALL XR), methylphenidate (RITALIN LA, RITALIN-SR, CONCERTA), and dextroamphetamine (DEXEDRINE SPANSULE). **Methylphenidate** is also available in a transdermal patch formulation (DAYTRANA).

Attention-deficit/hyperactivity disorder (ADHD) is a neurobehavioral disorder that afflicts about 5% of children. It is noted by inability to exercise age-appropriate inhibition of behavior. There are several diagnostic types of ADHD: a predominantly inattentive subtype, a predominantly hyperactive-impulsive subtype, and a combined subtype. ADHD is usually diagnosed and treated in childhood, although there is increasing recognition that the condition can continue into the adult years. It is estimated that more than 2.5 million children in the United States are treated with one of the following stimulants for ADHD on a daily basis. Treatment options include **amphetamine mixture, methylphenidate, dextroamphetamine, methamphetamine,** or **lisdexamfetamine. Atomoxetine** is a unique norepinephrine reuptake inhibitor approved for the treatment of ADHD. **Modafinil** has undergone large, multicenter clinical trials for safety and effectiveness in children; however, as of this writing, it is not approved for the treatment of ADHD. Nevertheless, modafinil appears to be used widely as an off-label drug for ADHD.

Narcolepsy is a sleep disorder characterized by excessive daytime sleepiness, even after sufficient nighttime sleep. Other symptoms include cataplexy, sleep paralysis, hypnagogic hallucinations, and automatic behavior; these are often triggered by sudden emotional reactions such as anger, surprise, or fear, and may last from seconds to minutes. **Amphetamine mixture, dextroamphetamine, methylphenidate, modafinil,** and **armodafinil** are indicated for the treatment of **narcolepsy,** as well as **obstructive sleep apnea/hypopnea syndrome** and **shift work sleep disorder.**

Obesity is commonly defined as being greater than 20% over one's ideal body weight, but more strict definitions are based on a body mass index greater than 30. In any event, there is no doubt that obesity is a major health concern in developed countries, and **amphetamines** were the first agents available for treatment of this growing disorder. **Methamphetamine** is still indicated for short-term use in treating exogenous obesity. The newer agents, **phentermine** and **sibutramine,** are amphetamine derivatives used as **appetite suppressants (anorectics)** in the treatment of obesity. The drugs act by stimulating the satiety center in the hypothalamus through similar sympathomimetic mechanisms. In comparison with amphetamine, they produce less CNS stimulation and have a **lower dependence liability.** Tolerance often develops to the anorectic effects of these drugs after a few weeks to a few months of use.

All of these CNS stimulants carry **risks of cardiovascular incidents**, ranging from high blood pressure to myocardial infarction and sudden death. In young children, their use is also associated with **decreases in growth and weight gain**. They are all controlled substances and, with the exception of atomoxetine and other newer drugs to treat ADHD, have a great potential for drug abuse (see Chapter 25).

SUMMARY OF IMPORTANT POINTS

■ Schizophrenia can result from abnormal function of the dopaminergic pathways in the brain. According to the dopamine hypothesis, this abnormality leads to dysfunctional dopamine neurotransmission in the prefrontal lobe cortex.

■ Delusions, hallucinations, and other positive symptoms of schizophrenia can result from excessive dopamine neurotransmission in mesolimbic pathways. Apathy, withdrawal, lack of motivation and pleasure, and other negative symptoms can result from impaired dopamine neurotransmission in mesocortical pathways.

■ Typical antipsychotic drugs are believed to act by blocking dopamine D_2 receptors in mesolimbic pathways. Atypical antipsychotic drugs act by blocking serotonin 5-HT_2 and D_2 receptors. Both classes of drugs alleviate the positive symptoms of schizophrenia, but the typical drugs cause a higher incidence of extrapyramidal side effects (akathisia, pseudoparkinsonism, dystonia, and tardive dyskinesia) and are less effective against the negative symptoms of schizophrenia.

■ Low-potency antipsychotics (chlorpromazine and thioridazine) produce more autonomic side effects and sedation than do high-potency drugs (fluphenazine and haloperidol), but the high-potency drugs cause more extrapyramidal side effects. Clozapine sometimes causes agranulocytosis, so leukocyte counts must be monitored.

■ Depression is believed to result from inadequate serotonergic and noradrenergic neurotransmission in limbic structures and elsewhere in the brain.

■ The TCAs block serotonin and norepinephrine reuptake. They effectively treat depression, but they have significant autonomic and cardiovascular side effects. When taken in an overdose, they can cause seizures and cardiac arrhythmia.

■ The SSRIs are antidepressants that have fewer autonomic and cardiovascular side effects and cause less sedation than do the TCAs. In comparison with other SSRIs, fluoxetine has a longer half-life and causes more drug interactions. Sertraline causes fewer drug interactions.

■ Other antidepressants (e.g., bupropion, mirtazapine, nefazodone, trazodone, and venlafaxine) have different pharmacologic profiles that lead to increased biogenic amines in the brain.

■ Nonselective MAOIs (e.g., phenelzine and tranylcypromine) bind to and inhibit MAO type A and type B. These drugs prevent the breakdown of serotonin, norepinephrine, dopamine, sympathomimetic drugs, and amines contained in certain foods. To prevent a hypertensive crisis in patients who are taking MAOIs, the use of interacting drugs and the consumption of particular foods must be avoided.

■ Lithium is a mood-stabilizing drug that is used primarily to treat and prevent the manic phase of bipolar disorder. It has a narrow therapeutic range, so its serum concentrations must be carefully monitored. Overdose can result in neurotoxicity and cardiac toxicity. Lithium produces many side effects, including tremor, weight gain, and polydipsia. Alternatives to lithium include carbamazepine and valproate.

■ Amphetamine, dextroamphetamine, methylphenidate, modafinil, and other amphetamine-like stimulants are indicated for treatment of ADHD, narcolepsy and other sleep disorders, and obesity. Atomoxetine is a unique nonstimulant agent for ADHD which acts by selective norepinephrine reuptake inhibition.

Review Questions

1. Clinical antipsychotic potency for "typical" antipsychotics correlate with actions at which receptor?
   (A) dopamine D_2
   (B) α_2-adrenergic
   (C) muscarinic
   (D) histamine
   (E) serotonin

2. Which agent listed below is an antipsychotic that can improve both positive and negative symptoms of schizophrenia?
   (A) chlorpromazine
   (B) haloperidol
   (C) thiothixene
   (D) risperidone
   (E) thioridazine

3. Which one of the following is not a class of antidepressant medications?
   (A) heterocyclic antidepressants
   (B) TCAs
   (C) MAOIs
   (D) acetylcholinesterase inhibitors
   (E) SSRIs

4. The older TCAs share all of the following adverse effects except which one?
   (A) orthostatic hypotension
   (B) sedation
   (C) seizures
   (D) weight gain
   (E) sexual dysfunction

5. Foods containing tyramine should be avoided when taken with which class of medications?
   (A) TCAs
   (B) MAOIs
   (C) SSRIs
   (D) atypical antidepressants
   (E) antihypertensive medications

Answers and Explanations

1. The correct choice is A: dopamine D_2. Antipsychotic agents are classified as typical, generally the older agents with actions at dopamine receptors, and the atypical antipsychotics, which can have multiple receptor action but primarily interact at 5-HT receptors. Answers (B), α_2-adrenergic receptors (α_2-adrenoceptors), and (C), muscarinic receptors, mediate some of the adverse effects of typical antipsychotic agents. There is no evidence for answer (D), histamine receptors, in the clinical effects of typical antipsychotics, but they can be involved in sedative effects of the older, less-selective agents. Answer (E), serotonin receptors, is correlated to the efficacy of the atypical agents and not the typical ones.

2. The correct answer is D: risperidone. Risperidone is a unique dual-acting antipsychotic agent that is an antagonist at both D_2 receptors and 5-HT$_2$ receptors and is effective in treating both positive and negative symptoms of schizophrenia. Answers (A), chlorpromazine, (B), haloperidol, (C), thiothixene, and (E), thioridazine, are all older, typical antipsychotics that block dopamine receptors (among other receptors) but with no appreciable affinity for 5-HT receptors.

3. The correct answer is D: acetylcholinesterase inhibitors. Acetylcholinesterase inhibitors, also known as indirect-actingcholinergic agonists, increase the synaptic concentration of acetylcholine. This has utility in the treatment of the dementia of Alzheimer's disease, but does not have antidepressant activity. The other answers are types of antidepressants.

4. The correct answer is E: sexual dysfunction. Whereas the older TCAs can cause all of the adverse effects listed from (A) through (D), it is the newer SSRIs, such as fluoxetine, that are noted for sometimes causing sexual dysfunction including priapism and impotency.

5. The correct choice is B: MAOIs. The MAOIs irreversibly inhibit monoamine oxidase, the enzyme that degrades biogenic amines neurotransmitters. This elevates the levels of the amine neurotransmitter available for synaptic release. Tyramine in food is not degraded because the MAO enzyme is blocked and a hypertensive crisis might ensue. Answers (A) and (C) through (E) are agents that do not interfere with the catabolism of dietary amines.

SELECTED READINGS

Alessandro, S., and M. Kato. The serotonin transporter gene and effectiveness of SSRIs. Expert Rev Neurother 8:111–120, 2008.

Bratti, I.M., J.M. Kane, and S.R. Marder. Chronic restlessness with antipsychotics. Am J Psychiatry 164:1648–1654, 2007.

Duman, R.S. Depression: a case of neuronal life and death? Biol Psychiatry 56:140–145, 2004.

Reynolds, G.P. The impact of pharmacogenetics on the development and use of antipsychotic drugs. Drug Discov Today 12:953–959, 2007.

Sink, K.M, K.F. Holden, and K. Yaffe. Pharmacological treatment of neuropsychiatric symptoms of dementia: a review of the evidence. JAMA 293: 596–608, 2005.

CHAPTER 23

Opioid Analgesics and Antagonists

CLASSIFICATION OF OPIOID ANALGESICS AND ANTAGONISTS

Strong Opioid Agonists
- Morphine
- Methadone
- Meperidine (DEMEROL)
- Oxycodone (OXYCONTIN, ROXICODONE)
- Hydromorphone (DILAUDID)
- Fentanyl (SUBLIMAZE)
- Sufentanil (SUFENTA)
- Alfentanil (ALFENTA)
- Remifentanil (ULTIVA)

Moderate Opioid Agonists
- Codeine
- Hydrocodone (VICODIN, LORTAB)
- Propoxyphene (DARVON)

Other Opioid Agonists
- Tramadol (ULTRAM)
- Dextromethorphan
- Diphenoxylate (LOMOTIL)
- Loperamide (IMODIUM)

Mixed Opioid Agonist-Antagonists
- Buprenorphine (BUPRENEX)
- Butorphanol (STADOL)
- Nalbuphine (NUBAIN)
- Pentazocine (TALWIN)

Opioid Antagonists
- Naloxone (NARCAN)
- Naltrexone (TREXAN, REVIA)

OVERVIEW

The relief of pain by the use of opioid analgesics is an ancient pharmacotherapy still very much in use today. As pain is a symptom associated with many disease states, trauma, and childbirth, this chapter begins with the definition of pain and a review of neural pathways that transmit nociceptive information in the central nervous system (CNS), as well as endogenous systems that are activated to suppress pain transmission. General characteristics of opioid analgesics are presented followed by key features of specific agonists, mixed opioid agonists-antagonists, and pure opioid antagonists. The chapter closes with treatment consideration for various acute and chronic pain states.

PAIN AND ANALGESIC AGENTS

Pain is an unpleasant sensory and emotional experience that serves to alert an individual to actual or potential tissue damage. This damage can be caused by exposure to noxious chemical, mechanical, or thermal stimuli (e.g., acids, pressure, percussion, and extreme heat) or by the presence of a pathologic process (e.g., a tumor, muscle spasm, inflammation, nerve damage, organ distention, or other mechanism that activates nociceptors on sensory neurons). Although pain serves a protective function by alerting a person to the presence of a health problem, its unbridled expression often leads to considerable morbidity and suffering. For this reason, **analgesics** or drugs that relieve pain are used for symptomatic treatment of pain from a wide variety of disease states, ranging from acute and chronic physical injuries to terminal cancer.

Based on their mechanisms of action, analgesics can be classified as **opioid analgesics** or **nonopioid analgesics**. Opioid analgesics act primarily in the spinal cord and brain to **inhibit the neurotransmission of pain.** In contrast, nonopioid analgesics act primarily in peripheral tissues to inhibit the formation of **algogenic** or **pain-producing substances** such as **prostaglandins.** Because most of the nonopioid analgesics also exhibit significant anti-inflammatory activity, they are called **nonsteroidal anti-inflammatory**

drugs (NSAIDs). The NSAIDs are described in greater detail in Chapter 30.

To facilitate the selection of an appropriate analgesic or anesthetic medication, patients are usually asked to describe their pain in terms of its intensity, duration, and location. In some cases, patients complain of an **intense, sharp,** or **stinging pain.** In other cases, they describe a **dull, burning,** or **aching pain.** These two types of pain are transmitted by different types of neurons and their primary afferent fibers (Box 23–1). Pain can be further distinguished on the basis of whether it is somatic, visceral, or neuropathic in origin. **Somatic pain** is often well localized to specific dermal, subcutaneous, or musculoskeletal tissue. **Visceral pain** originating in thoracic or abdominal structures is often poorly localized and may be referred to somatic structures. For example, cardiac pain is often referred to the chin, neck, shoulder, or arm. **Neuropathic pain** is usually caused by nerve damage, such as that resulting from nerve compression or inflammation, or from diabetes. Neuropathic pain is characteristic, for example, of **trigeminal neuralgia** *(tic douloureux),* **postherpetic neuralgia, and certain types of back and limb injuries.**

PAIN PATHWAYS

Exposure to a **noxious stimulus activates nociceptors** on the peripheral free nerve endings of **primary afferent neurons.** The cell bodies of these neurons sit alongside the spinal cord in the dorsal root ganglia and send one axon to the periphery and one to the dorsal horn of the spinal cord. With noxious stimulation, **substance P, glutamate,** and other excitatory neurotransmitters are released from the central terminations of the primary afferent fibers onto neurons of the spinal cord. Many of these terminals synapse directly on **spinothalamic tract neurons** in the dorsal horn, which send long fibers up the contralateral side of the spinal cord to transmit pain impulses via **ascending pain pathways** to the medulla, midbrain, thalamus, limbic structures, and cortex.

As shown in Box 23–1, the primary afferent fibers transmitting **nociceptive** information are **Aδ fibers** and **C fibers,** which are responsible for sharp pain and dull pain, respectively. Spinal reflexes activated by these fibers can lead to withdrawal from a noxious stimulus before pain is perceived by higher structures. Ascending pain pathways consist of two main anatomical-functional projections: the **sensory-discriminative** component, to the cerebral cortex, and the **motivational-affective** component, to the limbic cortex. Projections to the sensory cortex alert an individual to the presence and anatomic location of pain, whereas projections to limbic structures (e.g., the amygdala) enable the individual to experience discomfort, suffering, and other emotional reactions to pain.

The activation of spinothalamic neurons in the spinal cord are modulated by **descending inhibitory pathways** from the midbrain and by sensory Aβ fibers arising in peripheral tissues. These two systems constitute the neurologic basis of the **gate-control hypothesis.** According to this hypothesis, pain transmission by spinothalamic neurons can be modulated, or gated, by the inhibitory activity of other types of large fibers impinging on them. The activation of spinothalamic neurons is also inhibited by peripheral Aβ sensory fibers that stimulate the release of **met-enkephalin** from spinal cord interneurons. The Aβ fibers are thought to also mediate the analgesic effect produced by several types of tissue stimulation, including **acupuncture** and **transcutaneous electrical nerve stimulation (TENS).** These mechanisms explain the pain relief that may be produced by simply rubbing or massaging a mildly injured tissue.

The **descending inhibitory pathways** arise from **periaqueductal gray (PAG)** in the midbrain and they project to medullary nuclei that transmit impulses to the spinal cord (see Box 23–1). The medullary neurons include serotonergic nerves arising in the **nucleus magnus raphae (NMR)** and noradrenergic nerves arising in the **locus ceruleus (LC).** When these nerves release **serotonin** and **norepinephrine** in the spinal cord, they inhibit dorsal spinal neurons that transmit pain impulses to supraspinal sites. Nerve fibers from the PAG also activate spinal interneurons that release an endogenous opioid peptide, **met-enkephalin.** The enkephalins act presynaptically to decrease the release of pain transmitters from the central terminations of primary afferent neurons. They also act on postsynaptic receptors on spinothalamic tract neurons in the spinal cord to decrease the rostral transmission of the pain signal. Opioid analgesics **activate the descending PAG, NMR, and LC neuronal pathways,** and they also **directly activate opioid receptors** in the spinal cord.

OPIOID PEPTIDES AND RECEPTORS

Since ancient times, **opium,** the raw extract of the poppy plant, *Papaver somniferum,* has been used for the treatment of pain and diarrhea. During the 19th century, **morphine** was isolated from opium, and its pharmacologic effects were characterized. Later, specific sites in CNS tissue were discovered that bound morphine and other opioid agonists. The presence of stereoselective receptors for morphine in brain tissue indicated the likelihood of an **endogenous ligand** for these receptors, and this eventually led to the discovery of the three major families of endogenous opioid peptides: **enkephalins, β-endorphins,** and **dynorphins.**

The opioid peptides are derived from larger precursor proteins that are widely distributed in the brain. Endorphins and dynorphins are large peptides, whereas the two types of enkephalins are small pentapeptides containing Tyr-Gly-Gly-Phe-Met/Leu. Hence, the two types of enkephalins are called **met-enkephalin** and **leu-enkephalin.**

The **enkephalins are released** from neurons throughout the pain axis, including those in the PAG, medulla, and spinal cord. Enkephalins activate opioid receptors in these areas and thereby block the transmission of pain impulses. The enkephalins appear to act as neuromodulators in that they exert a long-acting inhibitory effect on the release of excitatory neurotransmitters by several neurons.

Opioid agonists mediate their effects at three types of opioid receptors; *mu* (μ) **opioid receptors,** *delta* (δ) **opioid receptors,** or *kappa* (κ) **opioid receptors.** Most of the clinically useful opioid analgesics, however, have preferential or strong **selectivity for *mu* opioid receptors.** Some

BOX 23–1. PAIN PATHWAYS AND SITES OF DRUG ACTION

Pain activates primary afferent neurons that enter the spinal cord, where they synapse with interneurons directly onto spinothalamic tract neurons (STTs). The neospinothalamic tract projects to the primary sensory cortex, which alerts the individual to the presence and location of pain, the **sensory-discriminative** component. The paleospinothalamic tract projects to limbic structures, which mediate the **motivational-affective** response to pain. Descending neuronal tracts from the periaqueductal gray matter activate neurons that release norepinephrine (NE), serotonin (5-hydroxytryptamine, or 5-HT), and enkephalin (Enk) in the spinal cord and thereby block ascending pain transmission. Opioid analgesics activate the descending pathways and directly activate opioid receptors on afferent nerve terminals and on STT neurons in the spinal cord. Nonopioid analgesics reduce the activation of primary afferent neurons via inhibition of prostaglandin synthesis. Glu = glutamate; LC = locus ceruleus; NMR = nucleus magnus raphae; SP = substance P.

Primary Afferent Neuron	Ascending Pathway	Projections	Type of Pain	Functions
Aδ (fast)	Neospinothalamic	Reticular formation, thalamus, and sensory cortex	Intense, sharp, stinging pain	Pain localization and withdrawal reflexes
C (slow)	Paleospinothalamic	Thalamus, periaqueductal gray matter, and limbic structures	Dull, burning, aching pain	Autonomic reflexes, pain memory, and pain discomfort

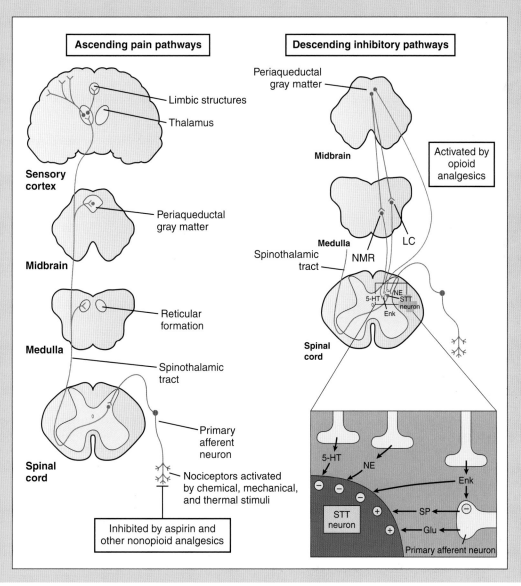

CASE PRESENTATION: A retired pharmacology professor presents to his primary care physician complaining of an itching and painful rash on his abdomen that is distributed like a band across both sides. The physician asks him whether he had chicken pox as a child, to which the professor replies that he did. His physician diagnoses him with shingles and tells him the rash will go away in about a week. Later that same month, the professor returns to the doctor's office complaining of pain on his stomach when his clothes rub against it, and sometimes when he is lying in bed. The doctor tells him he has postherpetic neuralgia and prescribes tramadol for the pain.

CASE DISCUSSION: Postherpetic neuralgia is a painful condition that develops after a case of the shingles. Shingles is the name given to a rash that develops from reactivation of chicken pox, the herpes varicella-zoster virus that lay dormant in the cell bodies of the dorsal root ganglia. It is estimated that in the United States nearly 1 million cases of shingles occur every year, mostly in the elderly with 40% to 50% of cases occurring in people that are 60 years of age and older. This may be due to waning immunological defenses or activation by drugs or other disease states. For reasons that are unclear, a number of these cases convert to postherpetic neuralgia. Drug treatment for this neuropathic pain condition includes antidepressants, opioids, and pregabalin. Tramadol is a unique dual-acting opioid agent and acts as an agonist at *mu* opioid receptors and inhibits the neuronal reuptake of serotonin and norepinephrine. It has shown effectiveness in a number of neuropathic pain states including postherpetic neuralgia.

of the mixed opioid agonist-antagonist agents have *kappa* opioid receptor selectivity, but attempts to develop useful opioid analgesics selective for *delta* receptors have not been successful.

OPIOID DRUGS

Classification

The opioid drugs can be classified as full agonists, mixed agonist-antagonists, or pure antagonists.

Based on their maximal clinical effectiveness, the **full agonists** can be characterized as strong or moderate agonists. In experimental pain models, all of the full agonists exert a maximal analgesic effect. In humans, the **strong opioid**

agonists are well tolerated when they are given in a dosage sufficient to relieve severe pain. The **moderate opioid agonists**, however, will cause intolerable adverse effects if they are given in a dosage sufficient to alleviate severe pain. For this reason, the moderate opioid agonists are administered in submaximal doses to treat moderate to mild pain, and they are usually formulated in combination with NSAIDs to enhance their clinical effectiveness.

The **mixed opioid agonist-antagonists** are analgesic drugs that have varying combinations of agonist, partial agonist, and antagonist activity and varying degrees of affinity for the different opioid receptor types.

The **opioid antagonists** have no analgesic effects. They are used to counteract the adverse effects of opioids taken in **overdose** and for the treatment of **drug dependence**.

Drug Properties

Mechanism of Action

The opioid receptors are prominent members of the **G protein–coupled receptor** superfamily. Activation of opioid receptors leads to **inhibition of adenylyl cyclase** and a decrease in the concentration of cyclic adenosine monophosphate, an increase in K^+ conductance, and a decrease in Ca^{2+} conductance (Fig. 23–1). The activated $G_{\alpha i}$ subunit of the G protein directly inhibits the adenylyl cyclase enzyme, and the $G_{\beta \gamma}$ subunits are thought to mediate the changes at the Ca^{2+} and K^+ channels. These actions cause both **presynaptic inhibition of neurotransmitter release** from the central terminations of small-diameter primary afferent fibers and **postsynaptic inhibition of membrane depolarization** of dorsal horn nociceptive neurons.

Pharmacologic Effects

CENTRAL NERVOUS SYSTEM. Morphine acts in the CNS to produce analgesia, sedation, euphoria or dysphoria, miosis, nausea, vomiting, respiratory depression, and inhibition of the cough reflex (Table 23–1).

Analgesia is produced by activation of opioid receptors in the spinal cord and at several supraspinal levels, as illustrated in Box 23–1. Sedation and euphoria can be caused by effects on midbrain dopaminergic, serotonergic, and noradrenergic nuclei. Surprisingly, many patients experience **dysphoria** after administration of opioids. **Miosis** or constricted pupils is produced by the direct stimulation of the Edinger-Westphal nucleus of the oculomotor nerve (cranial nerve III), which activates parasympathetic stimulation of the iris sphincter muscle. Because little or no tolerance develops to miosis, this sign can be **diagnostic of an opioid overdose**.

Codeine and other opioids inhibit the cough reflex at sites in the medulla where this reflex is integrated. The **antitussive actions of opioids** are discussed in greater detail in Chapter 27.

CARDIOVASCULAR SYSTEM. The most prominent cardiovascular effect of morphine and many other opioids is **vasodilation**, which is partly caused by histamine release from mast cells in peripheral tissues. Morphine can cause orthostatic hypotension from decreased peripheral resistance and a reduction in

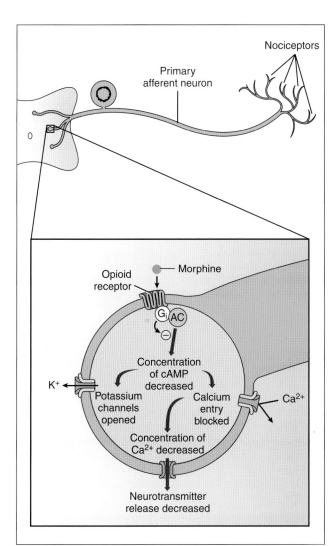

Figure 23-1. Mechanisms of opioid action in the spinal cord. Morphine and other opioid agonists activate presynaptic *mu, delta,* or *kappa* **opioid receptors** on primary afferent neurons. These receptors are coupled negatively to adenylyl cyclase (AC) via G proteins ($G_{\alpha i}$). Inhibition of cyclic adenosine monophosphate (cAMP) formation leads to opening of potassium channels and closing of calcium channels. $G_{\beta\gamma}$ subunits may also participate in the modulation of ion channels. Potassium efflux causes membrane hyperpolarization. The closing of calcium channels inhibits the release of neurotransmitters, such as substance P.

baroreceptor reflex activity. In patients with coronary artery disease, the decreased peripheral resistance leads to a **reduction of cardiac work** and myocardial oxygen demand.

GASTROINTESTINAL, BILIARY, AND GENITOURINARY SYSTEM. Morphine and most other opioids act to **increase smooth muscle tone** in the gastrointestinal, biliary, and genitourinary systems. In the gastrointestinal tract, increased muscle tone leads to inhibition of peristalsis and causes **constipation**. For this reason, the opioids are the oldest and most widely used medication for the treatment of diarrhea (see Chapter 28). Unfortunately, chronic pain patients do not appear to become tolerant to the constipating effects of opioids, necessitating a continual need for laxatives and other agents.

TABLE 23-1. Major Pharmacologic Effects of Opioid Agonists

CNS Effects

Analgesia
Dysphoria or euphoria
Inhibition of cough reflex
Miosis
Physical dependence
Respiratory depression
Sedation

Cardiovascular Effects

Decreased myocardial oxygen demand
Vasodilation and hypotension

Gastrointestinal and Biliary Effects

Constipation (increased intestinal smooth muscle tone)
Increased biliary sphincter tone and pressure
Nausea and vomiting (via CNS action)

Genitourinary Effects

Increased bladder sphincter tone
Prolongation of labor
Urinary retention

Neuroendocrine System Effects

Inhibition of release of luteinizing hormone
Stimulation of release of antidiuretic hormone and prolactin

Immune System Effects

Suppression of function of natural killer cells

Dermal Effects

Flushing
Pruritus
Urticaria (hives) or other rash

CNS = central nervous system.

Morphine and other opioids also **increase the tone of the biliary sphincter** (sphincter of Oddi), and can cause an exacerbation of pain in patients with biliary dysfunction or a gall bladder attack. Opioids also increase the tone of the bladder sphincter and can cause urinary retention in some patients. Because the opioid agonist, **meperidine**, has **less pronounced action on smooth muscle**, it is the drug of choice for these patients and for the pain associated with labor.

OTHER EFFECTS. Opioids have an effect on neuroendocrine and immunologic function. In the hypothalamus, they stimulate the **release of antidiuretic hormone** and **prolactin** and **inhibit** the release of **luteinizing hormone**. Opioids also **suppress** the activity of certain types of lymphocytes, including natural killer cells, and this action may contribute to the high rate of infectious diseases in heroin addicts.

Adverse Effects

The **major adverse effect** of morphine and other opioids is **respiratory depression**, which is usually the cause of death in severe overdoses. Opioids reduce the hypercapnic drive (the stimulation of respiratory centers by increased carbon dioxide levels) while producing relatively little effect on the hypoxic drive. Opioids reduce the respiratory tidal volume and rate, causing the rate to fall to three or four breaths per minute after an opioid overdose. As the cerebral circulation is exquisitely sensitive to CO_2 levels and responds with an increase in cerebral blood flow, leading to **increased intracranial pressure**, opioids should not be used in the case of a **closed-head injury**. The respiratory depressant effects of opioids are rapidly reversed by the intravenous administration of an opioid antagonist such as naloxone (see later text).

By stimulating the chemoreceptor trigger zone in the medulla, the opioids also cause **nausea and vomiting**. This is seen most often in ambulatory patients as opioids increase the sensitivity of the vestibular organ of the inner ear.

Opioids cause mast cells throughout the body to release histamine, which can cause itching, or **pruritus**. A flushing reaction, noted by redness and a feeling of warmth over the upper torso, may also occur from histamine release.

Allergic reactions to opioid analgesics are not uncommon. In most cases, however, a patient who is allergic to a particular opioid can use an opioid from a different chemical class. For example, someone who is allergic to codeine will probably not be allergic to propoxyphene or fentanyl.

Tolerance and Physical Dependence

Tolerance is defined as a decrease in initial pharmacologic effect observed following chronic or long-term administration. Repeated administration of an opioid agonist will lead to **pharmacodynamic tolerance** for both the administered opioid and other opioid analgesics. Tolerance primarily results from **down-regulation of opioid receptors**. Interestingly, in animal models, the magnitude of tolerance is inversely proportional to the efficacy of the opioid analgesic. This is because at equi-analgesic doses, a more efficacious opioid will occupy a lesser fraction of available opioid receptors than a less efficacious agent. Tolerance develops to most of the effects of opioids but not to **miosis** and **constipation**. Although considerable tolerance to respiratory depression occurs, a sufficiently high dose of an opioid can still be fatal to highly opioid tolerant individuals.

Opioid tolerance is usually accompanied by a similar degree of **physical dependence**. Physical dependence is defined as a physiologic state in which a person's continued use of a drug is required for his or her well-being. Tolerance and physical dependence appear with many drug classes and represent the establishment of a new equilibrium between the neuron and its environment (**neuroadaptation**), wherein the neuron becomes less responsive to the drug while requiring continued drug effect to maintain cellular homeostasis. If the chronic drug is abruptly withdrawn, the equilibrium is disturbed and a **rebound hyperexcitability** occurs owing to the loss of the inhibitory influence of the drug. This produces a withdrawal syndrome, the manifestations of which depend on the particular type of drug (see Chapter 25).

Because opioids demonstrate **cross-tolerance**, one opioid drug can substitute for another opioid drug and prevent symptoms of withdrawal in a physically dependent person. This is the basis for outpatient treatment of opioid dependence by the use of **methadone** or **buprenorphine** (see Chapter 25).

SPECIFIC AGENTS

STRONG OPIOID AGONISTS

The strong opioid agonists include naturally occurring drugs, such as **morphine,** and a number of synthetic drugs, including **fentanyl, meperidine,** and **methadone.** These drugs have equivalent analgesic effects but differ in their pharmacokinetic properties (Table 23–2), adverse effects, and uses.

Morphine

Morphine is the principal alkaloid of the opium poppy, *Papaver somniferum,* and constitutes about 10% of dried opium. Opium also contains **papaverine**, a drug sometimes used to relax smooth muscle and treat vasospastic disorders; **noscapine,** used as a cough suppressant, and minor amounts of **codeine**. The diacetic acid ester of morphine is heroin, a drug that is frequently abused (see Chapter 25).

Morphine is well absorbed from the gut, but it undergoes considerable **first-pass metabolism** in the liver, where a significant fraction of the drug is converted to glucuronides. For this reason, larger doses are required when the drug is administered orally than when it is administered parenterally. The principal metabolite of morphine is the 3-glucuronide, which is pharmacologically inactive. A significant amount of the **6-glucuronide** is also formed; it is **more active than morphine** and has a longer half-life. Hence, the 6-glucuronide contributes significantly to the analgesic effectiveness of morphine. Morphine is primarily excreted in the urine in the form of glucuronides. A small amount is excreted in the bile and undergoes enterohepatic cycling.

Morphine remains the standard of comparison for opioid analgesic drugs. It is primarily used to treat **severe pain associated with trauma, myocardial infarction, and cancer.** In patients with myocardial infarction, it relieves pain and anxiety while also dilating coronary arteries and reducing the myocardial oxygen demand. Morphine is available in both parenteral and oral formulations, including **long-acting oral formulations** (Kadian, Avinza) that are useful in patients with chronic pain.

Fentanyl and Its Derivatives

Fentanyl is a synthetic and highly potent opioid agonist. Fentanyl and its derivatives, including **sufentanil, alfentanil,** and **remifentanil,** are the most potent opioid agonists available. Indeed, tranquilizing darts used to sedate elephants and other large animals in zoos and in the wild are done using a fentanyl derivative called carfentanil (Wildnil). Because of its high potency and lipid solubility, **fentanyl** has been formulated in a **long-acting transdermal skin patch** (Duragesic) to provide continuous pain relief for patients with **severe or chronic pain**. It is also available for parenteral administration preoperatively and postoperatively and as an **adjunct to general anesthesia**. Fentanyl produces less nausea than does morphine, but is often associated with truncal rigidity when used as an adjunct parenteral anesthesia.

Alfentanil and **remifentanil** are used as part of anesthesia procedures and are available for intravenous administration.

TABLE 23-2.	Pharmacokinetic Properties of Opioid Drugs*			
Drug	**Route of Administration**	**Duration of Action (Hours)**	**Elimination Half-Life (Hours)**	**Active Metabolite**
Strong Opioid Agonists				
Fentanyl	Parenteral, transdermal, and transmucosal†	1	4	No
Meperidine	Oral and parenteral	3	3	Yes
Methadone	Oral and parenteral	8	24	No
Morphine	Oral and parenteral	4	3	Yes
Oxycodone	Oral	4	Unknown	No
Sufentanil	Parenteral	1	2	No
Remifentanil	IV infusion only	While infused	4 minutes	No
Moderate Opioid Agonists				
Codeine	Oral	4	3	Yes
Hydrocodone	Oral	4	4	No
Propoxyphene	Oral	4	9	Yes
Other Opioid Agonists				
Dextromethorphan	Oral	6	11	No
Diphenoxylate	Oral	6	12	Yes
Loperamide	Oral	6	10	No
Tramadol	Oral	4	6	Yes
Mixed Opioid Agonist-Antagonists				
Buprenorphine	Parenteral	5	5	No
Butorphanol	Intranasal and parenteral	3	3	No
Nalbuphine	Parenteral	4	5	No
Pentazocine	Oral and parenteral	4	4	No
Opioid Antagonists				
Naloxone	Parenteral	2	4	No
Naltrexone	Oral	24	12	Yes

*Values shown are the mean of values reported in the literature.
†Fentanyl lozenges are available for pediatric preanesthetic use.

Remifentanil is especially useful for short-term procedures and out-patient surgery as it is considered to have an **ultrarapid onset of action**, reaching blood-brain equilibrium and peak effect within 1 minute after the start of an intravenous infusion. It is also rapidly cleared by nonspecific **esterases** in tissue and blood, therefore recovery occurs within 5 to 10 minutes after the infusion stops.

Meperidine

Meperidine is a synthetic opioid agonist with an unusual profile of pharmacologic properties. It has no antitussive activity and has variable effects on pupil size. Because its effect on gastrointestinal, biliary, and uterine **smooth muscle is less pronounced** than that of morphine, it is less likely than morphine to cause constipation or an increase in biliary pressure. Meperidine **does not prolong labor** as much as morphine does, so it can be used for analgesia in obstetrics.

The parenteral formulation of meperidine is often used as an **obstetric or postsurgical analgesic**. The oral formulation is used to treat **moderate to severe pain** in the outpatient setting. The drug is converted to a toxic metabolite, **normeperidine**, which can cause CNS excitation, convulsions, and tremors when meperidine is administered in large doses or for a prolonged period. Hence, the drug is usually used for the **short-term treatment of acute pain syndromes**.

Methadone

Methadone is a long-acting synthetic opioid agonist. Although it is available in parenteral formulations, it is most often administered orally to ambulatory patients to treat **opioid dependence** or **chronic pain**. Use of the oral formulation by opioid-dependent patients can prevent their craving for heroin or other opioids, but it does not cause significant euphoria or other reinforcing effects. Because of its long duration of action, it can be administered once a day for this purpose. The treatment for opioid-dependent patients in this fashion is called a **methadone maintenance program**.

Oxycodone

Oxycodone is one of several semisynthetic morphine derivatives that are available as analgesics. Oxycodone is usually administered orally in combination with a nonopioid analgesic (e.g., acetaminophen) to treat **moderate or severe pain**. It is available as a single agent for acute treatment of pain (Roxicodone) and as **sustained-release oral form of oxycodone** (Oxycontin) for long-term treatment of chronic pain syndromes. The Oxycontin formulation is linked to several deaths of opioid abusers after they crushed the pills and dissolved the drug for intravenous administration.

MODERATE OPIOID AGONISTS

The moderate opioid agonists are less potent than the strong opioid agonists. Because they do not produce maximal analgesia at doses that are well tolerated by patients, the moderate agonists are used at submaximal doses, almost always in combination with an NSAID analgesic. Fixed-dose combination products containing one of the **moderate opioid agonists** and **acetaminophen, aspirin,** or **ibuprofen** are available for the treatment of moderate pain.

Codeine and Hydrocodone

Codeine is a naturally occurring opioid obtained from the opium poppy. Structurally, it is the 3-O-methyl derivative of morphine. Because codeine contains a methyl group at the 3 position, the principal site of morphine metabolism, codeine undergoes a **lesser degree of first-pass metabolism**. Thus, codeine has greater oral **bioavailability** than morphine.

Codeine is converted to morphine by cytochrome P450 isozyme CYP2D6, and persons with deficient variations of this isozyme obtain little pain relief from the drug. Conversely, pregnant and nursing mothers who are ultrarapid metabolizers of codeine may pose a risk of lethal morphine exposure to the fetus or nursing infant. An FDA warning in 2007 noted that a published case report of an infant death raises concern that breast-fed babies may be at increased risk of **morphine overdose** if their mothers are taking codeine and are ultra-rapid metabolizers of the drug.

Codeine is a less potent analgesic than morphine, and the doses required to obtain maximal analgesia produce intolerable side effects, such as constipation. For this reason, codeine is only available in combination with other agents (e.g., NSAIDs) to treat **mild to moderate pain**. Codeine also produces a significant antitussive effect and is included in many cough syrups to **alleviate** or **prevent coughing**.

The uses of **hydrocodone** are similar to those of codeine. Like codeine, it is only available in **combination** medicines, primarily with an NSAID such as aspirin or acetaminophen, in more than 15 different formulations.

Propoxyphene

Propoxyphene, a chemical analogue of methadone, has much weaker opioid agonist properties. Propoxyphene has about half the analgesic activity of codeine when administered in usual therapeutic doses. It is most frequently used in combination with acetaminophen to treat **mild to moderate somatic and visceral pain**. Propoxyphene is usually well tolerated, but prolonged administration can lead to the accumulation of a **toxic metabolite**.

OTHER OPIOID AGONISTS

Tramadol is a unique dual-action analgesic. It is an agonist at *mu* **opioid receptors** and inhibits the neuronal **reuptake of serotonin and norepinephrine**. The relationship between neuronal reuptake inhibition and analgesia is not certain. Reuptake inhibition, however, may **potentiate** the inhibitory effects of serotonin and norepinephrine on pain transmission in the spinal cord (see Box 23–1). Tricyclic antidepressants and other neuronal reuptake inhibitors also have analgesic effects, and some **antidepressants** are used to treat **chronic pain** syndromes. For this reason, investigators believe that neuronal reuptake inhibition by tramadol contributes to the drug's analgesic activity. Accordingly, the analgesic effect of tramadol is only partly inhibited by opioid antagonists like naloxone.

Tramadol is administered orally to treat **moderate pain**. It has a definite but limited drug dependence liability. Nevertheless, it has been used successfully in the treatment of **chronic pain syndromes** and produces minimal cardiovascular and respiratory depression. The drug lowers the seizure threshold, and the risk of seizures is increased if tramadol is used concurrently with antidepressants.

Several other opioid agents are available but have little analgesic activity. These include **dextromethorphan**, which has significant antitussive activity and is used in the treatment of **cough** (see Chapter 27), and **diphenoxylate** and **loperamide**, which activate opioid receptors in gastrointestinal smooth muscle and are used in the treatment of **diarrhea** (see Chapter 28).

MIXED OPIOID AGONIST-ANTAGONISTS AND PARTIAL AGONISTS

The mixed opioid agonist-antagonists are drugs that exhibit partial agonist or antagonist activity at *mu* receptors and show agonist or antagonist activity at *kappa* receptors. Examples are buprenorphine, butorphanol, nalbuphine, and pentazocine.

Drug Properties

Pharmacokinetics

The mixed opioid agonist-antagonists have a large chemical group on the nitrogen atom of the morphine molecule, which is responsible for their partial agonist or antagonist activity at opioid receptors. Their pharmacokinetic and pharmacologic properties are shown in Table 23–2. All of the agonist-antagonists can be given parenterally. In addition, pentazocine is available for oral use and butorphanol is available as a nasal spray. Butorphanol is rapidly absorbed from the nasal mucosa, which thereby enables the use of the drug on an as-needed basis.

MECHANISMS AND EFFECTS. The most important pharmacologic property of these drugs with respect to their clinical activity is the lack of full agonist effects at *mu* **opioid receptors**. Because of this, the mixed opioid agonist-antagonists produce **less respiratory depression** as the doses are increased than do strong opioid agonists such as morphine. Hence, the mixed opioid agonist-antagonists are safer to use with regard to respiratory depression and overdose. They also appear to have a lower liability for drug dependence and abuse than do full opioid agonists. The mixed opioids produce less constipation than do most of the full agonists. However, these sometimes cause anxiety, nightmares, and **psychoto-mimetic effects**, including hallucinations, as a result of the activation of *kappa* opioid receptors. They can also **precipitate withdrawal** in a person physically dependent on a full opioid agonist.

Indications

The parenterally administered agonist-antagonist drugs are primarily used for **preoperative and postoperative analgesia** and for **obstetric analgesia during labor and delivery**. The orally and nasally administered drugs are used to alleviate **moderate to severe pain**.

Specific Drugs

Buprenorphine, which is a **partial agonist at mu receptors**, is noted for a slow dissociation from the *mu* opioid receptor after binding. It is somewhat longer acting than most parenterally administered opioid analgesics and can be administered intramuscularly or intravenously. It was recently approved for outpatient treatment of opioid dependence (Chapter 25). It is available in an oral and sublingual formulation combined with naloxone to prevent intravenous abuse.

Butorphanol and **nalbuphine,** which are *kappa* **opioid receptor agonists**, have **partial agonist or antagonist** activity at *mu* **opioid receptors**. Both drugs are administered parenterally, and butorphanol is also available as a nasal spray.

Pentazocine is a *kappa* **opioid receptor** agonist with additional activity at *sigma (σ)* **receptors**. Sigma receptors were once considered a type of opioid receptor; it is now known that they are a **distinct class of receptors** mediating the psychotomimetic effects of phencyclidine (PCP) and ketamine (see Chapter 25). Pentazocine is available for parenteral and oral use. The parenteral formulation is primarily used as a preanesthetic medication and as a supplement to surgical anesthesia. The oral formulations are used to treat moderate to severe pain, and one of them contains **naloxone**, a pure opioid antagonist, to discourage parenteral abuse of the drug. Parenteral use of an oral pentazocine formulation can cause **severe cardiovascular effects**, especially in patients with existing cardiovascular disease. Pentazocine is also available in combination with aspirin or acetaminophen for oral administration.

OPIOID ANTAGONISTS

Naloxone and **naltrexone** are **competitive opioid receptor antagonists** that can rapidly reverse the effects of morphine and other opioid agonists. These pure opioid antagonists have two primary clinical uses: the treatment of **opioid overdose** and the treatment of **alcohol and opioid dependence.**

Naloxone and naltrexone are chemical analogs of morphine, with bulky chemical groups attached to the morphine molecule. This modification allows the molecule to bind to the opioid receptor but prevents the conformation change in the receptor required for agonist activity.

In cases of **opioid overdose**, naloxone is administered intravenously to rapidly terminate respiratory depression and other toxic effects of opioid agonists. Because naloxone has a relatively **short half-life** (see Table 23–2), repeated doses of the drug may be needed to counteract the effects of the longer-lasting opioid agonists. Naloxone is also formulated with opioid agonists in oral medications to prevent crushing of the pill and intravenous abuse. Because naloxone has low bioavailability and is not effective when given orally, it does not block the effects of the oral opioid but would block opioid effects or even precipitate withdrawal if used by the intravenous route.

Naltrexone, in oral (REVIA, DEPADE) and extended-release injectable suspension (once-a-month, VIVITROL) formulations, is also used to treat **alcohol and opioid dependence**. In contrast to naloxone, naltrexone has **high oral bioavailability** and can be used on a long-term basis by opioid addicts who have undergone detoxification and are no longer using opioids (see Chapter 25).

THE TREATMENT OF PAIN

CHOICE OF ANALGESIC

The location, cause, and severity of pain and the risk of producing drug dependence are all factors that influence the way in which pain is managed. As a general rule, patients with acute or chronic pain should be treated with the least potent analgesic that will control their pain. Mild pain usually responds to a nonopioid analgesic, usually an NSAID (Chapter 30). Moderate to severe pain is often treated with **codeine, hydrocodone,** or **oxycodone** in combination with a nonopioid analgesic. Severe pain usually requires the use of a strong opioid agonist (e.g., **fentanyl, meperidine, methadone,** or **morphine**). Although meperidine can be used for acute postsurgical pain and in other situations in which the duration of treatment is limited to a few days, it should not be used for longer durations, because of the possible accumulation of a toxic metabolite (normeperidine).

Acute pain caused by trauma, surgery, or short-term medical conditions can be effectively managed with an analgesic and appropriate treatment of the underlying condition. In patients with acute pain, the risk of producing drug dependence is extremely low. Hence, physicians and other health care professionals should not hesitate to administer adequate doses of a sufficiently strong analgesic to control pain.

Pain associated with **arthritis, neuropathy,** and other **chronic but nonterminal conditions** is more difficult to treat and is often managed with a combination of analgesics, co-analgesics, psychotherapy, physical therapy, and other treatment modalities. Use of opioid analgesics in the treatment of chronic pain is associated with a risk of opioid tolerance and physical dependence, so care must be exercised to prevent dosage escalation, drug dependence, and prescription drug abuse. Strict guidelines for prescription refills should be in place, and a prescription refill flowchart can be used to monitor drug usage and prevent dosage escalation. In some clinics, patients are asked to sign an "opioid contract" in which they agree to procedures that will ensure proper utilization of opioid drugs, including random drug testing.

Patients with **terminal illnesses**, such as metastatic cancer, should receive sufficient doses of opioid analgesics to control their pain, irrespective of any concerns about the development of tolerance and physical dependence.

ACUTE PAIN

Giving analgesics on an as-needed basis sometimes produces wide swings in pain and sedation during the early phase of treatment. Therefore, in the initial stages of acute pain, analgesics should be given around the clock at regular intervals. The dosage should be titrated to control pain while minimizing sedation and other side effects. As the pain subsides over time and the need for analgesia decreases, the patient can be transferred to an as-needed schedule of medication.

Patient-controlled analgesia is a method of intravenous administration that permits the patient to self-administer preset amounts of an analgesic (e.g., fentanyl) via a syringe pump that is interfaced with a timing device. The method enables the patient to balance pain control with sedation. Its use depends on the patient's ability to activate the device, so it may not be suitable for elderly patients or for patients immediately after surgery or trauma.

CHRONIC PAIN

Treatment of chronic pain varies greatly with the underlying cause. Although the discussion of specific chronic pain syndromes is beyond the scope of this text, a few general guidelines and comments will be offered.

Both **opioid analgesics** and **nonopioid analgesics** are useful in the management of chronic pain syndromes. If pain is associated with inflammation, nonopioid drugs with anti-inflammatory activity can be especially useful. If pain is associated with peripheral nerve or nerve root sensitization, treatment with **transcutaneous nerve stimulation** or a **local anesthetic** may help. In some cases, cream containing **capsaicin** is effective. Capsaicin activates peripheral nociceptors on primary sensory neurons, thereby leading to increased release of substance P and eventually to the depletion of substance P in the CNS. Capsaicin produces a burning sensation for the first few days of application, but this is gradually replaced by an analgesic effect.

Chronic pain is frequently seen in association with systemic disorders (e.g., diabetes). When pain has been present for a period of time, the responsiveness of dynamic wide-range nociceptive neurons in the spinal cord increases in a way that increases pain perception and memory. As these neurons become "wound up," their receptive fields increase so that pain is felt over a larger area. These changes appear to contribute to the maintenance of chronic neuropathic pain. Patients with this type of pain may benefit from a combination of nonpharmacologic therapies (e.g., TENS, acupuncture, and physical therapy), analgesic medications, and co-analgesic drugs. The most widely used **co-analgesics** are the **antiepileptic drugs** and the **antidepressant drugs**. These drugs provide pain relief in chronic pain syndromes and may potentiate the effects of opioid and nonopioid analgesics.

Antiepileptic drugs (e.g., **carbamazepine, gabapentin, phenytoin**, and **valproate**) are particularly effective in treating pain syndromes with an intermittent lancinating quality, such as **trigeminal neuralgia** and **postherpetic neuralgia**. They are also useful in syndromes characterized by continuous, burning neuropathic pain. They probably act by inhibiting the conduction of pain impulses in the CNS, but their exact mechanism is unknown. The general properties of these drugs are described in Chapter 20.

The **tricyclic antidepressants** are the most widely used type of antidepressants for the treatment of chronic pain, as they may be more effective than the selective serotonin reuptake inhibitors in this respect. **Amitriptyline, desipramine,** and other tricyclic antidepressants are particularly effective in the management of postherpetic neuralgia, diabetic neuropathy, migraine headache, and neuropathic pain syndromes. They can also be beneficial in the management of pain associated with chronic fatigue syndrome. The properties of these drugs are described in Chapter 22.

Tramadol is a dual-action analgesic that combines opioid receptor activation with inhibition of neuronal reuptake of neurotransmitters in a manner similar to tricyclic antidepressants. As noted above, tramadol is effective in many chronic pain syndromes and causes little constipation, respiratory depression, or drug dependence.

CANCER PAIN

Pain is the most common symptom of cancer, and it can be acute, chronic, or intermittent. Cancer-related pain is frequently undertreated. Most patients can be managed with oral medications, including opioid and NSAID analgesics, antidepressant drugs, and antiepileptic drugs. Acupuncture, TENS, and other modalities are also useful. Severe cancer pain usually requires the administration of a strong opioid agonist (e.g., fentanyl, methadone, or morphine). To maintain stable serum drug levels and prevent breakthrough pain, it may be helpful to use a long-acting preparation (e.g., sustained-release morphine tablets or transdermal fentanyl skin patches), either alone or in combination with a rapid-acting preparation, such as morphine oral solution.

SUMMARY OF IMPORTANT POINTS

■ Pain impulses are transmitted by primary afferent neurons to the spinal cord, where ascending connections from the spinothalamic tract neurons project to limbic structures and the cortex.

■ Descending inhibitory fibers from the periaqueductal gray matter activate midbrain and spinal cord neurons that release enkephalins, serotonin, and norepinephrine. Opioids activate these pathways and thereby inhibit ascending pain impulses.

■ Opioid drugs include strong and moderate agonists, mixed agonist-antagonists, and pure antagonists.

■ In addition to analgesia, opioid agonists can cause sedation, euphoria, miosis, respiratory depression, peripheral vasodilation, constipation, and drug dependence.

■ Opioid receptors can be divided into three types: *mu, delta,* or *kappa* opioid receptors. All types mediate analgesia, but *mu* opioid receptors are primarily responsible for analgesic effects, as well as respiratory depression and opioid dependence of most clinical agents.

■ The strong opioid agonists include morphine, fentanyl, meperidine, and methadone, which act primarily at *mu* opioid receptors. The first three of these agents are used to alleviate severe or moderate pain. Methadone is usually used in the treatment of opioid addiction (methadone maintenance programs).

■ The moderate agonists produce maximal analgesia at doses that cannot be tolerated, so they are usually combined with a nonopioid analgesic. The moderate agonists, codeine, hydrocodone, and propoxyphene, are used to treat moderate or mild pain.

■ Other agonists include tramadol, a dual-action analgesic that activates opioid receptors and blocks neuronal reuptake of serotonin and norepinephrine.

■ Buprenorphine, butorphanol, nalbuphine, and pentazocine are mixed opioid agonist-antagonists. These drugs exhibit partial agonist or antagonist activity at *mu* opioid receptors and exhibit agonist or antagonist activity at *kappa* opioid receptors. They produce less respiratory depression and are associated with a lower risk of drug dependence than are full opioid agonists.

■ Naloxone and naltrexone are opioid antagonists. These antagonists are used to counteract the adverse effects of opioids in overdose or to prevent and treat alcohol and opioid dependence.

Review Questions

1. Most clinically used opioid analgesics are selective for which type of opioid receptor?
   (A) *kappa (κ)*
   (B) *alpha (α)*
   (C) *beta (β)*
   (D) *mu (μ)*
   (E) *delta (δ)*

2. Codeine has a greater oral bioavailability compared with morphine because of which reason?
   (A) codeine undergoes less first-pass metabolism
   (B) morphine is conjugated more quickly
   (C) morphine directly passes into systemic circulation
   (D) codeine is only available in liquid formulation
   (E) codeine is metabolized more by hepatic enzymes

3. Which of the following statements best explains the observation that morphine is more likely to cause nausea and vomiting in ambulatory patients?
   (A) morphine inhibits "chemoceptor trigger zone" neurons
   (B) morphine sensitizes medulla cough center neurons
   (C) opioids cause sedation, which makes walking more difficult
   (D) patients on opioids eat more
   (E) opioids increase vestibular sensitivity

4. Which of the following opioids is so lipophilic that it is marketed in a skin patch used to treat chronic pain?
   (A) morphine
   (B) naltrexone
   (C) scopolamine
   (D) methadone
   (E) fentanyl

5. In a case of an opioid overdose, naloxone can be given in repeated doses because of which property of naloxone?
   (A) may have a shorter half-life than the opioid agonist
   (B) is only effective at high cumulative doses
   (C) is needed to stimulate the respiratory center
   (D) is safe only in extremely small doses
   (E) is only a partial opioid agonist

Answers and Explanations

1. The correct choice is D: *mu (μ)* receptors. Although there are three homologous opioid receptor proteins, most clinical opioid analgesics are agonists at the μ receptors. Answer (A), *kappa (κ)*, is also a type of opioid receptor that can mediate analgesia, but only plays a minor role with the action of some mixed agonist-antagonist opioids. Answer (B), *alpha (α)*, is part of the adrenoceptor family. Answer (C), *beta (β)*, is a type of adrenoceptor. Answer (E), *delta (δ)*, is also a type of opioid receptor and does mediate analgesic in preclinical models but δ-selective agents have not surfaced in the clinic.

2. The correct answer is A: codeine undergoes less first-pass metabolism. Codeine is methylmorphine with the methyl group at the 3 position. As this is the principal site of glucuronide metabolism of morphine, the codeine molecule is somewhat protected from the first-pass effect of hepatic metabolism. Answer (B), morphine is conjugated more quickly, is true but is not the best answer because codeine is not conjugated initially but first metabolized to morphine. Answers (C), morphine directly passes into systemic circulation, (D), codeine is only available in liquid formulation, and (E), codeine is metabolized more by hepatic enzymes, are not accurate statements.

3. The correct answer is E: opioids increase vestibular sensitivity. Ambulatory patients report more instances of nausea and vomiting than recumbent patients administered morphine. In vitro studies show that opioids modulate the inner ear vestibular complex to increase its sensitivity. Answers (A), morphine inhibits "chemoceptor trigger zone" neurons, and (B), morphine sensitizes medulla

cough center neurons, are both wrong because morphine has the opposite effects and stimulates the chemoreceptor trigger zone neurons in the medulla and inhibits cough center neurons. Answer (C), opioids cause sedation that makes walking more difficult, may be true but does not affect the onset of nausea and vomiting. Answer (D), patients on opioids eat more, has no support from the literature although fasting does appear to increase endogenous opioid peptides in the CNS and has been implicated in the pathology of the eating disorder anorexia nervosa.

4. The correct answer is E: fentanyl. This potent opioid is available as a transdermal patch for the treatment of chronic pain. Answer (A), morphine, is not so lipophilic to allow transdermal administration. Answer (B), naltrexone, is an opioid antagonist that does come in a patch formulation but would not help with chronic pain. It is used to treat opioid and alcohol dependence. Answer (C), scopolamine, does also come in a patch but is used for motion sickness. Answer (D), methadone, is a long-acting opioid agonist but is not available in a patch.

5. The correct choice is naloxone A: may have a shorter half-life than the opioid agonist. Treatment of opioid overdose often requires repeated doses of naloxone or continuous infusion to compete with the agonist at the receptor. Answer (B), naloxone, is only effective at high cumulative doses, is not true and even the first dose of naloxone may provide miraculous reversal of opioid overdose. Answers (C) through (E) are not true.

SELECTED READINGS

Craft, R.M. Sex differences in opioid analgesia: "from mouse to man." Clin J Pain 19:175–186, 2003.

Evans, C.J. Secrets of the opium poppy revealed. Neuropharmacol 47 (Suppl 1):293–299, 2004.

Katz, N. Opioids: after thousands of years, still getting to know you. Clin J Pain 23:303–306, 2007.

Riley, J., E. Eisenberg, G. Müller-Schwefe, A.M. Drewes, and L. Arendt-Nielsen. Oxycodone: a review of its use in the management of pain. Curr Med Res Opin 24:175–192, 2008.

Skaer, T.L. Practice guidelines for transdermal opioids in malignant pain. Drugs 64(23):2629–2638, 2004.

CHAPTER 24

Drugs for Neurodegenerative Diseases

CLASSIFICATION OF DRUGS FOR NEURODEGENERATIVE DISEASES*

Drugs for Parkinson's Disease
Drugs That Increase Dopamine Levels
- Levodopa (L-DOPA, LARODOPA)
- Carbidopa (WITH L-DOPA IN SINEMET)
- Amantadine (SYMMETREL)
- Selegiline (ELDEPRYL)
- Rasagiline (AZILECT)
- Tolcapone (TASMAR)
- Entacapone (COMTAN)

Dopamine Receptor Agonists
- Bromocriptine (PARLODEL)
- Pramipexole (MIRAPEX)
- Ropinirole (REQUIP)
- Rotigotine (NEUPRO)
- Apomorphine (APOKYN)

Cholinergic Receptor Antagonists
- Benztropine (COGENTIN)
- Trihexyphenidyl (ARTANE)

Drugs for Huntington's Disease
- Diazepam (VALIUM)
- Haloperidol (HALDOL)

Drugs for Alzheimer's Disease
- Donepezil (ARICEPT)
- Tacrine (COGNEX)
- Rivastigmine (EXELON)
- Galantamine (RAZADYNE)
- Memantine (NAMENDA)

Drugs for Multiple Sclerosis
- Baclofen (LIORESAL)
- Tizanidine (ZANAFLEX)
- Prednisone (PREDNISONE INTENSOL)
- Interferon Beta-1b (BETASERON)[a]

Drugs for Amyotrophic Lateral Sclerosis
- Riluzole (RILUTEK)
- Baclofen (LIORESAL)
- Gabapentin (NEURONTIN)

[a]Also interferon beta-1a (AVONEX), natalizumab (TYSABRI), mitoxantrone (NOVANTRONE), and glatiramer acetate (COPAXONE).
*Note that baclofen is listed more than once.

OVERVIEW

Parkinson's disease, Huntington's disease, Alzheimer's disease, multiple sclerosis, and amyotrophic lateral sclerosis (ALS, or Lou Gehrig's disease) are neurodegenerative diseases characterized by the progressive loss of neuronal function in a particular part of the central nervous system. The signs and symptoms of neurodegenerative diseases do not reflect a normal age-related loss of brain neurons. Instead, these progressive disease states are the result of an underlying pathologic process.

Although the cause of these diseases is unknown, evidence suggests the involvement of heredity, autoimmunity, and environmental factors. Substantial progress is noted for the development of drugs to treat Parkinson's disease, and somewhat for Alzheimer's disease, however drug therapy for the other neurodegenerative diseases is limited. New research findings elucidating the pathogenesis of neurodegenerative diseases will enable the development of more successful drugs in the near future.

PARKINSON'S DISEASE

Parkinson's disease, or **paralysis agitans**, is characterized by a **resting tremor** (involuntary trembling when a limb is at rest), **rigidity** (inability to initiate movements), and bradykinesia (slowness of movement). The disease results from the degeneration of **dopaminergic neurons** that arise in the **substantia nigra** and project to other structures in the **basal ganglia**.

ETIOLOGY AND PATHOGENESIS

The causes of neuron degeneration in Parkinson's disease remain largely unknown. In most cases, heredity appears to have a limited role. Scientists, however, have identified a defective gene responsible for a rare condition called **autosomal recessive juvenile parkinsonism**, which usually affects people in their teens and 20s.

One of the better-known theories for the cause of Parkinson's disease is called the **oxidative stress theory**. According to this theory, metabolic oxidation of **dopamine** in the basal ganglia yields highly reactive **free radicals** that are toxic to dopaminergic neurons and lead to their degeneration. Free radicals are molecules that lack an electron in their outer orbits and are capable of extracting an electron from other molecules and thereby causing cell damage. It is not understood, however, why some individuals would be more susceptible to oxidative stress than others.

The **basal ganglia** are a group of interconnected subcortical nuclei that include the striatum (caudate and putamen), substantia nigra, globus pallidus, and subthalamus. In healthy individuals, the basal ganglia receive input from the cerebral cortex, process this information, and send feedback to the motor area of the cortex in a way that leads to the smooth coordination of body movements. Even simple movements, such as walking, involve a complex sequence of motor acts whose smooth execution requires the continuous interplay of the cortex and basal ganglia. In patients with Parkinson's disease, **neuronal degeneration** interrupts this interplay. Because the basal ganglia also participate in procedural memory and other cognitive functions, patients with Parkinson's disease may have difficulty remembering how to perform learned motor skills, such as driving a car.

The basal ganglia function via a series of reciprocal innervations among themselves and the cortex (Fig. 24–1). The striatum receives input from the cerebral cortex and substantia nigra, and then sends output to the thalamus via the globus pallidus. The thalamus then feeds information back to the motor area of the cortex. Two pathways connect the striatum and the thalamus: a **direct pathway**, which is excitatory, and an **indirect pathway**, which is inhibitory. In patients with Parkinson's disease, the degeneration of dopaminergic neurons results in decreased activity in the direct pathway and increased activity in the indirect pathway. As a result, thalamic feedback to the

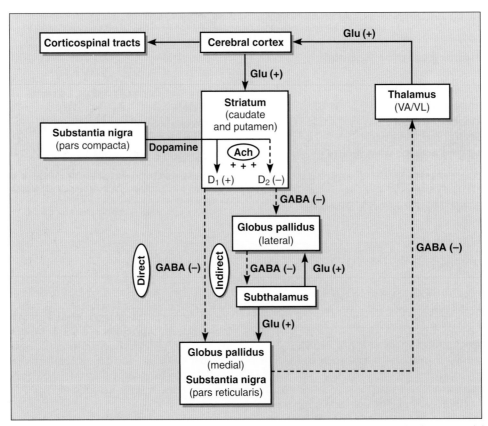

Figure 24-1. Pathophysiology of Parkinson's disease. The striatum receives input from the entire cerebral cortex and the substantia nigra and sends projections to the thalamus via direct and indirect pathways through the globus pallidus, substantia nigra, and subthalamus. Striatal dopamine D_1 receptors excite the direct pathway, whereas D_2 receptors inhibit the indirect pathway. In Parkinson's disease, the degeneration of dopaminergic neurons leads to decreased activity in the direct pathway and increased activity in the indirect pathway. As a result of these changes, thalamic input to the motor area of the cortex is reduced, and the patient exhibits rigidity and bradykinesia. GABA = γ-aminobutyric acid; Glu = glutamate; VA/VL = ventral anterior and ventral lateral nuclei; (+) = excitatory; (–) = inhibitory.

cortex is reduced, and patients exhibit bradykinesia and rigidity.

Excitatory **cholinergic neurons** also participate in the interconnections between structures in the basal ganglia. In Parkinson's disease, the degeneration of inhibitory dopaminergic neurons leads to a relative excess of cholinergic activity in these pathways. For this reason, patients with Parkinson's disease can be treated effectively with drugs that **inhibit cholinergic activity** or with drugs that **increase dopamine levels** in the basal ganglia.

DRUGS THAT INCREASE DOPAMINE LEVELS

Dopamine levels in the basal ganglia can be increased by various drugs in different ways. **Levodopa** increases dopamine levels by increasing dopamine synthesis; **selegiline** by inhibiting dopamine breakdown; and **amantadine** by increasing dopamine release from neurons. **Carbidopa** and **tolcapone** increase the amount of levodopa that enters the brain and thereby enhance dopamine synthesis. The sites of action of these drugs are illustrated in Figure 24–2.

Levodopa

Pharmacokinetics. Levodopa, also called L-**dopa** or **dihydroxyphenylalanine**, is the biosynthetic precursor of **dopamine**. Levodopa increases the concentration of dopamine in the brain and is the main treatment used to alleviate motor dysfunction in patients with Parkinson's disease. Dopamine itself is not effective in the treatment of Parkinson's disease when administered systemically, because it does not cross the blood-brain barrier to a significant extent.

Levodopa is absorbed from the proximal duodenum by the same process that absorbs large neutral amino acids (see Fig. 24–2). **Dietary amino acids** compete with levodopa for transport into the circulation, and amino acids can also reduce the transport of levodopa into the brain. For these reasons, the ingestion of high-protein foods can decrease the effectiveness of levodopa, and a protein-restricted diet may improve the response to levodopa in some patients.

Levodopa is metabolized by two pathways in peripheral tissues. It is converted to **dopamine** by L-**aromatic amino acid decarboxylase (LAAD)**, and it is metabolized to 3-O-methyldopa (3OMD) by **catechol-O-methyltransferase (COMT)**. A drug that inhibits LAAD (e.g., **carbidopa**) or

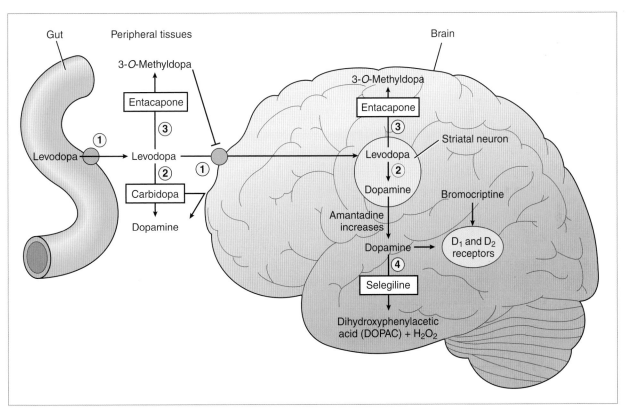

Figure 24–2. **Mechanisms of dopaminergic drugs used in the treatment of Parkinson's disease.** Levodopa is transported across the gut wall and the blood-brain barrier and is converted to dopamine in striatal neurons. Carbidopa inhibits the peripheral decarboxylation of levodopa and thereby increases the amount of levodopa that enters the brain. Carbidopa does not cross the blood-brain barrier and does not inhibit dopamine synthesis in the brain. Tolcapone and entacapone inhibit the methylation of levodopa in both peripheral tissues and the brain. Tolcapone and entacapone increase levodopa bioavailability and increase brain uptake of levodopa. Selegiline inhibits the degradation of dopamine to dihydroxyphenylacetic acid (DOPAC) and hydrogen peroxide (H_2O_2). By this action, selegiline increases dopamine levels in the striatum, and it may reduce the formation of free radicals that are derived from H_2O_2. Amantadine increases the release of dopamine from striatal neurons. Bromocriptine and other dopamine-receptor agonists activate dopamine receptors in the striatum. Numbered structures and enzymes are as follows: 1 = pump that transports large neutral amino acids; 2 = L-aromatic amino acid decarboxylase (LAAD); 3 = catechol-O-methyltransferase (COMT); 4 = monoamine oxidase type B (MAO-B).

inhibits COMT (e.g., **tolcapone**) is used in combination with levodopa to increase the amount of levodopa that enters brain tissue. LAAD requires **vitamin B$_6$ (pyridoxine)** as a cofactor. For this reason, vitamin B$_6$ supplements may enhance the peripheral decarboxylation of levodopa and should not be co-administered with levodopa.

Levodopa exhibits a large **first-pass effect**, and about 95% of an administered dose is metabolized in the gut wall and liver before it reaches the systemic circulation. Additional amounts of levodopa are converted to dopamine and 3OMD before the drug enters the CNS. Therefore, only about 1% of the administered dose of levodopa reaches brain tissue.

MECHANISMS AND PHARMACOLOGIC EFFECTS. In the brain, levodopa is taken up by dopaminergic neurons in the striatum and is converted to dopamine by LAAD. Levodopa thereby increases the amount of dopamine released by these neurons in patients with Parkinson's disease, and it serves as a form of **replacement therapy**. Levodopa can counteract all of the signs of parkinsonism, although the degree and duration of its effectiveness usually are not optimal. As the disease progresses and more dopaminergic neurons are lost, the conversion of levodopa to dopamine declines.

About 60% to 70% of nigrostriatal dopaminergic neurons are lost before the clinical symptoms of Parkinson's disease are first observed, and the degeneration of these neurons continues throughout the course of the disease. Over time, patients begin to experience two types of fluctuation in the effectiveness of levodopa, both of which are probably related to a reduced concentration of dopamine in the striatum. The first type, a "**wearing off**" effect, occurs toward the end of a dosage interval. The second type, the "**on-off**" **phenomenon**, is characterized by severe motor fluctuations that occur randomly.

ADVERSE EFFECTS. When levodopa is used alone, **nausea and vomiting** occur in about 80% of patients, **orthostatic hypotension** is reported in 25%, and **cardiac arrhythmias** occur in 10%. These effects, which are caused by the action of dopamine on β-adrenoceptors in the case of cardiac arrhythmias, are substantially reduced when **carbidopa** (see below) is administered with levodopa to block the peripheral formation of dopamine.

About 30% of patients who are treated with levodopa on a long-term basis eventually develop involuntary movements, or dyskinesias, as a result of excessive dopamine concentrations in the striatum. Dyskinesias most often occur when levodopa concentrations are highest, in which case they are called **peak-dose dyskinesias**. The dyskinesias often involve the oral and facial musculature, and patients can appear as if they are chewing on large pieces of food while protruding their lips. Other common dyskinesias involve writhing and flinging movements of the arms and legs. Less commonly, levodopa causes **psychotic effects**, including hallucinations and distorted thinking, which are probably caused by excessive dopamine concentrations in mesolimbic and mesocortical pathways. Although **dyskinesias** and psychotic effects could be managed by reducing the levodopa dosage, the therapeutic efficacy of the drug would be reduced as well.

Some patients treated with levodopa complain of sedative effects, agitation, delirium, vivid dreams, or nightmares. Others, however, report a pleasant euphoria after taking the drug.

INTERACTIONS. Levodopa has important interactions with a number of medications. Drugs that delay gastric emptying, such as anticholinergic drugs, can slow levodopa absorption and reduce its peak serum concentration. Drugs that promote gastric emptying (e.g., antacids) can increase levodopa bioavailability. Nonselective **monoamine oxidase inhibitors (MAOIs)**, for example the antidepressant **phenelzine,** inhibit the breakdown of dopamine and sometimes cause a hypertensive crisis in patients receiving levodopa. **Antipsychotic drugs** block dopamine receptors and can reduce the effectiveness of levodopa and exacerbate motor dysfunction. Because **clozapine** is much less likely to do this than other antipsychotic drugs, it is often used to manage psychotic reactions in patients receiving levodopa (see Chapter 22).

INDICATIONS. Levodopa is effective in the management of patients with **idiopathic Parkinson's disease** and in the treatment of patients with **postencephalitic parkinsonism**, a disorder portrayed in the movie *Awakenings*. It is also used to treat **parkinsonian symptoms** caused by carbon monoxide poisoning, manganese intoxication, or cerebral arteriosclerosis.

Carbidopa

Carbidopa, a structural analogue of levodopa, **inhibits LAAD** thereby reducing the conversion of levodopa to dopamine in peripheral tissues and so increasing the amount of levodopa that enters the brain (see Fig. 24–2). Carbidopa is highly ionized at physiological pH, and it does not cross the blood-brain barrier. For this reason, it does not inhibit the formation of dopamine in the CNS.

Carbidopa substantially reduces the gastrointestinal and cardiovascular side effects of levodopa and enables about a 75% reduction in the dosage of levodopa. A **levodopa-carbidopa combination** is available in immediate-release and sustained-release formulations that contain different ratios of the two drugs. The sustained-release formulations are designed to reduce the "wearing off" effect described above.

Amantadine

Amantadine is an antiviral drug that is used in the prevention and treatment of influenza but also has a beneficial effect on Parkinson's disease. Amantadine appears to work by increasing the **release of dopamine** from nigrostriatal neurons, but it may also inhibit the reuptake of dopamine by these neurons. Amantadine is generally better tolerated than levodopa or dopamine agonists, but it is also less effective.

Amantadine is used to treat early or mild cases of Parkinson's disease and as an adjunct to levodopa. Its adverse effects include sedation, restlessness, vivid dreams, nausea, dry mouth, and hypotension. It can also cause **livedo reticularis**, which is a reddish-blue mottling of the skin with edema. CNS side effects are more likely to occur in the elderly because of their reduced capacity to excrete the drug by the kidneys.

Selegiline

PHARMACOKINETICS. Selegiline, also known as deprenyl, is a modified phenylethylamine compound. The drug is well absorbed from the gut and is partly metabolized to amphetamine.

MECHANISMS AND PHARMACOLOGIC EFFECTS. Selegiline inhibits monoamine oxidase type B (MAO-B) and thereby prevents the oxidation of dopamine to dihydroxyphenylacetic acid and hydrogen peroxide, as shown in Figure 24–2. By this action, selegiline increases dopamine levels in the basal ganglia and decreases the formation of hydrogen peroxide. In the presence of iron, hydrogen peroxide is converted to hydroxyl and hydroxide free radicals that may participate in the degeneration of nigrostriatal neurons in patients with Parkinson's disease.

There is evidence that selegiline inhibits the progression of Parkinson's disease either by inhibiting the formation of free radicals or by inhibiting the formation of an active metabolite of an environmental toxin. However, the ability of selegiline to inhibit disease progression is controversial. It was initially suggested by studies showing that selegiline could prevent a form of parkinsonism that is induced by **1-methyl-4-phenyl-1,2,3,6-tetrahydropyridine (MPTP)**. MPTP is a toxic byproduct of the synthesis of "designer" street drugs; in the 1980s, people who took what they thought was a **meperidine** analogue ingested drugs contaminated with MPTP and developed classic signs of parkinsonism. MPTP must be converted to 1-methyl-4-phenylpyridium by MAO-B before it can damage dopaminergic neurons, and studies demonstrated that selegiline blocked this reaction. The results of these studies have led some investigators to postulate that idiopathic Parkinson's disease is caused by an environmental toxin whose action resembles that of MPTP. Although unfortunate for the drug abusers who were exposed to MPTP, it did lead to an important **animal model for parkinsonism** and the development of new agents.

ADVERSE EFFECTS AND INTERACTIONS. Adverse effects are listed in Table 24–1. Unlike the nonselective MAOIs used in treating mood disorders, selegiline does not inhibit monoamine oxidase type A (MAO-A), an enzyme that catalyzes the degradation of catecholamines. For this reason, selegiline is much less likely to cause hypertension when it is administered in combination with sympathomimetic amines or when it is taken with foods that contain **tyramine**. The drug's selectivity for MAO-B, however, is lost when it is given in higher doses, so the potential for food interaction still exists. Selegiline can cause adverse effects if it is administered with meperidine or with selective serotonin reuptake inhibitors (SSRIs; e.g., fluoxetine) as noted in Chapter 22.

INDICATIONS. Selegiline can be used as a single drug for the treatment of **early or mild Parkinson's disease**, and it is used as an adjunct with levodopa-carbidopa for **advanced disease**. Selegiline reduces the dosage requirement for levodopa, and it may improve motor function in patients who experience "wearing off" and "on-off" difficulties with levodopa.

The most controversial role of selegiline is its use as a **neuroprotective agent**. Although some clinical studies have indicated that selegiline slows the progression of Parkinson's disease, others have indicated that it does not.

Recently a second MAO-B inhibitor, **rasagiline**, was approved as a monotherapy or adjunct medication in the treatment of parkinsonism. It has the same potential adverse effects as selegiline, due to interactions with tyramine, meperidine, and SSRIs.

Tolcapone

Tolcapone is a drug used to enhance the effectiveness of levodopa in the treatment of Parkinson's disease. It inhibits **COMT**, the enzyme that metabolizes levodopa to 3OMD in the gut and liver. By this action, tolcapone produces a twofold increase in the oral bioavailability and half-life of levodopa. Because 3OMD competes with levodopa for transport into brain tissue, it may contribute to the "wearing off" and "on-off" effects that occur during long-term levodopa therapy. By inhibiting 3OMD formation, tolcapone may **stabilize dopamine levels** in the striatum and contribute to a more sustained improvement in motor function.

In clinical studies, tolcapone was found to increase the efficacy of levodopa while reducing the dosage requirement. Tolcapone was well tolerated, and most of the side effects were similar in frequency to those reported with use of a placebo. Although tolcapone caused diarrhea and nausea in some patients, these side effects decreased over time. A few reports were made of rare, but **fatal hepatitis** following administration of tolcapone.

Entacapone

Entacapone has the same mechanism of action as tolcapone but is more peripherally restricted in its distribution. It may be safer to use for the treatment of parkinsonism than tolcapone as there have yet to be reports of hepatic toxicity.

Dopamine Receptor Agonists

The dopamine-receptor agonists **directly activate dopamine receptors** in the striatum. Because they do not require a functional dopaminergic neuron to produce their effects, they are sometimes helpful in advanced cases of Parkinson's disease, in which few dopaminergic neurons remain. The drugs work primarily by activating D_2 receptors. As shown in Figure 24–1, activation of these receptors leads to inhibition of the indirect neuronal pathway from the striatum to the thalamus and increases thalamic stimulation of the motor area of the cortex.

Bromocriptine

Bromocriptine is an **ergot alkaloid**, in the same chemical class as the hallucinogen LSD. Other ergot alkaloids used to treat migraine headaches are discussed in Chapter 29. Bromocriptine is a D_2**-receptor agonist** and a D_1**-receptor antagonist**. Bromocriptine can serve as a useful adjunct to levodopa in patients who have advanced Parkinson's disease and experience "wearing off" effects and "on-off" motor fluctuations.

Dopamine-receptor agonists produce **adverse effects** that are similar to those of levodopa. Nausea, which occurs in as many as 50% of patients when they are first treated with a receptor agonist, primarily results from stimulation of dopamine receptors in the vomiting center located in the medulla. Dose-related CNS effects of the receptor agonists include confusion, dyskinesias, sedation, vivid dreams, and **hallucinations**. Other adverse effects include orthostatic hypotension, dry mouth, and decreased prolactin levels. Nausea and many other adverse effects subside over time. To enable patients to develop tolerance to the effects, treatment should begin with a low dose, and the dosage should be increased gradually.

Pergolide (PERMAX), is also an ergot alkaloid and direct-acting dopamine agonist, but was withdrawn from the market in 2007 due to increased risk of **damage to heart valves**.

Pramipexole and Ropinirole

In contrast to the older dopamine-receptor agonists, **pramipexole** and **ropinirole** are not ergot alkaloids. Both act as selective **D_2-receptor agonists**. In addition, pramipexole activates **D_3-receptors**, and this may contribute to its effectiveness in Parkinson's disease. The adverse effects, contraindications, and drug interactions of pramipexole and ropinirole are summarized in Table 24–1.

Clinical studies have shown that pramipexole or ropinirole can delay the need for levodopa when used in early stages of Parkinson's disease. In advanced stages, they can reduce the "off" period and **decrease the levodopa dosage requirement**. Thus, although the bromocriptine is primarily used as adjunct therapy in advanced Parkinson's disease, the newer agonists may prove effective as monotherapy in both early and advanced disease.

Pramipexole and **ropinirole** are also indicated for the treatment of **restless-legs syndrome**, a condition characterized by as an urge to move the legs at night in bed, often coupled with unpleasant sensations (**paraesthesia**) in the legs that are reduced by movement.

Rotigotine (NEUPRO) is a newer, nonergot dopamine agonist that is formulated as a **transdermal** patch preparation. Like pramipexole, rotigotine has selectivity for D_2 over D_1 receptors and additional activity at D_3 receptors which has been linked to slowing progression of neurodegenerative diseases.

Apomorphine

Apomorphine, which is chemically related to morphine, does not bind to opioid receptors but rather is a **dopamine receptor agonist**. It is actually an old drug put to a new use and was recently approved for the treatment of acute, intermittent **hypomobility** ("freezing") episodes associated with advanced Parkinson's disease. It is available for injection only and produces a rapid (within 5–10 min) reversal of the hypomobility state.

Acetylcholine Receptor Antagonists

Several centrally acting **anticholinergic drugs** are used in the management of Parkinson's disease. Two examples are **benztropine** and **trihexyphenidyl,** which are antagonists at cholinergic **muscarinic receptors**, and also exhibit some antihistamine activity. The anticholinergic drugs are generally less effective than the dopaminergic drugs, but they may be helpful as adjunct therapy in combination with levodopa and other drugs that augment dopaminergic activity. The anticholinergic drugs are more effective in reducing **tremor** than in reducing other manifestations of Parkinson's disease, although they may provide some reduction of bradykinesia and rigidity in patients with mild dysfunction. **Benztropine** may also inhibit the neuronal reuptake of dopamine by central dopaminergic neurons and thereby prolong the action of dopamine.

In addition to being useful in the treatment of **early** and **advanced Parkinson's disease**, the anticholinergic drugs can also reduce parkinsonian symptoms caused by dopamine receptor antagonists, such as **haloperidol** (see Chapter 22).

Treatment Considerations

Optimal management of Parkinson's disease requires that the disabilities of each patient be carefully assessed before drug treatment is recommended. Early disease of mild intensity can be best managed with exercise, nutrition, and education. Speech, occupational, and physical therapies can also be helpful.

For patients whose clinical manifestations are limited to mild tremor and slowness, anticholinergic drugs or amantadine may be helpful.

For patients with more severe functional disabilities, the dopaminergic drugs are the most effective treatment. Combination therapy with **levodopa and carbidopa** is usually prescribed for these patients, but monotherapy with a new dopamine receptor agonist (e.g., pramipexole or ropinirole) may provide an effective alternative for patients who have either early or advanced Parkinson's disease. Clinicians should remember that dopaminergic drugs have a delayed onset of action, so improvement in the patient's condition may not be noted until 2 to 3 weeks after therapy is started.

Tolcapone and **entacapone** inhibit the metabolism of levodopa, and **selegiline** inhibits the metabolism of dopamine, and these agents can be used to enhance the effectiveness of levodopa in patients with early or advanced disease. Some clinicians begin selegiline treatment early in the disease in an effort to retard disease progression.

For patients who have more advanced disease and begin to experience the "wearing off" and "on-off" fluctuations of levodopa-carbidopa, it is sometimes helpful to change the drug dosage or formulation. For example, the "wearing off" effect can be minimized by increasing the frequency of doses or using a combination of sustained-release and immediate-release formulations. Alternatively, an additional dopaminergic drug can be added to the treatment regimen. The addition of tolcapone, for example, may reduce motor fluctuations by increasing and stabilizing levodopa concentrations in the striatum. **Apomorphine**, a nonergot dopamine agonist, may provide quick relief from periods of hypomobility.

HUNTINGTON'S DISEASE

Etiology and Pathogenesis

Huntington's disease, or **Huntington's chorea**, is an autosomal dominant hereditary disorder that is characterized by abnormally expansive or choreoathetoid movements (dance-like movements) of the limbs, rhythmic movements of the

TABLE 24-1. Adverse Effects, and Interactions of Selected Drugs for Neurodegenerative Diseases

Drug	Major Adverse Effects	Major Drug Interactions
Drugs for Parkinson's Disease		
Drugs that increase dopamine levels		
Amantadine	Dry mouth; hypotension; livedo reticularis; nausea; restlessness; sedation; and vivid dreams.	Benztropine and trihexyphenidyl potentiate CNS side effects.
Levodopa-carbidopa	Agitation; arrhythmias; delirium; distorted thinking, hallucinations, and other psychotic effects; dyskinesias; hypotension; nausea and vomiting; nightmares or vivid dreams; and sedation.	Antacids and cisapride may increase bioavailability. Anticholinergic drugs may reduce peak serum level. Antipsychotic drugs, such as haloperidol, may decrease effects. Nonselective MAOIs, such as phenelzine, may cause a hypertensive crisis.
Selegiline	Confusion; dyskinesias; hallucinations; hypotension; insomnia; and nausea.	Severe reactions may result if taken with meperidine or with fluoxetine or other SSRIs.
Rasagiline	Same as selegiline.	Same as selegiline.
Tolcapone	Diarrhea and nausea.	Unknown.
Entacapone	Diarrhea and nausea.	Unknown.
Dopamine receptor agonists		
Bromocriptine	Confusion; decreased prolactin levels; dry mouth; dyskinesias; hallucinations; nausea; orthostatic hypotension; sedation; and vivid dreams.	Dopamine antagonists may reduce effects.
Pramipexole	Dizziness; hallucinations; insomnia; nausea and vomiting; and sedation.	Cimetidine inhibits renal excretion and increases serum levels.
Ropinirole	Same as pramipexole.	Ciprofloxacin increases serum levels.
Rotigotine	Somnolence; slight BP/HR increase; site irritation	Sulfite sensitivity; no major drug interactions.
Acetylcholine receptor antagonists		
Benztropine	Agitation; confusion; constipation; delirium; dry mouth; memory loss; urinary retention; and tachycardia.	Additive anticholinergic effect with antihistamines and phenothiazines.
Trihexyphenidyl	Same as benztropine.	Same as benztropine.
Drugs for Huntington's Disease		
Diazepam	Arrhythmias; CNS depression; drug dependence; hypotension; and mild respiratory depression.	Alcohol and other CNS depressants potentiate effects. Cimetidine increases and rifampin decreases serum levels.
Haloperidol	Extrapyramidal side effects and increased prolactin levels.	Barbiturates and carbamazepine decrease and quinidine increases serum levels.
Drugs for Alzheimer's Disease		
Donepezil	Bradycardia; diarrhea; gastrointestinal bleeding; and nausea and vomiting.	Anticholinergic drugs inhibit effects.
Tacrine	Bradycardia; diarrhea; gastrointestinal bleeding; hepatotoxicity; nausea and vomiting; and urinary incontinence.	Anticholinergic drugs inhibit effects. Cimetidine increases serum levels. Smoking decreases serum levels. Tacrine increases effects of succinylcholine and theophylline.
Rivastigmine	Risk of bradycardia and AV block; nausea and vomiting; anorexia; weight loss.	Anticholinergic drugs inhibit effects. Nicotine use increases oral clearance.
Galantamine	Risk of bradycardia and AV block; nausea and vomiting.	Anticholinergic drugs inhibit effects. Inhibitors of CYP2D6 increase serum levels.
Memantine	Confusion; dizziness; drowsiness; headache; insomnia.	Carbonic anhydrase inhibitors reduce renal elimination of memantine.
Drugs for Multiple Sclerosis		
Baclofen	Dizziness; fatigue; and weakness.	Unknown.
Interferon beta-1b	Chills; diarrhea; fever; headache; hypertension; myalgia; pain; and vomiting.	Increases serum levels of zidovudine.
Prednisone	Aggravation of diabetes mellitus; gastrointestinal bleeding; mood changes; pancreatitis; and seizures.	Barbiturates, carbamazepine, phenytoin, and rifampin decrease serum levels.
Drugs for Amyotrophic Lateral Sclerosis		
Baclofen	Dizziness; fatigue; and weakness.	Unknown.
Gabapentin	Ataxia; dizziness; drowsiness; nystagmus; and tremor.	Antacids decrease serum levels.
Riluzole	Asthenia; diarrhea; dizziness; drowsiness; increased hepatic enzyme levels; nausea and vomiting; paresthesias; and vertigo.	Quinolones and theophylline can increase serum levels. Omeprazole, rifampin, and smoking can decrease serum levels.

AV = atrioventricular; BP/HR = blood pressure/heart rate; CNS = central nervous system; MAOI = monoamine oxidase inhibitor; SSRI = selective serotonin reuptake inhibitor.

tongue and face, and mental deterioration that leads to personality disorders, psychosis, and dementia. Patients are usually in their late 30s when the disease begins, and progressive respiratory depression usually causes death in 10 to 15 years.

Huntington's disease is caused by the degeneration of **γ-aminobutyric acid (GABA) neurons** in the **striatum** and elsewhere in the brain. This degeneration may be fueled by excessive release of the excitatory amino acid glutamate and **glutamate-induced neurotoxicity**. The loss of GABA neurons that project from the striatum to the lateral globus pallidus leads to disinhibition of thalamic nuclei and to an increase in thalamic input to the motor area of the cortex (see Fig. 24–1).

Treatment

The symptoms of Huntington's disease are consistent with excessive dopaminergic activity in the basal ganglia. Therefore, drugs that block dopamine receptors (e.g., **haloperidol**) and other antipsychotic drugs (see Chapter 22) produce some improvement in motor function and are also helpful in relieving the psychosis that accompanies the disease. **Diazepam** and other benzodiazepine drugs (see Chapter 19) potentiate GABA and can also reduce excess movements in patients with Huntington's disease. The efficacy of benzodiazepines, however, declines significantly with disease progression.

In the future, new treatments may result from identification of the function of *huntingtin*, the abnormal gene product that is synthesized in Huntington's disease. Drugs that inhibit glutamate neurotoxicity might also prove useful in the treatment of this disease.

ALZHEIMER'S DISEASE

Etiology and Pathogenesis

Alzheimer's disease is a type of **progressive dementia** for which no cause is known and no cure has been found. In the United States, Alzheimer's disease accounts for about 60% of all cases of dementia in patients over 65 years of age and is associated with more than 100,000 deaths each year. The disease has a tremendous negative impact on patients and their families because of its devastating effects on the cognitive, emotional, and physical function of the patient with Alzheimer's disease (Box 24–1).

Alzheimer's disease results from the destruction of **cholinergic and other neurons** in the **cortex** and **limbic structures of the brain**, particularly the amygdala, basal forebrain, and hippocampus. Major changes in these structures include cortical atrophy, neurofibrillary tangles, and neuritic plaques containing β-amyloid protein. The cholinergic neurons destroyed in Alzheimer's disease originate in **Meynert's nucleus (nucleus basalis)** in the forebrain. These neurons project to the frontal cortex and hippocampus, and they have a critical role in memory and cognition.

Treatment

In patients with Alzheimer's disease, treatment with **donepezil** or **tacrine** is administered in an effort to improve cholinergic neurotransmission in affected areas of the brain.

BOX 24–1. THE CASE OF THE FORGETFUL FATHER

CASE PRESENTATION: A 59-year-old male is encouraged to see a physician by his family members, who have noticed that he has recently become more forgetful. He has been repeating himself and asking the same question over and over, has trouble finding the words to finish his sentences, and even forgot to attend his son's soccer game, which he had never done before. At a recent family gathering, when he couldn't remember the name of a new neighbor that he met a few days earlier, he became agitated. A visit to a neurologist ruled out stroke or other detectable changes on an MRI. The neurologist diagnosed him with early-stage or mild Alzheimer's disease and prescribed donepezil.

CASE DISCUSSION: An estimated 10% of individuals over age 65 and nearly half of those 85 or older have Alzheimer's disease, currently afflicting more than 5 millions people in the United States. By 2050, it is estimated that there will be 16 million patients with Alzheimer's disease, with the risk of Alzheimer's disease doubling every 5 years beyond age 65. Present treatments only provide lessening of symptoms in the best cases; there is no cure for this neurodegenerative disease. Donepezil is commonly prescribed as it is a central cholinesterase inhibitor and increases the availability of acetylcholine in the brain of patients with Alzheimer's disease. Other treatments include tacrine, which is less favored due to the risk of hepatotoxicity, and the newer agents rivastigmine, galantamine, and memantine.

Although these **centrally acting cholinesterase inhibitors** may slow the deterioration of cognitive function, they do not affect the underlying neurodegenerative process, so the disease is eventually fatal. The adverse effects, and drug interactions of donepezil and tacrine are outlined Table 24–1.

Studies in patients with Alzheimer's disease have demonstrated that those treated with donepezil for 24 weeks had significantly better cognitive function than those treated with a placebo. Donepezil is a **reversible cholinesterase inhibitor** that selectively inhibits cholinesterase in the CNS and increases acetylcholine levels in the cerebral cortex. The drug is well absorbed after oral administration and crosses the blood-brain barrier. Because it has a long half-life of about 70 hours, it is administered once a day. The adverse effects of donepezil include diarrhea, nausea, and vomiting, but these are usually mild and transient. Unlike tacrine, donepezil is not associated with **hepatotoxicity**.

Tacrine was the first centrally acting cholinesterase inhibitor approved for the treatment of Alzheimer's disease.

It has a lower bioavailability and a shorter half-life than does donepezil, and it must be administered several times a day. Tacrine, an acridine compound, is associated with a significant incidence of **hepatotoxicity** and with peripheral cholinergic side effects such as diarrhea, nausea, and urinary incontinence. Because of these adverse effects, few patients can tolerate the higher doses required to demonstrate cognitive improvement in Alzheimer's disease.

Rivastigmine and **galantamine** are newer centrally acting, **reversible cholinesterase inhibitors**. Taken in divided doses, they are shown to significantly delay the global cognitive impairment associated with Alzheimer's disease for at least 6 months in clinical trials. Recently, a **transdermal** formulation of rivastigmine (EXELON PATCH) was introduced which is applied every 24 hours, increasing patient compliance and simplifying caregiver administration.

Memantine is a recently approved agent with a new mechanism of action for the treatment of the dementia of Alzheimer's disease. Memantine is a low potency, **noncompetitive antagonist** at the N-methyl-D-aspartate (**NMDA**) receptor. It is hypothesized to work by attenuating the excitotoxic effects of glutamate that may underlie the pathologic process of neuronal loss in Alzheimer's disease. It is excreted largely unchanged as the parent molecule.

MULTIPLE SCLEROSIS

Etiology and Pathogenesis

Multiple sclerosis (MS) is a chronic disease characterized by the **demyelination of neurons** in the CNS. Although its etiology is unknown, the disease is postulated to have an **autoimmune** or **viral** origin. Demyelination leads to disruption of nerve transmission and is accompanied by an inflammatory response and the formation of plaques in the brain and spinal cord. These plaques typically contain decreased numbers of **oligodendrocytes** (myelin-forming cells). The neurologic symptoms of multiple sclerosis, which depend on the area of the brain that is affected, can include pain, spasticity, weakness, ataxia, fatigue, and problems with speech, vision, gait, and bladder function. Many patients experience relapses and remissions, but some have a more severe and unremitting progression of disease.

Treatment

Interferon beta-1b was the first drug to demonstrate an ability to halt and even reverse the progression of MS in some cases. In clinical studies, the drug was found to reduce the frequency of relapses and the number of new lesions detected by magnetic resonance imaging in patients who were ambulatory, had a relapsing-remitting type of multiple sclerosis, and had experienced at least two exacerbations during the last 2 years. Interferon beta-1b is a synthetic analogue of a **recombinant interferon-beta** produced in *Escherichia coli*. Although the drug's exact mechanism of action is unknown, its effects in patients with MS may be caused by its immunomodulating properties. Interferon beta-1b increases the cytotoxicity of natural killer cells and increases the phagocytic activity of macrophages. In addition, it reduces the amount of interferon-gamma secreted by activated lymphocytes. Because interferon-gamma has been shown to exacerbate the symptoms of MS, a reduction in its secretion may halt the disease. The pharmacologic effects and uses of various interferons are discussed more thoroughly in Chapter 45.

Recently, another interferon product, **interferon beta-1a** was approved to treat the relapsing forms of MS. As with its predecessor, it works as an immunomodulator and is synthesized by recombinant protein pathways.

A monoclonal preparation called **natalizumab** works by blocking the molecular pathway involving cell adhesion that draws lymphocytes into the CNS. The presence of lymphocytes around neuronal fibers is implicated in the immune processes that contribute to the pathology of MS. **Mitoxantrone** belongs to the class of antineoplastic agents and was recently approved for the treatment of MS. It acts by suppressing the activity of T cells, B cells, and macrophages that are thought to lead the attack on the myelin sheath. **Glatiramer acetate** is a synthetic protein that mimics the structure of **myelin basic protein**, a component of the myelin covering nerve fibers. This drug blocks myelin-damaging T cells by acting as a **myelin decoy**. In placebo-controlled clinical trials with relapsing-remitting MS, those taking the glatiramer acetate drug had significantly reduced episodes of relapse compared with control subjects.

Spasticity is frequently treated with physical therapy, but **antispastic drugs**, such as **baclofen** (see Table 24–1) may be useful in severe cases. **Tizanidine**, a centrally acting α_2-receptor agonist, is indicated for the management of spasticity. It is thought to reduce spasticity by blocking nerve impulses through presynaptic inhibition of motor neurons, resulting in decreased spasticity without a reduction in muscle strength.

Acute exacerbations are treated with **adrenal corticosteroid drugs** (e.g., **prednisone**). These drugs have anti-inflammatory activity and are discussed in Chapter 33. In patients with multiple sclerosis, corticosteroids shorten the duration of exacerbations and ameliorate symptoms, possibly by decreasing edema. They are administered orally in milder cases and are given parenterally in high doses in more severe cases.

AMYOTROPHIC LATERAL SCLEROSIS

Etiology and Pathogenesis

Amyotrophic lateral sclerosis (**ALS**), also called **Lou Gehrig's disease**, is a progressive disease of the **motor neurons**. It is characterized by muscle wasting, weakness, and respiratory failure leading to death in 2 to 5 years. The cause of ALS is unknown, but evidence suggests a defect in **superoxide dismutase**, an enzyme that scavenges superoxide radicals.

Treatment

The current treatment for ALS is largely symptomatic. Spasticity can be partly controlled with **baclofen**, a $GABA_B$ agonist whose properties are outlined in Table 24–1. The decline in muscle strength may be slowed by **gabapentin**, an antiepileptic drug discussed in Chapter 20.

Although many drugs have been studied for their potential to reduce the progression of ALS and prolong the length of survival, the first drug that has been specifically approved for use in the treatment of ALS is **riluzole**. This drug has been shown to prolong the time before patients require a tracheotomy and also to prolong life by approximately 3 months. Riluzole is believed to protect motor neurons from the neurotoxic effects of excitatory amino acids (e.g., glutamate) and to prevent the anoxia-related death of cortical neurons. Its exact mechanism of action is unclear, but it may inhibit voltage-gated sodium channels that mediate the release of glutamate from neurons. Clinical studies in patients with ALS indicate that riluzole is more effective in those with bulbar-onset disease than in those with limb-onset disease.

SUMMARY OF IMPORTANT POINTS

■ Parkinson's disease is a chronic disease caused by degeneration of dopaminergic neurons that arise in the substantia nigra. It is characterized by resting tremor, rigidity, and bradykinesia.

■ Parkinson's disease is primarily treated with drugs that increase dopamine levels in the basal ganglia or activate dopamine receptors.

■ Levodopa is converted to dopamine by LAAD. It is often co-administered with carbidopa, which inhibits the peripheral decarboxylation of levodopa and increases its brain uptake.

■ Other drugs that increase dopamine levels in the basal ganglia include tolcapone and entacapone, which inhibit methylation of levodopa, and selegiline and rasagiline, which inhibit the breakdown of dopamine catalyzed by MAO-B. Amantadine increases dopamine release and may inhibit its neuronal reuptake.

■ Direct-acting dopamine-receptor agonists include bromocriptine, pramipexole, ropinirole, and rotigotine. These drugs are often used as adjuncts to levodopa in the treatment of patients whose response to levodopa is inadequate.

■ Levodopa and other dopaminergic drugs can cause significant adverse effects, including nausea, dyskinesias, nightmares, and orthostatic hypotension.

■ Acetylcholine receptor antagonists (anticholinergic drugs) can reduce the tremor seen in Parkinson's disease, but their effectiveness is limited.

■ Huntington's disease is caused by degeneration of GABA neurons in the striatum and other parts of the brain. Degeneration of neurons leads to excessive dopamine neurotransmission and choreoathetoid movements. Dopamine-receptor antagonists can provide some improvement in affected patients.

■ Alzheimer's disease is a progressive dementia partly caused by loss of cholinergic neurons in the cortex and limbic structures of the brain. Donepezil and tacrine, two centrally acting cholinesterase inhibitors, and rivastigmine and galantamine, reversible inhibitors, as well as memantine, an NMDA antagonist, produce some cognitive improvement in patients with this disease.

■ Multiple sclerosis is a demyelinating disease whose exacerbations may be attenuated with corticosteroid drugs. Treatment with interferon beta-1b, and other immunomodifiers, retards disease progression in some patients.

■ Amyotrophic lateral sclerosis is a progressive disease of the motor neurons. Riluzole, the first drug approved for its treatment, has a limited effect on patient survival.

Review Questions

1. Which of the following is not a mechanism of action for antiparkinsonism agents?
   (A) direct dopamine agonist
   (B) precursor loading
   (C) inhibit dopamine metabolism
   (D) block cholinergic receptors
   (E) selective dopamine reuptake inhibition

2. Cardiac arrhythmias following initial doses of levodopa (L-dopa) are occasionally observed. Which of the following explanations most likely explain this occurrence?
   (A) direct action on cardiac dopamine receptors
   (B) decreased release of catecholamines
   (C) direct β-adrenoceptor stimulation
   (D) increased release of dopamine
   (E) interaction with vagal cholinergic receptors

3. Anticholinergic agents are useful in the treatment of parkinsonism because of which one of the following mechanisms?
   (A) decreased levels of acetylcholine from loss of neurons
   (B) continuing degeneration of dopamine neurons
   (C) neurotransmitter imbalance in the basal ganglia
   (D) increased activity of acetylcholinesterase
   (E) increased release of dopamine in basal ganglia

4. Selegiline, an antidepressant also used for the treatment of Parkinson's disease, has which one of the following mechanisms of action?
   (A) it is a selective MAO-B inhibitor
   (B) it blocks the reuptake of dopamine
   (C) it irreversibly binds to COMT
   (D) increases release of dopamine vesicles
   (E) blocks muscarinic cholinergic receptors

5. Baclofen is used to treat muscle spasticity because of which of the following effects?
   (A) is a receptor agonist at $GABA_B$ receptors
   (B) blocks acetylcholine receptors
   (C) enhances the release of GABA vesicles
   (D) is an antagonist as glutamate receptors
   (E) increases GABA action at Cl^- ion channel

Answers and Explanations

1. **The correct answer is E:** selective dopamine reuptake inhibition. Although this mechanism of action would be beneficial in the treatment of parkinsonism because it would lead to an increase in synaptic levels of dopamine, no such agents are currently available. Answer (A), direct dopamine agonist, is a mechanism used by dopamine agonists such as bromocriptine. Answer (B), precursor loading, is the mechanism of L-dopa. Answer (C), inhibit dopamine metabolism, is used by selegiline. Answer (D), block cholinergic receptors, is a mechanism also used for the treatment of parkinsonism by such agents as benztropine.

2. **The correct answer is C:** direct β-adrenoceptor stimulation. Metabolism of L-dopa in the periphery to dopamine can lead to cardiac arrhythmias by direct action of dopamine on cardiac β-adrenoceptors. Administration of L-dopa with carbidopa will decrease the formation of dopamine in the periphery and decrease the likelihood of cardiac abnormalities. Answer (A), direct action on cardiac dopamine receptors, may be a possible mechanism if there were significant dopamine receptors in the heart modulating cardiac rhythm, which there are not. Answer (B), decreased release of catecholamines, would decrease cardiac stimulation. Answer (D), increased release of dopamine, is not the best answer because increased peripheral formation is not the same as increased neuronal release. Answer (E), interaction with vagal cholinergic receptors, might affect cardiac function but dopamine or L-dopa has no interaction with cholinergic receptors.

3. **The correct answer is C:** neurotransmitter imbalance in the basal ganglia. The decrease of dopamine projections to the striatum results in a relative abundance of acetylcholine activity in the striatum. Acetylcholine (muscarinic) antagonists rebalance this abnormality. Answer (A), decreased levels of acetylcholine from loss of neurons, would not be a reason to give an antagonist to correct this condition. Answer (B), the continuing degeneration of dopamine neurons, is a fact of the progression of the disease state but antimuscarinic agents do not retard the progression of parkinsonism. Answer (D), the increased activity of acetylcholinesterase, is not correct because no evidence of enzyme up-regulation in parkinsonism exists. Answer (E), the increased release of dopamine in basal ganglia, is clearly wrong because the disease is caused by the degeneration of dopamine neurons.

4. **The correct answer is A:** it is a selective MAO-B inhibitor. Selegiline does retard the progress of parkinsonism by inhibiting the formation of free radicals from the action of MAO-B on dopamine. Answer (B), it blocks the reuptake of dopamine, would be a possible treatment but no drug like this has been tried in the treatment of parkinsonism. Answer (C), it irreversibly binds to COMT, may cause increased dopamine, but this is not the mechanism of selegiline. Answer (D), increases release of dopamine vesicles, is the mechanism of amantadine. Answer (E), blocks muscarinic cholinergic receptors, is the mechanism of anticholinergic agents used for the treatment of parkinsonism.

5. **The correct answer is A:** is a receptor agonist at GABA$_B$ receptors. Baclofen is presently the only GABA$_B$-receptor agonist approved for the treatment of spasticity. Answers (B) through (E) are incorrect because they are the mechanisms of anticholinergics, amantadine, memantine, and sedative-hypnotic agents, respectively.

SELECTED READINGS

Fernandez, O. Interferons in relapsing-remitting multiple sclerosis: are there benefits from long-term use? CNS Drugs 18:1057–1070, 2004.

Lichtlen, P., M.H. Mohajeri. Antibody-based approaches in Alzheimer's research: safety, pharmacokinetics, metabolism, and analytical tools. J Neurochem 104:859–874, 2008.

Steiger, M. Constant dopaminergic stimulation by transdermal delivery of dopaminergic drugs: a new treatment paradigm in Parkinson's disease. Eur J Neurol 15:6–15, 2008.

Weiss, M.D., P. Weydt, G.T. Carter. Current pharmacological management of amyotrophic lateral sclerosis and a role for rational polypharmacy. Expert Opin Pharmacother 5:735–746, 2004.

Winklhofer, K.F. The parkin protein as a therapeutic target in Parkinson's disease. Expert Opin Ther Targets 11:1543–1552, 2007.

Drugs of Abuse

CLASSIFICATION OF DRUGS OF ABUSE

Central Nervous System Depressants
Alcohols and Glycols
- Ethanol
- Methanol
- Ethylene glycol
- Isopropyl alcohol
- Fomepizole (ANTISOL)[a]

Barbiturates and Benzodiazepines
- Pentobarbital (NEMBUTAL)
- Flunitrazepam (ROHYPNOL)
- γ-Hydroxybutyrate (GHB)

Opioids
- Heroin
- Oxycodone (OXYCONTIN)

Central Nervous System Stimulants
Amphetamine and Its Derivatives
- Amphetamine
- Methamphetamine
- 3,4-Methylenedioxy-Methamphetamine (MDMA)

Other Stimulants
- Cocaine
- Caffeine
- Nicotine

Other Psychoactive Drugs
Cannabis and Its Derivatives
- Marijuana
- Dronabinol (MARINOL)
- Nabilone (CESAMET)

Hallucinogens
- Lysergic Acid Diethylamide (LSD)
- Mescaline And Psilocybin
- Phencyclidine (PCP)

Drugs for Treating Drug Dependence
- Methadone
- Disulfiram (ANTABUSE)
- Acamprosate Calcium (CAMPRAL)
- Naltrexone (REVIA, DEPADE, VIVITROL)
- Buprenorphine (SUBUTEX, SUBOXONE)
- Nicotine (NICORETTE, NICODERM)
- Bupropion (ZYBAN)
- Varenicline (CHANTIX)

[a] Used for methanol or ethylene glycol poisoning.

OVERVIEW

This chapter addresses the grave medical, legal, and social problems of drug abuse, also called substance abuse. It begins with a review of general concepts and mechanisms of drug abuse, moves on to specific classes and agents that are likely to be abused, and follows with an update on prescription drug, steroid, and inhalant abuse. The chapter ends with a discussion of pharmacologic agents used to treat drug dependence and the agents' mechanisms of action.

Drug Abuse

It is human nature that some individuals will experiment with occasional use or become dependent on **mind-altering substances.** Nearly every society in recorded history sanctioned the use of certain drugs while banning the use of others. In many Western countries, for example, products containing ethanol, nicotine, or caffeine are socially acceptable or at least tolerated by the majority of the population, whereas the use of cocaine, marijuana, hallucinogens, and other psychoactive drugs is illegal. In other countries, use

of alcohol is discouraged, but the use of other psychoactive drugs, such as marijuana, is socially acceptable. Hence, what constitutes drug abuse from a social or political perspective is highly dependent on cultural attitudes and legal restrictions.

From a medical and psychological perspective, drug abuse can be defined as the use of a drug in a manner that is **detrimental** to the health or well-being of the drug user, other individuals, or society as a whole. Drug abuse is not restricted to the use of illegal drugs, as the cumulative health and social effects caused by the use of alcoholic beverages and tobacco products in the United States far outweigh the negative effects of all illicit drug use.

Drug Dependence

Drug dependence is a condition in which an individual feels compelled to repeatedly administer a psychoactive drug. When this is done to avoid physical discomfort or withdrawal, it is known as **physical dependence**; when it has a psychological aspect (the need for stimulation or pleasure, or to escape reality) then it is known as **psychological dependence**. Repeated drug use is a learned behavior that is reinforced, both by the pleasurable effects of the drug and by the negative effects of drug abstinence (withdrawal). These effects are the basis of drug craving in drug-dependent individuals. **Psychological dependence** is caused by the positive reinforcement of drug use that results from the activation of neurons located in the nucleus accumbens. **Physical dependence** is a state in which continued drug use is required to prevent an unpleasant **withdrawal syndrome**. Hence, physical dependence leads to negative reinforcement of drug use. Both psychological and physical dependence appear to result from **neuronal adaptation** to the presence of the drug, albeit in different areas of the brain.

Psychological Dependence

The craving for **alcohol, barbiturates, caffeine, cocaine, opioids**, and **tobacco** is remarkably similar, despite the varied behavioral and physiological effects that these drugs produce. This similarity supports the hypothesis that psychological dependence is mediated by a **common neuronal pathway** that leads to **behavioral reinforcement** of drug use. Psychoactive drugs that evoke behavioral reinforcement of their use appear to sensitize dopaminergic neurons that project from the ventral tegmental area to the **nucleus accumbens**. Other psychoactive drugs that are used for their mind-altering effects, including **lysergic acid diethylamide (LSD)**, have a much smaller effect on the dopamine pathway and cause little reinforcement, resulting in less compulsive use of LSD and other such agents.

Much evidence indicates that **dopamine** mediates drug reinforcement by binding to dopamine D_1-receptors in the **nucleus accumbens**. This signal transduction pathway activates adenylyl cyclase, increasing cyclic adenosine monophosphate (cAMP) levels and activating cAMP-dependent kinases. The kinases, in turn, activate other proteins in the signal transduction pathway, including **transcription factors**. In the accumbens, the transcription factor, cAMP-response element binding protein, increases the synthesis of G proteins, cAMP-dependent protein kinases, and

other cell transduction molecules that **amplify** responses to dopamine. Dopamine release onto accumbens neurons also increases the expression of **glutamate receptors**, which strengthens synaptic pathways for dopamine neurotransmission much like the molecular mechanisms of learning discovered in the hippocampus. These mechanisms lead to **sensitization** to dopamine, which underlies the behavioral reinforcement of drug use.

The peak of dopamine release in the nucleus accumbens occurs at the time of the drug's **peak effect** on the central nervous system (CNS). The degree of short-term reinforcement of drug use is linked to the **rate of increase of dopamine levels** in the nucleus accumbens. This relationship appears to account for the propensity of some drugs to produce drug dependence. It also appears to explain the difference in reinforcement effects produced by different routes of administration of a particular drug. For example, the oral administration of an opioid or cocaine causes less reinforcement and psychological dependence than does the intravenous administration or inhalation of an equivalent dose of the same drug. The differences in effect are determined by the rate at which the drug is distributed to the brain and the rate at which dopamine levels in the nucleus accumbens are increased.

Physical Dependence

Physical dependence, also called **neuroadaptation**, results from the adaptations of specific neurons or areas of the brain to the continued presence of a drug. **Physical dependence** is only observed outwardly by the development of a drug-specific withdrawal syndrome if the drug is discontinued or blocked, as during **drug abstinence**. For this reason, physical dependence contributes to the continued use of a drug to avoid unwanted symptoms. The negative effects of nicotine withdrawal, for example, are responsible for the high relapse rate in persons trying to stop smoking cigarettes. The withdrawal symptoms are often opposite to the drug's acute effect, unmasking the neuroadaptation that acted to balance the effects of chronic drug administration. For example, opioids inhibit neurons regulating the peristaltic tone of the gastrointestinal tract and cause constipation; diarrhea is a classic sign of opioid withdrawal.

Drug Addiction

Drug addiction usually refers to an extreme pattern of drug abuse in which an individual is continuously preoccupied with drug procurement and use and thus neglects other responsibilities and personal relationships. Addiction is usually associated with a high level of drug dependence. The term *addict* has a pejorative connotation, however, and the modern treatment of substance abuse as a disease state calls for use of the term *drug-dependent individuals* or *patients*. Such patients are afflicted with a **substance abuse disorder**, as outlined in the *Diagnostic and Statistical Manual of Mental Disorders*, used by psychiatrists.

Classification of Drugs of Abuse

The psychoactive drugs that are used by some individuals for nonmedicinal purposes can be classified as CNS depressants, CNS stimulants, and miscellaneous agents, with the latter group including marijuana, hallucinogens,

TABLE 25-1. **Common Signs and Symptoms of Drug Intoxication**

Drug	Motor and Speech Impairment	Emotional and Perceptual Manifestations	Cardiovascular Manifestations	Other Manifestations
Alcohol	Ataxia, incoordination, loquacity, and slurred speech	Euphoria, impaired attention, irritability, mood changes, and sedation	Flushed face	Nystagmus
Amphetamines	Agitation and loquacity	Decreased fatigue, euphoria, grandiosity, hypervigilance, and paranoia	Hypertension or hypotension and tachycardia	Chills, mydriasis, nausea, nystagmus, sweating, and vomiting
Barbiturates	Same as alcohol	Same as alcohol	Hypotension	Nystagmus
Benzodiazepines	Same as alcohol	Same as alcohol	Hypotension	Nystagmus
Cocaine	Same as amphetamines	Altered tactile sensation ("cocaine bugs"), decreased fatigue, euphoria, grandiosity, hypervigilance, and paranoia	Same as amphetamines	Same as amphetamines
Hallucinogens	Dizziness, incoordination, tremor, and weakness	Depersonalization, derealization, hallucinations, illusions, and synesthesia	Tachycardia	Blurred vision, mydriasis, and sweating
Marijuana	Loquacity and rapid speech	Euphoria, hallucinations (with high doses), jocularity, and sensory intensification	Hypertension and tachycardia	Conjunctivitis, dry mouth, increased appetite, and tightness in chest
Opioids	Motor slowness and slurred speech	Apathy, euphoria or dysphoria, impaired attention, and sedation	None	Miosis
Phencyclidine	Agitation, ataxia, muscle rigidity, and slurred speech	Anxiety, delusions, emotional lability, euphoria, and hallucinations	Hypertension and tachycardia	Hostility, miosis, nystagmus, and violent behavior

TABLE 25-2. **Emergency Treatment of Drug Intoxication**

Drug	Pharmacologic Treatment	Nonpharmacologic Treatment
Alcohol	None	Support vital functions
Amphetamines	Lorazepam for agitation and haloperidol for psychosis	Monitor and support cardiac function
Barbiturates	None	Support vital functions
Benzodiazepines	Flumazenil	Support vital functions
Cocaine	Lorazepam for agitation or seizures	Support vital functions
Hallucinogens	Lorazepam for agitation	Give reassurance and support vital functions
Marijuana	Lorazepam for agitation	Give reassurance and support vital functions
Opioids	Naloxone	Support vital functions
Phencyclidine	Lorazepam for agitation and haloperidol for psychosis	Minimize sensory input

and phencyclidine. In many cases, individuals with a substance-abuse disorder are using legal or illegal substances as self-medication for **comorbid disorders** such as anxiety or depression. After describing the pharmacologic effects of these drugs and any clinical use that they may have, this chapter discusses the treatment of substance abuse. Tables 25–1, 25–2, and 25–3 provide information about the manifestations and treatment of drug intoxication and withdrawal.

CENTRAL NERVOUS SYSTEM DEPRESSANTS

Alcohols and Glycols

In North America, about 12 million individuals have one or more symptoms of alcoholism, making **alcohol abuse** the number one substance abuse problem. In the United States

alone, the cost of health care, lost work hours, criminal activity, and other problems related to alcohol use is roughly $90 billion each year.

The alcohols and glycols most commonly ingested are ethanol, methanol, and ethylene glycol. Whereas ethanol selectively produces CNS depression at normal doses, even relatively small doses of methanol and ethylene glycol affect multiple organ systems and can produce severe or life-threatening toxicity, even when ingested in relatively small doses.

Ethanol

Ethanol, or **ethyl alcohol**, is classified as a CNS depressant and has pharmacologic effects similar to those of the barbiturates and benzodiazepines.

PHARMACOKINETICS. Ethanol has sufficient lipid solubility to enable rapid and almost complete absorption from the gut. It is more rapidly absorbed from the duodenum than from the

TABLE 25-3. Common Signs and Symptoms of Drug Withdrawal

Drug	Central Nervous System Manifestations	Musculoskeletal Manifestations	Cardiovascular Manifestations	Other Manifestations
Alcohol	Altered perceptions, insomnia, irritability, and seizures	Tremor	Hypertension and tachycardia	Delirium tremens, nausea, and sweating
Amphetamines	Depression, drowsiness, dysphoria, fatigue, increased appetite, and sleepiness	None	Bradycardia	None
Barbiturates	Anxiety, insomnia, irritability, and seizures	Muscle twitches	Hypertension and tachycardia	None
Benzodiazepines	Agitation, anxiety, dizziness, and insomnia	Muscle cramps and myoclonic contractions	Hypertension and tachycardia	None
Cocaine	Same as amphetamines	None	Bradycardia	None
Marijuana	Irritability, mild agitation, and sleep disturbances	None	None	Nausea and stomach cramps
Nicotine	Anxiety, dysphoria, hostility, impatience, irritability, and restlessness	None	Decreased heart rate	Increased appetite
Opioids	Anxiety, dysphoria, irritability, restlessness, and sleep disturbances	Muscle aches	Hypertension and tachycardia	Diarrhea, fever, mydriasis, piloerection,* sweating, vomiting, and yawning

*Because piloerection causes "goose bumps" or "gooseflesh," patients withdrawing from opioids are sometimes described as "going cold turkey."

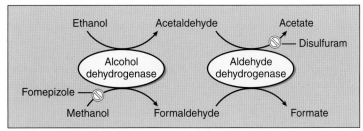

Figure 25–1. Metabolism of ethanol and methanol. Alcohols are oxidized to aldehydes by alcohol dehydrogenase. The aldehydes are oxidized to acetate or formate by aldehyde dehydrogenase. Disulfiram inhibits aldehyde dehydrogenase and leads to the accumulation of acetaldehyde during ethanol ingestion. Fomepizole inhibits alcohol dehydrogenase and is used in methanol or ethylene glycol poisoning.

stomach, and food slows its absorption by slowing the rate of gastric emptying. Ethanol is widely distributed throughout the body and has a volume of distribution that is roughly equivalent to the total body water, or about 38 L/70 kg of body weight.

As shown in Figure 25–1, ethanol is primarily oxidized by **alcohol dehydrogenase** to form acetaldehyde and is then oxidized by **acetaldehyde dehydrogenase** to form acetate. The acetate derived from ethanol enters the citric acid cycle for further oxidation to carbon dioxide and water. The oxidation of ethanol utilizes significant quantities of nicotinamide adenine dinucleotide (NAD), and the depletion of NAD is responsible for some of the metabolic effects of ethanol that are described below. Ethanol at higher or chronic doses also undergoes oxidation by cytochrome P450 enzymes, namely the **CYP2E1** isozyme. Unlike alcohol dehydrogenase metabolism, CYP2E1 metabolism is induced by long-term alcohol use, contributing to alcohol tolerance in heavy drinkers.

About 2% of ethanol is excreted unchanged by the kidneys and lungs. The concentration of ethanol in alveolar air is about 0.05% of that in the blood, and this relationship is used to estimate the **blood alcohol concentration (BAC)** in exhaled air when the **breathalyzer test** is administered.

Because ethanol can markedly impair the psychomotor skills required to safely drive a vehicle, nearly all nations prohibit the operation of motor vehicles while under the influence of alcohol. As of July 2004, the legal limit of blood alcohol is a BAC less than 0.08% (80 mg/dL) in all states and federal territories of the United States.

The capacity of alcohol dehydrogenase to metabolize ethanol is limited because the enzyme is saturated at relatively low ethanol concentrations. Hence, ethanol metabolism exhibits **zero-order kinetics**, except when serum concentrations of ethanol are very low. For this reason, the BAC is largely determined by the rate of ethanol ingestion. An adult weighing 70 kg usually metabolizes only about 10 mL of absolute ethanol per hour, which is roughly equivalent to the amount of ethanol contained in one alcoholic drink. A BAC of 0.08% to 0.10% in most cases is reached after an adult consumes from two to four drinks (bottles of beer, glasses of wine, or 6 ounces of distilled liquor) within an hour.

CENTRAL NERVOUS SYSTEM EFFECTS, MECHANISMS, AND INTERACTIONS. Ethanol potentiates the actions of γ-aminobutyric acid **(GABA)** in a manner similar to that of benzodiazepines and barbiturates (see Chapter 19). It thereby produces sedative-hypnotic, anxiolytic, amnesic, and anticonvulsant effects.

However, long-term ethanol use or ethanol withdrawal may lower the seizure threshold and thereby cause seizures. Predictably, ethanol **potentiates** the effects of benzodiazepines and barbiturates, so the combination of any of these drugs with ethanol can produce fatal CNS depression.

Ethanol at low doses produces **disinhibition** and **mild euphoria**, which facilitate social interactions by reducing behavioral inhibitions and self-consciousness. These reinforcing effects are correlated to the rise of the BAC, which probably determines the rate at which **dopamine increases** in the nucleus accumbens. In many individuals, reinforcement leads to the continued consumption of alcoholic beverages and to ethanol intoxication. This problem is exacerbated by the limited rate at which ethanol can be eliminated from the body.

Ethanol inhibits the release of acetylcholine from CNS neurons, and this action may contribute to the sedation and delirium that occur during alcohol intoxication. Ethanol also **inhibits the release of antidiuretic hormone** from the pituitary gland and thereby produces a diuretic effect. This diuretic effect is augmented by the consumption of large volumes of alcoholic beverages, such as a six-pack of beer.

Ethanol produces vasodilation and increases heat loss from the body, partly by interfering with temperature regulation by the hypothalamus. Hence, alcohol consumption can contribute to **hypothermia** during cold weather.

OTHER EFFECTS, MECHANISMS, AND INTERACTIONS. In addition to producing CNS effects, ethanol ingestion produces a variety of short-term and long-term **cardiovascular** and **autonomic** effects.

Blood pressure fluctuations are caused by the combination of peripheral vasodilation, depression of regulatory centers in the medulla, and the release of norepinephrine from sympathetic neurons. Consumption of large amounts of ethanol on a long-term basis can eventually lead to alcoholic cardiomyopathy and cardiac arrhythmias.

In alcoholic patients, thiamine deficiency secondary to a poor diet is commonly observed, which leads to nerve demyelination. This, in turn, causes peripheral neuropathies, characterized by paresthesias and reduced sensory acuity. Thiamine deficiency can also cause Wernicke-Korsakoff syndrome, a behavioral disorder characterized by confusion, severe anterograde and retrograde amnesia, ataxia, nystagmus, and ophthalmoplegia. The administration of thiamine substantially reverses all but the amnesic effects seen in patients with this syndrome.

Alcoholic patients can also develop several metabolic disorders. The depletion of NAD causes several citric acid cycle metabolites and lactate to accumulate and eventually contributes to liver degeneration (**cirrhosis**) and impaired glycogenolysis. The resulting hypoglycemia exacerbates the effects of ethanol on the CNS. A dietary deficiency of folate can lead to megaloblastic anemia, whereas a deficiency of other vitamins and antioxidants contributes to the overall tissue damage observed in alcoholism.

The consumption of significant quantities of ethanol during pregnancy is responsible for the occurrence of the **fetal alcohol syndrome**, which is characterized by low birth weight, **microcephaly**, facial abnormalities (flattening), mental retardation, heart defects, and other abnormalities.

Other Alcohols and Glycols

Methanol, also called **methyl alcohol** or **wood alcohol**, is a highly toxic form of alcohol that can cause profound **anion gap metabolic acidosis** and severe damage to the eyes. As shown in Figure 25–1, methanol is converted to formaldehyde and then to formate. Formate is primarily responsible for **optic nerve damage**, which can result in visual field impairment or permanent blindness. In cases of methanol poisoning, patients are treated with ethanol, which serves to saturate alcohol dehydrogenase and thereby prevent the formation of formaldehyde and formate. Ethanol has a greater affinity for alcohol dehydrogenase than does methanol. Hemodialysis is also used to reduce methanol levels in severe intoxication. **Fomepizole**, an inhibitor of alcohol dehydrogenase can also be administered, which prevents the formation of toxic metabolites in cases of methanol and ethylene glycol poisoning.

Isopropyl alcohol, which is contained in many formulations of rubbing alcohol, produces more CNS depression than does ethanol or methanol. Isopropyl alcohol is converted to **acetone**, a substance that can be smelled on the breath. The treatment of intoxication is largely supportive.

Ethylene glycol is contained in automobile antifreeze and de-icing fluids, and its ingestion can cause anion gap metabolic acidosis and serious toxicity to the kidneys, lungs, and CNS. Due to its sweet taste and appealing color, children often succumb to ethylene glycol poisoning from automobile antifreeze left accessible in the garage. Ethylene glycol is metabolized to oxalic acid, and calcium oxalate crystals may be found in the urine of patients after ethylene glycol ingestion. Treatment consists of supporting vital functions, giving **ethanol** or **fomepizole**, managing acidosis, and performing hemodialysis.

Barbiturates and Benzodiazepines

The pharmacologic properties of barbiturates and benzodiazepines are discussed in Chapter 19. These drugs are sedative-hypnotic agents that are prescribed for the treatment of anxiety disorders, insomnia, and other conditions. They are used recreationally for their euphoric and anxiolytic effects, and some polydrug users use them to reduce the irritability and anxiety associated with cocaine or amphetamine use.

The short-acting barbiturates (e.g., **pentobarbital**) are among the most widely abused sedative-hypnotic drugs. Several benzodiazepines have also been used illicitly, including **flunitrazepam**. Although this drug is not approved for use in the United States, it is used throughout much of the world as an anxiolytic or hypnotic drug. In the United States, it is widely available from street dealers and is sometimes referred to as **roofies**, derived from its trade name, ROHYPNOL. Flunitrazepam has gained notoriety as a party drug, a club drug, and a drug that contributes to **date rape**. It is an extremely potent benzodiazepine that is tasteless when dissolved in a beverage. Flunitrazepam produces drowsiness, impaired motor skills, and anterograde amnesia. Hence, victims do not recall events that happened the night before.

The long-term use of barbiturate or benzodiazepine drugs can lead to psychological and physical dependence, and their abrupt withdrawal produces symptoms that are similar to those caused by alcohol withdrawal (see Table 25–3).

Gamma hydroxybutyrate (GHB) usually comes as an odorless liquid, slightly salty to the taste, and is sold in small bottles. It has also been found in powder and capsule form. The use of this club drug has resulted in deaths from CNS depression and to synergistic effects when mixed with alcohol. It is also listed by the Drug Enforcement Administration as a **predatory** or **date-rape drug**. Its exact mechanism of action is unknown, but it has agonist activity at **GABA$_B$-receptors** in the brain.

Opioids

The most commonly abused opioid street drug is **heroin**. This drug is prepared from morphine by the addition of acetyl groups, so structurally it is known as **diacetylmorphine**. Heroin is highly potent and water soluble and thus can be injected intravenously. Because it rapidly enters the brain following injection, heroin can produce an intense euphoric sensation called a **rush**. Long-term heroin users develop considerable drug tolerance and physical dependence, and they undergo a wide variety of withdrawal symptoms (see Table 25–3) if they abruptly discontinue their use of the drug (Box 25–1).

Other opioids produce effects similar to those of heroin, but usually to a lesser degree. These effects vary with the potency and pharmacokinetic properties of the opioid and with the route of administration. Opioids administered orally tend to produce less euphoria and dependence than do opioids administered by other routes. For this reason, an orally administered drug such as methadone (see Chapter 23) can be used to prevent the craving for heroin as well as the opioid withdrawal reaction without causing significant reinforcement or exacerbating drug dependence. **Oxycodone**, in the slow-release formulation marketed as OxyContin, gained notoriety among street users because a dose intended for 24-hour pain relief in patients with chronic pain could be crushed and injected intravenously for a powerful rush. This has led to an increase in the number of deaths caused by opioid overdose. It is also a leading **prescription abuse** drug (see below).

CENTRAL NERVOUS SYSTEM STIMULANTS

The CNS stimulants include **amphetamine, amphetamine derivatives, cocaine, caffeine,** and **nicotine**. The amphetamine compounds and cocaine increase the synaptic concentration of norepinephrine and dopamine and exert sympathomimetic effects. They also induce a release of dopamine in the nucleus accumbens because this is the final common pathway for all chronically abused drugs and reinforced behaviors.

Amphetamine and Its Derivatives

Amphetamine and its derivatives **increase the synaptic concentration** of **norepinephrine** and **dopamine** by gaining entry into the presynaptic terminal through the reuptake

---

BOX 25-1. THE CASE OF THE OVERDOSED OPIOID ADDICT

CASE PRESENTATION: An 18-year-old male is brought to the emergency room in an unresponsive state with depressed respiration, pinpoint pupils, and cold, clammy skin. His pulse rate is 40 beats per minute. There are multiple needle tracks on both his arms. He is administered 2 mg of naloxone in an intravenous bolus and within minutes is sitting up and acting bellicose, complaining to the emergency room staff that they "ruined his high."

CASE DISCUSSION: The needle tracks and the triad of apnea or depressed respiration, miosis (pinpoint pupils), and a comatose state indicate that the patient arrived at the hospital in an opioid overdose condition. Needle tracks in his arms suggest heroin use, although prescription opioids are also increasingly injected intravenously in opioid-dependent individuals. Naloxone is a pure opioid receptor antagonist and can quickly reverse the near-death condition of an opioid overdose, a phenomenon sometimes called the Lazarus effect, from the biblical story. As the elimination half-life of naloxone is sometimes shorter than the opioid that caused the overdose, patients may be given multiple doses of naloxone and monitored so that a relapse does not occur. It is recommended that patients who receive naloxone be continuously observed for a minimum of 2 hours after the last dose. It is not uncommon that the overdosed individual will be angry at the hospital staff for reversing the opioid effect, and naloxone may precipitate an opioid withdrawal syndrome.

---

transporter protein and releasing the catecholamines from vesicles. Amphetamine also facilitates the reverse transport of the catecholamines inside the terminal out through the reuptake transporter into the synapse. At high concentrations, amphetamine, but not all derivatives, can also **inhibit monoamine oxidase** and, by this second mechanism, can increase the levels of catecholamines.

The use of amphetamines produces a constellation of central and peripheral effects, including euphoria, insomnia, psychomotor stimulation, anxiety, loss of appetite, increased concentration, decreased fatigue, respiratory stimulation, and hyperthermia. It also produces **sympathomimetic effects** such as mydriasis, tachycardia, and hypertension. The euphoria and other reinforcing effects are caused by increased dopamine levels in the nucleus accumbens, whereas the jittery and anxious feelings produced by amphetamines primarily result from enhanced release of norepinephrine in the central and peripheral nervous systems.

The amphetamines, including methamphetamine, have legitimate medical indications such as **attention-deficit/hyperactivity disorder (ADHD)**, **narcolepsy** and other **sleep disorders**, and **obesity** (see Chapter 22).

Methamphetamine

Amphetamine and methamphetamine are closely related sympathomimetic amines, and both are drugs of abuse. Of the two, **methamphetamine** is often preferred by abusers because it causes less norepinephrine to be released and can be more easily pyrolyzed (burned) and smoked. When methamphetamine free base is extracted by ether, pyrolyzed, and smoked, it is called **ice** or **crystal meth**. The euphoria produced by smoking "ice" is much greater than that produced by taking methamphetamine orally, presumably because of the faster rate at which dopamine levels are increased by inhaling the drug. The inexpensive cost and relative ease of making methamphetamine from precursor drugs found in nonprescription cold medicines enabled an illicit cottage industry in small-scale meth labs.

Other Amphetamine Derivatives

Several other amphetamine derivatives have been clandestinely synthesized and sold as **designer drugs** on the street. These include **3,4-methylenedioxymethamphetamine (MDMA)**, a drug called **ecstasy** or **X**. **MDMA** produces both psychostimulant and psychotomimetic effects by increasing dopamine and serotonin levels in the brain.

Users of MDMA report that the drug causes euphoria, increases empathy, enhances pleasure, heightens sexuality, and expands consciousness without loss of control. MDMA, however, causes various unpleasant effects (e.g., nausea, anorexia, and anxiety), and its use can be life threatening. A number of deaths have occurred in MDMA users due to **cardiac arrhythmias**, **hyperthermia**, **rhabdomyolysis**, and **disseminated intravascular coagulation**. MDMA is **neurotoxic** to serotonergic neurons, with clear degeneration of serotonergic pathways in animal models. Use of MDMA in humans likely destroys serotonergic brain neurons, which can contribute to some of the associated psychiatric complications, including panic reactions, psychosis, depression, and suicide. These disorders are prevalent in MDMA users today and will probably be observed to a greater extent later in these individuals when neuronal injury is compounded by loss of neurons during aging.

Other Stimulants

Cocaine

Cocaine produces both psychostimulant and local anesthetic activity and has limited clinical use as a local anesthetic (see Chapter 21). Thus, unlike many of the other drugs discussed in this chapter, it is a Schedule II drug under the Controlled Substances Act. The stimulant effects are caused by **inhibition of the neuronal reuptake** of norepinephrine and dopamine. Cocaine binds to the neurotransmitter transport proteins and causes them to undergo a conformational change that reduces their capacity to transport dopamine or norepinephrine. It is a reuptake blocker in the same manner as an antidepressant. By this mechanism, cocaine increases the synaptic concentration of these neurotransmitters.

Cocaine is an alkaloid derived from the leaves of a plant indigenous to South America, *Erythroxylon coca*. When native South Americans chew the leaves to relieve fatigue, relatively few adverse effects are seen. Use of the purified forms of cocaine, however, is associated with significant drug dependence, as well as cardiovascular, pulmonary, and neural toxicity.

In the past, many cocaine users took powdered cocaine hydrochloride by insufflation (snorting). Cocaine taken in this manner is absorbed across the nasal mucosa and into the circulation. More recently, cocaine free base became available in the form of pellets or rocks, called crack, because of the cracking sound made during the processing of cocaine powder to the base form. Unlike cocaine powder, crack cocaine can be smoked. Crack cocaine becomes aerosolized when it is heated, and inhaling the substance into the lungs causes it to be rapidly absorbed into the circulation. Inhalation of crack cocaine produces serum levels that are comparable to those obtained by intravenous administration of the drug. For this reason, crack cocaine produces a euphoric effect that is more intense than that obtained by snorting cocaine. The higher serum levels achieved with crack cocaine use also increase the potential for overdose toxicity, particularly during repeated administration.

The common signs and symptoms of cocaine intoxication are listed in Table 25–1. Unlike other drugs of abuse, cocaine can **alter tactile sensation**, causing its users to feel as if insects are crawling under their skin (**cocaine bugs**) and causing them to scratch and produce self-inflicted skin lesions. Cocaine often stimulates respiration at lower doses, and high doses can produce irregular breathing and apnea known as **Cheyne-Stokes respiration**. The local anesthetic actions of cocaine probably contribute to the drug's **cardiac toxicity** when high doses are administered.

With frank overdoses, the potential for neurotoxicity and cardiac toxicity increases. Cocaine overdose victims often suffer from delirium and can become aggressive and violent. The pulse can become rapid, weak, and irregular. In some cases, cocaine overdose causes **tonic-clonic seizures** (including status epilepticus), **malignant encephalopathy**, or **myocardial infarction**. When fatalities occur, they typically result from ventricular fibrillation or cardiac arrest. For this reason, the management of cocaine overdose must include cardiovascular and pulmonary support, as well as the administration of a benzodiazepine (e.g., lorazepam) to control agitation or seizures.

Cocaine withdrawal produces fatigue, depression, nightmares or other sleep disturbances, and increased appetite. The management of cocaine withdrawal is largely supportive. **Bromocriptine**, a dopamine receptor agonist, has been used to reduce craving for the drug, but the effectiveness of this treatment for withdrawal has not been firmly established.

Nicotine

Nicotine, the principal alkaloid of plants of the genus *Nicotiana*, is widely available in the form of various tobacco products that can be chewed or smoked.

Nicotine is a lipid-soluble tertiary amine. It is rapidly absorbed into the circulation from the mouth or the respiratory tract and is then quickly distributed to the brain. The drug's CNS effects are rapidly terminated by redistribution from the brain to the peripheral tissues. Although nicotine has a half-life of about 30 minutes, it is metabolized to the

active metabolite, **cotinine**, which has a half-life of about 2 hours. The induction of cytochrome P450 enzymes by tars contained in cigarette smoke accelerates the metabolism of nicotine, and this leads to the development of **pharmaco-kinetic tolerance** to the drug. Because the use of cigarettes accelerates the metabolism of β-adrenoceptor antagonists, benzodiazepines, opioids, and theophylline, cigarette smokers may require higher doses of these drugs to maintain therapeutic serum levels.

Nicotine activates cholinergic **nicotinic receptors** in the central and peripheral nervous systems and produces a complex constellation of subjective and physiologic effects. The CNS effects of nicotine are similar to those of the psychostimulants and include **mild euphoria**, **increased arousal and concentration**, **improved memory**, and **appetite suppression**. In addition to activating nicotinic receptors, nicotine **inhibits monoamine oxidase**. The drug's ability to inhibit this enzyme partly explains its ability to activate dopaminergic neurotransmission and its dependence liability. The monoamine oxidase inhibitors used in treating depression, however, do not cause significant drug dependence or the intense drug craving associated with nicotine use. More directly, nicotine increases the release of dopamine in the nucleus accumbens, as with all other addictive drugs and behaviors, and strongly initiates drug dependence.

Caffeine

Caffeine citrate is occasionally administered intravenously to treat **apnea in neonates**. It is also available in nonprescription tablets to prevent **fatigue**.

Caffeine is a methylxanthine that produces mild stimulation by **blocking adenosine receptors** on neurons throughout the CNS. Because adenosine inhibits dopamine release, caffeine indirectly enhances dopamine neurotransmission. This action is probably responsible for the drug's stimulant effects and dependence liability.

Caffeine is the most widely ingested drug in the world; it is contained in coffee, cola beverages, teas, and many other products. Caffeine use **combats fatigue; elevates mood;** and **increases alertness, concentration, motivation,** and **talkativeness**. By arousing the sympathetic system, it causes a **mild stimulation** of heart rate and blood pressure. Caffeine also relaxes most smooth muscles and causes diuresis by increasing renal blood flow.

Because caffeine **increases the secretion** of gastric acid and pepsin, it can contribute to gastritis and peptic **ulcers**. High doses of caffeine produce nausea, vomiting, increased muscle tone, and tremors. Although extremely high doses of caffeine can cause delirium, seizures, and even death, these doses are almost impossible to reach by ingesting a caffeinated beverage such as coffee. They can be reached by ingesting caffeine tablets, but abuse of caffeine tablets is limited by the fact that large doses of them produce such unpleasant symptoms.

The manifestations of caffeine withdrawal are **relatively mild**; they include headache, impaired concentration, irritability, depression, anxiety, flu-like symptoms, and blurred vision. The withdrawal symptoms can be lessened by reducing caffeine consumption gradually over a period of several weeks.

OTHER PSYCHOACTIVE DRUGS

Cannabis and Its Derivatives

The best-known form of cannabis is **marijuana**, which consists of the dried flowers and leaves of *Cannabis sativa* and is a popular and illegal drug of abuse. The primary cannabinoid in marijuana is Δ^9-**tetrahydrocannabinol (THC).** When cannabis is inhaled, about 20% of the THC is absorbed into the circulation. In contrast, when cannabis is ingested orally, only about 6% of the THC is absorbed from the gut, owing to the extensive first-pass metabolism. THC has multiple effects on neuronal function. It binds stereospecifically to membrane **cannabinoid receptors** in neurons, and this action is linked with inhibition of adenylyl cyclase and cAMP production. The recently discovered endogenous ligand for cannabinoid receptors is called **anandamide** (from *ananda*, the Sanskrit word for "bliss"). Anandamide binds to cannabinoid receptors, decreases the level of cAMP via G proteins, and inhibits voltage-gated calcium channels that regulate neurotransmitter release. Through these and other actions, THC appears to modulate the activity of acetylcholine, dopamine, and serotonin.

When marijuana is smoked, pyrolysis releases THC and other substances. The plasma level of THC peaks within several minutes, then it falls rapidly during the first hour, as the drug is redistributed to adipose tissue. Thereafter, it declines slowly, owing to metabolism and excretion in the urine and feces. Because of its **high lipophilicity**, THC is stored in fat, and the drug and its metabolites can be detected in the body for weeks.

Marijuana use initially causes mild stimulation followed by a depressive phase. The stimulant phase is described as a dream-like **euphoric state** characterized by an **altered sense of time, increased visual acuity, difficulty in concentrating,** and **impaired short-term memory**. The depressive phase is characterized by **drowsiness, lethargy,** and **increased appetite**. The psychoactive effects of marijuana depend somewhat on the environment and the extent of prior use of the drug. For example, first-time users are more likely to experience anxiety than are habitual users.

Marijuana has been implicated as the cause of an **amotivational syndrome** that is characterized by a lack of desire to work or excel in any part of life. It has also been described as a **gateway drug** whose initial use leads to the subsequent use of other drugs (e.g., cocaine or heroin). Little scientific evidence supports either of these claims. Marijuana, however, causes minor **decreases in the levels of testosterone** in men, **low birth weight in neonates**, increased **fetal malformations**, and **decreased ovulation** in females. Studies in humans have consistently demonstrated that marijuana reduces aggressive behavior, even though animals injected with THC may show aggression. There is also some evidence linking marijuana use in adolescents to **schizophrenia**, although these data are controversial.

Experimental studies have demonstrated that cannabinoids are effective in the treatment of **asthma, glaucoma,** and **nausea and vomiting**. This is because their use causes bronchodilation, decreased intraocular pressure, and inhibition of nausea. Their use can also cause tachycardia. In the United States, a synthetic cannabis

derivative called **dronabinol** (MARINOL) is approved for the **treatment of nausea** caused by cancer chemotherapy and for the **stimulation of appetite** in patients who have acquired immunodeficiency syndrome (AIDS) and are suffering from anorexia. The drug is administered orally for these purposes. More recently, **nabilone** (CESAMET), another cannabinoid agonist, was also approved for the same indications.

The common signs and symptoms of marijuana intoxication and withdrawal are listed in Tables 25–1 and 25–3.

Hallucinogens

Prescription drugs, fever, and disorders such as schizophrenia are all capable of causing hallucinations, which are false perceptions that result from abnormal sensory processing. Unlike prescription drugs, however, drugs such as **LSD, mescaline,** and **psilocybin** can produce **hallucinations without causing delirium**. LSD is a synthetic ergot derivative, **mescaline** is found in the *Peyote* cactus, and **psilocybin** in mushrooms (*Psilocybe coprophilia*) that grow on cow excrement. These street drugs are taken orally and usually begin to produce hallucinations within an hour. The effects of LSD can last as long as 12 hours, whereas the effects of mescaline and psilocybin last about 6 hours. The mechanisms responsible for the effects are incompletely understood. Some evidence indicates that LSD selectively activates certain subtypes of **serotonin (5-HT) receptors** in the neocortex, limbic system, and brain stem. According to one hypothesis, the activation of **5-HT$_2$ receptors in the reticular formation** leads to the generalization of sensory stimuli to evoke hallucinations.

Although the use of LSD or mescaline usually causes **visual hallucinations**, it can also cause auditory, tactile, olfactory, gustatory, kinesthetic, and synesthetic hallucinations. Visual hallucinations often follow a temporal pattern in which amorphous bursts of light are followed by geometric forms and then by faces or scenes. Some users also report the occurrence of **synesthesia**, a condition in which one sensory modality assumes the characteristics of another. In a synesthetic hallucination, for example, sounds may be seen or colors may be heard.

The hallucinogens have little effect on cognitive function or arousal. If mood changes occur, they are generally an exaggeration of the predrug mood and are highly context-dependent. They are usually pleasant, but they can be terrifying and cause sufficient anxiety to resemble a panic attack. Mood changes are accompanied by somatic signs of sympathetic activation, including increased heart rate, increased blood pressure, and dilated pupils. Nausea and vomiting can occur, particularly with mescaline use.

Overdoses are rarely serious, but the occasional **panic attack (bad trip)** may require intervention that consists of removing the patient to a quiet room and having someone remain with the patient for reassurance.

Phencyclidine

Phencyclidine (PCP) is a widely used street drug, despite its reputation for causing dangerous side effects and efforts to reduce its supply by limiting the sale of chemicals used in its synthesis. PCP was originally developed as a **dissociative anesthetic** similar to ketamine, but the occurrence of a high incidence of postanesthetic hallucinations and delirium forced its removal from the market.

Sometimes called **angel dust**, PCP can be taken via various routes. The drug is incompletely and erratically absorbed from the gut, so it is usually smoked. In some cases, it is sprinkled on tobacco or marijuana and then smoked. In other cases, it is combined with cocaine and heroin before it is used.

Use of PCP produces a unique spectrum of effects that probably result from **blockade of glutamate N-methyl-D-aspartate (NMDA) receptors** and action at less characterized receptors called **sigma receptors**. As shown in Table 25–1, these effects include euphoria, hallucinations, and psychotomimetic activity, sometimes accompanied by **hostility** and **violent behavior**. PCP causes little tolerance, physical dependence, or withdrawal effects.

PRESCRIPTION DRUG ABUSE

The **nonmedical use** or **abuse of prescription drugs** is a serious and growing public health problem. It is estimated that 48 million people (ages 12 and older) used prescription drugs for nonmedical reasons. This represents about 20% of the U.S. population. Most alarming is the fact that recent government data showed that nearly 15% of young teenagers reported using opioids (VICODIN or OXYCONTIN) without a prescription, making these medications among the most commonly abused drugs by adolescents, second only to marijuana. **Accessibility** is likely a contributing factor, with a growing number of medications available in the home medicine cabinet and through some **online pharmacies** that dispense medications without prescriptions and without identity verification, allowing minors to order the medications easily over the Internet. **Unintentional fatal drug overdoses** nearly doubled from 1999 to 2004 and were the **second leading cause of accidental death** in the United States in 2004, with only automobile crashes accounting for a greater number of deaths. For the first time since records were kept, almost half of drug overdose admissions to hospital emergency rooms were due to prescription drugs, gaining rapidly on the number of admissions for illicit drug overdose.

STEROID DRUG ABUSE

Anabolic steroids are synthetic drugs similar to the male hormone, **testosterone**. They are available in tablets, powder, or by intramuscular injection and are abused to improve muscle growth (**bulking**), endurance, and strength. They are classified as controlled substances, making it illegal to possess an anabolic steroid without a prescription. In response to a growing clandestine industry manufacturing precursors and designer steroids, the Anabolic Steroid Control Act of 2004 listed an additional 32 steroid agents as Schedule III controlled substances.

Unlike other drugs of abuse, there is not an immediate rush or euphoria experienced by the steroid abuser. Abuse

of steroids is driven by desires to change physical appearance and increase athletic ability. Anabolic steroids can lead to **heart attack, stroke, hepatic toxicity, renal failure,** and **serious psychiatric problems**. Use in males leads to reduction of the testes and sperm production. In females, steroid abuse results in growth of facial hair, menstrual cycle dysfunction, enlargement of the clitoris, and reduced breast size.

There is also evidence that steroid abuse contributes to violent crime due to **increased aggression** associated with users of anabolic steroids. Most unfortunate, media reports of a number of celebrity athletes exposed using steroids send a dangerous message to youth who often revere these athletes as role models.

INHALANT ABUSE

Although attention in the drug abuse field is focused on the nonmedical use of prescription drugs, alcohol, tobacco, or illegal drugs, there are increasing numbers of children and adolescents abusing the most easily obtained mind-altering substances: **household solvents**, **sprays**, and **cleaners**. Nationwide studies report over 15% of 8th graders reported using inhalants to "get high". Inhalants are also among the most deadly of abused substances, with even a single session of inhalant abuse causing mortality from **cardiac arrest**. Regular inhalant abuse results in toxicity to the brain, heart, kidneys, and liver.

Products such as nail polish remover, lighter fluid, spray paints, deodorant and hair sprays, pressurized air cleaners, and any type of liquid fuel are soaked in rags or emptied in plastic bags and their concentrated vapors inhaled, a practice called **huffing** or **sniffing**. The latest reports indicate that the organic solvents in these products, such as **toluene**, activate the dopamine system much like any other abused drug, leading to repeated administration and drug dependence.

MANAGEMENT OF DRUG ABUSE

Use of psychoactive drugs can cause several distinct clinical problems, including drug intoxication or overdose, drug withdrawal, and drug dependence. The severity of these problems varies markedly among different classes of drugs and patterns of drug use. A diagnosis of drug intoxication or dependence in a particular individual is based on the individual's history, psychological assessment, physical examination, and laboratory findings.

Drug Intoxication and Withdrawal

The initial treatment of drug intoxication or overdose consists of supporting cardiovascular and pulmonary functions. **Naloxone** or **flumazenil** can be administered to counteract the acute CNS depression caused by toxic doses of an opioid or a benzodiazepine, respectively (see Table 25–2). **Lorazepam** can be used to control agitation, and an antipsychotic drug (e.g., **haloperidol**) can be administered for psychosis, which can occur with PCP overdose. Haloperidol should not be used in cases of cocaine overdose, however,

because it lowers the seizure threshold and can exacerbate or precipitate seizures.

The next stage of treatment is the management of withdrawal reactions that occur as the drug is eliminated from the body. The pharmacologic treatment of withdrawal consists primarily of substitution therapy and symptomatic relief.

A benzodiazepine (e.g., **lorazepam** or **chlordiazepoxide**) can be administered to suppress the acute manifestations of withdrawal from alcohol, including delusions, hallucinations, a coarse tremor, and agitation (**delirium tremens**). The benzodiazepine is then gradually withdrawn over several weeks.

Methadone is usually used to suppress withdrawal reactions in opioid users because it is long-acting and orally effective. Methadone is also given on a long-term basis in the out-treatment of heroin dependence.

Clonidine, an α_2-adrenoceptor agonist, is effective in reducing the sympathetic nervous system symptoms of alcohol, opioid, or nicotine withdrawal, and it may facilitate continued abstinence in persons who are dependent on these drugs.

Treatment of Drug Dependence

After treatment of drug intoxication and withdrawal, attention can be directed to the more difficult problem of treating drug dependence. In this endeavor, behavioral therapy and personal motivation are as important as subsequent pharmacologic treatments. Patients are rarely cured, and most clinicians view treatment as a **life-long process** in which patients are continually recovering. Twelve-step groups, such as Alcoholics Anonymous and Narcotics Anonymous, have been successful in reducing recidivism, partly because they recognize that the individual is always in a state of remission from drug or alcohol dependence and that an ever-present possibility exists of slipping into drug use again.

Among the pharmacologic agents used for the treatment of drug dependence is **disulfiram,** a drug that inhibits acetaldehyde dehydrogenase. When disulfiram is taken and ethanol subsequently ingested, the accumulation of acetaldehyde causes nausea, profuse vomiting, sweating, flushing, palpitations, and dyspnea. Because of its ability to cause these extremely unpleasant symptoms, disulfiram is sometimes prescribed to encourage alcoholic patients to abstain from ethanol use. Other drugs that can cause disulfiram-like effects when administered concurrently with ethanol include metronidazole (a drug used in the treatment of protozoal infections) and some of the third-generation cephalosporin antibiotics.

Recently, a new dependence medication for alcohol was approved called **acamprosate calcium.** It is a synthetic compound with a chemical structure similar to that of the endogenous amino acid homotaurine, which is a structural analogue of the amino acid neurotransmitter GABA and the amino acid neuromodulator taurine. The mechanism of action of acamprosate in maintenance of alcohol abstinence is not completely understood. Chronic alcohol exposure is hypothesized to alter the normal balance between neuronal excitation and inhibition. In vitro and in vivo studies in animals have provided evidence to suggest acamprosate can interact with glutamate and GABA neurotransmitter systems centrally, and has led to the hypothesis that acamprosate restores this balance.

Buprenorphine was recently approved for physician outpatient treatment of opioid dependence. It is formulated in a sublingual tablet or oral form in combination with naloxone to prevent intravenous abuse. **Naltrexone** is available in oral (REVIA, DEPADE) and extended-release injectable suspension (once-a-month; VIVITROL) formulations and is used to treat **alcohol and opioid dependence.** For opioid-dependent patients, naltrexone directly blocks opioid receptors and prevents the euphoria associated with opioid abuse. It is effective for the treatment of alcohol dependence because endogenous opioid systems play a key role in the pathway that leads to reinforcement of alcohol and other drugs. **Clonidine**, a centrally acting α_2-agonist, is used to facilitate withdrawal from opioids and nicotine.

Nicotine chewing gum, lozenges, and skin patches have been developed to mitigate nicotine withdrawal reactions in persons who are trying to quit smoking. Another drug used to treat nicotine dependence is the antidepressant **bupropion** (ZYBAN), now available in a long-acting formulation for this purpose. The ability of bupropion to block the reuptake of dopamine may contribute to its effectiveness in treating drug dependence. The combined use of bupropion and nicotine patches is currently being investigated.

Recently, **varenicline** (CHANTIX) was approved for smoking cessation and shows a relatively high degree of success. Varenicline is selective for nicotinic receptors containing $\alpha_4\beta_2$ subunits. The efficacy of varenicline is believed to be the result of **partial agonist** activity, while simultaneously preventing the full agonist nicotine binding to $\alpha_4\beta_2$-receptors. However, in 2008, the U.S. Food and Drug Administration issued a warning that in patients taking **varenicline,** cases of serious **neuropsychiatric symptoms** have occurred, including agitation, depressed mood, suicidal ideation, and attempted and successful suicide.

Spurred on by both the commercial and medical success of **bupropion** and **varenicline** for smoking cessation, government and industry leaders are awakening to the treatment needs of drug-dependent individuals. Many anti-craving agents and pharmacologic approaches are currently in development. For example, treatment of cocaine dependence by vaccinations to produce **anticocaine antibodies** is in clinical trials. Other approved agents (e.g., clonidine and bromocriptine) are being tested in drug-dependent populations. Progress on the prevention and management of drug abuse and drug dependence will soon lead to more effective pharmacotherapy for these difficult but treatable CNS disorders.

SUMMARY OF IMPORTANT POINTS

■ Drug dependence is a condition in which an individual feels compelled to repeatedly administer a psychoactive drug. The condition is caused by positive reinforcement (psychological dependence) and negative reinforcement (physical dependence) from continued drug use.

■ Reinforcement of drug use results from increased levels of dopamine in the nucleus accumbens and dopamine sensitization of these pathways.

■ Physical dependence, which results from neuronal adaptation to the continued presence of a drug, is usually associated with drug tolerance. Physical dependence results in a characteristic withdrawal syndrome when drug use is discontinued.

■ Alcohol and other CNS depressants produce motor and cognitive impairment, sedation, euphoria, and behavioral disinhibition.

■ Amphetamines, cocaine, and other CNS stimulants produce euphoria, agitation, hypervigilance, mydriasis, and sympathetic nervous system arousal. Cocaine also produces altered tactile sensation, and cocaine overdose can cause severe cardiovascular and neural toxicity.

■ Marijuana and cannabis derivatives produce a mild euphoria, talkativeness, conjunctivitis, and increased appetite.

■ LSD and other hallucinogens cause hallucinations without producing delirium.

■ Prescription drug abuse, steroid drug abuse, and inhalant abuse are major substance-abuse problems that affect a growing number of children, adolescents, and adults.

■ The treatment of drug dependence and withdrawal can include some type of substitution therapy: a benzodiazepine substituted for alcohol, methadone substituted for an opioid, and nicotine chewing gum or skin patches substituted for cigarettes.

■ The treatment of alcohol- and opioid-dependent individuals can include naltrexone transdermal patches. Naltrexone is an opioid antagonist that blocks the opioid receptor link in the dopamine reinforcement pathway in the nucleus accumbens.

Review Questions

1. Disulfiram effectively treats alcohol (ethanol) dependence by which of the following mechanisms?
   (A) increasing plasma ethanol concentration
   (B) preventing the conversion of ethanol to methanol in the liver
   (C) increasing circulating acetaldehyde concentrations
   (D) blocking the action of ethanol at its cell membrane receptor
   (E) stabilizing the cell membrane to prevent ethanol disruption

2. The fact that the degree of reinforcement for morphine is less than that of heroin is best explained by which one of the following statements?
   (A) morphine is a partial agonist
   (B) heroin binds tighter to opioid receptors
   (C) morphine is metabolized faster than heroin

(D) morphine is first metabolized to heroin

(E) heroin is distributed more rapidly to the brain

3. Synesthesia is an acute pharmacologic effect of which drug of abuse?

(A) marijuana

(B) LSD

(C) cocaine

(D) PCP

(E) alcohol

4. Which of the following has not been reported as a health hazard of chronic marijuana abuse?

(A) low birth weight in neonates

(B) decreased testosterone in men

(C) anovulatory cycle in females

(D) increased fetal malformations

(E) increased intraocular pressure

5. Crack cocaine in the 1990s became more problematic than the powder cocaine of the 1980s because of which difference between the two forms of cocaine?

(A) cocaine in crack is more potent than cocaine in powder form

(B) crack cocaine is not metabolized in humans

(C) reinforcement is greater with inhalation versus insufflation

(D) powder cocaine reaches the brain more rapidly than crack cocaine

(E) coca plants in the 1990s were bred for greater cocaine content

Answers and Explanations

1. **The correct answer is C:** increasing circulating acetaldehyde concentrations. Disulfiram inhibits the acetaldehyde dehydrogenase, a step in the metabolism of alcohol. Concurrent administration of disulfiram and ethanol causes increased acetaldehyde blood levels, which is associated with flushing, nausea and vomiting, and other ill effects. Answer (A), increasing plasma ethanol concentration, would not be a good ethanol treatment plan because disulfiram is approved for the treatment of alcohol dependence. Answer (B), preventing the conversion of ethanol to methanol in the liver, is simply not true, and answer (D), blocking the action of ethanol at its cell membrane receptor, is also incorrect. Answer (E), stabilizing the cell membrane to prevent ethanol disruption, refers to an older hypothesis of ethanol action in which it was thought that ethanol fluidizes neuronal membranes and thereby disrupts ion channels and neurotransmission. This is clearly not an action of disulfiram.

2. **The correct answer is E:** heroin is distributed more rapidly to the brain. Heroin is an illicit opioid made by the addition of two acetyl groups at the 3 and 6 position of the morphine molecule. Because of this, diacetylmorphine (heroin) is more lipophilic and crosses the blood-brain barrier quite rapidly to exert its reinforcing effects. Although answer (A), morphine, is a partial agonist, and answer (B), heroin, binds tighter to opioid receptors, are

wrong, answer (C), morphine, is metabolized faster than heroin, may be generally true because heroin has extra groups to demethylate, but the degree of reinforcement is greater with more rapid acting agents. Answer (D), morphine is first metabolized to heroin, is simply wrong.

3. **The correct answer is B:** LSD. This potent ergot derivative is noted for synesthesia, the phenomenon whereby the perception of sensory modalities crosses over; for example, sounds can be seen and sights can be heard. The drugs of abuse listed as answers (A) and (C) through (E) are not known for such a bizarre CNS effect.

4. **The correct answer is E:** increased intraocular pressure. This is not an effect of marijuana use and indeed THC, the active ingredient in marijuana, shows promise as a treatment for glaucoma, which is increased intraocular pressure. The other adverse effects listed as answers (A) through (D) are true concerning the chronic use of marijuana.

5. **The correct answer is C:** reinforcement is greater with inhalation versus insufflation. The crack epidemic is caused by the switch from insufflation (snorting) to inhalation (smoking) because of the change in cocaine formulation from powder to the free base forms (crack). Answer (A), cocaine in crack is more potent than cocaine in powder form, is not true; the cocaine molecule itself has the same potency regardless of form. Answers (B), crack cocaine is not metabolized in humans, and (D), powder cocaine reaches the brain more rapidly than crack cocaine, are simply not true. Answer (E), coca plants in the 1990s were bred for greater cocaine content, may be true, but the cocaine molecule itself would not be altered.

SELECTED READINGS

Brady, K.T., M.L. Verduin, and B.K. Tolliver. Treatment of patients comorbid for addiction and other psychiatric disorders. Curr Psychiatry Rep 9:374–380, 2007.

Fudala, P.J., and G.W. Woody. Recent advances in the treatment of opiate addiction. Curr Psychiatry Rep 6(5):339–346, 2004.

Johnson, B.A., Update on neuropharmacological treatments for alcoholism: scientific basis and clinical findings. Biochem Pharmacol 75:34–56, 2008.

Karlsen, S.N., O. Spigset, and L. Slørdal. The dark side of ecstasy: neuropsychiatric symptoms after exposure to 3,4-methylenedioxymethamphetamine. Basic Clin Pharmacol Toxicol 102:15–24, 2008.

Pauly, J.R. Gender differences in tobacco smoking dynamics and the neuropharmacological actions of nicotine. Front Biosci 13:505–516, 2008.

Rounsaville, B.J. Treatment of cocaine dependence and depression. Biol Psychiatry 56(10):803–809, 2004.

PHARMACOLOGY OF THE RESPIRATORY AND OTHER SYSTEMS

CHAPTER 26

Autacoid Drugs

CLASSIFICATION OF AUTACOID DRUGS

Histamine H$_1$ Receptor Antagonists
First-generation Antihistamines
- Promethazine (PHENERGAN)
- Diphenhydramine (BENADRYL)
- Chlorpheniramine (CHLOR-TRIMETON)
- Clemastine (TAVIST)
- Dimenhydrinate (DRAMAMINE)
- Hydroxyzine (ATARAX)
- Meclizine (ANTIVERT)

Second-generation Antihistamines
- Fexofenadine (ALLEGRA)
- Loratadine (CLARITIN)
- Desloratadine (CLARINEX)
- Cetirizine (ZYRTEC)

Intranasal Antihistamines
- Azelastine (ASTELIN)

Opthalmic Antihistamines
- Ketotifen (ZADITOR)
- Levocabastine (LIVOSTIN)[a]

Serotonergic Drugs
Serotonin Agonists
- Buspirone (BUSPAR)
- Sumatriptan (IMITREX)[b]

Serotonin Antagonists
- Clozapine (CLOZARIL)
- Cyproheptadine (PERIACTIN)
- Methysergide (SANSERT)
- Ondansetron (ZOFRAN)[c]

Prostaglandin Drugs
- Alprostadil (CAVERJECT, MUSE)
- Carboprost Tromethamine (HEMABATE)
- Dinoprostone (CERVIDIL)
- Misoprostol (CYTOTEC)
- Epoprostenol (FLOLAN)
- Treprostinil (REMODULIN)
- Latanoprost (XALATAN)[d]

Endothelin-1 Antagonists
- Bosentan (TRACLEER)
- Ambrisentan (LETAIRIS)

[a]Also epinastine (ELESTAT) and olopatadine (PATANOL).
[b]Also zolmitriptan (ZOMIG), rizatriptan (MAXALT), naratriptan (AMERGE), frovatriptan (FROVA), almotriptan (AXERT), and eletriptan (RELPAX).
[c]Also granisetron (KYTRIL), palonosetron (ALOXI), alosetron (LOTRONEX), and dolasetron (ANZEMET).
[d]Also bimatoprost (LUMIGAN) and travoprost (TRAVATAN).

OVERVIEW

Autacoids (also spelled autocoids) are substances produced by neural and non-neural tissues throughout the body and act locally to modulate the activity of smooth muscles, nerves, glands, platelets, and other tissues (Table 26–1). Several autacoids also serve as neurotransmitters in the central nervous system (CNS) or enteric nervous system.

Autacoids regulate certain aspects of gastrointestinal, uterine, and renal function, and they are involved in pain, fever, inflammation, allergic reactions, asthma, thromboembolic disorders, and other pathologic conditions. Drugs that inhibit autacoid synthesis or block autacoid receptors are helpful in treating these conditions, whereas drugs that activate autacoid receptors are useful for inducing labor, alleviating migraine headaches, counteracting drug-induced peptic ulcers, and other purposes.

Autacoids include monoamines, such as **histamine** and **serotonin**, as well as fatty acid derivatives, including **prostaglandins** and **leukotrienes**. Autacoids activate specific membrane receptors in target tissues, mostly of the G protein–coupled receptor type. Their effects are usually restricted to the tissue in which they are formed, but under pathologic conditions, extraordinarily large amounts of autacoids can be released into the systemic circulation. These disorders include **carcinoid tumor** and **anaphylactic shock**, which cause the release of copious amounts of serotonin and histamine, respectively, and exert systemic effects including CNS effects. Most

TABLE 26-1.	**Effects of Selected Autacoids**		
Autacoid	**Effects on VSM**	**Effects on NVSM**	**Other Effects**
Histamine	Vasodilation and edema	Contraction of bronchial and other NVSMs	Itching; increase in gastric acid secretion
Serotonin	Vasoconstriction in most vascular beds	Contraction of gastrointestinal and other NVSMs	Central nervous system neurotransmission; stimulation of platelet aggregation
Eicosanoids			
Leukotrienes	Vasoconstriction or vasodilation	Contraction of bronchial and other NVSMs	Inflammatory effects; increase in vascular permeability
Prostaglandin E	Vasodilation	Relaxation of bronchial muscle and contraction of uterine muscle	Inhibition of gastric acid secretion
Prostaglandin F	Vasoconstriction in most vascular beds	Contraction of bronchial and uterine muscle	Increase in aqueous humor outflow
Prostaglandin I	Vasodilation	Contraction	Inhibition of platelet aggregation
Thromboxane A_2	Vasoconstriction	Contraction	Stimulation of platelet aggregation

NVSM = nonvascular smooth muscle; VSM = vascular smooth muscle.

autacoids are rapidly metabolized to inactive compounds, as seen with prostaglandins, and some autacoids undergo tissue reuptake, as evidenced by 5-hydroxytryptamine (5-HT) reuptake transporter proteins in neurons and peripheral cells.

This chapter provides basic information about autacoids and reviews the many types of drugs that influence their effects. Some autacoid drugs are covered completely here, whereas other chapters provide more details on other agents.

HISTAMINE AND RELATED DRUGS

Histamine Biosynthesis and Release

Histamine is a biogenic amine produced primarily by mast cells and basophils, which are particularly abundant in the skin, gastrointestinal tract, and respiratory tract. Histamine is also produced by paracrine cells in the gastric fundus, where it stimulates acid secretion by parietal cells. Histamine also functions as a neurotransmitter in the CNS (see Chapter 18).

Histamine is formed when the amino acid **histidine** is decarboxylated in a reaction catalyzed by the enzyme, L-histidine decarboxylase. Histamine is stored in granules (vesicles) in mast cells and basophils until it is released. It is released from mast cells when membrane-bound **immunoglobulin E (IgE)** interacts with an IgE antigen to cause mast cell degranulation. This process can be blocked by **cromolyn sodium** and related respiratory drugs, as described in Chapter 27. A number of other stimuli can also cause the release of histamine from mast cells (Fig. 26–1). Stimuli that increase cyclic guanosine monophosphate increase histamine release, whereas those that increase cyclic adenosine monophosphate oppose this action.

Mast cell degranulation can also be triggered by bacterial toxins and by drugs such as **morphine** and **tubocurarine**. Some of these stimuli result in the formation of inositol triphosphate (IP_3) and diacylglycerol (DAG). As with neurons, this causes the release of intracellular calcium and the fusion of granule membranes with the plasma membrane, thereby releasing **histamine** and other compounds. The release of histamine that can occur with morphine administration does not appear to be mediated by opioid receptors because the opioid antagonist, naloxone, does not inhibit morphine-induced histamine release from mast cells.

Histamine is inactivated by methylation and oxidation reactions that are catalyzed by a methyltransferase enzyme and diamine oxidase, respectively.

Histamine Receptors and Effects

Histamine receptors have been classified as H_1, H_2, and H_3. All three types are typical, seven-transmembrane G protein–coupled receptor proteins.

H_1 **receptors** are involved in allergic reactions that cause **dermatitis, rhinitis, conjunctivitis,** and **other forms of allergy.** Activation of H_1 receptors in the skin and mucous membranes causes vasodilation; increases vascular permeability; and leads to erythema (heat and redness), congestion, edema, and inflammation. Stimulation of H_1 receptors on mucocutaneous nerve endings can cause pruritus (itching), and in the lungs, it initiates the cough reflex. If sufficient histamine is released into the circulation, total peripheral resistance and blood pressure fall and the individual may progress to **anaphylactic shock.** Activation of H_1 receptors also causes bronchoconstriction and contraction of most gastrointestinal smooth muscles.

H_2 **receptors** are most noted for increasing **gastric acid secretion,** but they are also involved in **allergic reactions.** For this reason, H_2 receptor antagonists are sometimes used in combination with H_1 receptor antagonists in the treatment of allergies. Activation of H_2 receptors in the heart increases the heart rate and contractility, but the cardiac effects of histamine are not prominent under most conditions.

H_3 **receptors** are located in various tissues in the periphery and on nerve terminals. Activation of these presynaptic receptors in the brain inhibits the release of histamine and other neurotransmitters.

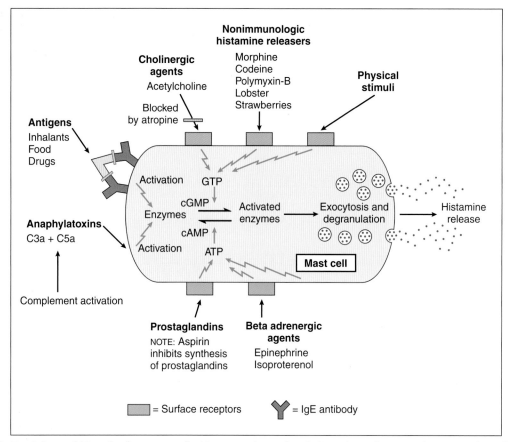

Figure 26-1. Release of histamine from mast cells. Numerous chemical and physical stimuli activate histamine release from mast cells. Complement activation from serum sickness or bacterial endotoxins produces the anaphylactic peptides C3a and C5a, allergic antigens bind to IgE antibodies, and chemicals and other substances increase guanosine triphosphate (GTP) and cyclic guanosine monophosphate (cGMP) to activate enzymes causing increased intracellular calcium and release of histamine granules. β-Adrenoceptor agents and some prostaglandins increase adenosine triphosphate (ATP) and cyclic adenosine monophosphate (cAMP) and reduce activated enzymes.

ANTIHISTAMINE DRUGS

Antihistamines, or **histamine receptor antagonists**, have been categorized on the basis of their receptor selectivity as H_1 receptor antagonists or H_2 receptor antagonists.

Histamine H_1 Receptor Antagonists

Classification

The following discussion focuses on the properties and uses of four groups of H_1 receptor antagonists. Chlorpheniramine, clemastine, dimenhydrinate, diphenhydramine, hydroxyzine, meclizine, and promethazine are examples of **first-generation** drugs. Cetirizine, fexofenadine, loratadine, and desloratadine are examples of **second-generation** drugs. Drugs in these two groups are administered orally or parenterally. A major difference in the two groups is that the first-generation antihistamines are distributed to the CNS and can cause **sedation**, whereas the second-generation antihistamines do not cross the **blood-brain barrier** significantly. Azelastine is an example of an **intranasal antihistamine**, and levocabastine, ketotifen, epinastine, and olopatadine are used for **ophthalmic** treatment.

MECHANISMS AND PHARMACOKINETICS. The H_1 antihistamines contain an alkylamine group that resembles the side chain of histamine and permits them to bind to the H_1 receptor and act as competitive receptor **antagonists**. The drugs can block most of the effects of histamine on vascular smooth muscles and nerves and thereby prevent or counteract allergic reactions.

When antihistamines are administered orally, they are rapidly absorbed and are widely distributed to tissues. Many of them are extensively metabolized in the liver by cytochrome P450 enzymes. Hydroxyzine has an active metabolite that is also available as the drug, cetirizine, and this drug is excreted unchanged in the urine and feces.

Azelastine is an H_1 antihistamine that is marketed as a nasal spray for the treatment of allergic rhinitis. It blocks H_1 receptors and inhibits the release of histamine from mast cells, and it is much more potent than either **sodium cromoglycate** or **theophylline** in its inhibition. The systemic bioavailability of azelastine following intranasal administration is about 40%, and the plasma half-life is about 22 hours. Azelastine is metabolized by cytochrome P450 enzymes to an active metabolite, **desmethylazelastine**, a substance whose plasma concentrations are 20% to 30% of azelastine concentrations. Azelastine and its principal metabolite are both H_1 receptor antagonists. The unchanged drug and its active metabolite are excreted primarily in the feces.

TABLE 26-2. Pharmacologic Properties of Selected Histamine H₁ Receptor Antagonists

Drug	Duration of Action (Hours)	Sedative Effects	Antiemetic Effects	Anticholinergic Effects
First-generation Antihistamines				
Chlorpheniramine	6	Medium	None	Medium
Dimenhydrinate	8	High	Medium	High
Diphenhydramine	8	High	Medium	High
Hydroxyzine	6	High	High	Medium
Meclizine	12	Medium	High	Medium
Promethazine	12	High	High	High
Second-generation Antihistamines				
Cetirizine	24	Low	None	Very low
Fexofenadine	12	Very low	None	Very low
Loratadine	24	Very low	None	Very low
Intranasal Antihistamines				
Azelastine	12	Low	None	Very low

PHARMACOLOGIC EFFECTS AND INDICATIONS. The H₁ antihistamines are all equally effective in treating **allergies**, but they differ markedly in their sedative, antiemetic, and anticholinergic properties (Table 26–2). The second-generation antihistamines cause little or no sedation, so they are often preferred for the treatment of allergies. Antihistamines are usually more effective when administered before exposure to an allergen than afterward. Hence, persons with seasonal allergies, such as **allergic rhinitis** (see Chapter 27), should take them on a regular basis throughout the allergy season.

First-Generation Antihistamines

Because the first-generation antihistamines have sedative effects, they are occasionally used to produce **sedation**. They are also used to treat **nausea and vomiting**, to prevent **motion sickness** in persons traveling by plane or boat, or to treat **vertigo** (an illusory sense that the environment or one's own body is revolving).

The most sedating drugs are **diphenhydramine, hydroxyzine**, and **promethazine**. These drugs have been used to induce sleep or for preoperative sedation. Their sedating properties can also be useful in relieving distress caused by the severe pruritus associated with some allergic reactions. Persons taking these drugs should be cautioned against driving or operating machinery.

Pheniramine drugs (e.g., **chlorpheniramine**), are less sedating than other first-generation drugs and are used primarily in the treatment of allergic reactions to pollen, mold spores, and other environmental allergens.

Meclizine, diphenhydramine, hydroxyzine, and **promethazine** have higher **antiemetic activity** than other antihistamines. Meclizine is less sedating than diphenhydramine, hydroxyzine, and promethazine, so it is frequently used to prevent **motion sickness** or treat vertigo. **Dimenhydrinate** is a mixture of diphenhydramine and 8-chlorotheophylline and is also used for these purposes. Promethazine suppositories are often used to relieve **nausea** and **vomiting** associated with various conditions (see Chapter 28).

Second-Generation Antihistamines

The second-generation drugs lack antiemetic activity, so their use is limited to the treatment of **allergies**. None of these drugs causes substantial sedation; however, **cetirizine** is more likely than astemizole, fexofenadine, or loratadine to cause some sedation. Because **fexofenadine** has a shorter half-life, it must be taken twice a day, whereas the other second-generation drugs are taken once a day. Fexofenadine and cetirizine are eliminated primarily as the unchanged drug in the feces and urine, respectively. **Loratadine** and **desloratadine** are metabolized to **active metabolites**, which are excreted in the urine and feces.

Intranasal Antihistamines

Azelastine is indicated for the treatment of symptoms of **allergic rhinitis**, including sneezing, nasal itching, and nasal discharge. It is administered as two sprays per nostril twice daily. The drug can cause drowsiness so should be used cautiously when patients are driving or operating machinery.

Opthalmic Antihistamines

Currently, four antihistamine eyedrop formulations are available. **Levocabastine, epinastine**, and **olopadine** are selective H₁ antagonists for topical ophthalmic use. They are indicated for the temporary relief of the signs and symptoms of seasonal allergic conjunctivitis. **Ketotifen** is a selective, **noncompetitive H₁ antagonist** and **mast cell stabilizer**. The action of ketotifen occurs rapidly with an effect seen within minutes after administration and, because of the noncompetitive nature of the receptor antagonism, it has a longer duration of action than the other agents. It is indicated for the temporary prevention of itching of the eye caused by allergic conjunctivitis.

ADVERSE EFFECTS AND INTERACTIONS. The H₁ antihistamines produce few serious side effects.

CASE PRESENTATION: A 35-year-old male working as a stockbroker complains to his physician that he is constantly sneezing and has a runny nose and itchy, watery eyes whenever he is at his home in the country. He tells his physician that he tried an over-the-counter allergy medicine but that it made him drowsy and feel "like he was living in a fog." His doctor tells him that he suffers from allergic rhinitis, or "hay fever," and prescribes a nasal spray containing azelastine.

CASE DISCUSSION: The most common symptom of seasonal allergies is allergic rhinitis, otherwise known as hay fever. Symptoms of allergic rhinitis closely mimic those of the common cold, but with a cold, nasal discharge may be thick and yellow. With allergies, it is generally thin and clear. An allergy is also often accompanied by itchy, watery eyes. Most over-the-counter medications include diphenhydramine, a first-generation antihistamine, but these preparations are known to cause drowsiness. The newer, second-generation antihistamines are fexofenadine and loratadine, which do not cause drowsiness, as they do not readily gain access into the CNS. Among the different types of nose sprays, there is azelastine, an antihistamine, and those that contain steroids, such as beclomethasone, fluticasone, or triamcinolone. The drawback to steroid medications is that they may take a week or so to be maximally effective. There is also a nasal spray containing cromolyn sodium, a mast cell stabilizer, available without a prescription.

FIRST-GENERATION ANTIHISTAMINES. **Sedation** is the most common side effect of the first-generation antihistamines. Paradoxically, however, the drugs can produce **excitement** in infants and children and should be used with caution in these patients.

Diphenhydramine and **promethazine** have the highest **anticholinergic activity** (see Table 26–2), but other first-generation drugs also block cholinergic muscarinic receptors. As a result, the drugs can cause dry mouth, blurred vision, tachycardia, urinary retention, and other atropine-like side effects.

Anticholinergic toxicity is the principal manifestation of an overdose of first-generation antihistamines. Administration of **physostigmine**, a **cholinesterase inhibitor** that crosses the blood-brain barrier, may be required to counteract the anticholinergic effects of antihistamines in the CNS.

SECOND-GENERATION ANTIHISTAMINES. **Astemizole** (HISMANAL) also caused prolongation of the QT interval and was removed from the market. Fexofenadine, is the active metabolite of **terfenadine** (SELDANE). Terfenadine was the first nonsedating H_1 blocker, but was withdrawn from the market by the U.S. Food and Drug Administration because it prolonged the QT interval on the electrocardiogram, leading to a type of **cardiac arrhythmia** called *torsades de pointes*. **Fexofenadine** does not appear to cause cardiac abnormalities. **Cetirizine** and **loratadine** also lack cardiac effects (Box 26–1).

INTRANASAL ANTIHISTAMINES. Adverse effects of azelastine are rare and include dizziness, fatigue, headache, nasal irritation, dry mouth, and weight gain.

OPTHALMIC ANTIHISTAMINES. Adverse effects of levocabastine, epinastine, olopatadine, and ketotifen are usually limited to the eyes and include transient stinging and burning. These occur in less than 5% of patients.

Histamine H_2 and H_3 Receptor Antagonists

Chapter 28 outlines the properties of H_2 receptor antagonists, which are used primarily to treat **peptic ulcer disease**. There are presently no approved H_3 receptor agents, although clinical trials are under way (see Selected Readings).

SEROTONIN AND RELATED DRUGS

Serotonin Biosynthesis and Release

Serotonin, or **5-hydroxytryptamine** (5-HT), is an autacoid and a neurotransmitter that is produced primarily by platelets, enterochromaffin cells in the gut, and neurons. The greatest concentration of serotonin is in the enterochromaffin cells of the gastrointestinal tract. As illustrated in Figure 18–3C, serotonin is synthesized from the amino acid **tryptophan** and is converted to **5-hydroxyindoleacetic acid** (5-HIAA) by monoamine oxidase and aldehyde dehydrogenase. 5-HIAA is then excreted in the urine. Serotonin is concentrated in vesicles within the cell and released by calcium-mediated exocytosis.

Serotonin Receptors and Effects

The four main types of **serotonin receptors** are designated as $5\text{-}HT_1$ through $5\text{-}HT_4$. The $5\text{-}HT_1$ and $5\text{-}HT_2$ receptors have several subtypes that are designated by letters (e.g., $5\text{-}HT_{1A}$ and $5\text{-}HT_{1D}$). Although most serotonin receptors are G protein–coupled receptors, the **$5\text{-}HT_3$ receptor** is a ligand-gated ion channel. The mechanisms of signal transduction for serotonin receptors are outlined in Table 18–1.

In the peripheral tissues, the physiologic effects of serotonin include platelet aggregation, stimulation of gastrointestinal motility, and modulation of vascular smooth muscle contraction. Serotonin causes **vasoconstriction** in most vascular beds and contraction of most smooth muscles. In the CNS, serotonin is involved in the regulation of mood, appetite, sleep, emotional processing, and pain processing (see Chapter 18).

Drugs that affect serotonin activity are classified as serotonin agonists, serotonin antagonists, and serotonin reuptake inhibitors. Examples are mentioned later in this chapter and discussed in detail in other chapters.

5-HT Agonists

Serotonin agonists have been developed for use in the management of several specific disorders (Table 26–3). **Buspirone**, a partial agonist that acts at the 5-HT$_{1A}$ receptor, is used to treat **anxiety** and **depression** (see Chapter 19). **Sumatriptan** and related **triptan** compounds, and some **ergot drugs**, are 5-HT$_{1D/1B}$ receptor agonists that are used to treat **migraine headaches** (see Chapter 29).

Cisapride was the first 5-HT$_4$ receptor agonist used for the treatment of **gastroesophageal reflux disease** and **gastrointestinal hypomotility** (see Chapter 28). Activation of 5-HT$_4$ receptors increases the peristaltic action of the gastrointestinal tract, which is helpful in the treatment of both gastroesophageal reflux disease and gastrointestinal hypomotility. However, **cisapride** (PROPULSID) was pulled from the market in the United States in 2000 after postmarketing surveillance revealed a risk of rare but sometimes fatal prolongation of the QT interval on electrocardiogram records ('long QT syndrome'). A newer 5-HT$_4$ agonist, **tegaserod** (ZELNORM), was approved for a narrower indication for women who have **irritable bowel syndrome** with constipation as their main symptom, but it was recently withdrawn from the market due to **increased risk of heart attack** or **stroke**.

5-HT Antagonists

Examples of serotonin antagonists include clozapine, cyproheptadine, methysergide, and ondansetron (see Table 26–3).

Clozapine and other drugs are classified as **atypical antipsychotics** that act partly by blocking 5-HT$_2$ receptors in the CNS. They are used in the treatment of **schizophrenia** (see Chapter 22).

Cyproheptadine is a 5-HT$_2$ receptor antagonist that also has H$_1$ antihistamine activity. This makes it useful in managing **urticaria** (hives) and other allergic reactions in which **pruritus** is a prominent feature. Cyproheptadine is administered orally every 8 to 12 hours and can cause slight to moderate drowsiness.

Methysergide is a 5-HT$_2$ receptor antagonist that is used to **prevent migraine headaches** (see Chapter 29).

Cyproheptadine and **methysergide** are both useful in the care of patients with **carcinoid tumor**. This tumor can produce huge quantities of serotonin, histamine, and other vasoactive substances that cause a constellation of clinical effects called the **carcinoid syndrome**. Affected patients suffer from malabsorption, violent attacks of watery diarrhea and cramping, and paroxysmal vasomotor attacks characterized by sudden red to purple flushing of the face and neck. The malabsorption and diarrhea can be managed by giving cyproheptadine or methysergide in combination with opioid antidiarrheal drugs.

Ondansetron was the first selective **5-HT$_3$ receptor antagonist** used as an antiemetic agent in cancer chemotherapy as well as treating nausea and vomiting from other causes. It prevents **nausea and vomiting** by blocking the effects of serotonin in the chemoreceptor trigger zone and in vagal afferent nerves in the gastrointestinal tract (see Chapter 28). Closely related gastrointestinal agents sharing the same mechanism of action include **granisetron**, **alosetron**, **palonosetron**, and **dolasetron**. Granisetron, as with ondansetron, is used to **prevent nausea and vomiting** caused by cancer chemotherapy and radiation therapy. **Alosetron** is indicated for treatment of women with irritable bowel syndrome whose predominant bowel symptom is diarrhea. **Palonosetron** is an injectable-only formulation for the prevention of acute or delayed nausea and vomiting associated with initial and repeat courses of emetogenic cancer chemotherapy.

Serotonin Reuptake Inhibitors

Serotonin reuptake inhibitors are used in the treatment of **depression** and **other CNS disorders** (see Chapter 22).

EICOSANOIDS AND RELATED DRUGS

Eicosanoids are autacoids derived from **arachidonic acid** (eicosatetraenoic acid) and other 20-carbon fatty acids (*eicos* in Greek means "twenty").

Eicosanoid Biosynthesis and Release

Eicosanoids are made from arachidonic acid and other polyunsaturated fatty acids in the cell membrane. They are freed from their esteric attachment to membrane phospholipids by **phospholipase A$_2$**, an enzyme that is activated by numerous chemical stimuli and by physical stimuli such as cell damage. The two main groups of eicosanoids are the **prostaglandins** and the **leukotrienes**, whose formation begins with

TABLE 26–3. Serotonin Receptors and Clinical Uses of Serotonin Agonists and Antagonists

Drug	5-HT Receptor	Clinical Use
Serotonin Agonists		
Buspirone	5-HT$_{1A}$	Anxiety; depression
(In development)	5-HT$_4$	Irritable bowel syndrome with constipation
Sumatriptan	5-HT$_{1D/1B}$	Migraine headaches
Serotonin Antagonists		
Clozapine	5-HT$_2$	Schizophrenia
Cyproheptadine	5-HT$_2$	Carcinoid syndrome; pruritus; urticaria
Methysergide	5-HT$_2$	Carcinoid syndrome; migraine headaches
Ondansetron	5-HT$_3$	Nausea and vomiting

5-HT = 5-hydroxytryptamine (serotonin).

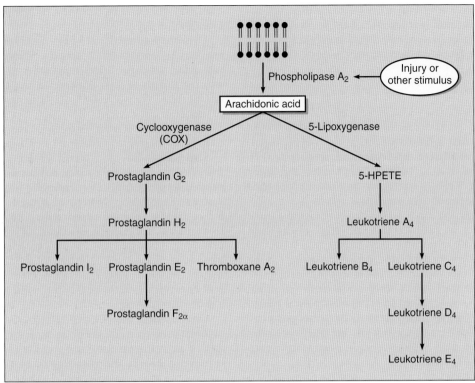

Figure 26–2. Synthesis of eicosanoids. When phospholipase A_2 is activated by an injury or other stimulus, it catalyzes the hydrolysis of arachidonic acid and other 20-carbon fatty acids from cell membrane phospholipids. Arachidonic acid is converted to prostaglandins and leukotrienes by cyclooxygenase and 5-lipoxygenase, respectively. Other enzymes complete the synthesis of specific eicosanoids. 5-HPETE= 5-hydroperoxyeicosatetraenoic acid.

reactions catalyzed by **cyclooxygenase** and **5-lipoxygenase**, respectively. As shown in Figure 26–2, subsequent reactions convert the products of these reactions to specific prostaglandins and leukotrienes.

Each prostaglandin (PG) and leukotriene is assigned a letter and subscript number (e.g., PGE_2). The letter refers to the specific ring structure of the substance, and the subscript number indicates the **number of double bonds** in the fatty acid chains.

Eicosanoid end products made in individuals consuming a typical Western diet come primarily from arachidonic acid, containing four carbon double bonds. Because the first double bond is located at the sixth carbon, arachidonic acid is known as an **omega-6 fatty acid**. In diets rich in coldwater fish or plants, cell membranes contain an **omega-3 fatty acid**, eicosapentaenoic acid, with five double bonds starting at the third carbon position. Eicosapentaenoic acid is also a precursor to eicosanoid products but these products have different biological activities than eicosanoids generated from arachidonic acid. For example, prostaglandins derived from omega-6 fatty acids have different vasoactive and platelet-aggregating properties than do prostaglandins derived from omega-3 fatty acids (see below).

After synthesis, **eicosanoids are released** from the cell to exert local effects on surrounding tissues. Unlike other autacoids, no evidence exists of vesicular storage or calcium-mediated exocytosis for eicosanoid substances within the cell. Because of this, the synthesis of eicosanoids coincides with its release though the cell membrane and into the surrounding tissue.

Eicosanoid Receptors and Effects

All of the naturally released eicosanoids are **short-lived** and locally acting. Eicosanoid drugs exist as either purified preparations of the same naturally occurring substance or closely related synthetic analogues. **Prostaglandins** exert their effects on smooth muscle, platelet aggregation, neurotransmission, glandular secretion, and other biologic activities by activating specific **prostanoid receptors** in target tissues. These receptors are G protein–coupled receptor proteins named by the prostaglandin that binds with the highest affinity and selectivity. Accordingly, the prostanoid receptor for PGD_2 is DP, the receptor for PGE_2 is EP, and so forth, to identify the ligands for the FP, IP, and TP (**thromboxane**) receptors. To date, four types of EP receptors are identified, designated EP_1 through EP_4; two types of DP receptors (D_1 and D_2); and one type each of FP, IP, and TP receptors. The signal transduction pathways of prostanoid receptors are diverse and mediated by of G proteins that increase or decrease cyclic adenosine monophosphate, or the DAG/IP_3 pathway (see Chapter 3). **Thromboxanes**, which are substances derived from prostaglandin synthesis (see Fig. 26–2), also act on smooth muscle and platelet aggregation. Different types of thromboxanes and prostaglandins have different physiologic effects, and often have apposing effects. The eicosanoid released from a tissue or cell will depend on the particular set of synthetic enzymes contained within the cell.

Whereas **platelet aggregation** is stimulated by **thromboxane A_2 (TXA_2)**, it is inhibited by **prostacyclin** (prostaglandin I_2 [PGI_2]). Prostacyclin is released primarily from

vascular endothelial cells and serves to prevent platelet aggregation under normal conditions. In contrast, TXA_2 is produced and released only when a blood vessel is injured, at which time the adherence of platelets to vascular endothelium activates the platelets and leads to the synthesis and release of TXA_2 (see Chapter 16 and Fig. 16–5).

In some cases, the fatty acid precursor of a prostaglandin or thromboxane has a major impact on its biologic activity. For example, thromboxane A_3 (TXA_3), which is synthesized from eicosapentaenoic acid, an omega-3 fatty acid found in fish oils, produces relatively little platelet aggregation or vasoconstriction in comparison with TXA_2. This difference can largely explain the correlation between **increased fish oil consumption** and a **decreased incidence of thrombotic events** (strokes and heart attacks) in certain native populations.

Both PGE_2 and PGI_2 cause **vasodilation** in several vascular beds. These prostaglandins appear to play a role in maintaining **pulmonary blood flow**, and they also serve to maintain the **patency of the ductus arteriosus** until it is time for its closure. In the kidneys, PGE_2 and PGI_2 produce vasodilation and have important roles in modulating **renal blood flow** and **glomerular filtration**. These actions are particularly important in persons with renal insufficiency and in the elderly. The renal actions of prostaglandin also appear to exert an **antihypertensive effect**, partly by increasing water and sodium excretion. Because **nonsteroidal anti-inflammatory drugs** (NSAIDs) inhibit prostaglandin synthesis, their use can cause or exacerbate renal disorders and may counteract the antihypertensive effect of antihypertensive medications taken concurrently.

Many prostaglandins, including PGE_2 and prostaglandin $F_{2\alpha}$ ($PGF_{2\alpha}$), stimulate **uterine contractions** and increase **gastrointestinal motility**. Their uterine activity is the basis for several therapeutic applications, whereas their gastrointestinal actions can lead to adverse effects (e.g., diarrhea and intestinal cramping). Several prostaglandins also produce a **cytoprotective effect on the gastrointestinal mucosa**.

The **leukotrienes** are produced primarily in inflammatory cells, including mast cells, basophils, eosinophils, macrophages, and polymorphonuclear leukocytes. Leukotrienes C_4 and D_4 (LTC_4 and LTD_4) are the main components of the **slow-reacting substance of anaphylaxis**. These two leukotrienes are secreted in the presence of asthma and anaphylaxis and play a major role in bronchospastic disease.

EICOSANOID DRUGS

The effects and clinical uses of prostaglandin drugs are outlined in Table 26–4, and summarized in the following paragraphs.

Eicosanoid Synthesis Inhibitors

Among the groups of drugs that inhibit eicosanoid synthesis are **leukotriene inhibitors** (see Chapter 27), **NSAIDs** (see Chapter 30), and **corticosteroids** (see Chapter 33).

Leukotriene inhibitors act either by inhibiting 5-lipoxygenase or by blocking leukotriene receptors. They are currently used in the management of **asthma**, but other therapeutic applications are being explored.

The **NSAIDs** act by inhibiting cyclooxygenase and are used primarily to alleviate **pain** and **inflammation**.

Corticosteroids block the formation of all eicosanoids, partly by inhibiting phospholipase A_2. They have **anti-inflammatory**, **antiallergic**, and **antineoplastic effects** and are used in the treatment of a wide variety of adrenal diseases and nonadrenal disorders.

Prostaglandin Drugs

Prostaglandin E_1 and Prostaglandin E_1 Derivatives

Alprostadil is identical to naturally occurring PGE_1 and is available in several formulations for specific clinical uses.

Alprostadil is given by continuous intravenous infusion to maintain the **patency of the ductus arteriosus** in neonates who are awaiting surgery for some types of congenital heart diseases. These include cyanotic heart defects (pulmonary atresia or stenosis, tricuspid atresia, tetralogy of Fallot, and transposition of the great vessels) and acyanotic heart defects (coarctation of the aorta and hypoplastic left ventricle).

Alprostadil is available in injectable, pellet, and cream formulations to treat **erectile dysfunction** in men. For this purpose, the drug is injected into the cavernosa of

TABLE 26–4. **Effects and Clinical Uses of Selected Prostaglandin Drugs**

Drug	PG Class	Effect	Clinical Use
Alprostadil	PGE_1	Vasodilation	Erectile dysfunction; patency of the ductus arteriosus
Carboprost tromethamine	$PGF_{2\alpha}$ analogue	Contraction of uterine muscle	Abortifacient; postpartum bleeding
Dinoprostone	PGE_2	Contraction of uterine muscle	Abortifacient; cervical ripening
Epoprostenol	PGI_2	Vasodilation	Pulmonary hypertension
Latanoprost	$PGF_{2\alpha}$ analogue	Increase in aqueous humor outflow	Glaucoma
Misoprostol	PGE_1 analogue	Gastric cytoprotection	Gastric and duodenal ulcers induced by use of NSAIDs

NSAIDs = nonsteroidal anti-inflammatory drugs; PG = prostaglandin.

the penis or slow-release pellets or drops of cream are inserted into the meatus of the urethra. Adverse effects in men treated with alprostadil include penile pain, penile fibrosis, **priapism** (persistent erection), flushing, diarrhea, headache, and fever. Given the rise in the use of oral drugs to treat erectile dysfunction—for example, **sildenafil** (VIAGRA), **tadalafil** (CIALIS), and **vardenafil** (LEVITRA)—it is likely that aprostadil will be limited to those patients for whom the aforementioned popular drugs are contraindicated.

Misoprostol is a synthetic PGE_1 analogue available in an orally administered formulation for the prevention of NSAID-induced **gastric ulcers** and **duodenal ulcers** (see Chapter 28). Misoprostol treatment is particularly useful in patients who take NSAIDs on a long-term basis to alleviate the symptoms of arthritis and other inflammatory conditions. Misoprostol acts locally on the gastrointestinal mucosa to exert a cytoprotective effect by inhibiting gastric acid secretion and by increasing bicarbonate secretion from mucosal cells. Diarrhea, one of the most common adverse effects of misoprostol use, can be minimized by starting patients on a low dose of the drug and then gradually increasing the dose. In pregnant women, misoprostol is absolutely contraindicated because it can stimulate uterine contractions and cause premature labor.

Misoprostol is also approved for use as an abortifacient in combination with the progesterone receptor antagonist, **mifepristone** (RU86, MIFEPREX). When used in combination, mifepristone and misoprostol are 95% to 97% effective within the first 2 weeks of pregnancy.

Prostaglandin E_2 and Prostaglandin $F_{2\alpha}$ Derivatives

Dinoprostone and **carboprost tromethamine** are prostaglandin drugs that have oxytocic activity and increase the uterine contractions of pregnant women. Dinoprostone is a formulation of naturally occurring PGE_2, whereas carboprost is a synthetic derivative of $PGF_{2\alpha}$.

Dinoprostone is available as a vaginal insert, gel, or suppository. In pregnant women, the vaginal insert or gel is applied to the vagina or cervix to produce **cervical ripening** before labor induction. The insert may provide more accurate dosing than the gel. The suppository is used to **evacuate the uterine contents** in cases of intrauterine fetal death, benign hydatidiform mole, or second-trimester termination of pregnancy.

Carboprost is administered intramuscularly to **control postpartum bleeding** when other measures have failed and to **terminate pregnancy (abortifacient)**. It can cause flushing, diarrhea, vomiting, altered blood pressure, blurred vision, respiratory distress, and other adverse reactions.

Latanoprost was the first prostaglandin drug indicated for the treatment of **glaucoma**. It is administered topically as eyedrops and is used to treat open-angle glaucoma that is resistant to other pharmacologic treatments. Latanoprost is a $PGF_{2\alpha}$ analogue that acts on FP receptors to increase aqueous humor outflow via the uveoscleral pathway (see Box 6–1). It can alter the color of the iris and cause a **permanent eye color change** by increasing the amount of melanin in melanocytes. Other synthetic FP receptor agonists developed for the reduction of intraocular pressure in patients

with open-angle glaucoma or ocular hypertension are **bimatoprost** and **travoprost**.

Prostaglandin I_2 and Prostaglandin I_2 Derivatives

Epoprostenol is a formulation of naturally occurring PGI_2 (prostacyclin) that is used to treat **pulmonary arterial hypertension**. Epoprostenol acts on IP receptors to dilate pulmonary blood vessels and increase pulmonary blood flow, thereby counteracting the pathophysiologic consequences of pulmonary hypertension. The drug is administered by continuous intravenous infusion, and the dosage is titrated on the basis of clinical improvement and adverse effects. The most common adverse reactions include flushing, tachycardia, hypotension, diarrhea, nausea, vomiting, and flulike symptoms.

Treprostinil is a stable analogue of prostacyclin which has a half-life of between 2 and 4 hours and can be safely administered by a continuous subcutaneous infusion, via a self-inserted subcutaneous catheter using a microinfusion pump designed specifically for subcutaneous drug delivery. It is approved to diminish the symptoms (e.g., shortness of breath) associated with physical activity in patients with pulmonary arterial hypertension.

ENDOTHELIN-1 ANTAGONISTS

Endothelin-1 (**ET-1**) is a peptide autacoid produced by vascular endothelial cells. It activates ET_A and ET_B **receptors** in vascular smooth muscle and other tissues. The results of ET_A receptor activation are vasoconstriction and cell proliferation, while ET_B receptors mediate vasodilation, antiproliferation, and increased ET-1 clearance. ET-1 may serve physiologically to counteract the vasodilation produced by the endothelin-relaxing factor (nitric oxide), but levels of ET-1 peptide are increased 10-fold in pulmonary arteries of patients with **pulmonary arterial hypertension**. ET-1 also appears to contribute to cardiac dysfunction during reperfusion after thrombolytic treatment in patients suffering from acute myocardial infarction.

Bosentan (TRACLEER) is a **dual ET_A and ET_B receptor antagonist** that is approved for treating pulmonary arterial hypertension. Clinical trials have shown that bosentan significantly improves 6-minute walking distance in persons with class III or IV pulmonary arterial hypertension, while decreasing pulmonary vascular resistance and dyspnea.

Bosentan is administered orally and is generally well tolerated, but 11% of patients experienced elevated serum aminotransferase levels. For this reason, **liver function tests** should be monitored at baseline and then monthly in persons taking bosentan. Based on animal studies, bosentan is very likely to cause major **birth defects** if used by pregnant women, and it is contraindicated in pregnancy and in women of childbearing age who are not using hormonal contraceptives.

A second ET receptor antagonist, **ambrisentan**, was recently approved for the treatment of pulmonary arterial hypertension. Ambrisentan has much **greater selectivity for ET_A receptors** compared to ET_B receptors (>4000-fold), although the clinical impact of such high selectivity is not known. Like bosentan, similar warnings are made regarding

hepatic function and enzyme level monitoring. Although not an endothelin drug, **sildenafil** has been marketed under a new trade name, REVATIO, for the treatment of pulmonary arterial hypertension. As sildenafil inhibits phosphodiesterase type 5, an increase of cyclic guanosine monophosphate within pulmonary vascular smooth muscle cells results in relaxation and vasodilation of the pulmonary vascular bed.

SUMMARY OF IMPORTANT POINTS

■ Autacoids include histamine, serotonin, prostaglandins, and leukotrienes. These substances usually act on the same tissue in which they are produced.

■ Histamine is the primary mediator of allergic reactions. Stimulation of H_1 receptors causes vasodilation, edema, congestion, and pruritus. Stimulation of H_2 receptors mediates gastric acid secretion.

■ The first-generation H_1 receptor antagonists (chlorpheniramine, diphenhydramine, meclizine, promethazine, and others) produce varying degrees of sedation and also have anticholinergic side effects. The second-generation drugs (cetirizine, loratadine, fexofenadine, and desloratadine) are largely devoid of CNS effects.

■ The H_1 receptor antagonists are used primarily to treat allergies, but meclizine is used to prevent motion sickness and promethazine is used to treat nausea and vomiting.

■ Fexofenadine is the active metabolite of the now-banned terfenadine. Unlike terfenadine, fexofenadine does not prolong the QT interval or cause *torsades de pointes*. Cetirizine, desloratadine, and loratadine also lack cardiac effects.

■ Drugs that affect serotonin (5-hydroxytryptamine, or 5-HT) are classified as serotonin agonists, serotonin antagonists, and serotonin reuptake inhibitors.

■ Some $5-HT_1$ receptor agonists (e.g., sumatriptan) can be used to treat migraine headaches, whereas some $5-HT_2$ receptor antagonists (e.g., methysergide) can be used to prevent migraine headaches.

■ Cyproheptadine and methysergide, both of which are $5-HT_2$ receptor antagonists, are used in the management of carcinoid syndrome, which is caused by excessive production of serotonin and other vasoactive substances in patients with carcinoid tumors from enterochromaffin tissue.

■ Ondansetron, granisetron, and many others "setron" drugs are $5-HT_3$ receptor antagonists used in the treatment of nausea and vomiting.

■ Eicosanoids are derived from arachidonic acid and other precursor 20-carbon fatty acids. The two main groups of eicosanoids are prostaglandins and leukotrienes. The ratio of omega-6 and omega-3 fatty acids in the diet plays an important role in the activity of eicosanoid end products.

■ Alprostadil is PGE_1 and misoprostol is a PGE_1 derivative. Alprostadil is used to maintain patency of the ductus arteriosus in neonates awaiting surgery for heart defects. It is also used to treat erectile dysfunction in men. Misoprostol is used to prevent gastric and duodenal ulcers in persons taking NSAIDs.

■ Dinoprostone, the same as PGE_2, is used for cervical ripening before induction of labor and for evacuation of the uterine contents.

■ Carboprost and latanoprost are $PGF_{2\alpha}$ derivatives. Carboprost is used to control postpartum bleeding and to terminate pregnancy. Latanoprost and other prostaglandin antiglaucoma drugs that increase the aqueous humor outflow are used to treat glaucoma.

■ Epoprostenol is PGI_2 (prostacyclin) and treprostinil is a PGI_2 derivative; both are used to treat pulmonary arterial hypertension. Additionally, bosentan and ambrisentan, endothelin-1 receptor antagonists, and a new formulation of sildenafil are indicated for pulmonary arterial hypertension.

Review Questions

1. Which of the following antihistamines would be best used to treat mild nausea and vomiting due to motion sickness?
   (A) cetirizine
   (B) fexofenadine
   (C) loratadine
   (D) diphenhydramine
   (E) meclizine

2. Which of the following describes the major difference between a first- and second-generation antihistamine?
   (A) selectivity at H_1 receptors
   (B) ability to cross the blood-brain barrier
   (C) effectiveness in treating allergies
   (D) potency at blocking H_1 receptors
   (E) indications for use

3. Of the major serotonin (5-HT) receptors identified and used as targets for therapeutic agents, which one is the only one considered a ligand-gated ion channel?
   (A) $5-HT_{1B}$
   (B) $5-HT_{1D}$
   (C) $5-HT_2$
   (D) $5-HT_3$
   (E) $5-HT_4$

4. Which of the following drugs is the same as PGI_2 (prostacyclin) and is used for the treatment of pulmonary hypertension?
   (A) misoprostol
   (B) alprostadil
   (C) epoprostenol
   (D) treprostinil
   (E) travoprost

5. Latanoprost is an agonist at the PGF_2 receptors and is effective for the treatment of?
   (A) cornea abrasions
   (B) ocular hypertension and open-angle glaucoma
   (C) ocular albinism
   (D) closed-angle glaucoma
   (E) allergic conjunctivitis

Answers and Explanations

1. **The correct answer is E:** meclizine. Meclizine is a first-generation antihistamine with higher antiemetic activity than other agents and also less sedating. Answers (A) through (C) are second-generation antihistamines and gain little access to the CNS and thus are nonsedating and ideal for treating allergies but would be little help for motion sickness. Answer (D), diphenhydramine, has antiemetic effects but is more sedating than meclizine and thus not the ideal treatment agent. Dimenhydrinate, which is a mixture of diphenhydramine and 8-chlorotheophylline, is used for motion sickness, however.

2. **The correct answer is B:** ability to cross the blood-brain barrier. The major problem with treatment of allergies with the first-generation antihistamines is the adverse effects of sedation. Answer (A), selectivity at H_1 receptors, may be the case for select first-generation versus second-generation agents but is not the major difference between the classes. Answer (C), effectiveness in treating allergies, is not correct because both can effectively treat the symptoms of allergies but second-generation agents can do so without significant sedation. Answer (D), potency at blocking H_1 receptors, is another measure of antagonist affinity and is not correct for the same reasons that (A) is not correct. Answer (E), indications for use, is not correct because both types of agents are used for allergies.

3. **The correct answer is D:** $5-HT_3$. This type of receptor for serotonin is famous as the only biogenic amine receptor that is ionotropic. The other answers (A) through (C), and (E) are all types of metabotropic receptors, also known as G protein–coupled receptors.

4. **The correct answer is C:** epoprostenol. Epoprostenol is the same substance as PGI_2 (prostacyclin) and is used for the treatment of pulmonary hypertension. Answer (A) misoprostol, is a synthetic PGE_1 analogue that is available in an orally administered formulation for the prevention of NSAID-induced gastric ulcers and duodenal ulcers. Answer (B), alprostadil, is a naturally occurring prostaglandin but is known as PGE_1. Answer (D), treprostinil, is also used for pulmonary hypertension but is a stable analogue of prostacyclin, not the same as prostacyclin itself. Answer (E), travoprost, is a $PGF_{2\alpha}$ analogue and an agonist at FP receptors. It is used for the treatment of open-angle glaucoma.

5. **The correct answer is B:** ocular hypertension and open-angle glaucoma. Latanoprost, like bimatoprost and travoprost, is an agonist at the $PGF_{2\alpha}$ receptors and is among the most prescribed classes of antiglaucoma agents. Answer (A), cornea abrasions, might call for the use of an ocular antihistamine. Answer (C), ocular albinism, might make sense considering the bizarre adverse effect of latanoprost in darkening the color of the iris but is not approved by the U.S. Food and Drug Administration as an indication for latanoprost. Answer (D), closed-angle glaucoma, is usually treated by carbonic anhydrase inhibitors (e.g., acetazolamide) because the pressure rises very high inside the eye and needs to be dropped rapidly. Answer (E), allergic conjunctivitis, is best treated by one of the ocular antihistamines.

SELECTED READINGS

Domingo, J.L. Omega-3 fatty acids and the benefits of fish consumption: is all that glitters gold? Environ Int 33:993–998, 2007.

Driscoll, J.A., and M.M. Chakinala. Medical therapy for pulmonary arterial hypertension. Expert Opin Pharmacother 9:65–81, 2008.

Robertson, R.G., W.J. Geiger, and N.B. Davis. Carcinoid tumors. Am Fam Physician 74:429–434, 2006.

Simmons, D.L., R.M. Botting, and T. Hla. Cyclooxygenase isozymes: the biology of prostaglandin synthesis and inhibition. Pharmacol Rev 56(3):387–437, 2004.

Simons, F.E. Advances in H_1-antihistamines. N Engl J Med 351(21):2203–2217, 2004.

Wijtmans, M., R. Leurs, and I. de Esch. Histamine H_3 receptor ligands break ground in a remarkable plethora of therapeutic areas. Expert Opin Investig Drugs 16:967–985, 2007.

CHAPTER 27

Drugs for Respiratory Tract Disorders

CLASSIFICATION OF DRUGS FOR RESPIRATORY TRACT DISORDERS

Anti-inflammatory Drugs
Glucocorticoids
- Fluticasone (FLOVENT, FLONASE)[a]
- Prednisone[b]

Mast Cell Stabilizers
- Cromolyn Sodium[c]

Antileukotriene Drugs
- Montelukast (SINGULAIR)
- Zafirlukast (ACCOLATE)
- Zileution (ZYFLO)

Bronchodilators
Selective β₂-Adrenoceptor Agonists
- Albuterol (PROVENTIL, VENTOLIN)[d]
- Salmeterol (SEREVENT)
- Formoterol (FORADIL)
- Arformoterol (BROVANA)

Other Bronchodilators
- Ipratropium (ATROVENT)
- Tiotropiium (SPIRIVA)
- Theophylline (THEODUR)

Immunoglobulin Antagonist
- Omalizumab (XOLAIR)

Antitussives
- Codeine
- Dextromethorphan
- Hydrocodone

Expectorants
- Guaifenesin

Antihistamines
- Fexofenadine (ALLEGRA)[e]
- Diphenhydramine (BENADRYL)

[a]Also budesonide (PULMICORT, RHINOCORT), beclomethasone (BECLOVENT), triamcinolone (NASACORT), and ciclesonide (OMNARIS).
[b]Also prednisolone, methylprednisolone.
[c]Also lodoxamide (ALOMIDE) and nedocromil (TILADE).
[d]Also levalbuterol (XOPENEX), pirbuterol (MAXAIR), terbutaline (BRETHINE), and fenoterol (BEROTEC).
[e]Also loratadine (CLARITIN) and cetirizine (ZYRTEC).

OVERVIEW

Disorders of the respiratory tract include a wide range of conditions that can be divided into pulmonary disorders and upper respiratory tract disorders. Pulmonary disorders include asthma, chronic obstructive pulmonary disease (COPD), pneumonia, pulmonary fibrosis, and various other conditions. Upper respiratory tract disorders include allergic rhinitis and microbial infections of the nose, sinuses, and throat. This chapter is concerned primarily with the drugs used in the treatment of asthma, COPD, and rhinitis. Drugs used to treat cough and congestion are also discussed in this chapter.

Asthma

Asthma is characterized by airway inflammation and hyperresponsiveness to stimuli that produce bronchoconstriction. These stimuli include **cold air**, **exercise**, a wide variety of **allergens**, and **emotional stress** (see Box 27–1).

In susceptible persons, exposure to a stimulus triggers the release of substances from mast cells, eosinophils, basophils, neutrophils, and macrophages. Some of these substances are stored in cell granules, such as **histamine, adenosine, bradykinin**, and **major basic protein**. Other substances are formed and immediately released in response to asthmatic stimuli, including lipid mediators derived from arachidonic acid,

BOX 27–1.   A CASE OF COUGHING AND WHEEZING

CASE PRESENTATION: A 12-year-old boy is brought to his pediatrician after the recent onset of episodes of coughing, wheezing, and shortness of breath. These episodes have occurred two or three times a week while he was playing outdoors, and they gradually subsided after he came indoors and sat down to rest. The family has a history of allergies to molds and pollens, and the boy has been taking an antihistamine for allergic rhinitis. Examination shows an alert, well-developed boy of normal height and weight who is in no distress. His vital signs and breath sounds are normal except for fine wheezes during forced expiration, and there are no signs of infection. Spirometry tests show a forced expiratory volume in 1 second (FEV_1) that is 85% of the predicted value, and the boy's peak expiratory flow (PEF) variability is 20% (normal <20%). These findings are consistent with a diagnosis of mild asthma, which was probably precipitated by exposure to allergens and by exercise. After discussing treatment options with his parents, the boy is started on a daily dose of montelukast, and an albuterol inhaler will be used to control acute episodes. The patient and his parents receive further instructions and training concerning the use of the inhaler, and he is given prescriptions and scheduled for a follow-up evaluation in 3 weeks to determine the need for additional therapy.

CASE DISCUSSION: Asthma typically presents with wheezing, dyspnea, and coughing and is often associated with a history of respiratory allergies. The history, physical exam, and FEV_1 usually provide most of the information needed to diagnose and manage asthma. The patient appears to have mild asthma, which may be intermittent or persistent. Because the severity of his illness is uncertain, the patient is started on a leukotriene receptor antagonist because of its convenience, safety, and demonstrated effectiveness in children. The course of asthma is highly variable. His response to treatment and the future course of his illness will be monitored in order to determine the need for additional tests and treatments.

such as **leukotrienes** and **prostaglandins**. All of these substances contribute to inflammation of the airway, edema and desquamation of the bronchial epithelium, and hypertrophy of smooth muscles in the respiratory tract. These chemical mediators also increase the responsiveness of smooth muscles and the permeability of bronchioles to allergens, infectious agents, mediators of inflammation, and other irritants. As a result of these effects, mucus production increases and

leads to mucus plugging of the airways, thereby decreasing the ability of the airways to remove noxious substances. As a result, patients suffer from airway obstruction and must use accessory muscles to breathe.

Airway obstruction in asthma results from a combination of bronchial inflammation, smooth muscle constriction, and obstruction of the lumen with mucus, inflammatory cells, and epithelial debris. Symptoms of obstruction include dyspnea (difficulty in breathing), coughing, wheezing, headache, tachycardia, syncope, diaphoresis, pallor, and cyanosis. Patients experience a **biphasic reduction in pulmonary function**, with an **early phase** that occurs within 10 to 30 minutes of exposure to an allergen and lasts for 2 to 3 hours and then a **later phase** that occurs 2 to 8 hours after exposure. The late phase is believed to be responsible for inducing and maintaining bronchial hyperreactivity in asthmatic patients. Because of the circadian variation in bronchial responsiveness, some patients have up to an eightfold increase in airway hyperresponsiveness at night, and nearly 70% of asthma-related deaths happen at night.

The drugs used to treat asthma include anti-inflammatory drugs and bronchodilators. The pathophysiology of asthma and sites of anti-inflammatory drug action are shown in Figure 27–1.

Rhinitis

Rhinitis is most frequently caused by allergic reactions to **pollens**, **mold spores**, **dust mites**, and **other environmental allergens** or by infections with **viruses**, such as rhinoviruses and other agents of the common cold.

Allergic rhinitis can be seasonal or nonseasonal (perennial), whereas **viral rhinitis** is an acute, self-limiting condition. Both types of rhinitis are characterized by sneezing, nasal congestion, and rhinorrhea. Nasal pruritus and conjunctivitis are more commonly associated with allergic rhinitis than with viral rhinitis. Malaise, pain, and general discomfort are generally associated with viral rhinitis.

Table 27–1 shows the relative efficacy of various types of respiratory tract drugs, including those used in the treatment of allergic rhinitis and viral rhinitis.

Chronic Obstructive Pulmonary Diseases

COPDs include **chronic bronchitis** and **emphysema**. Chronic bronchitis is characterized by a productive cough associated with inflammation of the bronchioles, whereas emphysema is caused by permanent destruction and enlargement of the airspaces distal to the bronchioles. Both conditions result in airway obstruction, dyspnea (difficult breathing), decreased blood oxygen concentrations, and elevated blood carbon dioxide concentrations. Patients with these conditions have abnormal pulmonary function test values, such as a decreased forced expiratory volume in 1 second (FEV_1). Smoking and advanced age are the primary risk factors for COPD, and smoking cessation can slow disease progression. Although most of the airway obstruction in COPD is irreversible, a portion of the obstruction is caused by smooth muscle spasm and bronchiolar inflammation, and this portion can be reversed by bronchodilator drugs. Patients with COPD often require long-term

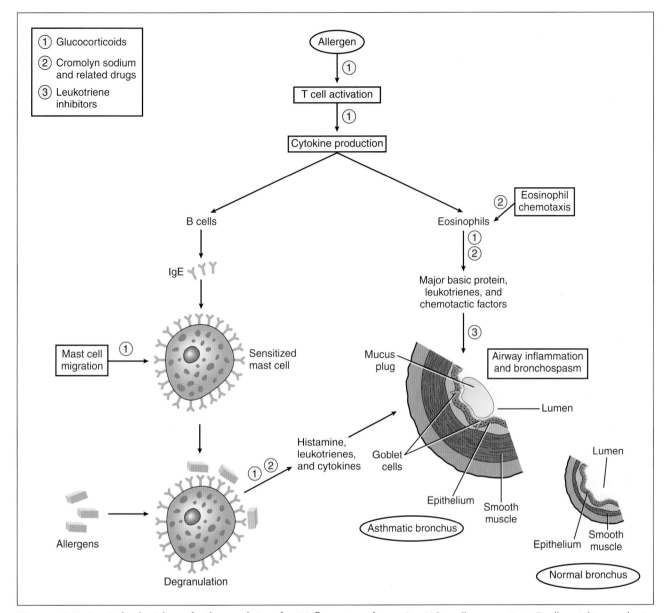

Figure 27–1. Pathophysiology of asthma and sites of anti-inflammatory drug action. When allergens activate T cells, cytokine production is stimulated. The cytokines, in turn, trigger the recruitment, activation, and release of a variety of cells and mediators. Glucocorticoids inhibit numerous steps in this process, including T-cell activation, cytokine production, eosinophil recruitment and activation, and mast cell migration. Glucocorticoids, cromolyn sodium, and other cromolyn-related drugs all inhibit the release of mediators from mast cells and eosinophils. Cromolyn and related drugs also inhibit eosinophil chemotaxis induced by cytokines and other mediators. Leukotriene inhibitors either block leukotriene receptors or inhibit leukotriene synthesis. IgE = immunoglobulin E.

oxygen therapy, and antibiotics can be used to treat acute exacerbations caused by bacterial infections.

ANTI-INFLAMMATORY DRUGS

Glucocorticoids

Glucocorticoids (corticosteroids) are effective in the treatment of a wide variety of inflammatory and other diseases. The discussion here focuses on the use of glucocorticoids for **asthma**, **allergic rhinitis**, and **COPD**. Chapter 33 provides a detailed description of their properties and use.

The recognition that asthma is primarily an inflammatory disease has increased the role of glucocorticoids in asthma therapy. For persons with moderate to severe asthma, glucocorticoids have become the cornerstone of therapy, and some patients with mild asthma may derive significant benefit from their use as well. Although glucocorticoids are the most efficacious anti-inflammatory drugs available for the treatment of both asthma and allergic rhinitis (see Table 27–1), they have the potential to cause a number of adverse effects if given systemically. The incidence of adverse effects is markedly reduced when these drugs are given by inhalation, so this route of administration is employed whenever possible. Systemic administration is usually reserved for the

TABLE 27–1. **Relative Efficacy of Anti-inflammatory Drugs, Bronchodilators, and Miscellaneous Agents in the Management of Respiratory Tract Disorders***

Drug	Asthma	COPD	Allergic Rhinitis	Viral Rhinitis
Anti-inflammatory Drugs				
Glucocorticoids	++++	0 to ++	++++	0
Mast cell stabilizers	+++	0 to ++	+++	0
Leukotriene inhibitors	+++	0 to +	Unknown	0
Bronchodilators				
Selective β₂-adrenoceptor agonists	++++	++	0	0
Other bronchodilators				
– Ipratropium	+	+++	++	++
– Theophylline	++ to +++	++ to +++	0	0
Miscellaneous Agents				
Analgesics	0	0	0	+++
Antihistamines	0 to ++	0	++++	+
Decongestants	0 to ++	0 to ++	+++	+++

*Ratings range from 0 (not efficacious) to ++++ (highly efficacious).
COPD = chronic obstructive pulmonary disease (e.g., emphysema).

treatment of severe asthma or for short-term treatment of severe allergic rhinitis.

Among the glucocorticoids available as metered-dose inhalers are **beclomethasone**, **budesonide**, **fluticasone**, and **triamcinolone**. Beclomethasone and triamcinolone are usually administered three or four times a day, whereas fluticasone and budesonide need to be administered only twice a day. The proper use of metered-dose inhalers requires considerable skill and the utilization of a spacer device between the mouth and the inhaler. The spacer decreases the amount of drug that is deposited in the mouth and upper airway and facilitates the delivery of the drug to the bronchioles.

As with other anti-inflammatory drugs, glucocorticoids are primarily used on a long-term basis to prevent asthmatic attacks, rather than to treat acute bronchospasm. The maximal response to glucocorticoids usually requires treatment for up to 8 weeks. Glucocorticoids can reduce the number and severity of symptoms and decrease the need for β₂-adrenoceptor agonists and other bronchodilators.

Adverse effects associated with inhaled glucocorticoids are usually mild. Excessive deposition of the drugs in the mouth and upper airway can lead to oral candidiasis (thrush). There has been some concern about the potential for glucocorticoids to suppress growth in children. This problem is difficult to evaluate because asthmatic children may have growth disturbances related to their disease. A meta-analysis of 21 studies, however, concluded that inhaled beclomethasone does not cause growth impairment. Another study showed that 95% of children who received inhaled budesonide for an average of 9 years reached their target adult height despite initial growth retardation.

Mast Cell Stabilizers

Cromolyn Sodium

CHEMISTRY AND MECHANISMS. Cromolyn sodium and related drugs are nonsteroidal compounds that stabilize the plasma membranes of mast cells and eosinophils and thereby prevent degranulation and release of histamine, leukotrienes, and other substances that cause airway inflammation (see Fig. 27–1). Hence, these drugs are often called **mast cell stabilizers**. Inhibition of mediator release by cromolyn and related drugs is thought to result from **blockade of calcium influx** into mast cells. Cromolyn and related drugs do not interfere with the binding of immunoglobulin E (IgE) to mast cells or with the binding of antigen to IgE. Their beneficial effects in asthma and other conditions are largely prophylactic.

PHARMACOKINETICS. Cromolyn and other mast cell stabilizers are rather insoluble in body fluids, and minimal systemic absorption occurs after oral administration or inhalation of these drugs. In fact, the oral bioavailability of cromolyn is about 1%. When cromolyn is administered by inhalation, its major effect is exerted on the respiratory tract and very little is absorbed into the circulation. Most of the drug is swallowed following inhalation, and about 98% is excreted in the feces.

INDICATIONS. Cromolyn is administered by inhalation to treat **asthma** or **allergic rhinitis** and is available in an ophthalmic solution to treat **vernal (seasonal) conjunctivitis**. Cromolyn and related compounds are primarily used for the long-term prophylaxis of asthmatic bronchoconstriction and allergic reactions, and they have no role in the treatment of acute bronchospasm. For perennial asthma, the drug is usually given several times a day at regular intervals until symptoms resolve. Improvement can require several weeks, and then the dosage can be reduced to the lowest effective level. For exercise-induced asthma, cromolyn is inhaled 1 hour or less before the anticipated exercise. For allergic rhinitis or vernal conjunctivitis, cromolyn is administered several times a day at regular intervals.

Cromolyn is administered orally before meals and at bedtime to treat **systemic mastocytosis**, a rare condition characterized by infiltration of the liver, spleen, lymph nodes, and gastrointestinal tract with mast cells. A similar dosage schedule has been used to treat **ulcerative colitis** and **food allergy**.

ADVERSE EFFECTS. Cromolyn and other mast cell stabilizers are remarkably nontoxic, partly because of their low solubility and systemic absorption. In some patients, however, inhaled cromolyn can irritate the throat and cause cough and bronchospasm. Administration of a β_2-adrenoceptor agonist can usually prevent or relieve this reaction. Nasal and ocular preparations can cause localized pain and irritation, but these effects are usually mild and transient. Cromolyn does not interact significantly with other drugs.

Lodoxamide and Nedocromil

Lodoxamide is formulated as an ophthalmic solution to treat ocular allergies, including **vernal keratitis** and **vernal conjunctivitis**. It can cause ocular discomfort but is generally well tolerated.

Nedocromil has properties that are similar to those of cromolyn, but it is only available as an aerosol for the prevention of bronchoconstriction in patients with **asthma**. It is initially administered as two inhalations four times a day, but the frequency of doses can be reduced in persons whose asthma is well controlled.

Leukotriene Inhibitors

Leukotrienes (*leuko* from leukocytes; *trienes* from three conjugated double bonds) are a group of arachidonic acid metabolites formed via the **5-lipoxygenase pathway** in mast cells and various types of leukocytes, as shown in Figure 27–2. **Cysteinyl leukotrienes C_4, D_4, and E_4** activate the **type 1 cysteinyl leukotriene receptor** (CysLT$_1$) and thereby increase recruitment of leukocytes, stimulate mucus secretion, increase vascular permeability, increase collagen, and cause smooth muscle proliferation and contraction. These effects lead to **airway inflammation** and to **sustained bronchoconstriction**. The effects of leukotrienes are mediated by activation of G protein–coupled receptors linked with G_q and G_i, which increase intracellular calcium, decrease cyclic adenosine monophosphate (cAMP), and lead to protein kinase activation and tissue responses.

Leukotriene Receptor Antagonists

MECHANISMS. Montelukast and zafirlukast have a structure that resembles that of the **cysteinyl leukotrienes**, and they compete with these substances for the CysLT$_1$ receptor. These drugs inhibit both the early and the late phases of bronchoconstriction induced by antigen challenge. However, they do not block the effects of leukotriene B_4, which appear to be important in severe asthma and asthma exacerbations.

PHARMACOKINETICS. Montelukast and zafirlukast are administered orally and are well absorbed from the gut. Montelukast is taken as a single daily dose in the evening and is available in dosage forms for treating adults and pediatric patients as young as 6 months old. Zafirlukast is indicated for patients aged 5 years and older and is given twice daily 1 to 2 hours before meals because food retards its absorption. These drugs are highly bound to plasma proteins (>99%) and are extensively metabolized by hepatic cytochrome P450 enzymes.

EFFECTS AND INDICATIONS. Montelukast and zafirlukast have been shown to improve pulmonary function, control symptoms, reduce the need for short-acting rescue β_2-agonists, decrease asthma exacerbations, and improve overall quality of life. Although inhaled glucocorticoids are more potent than leukotriene antagonists and are generally preferred for initial therapy, antileukotriene agents can be used in persons who are unable or unwilling to take glucocorticoids. Leukotriene receptor antagonists offer the advantages of convenient oral administration and minimal side effects, and they often benefit asthmatic patients not adequately controlled by inhaled steroids alone. They are probably not as effective as long-acting β_2-agonists as add-on therapy to glucocorticoids, but they may be safer (see below).

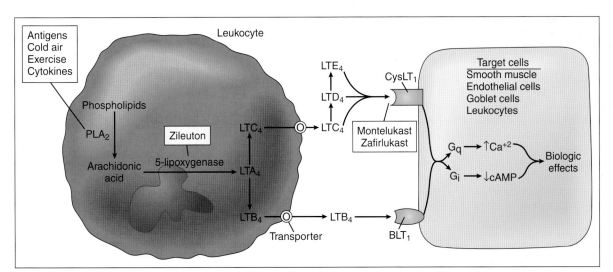

Figure 27-2. Synthesis and effects of leukotrienes and sites of drug action. Asthmatic stimuli (antigens, cold air, exercise, cytokines, and others) activate phospholipase A_2 (PLA$_2$), leading to formation of leukotriene A_4 (LTA$_4$) by 5-lipoxygenase, which is inhibited by zileuton. LTA$_4$ is converted to leukotriene B_4, which activates B leukotriene receptors, such as BLT$_1$. LTA$_4$ is also converted to the cysteinyl leukotrienes C_4, D_4, and E_4, which activate cysteinyl leukotriene receptors, such as CysLT$_1$. These receptors are blocked by montelukast and zafirlukast. Leukotriene receptors are coupled with G_q and G_i, leading to increased intracellular calcium, decreased cAMP, activation of protein kinases, and biologic effects.

Antileukotriene drugs are effective in persons with **allergic asthma**, including **aspirin-sensitive asthma**, and they may be used to prevent **exercised-induced asthma** when taken at least 2 hours before the precipitating event. The beneficial effects of these drugs are cumulative, and maximal effectiveness may require several weeks to months of therapy. Although they are not indicated for the treatment of acute bronchospasm, they do enhance the bronchodilating effect of β_2-agonists. In general, antileukotriene agents benefit children more than adults, and younger children more than older children.

ADVERSE EFFECTS AND INTERACTIONS. Leukotriene antagonists are relatively free of serious adverse effects, but hypersensitivity reactions and other adverse effects may occur in a small percentage of patients. Rare cases of liver injury have been reported, and a few cases of liver failure have occurred. Rarely, allergic granulomatous vasculitis (Churg-Strauss syndrome), a condition often treated with corticosteroids, has developed in patients being withdrawn from glucocorticoid therapy while substituting a leukotriene antagonist. In such cases, glucocorticoids should be withdrawn gradually and patients closely monitored.

Zafirlukast inhibits CYP2C9 and CYP3A4 and may interfere with the metabolism of phenytoin and warfarin (metabolized by CYP2C9) and of felodipine, lovastatin, and triazolam (metabolized by CYP3A4). Montelukast does not inhibit these isozymes or exhibit significant drug interactions, and its use may be preferred in patients receiving concomitant drug therapy.

Zileuton

EFFECTS AND INDICATIONS. Leukotriene synthesis increases during an asthmatic attack; this can be prevented by zileuton, which inhibits **5-lipoxygenase** and blocks the formation of all leukotrienes, including LTB_4. Because the $CysLT_1$ receptor antagonists do not block the leukocyte chemoattractant and other effects of LTB_4, zileuton might be more effective in severe cases of asthma where these effects may be particularly important.

Zileuton is indicated for the prophylaxis and treatment of asthma in adults and children 12 years of age and older. The immediate-release formulation should be taken orally four times a day, but a sustained-release preparation is now available for twice-daily administration. Zileuton undergoes some first-pass hepatic inactivation and is almost entirely eliminated as the glucuronide metabolite with a half-life of about 2 hours.

ADVERSE EFFECTS AND INTERACTIONS. Mild and transient adverse reactions to zileuton use include a flulike syndrome, headache, drowsiness, and dyspepsia. Zileuton may elevate **hepatic enzyme levels**, so patients taking the drug should be monitored for signs of hepatitis. Patients with transaminase levels greater than three times the upper limit of normal should discontinue zileuton, and it should be used cautiously in patients who consume substantial quantities of alcohol.

Zileuton **inhibits CYP1A2 and CYP3A4**, and it may elevate plasma concentrations of theophylline and warfarin.

Doses of these drugs may need to be reduced in individuals taking zileuton.

BRONCHODILATORS

The bronchodilators include selective β_2-adrenoceptor agonists, muscarinic receptor antagonists, and theophylline. All of these drugs relax bronchial smooth muscle and prevent or relieve bronchospasm. The β_2-agonists are the only type of bronchodilator used to counteract acute asthmatic attacks. Muscarinic antagonists, which are less useful in asthma, are primarily used to treat patients with COPD. Theophylline can be administered on a long-term basis to prevent bronchoconstriction in patients with either asthma or emphysema.

β_2-Adrenoceptor Agonists

The selective β_2-adrenoceptor agonists are the primary bronchodilators used in the treatment of **asthma.** By activating β_2-receptors, these drugs increase cAMP concentrations in smooth muscle and thereby cause the muscle to relax (Fig. 27–3; see also Fig. 11–3). The selective β_2-agonists relax bronchial smooth muscle without producing as much

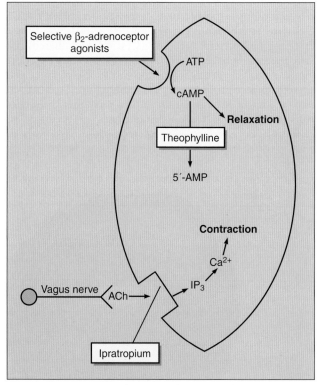

Figure 27-3. Mechanisms of action of bronchodilators. Selective β_2-adrenoceptor agonists activate β_2-receptors. This increases cAMP concentrations in smooth muscle and causes the muscle to relax. Theophylline inhibits phosphodiesterase isozymes and blocks the degradation of cAMP to 5′-AMP. Ipratropium and tiotropium block the stimulation of muscarinic receptors by acetylcholine (ACh) released from vagus nerves and thereby attenuate reflex bronchoconstriction. The effect of ACh is mediated by IP_3-induced calcium release and leads to smooth muscle contraction. ATP = adenosine triphosphate; IP_3 = inositol triphosphate.

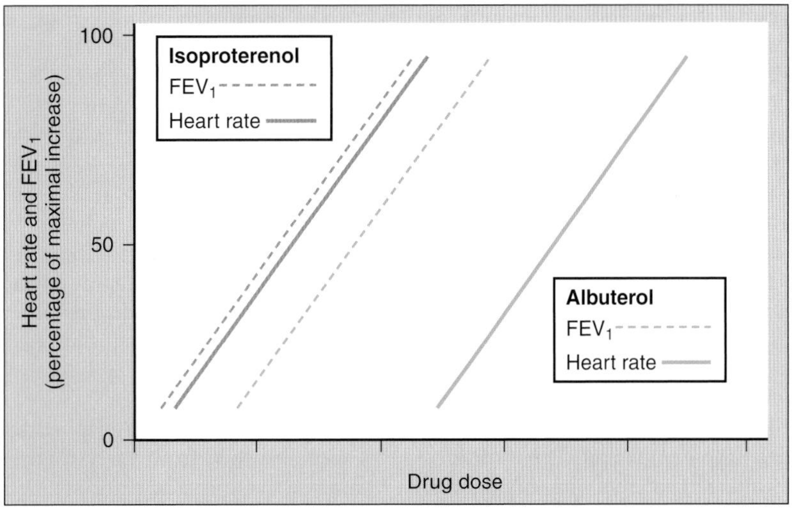

Figure 27-4. Effects of isoproterenol and albuterol on heart rate and pulmonary function in asthmatic patients. Albuterol, a selective β_2-adrenoceptor agonist, increases the forced expiratory volume in 1 second (FEV$_1$) at doses that produce relatively little cardiac stimulation. Isoproterenol, a nonselective β_1- and β_2-adrenoceptor agonist, has equipotent effects on heart rate and FEV$_1$.

cardiac stimulation as do the nonselective β-receptor agonists (Fig. 27–4). The selectivity of β$_2$-agonists is limited, however, and higher doses can activate cardiac β$_1$-receptors and thereby increase heart rate. Furthermore, the human heart contains some β-receptors, which may comprise 10% to 50% of the total cardiac β-receptors, and even highly selective β$_2$-agonists may thereby increase heart rate and contractility.

Chapter 8 describes the pharmacologic and other properties of various types of adrenoceptor agonists, and Table 27–2 compares the properties of selective β$_2$-adrenoceptor agonists that are administered by inhalation. All β$_2$-agonists can cause tachycardia, tremor, and nervousness.

Rapid-acting β$_2$-agonists (e.g., **albuterol**, **levalbuterol**, **fenoterol**, **pirbuterol**, and **terbutaline**) are usually given by the inhalational route to prevent or treat **acute bronchospasm**. Although oral formulations of albuterol and terbutaline are available for children or adults who are unable to use a metered-dose inhaler, the oral formulations have a slower onset of action and can cause more systemic side effects.

Levalbuterol, the (R)-enantiomer of racemic albuterol, is claimed to cause less tachycardia, fewer palpitations, and fewer tremors than albuterol, but a study found no significant difference in heart rates or number of emergency department visits between racemic albuterol and levalbuterol.

Salmeterol and formoterol are longer-acting β$_2$-receptor agonists that are given twice daily by inhalation for the long-term treatment of asthma and emphysema. They are particularly useful in preventing **nocturnal asthmatic attacks**, which are sometimes life-threatening. Salmeterol and formoterol inhibit the late phase of **allergen-induced bronchoconstriction**, which usually occurs after the bronchodilating effects of shorter-acting drugs have dissipated. These drugs are not indicated for the treatment of acute bronchospasm, for which a rapid-acting β$_2$-agonist should be used.

Arformoterol, the active (R,R)-isomer of formoterol, is available as a inhalation solution for the twice-daily treatment of bronchoconstriction in patients with **chronic bronchitis** or **emphysema**. Salmeterol and formoterol are

TABLE 27-2. Pharmacologic Properties of Selected β$_2$-Adrenoceptor Agonists Administered by Inhalation

Drug	Onset of Action (Minutes)	Duration of Action (Hours)	Dosage
Albuterol	5	3–8	2 puffs every 4–6 hours
Formoterol	5	12	1 inhalation every 12 hours
Pirbuterol	5	5	2 puffs every 4–6 hours
Salmeterol	20	12	2 puffs every 12 hours
Terbutaline	5–15	3–6	2 puffs every 4–6 hours

available as single ingredients and in combination products that contain fluticasone or budesonide, respectively.

A **black-box warning** has been added to products containing long-acting β$_2$-agonists, stating that these drugs may increase the **risk of asthma-related death**. However, the two studies on which this warning is based have been criticized as having not been well controlled, and recent asthma treatment guidelines still recommend use of long-acting β$_2$-agonists in combination with glucocorticoids for persons with moderate to severe asthma not controlled by glucocorticoids alone (see Oppenheimer and Nelson, 2008).

Other Bronchodilators

Ipratropium and Tiotropium

Ipratropium and tiotropium are muscarinic receptor antagonists. Ipratropium is the isopropyl derivative of atropine, whose properties are described in Chapter 7. The addition of the isopropyl group results in a quaternary ammonium compound that is not well absorbed into the circulation. Tiotropium is a synthetic quaternary ammonium compound. Both drugs are administered by oral inhalation for pulmonary disease and produce very few systemic side effects. Ipratropium is also available as a nasal spray for rhinitis. These drugs produce their bronchodilating effects by blocking the bronchoconstricting effect of vagus (parasympathetic) nerve stimulation (see Fig. 27–3).

In patients with a **COPD** (e.g., **chronic bronchitis** and **emphysema**), the bronchodilating effect of ipratropium is slower to develop than that of a β_2-agonist, but it lasts longer. In one study, for example, investigators found that the effect of ipratropium was sustained after 12 weeks of treatment, whereas the effect of albuterol on FEV_1 appeared to diminish over a 12-week period. Other studies have demonstrated that ipratropium improves the quality of life in patients with moderate to severe COPD, reduces rhinorrhea in patients with **allergic or viral rhinitis**, and benefits infants with **acute bronchitis**.

Ipratropium is typically less effective than a β_2-agonist in asthmatic patients, but combined therapy with ipratropium and a β_2-agonist has a greater bronchodilating effect than either drug alone, and this combination is beneficial in some cases of moderate to severe asthma. Ipratropium is useful as a "rescue" therapy, in combination with other drugs, for children with acute severe asthma.

Tiotropium is the first once-daily inhaled treatment for patients with COPD. It improves lung function for a full 24 hours and is a first-line treatment for patients with mild to severe COPD. Clinical studies found that tiotropium increased FEV_1 by 0.28 to 0.31 L (28% to 31%) after 1 week of therapy, and this improvement was maintained throughout the 6-month study period. As with ipratropium, the most common adverse effect of tiotropium is dry mouth.

Theophylline

CHEMISTRY, MECHANISMS, AND EFFECTS. As with caffeine, theophylline is a **methylxanthine drug**. These drugs produce varying degrees of central nervous system (CNS) stimulation, bronchodilation, and diuresis. In comparison with caffeine, theophylline produces less CNS stimulation and more bronchodilation.

Theophylline has several actions at the cellular level, including inhibition of phosphodiesterase (PDE) isozymes, antagonism of adenosine receptors, inhibition of calcium influx, and enhancement of catecholamine secretion. All of these effects are purported to contribute to the drug's beneficial bronchodilating effects in patients with asthma, yet each has also been subject to criticism. Recently, theophylline has also been found to elicit several anti-inflammatory and immunosuppressant effects that may contribute to its efficacy in asthma. It seems likely that theophylline exerts its beneficial effects through multiple actions and interactions involving numerous types of cells and receptors.

Theophylline is a nonspecific inhibitor of PDE isozymes found in bronchial smooth muscle and inflammatory cells, and it has been proposed that theophylline produces its bronchodilating effect by **inhibiting PDE isozymes** that catalyze the degradation of cAMP (see Fig. 27–3). Investigational drugs that selectively inhibit types III and IV PDE also relax human bronchial smooth muscle, and most authorities believe that inhibition of PDE remains a viable mechanism for the bronchodilating effect of theophylline.

Theophylline also exerts anti-inflammatory and other effects relevant to the treatment of asthma. Some of these actions are mediated by PDE inhibition, whereas others are caused by inhibition of T lymphocyte proliferation and cytokine production. In patients with asthma, theophylline reduces the number of eosinophils, lymphocytes, and monocytes that infiltrate the airway epithelium. It also impairs the release of **cationic basic protein** and **eosinophil-derived neurotoxin**, which are substances that contribute to asthma by damaging the epithelial lining of bronchioles.

PHARMACOKINETICS. After oral administration, theophylline is well absorbed from the gut and has relatively little first-pass inactivation. The drug is widely distributed and crosses the blood-brain barrier to enter the CNS. Theophylline is converted to inactive metabolites by CYP1A2, which are primarily excreted in the urine, along with 10% of the parent drug. The half-life of theophylline is about 8 hours in adults who do not smoke. In contrast, it is about 4.5 hours in adults who smoke and in **children from 1 to 9** years of age, because these populations metabolize the drug more rapidly. **Cigarette smoke** contains compounds that induce CYP1A2 enzyme synthesis. Hence, children and persons who smoke cigarettes may require larger theophylline doses per kilogram of body weight than do nonsmoking adults.

Because of theophylline's narrow margin of safety, theophylline serum levels should be monitored, especially when therapy is initiated. Therapeutic serum levels are considered to be in the range of 5 to 15 mg/L. Higher levels are associated with a greater risk of adverse reactions. The use of theophylline has declined with the advent of safer and more efficacious bronchodilators and with the increased emphasis on anti-inflammatory drug therapy for asthma. Today, theophylline is primarily used to treat patients not controlled by other drugs alone.

INDICATIONS. Theophylline is primarily used to treat chronic obstructive lung disorders and asthma, but it is also used to treat apnea.

In patients with **COPD**, theophylline is an effective bronchodilator whose long-term use is associated with a 20% increase in FEV_1 and with improvement in minute ventilation and gas exchange. Treatment with theophylline reduces dyspnea, increases diaphragmatic contractility, improves the exercise performance and sense of well-being of patients, and reduces fatigue. Theophylline can also increase the central respiratory drive and has favorable cardiovascular effects, including a reduction in pulmonary artery pressure and vascular resistance and an increase in right and left ventricular ejection fractions. The drug's other beneficial effects include increased mucociliary clearance and reduced airway inflammation. Hence, a good rationale exists for using theophylline to treat COPD in patients whose symptoms are not controlled with optimal doses of a β_2-agonist and ipratropium or tiotropium. Theophylline is most beneficial in patients with moderate to severe COPD.

Although the use of theophylline in the management of **asthma** is declining, recent studies support a continuing role for this drug in specific situations. It is useful in controlling nocturnal asthma, and it can improve pulmonary function in patients who require large doses of glucocorticoids. Patients who have moderate to severe asthma and are already being treated with glucocorticoids and β_2-agonists may benefit from the addition of theophylline to their regimen.

Theophylline is used for the treatment of **recurrent apnea in premature infants**, though **caffeine** is often preferred for this indication. In this setting, these drugs **block adenosine** and thereby increase both the sensitivity of respiratory centers to carbon dioxide and the contractility of respiratory muscles. Theophylline has also been used to treat **obstructive sleep apnea** and periodic breathing. The drug, however, can reduce sleep quality via CNS stimulation.

ADVERSE EFFECTS. Major adverse effects of theophylline include gastrointestinal distress, CNS stimulation, and cardiac stimulation.

Adverse gastrointestinal effects (e.g., abdominal pain, nausea, and vomiting) may be minimized by taking the drug with food or antacids or with a full glass of water or milk.

CNS effects include headache, anxiety, restlessness, insomnia, dizziness, and seizures. A reduction in dosage will often eliminate these problems.

Theophylline can affect the cardiovascular system, causing hypotension, bradycardia, extra systoles, premature ventricular contractions, and tachycardia. These events are usually mild and transient, but serious reactions occasionally develop. Seizures and serious arrhythmias can occur at concentrations over 25 mg/L.

INTERACTIONS. Cimetidine and erythromycin inhibit CYP1A2 and increase theophylline plasma concentrations, but the interaction is significant only when theophylline concentrations are already in the high therapeutic range. Other drugs that increase theophylline levels include fluoroquinolone antimicrobial drugs, isoniazid, and verapamil. Careful monitoring of patients is important, because it is difficult to predict which patients will require theophylline dosage adjustments when other drugs are given concurrently.

MANAGEMENT OF ASTHMA

The management of asthma is based on the severity and frequency of asthmatic episodes, as determined by the number of days and nights with symptoms per week, and by the FEV_1 expressed as a percentage of the predicted normal FEV_1. Based on these criteria, asthma can be classified as mild intermittent or as mild, moderate, or severe persistent asthma. The pharmacologic therapy for asthma falls into two categories. Some medications are administered daily to suppress airway inflammation and prevent bronchospasm, whereas others are used as rescue therapy to counteract bronchospasm when acute exacerbations occur.

For **mild, intermittent asthma**, no daily medications are required and acute asthma episodes are treated with a short-acting β_2-agonist. For mild, persistent asthma, a low dose of an inhaled corticosteroid administered with a nebulizer or a metered-dose inhaler is the preferred therapy for preventing asthma episodes. Alternatives include cromolyn compounds, antileukotriene drugs, or a sustained-release theophylline preparation.

The preferred treatment to prevent acute episodes in persons with **moderate, persistent asthma** is a low-dose or medium-dose inhaled corticosteroid. A long-acting β_2-agonist can be added if a corticosteroid alone is not adequate. Alternatively, a leukotriene antagonist or theophylline can be added to low to medium doses of an inhaled corticosteroid. Long-term preventive therapy for severe, persistent asthma is usually a medium dose of an inhaled corticosteroid plus a long-acting β_2-agonist.

Persons 12 years of age and older with moderate to severe allergic asthma may benefit from injections of an immunoglobulin E (IgE) antagonist known as **omalizumab**, which is given subcutaneously every 2 to 4 weeks in combination with inhaled corticosteroid therapy. Omalizumab, however, can cause various allergic reactions itself, including anaphylaxis.

Mild acute exacerbations of asthma are usually managed with one or two treatments of an inhaled β_2-agonist (e.g., albuterol or levalbuterol), given 4 to 6 hours apart. Medical attention is required if the patient does not respond to these treatments and may consist of multiple treatments of albuterol alone or in combination with ipratropium, oxygen, and possibly fluid replacement. In addition, short-course "burst" treatments of systemic corticosteroids (e.g., prednisone, prednisolone, or intravenous methylprednisolone) may be initiated for these episodes. Antibiotics should also be prescribed for documented bacterial infections. Severe attacks that do not respond to normal therapy, termed *status asthmaticus*, are more aggressively treated with oxygen, systemic steroids, and back-to-back or continuous β_2-agonist treatments.

ANTITUSSIVES

Coughing usually serves a beneficial purpose by expelling irritating substances such as dust, pollen, and accumulated fluids and inflammatory cells from the upper airways. An incessant nonproductive cough, however, can lead to loss of sleep, rib fractures, pneumothorax, rupture of surgical wounds, or even syncope. Antitussive drugs are frequently used to **suppress coughing**, but the first-line therapy consists of controlling the infection, allergy, or other condition responsible for the cough.

The **cough reflex** is initiated by stimulation of sensory receptors on afferent nerve endings located between mucosal cells of the pharynx, larynx, and larger airways. The impulses ascend via the vagus nerve to the dorsal medulla. The efferent limb of the reflex consists of somatic nerves innervating the larynx and thoracoabdominal muscles. Some antitussives act locally to anesthetize the afferent nerves that initiate the cough reflex, whereas others act by inhibiting the cough center in the medulla.

The locally acting antitussives include **menthol and related drugs** that are administered as throat sprays or lozenges. The centrally acting antitussives consist of **opioids**, and these are usually administered orally. Almost all of the opioid agonist drugs will exert an antitussive effect, but opioids that have a higher ratio of antitussive effects to analgesic and euphoric effects are usually used for this purpose. These include **dextromethorphan**, **codeine**, and **hydrocodone**.

Dextromethorphan is the D-isomer of a potent opioid agonist. Although dextromethorphan is an effective antitussive drug, it will not cause drowsiness, euphoria, analgesia, or other CNS effects, except at extremely high doses. For these reasons, it is available in many nonprescription products for cough and other respiratory tract conditions, and it is the most widely used opioid antitussive drug.

Codeine and hydrocodone are moderate opioid agonists whose analgesic effects are described in Chapter 23. These drugs exhibit excellent antitussive activity at doses that produce relatively little CNS depression or euphoria. They are available in a number of liquid cough preparations that may also include guaifenesin, antihistamines, and decongestants.

EXPECTORANTS

An expectorant is a drug that facilitates the coughing up of mucus and other material from the lungs. **Guaifenesin** is an oral nonprescription drug that has been used for this purpose for many years. It is purported to reduce the adhesiveness and surface tension of respiratory tract secretions and thereby facilitate their expectoration, but the exact mechanism by which the drug produces this effect is unknown. Through its expectorant effect, guaifenesin can also reduce the frequency of coughing. The drug may be useful in patients with **thick, tenacious respiratory tract secretions**; in patients with **dry, nonproductive coughing**; and in patients with **sinusitis** to increase airway hydration.

MANAGEMENT OF RHINITIS

Allergic Rhinitis

The effective management of allergic rhinitis includes environmental control of allergens, prophylactic use of antiinflammatory medications, and control of symptoms with antihistamine drugs and decongestants. Most patients with mild symptoms can be adequately treated with an antihistamine drug alone, but patients with moderate to severe rhinitis usually benefit from anti-inflammatory therapy.

Antihistamines are usually employed during peak seasonal exposure to pollens and mold spores. A long-acting, nonsedating drug such as **cetirizine, loratadine,** or **fexofenadine** is suitable for most patients (see Chapter 26). Diphenhydramine is highly effective but causes sedation and is best reserved for relief of nocturnal symptoms.

Glucocorticoids are the most efficacious anti-inflammatory drugs for allergic rhinitis (see Table 27–1), and inhalational formulations of **budesonide, fluticasone, ciclesonide,** and other glucocorticoids are available for this purpose. These products are convenient and effective, and they cause very few adverse reactions. **Cromolyn sodium** is slightly less effective but can be used in patients who do not tolerate glucocorticoids.

If anti-inflammatory drugs and antihistamines do not control nasal congestion, a decongestant drug such as **pseudoephedrine** (see Chapter 8) can also be added to the regimen. Decongestants, however, are often not needed if patients begin taking anti-inflammatory drugs before the onset of seasonal allergies and if they add an antihistamine drug at the first sign of allergic symptoms.

Ipratropium is used occasionally for the treatment of rhinorrhea associated with rhinitis. A nasal spray formulation is available for this purpose, but it does not relieve nasal itching or congestion.

Ocular inflammation, discomfort, and pruritus can be particularly troublesome aspects of seasonal allergies. **Cromolyn** and **lodoxamide** are available in topical ocular formulations that are effective in preventing symptoms of allergic conjunctivitis. Mild ocular symptoms can be treated with topical decongestants and oral or topical antihistamines, such as azelastine and olopatadine. More severe ocular symptoms may be controlled with a topical nonsteroidal anti-inflammatory drug such as **ketorolac** (see Chapter 30). Topical corticosteroids are not usually used for allergic conjunctivitis, because their long-term use is associated with adverse effects, such as increased intraocular pressure and cataracts.

Viral Rhinitis

Viral rhinitis (the common cold) is a self-limiting condition that is best treated conservatively. Analgesics such as **acetaminophen** or **ibuprofen** (see Chapter 30) can be used to relieve the aches and discomfort associated with viral rhinitis. Decongestants such as **pseudoephedrine** (see Chapter 8) can be used to relieve nasal congestion, and **ipratropium** is approved for the treatment of rhinorrhea in persons with viral or allergic rhinitis. Some clinicians advocate short-term use (≤10 days) of herbal products containing *Echinacea*, which stimulates the immune system and may shorten the duration and severity of viral rhinitis. Long-term use of *Echinacea* may suppress the immune system, however.

SUMMARY OF IMPORTANT POINTS

■ Drugs used in the management of asthma are classified as anti-inflammatory agents or bronchodilators, but some drugs exhibit both anti-inflammatory and bronchodilating action.

■ Glucocorticoids, the most efficacious anti-inflammatory drugs, are usually given by inhalation on a long-term basis to prevent asthmatic attacks. Orally or parenterally administered glucocorticoids are used for the management of chronic severe asthma or acute exacerbations of asthma.

■ Cromolyn sodium and related drugs are used prophylactically in the management of mild to moderate asthma, allergic rhinitis, and related disorders. They have few adverse effects.

■ Leukotriene inhibitors have anti-inflammatory and bronchodilating activity and offer convenient oral therapy for the prevention of asthmatic attacks. Montelukast and zafirlukast are leukotriene receptor antagonists, and zileuton is a leukotriene synthesis inhibitor.

■ Short-acting β_2-adrenoceptor agonists are the most efficacious bronchodilators for the treatment of acute bronchospasm. Examples are albuterol, pirbuterol, and terbutaline. Long-acting β_2-agonists, salmeterol and formoterol, are used to prevent bronchospasm.

■ Ipratropium and tiotropium are muscarinic receptor antagonists that are primarily used to treat COPD.

■ Theophylline has anti-inflammatory and bronchodilating activity and is useful for the treatment of asthma and COPD. The metabolism of theophylline is affected by smoking and by the concurrent administration of drugs that inhibit cytochrome P450. Children metabolize theophylline more rapidly than do adults.

■ Theophylline levels should be monitored to ensure efficacy and prevent toxicity. Adverse effects include gastrointestinal, central nervous system, and cardiac toxicity.

■ Antitussives are used to suppress dry, nonproductive coughing. Dextromethorphan is available without a prescription, whereas codeine and hydrocodone are contained in many prescription cough preparations.

■ Allergic rhinitis is managed with anti-inflammatory drugs (glucocorticoids and cromolyn compounds), antihistamines, and decongestants.

Review Questions

1. A 3-year-old boy with asthma is taking an antileukotriene drug. Which property is correctly associated with this drug?
   (A) blocks receptors for leukotrienes B_4, C_4, D_4, and E_4
   (B) inhibits cytochrome P450 enzymes
   (C) administered once daily in the evening
   (D) inhibits formation of leukotriene A_4
   (E) excreted unchanged in the urine

2. A 64-year-old woman with emphysema has been placed on a drug that inhibits degradation of cAMP. Which beneficial effect may result from taking this drug?
   (A) increased pulmonary artery pressure
   (B) increased diaphragmatic contractility
   (C) reduced minute ventilation and gas exchange
   (D) decreased central respiratory drive
   (E) decreased mucociliary activity

3. A woman with allergic conjunctivitis uses a drug that prevents the release of chemical mediators from mast cells. Which mechanism is responsible for this pharmacologic effect?
   (A) activation of β_2-adrenoceptors
   (B) decreased cytokine production
   (C) blockade of muscarinic receptors
   (D) inhibition of 5-lipoxygenase
   (E) blockade of calcium influx

4. A 15-year-old girl with asthma precipitated by seasonal pollens is receiving twice-monthly injections of a monoclonal antibody. Which mediator of asthma is antagonized by this drug?
   (A) immunoglobulin E
   (B) leukotriene C_4
   (C) major basic protein
   (D) histamine
   (E) interleukin-2

5. A man being treated for severe asthma experiences an episode of life-threatening tachycardia requiring emergency treatment. Which drug is most likely responsible for this adverse effect?
   (A) budesonide
   (B) ipratropium
   (C) formoterol
   (D) cromolyn
   (E) montelukast

Answers and Explanations

1. **The correct answer is C:** administered once daily in the evening. Montelukast is the only antileukotriene drug approved for use in children under 5 years of age. It is taken as a single daily dose in the evening. It blocks receptors for leukotrienes C_4, D_4, and E_4, but not for leukotriene B_4 (Option A). It does not inhibit cytochrome P450 enzymes (Option B), and it does not inhibit leukotriene synthesis (Option D). Montelukast is not excreted unchanged (Option E) but is extensively metabolized before excretion.

2. **The correct answer is B:** increased diaphragmatic contractility. The woman was most likely placed on theophylline, which produces a number of benefits in patients with COPD, including increased diaphragmatic contractility. Theophylline decreases rather than increases pulmonary artery pressure (Option A), and it increases rather than reduces minute volume and gas exchange (Option C). It also increases rather than decreases central respiratory drive (Option D), and it increases rather than decreases mucociliary clearance (Option E).

3. **The correct answer is E:** blockade of calcium influx. The patient is most likely using an ocular solution of lodoxamide, a drug that is related to cromolyn and acts by blocking calcium influx into mast cells and thereby preventing degranulation and release of histamine and other allergy mediators. Lodoxamide does not activate β_2-adrenoceptors (Option A), decrease cytokine production (Option B), block muscarinic receptors (Option C), or inhibit 5-lipoxygenase (Option D).

4. **The correct answer is A:** immunoglobulin E. The patient is most likely taking omalizumab, a monoclonal antibody that inactivates immunoglobulin-E and thereby prevents allergic asthma attacks. Antibodies to leukotriene C_4 (Option B), major basic protein or histamine (Options C and D), or interleukin-2 (Option E) are not used in treating asthma.

5. The answer is C: formoterol. Formoterol is a long-acting β_2-agonist that may cause tachycardia and may increase mortality in asthmatic patients. Although ipratropium (Option B) may occasionally cause tachycardia, the drug is poorly absorbed after inhalation and is less likely to cause severe tachycardia than are β_2-agonists. Budesonide, cromolyn, and montelukast (Options A, D, and E) are even less likely to cause tachycardia.

SELECTED READINGS

Bjermer, L. Time for a paradigm shift in asthma treatment: from relieving bronchospasm to controlling systemic inflammation. J Allergy Clin Immunol 120:1269–1275, 2007.

Fox, H. Anti-IgE in severe persistent allergic asthma. Respirology 12: S22–S28, 2007.

Oppenheimer, J., and H.S. Nelson. Safety of long-acting beta-agonists in asthma: a review. Curr Opin Pulm Med 14:64–69, 2008.

Prenner, B.M. Role of long-acting beta$_2$-adrenergic agonists in asthma management based on updated asthma guidelines. Curr Opin Pulm Med 14:57–63, 2008.

CHAPTER 28

Drugs for Gastrointestinal Tract Disorders

CLASSIFICATION OF DRUGS FOR GASTROINTESTINAL TRACT DISORDERS

Drugs for Peptic Ulcer Disease
Histamine H$_2$ Receptor Antagonists
- Famotidine (PEPCID)[a]

Proton Pump Inhibitors
- Omeprazole (PRILOSEC)[b]

Gastric Antacids
- Aluminum and Magnesium Hydroxides
- Calcium Carbonate

Cytoprotective Drugs
- Misoprostol (CYTOTEC)
- Sucralfate

Drugs for Inflammatory Bowel Diseases
- Mesalamine (ASACOL)
- Infliximab (REMICADE)
- Hydrocortisone

Prokinetic Drugs
- Metoclopramide (REGLAN)

Drugs for Constipation
- Bisacodyl (DULCOLAX)
- Magnesium Oxide and Sodium Phosphate

- Psyllium (METAMUCIL)
- Docusate (Colace, SURFAK)
- Lubiprostone (AMITIZA)

Antidiarrheal Agents
- Loperamide (IMODIUM)
- Diphenoxylate (LOMOTIL)
- Polycarbophil
- Alosetron (LOTRONEX)

Antiemetic Agents
Serotonin 5-HT$_3$ Receptor Antagonists
- Ondansetron (ZOFRAN)[c]

Neurokinin-1 (NK$_1$) Receptor Antagonists
- Aprepitant (EMEND)

Other Agents
- Meclizine (ANTIVERT)[d]
- Dronabinol (MARINOL)
- Dexamethasone (DECADRON)

[a]Also cimetidine (TAGAMET), ranitidine (ZANTAC), and nizatidine (AXID).
[b]Also rabeprazole (ACIPHEX), pantoprazole (PROTONIX), and esomeprazole (NEXIUM).
[c]Also granisetron (KYTRIL), palonosetron (ALOXI), and dolasetron (ANZEMET).
[d]Also promethazine (PHENERGAN) and dimenhydrinate (DRAMAMINE).

OVERVIEW

Gastrointestinal tract disorders are among the most common reasons that people seek assistance from health care providers. Many drugs are available to treat the causes and relieve the various symptoms of gastrointestinal diseases. This chapter focuses on drugs used in the management of peptic ulcer disease, inflammatory bowel diseases, gastrointestinal motility disorders, and nausea and vomiting.

DRUGS FOR PEPTIC ULCER DISEASE

Peptic ulcer disease is characterized by epigastric pain, loss of appetite, and weight loss caused by inflamed excavations (ulcers) of the mucosa and underlying tissue of the upper gastrointestinal tract. The ulcers result from damage to the mucous membrane that normally protects the esophagus, stomach, and duodenum from gastric acid and pepsin. This damage is often caused by *Helicobacter pylori* infection, but nonsteroidal anti-inflammatory drugs and other factors may cause or contribute to peptic ulcers.

In Western countries, the number of persons who harbor *H. pylori* increases from under 5% at birth to about 20% at the age of 45 years. Only a small proportion of persons harboring this bacterial organism, however, will develop peptic ulcer disease. Those at greatest risk include individuals who smoke, ingest excessive amounts of alcohol or nonsteroidal anti-inflammatory drugs (NSAIDs), are elderly, or have gastrointestinal ischemia. Prolonged use of glucocorticoids can also be a risk factor for peptic ulcer disease.

H. pylori are found in the gastrointestinal tract of almost all patients with **duodenal ulcers** and about 80% of patients with **gastric ulcers**. *H. pylori*–induced gastritis is believed to precede the development of peptic ulcers in most persons. The organism attaches to epithelial cells and releases enzymes that damage mucosal cells and cause inflammation and tissue destruction. Eradication of *H. pylori* heals most peptic ulcers and significantly reduces the recurrence rate for gastric and duodenal ulcers.

The agents used to treat peptic ulcer disease include drugs that eliminate *H. pylori*, drugs that reduce gastric acidity, and drugs that exert a cytoprotective effect on the gastrointestinal mucosa.

Drugs That Reduce Gastric Acidity

The physiology of gastric acid secretion and sites of drug action are illustrated in Figure 28–1.

The principal physiologic stimulants of gastric acid secretion are **gastrin**, **acetylcholine**, and **histamine**. Gastrin is a hormone secreted by G cells in the gastric antrum, whereas acetylcholine is released from vagus nerve terminals. Gastrin and acetylcholine directly stimulate acid secretion by parietal cells, and they also stimulate the release of histamine from paracrine (enterochromaffin-like) cells. Histamine stimulates H_2 receptors located on parietal cells and provokes acid secretion via cyclic adenosine monophosphate (cAMP) stimulation of the proton pump (H^+,K^+-ATPase).

The vagus nerve mediates the cephalic phase of gastric acid secretion evoked by the smell, taste, and thought of food. Gastrin mediates the gastric phase of acid secretion evoked by the presence of food in the stomach. Histamine contributes to the cephalic and gastric phases of acid secretion, and it also mediates basal acid secretion in the fasting state.

The level of gastric acidity can be reduced either by neutralizing gastric acid with antacids or by inhibiting gastric acid secretion with a histamine H_2 receptor antagonist or a proton pump inhibitor.

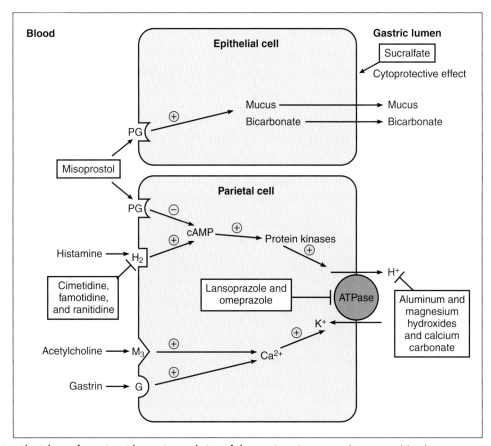

Figure 28–1. Physiology of gastric acid secretion and sites of drug action. Gastric acid is secreted by the proton pump (H^+,K^+-ATPase) located in the luminal membrane of parietal cells. H^+,K^+-ATPase is stimulated by histamine, acetylcholine, and gastrin, and it is irreversibly blocked by the proton pump inhibitors (lansoprazole and omeprazole). The effect of histamine is blocked by H_2 receptor antagonists (cimetidine, famotidine, and ranitidine). Prostaglandins (e.g., misoprostol) inhibit gastric acid secretion and stimulate secretion of mucus and bicarbonate by epithelial cells. Sucralfate binds to proteins of the ulcer crater and exerts a cytoprotective effect, whereas antacids (aluminum and magnesium hydroxides and calcium carbonate) neutralize acid in the gastric lumen. cAMP = cyclic adenosine monophosphate; G = gastrin receptor; H_2 = histamine H_2 receptor; M_3 = muscarinic M_3 receptor; PG = prostaglandin receptor.

Histamine H₂ Receptor Antagonists

The H_2 receptor antagonists, or **H₂ blockers**, include **cimetidine**, **famotidine**, and **ranitidine**.

CHEMISTRY, MECHANISMS, AND EFFECTS. The structure of H_2 blockers is similar to that of histamine (Fig. 28–2), and this enables the drugs to compete with histamine for binding to H_2 receptors on gastric parietal cells (see Fig. 28–1). The H_2 blockers have been shown to be potent inhibitors of both **meal-stimulated secretion** and **basal secretion** of gastric acid. When they reduce the volume and concentration of gastric acid, they produce a proportionate decrease in the production of **pepsin** because gastric acid catalyzes the conversion of inactive pepsinogen to pepsin. The H_2 blockers also reduce the secretion of **intrinsic factor**, but not enough to significantly reduce vitamin B_{12} absorption. They have no effect on gastric emptying time, esophageal sphincter pressure, or pancreatic enzyme secretion.

PHARMACOKINETICS. The H_2 blockers are well absorbed from the gut and undergo varying degrees of hepatic inactivation before being excreted in the urine. Although the half-life of most H_2 blockers is only 2 to 3 hours, their duration of action is considerably longer (Table 28–1), and these drugs are usually administered once or twice daily.

INDICATIONS

The H_2 blockers are used to treat conditions associated with excessive acid production, including dyspepsia, peptic ulcer disease, and gastroesophageal reflux disease (GERD). An H_2 blocker is also occasionally used in combination with an H_1 blocker for the treatment of **allergic reactions** that do not respond when an H_1 blocker is used alone.

Dyspepsia, or **heartburn**, is characterized by epigastric discomfort following meals. It is often associated with impaired digestion and excessive stomach acidity. Several low-dose formulations of H_2 receptor antagonists are available as nonprescription drugs for the prevention and treatment of dyspepsia. These formulations are most effective when taken 30 minutes before ingestion of a dyspepsia-provoking meal.

For the treatment of **peptic ulcer disease**, H_2 blockers are administered once or twice daily at doses that raise the gastric pH above 4 for at least 13 hours a day. Most authorities recommend giving a single daily dose at bedtime to ensure that acid secretion is suppressed all night. Proton pump inhibitors are usually preferred for treating peptic ulcer disease because they heal 80% to 100% of ulcers in 4 weeks, whereas H_2 blockers require 6 to 8 weeks to achieve this level of efficacy.

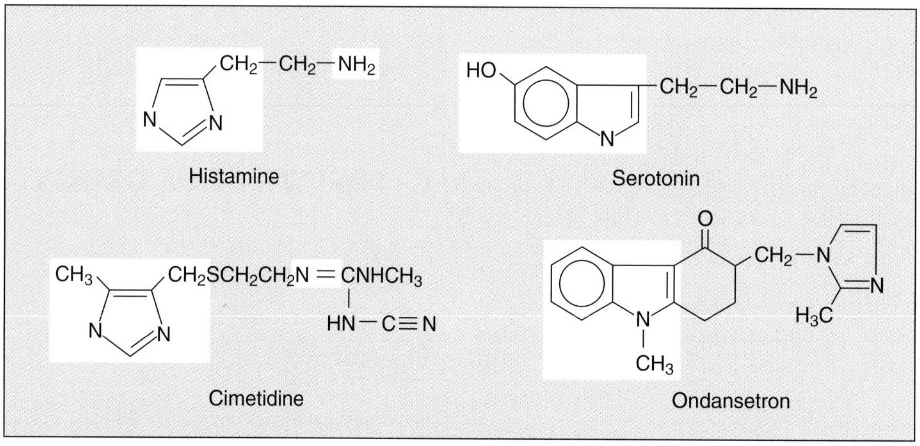

Figure 28–2. Structures of histamine and serotonin and their antagonists. Cimetidine is a histamine H_2 receptor antagonist whose structure is similar to that of histamine. Ondansetron is a serotonin 5-HT_3 receptor antagonist whose structure is similar to that of serotonin. The parts of the structures that are similar are unshaded.

TABLE 28–1. Properties of Selected Drugs for Peptic Ulcer Disease

Drug Class	Duration of Action (Hours)	Duration of Therapy (Weeks)	Recurrence Rate* (%)
Antimicrobial agents	Varies	1–2	<5
Cytoprotective drugs (sucralfate)	6–12	6–8	80–90
Gastric antacids	3–4	6–8	80–90
Histamine H_2 receptor antagonists	12	6–8	80–90
Proton pump inhibitors	24–48	2–6	80–90

*Recurrence rates are high when patients with peptic ulcer disease are not treated for *Helicobacter pylori* infection. To reduce the recurrence rate, patients should be treated concomitantly with two or three appropriate antimicrobial agents (e.g., amoxicillin, bismuth, clarithromycin, metronidazole, and tetracycline) for 2 weeks plus an inhibitor of gastric acid secretion (either a histamine H_2 receptor antagonist or a proton pump inhibitor) for 6 to 8 weeks.

ADVERSE EFFECTS AND INTERACTIONS. Cimetidine has weak **antiandrogenic activity** and can cause gynecomastia in elderly men, but this reaction is uncommon with other H_2 blockers. The fact that the H_2 blockers have proved remarkably nontoxic has led to their approval as nonprescription drugs.

Cimetidine is a well-known **inhibitor of cytochrome P450 isozymes** CYP2C9, CYP2D6, and CYP3A4. These isozymes are involved in the metabolism of numerous drugs, including alprazolam, carbamazepine, cisapride, disopyramide, felodipine, lovastatin, phenytoin, saquinavir, triazolam, and warfarin. The dosage of these drugs may need to be reduced in patients taking cimetidine. Other H_2 blockers do not inhibit P450 enzymes significantly and are preferred for patients receiving concomitant drug therapy.

Proton Pump Inhibitors

The proton pump inhibitors include esomeprazole, omeprazole, pantoprazole, and rabeprazole.

CHEMISTRY AND PHARMACOKINETICS. The proton pump inhibitors are acid-labile prodrugs that are administered orally as sustained-release, **enteric-coated** preparations. After they are absorbed from the gut, the drugs are distributed to the secretory canaliculi in the gastric mucosa and converted to **active metabolites** that bind to the proton pump. These drugs are eventually metabolized to inactive compounds in the liver, primarily by cytochrome P450 CYP2C19, and these compounds are excreted in the urine and feces. Persons with the CYP2C19 **extensive metabolizer phenotype** may require higher doses of proton pump inhibitors to cure peptic ulcer.

MECHANISMS AND EFFECTS. The active metabolites of proton pump inhibitors form a covalent disulfide link with a cysteinyl residue in the **proton pump (H^+,K^+-ATPase)** located in the luminal membrane of gastric parietal cells (see Fig. 28–1). The drugs irreversibly inhibit the proton pump and to prevent the secretion of gastric acid for an extended period of time. The drugs can produce a dose-dependent inhibition of up to 95% of gastric acid secretion, and a single dose can inhibit acid secretion for 1 to 2 days. Hence, the proton pump inhibitors are more efficacious than the H_2 blockers for most conditions (see Table 28–1).

INDICATIONS. Proton pump inhibitors (PPIs) are highly effective in treating **peptic ulcer disease**. They typically heal 80% to 100% of peptic ulcers in 4 weeks when used in combination with antibiotics, whereas H_2-blocker combinations heal 70% to 80% in 4 weeks.

PPIs are the drugs of choice for patients with **Zollinger-Ellison syndrome**, a condition characterized by severe ulcers resulting from **gastrin-secreting tumors (gastrinomas)**. Higher doses are required for treating patients with this condition than for treating patients with typical peptic ulcer disease.

PPIs are also the most effective drugs for treating **GERD**. Omeprazole is available in a nonprescription product for the treatment of **dyspepsia and heartburn**. Finally, PPIs can be used to prevent peptic ulcers and bleeding in persons receiving high-dose or long-term therapy with **NSAIDs** such as diclofenac.

ADVERSE EFFECTS. Proton pump inhibitors are usually well tolerated. Minor gastrointestinal and central nervous system (CNS) side effects have occurred in some patients, and skin rash and elevated hepatic enzyme levels have also been reported. Many patients with GERD have been treated for several years without significant side effects.

Gastric Antacids

Gastric antacids chemically neutralize stomach acid. This raises the gastrointestinal pH sufficiently to relieve the pain of dyspepsia and acid indigestion and to enable peptic ulcers to heal. The most commonly used antacids are **aluminum and magnesium hydroxides** and **calcium carbonate**. These substances are available in chewable tablets and in liquid suspensions. When used alone, aluminum hydroxide can cause constipation, whereas magnesium hydroxide often causes diarrhea. For this reason, the combination of aluminum and magnesium hydroxides usually has a relatively neutral effect on gastrointestinal motility. Calcium carbonate can also cause constipation, and large doses of calcium carbonate can lead to a rebound in acid secretion.

Antacids are available without a prescription and are commonly used to treat **acid indigestion** and **dyspepsia**. Nonprescription products containing a low dose of a histamine H_2 antagonist and an antacid are also available for this purpose. Antacids were formerly used to treat peptic ulcers, but they must be taken in large doses at frequent intervals for this purpose, and nocturnal acid secretion is particularly difficult to control with antacids. Hence, they are seldom used in treating peptic ulcer today.

CYTOPROTECTIVE DRUGS

Sucralfate and misoprostol both protect the gastrointestinal mucosa, but they do so by different means (see Fig. 28–1).

Sucralfate

CHEMISTRY, MECHANISMS, AND EFFECTS. Sucralfate is a viscous polymer of sucrose octasulfate and aluminum hydroxide. This sulfated polysaccharide adheres to ulcer craters and epithelial cells, and it inhibits pepsin-catalyzed hydrolysis of mucosal proteins. Sucralfate also stimulates prostaglandin synthesis in mucosal cells. These actions contribute to the formation of a protective barrier to acid and pepsin and thereby facilitate the healing of ulcers.

PHARMACOKINETICS. Sucralfate is administered orally as a tablet or suspension. The drug is not absorbed significantly from the gut, and it is primarily excreted in the feces. Patients absorb a small amount of aluminum from the drug, so sucralfate should be used cautiously in patients with renal impairment.

INDICATIONS. In the management of **peptic ulcer disease**, sucralfate can be used to treat active ulcers or to suppress the recurrence of ulcers. Because it is somewhat less effective than drugs that inhibit gastric acid secretion, it is primarily

used in patients who cannot tolerate H$_2$ blockers or proton pump inhibitors.

ADVERSE EFFECTS AND INTERACTIONS. Although sucralfate causes very few systemic adverse effects, constipation and other gastrointestinal disturbances and laryngospasm have been reported occasionally. The use of sucralfate can impair the absorption of other drugs (e.g., digoxin, fluoroquinolones, ketoconazole, and phenytoin). To prevent this problem, sucralfate should be ingested 2 hours before or after these other drugs are taken.

Misoprostol

As discussed in Chapter 26, misoprostol is a prostaglandin E$_1$ analogue. The drug exerts a cytoprotective effect by inhibiting gastric acid secretion and promoting the secretion of mucus and bicarbonate. It is primarily indicated for the prevention of **gastric and duodenal ulcers** in patients who are taking NSAIDs on a long-term basis for the treatment of arthritis and other conditions. Because misoprostol is expensive, it is usually reserved for patients at high risk of NSAID-induced ulcers, including the elderly and those with a history of peptic ulcer disease.

Misoprostol is administered orally 4 times daily with food for the duration of NSAID therapy. Diarrhea and intestinal cramping are the most common adverse effects, but other gastrointestinal reactions can also occur.

Misoprostol can stimulate uterine contractions and induce labor in pregnant women, so its use is **contraindicated during pregnancy**.

Muscarinic Receptor Antagonists

Historically, atropine was used to treat peptic ulcer disease, but large doses of the drug are required to inhibit gastric acid secretion, and these doses caused numerous side effects such as blurred vision, urinary retention, and many others. **Pirenzepine** is a selective muscarinic M$_1$ receptor antagonist that inhibits histamine release from gastric paracrine cells and causes fewer side effects than atropine. It is available in Canada but not in the United States for treating peptic ulcer disease.

Atropine, hyoscyamine, dicyclomine, and other muscarinic blockers are used as antispasmodic agents to temporarily relieve **intestinal cramping and pain** and other symptoms of intestinal hyperactivity.

DRUGS FOR *HELICOBACTER PYLORI* INFECTION

Studies show that 80% to 90% of patients who undergo monotherapy with a gastric acid inhibitor have an **ulcer recurrence** within 1 year after discontinuing this therapy. In contrast, less than 5% of patients who undergo therapy with both a gastric acid inhibitor and an agent to eliminate *H. pylori* have an ulcer recurrence. Hence, combination therapy is now the standard of care.

The currently recommended treatments for peptic ulcer disease consist of a gastric acid secretion inhibitor (usually a proton pump inhibitor) and two or more of the following agents: amoxicillin, bismuth, clarithromycin, metronidazole, tetracycline, or levofloxacin.

Short-course treatments of 10 to 14 days duration (and possibly 7 days or less) consist of twice daily omeprazole or lansoprazole plus amoxicillin and clarithromycin. Metronidazole may be substituted for amoxicillin in persons allergic to penicillins. Alternative short-course regimens include twice daily ranitidine bismuth citrate (a single drug), plus clarithromycin and tetracycline. Another regimen consists of pantoprazole plus amoxicillin and levofloxacin. These regimens eradicate *H. pylori* in 80% to 90% of cases of duodenal ulcers (see Box 28–1).

Four-week treatments for duodenal peptic ulcer consist of a once-daily proton pump inhibitor plus antimicrobial agents. Histamine H$_2$ blockers or sucralfate may also be effective in 4 weeks or longer when given in combination with antibiotics. Longer (8 weeks) treatments are usually required for treating gastric ulcers.

The properties of antimicrobial agents are discussed in the chapters of Section VII.

DRUGS FOR INFLAMMATORY BOWEL DISEASES

The two most common inflammatory bowel diseases are **ulcerative colitis** and **Crohn's disease**. In ulcerative colitis, inflammation of the gastrointestinal mucosa is limited to the colon and rectum. In Crohn's disease, inflammation is transmural and can occur in any part of the gastrointestinal tract.

Abdominal cramping and diarrhea are the most common complaints of patients with inflammatory bowel disease. Many patients experience acute exacerbations separated by periods of remission, but prolonged illness can occur in persons with severe disease. Ulcerative colitis and Crohn's disease are generally treated with glucocorticoids, mesalamine, and infliximab.

Glucocorticoids

Hydrocortisone and other glucocorticoids (see Chapter 33) have been extensively used for the treatment of both **ulcerative colitis** and **Crohn's disease**. In cases of mild ulcerative colitis, they may be effectively administered as rectal enemas. In cases of Crohn's disease and more severe ulcerative colitis, they are usually administered orally or parenterally.

Glucocorticoids are often able to induce the remission of ulcerative colitis or Crohn's disease, but they have proved less valuable in maintaining remission, particularly without causing significant toxicity.

Aminosalicylates

Sulfasalazine and its active metabolite, **mesalamine**, are used to induce and maintain the remission of ulcerative colitis, but they are less effective in maintaining remission of Crohn's disease.

Sulfasalazine is a modified sulfonamide compound that is not well absorbed from the gut. In the gastrointestinal tract, bacteria convert sulfasalazine to 5-aminosalicylic acid

(5-ASA, or mesalamine) and sulfapyridine. Although 5-ASA is believed to mediate the anti-inflammatory effects of sulfasalazine, the exact mechanism is uncertain. Some investigators hypothesize that 5-ASA acts by inhibiting prostaglandin synthesis or by inhibiting the migration of inflammatory cells into the bowel wall. Others hypothesize that 5-ASA is a superoxide-free radical scavenger.

Mesalamine can be administered as a rectal suppository, rectal suspension, or delayed-release oral tablet. It acts primarily in the gut, but about 15% of the drug is absorbed into the circulation.

Infliximab

Immunosuppressive agents may be useful in maintaining remission in patients with Crohn's disease and severe ulcerative colitis. Infliximab is a monoclonal antibody to **tumor necrosis factor-α,** a substance believed to play a role in the pathogenesis of these conditions (see Chapter 30). The drug appears to provide considerable benefit to patients with moderate to severe Crohn's disease or ulcerative colitis. Azathioprine and cyclosporine have also been used for these conditions (see Chapter 45).

GASTROINTESTINAL MOTILITY DISORDERS

A number of gastrointestinal tract disorders are characterized by abnormal gastrointestinal motility. These include constipation, diarrhea, GERD, gastroparesis, and irritable bowel syndrome (IBS).

GERD, which is characterized by esophagitis, is caused by the reflux of gastric acid into the esophagus. The disease is often associated with excessive secretion of gastric acid and decreased pressure in the lower esophageal sphincter. Pharmacologic agents used in the treatment of GERD include drugs that reduce gastric acidity (e.g., H_2 receptor antagonists and proton pump inhibitors) and drugs that increase esophageal sphincter pressure, such as metoclopramide. Also useful are nonpharmacologic measures that include avoidance of certain foods (e.g., chocolate), avoidance of bedtime snacks, and elevation of the upper body during sleep. Because obesity contributes to GERD, weight reduction can help alleviate symptoms.

Acute gastroparesis is a delay in gastric emptying that is typically seen in patients recovering from surgery, trauma, or abdominal infections. **Chronic gastroparesis** is seen in patients with neuropathies that affect the stomach, such as patients with diabetes mellitus. As with other forms of gastroparesis, **diabetic gastroparesis** can be treated with prokinetic drugs such as metoclopramide.

Metoclopramide

MECHANISMS AND EFFECTS. Metoclopramide is a prokinetic drug that is believed to increase **gastrointestinal tone and motility** by blocking dopamine D_2 receptors, which prevents relaxation of gastrointestinal smooth muscle produced by dopamine. Dopamine infusions have been found to reduce gastric muscle tone in human volunteers and to cause delayed gastric emptying. In addition to blocking the direct effects of dopamine, metoclopramide increases the release of acetylcholine from cholinergic motor neurons in the enteric nervous system by blocking presynaptic dopamine receptors whose activation inhibits acetylcholine release. This increases stimulation of acetylcholine muscarinic receptors and enhances propulsive activity, leading to increased tone and motility in the esophagus and stomach.

Metoclopramide accelerates gastric emptying by preventing relaxation of the gastric body and increasing phasic contractions of the antrum. At the same time, it relaxes the proximal duodenum so that it can accept gastric material as antral contractions arrive at the pyloric sphincter.

BOX 28–1. A CASE OF BURNING EPIGASTRIC PAIN

CASE PRESENTATION: A 50-year-old man complains to his physician of a burning epigastric pain that has awakened him at night for the past 3 weeks. The pain often begins in the late morning and is relieved by food or antacids, but reappears about 3 hours after a meal and during sleep. He has been otherwise healthy and his vital signs and physical exam are normal. Blood samples are taken for routine chemistries and blood cell counts. A rapid urease test for *H. pylori* is positive, and he is scheduled for gastrointestinal endoscopy, which reveals an inflamed ulcer in the wall of the duodenal bulb. A gastric mucosal biopsy confirms the presence of *H. pylori*. The patient denies any drug allergies and is placed on triple therapy with 40 mg/day of omeprazole, 2 g/day of amoxicillin, and 1000 mg/day of clarithromycin, all of which are divided into 2 daily doses and given for 2 weeks. His symptoms improve markedly after several days of therapy and endoscopy confirms ulcer healing after completion of his treatment.

CASE DISCUSSION: *Helicobacter pylori* infection is responsible for most cases of duodenal ulcer. Epigastric pain is the most common symptom, which is usually relieved by food but often awakens a patient at night. Several tests for *H. pylori* are available, including the rapid urease test. Endoscopy is a valuable tool for determining the type and location of a peptic ulcer and enables biopsy to distinguish simple gastric ulcers from stomach cancer. It can also identify a bleeding ulcer and permit laser probe coagulation to stop bleeding. The treatment of ulcers caused by *H. pylori* has been continuously improved and 1- or 2-week treatments using a proton pump inhibitor and two antibiotics are highly effective. Amoxicillin and clarithromycin are the antibiotics of choice for this indication.

Metoclopramide also increases the resting pressure of the **lower esophageal sphincter** and thereby **reduces reflux of acid** from the stomach into the esophagus.

PHARMACOKINETICS AND USE. Metoclopramide can be administered orally or parenterally. It is rapidly absorbed from the gut and has an average bioavailability of 85%. The drug is conjugated with sulfate and glucuronate, and these metabolites are excreted in the urine, along with 20% of the parent compound. The terminal half-life is about 4 hours.

Metoclopramide is used to treat **GERD, diabetic gastroparesis**, and **intractable hiccup**. It is sometimes used to facilitate **intubation of the small bowel** during radiologic examination. In addition, metoclopramide exerts **antiemetic effects** by blocking dopamine D_2 and serotonin 5-HT$_3$ receptors in the chemoreceptor trigger zone (below).

ADVERSE EFFECTS. The major adverse effects of metoclopramide are CNS reactions (e.g., drowsiness, extra-pyramidal effects, and seizures). Hyperprolactinemia, diarrhea, and hematologic toxicity have also been reported. Metoclopramide is contraindicated in persons with seizure disorders, mechanical obstruction of the gastrointestinal tract, gastrointestinal hemorrhage, or pheochromocytoma.

LAXATIVES

Constipation

Constipation can be an acute or chronic condition, and it is characterized by the difficult passage of hard, dry feces. The treatment of constipation rests on a foundation of increased dietary fiber ingestion, adequate fluid intake, and regular exercise. Patients should be encouraged to eat fruits, vegetables, and whole grain foods that add bulk to the diet. If dietary modifications are not sufficient to alleviate constipation, a laxative can be used to facilitate peristalsis. Bulk-forming laxatives can be used on a long-term basis without noticeable side effects, but the other types of laxatives should be used only to relieve acute constipation. **Lubiprostone** represents a new type of drug for the treatment of chronic constipation (see below).

Laxatives are drugs that stimulate intestinal peristalsis and increase the movement of material through the bowel. By these actions, laxatives decrease the intestinal transit time and facilitate defecation. Laxatives are used to **treat constipation** and to **evacuate the bowel before surgery or diagnostic examination.** They are also used to **eliminate drugs or poisons from the intestinal tract** in cases of drug overdose or poisoning.

Laxatives are classified according to their mechanism of action as bulk-forming, surfactant, osmotic, or stimulant. Lubricant laxatives, such as mineral oil, are essentially obsolete.

Bulk-Forming Laxatives

Bulk-forming laxatives are indigestible hydrophilic substances, such as **psyllium hydrophilic mucilloid** and **calcium polycarbophil** that resemble natural dietary fiber. They absorb and retain water in the intestinal lumen and thereby increase the mass of intestinal material. These actions cause mechanical distention of the intestinal wall and stimulate peristalsis. Bulk-forming laxatives are available in several preparations, including fiber tablets and packets of psyllium granules. They must be taken with a full glass of water to ensure adequate hydration of the preparation and avoid intestinal obstruction. Bulk-forming laxatives are the safest and most physiologic type of laxative, and they rarely cause adverse effects. For this reason, they are the preferred drugs for the management of chronic constipation. Because of their ability to absorb water and irritant substances such as bile salts, these drugs are also used in the treatment of diarrhea (see below).

Surfactant Laxatives

The surfactant laxatives include **docusate sodium** and docusate calcium. These laxatives are also called **stool softeners** because they facilitate the incorporation of water into fatty intestinal material and thereby soften the feces. Stool softeners are primarily beneficial when fecal materials are hard or dry and when their passage is irritating and painful (e.g., as occurs with anorectal conditions such as hemorrhoids). They are also useful when patients must avoid straining during defecation (e.g., after having abdominal or other surgery). Surfactants produce few adverse effects.

Osmotic (Saline) Laxatives

Osmotic laxatives consist of poorly absorbed inorganic salts, such as **magnesium oxide** (milk of magnesia) and **sodium phosphate**. These substances attract and retain water in the intestinal lumen and increase intraluminal pressure, thereby stimulating peristalsis. They can be taken orally as a liquid or chewable tablet, or they can be administered as an enema. Sufficient doses of osmotic laxatives act rapidly to stimulate defecation. Sodium phosphate is often used to **evacuate the bowel** in patients scheduled for surgery or diagnostic examination or in patients suffering from drug overdose or poisoning. Lower doses of magnesium oxide can be used to prevent constipation in some patients, such as those receiving opioid analgesics. Use of osmotic laxatives, however, can lead to excessive **loss of fluids and electrolytes**, so these laxatives are generally not well suited for the treatment of chronic constipation. Patients with renal impairment are particularly susceptible to these adverse effects, because they may not be able to properly excrete osmotic substances that are absorbed into the circulation.

Stimulant (Secretory) Laxatives

The stimulant laxatives include a large group of natural and synthetic compounds that act directly on the intestinal mucosa to alter fluid secretion and stimulate peristalsis. These compounds include natural products (e.g., castor oil, plant extracts of senna, or cascara), and synthetic compounds such as **bisacodyl**. Bisacodyl is available in oral and rectal suppository formulations that are used in **evacuating the bowel** before surgery or examination. The stimulant laxatives can cause a number of adverse effects, including abdominal cramping and significant electrolyte and fluid depletion. For this reason, the use of these drugs should be limited to the **short-term treatment of constipation**.

Lubiprostone

Chronic idiopathic constipation is a syndrome characterized by abdominal pain, bloating, and hard or lumpy stools that appears to result from colonic inactivity and impaired evacuation of feces. Lubiprostone activates the **chloride Cl-C$_2$ channel** in the apical (luminal) membrane of the intestinal epithelium and stimulates secretion of chloride-rich fluid into the intestinal lumen, thereby increasing intestinal motility. Lubiprostone has low systemic bioavailability after oral administration and appears to act directly on intestinal chloride channels. Clinical studies found that it increased the frequency of bowel movements in persons with chronic idiopathic constipation and relieved abdominal discomfort and bloating. The drug caused **nausea** in about 30% of patients, which is reduced by taking it with food, and **diarrhea** occurred in 13% of persons taking the drug.

ANTIDIARRHEAL AGENTS

Diarrhea

The frequency of elimination and consistency of stools vary from person to person. Diarrhea is a condition characterized by an increase in the number and liquidity of a person's stools. It can be acute or chronic, it can range in severity from mild to life-threatening, and it has many causes and pathophysiologic mechanisms. **Secretory diarrhea** can be caused by **microbial toxins**, laxatives, vasoactive intestinal polypeptide secreted by a pancreatic tumor, excessive bile acids, or unabsorbed fat in malabsorption syndromes (steatorrhea). Most of the mediators of secretory diarrhea act by **stimulating cAMP formation** or inhibiting membrane Na$^+$-K$^+$-ATPase, and this leads to an increase in the secretion of water and electrolytes by the intestinal mucosa. **Cholera toxin**, for instance, stimulates adenylyl cyclase activity and increases cAMP levels in intestinal cells which, in turn, cause active secretion of electrolytes and water into the intestinal lumen. Some mediators of diarrhea also inhibit ion absorption by intestinal cells.

Severe diarrhea caused by bacterial infections and other causes can lead to significant loss of fluids and electrolytes and should be treated promptly. If fever or systemic symptoms are present, patients with diarrhea should be examined for **microbial or parasitic infections**. If cultures are positive, an appropriate antimicrobial or antiparasitic drug should be given. **Chronic diarrhea** is defined as diarrhea lasting for 14 days or longer. This condition requires a more thorough diagnostic work-up to determine the underlying cause and enable the selection of appropriate therapy.

Most cases of **mild diarrhea** are self-limiting and subside within 1 or 2 days. Mild diarrhea can be managed with **dietary restrictions** and **fluid and electrolyte replacement**. Dietary guidelines consist of avoiding solid food and milk products for 24 hours after onset of illness, and preparations that contain the correct proportions of glucose and electrolytes for fluid and electrolyte replacement are available. An **antidiarrheal agent** can be given as adjunct treatment in older children and adults. As bowel movements decrease, a bland diet can be started.

A number of drugs can cause diarrhea, including antibiotics that eradicate the normal intestinal flora. Administration of *Lactobacillus* preparations can help restore the normal bowel flora and reduce diarrhea in these patients.

Opioid Drugs

The opioids are the most efficacious antidiarrheal drugs. They exert a nonspecific effect that can control diarrhea from almost any cause. Opioids act by inducing a sustained segmental contraction of intestinal smooth muscle, which prevents the rhythmic waves of contraction and relaxation of smooth muscle that occur with normal peristalsis.

The effects of opioids are mediated by activation of **opioid receptors** in smooth muscle. All of the more potent opioid receptor agonists are effective antidiarrheal compounds. In most cases, the opioid chosen for treatment of diarrhea is one that selectively activates intestinal opioid receptors while having relatively little effect on the CNS. **Diphenoxylate** and **loperamide** are the opioid agonists with the greatest ratio of intestinal smooth muscle activity to CNS activity, so they are the most widely used opioids for treating diarrhea. Loperamide is available without a prescription and can effectively control mild diarrhea. Excessive use of these drugs can cause constipation.

Locally Acting Drugs

Psyllium hydrophilic mucilloid and **calcium polycarbophil** control diarrhea by acting locally within the intestinal tract to adsorb water and irritant substances such as bile acids. These substances are suitable for the treatment of mild diarrhea.

Bismuth subsalicylate appears to produce its antidiarrheal effect by inhibiting intestinal secretions. It is most effective in treating **infectious diarrhea**, which often has a strong secretory component. In patients with traveler's diarrhea and other forms of infectious diarrhea, clinical studies demonstrated that bismuth subsalicylate caused a greater reduction in the number of diarrheal episodes than did a placebo. Bismuth subsalicylate suspension, however, must be given frequently and repeatedly for maximal efficacy (30 mL every 30 minutes for up to 8 doses per day). This preparation causes few side effects, but excessively large doses can expose the patient to bismuth or salicylate toxicity.

Alosetron and Tegaserod

Irritable bowel syndrome is a complex biopsychosocial disorder characterized by chronic abdominal pain that is relieved by defecation and is associated with altered bowel habits. Some patients complain primarily of **diarrhea**, whereas **constipation** predominates in others. Many patients with IBS also experience nausea, bloating, and flatulence.

Alosetron is a serotonin **5-HT$_3$ receptor antagonist** that is used to treat IBS in women whose predominant symptom is diarrhea. 5-HT$_3$ receptors are ligand-gated cation channels found on enteric neurons in the gastrointestinal tract. Activation of these receptors causes neuronal depolarization, which is believed to increase colonic transit, alter gastrointestinal secretions, and contribute to visceral pain in patients with IBS. Alosetron is employed in women whose symptoms have lasted 6 months or longer and which include diarrhea and abdominal pain or discomfort, as well as frequent bowel urgency or incontinence causing disability or restriction of daily activities. In these patients, alosetron increases colonic transit time and reduces pain and other symptoms of IBS.

Alosetron may infrequently cause adverse gastrointestinal effects, including **ischemic colitis**, that rarely require blood transfusions and surgery, and which have been fatal in a few cases. Hence, the drug is restricted to treating patients that don't respond to conventional antidiarrheal and antispasmodic medications.

Tegaserod has been used for treating women with IBS whose predominant symptom is constipation, but it has been removed from the market because of a small but statistically significant increase in **angina**, **myocardial infarction**, and **stroke** associated with the drug. It is still available under a treatment IND (Investigational New Drug) protocol for patients who cannot be effectively treated with any other agent.

ANTIEMETICS

Nausea and Vomiting

Emesis, or vomiting, is a physiologic response to the presence of irritating and potentially harmful substances in the gut or bloodstream. It sometimes occurs as a result of excessive vestibular stimulation (motion sickness) or psychological stimuli such as fear, dread, or obnoxious sights and odors. Vomiting is frequently preceded by nausea.

Vomiting is initiated by a nucleus of cells located in the medulla that is called the **vomiting** or **emesis center**. This center coordinates a complex series of events involving pharyngeal, gastrointestinal, and abdominal wall contractions that lead to expulsion of the gastric contents. These include orally migrating intestinal contractions (reverse peristalsis), gastric contractions, contractions of the diaphragm and abdominal wall, and relaxation of the esophageal sphincter and wall. The reverse intestinal contractions are associated with **nausea**, which is an intensely unpleasant feeling of the imminent need to vomit. Nausea can also occur in the absence of vomiting.

The neural pathways involved in emesis and the sites of antiemetic drug action are shown in Figure 28–3. The vomiting center can be activated by afferent fibers arising from the gut, **chemoreceptor trigger zone** (CTZ), cerebral cortex, or vestibular apparatus. The CTZ is located in the area postrema and responds to blood-borne substances, including cytotoxic cancer chemotherapy drugs. These substances activate the CTZ via stimulation of **serotonin 5-HT$_3$, dopamine D$_2$, or muscarinic M$_1$ receptors**. The vestibular apparatus activates the vomiting center via fibers that project to the cerebellum and release acetylcholine or histamine. Noxious substances in the gut can activate vagal afferent pathways to the solitary tract nucleus, which projects to the vomiting center, as well as pathways to the nerve tracts that stimulate the CTZ. The D$_2$, 5-HT$_3$, and **neurokinin 1 (NK$_1$) receptors** also have a major role in these pathways.

Most antiemetic drugs act by blocking **dopamine, serotonin, muscarinic, or histamine receptors**. Some drugs appear to inhibit several pathways that lead to vomiting center activation. The D$_2$ and 5-HT$_3$ receptor antagonists inhibit activation of both the CTZ and the solitary tract nucleus. Muscarinic receptor antagonists can block the CTZ, solitary tract, and vestibular pathways involved in emesis. **Dexamethasone** is an effective antiemetic whose mechanism is not well understood. It is particularly effective for preventing delayed nausea and vomiting in persons receiving cancer chemotherapy.

Serotonin 5-HT$_3$ Receptor Antagonists

Ondansetron was the first selective 5-HT$_3$ receptor antagonist to be developed for the treatment of cancer chemotherapy-induced nausea and vomiting. It was found to significantly reduce the number of episodes of emesis in patients treated with cisplatin, which is one of the most highly emetogenic chemotherapy agents. Other first-generation 5-HT$_3$ antagonists were subsequently developed and include **granisetron** and **dolasetron**. All of the first-generation 5-HT$_3$ antagonists have similar pharmacologic properties and clinical efficacies. **Palonosetron** is a newer drug that has been called a second-generation 5-HT$_3$ antagonist because of its greater affinity for 5-HT$_3$ receptors and its much longer half-life and duration of action.

CHEMISTRY, MECHANISMS, AND EFFECTS. The 5-HT$_3$ antagonists (e.g., ondansetron) have structures that resemble the structure of serotonin (see Fig. 28–2). Cancer chemotherapy is associated with nausea and vomiting when serotonin released from enterochromaffin cells of the small intestine activates 5-HT$_3$ receptors located on vagal afferents and activates the vomiting reflex (see Fig. 28–3). Anticancer drugs also stimulate the CTZ that activates the vomiting center in the medulla. Ondansetron and related drugs competitively block 5-HT$_3$ receptors located on visceral afferent nerves in the gastrointestinal tract, in the solitary tract nucleus, and in the CTZ. This enables these drugs to prevent both peripheral and central stimulation of the vomiting center.

PHARMACOKINETICS AND INDICATIONS. Some of the 5-HT$_3$ receptor antagonists (e.g., ondansetron) can be administered orally or intravenously, whereas others (e.g., palonosetron) are only given intravenously. These drugs are metabolized by cytochrome P450, and the metabolites are primarily eliminated in the urine. The half-lives of granisetron, ondansetron, and dolasetron are 4, 6, and 7 hours, respectively. Palonosetron has a half-life of about 40 hours, which confers a much longer duration of action than other 5-HT$_3$ antagonists.

All of the 5-HT$_3$ antagonists are primarily used for the prevention of **cancer chemotherapy-induced emesis**. Ondansetron and dolasetron are also approved for the prevention and treatment of **postoperative emesis**, whereas ondansetron and granisetron are used to prevent **nausea and vomiting caused by radiation therapy**.

First-generation 5-HT$_3$ antagonists are usually administered just before chemotherapy and continued for 3 to 5 days

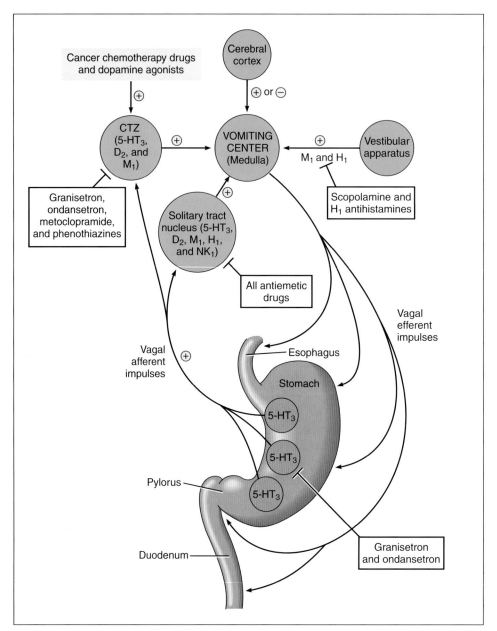

Figure 28-3. Physiology of emesis and sites of drug action. Emetic stimuli travel from the gastrointestinal tract via the solitary tract nucleus to arrive at the vomiting center in the medulla. Emetic stimuli also reach the vomiting center via afferent fibers from the chemoreceptor trigger zone (CTZ), cerebral cortex, and vestibular apparatus. Granisetron and ondansetron prevent emesis by blocking serotonin 5-HT_3 receptors in the gastrointestinal tract, solitary tract nucleus, and CTZ. Metoclopramide and phenothiazines prevent emesis by blocking dopamine D_2 receptors in the solitary tract nucleus and CTZ. Aprepitant blocks neurokinin 1 (NK_1) receptors in the solitary tract. Scopolamine and the H_1 antihistamines prevent emesis by blocking muscarinic M_1 receptors, histamine H_1 receptors, or both types of receptors in the vestibular tracts that project to the vomiting center and in the solitary tract nucleus and CTZ. Note that cancer chemotherapy drugs and dopamine agonists cause emesis, in part, by stimulating the CTZ.

after the course of chemotherapy is completed. Because of its longer duration of action, a single dose of palonosetron may prevent nausea and vomiting for up to 7 days following chemotherapy. One study found that a single intravenous dose of 0.25 mg **palonosetron** was significantly superior to 32 mg of intravenous ondansetron in the prevention of acute and delayed chemotherapy-induced nausea and vomiting. Palonosetron is approved for treating both acute and delayed nausea and vomiting in persons receiving emetogenic chemotherapy.

Other antiemetic drugs appear to exert an additive or synergistic effect in combination with 5-HT_3 antagonists, and **dexamethasone** is often employed in combination with a 5-HT_3 antagonist for preventing chemotherapy-induced emesis (see "Guidelines").

Studies have also confirmed the usefulness of ondansetron in controlling postoperative nausea and vomiting. In patients who underwent laparoscopic cholecystectomy, for example, ondansetron was found to be more effective than metoclopramide or a placebo in controlling emesis.

ADVERSE EFFECTS AND INTERACTIONS. The serotonin 5-HT$_3$ antagonists are well tolerated and usually produce few adverse effects. The most common side effects are headache, constipation, and diarrhea. Less common reactions include hypertension and elevated hepatic enzyme levels. In several cases, use of ondansetron resulted in an anaphylactoid reaction consisting of bronchospasm, angioedema, hypotension, and urticaria. Clinically significant drug interactions with 5-HT$_3$ receptor antagonists have not been identified.

Dopamine D$_2$ Receptor Antagonists

The D$_2$ receptor antagonists include **metoclopramide** and a large number of **phenothiazine drugs** such as **prochlorperazine**. All of the D$_2$ receptor antagonists appear to act primarily on the CTZ to inhibit stimulation of the vomiting center, but they may also inhibit afferent impulses from the gut by antagonizing receptors in the solitary tract nucleus.

The phenothiazines have antiemetic, antipsychotic, anticholinergic, antihistamine, and sedative properties (see Chapter 22). Prochlorperazine and other phenothiazines have been used in treating emesis due to a wide range of medical conditions. They can be administered parenterally or as a rectal suppository in patients who are unable to take oral medication. Phenothiazines are not as effective as other drugs in treating chemotherapy-induced emesis. Likewise, metoclopramide is less effective than 5-HT$_3$ antagonists for this purpose.

Aprepitant

Substance P is a peptide of the **tachykinin** family that acts as a neurotransmitter in the gut and brain. Substance P is released from vagal afferent fibers in the solitary tract where it activates **neurokinin 1** receptors and thereby produces emesis (see Fig. 28–3). **Aprepitant** is a nonpeptide NK$_1$ receptor antagonist that prevents emesis induced by various stimuli in animal models. The drug is intended to be used in combination with a 5-HT$_3$ antagonist (e.g., ondansetron) and dexamethasone to prevent acute and delayed nausea and vomiting occurring with highly emetogenic cancer chemotherapy, including cisplatin (see below).

Aprepitant is administered orally and is metabolized primarily by cytochrome P450 CYP3A4 with a terminal half-life of 9 to 13 hours. Drugs that inhibit CYP3A4 can elevate plasma concentrations of aprepitant. The drug has a low incidence of adverse effects.

Guidelines for Chemotherapy-Induced Emesis

The current Multinational Association for Supportive Care in Cancer guidelines for antiemetic therapy recommend a serotonin antagonist plus dexamethasone plus aprepitant for preventing acute emesis due to highly emetogenic drugs such as cisplatin, dacarbazine, and cyclophosphamide. Aprepitant and dexamethasone are recommended to be given on days 2 and 3 for preventing delayed emesis. For moderately emetogenic chemotherapy, a serotonin antagonist and dexamethasone are recommended for acute emesis, and dexamethasone alone for delayed emesis. For minimally emetogenic chemotherapy, a low dose of dexamethasone is recommended.

Other Antiemetics

Dronabinol, an oral formulation of Δ^9-tetrahydrocannabinol, is approved for the treatment of **cancer chemotherapy-induced emesis** when conventional antiemetic drugs have failed. Dronabinol is usually administered several hours before chemotherapy and is then administered every 4 to 6 hours during a 12-hour period after chemotherapy. The drug probably acts on the vomiting center in the medulla. It is less effective than serotonin antagonists and has about the same antiemetic efficacy as the phenothiazines. Dronabinol is also approved as an **appetite stimulant** for anorexic patients with acquired immunodeficiency syndrome (AIDS).

Several histamine H$_1$ receptor antagonists (H$_1$ antihistamines) have antiemetic actions and are discussed in Chapter 26. Two of these agents, **dimenhydrinate** and **meclizine**, are used in the management of **motion sickness.** Another of these agents, **promethazine**, is an H$_1$ antihistamine that also has significant antimuscarinic activity and is used to prevent and treat **nausea and vomiting** induced by medications, anesthetics, and a wide variety of neurologic, psychogenic, and gastrointestinal stimuli. Promethazine is usually administered as a rectal suppository or by injection.

Scopolamine is a muscarinic receptor antagonist that is similar to atropine and is primarily used to prevent **motion sickness.** In addition to being used by persons traveling in cars, planes, or boats for extended times, it has been used by astronauts in space. Scopolamine is available as a skin patch that slowly releases the drug over 72 hours.

SUMMARY OF IMPORTANT POINTS

■ Drugs used to treat peptic ulcers include inhibitors of gastric acid secretion, cytoprotective agents, and antibiotics for *H. pylori* infection. The histamine H$_2$ receptor antagonists (cimetidine, famotidine, ranitidine, and others) and the proton pump inhibitors (omeprazole and others) are the primary gastric acid inhibitors. Gastric antacids (aluminum and magnesium hydroxides and calcium carbonate) are used to relieve heartburn and dyspepsia.

■ The H$_2$ receptor antagonists inhibit basal and meal-stimulated acid secretion and can be used to treat GERD and dyspepsia as well as peptic ulcer disease. Cimetidine inhibits cytochrome P450 isozymes and may increase the plasma concentrations of many other drugs, leading to potential toxicity.

■ Omeprazole and related drugs irreversibly inhibit the proton pump (H$^+$, K$^+$-ATPase) and acid secretion. They are the most efficacious drugs for treating GERD and peptic ulcers, and they are the drugs of choice for use in patients with gastrin-secreting tumors (gastrinomas) and Zollinger-Ellison syndrome.

■ Sucralfate is a cytoprotective drug that binds to the ulcer crater and forms a barrier to acid and pepsin. Misoprostol is a prostaglandin E$_1$ analogue that increases the production of mucus and bicarbonate while reducing the secretion of gastric acid. Misoprostol is used to prevent ulcers caused by long-term therapy with NSAIDs.

■ Inflammatory bowel diseases (ulcerative colitis and Crohn's disease) are primarily treated with glucocorticoids, aminosalicylates (sulfasalazine and mesalamine), and infliximab (an antibody to tumor necrosis factor-α).

■ Metoclopramide inhibits dopamine D_2 receptors and blocks dopamine-induced smooth muscle relaxation while increasing acetylcholine release in the gut. It is used to increase gastrointestinal motility in gastroparesis and to increase lower esophageal pressure in GERD.

■ Alosetron is a serotonin 5-HT_3 antagonist that decreases gastrointestinal motility and relieves diarrhea and other symptoms in women with irritable bowel disease.

■ Laxatives are drugs used to facilitate defecation and evacuate the bowels. They include bulk-forming laxatives (psyllium), surfactant laxatives (docusate sodium), osmotic laxatives (magnesium oxide and sodium phosphate), and stimulant laxatives (bisacodyl and others). Bulk-forming laxatives are preferred for the treatment of chronic constipation. Osmotic and stimulant laxatives are used to clear the bowels of patients preparing for intestinal surgery or diagnostic examination and patients being treated for a drug overdose or poisoning.

■ Opioids are the most efficacious antidiarrheal drugs. Loperamide and diphenoxylate cause little or no central nervous system effects at doses that control diarrhea.

■ Serotonin 5-HT_3 receptor antagonists (ondansetron and others) are the most efficacious antiemetics for the management of cancer chemotherapy-induced nausea and vomiting. Aprepitant, a neurokinin 1 receptor antagonist, also prevents chemotherapy-induced emesis. Metoclopramide and other D_2 receptor antagonists (e.g., prochlorperazine) are also effective antiemetics.

■ Promethazine is used for mild nausea and vomiting caused by drugs, infections, and other stimuli. Motion sickness can be prevented by meclizine and dimenhydrinate (H_1 receptor antagonists), or by scopolamine, a muscarinic receptor antagonist.

Review Questions

1. A woman is using a skin patch medication to prevent motion sickness while on a cruise ship. Which adverse effect may result from taking this drug?
   (A) flatulence
   (B) heartburn
   (C) headache
   (D) diarrhea
   (E) dry mouth

2. A woman with IBS has recurrent episodes of abdominal pain, flatulence, and diarrhea that are not relieved by loperamide. Which adverse effect may result from taking the drug approved for this condition?
   (A) pulmonary fibrosis
   (B) ischemic colitis

   (C) ischemic heart disease
   (D) gastric ulcer
   (E) muscle rigidity and tremor

3. A woman is found to have a duodenal ulcer caused by *H. pylori* infection, and she desires the shortest effective treatment available. Which drug combination would most likely achieve this goal?
   (A) once daily lansoprazole, amoxicillin, and metronidazole
   (B) twice daily omeprazole, bismuth subsalicylate, and tetracycline
   (C) once daily famotidine, amoxicillin, and clarithromycin
   (D) twice daily lansoprazole, amoxicillin, and clarithromycin
   (E) twice daily rabeprazole, cimetidine, and bismuth subsalicylate

4. A man with chronic heartburn caused by gastric acid reflux is placed on a drug that increases lower esophageal sphincter tone. Which mechanism is responsible for this pharmacologic effect?
   (A) histamine H_2 receptor blockade
   (B) muscarinic receptor blockade
   (C) dopamine D_2 receptor blockade
   (D) α-adrenoceptor activation
   (E) chloride $Cl-C_2$ channel activation

5. A man undergoing cancer chemotherapy with cisplatin is placed on medication to prevent acute emesis. Which combination of drugs is recommended for this purpose in current guidelines?
   (A) palonosetron, dexamethasone, and aprepitant
   (B) dexamethasone only
   (C) dexamethasone and aprepitant
   (D) aprepitant only
   (E) palonosetron only

Answers and Explanations

1. **The correct answer is E:** dry mouth. The woman is most likely taking scopolamine, a muscarinic receptor antagonist that may cause dry mouth. It could also cause constipation, rather than diarrhea (Option D). It is unlikely to cause flatulence, heartburn, or headache (Options A, B, and C).

2. **The correct answer is B:** ischemic colitis. Alosetron is used to treat diarrhea-predominant IBS, but it may uncommonly cause ischemic colitis. It is not associated with pulmonary fibrosis, ischemic heart disease, gastric ulcer, or muscle rigidity and tremor (Options A, C, D, and E).

3. **The correct answer is D:** twice daily lansoprazole, amoxicillin, and clarithromycin. Effective short-course treatments, some as short as 7 days, include twice daily administration of a proton pump inhibitor and two antimicrobial agents. Amoxicillin and clarithromycin are highly effective for this purpose. Once daily drug administration requires 4 or more weeks for eradication of *H. pylori*.

4. **The correct answer is C:** dopamine D_2 receptor blockade. Metoclopramide increases lower esophageal sphincter tone by directly blocking dopamine D_2 receptors and increasing acetylcholine release, thereby activating muscarinic receptors in esophageal muscle. Metoclopramide does not block muscarinic or histamine receptors (Options A and B), and it does not activate α-adrenoceptors or chloride channels (Options D and E).

5. **The correct answer is A:** palonosetron, dexamethasone, and aprepitant. Current guidelines of the Multinational Association of Supportive Care in Cancer recommend a three-drug combination for prevent acute emesis to highly emetogenic drugs such as cisplatin. The combination should include a serotonin 5-HT$_3$ antagonist along with dexamethasone and aprepitant. Single- and dual-drug therapy is less effective for this purpose (Options B, C, D, and E).

SELECTED READINGS

Baker, D.E. Lubiprostone: a new drug for the treatment of chronic idiopathic constipation. Rev Gastroenterol Disord 7:214–222, 2007.

Herrstedt, J. Antiemetics: an update and the MASCC guidelines applied in clinical practice. Nat Clin Pract Oncol 5:32–43, 2008.

Krause, R., V. Ameen, S.H. Gordon, M. West, A.T. Heath, et al. A randomized, double-blind, placebo-controlled study to assess the efficacy and safety of 0.5 mg and 1 mg alosetron in women with severe diarrhea-predominant IBS. Am J Gastroenterol 102:1709–1719, 2007.

Langan, R.C., P.B. Gotsch, and M.A. Krafczyk. Ulcerative colitis: diagnosis and treatment. Am Fam Physician 76:1323–1330, 2007.

Ramakrishnan, K., and R.C. Salinas. Peptic ulcer disease. Am Fam Physician 76:1005–1012, 2007.

Wald, A. Appropriate use of laxatives in the management of constipation. Curr Gastroenterol Rep 9:410–414, 2007.

CHAPTER 29

Drugs for Headache Disorders

CLASSIFICATION OF DRUGS FOR HEADACHE DISORDERS*

Drugs for Migraine Headaches
Drugs for Preventing Migraine Headaches
Anticonvulsants and Antidepressants
- Divalproex Sodium (DEPAKOTE)
- Amitriptyline (ELAVIL)
- Fluoxetine (PROZAC)
- Phenelzine (NARDIL)

Nonsteroidal Anti-inflammatory Drugs
- Aspirin
- Naproxen (NAPROSYN, ALEVE)
- Fenoprofen (NALFON)[a]

β-Adrenoceptor Antagonists
- Propranolol (INDERAL)
- Timolol (TIMOLIDE)

Calcium Channel Blockers
- Verapamil (CALAN)
- Nimodipine (NIMOTOP)

Serotonin 5-HT$_2$ Receptor Antagonists
- Methysergide (SANSERT)

Other Drugs or Agents for Preventing Migraine
- Gabapentin (NEURONTIN)
- Feverfew/Ginger (GELSTAT MIGRAINE)
- Vitamin B$_2$ (RIBOFLAVIN)

Drugs for Aborting Migraine Headaches
Serotonin 5-HT$_{1D/1B}$ Receptor Agonists
- Dihydroergotamine (DHE 45, MIGRANAL)
- Ergotamine (ERGONAL)
- Sumatriptan (IMITREX)
- Zolmitriptan (ZOMIG)
- Rizatriptan (MAXALT)
- Naratriptan (AMERGE)[b]

Other Drugs for Aborting Migraine
- Isometheptene (MIDRID)
- Tramadol (ULTRAM)
- Butorphanol (STADOL NS)
- Acetaminophen/Codeine (TYLENOL WITH CODEINE #3)
- Acetaminophen/Caffeine/Butalbital (FIORICET)
- Naproxen (NAPROSYN, ALEVE)
- Prochlorperazine (COMPAZINE)

Drugs for Cluster and Tension Headaches
See Table 29–1.

*Note that some drugs are listed more than once.
[a]Also flurbiprofen (ANSAID), ketoprofen (ORUDIS), and mefenamic acid (PONSTEL).
[b]Also frovatriptan (FROVA), almotriptan (AXERT), and eletriptan (RELPAX).

OVERVIEW

An occasional headache suffered by most people is easily remedied by a couple of aspirin or ibuprofen pills and a glass of water. However, for many people, headaches are unremitting, severe, and recurring. The International Headache Society divides headache disorders into two large groups. The first group, primary headache disorders, includes cluster, migraine, and tension headaches. The characteristics and management of these three types of headaches, which

together account for about 95% of all headaches, are compared in Table 29–1. The second group, secondary headache disorders, arises from organic disorders (e.g., hemorrhage, infection, neuropathy, stroke, and tumor). In patients with secondary headaches, management focuses on treating the underlying disorder.

Because migraine is the most serious and common type of headache in patients afflicted with a headache disorder, it is the main focus of the discussion. The chapter closes with a brief review of treatment options for cluster and tension headaches.

TABLE 29–1. **Classification and Pharmacologic Management of Headache Disorders**

Classification	Characteristics	Drugs for Preventing Headaches	Drugs for Aborting Headaches
Primary Headaches			
Cluster headaches	Severe, unilateral, retro-orbital; clustered over time	Lithium, methysergide, and verapamil	DHE, ergotamine, glucocorticoids, lidocaine, oxygen, and sumatriptan
Migraine headaches	Moderate or severe, often unilateral, usually pulsatile; occur with or without aura	β-Adrenoceptor antagonists, anticonvulsants, antidepressants, calcium channel blockers, NSAIDs, and serotonin 5-HT$_2$ receptor antagonists	DHE, ergotamine, isometheptene, NSAIDs, tramadol, and triptans*
Tension headaches	Mild or moderate, bilateral, nonpulsatile; exert band-like pressure	Amitriptyline	Muscle relaxants and NSAIDs
Secondary Headaches	Characteristics vary, depending on the underlying cause†	None	None (treat underlying disorder)

*Triptans include naratriptan, rizatriptan, sumatriptan, and zolmitriptan.
†Examples of causes are hemorrhage, infection, neuropathy, stroke, and tumor.
DHE = dihydroergotamine; NSAIDs = nonsteroidal anti-inflammatory drugs.

CHARACTERISTICS AND PATHOGENESIS OF MIGRAINE HEADACHES

In the United States, approximately 24 million people suffer from migraine headaches (Box 29–1). The pathophysiological mechanisms of migraines are not completely understood, but migraine headaches appear to result from neurovascular dysfunction caused by an imbalance between excitatory and inhibitory neuronal activity at various levels in the central nervous system (CNS). This imbalance can be triggered by hormones, stress, fatigue, hunger, diet, or drugs.

About 15% of patients who have migraine headache disorder report that they experience an **aura** that precedes each headache attack and lasts for about 15 to 20 minutes. A **visual aura** can take the form of brightly flashing lights or rippling images that spread from the corner of the visual field (teichopsia). A **sensory aura** can take the form of paresthesias that involves the arm and face and tends to "march" sequentially from the fingers to the hand and then to the body. Auras are believed to result from the cerebral vasoconstriction and ischemia that precipitate migraine attacks. A migraine without an aura (previously known as a **common migraine**) is often accompanied by an attack of photophobia, phonophobia, nausea, or vomiting.

Each migraine attack has two phases. The **first phase** is characterized by **cerebral vasoconstriction** and **ischemia.** The release of **serotonin** from CNS neurons and circulating platelets contributes to this first phase. Hence, antiplatelet drugs and serotonin receptor antagonists are efficacious in the prevention of migraine headaches. The **second phase,** which is longer than the first one, is characterized by **cerebral vasodilation** and **pain.** The trigeminal neurovascular system appears to play a central role in the second phase. Neurons in the trigeminal complex release vasoactive peptides, including **substance P** and **calcitonin gene-related peptide** (CGRP). These peptides trigger vasodilation and inflammation of pial and dural vessels which, in turn, stimulate nociceptive fibers

of the trigeminal nerve and cause pain. Figure 29–1 depicts these events and the mechanisms of drugs that are used to terminate migraine headaches.

DRUGS FOR MIGRAINE HEADACHES

The drugs used to manage patients with migraine headaches can be classified as **prophylactic drugs** and **abortive (symptomatic) drugs.** Many prophylactic drugs act by preventing the vasoconstrictive phase of the disorder, whereas abortive drugs reverse the vasodilative phase of migraine or relieve pain and inflammation.

Several drugs for migraine are antagonists or agonists at specific types of **serotonin receptors.** These receptors have been classified into four main types, 5-HT$_1$ through 5-HT$_4$.

The **5-HT$_2$ receptors** are widely distributed in the CNS, smooth muscle, and platelets, where they mediate vasoconstriction and platelet aggregation. Drugs that block 5-HT$_2$ receptors, such as **methysergide,** can prevent the vasoconstrictive phase of migraine and are used as migraine prophylactics.

The **5-HT$_1$ receptors** are the predominant serotonin receptors in the CNS, and many of them function as presynaptic autoreceptors whose activation inhibits the release of serotonin and other neurotransmitters. The 5-HT$_1$ receptors also mediate cerebral vasoconstriction. Drugs that activate these receptors, like **sumatriptan,** are used to terminate a migraine attack.

DRUGS FOR MIGRAINE PREVENTION

Numerous classes of drugs are used to prevent migraine headaches in persons who experience frequent attacks. These include anticonvulsants, antidepressants, anti-inflammatory drugs, β-adrenoceptor antagonists, calcium channel blockers,

and serotonin-receptor antagonists. A trial of several different types of drugs may be useful to determine the most effective drug for a particular patient. Each drug requires several weeks of therapy before its effectiveness can be determined.

Anticonvulsants and Antidepressants

The properties of anticonvulsants and antidepressants are described in Chapters 20 and 22, respectively. Studies have shown that these two classes of drugs can prevent migraine in some patients, but the precise mechanisms underlying their effects are poorly understood.

Valproate (DIVALPROEX) is the most widely used anticonvulsant for migraine prophylaxis. Its onset of efficacy (2–3 weeks) is somewhat shorter than that of other prophylactic drugs. Its common adverse effects include sedation, tremor, and weight gain.

Three types of antidepressants can be used to prevent migraine. The first consists of selective serotonin reuptake inhibitors (SSRIs), such as **fluoxetine.** The second consists of tricyclic antidepressants (TCAs). In this second group, tertiary amines such as **amitriptyline** are more potent inhibitors of serotonin reuptake and may be more effective in preventing migraine than are secondary amines such as **desipramine.** The third group consists of monoamine oxidase inhibitors (MAOIs), such as **phenelzine.** MAOIs can block serotonin degradation and are occasionally used in persons who fail to respond to other antidepressants.

Patients must take antidepressants for 3 to 4 weeks before the drugs become effective in preventing headaches, as is the case for alleviating the symptoms of depression. The inhibition of serotonin reuptake by the antidepressants leads to **down-regulation** of postsynaptic serotonin receptors and a compensatory increase in the firing rate of serotonin neurons. The relationship between these actions and migraine prophylaxis, however, is not clearly established.

Serotonin reuptake inhibitors sometimes cause anxiety, insomnia, tremor, anorexia, and sexual dysfunction. TCAs can cause drowsiness, tremor, and anticholinergic effects such as dry mouth, blurred vision, and urinary retention. MAOIs can cause a hypertensive crisis if they are taken with tyramine-containing foods or with sympathomimetic amine drugs (Chapter 22).

Nonsteroidal Anti-inflammatory Drugs

Nonsteroidal anti-inflammatory drugs (NSAIDs), including **naproxen**, can be used for the prevention and treatment of migraine. As discussed in Chapter 30, these drugs act by blocking thromboxane synthesis and platelet aggregation and thereby reducing the release of serotonin. NSAIDs can be used continuously or on an intermittent basis to prevent predictable headaches. For example, administration beginning 1 week before menses and continuing through menstruation may prevent migraine headaches associated with the menstrual cycle.

β-Adrenoceptor Antagonists

Of the various types of β-adrenoceptor antagonists that are available (see Chapter 9), only the β-blockers that lack intrinsic sympathomimetic activity are effective for the prevention of migraine headaches. One example of effective β-blockers is **timolol.** Another example, **propranolol**, is widely used for migraine prophylaxis but can cause more CNS side effects than timolol.

The mechanism of action of β-blockers in migraine prophylaxis is uncertain. These drugs may attenuate the **second phase** of migraine by **blocking vasodilation** mediated by β₂-adrenoceptors. They may also reduce platelet aggregation and thereby decrease the release of serotonin from platelets.

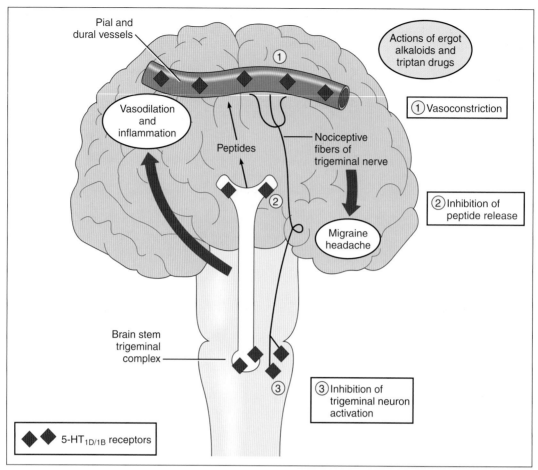

Figure 29-1. **Mechanisms of ergot alkaloids and triptan drugs used in the treatment of migraine headache disorder.** Migraine attacks are thought to result from trigeminal neurovascular dysfunction. When neurons in the trigeminal complex release peptides such as substance P and calcitonin gene-related peptide (CGRP), this causes vasodilation and inflammation of pial and dural vessels. These events activate nociceptive trigeminal fibers and cause the moderate to severe pain that is characteristic of migraine headaches. Ergot alkaloids and triptan drugs terminate the pain by activating serotonin 5-HT$_{1B/1D}$ receptors at several sites: (1) They activate receptors on pial and dural vessels and thereby cause vasoconstriction. (2) They activate presynaptic receptors to inhibit the release of peptides and other mediators from trigeminal neurons. (3) They activate receptors in the brain stem, which is believed to inhibit activation of trigeminal neurons responsible for migraine attacks.

Calcium Channel Blockers

Although **verapamil** and other calcium channel blockers are used for migraine prophylaxis, there is evidence that the calcium channel blockers are less effective in preventing migraine attacks than are other classes of drugs.

Calcium channel blockers may be effective in migraines by preventing the **vasoconstrictive phase** of migraine headaches. The properties of these drugs are described in Chapter 10.

5-HT$_2$ Receptor Antagonists

Methysergide is a drug that blocks 5-HT$_2$ receptors and thereby prevents the vasoconstrictive phase of migraine from occurring. Because of the potential toxicity of methysergide, however, other prophylactic drugs are usually chosen initially for migraine prophylaxis.

The drug is associated with a number of relatively mild adverse effects, including abdominal pain, weight gain, and hallucinations. It is also associated with a risk of life-threatening retroperitoneal, pleural, and cardiac valve **fibrosis**. For this

reason, it should not be used longer than 6 months without a drug-free period of one month that begins with a 2-week period of decreasing dosage. Serum creatinine measurements should be monitored and a chest x-ray taken periodically to detect early signs of fibrosis in patients treated with methysergide.

Other Agents for Migraine Prevention

Gabapentin is an agent approved for the treatment of seizure disorders (see Chapter 20) and postherpetic neuralgia. It is moderately effective with little adverse effects in preventing occurrence of migraines. Although gabapentin is known to enhance γ-aminobutyric acid (GABA) action in the treatment of seizure disorder, its actions in migraine treatment are unclear.

The result of a double-blind, placebo-controlled study of patients with migraines showed that **riboflavin (vitamin B$_2$)** can significantly reduce the frequency and duration of migraine attacks. This study found that a daily dose of riboflavin

at 400 mg produced a significant decrease in the number of migraine attacks as well as the total days with headache pain. The effect was not evident until after 2 months of administration, however, and the mechanism of action is unknown.

Feverfew is an herbal remedy that has low to moderate efficacy in preventing migraines with little side effects. It is available without a prescription as a combination of the extracts of *Pyrethrum parthenium* (feverfew) and *Zingiber officinale* (ginger) in a rapidly dissolving formulation. The active ingredient in feverfew is **parthenolide**, which has anti-inflammatory activity. As with NSAIDs, parthenolide may prevent inflammation associated with migraine headaches.

DRUGS FOR MIGRAINE TERMINATION

Numerous drugs can be used to terminate a migraine headache after it has begun. Most of these drugs are serotonin 5-HT$_{1D/1B}$ receptor agonists, and their sites of action are shown in Figure 29–1.

5-HT$_{1D/1B}$ Receptor Agonists

Ergot Agents

Ergotamine and **dihydroergotamine (DHE)** are **ergot alkaloids** and are effective in the treatment of migraine headaches and cluster headaches. A number of other ergot alkaloids are available and are used in the treatment of Parkinson's disease, hyperprolactinemia, and other disorders. The potent hallucinogen lysergic acid diethylamide (LSD) is also an ergot derivative.

MECHANISM OF ACTION. Ergotamine and DHE are isolated from substances produced by *Claviceps purpurea*, a fungus first discovered growing on rye grain. Ergotamine and DHE relieve migraine primarily by activating **serotonin 5-HT$_{1D/1B}$ receptors** at several levels in the trigeminal neurovascular system. Agonist activity at 5-HT$_{1D/1B}$ receptors in cerebral blood vessels produces **vasoconstriction**, thereby reversing the vasodilation that contributes to the throbbing migraine headache. Stimulation of presynaptic 5-HT$_{1D/1B}$ receptors on trigeminal nerve endings also inhibits the release of peptides that cause vasodilation, neurogenic inflammation, and pain. Finally, stimulation of 5-HT$_{1D/1B}$ receptors in the brain stem prevents activation of pain fibers in trigeminal nerves involved in migraine headache.

PHARMACOKINETIC AND PHARMACOLOGIC EFFECTS. The ergot alkaloids are most effective when they are given early in a migraine attack.

Ergotamine is marketed in parenteral, oral, and rectal formulations. When it is given orally, it has a relatively slow onset of action because of its poor oral bioavailability. Although it is available as a rectal suppository for use by patients with nausea and vomiting, it can actually worsen these symptoms by stimulating the vomiting center. Some oral and rectal ergotamine preparations contain caffeine, which appears to increase the absorption of ergotamine

and may also exert a mild vasoconstrictive effect that helps relieve migraine.

Dihydroergotamine is available in intranasal and injectable preparations. The intranasal preparation, which was recently approved by the FDA, offers patients a convenient method of administering DHE and has a moderately rapid onset of action. The injectable DHE preparation, which is usually more rapid acting and reliable than the various ergotamine preparations, can be administered subcutaneously, intramuscularly, or intravenously. When administered parenterally, DHE is often given with an antiemetic drug, such as the dopamine receptor antagonist, **metoclopramide**, to prevent drug-induced nausea and vomiting.

ADVERSE EFFECTS. The relatively mild adverse effects of ergot alkaloids include nausea and vomiting, diarrhea, muscle cramps, cold skin, paresthesias, and vertigo.

Ergotamine and DHE can cause peripheral vasoconstriction by stimulating α_1-adrenoceptors and by directly stimulating vascular smooth muscle. These drugs, therefore, are contraindicated in persons with coronary artery disease or peripheral vascular disease. Excessive doses of ergotamine or DHE can cause severe cerebral vasoconstriction, ischemia, and rebound vasodilation and headache. A rebound headache can last several days, and hospitalization may be required to wean the patient from ergotamine and alleviate the pain. Strict dosage guidelines must be followed to prevent rebound headache and other forms of toxicity. To prevent cumulative toxicity, daily use of ergotamine should be avoided.

INTERACTIONS. Concomitant use of **ergot alkaloids** and **β-adrenoceptor antagonists** can cause severe peripheral ischemia resulting from α-adrenoceptor–mediated vasoconstriction that is unopposed by β_2-adrenoceptor–mediated vasodilation. Hence, this drug combination should be avoided.

Triptan Agents

Sumatriptan was the first of a new group of selective serotonin 5-HT$_{1D/1B}$ agonists to be developed for the treatment of migraines. The class of **triptan drugs** is now quite numerous and includes **naratriptan, rizatriptan,** and **zolmitriptan.** Although these four triptans have amassed the most data on their effectiveness in aborting a migraine attack, newer agents, such as **frovatriptan, almotriptan,** and **eletriptan,** are also available. The newer triptans are similar to sumatriptan, but their improved pharmacokinetic properties may be advantageous in some cases.

MECHANISM OF ACTION. Sumatriptan and other 5-HT$_{1D/1B}$ agonists are structural analogues of serotonin. Their mechanisms for terminating migraine headaches appear to be similar to those of ergotamine and DHE (see above).

PHARMACOKINETIC AND PHARMACOLOGIC EFFECTS. A sumatriptan preparation for subcutaneous administration was introduced in 1992, and oral and intranasal preparations were introduced several years later. Peak plasma levels of sumatriptan are achieved most rapidly with subcutaneous administration and least rapidly with oral administration. Relief of migraine usually takes an hour when the drug is given subcutaneously but can take up to 2 hours when it is given orally.

Naratriptan, **rizatriptan**, and **zolmitriptan** are currently limited to oral administration. In comparison with sumatriptan, these newer triptan drugs are more lipophilic, have higher oral bioavailabilities, and achieve higher concentrations in the CNS. The finding that they penetrate the CNS more readily may enable them to inhibit the brain stem mechanisms involved in migraine more effectively than does sumatriptan.

In a clinical trial comparing the effects of sumatriptan treatment with those of DHE treatment in patients who suffer from migraine headache disorder, subcutaneously administered sumatriptan was found to relieve 85% of migraine attacks and to be slightly superior to DHE in this regard. Nevertheless, studies show that sumatriptan is not efficacious in 10% to 20% of patients who have migraine headache disorder, and about 40% of patients who initially obtain relief with sumatriptan have a **recurrence** of their headache on the same day. Recurrences are more prevalent in patients who have more severe and longer attacks. If a headache recurs, treatment can be repeated at specified intervals until a maximal daily dose of sumatriptan has been administered. Because sumatriptan and other triptan drugs cost more than ergotamine alkaloids, the need to repeat doses may be a factor in drug selection.

According to some clinical trials, the newer triptans have a 10% to 20% greater efficacy than sumatriptan, and their rates of headache recurrence are lower (30% for newer triptans vs. 40% for sumatriptan). **Naratriptan** has a **longer half-life** than sumatriptan, and this may explain its lower rate of headache recurrence. Further clinical studies are needed to confirm these differences.

ADVERSE EFFECTS AND INTERACTIONS. In clinical trials, the incidence of chest tightness, weakness, somnolence, and dizziness in subjects treated with a triptan agent was nearly 50%, whereas the incidence in subjects treated with a placebo was about 30%. The incidence of adverse effects appears to be similar for all triptan drugs.

The triptans have been reported to cause abnormal tingling or burning sensations (paresthesias) in the skin on various parts of the body. These sensations are benign, but they can be mistaken for a serious adverse effect by the patient.

Triptan drugs can cause **coronary vasospasm** and should not be used in patients with a history of angina pectoris, myocardial infarction, or other coronary artery disease. As with ergots, triptan agents can increase blood pressure so they should not be given to patients with uncontrolled hypertension. The triptans should not be used concurrently with MAOI, nor should they be used within 24 hours of administering an ergot alkaloid or methysergide. Use of triptans with SSRI antidepressant agents, such as **duloxetine** or **fluoxetine**, increases the risk of triggering a **serotonin syndrome** (see Chapter 22).

Other Drugs for Migraine Termination

An NSAID, such as **naproxen**, can be used either to prevent or to abort a migraine attack. Combination formulations of acetaminophen, butalbital (a barbiturate), and caffeine are also effective in aborting migraine headaches.

Isometheptene, an agent that acts as a sympathomimetic, can terminate migraine headaches. It is available in a preparation that also contains acetaminophen and a mild sedative drug.

Opioid analgesics can relieve the pain of migraine headaches, but their use should be reserved for patients in whom other agents are contraindicated or ineffective. **Tramadol** has been particularly useful in chronic pain syndromes (see Chapter 23) and is one of the most widely used opioid drugs for the treatment of migraine. Tramadol is an agonist at *mu* opioid receptors, and it also inhibits norepinephrine and serotonin reuptake in the CNS. The latter action may contribute to the drug's analgesic effect. **Butorphanol** acts as an agonist at *kappa* opioid receptors and a mixed agonist-antagonist at *mu* opioid receptors. It is available in a nasal spray formulation for rapid onset of action. **Acetaminophen with codeine**, or other NSAID-opioid combinations, is also effective in patients resistant to other drug treatments.

The antipsychotic agent **prochlorperazine** is effective in aborting unremitting migraine headache when given intravenously.

GUIDELINES FOR MANAGING MIGRAINE HEADACHES

Prophylactic Treatment of Migraines

Nonpharmacologic measures can play a significant role in the prevention of migraine attacks. These measures include appropriate patient education; the identification and avoidance of factors that contribute to migraine attacks, including particular foods, beverages, and environmental factors; biofeedback and relaxation therapy; and psychotherapy. Acupuncture and physiotherapy may be beneficial, but their efficacy is not established in controlled, clinical trials.

Many pharmacologic agents are known to **prevent migraine attacks**. The efficacy of these agents varies from patient to patient, however, so finding a drug that works well is largely a matter of trial and error. The characteristics of individual patients should help guide drug selection. For example, β-blockers have negative effects on cardiac output, so they are usually less suitable than other drugs for competitive athletes. The goal of prophylactic drug use is to reduce the frequency of migraine attacks by at least 50%, and the criteria for evaluating the efficacy of particular drugs should be clearly established and understood by the physician and patient. It usually takes 3 to 4 weeks of therapy before the benefit of a given drug is observed, so authorities recommend a trial of 4 to 6 weeks before switching to another drug.

Acute Treatment of Migraines

The ideal drug to terminate migraine headaches would act rapidly, be highly efficacious, and have a low potential to cause serious adverse effects. No available drug meets all of these criteria. The newer serotonin agonists (triptans) appear to be **less toxic** and slightly more effective than the ergot preparations. DHE, however, has the advantage of a longer duration of action than the triptan drugs. Intranasal preparations of sumatriptan and DHE offer a more rapid onset of action than do oral preparations, and they are more convenient than parenteral therapy.

The optimal use of abortive treatment requires prudent drug selection and reasonable restrictions on drug use to avoid **toxicity** or **habituation**. The effectiveness of a given drug varies widely from patient to patient, so a judicious trial of several drugs is usually required to determine the most effective drug for a particular patient. Some authorities recommend starting abortive therapy with an NSAID (e.g., naproxen). If use of an NSAID consistently fails to relieve pain within an hour, then the patient should be encouraged to switch to a different agent, such as a triptan drug or DHE. Although this approach may work well for some patients, others may derive more benefit from the initial use of a triptan or DHE. To evaluate the effects of drug therapy, the patient should be instructed to keep an accurate log of drug dosage and symptom severity, especially during a trial period.

The overuse of abortive drugs can lead to serious toxicity, so patients must be properly instructed about limiting their use of these drugs. According to the guidelines of the National Headache Foundation, patients should limit their use of **ergotamine** to 8 treatment days per month, with an ample interval between treatment days. They should limit their use of **sumatriptan** and other triptan drugs to 6 treatment days per month and 2 treatment days per week, and they should limit their use of opioid drugs to 2 treatment days per week.

CHARACTERISTICS AND TREATMENT OF CLUSTER HEADACHES

Cluster headaches are severe, unilateral, **retro-orbital headaches** that tend to group or cluster over time. Patients often describe a searing or burning pain that arises behind one eye, occurs without warning, and can be excruciating. Pain often lasts from 15 minutes to 3 hours and usually occurs at the same time each day. Unlike patients with migraine headaches, who are highly sensitive to movement and external stimuli, those with cluster headaches often pace in an agitated fashion, apply pressure to the orbit, or even strike the face to provide distraction from the pain. The incidence of cluster headache disorder is low, however, affecting less than 0.5% of the population.

Drugs to prevent cluster headaches include **lithium** (see Chapter 22), **methysergide**, and **verapamil**. As with migraine headaches, cluster headaches can be aborted by administering DHE, ergotamine, or sumatriptan. Other agents that are effective in aborting cluster headaches include inhaled oxygen, intranasal lidocaine, and glucocorticoids. Guidelines for selecting drugs to manage cluster headaches are similar to those outlined above for migraine headaches.

CHARACTERISTICS AND TREATMENT OF TENSION HEADACHES

Tension headaches are characterized by bilateral, nonpulsatile, **band-like** pressure that is mild or moderate in intensity. This common type of headache often responds to physiological approaches that correct cervical or dental alignment or visual refractive error. Nonpharmacologic therapies (e.g., biofeedback, acupuncture, and physiotherapy) are also useful in controlling both episodic and chronic tension headaches. Pharmacological therapy usually consists of NSAIDs and muscle relaxants, but patients with chronic tension headaches may also respond to prophylactic use of **amitriptyline**. This drug is usually tolerated well when therapy is initiated with a low dose at bedtime, and the dosage is gradually increased over a period of several weeks.

SUMMARY OF IMPORTANT POINTS

■ Migraine, the most common headache disorder, is believed to result from neurovascular dysfunction at several levels in the CNS. Cerebral vasoconstriction and ischemia are followed by vasodilation, inflammation, and a unilateral, pulsatile headache.

■ Drugs for migraine prophylaxis should aim to reduce the frequency of migraine attacks by 50%. These include anticonvulsants (valproate), antidepressants (amitriptyline and fluoxetine), NSAIDs (naproxen), β-adrenoceptor antagonists (propranolol, timolol), calcium channel blockers (verapamil, nimodipine), and serotonin 5-HT$_2$ receptor antagonists (methysergide).

■ Prophylactic drugs often must be taken for 3 to 4 weeks before benefits are observed.

■ Drugs for aborting migraine headaches include ergot alkaloids (ergotamine and dihydroergotamine) and so-called triptan drugs (sumatriptan and others). These drugs act primarily by stimulating serotonin 5-HT$_{1D/1B}$ receptors. This stimulation causes cerebral vasoconstriction, inhibits the release of peptides and other mediators of inflammation and vasodilation from trigeminal neurons, and inhibits activation of the trigeminal nucleus in the brain stem.

■ Ergot alkaloids and triptan drugs can cause marked vasoconstriction, so their dosage and frequency of use must be restricted to avoid rebound headache and adverse effects. Common adverse effects of ergots include nausea, vomiting, and muscle cramps; those of triptans include chest tightness and drowsiness. Use of ergots or triptans is contraindicated in patients with coronary artery disease.

■ Other agents for aborting migraine headaches include NSAIDs (e.g., naproxen), opioid analgesics (e.g., tramadol), and a sympathomimetic drug called isometheptene.

■ Cluster headaches can be prevented with lithium, methysergide, or verapamil. They can be terminated with ergot alkaloids, sumatriptan, inhaled oxygen, intranasal lidocaine, or glucocorticoids.

■ Tension headaches often respond to NSAIDs and muscle relaxants. Nonpharmacologic therapies (e.g., biofeedback and physiotherapy) are also useful.

Review Questions

1. Which of the following agents has not shown effectiveness in the prophylactic treatment of migraine headache?
   (A) zolmitriptan
   (B) methysergide
   (C) verapamil
   (D) naproxen
   (E) amitriptyline

2. Use of sumatriptan is contraindicated in which one of the following conditions?
   (A) postpartum women
   (B) uncontrolled hypertension
   (C) moderate to unresponsive severe migraines
   (D) hepatic insufficiency
   (E) renal dysfunction

3. The therapeutic effect of the triptan class of drugs is caused by which mechanism of action?
   (A) antagonism at serotonin 5-HT$_2$ receptors
   (B) stimulation of serotonin 5-HT$_{1D}$ receptors
   (C) antagonism at dopamine receptors
   (D) antagonism at α-adrenoceptors
   (E) direct inhibition of substance P receptors in the vasculature

4. Methysergide is indicated for the treatment of migraine because it has which one of the following effects?
   (A) it prevents the release of serotonin
   (B) it is a 5-HT$_{1B/D}$ agonist
   (C) it inhibits the COX-2 enzyme
   (D) it is an antagonist at 5-HT$_2$ receptors
   (E) it blocks calcium channels

5. A 35-year-old woman with a history of migraine reports to her physician that the last time she used her medicine to stop an acute attack, she felt numbness and tingling in her extremities and blanching and cyanosis of her fingers. Which one of the following medications did she take?
   (A) methysergide
   (B) sumatriptan
   (C) dihydroergotamine
   (D) tramadol
   (E) naproxen

Answers and Explanations

1. **The correct answer is A:** zolmitriptan. The triptan agents are only effective in the acute treatment of a migraine headache. They are agonists at 5-HT$_{1B/1D}$ receptors in cerebral blood vessels that produce vasoconstriction, on trigeminal nerve endings inhibiting the release of inflammatory substances, and in the brain stem to prevent activation of trigeminal nerves. Answers (B) through (E) have shown various degrees of effectiveness in preventing migraines in controlled studies.

2. **The correct choice is B:** uncontrolled hypertension. Triptans can increase blood pressure by constriction of peripheral smooth muscle. This is also a contraindication for using ergot agents such as DHE and ergotamine. Answers (A), (C), (D), and (E) are not conditions warranting contraindications for triptan use.

3. **The correct answer is B:** stimulation of serotonin 5-HT$_{1D}$ receptors. These agents are agonists at 5-HT$_{1B/1D}$ receptors. Answers (A) and (C) through (E) are mechanisms of other agents unrelated to the clinically used triptan drugs.

4. **The correct answer is D:** it is an antagonist at 5-HT$_2$ receptors. Methysergide is indicated for the treatment of migraine or, better stated, the prophylactic treatment to prevent migraine attacks because of its antagonist activity at serotonin receptors. Other answer choices are not the primary mechanism of action of methysergide.

5. **The correct choice is C:** dihydroergotamine. DHE is an ergot alkaloid, and these agents are known to cause vasoconstriction and paresthesia in the extremities, especially at high doses. Answer (A), methysergide, is also an ergot but is not used for acute treatment of migraine attacks. Answer (B), sumatriptan, is a triptan also used for acute attacks and can cause vasoconstriction, but not as commonly as observed with DHE. Answer (D), tramadol, is a dual-action opioid-antidepressant agent, helpful in the acute treatment of migraine but not producing the patient's constellation of adverse effects. Answer (E), naproxen, is an NSAID agent that can cause increased release of norepinephrine and possible vasoconstriction, but it does not produce these effects as commonly as DHE.

SELECTED READINGS

Ashkenazi, A., and S. Silberstein. Botulinum toxin type A for the treatment of headache: why we say yes. Arch Neurol. 65:146–149, 2008.

Beck, E., W.J. Sieber, and R. Trejo. Management of cluster headache. Am Fam Physician 71(4):717–724, 2005.

Colombo, B., P.O. Annovazzi, and G. Comi. Therapy of primary headaches: the role of antidepressants. Neurol Sci 25(Suppl 3):S171–S175, 2004.

Lipton, R.B., and M.E. Bigal. Headache: triumphs in translational research. Lancet Neurol 4(1):11–12, 2005.

Peres, M.F., A.L. Gonçalves, and A. Krymchantowski. Migraine, tension-type headache, and transformed migraine. Curr Pain Headache Rep 11:449–453, 2007.

CHAPTER 30

Drugs for Pain, Inflammation, and Arthritic Disorders

CLASSIFICATION OF DRUGS FOR PAIN, INFLAMMATION, AND ARTHRITIC DISORDERS*

Nonsteroidal Anti-inflammatory Drugs (NSAIDS)
Nonselective Cyclooxygenase Inhibitors
- Aspirin and Other Salicylates
- Acetaminophen (Tylenol)
- Ibuprofen (Motrin, Advil)
- Ketoprofen (Orudis)
- Naproxen (Naprosyn, Aleve)[a]

Selective Cyclooxygenase-2 Inhibitors
- Celecoxib (Celebrex)

Disease-modifying Antirheumatic Drugs (DMARDS)
Gold Salts
- Auranofin (Ridaura)
- Gold Sodium Thiomalate (Myochrysine, Aurolate)
- Aurothioglucose (Solganal)

Glucocorticoids
- Prednisone (Deltasone)

Other Disease-Modifying Antirheumatic Drugs
- Methotrexate (Rheumatrex)
- Leflunomide (Arava)
- Hydroxychloroquine (Plaquenil)
- Penicillamine (Cuprimine)
- Sulfasalazine (Azulfidine)
- Etanercept (Enbrel)[b]

Drugs for Gout
Drugs to Prevent Gout Attacks
- Probenecid (Benemid)
- Sulfinpyrazone (Anturane)
- Allopurinol (Zyloprim)

Drugs to Treat Gout Attacks
- Colchicine
- Indomethacin and Other Nsaids

*Note that some drugs are listed more than once.
[a]Also indomethacin (Indocin), sulindac (Clinoril), ketorolac (Toradol), piroxicam (Feldene), nabumetone (Relafen), etodolac (Lodine), meloxicam (Mobic), and diclofenac (Flector, Voltaren Gel).
[b]Also infliximab (Remicade), adalimumab (Humira), anakinra (Kineret), and abatacept (Orencia).

OVERVIEW

A variety of medical disorders and injuries are characterized by pain and inflammation. This chapter describes the pharmacologic properties of nonsteroidal anti-inflammatory drugs (NSAIDs), which are widely used to alleviate the symptoms of rheumatoid arthritis, osteoarthritis, and gout, as well as to relieve the pain and fever that accompany many nonarthritic disorders. They are also used by millions on a daily basis for the occasional headache. The chapter also discusses disease-modifying antirheumatic drugs (DMARDs) and drugs for the prevention and treatment of gout.

RHEUMATOID ARTHRITIS

Rheumatoid arthritis (RA) is an **autoimmune disorder** of unknown etiology. The hallmark symptom of RA is joint inflammation, and most patients with RA experience a chronic, fluctuating course of disease that, despite therapeutic measures, can result in progressive joint destruction, deformity, disability, and premature death. RA affects 2% to 3% of the U.S. population, making it the **most common systemic inflammatory disease** (Box 30–1). It is three times more common in women than in men. RA is characterized by **symmetrical joint inflammation** that most frequently affects the small joints of the hands, wrists, and feet, but also the joints of the ankles, elbows, hips, knees, and shoulders. Cardiopulmonary, neurologic, and ocular inflammation are also often found in patients with RA, and many patients develop **rheumatoid nodules** on the extensor surfaces of the elbows, forearms, and hands. In addition, many patients have extra-articular manifestations, such as vasculitis, lymphadenopathy, and splenomegaly.

As shown in Figure 30–1, RA is triggered by **autoimmune mechanisms** that lead to the destruction of synovial tissue and other connective tissue. Both humoral and cellular immune mechanisms are involved in the pathogenesis of the disease. These mechanisms include the cytokine-mediated activation of T and B lymphocytes and the recruitment and activation of macrophages. The inflammatory

leukocytes then release a variety of prostaglandins, cytotoxic compounds, and free radicals that cause joint inflammation and destruction. Patients with RA show elevated levels of immunoglobulin G-rheumatoid factor (IgG-RF) complexes; extracorporeal filtering of these complexes using immuno-absorption **apheresis** has helped some patients.

In patients with RA, NSAIDs are used to relieve pain and inflammation, and DMARDs are used to suppress the underlying disease process and slow the progression of joint destruction. The sites of action of selected antirheumatic drugs are depicted in Figure 30–1 and discussed below.

OSTEOARTHRITIS

Osteoarthritis, also called **degenerative joint disease**, is the most common joint disease in the world. It affects about 10% of persons over 60 years of age, and radiographic evidence of osteoarthritis can be found in most persons over 65. However, the disease is not simply associated with the aging process. Other factors that increase the risk for osteoarthritis include obesity, osteoporosis, smoking, heredity, repetitive use of joints through work or leisure activities, and joint trauma.

Osteoarthritis primarily affects **weight-bearing joints** and causes deformity, limitation of motion, and progressive disability. The cartilage undergoes thickening, inflammation, splitting, and thinning. Eventually, the cartilaginous layer is completely destroyed, leading to erosion and microfractures in the underlying bone. The major symptoms of osteoarthritis are **pain**, **stiffness**, and **muscle weakness** around affected joints.

Nonpharmacologic measures for treating osteoarthritis include joint protection and splinting, physiotherapy, orthotic prostheses to support the feet, and joint replacement surgery. Pharmacologic measures include NSAIDs, local glucocorticoid injections, and experimental chondroprotective drugs (e.g., chondroitin sulfate and glucosamine). Recently, sodium **hyaluronate** (Supartz) was approved for intra-articular injection as a type of joint fluid replacement in the treatment of osteoarthritis. It is a sterile, viscoelastic solution prepared from chicken combs (the fleshy growths on top of chicken heads).

GOUT

Gout is an arthritic syndrome caused by an inflammatory response to crystals of **monosodium urate monohydrate** in joints, renal tubules, and other tissues. The deposition of these crystals occurs as a consequence of **hyperuricemia**, which can result from overproduction or underexcretion of uric acid. Other risk factors for gout include **obesity, alcohol consumption**, and **hypertension**.

Acute gout is treated with an NSAID or colchicine to relieve joint inflammation. Subsequent attacks of gout can be prevented by long-term therapy with a drug that either increases uric acid excretion or inhibits uric acid formation and thereby reduces the serum level of uric acid.

> ### BOX 30–1. THE CASE OF THE ACHING ARTHRITIC
>
> **CASE PRESENTATION:** A 52-year-old woman complains of sore knees and wrists that are not related to physical activity. Her physician notes that both right and left joints are affected and appear reddened and swollen. She has round, painless nodules under the skin and tells her physician that the pain is worse in the morning. The physician orders joint x-rays, a synovial fluid draw, and a blood test for rheumatic factor. All three studies come back positive for RA, so the doctor prescribes celecoxib for the pain and inflammation and methotrexate to slow the progression of the disease.
>
> **CASE DISCUSSION:** Rheumatoid arthritis (RA) is a common disease, affecting more than two million people in the United States; it is three times more likely to be found in women than in men. RA is an autoimmune disease that causes chronic, symmetrical inflammation of the joints. The disease can begin at any age, but most often starts after age 40 and before age 60. There are two main classes of medications used in treating RA: the anti-inflammatory agents, such as celecoxib, aspirin, or cortisone, used to reduce pain and inflammation; and the DMARD agents, such as methotrexate, leflunomide, hydroxychloroquine, and others, which promote disease remission and prevent progressive joint destruction. Newer immunomodulating DMARD agents are administered by the intravenous route and include infliximab, anakinra, adalimumab, and others. Methotrexate is the most common DMARD used to treat RA, and the use of the selective COX-2 inhibitor, celecoxib, is warranted given no stated history of cardiovascular disease in the patient.

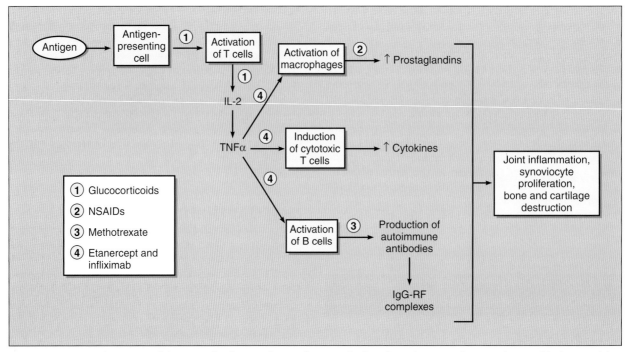

Figure 30–1. **Pathogenesis of rheumatoid arthritis and sites of action of selected antirheumatic drugs.** In this simplified view of the immune system, antigen-presenting cells phagocytose antigens and present them to T cells, thereby activating the T cells. Activated T cells produce cytokines (IL-2, IL-1, TNF-α, and others) that stimulate the production of B and T cells. B cells produce plasma cells that form antibodies. Helper T cells activate macrophages and cytotoxic T cells. Together, T cells, macrophages, and cytotoxic T cells produce cytotoxic cytokines and prostaglandins that cause joint inflammation, synovial proliferation, and bone and cartilage destruction. Glucocorticoids inhibit T-cell activation and interleukin-2 (IL-2) production by regulation of gene transcription. Glucocorticoids and nonsteroidal anti-inflammatory drugs (NSAIDs) inhibit the formation of prostaglandins. Methotrexate inhibits the proliferation and activity of T cells and B cells. Etanercept and infliximab inactivate a cytokine called tumor necrosis factor-α (TNF-α). Immunoglobulin G-rheumatoid factor (IgG-RF) complexes are detected in the blood of patients with rheumatoid arthritis.

NONSTEROIDAL ANTI-INFLAMMATORY DRUGS

MECHANISM OF ACTION

The nonsteroidal anti-inflammatory drugs comprise a large family of weak acidic drugs whose pharmacological effects result primarily from the inhibition of **cyclooxygenase (COX)**, an enzyme that catalyzes the first step in the synthesis of **prostaglandins** from arachidonic acid and other precursor fatty acids (see Chapter 26). COX is a microsomal enzyme, existing as a dimer (two molecules linked to form a functional unit) in the lumen and membrane of the endoplasmic reticulum. NSAIDs decrease COX activity primarily by competitive inhibition; however, aspirin forms a covalent, irreversible inhibition of COX (Fig. 30–2). The net effect of NSAID administration is a decrease in the production of prostaglandins and other autacoids.

Prostaglandin Effects

Prostaglandins play an important role in the development of pain, inflammation, and fever. Prostaglandins are released from cells in response to chemical stimuli or physical trauma. They sensitize sensory nerve endings to nociceptive stimuli and thereby amplify the generation of pain impulses. They also promote tissue **inflammation** by stimulating inflammatory cell chemotaxis, causing vasodilation and increasing capillary permeability and edema.

Fever, defined as the elevation of body temperature to a level above 37° C (98.6° F), often results from an alteration of hypothalamic thermoregulatory mechanisms. Bacterial toxins and other **pyrogens** stimulate the production of cytokines by leukocytes, and these cytokines increase prostaglandin synthesis in the preoptic area of the hypothalamus. The prostaglandins then act to reset the body's thermostat to a new point above 37° C. This, in turn, activates temperature-raising mechanisms, such as a reduction in heat loss via cutaneous vasodilation, and causes the temperature to rise. All NSAIDs relieve fever by inhibiting prostaglandin synthesis in the hypothalamus, but these drugs are not capable of reducing body temperature below normal.

Cyclooxygenase Isozymes

Cyclooxygenase is now known to occur in two major isoforms: **cyclooxygenase-1 (COX-1)** and **cyclooxygenase-2 (COX-2)**. COX-1 is a **constitutive** or "housekeeping" enzyme that is found in relatively constant levels in various tissues. COX-1 participates in the synthesis of prostaglandins that have a cytoprotective effect on the gastrointestinal (GI) tract. It also catalyzes the formation of thromboxane A_2 in platelets, leading to platelet aggregation and hemostasis. In contrast, COX-2 is an **inducible** enzyme. Its levels are normally very low in most tissues but are rapidly up-regulated during the inflammatory process by proinflammatory substances (e.g., cytokines, endotoxins, and tumor promoters). Both COX-1 and COX-2 appear to participate in renal homeostasis.

Most of the NSAIDs available today are nonselective inhibitors of COX-1 and COX-2. The discovery of COX isozymes led to the development of selective COX-2 inhibitors, the first one being **celecoxib**. These selective inhibitors are effective anti-inflammatory drugs, and they produce less GI bleeding and ulcers than do the nonselective COX inhibitors.

A third COX isozyme (**COX-3**), which was recently discovered, appears to be an alternative splice variant of COX-1. **Acetaminophen** potently inhibits COX-3, and this finding likely explains the reason that acetaminophen has little anti-inflammatory action.

SPECIFIC AGENTS

Nonselective Cyclooxygenase Inhibitors

Among the nonselective COX inhibitors are many well-known NSAIDs that are available without a prescription, including aspirin, ibuprofen, ketoprofen, and naproxen. Acetaminophen is a **weak anti-inflammatory** agent, but it is also included in this class of drugs because it exerts **analgesic** and **antipyretic** effects via inhibition of COX. As shown in Table 30–1, NSAIDs vary greatly in potency and half-life, but most of them are administered from two to four times a day with food.

Lower doses of NSAIDs are usually sufficient to treat **mild to moderate pain** and counteract **fever**, whereas higher doses are generally needed to relieve **inflammation** associated with arthritic disorders and injuries. NSAIDs are particularly effective in **relieving pain** caused by **tissue inflammation** or bone or joint trauma, and they can be combined with opioid analgesics to obtain a greater analgesic effect and reduce the need for higher doses of opioids. For example, NSAIDs are widely used in the treatment of postoperative pain, either alone or in combination with an **opioid**.

Although NSAIDs are effective in relieving the pain of chronic disorders, their long-term use is associated with a number of **adverse effects**, including GI bleeding, peptic ulcers, and renal and hepatic dysfunction. **Acetaminophen**

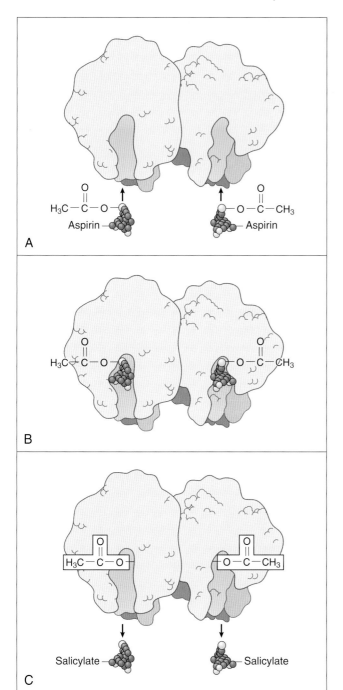

Figure 30-2. **Mechanism of action for aspirin.** (A) The COX enzyme exists as a homodimer with two interlocking identical molecules each providing an active channel for its substrates. Aspirin is chemically known as acetylsalicylic acid. (B) Aspirin molecules enter the active channel of COX and add an acetyl group to an amino acid R-group in the active site of COX. The acetyl group is attached to serine at the 530 position in COX-1 and to serine at the 516 position in COX-2. This produces irreversible or noncompetitive inhibition. (C) The aspirin molecule without the acetyl group is called salicylic acid or salicylate, which is a competitive inhibitor of COX.

TABLE 30-1.	Properties of Nonsteroidal Anti-inflammatory Drugs		
Drug	**Relative Potency**	**Half-Life (Hours)**	**Daily Doses**
Nonselective COX Inhibitors			
Acetaminophen	1	3	4
Aspirin	1	2*	4
Ibuprofen	4	2	2–4
Indomethacin	40	4	1–3
Ketoprofen	20	2	2–4
Ketorolac	100	7	4
Naproxen	4	14	2
Selective COX-2 Inhibitors			
Celecoxib	20	11	2

*For aspirin, the value shown is the half-life of the active metabolite, salicylic acid.
COX = cyclooxygenase.

produces fewer GI problems than do other nonselective COX inhibitors, but it also lacks significant antiplatelet and anti-inflammatory activity. Although acetaminophen can be used concurrently with another NSAID for supplemental analgesia, alternative combinations of two NSAIDs should generally be avoided, not only because they increase the risk of GI and other side effects but also because they sometimes have **adverse interactions**. For example, aspirin and other salicylates displace some NSAIDs (e.g., ketorolac) from plasma proteins and thereby increase their serum levels significantly.

The NSAIDs can interact with a large number of other drugs through pharmacokinetic and pharmacodynamic mechanisms. Most NSAIDs inhibit the renal excretion of **lithium** and can increase lithium serum levels and toxicity. NSAIDs can **reduce the clearance** of methotrexate and aminoglycoside drugs. NSAIDs can also interfere to varying degrees with the antihypertensive effect of diuretics, β-adrenoceptor antagonists, angiotensin inhibitors, and other antihypertensive drugs. When given with potassium-sparing diuretics, NSAIDs can cause potassium retention and lead to **hyperkalemia**. Some drug interactions are only associated with a particular NSAID. For example, high doses of salicylates exert a **hypoglycemic effect** that can alter the effects of antidiabetic drugs. Indomethacin reduces the **natriuretic effect** of diuretics and can cause nephrotoxicity when given with triamterene.

Low doses of acetaminophen can be safely used for analgesia and antipyresis during pregnancy. The use of other NSAIDs during the second half of pregnancy is generally not recommended, however, because of potential **adverse effects to the fetus**. These effects result from prostaglandin inhibition and include GI bleeding, platelet inhibition, renal dysfunction, and premature closure of the ductus arteriosus.

Aspirin and Other Salicylates

The therapeutic value of salicylates was originally recognized when they were identified as the active ingredients of willow bark and other plant materials used in folk medicine to relieve pain and fever. Aspirin was synthesized in 1899 during a search for a salicylate derivative that would be less irritating to the stomach than salicylic acid. Aspirin soon became widely used around the world as an **analgesic**, **antipyretic**, and **anti-inflammatory** drug.

Salicylic acid derivatives include **aspirin (acetyl-salicylic acid)** and several nonacetylated drugs, such as **salsalate**, **choline magnesium salicylate**, and **methyl salicylate** (oil of wintergreen).

PHARMACOLOGICAL EFFECTS AND INDICATIONS. In adults, the salicylates can be used in the management of **pain, fever**, and **inflammation**, as well as in the prophylaxis of **myocardial infarction, stroke, and other thromboembolic disorder**. In children, the use of salicylates should be avoided, because the risk of **Reye's syndrome** appears to be increased in virus-infected children who are treated with these drugs.

The analgesic, antipyretic, and anti-inflammatory effect of aspirin and other salicylates result from nonspecific **inhibition of COX** in peripheral tissues and the CNS. Aspirin **irreversibly** acetylates platelet COX and has a longer-lasting effect on thromboxane synthesis than do other salicylates. The **antiplatelet effect** of aspirin persists for about 14 days,

whereas that of most other NSAIDs is much shorter. The effect is long-lived, because platelets lack a nucleus and do not make new COX enzyme.

The salicylates are usually administered orally, but formulations are also available for topical and rectal administration. The oral dosage of aspirin that is needed to inhibit platelet aggregation is somewhat lower than the oral dosage needed to obtain analgesic and antipyretic effects, and it is much lower than the oral dosage needed to relieve inflammation caused by arthritic and other inflammatory disorders. Figure 30–3 shows the relationship between the dosage of aspirin and the pharmacologic and toxic effects of the drug.

PHARMACOKINETICS. Aspirin is well absorbed from the gut. Although its concurrent administration with antacids may slow its absorption rate, it does not significantly reduce its bioavailability. Aspirin is rapidly hydrolyzed to salicylic acid (**salicylate**) by **plasma esterase**, and this accounts for its short plasma half-life (about 15 minutes). Most of the pharmacologic effects of aspirin are attributed to its **salicylate metabolite**, which has a half-life of about 2 hours. Aspirin itself, however, is responsible for irreversible inhibition of platelet COX and platelet aggregation.

Most of the salicylic acid formed from aspirin and other salicylate drugs is **conjugated with glycine** to form salicyluric acid. This substance is then excreted in the urine, along with about 10% of free salicylate and a similar amount of glucuronide conjugates. The rate of excretion of salicylate is affected by urine pH. For this reason, **alkalinization** of the urine by administration of sodium bicarbonate has been used to increase the ionization and elimination of salicylic acid in cases of drug overdose (see Chapter 2).

When a therapeutic dose of aspirin or other salicylate drug is ingested, the rate of metabolism and the rate of excretion of salicylate are proportional to the drug's plasma concentration (**first-order elimination**). When an excessive dose is taken, the elimination pathways become saturated, giving rise to **zero-order elimination**. For this reason, larger doses can rapidly elevate plasma salicylate concentrations to toxic levels, especially in the elderly, who are at greatest risk of aspirin toxicity.

ADVERSE EFFECTS. The use of aspirin in children with chickenpox and other viral infections has been associated with **Reye's syndrome**. As mentioned, treatment with salicylates, therefore, should be avoided in children.

Therapeutic doses of aspirin can cause **gastric irritation** and contribute to **GI bleeding and peptic ulcers**. Moderately high therapeutic doses can cause **tinnitus**, which is described as an abnormal auditory sensation or buzzing noise, and considered an early sign of salicylate toxicity.

Excessive doses of aspirin produce the toxic effects shown in Figure 30–3. **Hyperventilation** is caused by direct and indirect stimulation of the respiratory center in the medulla, and it often leads to increased exhalation of carbon dioxide and respiratory alkalosis. Higher plasma salicylate concentrations can cause fever, dehydration, and severe metabolic acidosis. If not treated promptly, these events can culminate in shock, coma, organ system failure, and death. Excessive doses of aspirin also cause **hypoprothrombinemia**, which is an impairment of **hemostasis** and causes bleeding.

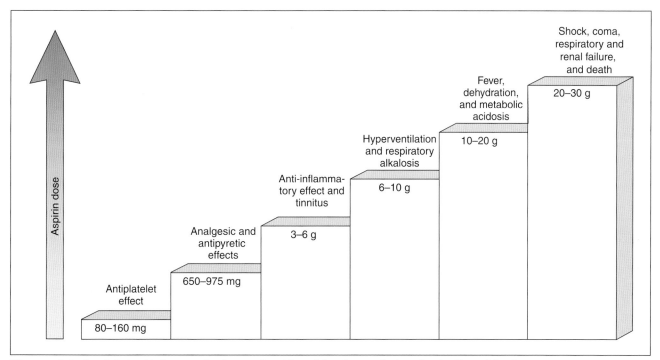

Figure 30-3. Relationship between the dosage of aspirin and the pharmacologic and toxic effects of the drug.

Aspirin **hypersensitivity** is an uncommon but serious condition that can result in severe and potentially fatal anaphylactic reactions. Symptoms of aspirin intolerance include vasomotor rhinitis, angioedema, and urticaria (hives). Aspirin sensitivity occurs most frequently in persons with asthma, nasal polyps, or chronic urticaria. Persons who have had a severe hypersensitivity reaction to aspirin or another salicylate should not be treated with another type of NSAID, because a 5% risk of cross-sensitivity exists between salicylates and other NSAIDs.

TREATMENT OF SALICYLATE OVERDOSE. The treatment of salicylate poisoning may include the following: (1) induction of vomiting and gastric lavage to remove unabsorbed drug; (2) intravenous administration of **sodium bicarbonate** to counteract metabolic acidosis, increase the ionization of salicylate in the kidneys, and thereby enhance the rate of excretion of salicylate; and (3) administration of fluids, electrolytes, and other supportive care, as needed.

Acetaminophen

PHARMACOLOGICAL EFFECTS AND INDICATIONS. For more than 100 years, acetaminophen has been available for the treatment of **mild pain and fever**. The drug is a *p*-aminophenol derivative that exerts analgesic and antipyretic effects at doses that are well tolerated and produce remarkably few adverse effects during short-term administration. Unlike aspirin use, acetaminophen use has not been associated with Reye's syndrome, so acetaminophen can be safely given to children with fever caused by viral illnesses.

Acetaminophen has only **weak anti-inflammatory activity**, partly because it is inactivated by peroxides produced in the cells of inflamed tissue. Recent evidence suggests the existence of a third COX isoform, designated **COX-3**, with roles in mediating pain and fever, and subject to inhibition by acetaminophen. Acetaminophen has little effect on COX-1 or COX-2 and, thus, **lacks anti-inflammatory activity**. Although acetaminophen is not considered a first-line drug for patients with arthritic disorders, it is sometimes used as an analgesic in those with **mild arthritis**. Because acetaminophen lacks the ability to inhibit thromboxane synthesis and platelet aggregation, it is not used for the prophylaxis of myocardial infarction, stroke, or other thromboembolic disorders.

PHARMACOKINETICS. Acetaminophen is rapidly absorbed from the gut, exhibits minimal binding to plasma proteins, and is widely distributed to peripheral tissues and the CNS.

As shown in Figure 30–4, acetaminophen is extensively metabolized by several pathways in the liver. Most of the drug is conjugated with sulfate and glucuronide, and these metabolites are excreted in the urine. A small amount of acetaminophen is converted by cytochrome P450 to a potentially hepatotoxic quinone intermediate. When a therapeutic dose of acetaminophen is taken, the quinone intermediate is rapidly inactivated by conjugation with glutathione. Toxic doses of acetaminophen, however, **deplete hepatic glutathione**, cause accumulation of the quinone intermediate, and lead to hepatic necrosis. To prevent liver damage, patients who ingest an overdose and are determined to be at risk for hepatotoxicity can be given **acetylcysteine**, a sulfhydryl compound that conjugates the quinone intermediate and renders it harmless.

ADVERSE EFFECTS. Some epidemiologic evidence indicates that long-term use of acetaminophen is associated with an increased risk of **renal dysfunction**.

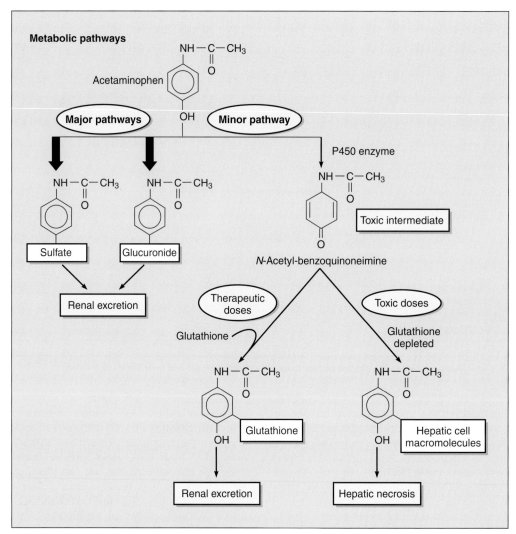

Figure 30–4. Acetaminophen metabolism and hepatotoxicity. Acetaminophen is primarily metabolized by conjugation with sulfate and glucuronide. A minor pathway involves oxidation of acetaminophen by cytochrome P450 enzymes (CYP1A2, CYP2E1, and CYP3A isozymes) to form a potentially toxic intermediate, N-acetyl-benzoquinoneimine. When a therapeutic dose of acetaminophen is taken, this quinone intermediate is conjugated with glutathione and excreted in the urine. When a toxic dose of acetaminophen is taken, glutathione stores are depleted, and the quinone intermediate attacks hepatic cell macromolecules. This process results in hepatic necrosis. Acetylcysteine (MUCOMYST) given to treat acetaminophen overdose protects the liver by maintaining or restoring the glutathione levels, or by acting as an alternate substrate for conjugation with, and thus, detoxification of the reactive metabolite.

Although therapeutic doses of acetaminophen are remarkably nontoxic, the ingestion of 20 to 30 tablets is sufficient to cause life-threatening **hepatotoxicity**.

TREATMENT OF ACETAMINOPHEN OVERDOSE. Because hepatotoxicity gradually progresses over several days following an acetaminophen overdose, prompt treatment with **acetylcysteine** can prevent or significantly reduce hepatotoxicity.

Ibuprofen, Ketoprofen, and Naproxen

PHARMACOLOGICAL EFFECTS AND INDICATIONS. Ibuprofen, ketoprofen, and naproxen are among the most widely used NSAIDs for pain and inflammation caused by trauma, infection, autoimmune disorders, neoplasms, joint degeneration, and other causes. By reversibly and nonselectively **inhibiting COX isozymes**, these drugs exert analgesic, antipyretic, and anti-inflammatory effects. Low-dose formulations of the

drugs are available without prescription for the treatment of mild pain and inflammation. Formulations with higher doses are used to treat most arthritic disorders and still require a prescription.

PHARMACOKINETICS. Ibuprofen, ketoprofen, and naproxen are administered orally, are widely distributed, and are extensively metabolized to inactive metabolites in the liver before undergoing renal excretion. Naproxen has a **longer half-life** (14 hours) than does ibuprofen or ketoprofen (2 hours each). For this reason, naproxen is given twice daily, whereas ibuprofen or ketoprofen is usually administered from two to four times a day.

ADVERSE EFFECTS. Ibuprofen and related drugs produce dose-dependent gastric irritation, nausea, dyspepsia, and bleeding. Long-term administration of high doses has been associated with peptic ulcer disease, but short-term use of low doses causes very few serious adverse effects. Among the serious effects that have been reported are hepatic toxicity and renal toxicity. In some cases, acute renal failure occurred following short-term use of therapeutic doses by patients who failed to ingest adequate fluids and became dehydrated.

Indomethacin, Sulindac, and Ketorolac

Indomethacin, an indoleacetic acid derivative, is one of the most potent inhibitors of COX isozymes. Because of its greater tendency to cause adverse effects, this drug is usually reserved for the management of **moderate to severe acute inflammatory conditions**. It is also used to treat infants with a **patent ductus arteriosus**. In these infants, indomethacin inhibits the synthesis of prostaglandins and thereby causes closure of the ductus arteriosus.

The incidence of GI and CNS side effects is higher with the use of indomethacin than with the use of many other NSAIDs. Indomethacin therapy is also associated with a risk of serious **hematological toxicity**. Hence, therapy should be limited to **short-term use** whenever possible, and patients should be closely monitored.

Sulindac, which is structurally related to indomethacin, is actually a **prodrug** converted to an active sulfide metabolite. The parent compound, sulindac sulfoxide, is inactive in COX inhibition assays done in vitro as biotransformation in the liver produces the active metabolite. It is noted for having a "renal-sparing" effect such that moderate doses alter renal prostaglandin production less than other NSAIDs. Besides sulindac use in the treatment of RA, it is also administered to treat adenomas in polyp disease.

Ketorolac is an arylacetic acid derivative. It has potent analgesic activity and is one of the few NSAIDs that is available for **parenteral** use for either intravenous or intramuscular administration. In studies of mild to moderate postoperative pain, ketorolac produced a level of analgesia comparable to that produced by morphine but caused less nausea, vomiting, and drowsiness. Ketorolac, therefore, has been widely used for the short-term management of **moderate pain**, such as **postoperative pain associated with dental surgery**. Although the drug has also been used to treat **migraine headaches**, it does not appear to be superior to ibuprofen for treatment of musculoskeletal pain. The ophthalmic solution for ketorolac is used to treat **allergic conjunctivitis** and **postoperative ocular inflammation**.

Ketorolac causes fewer adverse GI and CNS effects than do opioid analgesics, but it poses a significant risk of hematologic toxicity and other adverse effects. For this reason, oral or parenteral therapy with the drug must be limited to 5 or fewer days. In patients with renal or hepatic disease, ketorolac should be used with caution because it is associated with an increased risk of severe renal or hepatic impairment. A similar drug, **bromfenac** (DURACT), was withdrawn from the market in 1998, following postmarketing reports of hepatic failure and death.

Piroxicam and Nabumetone

Piroxicam is an effective anti-inflammatory agent with potency equal to aspirin or naproxen for the chronic treatment of RA. The main advantage of piroxicam is its 50-hour plasma half-life. This allows a single daily dose in most patients, although it can take up to 2 weeks to achieve maximal therapeutic effect.

One of the few nonacid NSAIDs, **nabumetone**, is a ketone **prodrug** with weak COX inhibitory activity in vitro. It is converted to one or more active metabolites in vivo and a potent inhibition of COX activity occurs with these metabolites. It also has the advantage that a half-life of 20 hours allows once-daily dosing in most patients.

Etodolac and Meloxicam

Other NSAIDs, including **meloxicam** and **etodolac**, which have been marketed in Europe or the United States as safer NSAIDs, were found after the discovery of COX-2 to be preferential inhibitors of this enzyme. They are more selective for COX-2 than typical NSAIDs but not as selective as the remaining COX-2 inhibitor, **celecoxib**.

Diclofenac

Diclofenac is available in a number of preparations including immediate-release, extended-release, a transdermal patch (FLECTOR), and a new formulation for topical administration (VOLTAREN GEL). The latter formulation contains 1% diclofenac sodium indicated for treating pain associated with osteoarthritis in joints amenable to topical treatment.

Selective Cyclooxygenase-2 Inhibitors

Celecoxib, Rofecoxib, and Valdecoxib

The selective COX-2 inhibitors are a new group of drugs that provide potent anti-inflammatory activity without causing significant GI toxicity. **Celecoxib** (CELEBREX), the first selective COX-2 inhibitor to be marketed, was soon followed by the release of **rofecoxib** (VIOXX) and **valdecoxib** (BEXTRA). Together, these agents are known as "**coxibs**."

In late 2004, the makers of **rofecoxib voluntarily withdrew the drug** from the market after data were analyzed from a clinical trial testing rofecoxib's effectiveness in preventing recurrence of colorectal polyps. This study found an increased relative risk for confirmed cardiovascular events (e.g., heart attack and stroke) beginning after 18 months of treatment in the patients taking rofecoxib compared with those taking placebo.

Valdecoxib also showed an increased risk for cardiovascular events in patients after heart surgery. Serious skin reactions (e.g., toxic epidermal necrolysis, **Stevens-Johnson syndrome**, and erythema multiforme) were reported in patients receiving valdecoxib. Some of these reactions resulted in fatalities. For these reasons, the U.S. Food and Drug Administration (FDA) **removed valdecoxib from the market** in 2005.

With regard to **celecoxib**, patients in a colon cancer clinical trial taking 400 mg of celecoxib twice daily had a 3.4 times greater risk of cardiovascular events compared with those taking placebo. For patients in the trial taking 200 mg of celecoxib twice daily, the risk was 2.5 times greater. As a result, the FDA recently strengthened the warnings for cardiovascular risk of the only remaining selective COX-2 inhibitor, **celecoxib**, and for **all NSAID agents except aspirin**.

While cardiovascular risk may dampen wider use of coxibs and other NSAID agents, recent studies show that NSAIDs can delay or slow the progress of **Alzheimer's disease**. The neurodegeneration that occurs in this disease is accompanied by inflammatory mechanisms that involve COX and the activation of the complement cascade. Additionally, increased expression of COX-2 is seen in some cancer cells and the angiogenesis essential to tumor growth requires COX-2 activity. Overexpression of COX-2 leads to increased expression of vascular endothelial growth factor, a factor vital to tumor angiogenesis. Regular use of NSAIDs may therefore **decrease the risk of developing cancer** (particularly colon cancer), and especially so with the use of a COX-2 selective inhibitor.

PHARMACOLOGICAL EFFECTS AND INDICATIONS. Celecoxib is a potent analgesic, antipyretic, and anti-inflammatory agent. This drug does not inhibit platelet aggregation, because platelets contain only the COX-1 isozyme.

In clinical studies of **osteoarthritis** and **rheumatoid arthritis**, celecoxib was shown to be as efficacious as naproxen without causing significant side effects. In a study of postoperative pain management, however, celecoxib was reported to provide insufficient analgesia to control pain after general surgery. In laboratory studies, investigators found that celecoxib was more effective than nonselective COX inhibitors in protecting against **colon carcinogenesis**. This finding suggested a role for prophylactic coxib use in persons with a high risk of colon cancer; however, clinical trials were halted because of cardiovascular events (see above).

PHARMACOKINETICS. Celecoxib is available for oral administration and is usually taken twice daily. The drug is rapidly absorbed from the gut, is metabolized by cytochrome P450 isozyme CYP2C9, and is excreted in the feces and urine. The half-life is about 11 hours.

ADVERSE EFFECTS AND INTERACTIONS. Besides the risk of cardiovascular events, celecoxib appears to cause a **low incidence of adverse reactions**, the most common of which are diarrhea, dyspepsia, and abdominal pain. This drug is associated with a much lower incidence of gastroduodenal ulcers than the nonselective NSAIDs (e.g., ibuprofen and naproxen).

Because celecoxib is metabolized by CYP2C9, drugs such as fluconazole, fluvastatin, and zafirlukast may inhibit its metabolism and increase its serum concentration. Lower doses of celecoxib should be used in patients treated concurrently with these interacting drugs.

DISEASE-MODIFYING ANTIRHEUMATIC DRUGS

DMARDs are agents capable of slowing the progression of joint erosions in patients with RA. Examples of DMARDs are gold salts, glucocorticoids, hydroxychloroquine, methotrexate, and a number of newer immunologic agents, including leflunomide, etanercept, and infliximab. These drugs have a delayed onset of action and require several weeks to months before their antirheumatic benefits are observed. Several studies suggest that using a **combination** of DMARDs is more effective than using a single DMARD in many patients with RA.

Disease-modifying antirheumatic drugs act by various mechanisms to suppress the proliferation and activity of lymphocytes and polymorphonuclear leukocytes and thereby counteract their ability to cause joint inflammation and destruction. Because joint erosion is usually found within the first 2 years of RA, many rheumatologists prescribe DMARDs at the time of diagnosis. The utility of DMARDs, however, is often limited by their toxicity or by their loss of efficacy over time, and many patients must cease taking them within 5 years of commencing therapy.

GOLD SALTS

Gold salts were first used to treat RA in the late 1920s, from the finding of Robert Koch in 1890 that elemental gold inhibited the growth of *Mycobacterium tuberculosis* and the mistaken belief that the swollen joints characteristic of RA were caused by these bacteria. They were once used extensively in the management of this disease, but their popularity has declined with the introduction of newer DMARDs, which tend to be more efficacious and less toxic. However, both oral and parenteral gold preparations are still available. The oral compound, **auranofin**, is poorly absorbed from the gut, however, and may be less efficacious than parenteral preparations, such as **gold sodium thiomalate** (also called **sodium aurothiomalate**). A second preparation of gold for intravenous administration is available as **aurothioglucose**. The antirheumatic effects of gold salts are usually not observed until 3 to 6 months after starting therapy.

Gold salts can cause a variety of adverse hematologic, dermatologic, GI, and renal effects. Flushing, hypotension, and tachycardia are sometimes observed. Skin rash and stomatitis are commonly observed and require discontinuation of treatment until they resolve.

GLUCOCORTICOIDS

For many years, **prednisone** and **other glucocorticoids** have played an important role in the treatment of RA. These drugs induce the formation of lipocortin, a protein that inhibits phospholipase A_2 activity. By this mechanism, they inhibit the release of arachidonic acid from cell membranes and the formation of prostaglandins. Glucocorticoids also inhibit the production of numerous cytokines, including interleukins and tumor necrosis factor, by synthesis of proteins that inhibit their action.

Glucocorticoids act more **rapidly than other DMARDs**, but their long-term use is limited by the development of serious adverse effects. In light of these facts, glucocorticoids have been used in various ways to manage patients with RA or other inflammatory joint diseases. For example, they have been used to induce a remission in the disease at the time that therapy with another (slower-acting) DMARD is started; to provide short courses of therapy during disease flare-ups; and to provide continuous low-dose background therapy in patients being treated with other DMARDs and NSAIDs.

OTHER DISEASE-MODIFYING ANTIRHEUMATIC DRUGS

Methotrexate

Methotrexate is an antineoplastic and immunomodulating drug whose properties are discussed in detail in Chapter 45. The drug was first used to treat RA in the 1980s, and it remains the single most effective DMARD available today.

Methotrexate has several mechanisms of action. It **inhibits human folate reductase** and thereby reduces the availability of active forms of folate that are required for thymidylate and DNA synthesis. It also **inhibits lymphocyte proliferation** and the production of cytokines and rheumatoid factor. In addition, it interferes with polymorphonuclear leukocyte chemotaxis and reduces the production of cytotoxins and free radicals that damage the synovial membrane and bone.

Methotrexate is considered the **DMARD of choice** for most patients with RA. The drug can be given orally or intramuscularly and has a fairly rapid onset of action, with benefits observed as early as 2 to 3 weeks after therapy is started. From 45% to 55% of patients continue therapy for at least 5 to 7 years, and sustained efficacy for up to 15 years has been demonstrated in some patients. The combined use of methotrexate and other DMARDs is often more effective than single-drug therapy.

Treatment with methotrexate is generally well tolerated by patients with RA, but it can cause adverse GI, hematologic, hepatic, and pulmonary reactions. **Elevated liver enzyme** levels are found in up to 15% of patients treated with methotrexate, but serious hepatotoxicity is rare. The administration of folic acid supplements does not reduce the drug efficacy and may prevent some of these adverse effects. The use of methotrexate is **contraindicated in pregnancy**.

Leflunomide

Leflunomide is a newer immunosuppressive drug that acts as a **powerful inhibitor of leukocyte** and **T-cell proliferation**. The active metabolite of leflunomide inhibits a key enzyme in pyrimidine synthesis, **dihydroorotate dehydrogenase**, and thereby prevents replication of DNA and synthesis of RNA and protein in immune cells. Leflunomide is converted to its active metabolite in the intestinal wall and liver. The active metabolite is further metabolized and excreted in the urine and feces, with an elimination half-life of about 2 weeks.

Leflunomide is marketed as an alternative to methotrexate for the first-line management of RA. In a controlled trial, 41% of patients treated with leflunomide showed significant improvement in tender and swollen joints, compared with 35% of those treated with methotrexate and 19% given a placebo.

The adverse effects of leflunomide include **diarrhea** and **reversible alopecia** (baldness). The drug can increase serum levels of hepatic enzymes and increase the risk of hepatotoxicity when it is used in combination with methotrexate. The active metabolite of leflunomide inhibits CYP2C9 and may thereby increase the serum level of many drugs, including ibuprofen and some of the other NSAIDs. Leflunomide is teratogenic, so its use is **contraindicated in pregnancy**.

Hydroxychloroquine

Hydroxychloroquine, an antimalarial drug related to chloroquine, is extensively used as a DMARD. It **reduces the chemotaxis** and **phagocytosis** of polymorphonuclear leukocytes and decreases the production of **superoxide radicals** by these cells. The drug has a slow onset of action and can require 6 months of therapy before benefits are observed. It does not produce the myelosuppressive, hepatic, and renal toxicities that many other DMARDs produce. Hydroxychloroquine occasionally causes GI disturbances, and patients undergoing hydroxychloroquine treatment must be monitored for **adverse ocular effects**, including blurred vision, scotomas, and night blindness.

Immunomodulators

Etanercept, Infliximab, Adalimumab, Anakinra and Abatacept

Etanercept, **infliximab**, and **adalimumab** are immunomodulating agents that exert their effects by binding to and inactivating **tumor necrosis factor** (TNF). TNF is one of the proinflammatory cytokines produced by macrophages and activated T cells. Elevated levels of TNF are found in the synovial fluid of joints and play an important role in both the pathologic inflammation and the joint destruction that are hallmarks of RA (see Fig. 30–1). **Anakinra** and **abatacept** have novel mechanisms of action and prevent interleukin binding T-cell activation (see below) respectively.

Etanercept is a protein formed by recombining human p75 (75-kd) TNF receptors with Fc fragments of human immunoglobulin G1 (IgG1). In comparison with the original protein, the recombined protein can **antagonize TNF** to a greater extent and has a longer half-life. Experimental studies in several animal models of RA have found etanercept treatment to be effective, as have subsequent clinical trials in patients with this disease. According to a 3-month clinical study, 75% of patients with RA had a significant improvement in the signs and symptoms of their disease. The drug was generally well tolerated, although injection site reactions were common.

Etanercept must be administered subcutaneously twice a week and is expensive (a 6-month supply costs about $6300 in the United States). The drug is currently intended for use in patients whose RA is refractory to treatment with methotrexate or other DMARDs. Etanercept can be used alone or in combination with methotrexate in these patients.

Infliximab is a chimeric human-murine (mouse) monoclonal antibody that inactivates TNF. It is used in the treatment of **Crohn's disease** and RA. In one clinical trial, infliximab treatment resulted in an improvement of RA manifestations in 80% of patients whose disease was refractory to other drugs. In another study, infliximab was found to be more effective when combined with methotrexate than when used alone. Infliximab is administered intravenously at 4- to 12-week intervals.

Adalimumab is a human IgG1 monoclonal antibody specific for **human TNF**. It is made by recombinant DNA technology in a mammalian cell expression system and purified to exclude viral particles. For adult patients, adalimumab (40 mg) is administered every other week as a subcutaneous injection. During adalimumab treatment, administration of methotrexate, glucocorticoids, salicylates, NSAIDs, analgesics or other DMARDs can continue safely. Some patients not taking concomitant methotrexate may see additional benefits by increasing the frequency of adalimumab to 40 mg every week.

All TNF blocking agents, including adalimumab, produced serious **infections** and **sepsis**, some fatal, during clinical trials. Many of the serious infections were seen in patients on concomitant immunosuppressive therapy that, in addition to their RA, could predispose them to infections. Tuberculosis and invasive opportunistic fungal infections were also noted during treatment with TNF blockers.

Lymphomas were also reported in patients treated with TNF blocking agents. In clinical trials, patients with RA, particularly those with highly active disease, were at increased risk for the development of lymphoma. The role of TNF blockers in the development of this malignancy is not known.

Anakinra

Anakinra is a recombinant form of the human **interleukin-1 receptor antagonist** (IL-1Ra), differing only by the addition of a single methionine residue at its amino terminus. It blocks the biologic activity of IL-1 by competitively **inhibiting IL-1 binding** to the interleukin-1 type I receptor (IL-1RI). IL-1 production is induced in response to inflammatory stimuli and mediates inflammatory and immunologic responses. IL-1 has a broad range of activities, including cartilage degradation by its induction of the rapid loss of proteoglycans, as well as stimulation of bone resorption. The levels of the naturally occurring IL-1Ra in synovial fluid of patients with RA are not sufficient to compete with the increased production of IL-1.

The recommended dose of anakinra is 100 mg/day administered daily by subcutaneous injection. The adverse effects are the same as for the TNF blockers, with serious infections and lymphoma of most concern.

Abatacept

Abatacept is a selective **costimulation modulator** and inhibits T-cell activation by binding to **cell surface markers** (proteins) on leukocytes. Activated T lymphocytes are involved in the etiology of RA and are found in the synovial fluid of patients with RA. Abatacept is a recombinant protein made by joining the extracellular domain of human cytotoxic T-lymphocyte-associated antigen 4 (CTLA-4) to the modified Fc portion of human IgG1. It is the CTLA part of the molecule that binds to specific cell surface proteins of T-lymphocytes to prevent their activation.

Sulfasalazine and Penicillamine

Sulfasalazine was originally used in the treatment of RA in the 1930s, but only recently was it approved for this indication by the FDA. In the 1920s and 1930s, scientists theorized that RA was an inflammatory disease caused by an infection in the GI tract. Consistent with that hypothesis, sulfasalazine was developed and is a formulation combining an **anti-inflammatory** drug, 5-amino salicylic acid, with an **antibacterial drug**, sulfapyridine. Recent experiments suggest that it is sulfapyridine that is active against RA, but the exact mechanism is not known. Because sulfasalazine is a sulfa drug, people who are allergic to sulfa compounds should not take it.

D-penicillamine is a penicillin-derived compound used frequently in the past, but its use today has declined with the increasing use of other disease modifying anti-rheumatic drugs (e.g., methotrexate). It is not understood exactly how penicillamine provides a benefit in RA, but it is known to reduce the blood levels of **inflammatory cytokines**. Penicillamine effects can take up to 3 months to manifest; however, if no effect is seen in a year, it should be stopped.

DRUGS FOR THE TREATMENT OF GOUT

The effective management of gout often requires the use of various agents to prevent and treat acute attacks.

DRUGS FOR PREVENTING GOUT ATTACKS

Gout attacks can be prevented by lowering the **serum concentration of uric acid**. Probenecid and sulfinpyrazone accomplish this goal by **increasing the excretion of uric acid**, whereas allopurinol does so by **inhibiting the synthesis of uric acid**. Uric acid metabolism and sites of drug action are depicted in Figure 30–5.

Probenecid

A **uricosuric drug**, such as probenecid, is used to prevent gout attacks in persons who under-excrete uric acid, as indicated by a 24-hour uric acid excretion that is less than 800 mg.

Probenecid is a weak acid that competitively inhibits the reabsorption of uric acid by renal tubules and thereby **increases the excretion of uric acid**. The drug is taken orally and should be swallowed with a full glass of water to ensure adequate fluid intake. Treatment should begin with a low dose, and the dosage should be gradually increased until an adequate uricosuric effect is obtained or the maximal dosage is reached. Probenecid treatment is usually well tolerated.

The use of aspirin and other salicylates can alter or interfere with the **uricosuric effect** of probenecid, so patients should avoid concurrent use of these agents. High doses of salicylates inhibit uric acid reabsorption and exert a uricosuric effect. Low doses of salicylates, however, inhibit uric acid secretion by renal tubules and thereby increase serum concentrations of uric acid.

Sulfinpyrazone

Sulfinpyrazone is another **uricosuric agent** that competitively inhibits the active reabsorption of urate at the proximal renal tubule. As with probenecid, it increases the

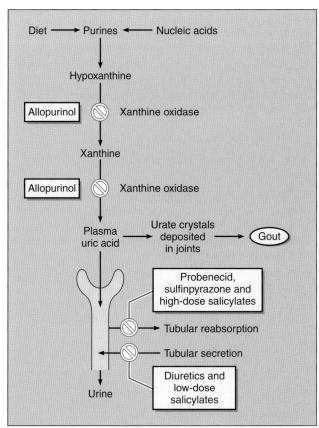

Figure 30–5. Uric acid metabolism and sites of drug action. Purines obtained from the diet or from catabolism of nucleic acids are converted to hypoxanthine. Under normal conditions, xanthine oxidase converts hypoxanthine to xanthine and then to uric acid. Allopurinol acts by inhibiting xanthine oxidase. Probenecid, sulfinpyrazone, and high-dose salicylates inhibit the renal tubular reabsorption of uric acid, whereas diuretics and low-dose salicylates inhibit the renal tubular secretion of uric acid.

urinary excretion of uric acid and lowers serum urate concentrations. Although sulfinpyrazone lacks clinically useful anti-inflammatory or analgesic activity, it inhibits prostaglandin synthesis and shares some of the risks associated with NSAIDs, including the potential for causing GI, renal, or hematologic adverse effects.

Allopurinol

Allopurinol is used to prevent gout attacks in persons who **overproduce uric acid**, as indicated by a 24-hour uric acid excretion that is greater than 800 mg. It is also sometimes used to prevent **hyperuricemia** and **gout** in persons who are having cancer chemotherapy and whose rate of purine catabolism is high because of the death of neoplastic cells.

Allopurinol and its active metabolite, **oxypurinol** (also called alloxanthine), decrease the production of uric acid by **inhibiting xanthine oxidase**, the enzyme that converts hypoxanthine to xanthine and xanthine to uric acid. Allopurinol is a competitive inhibitor of **xanthine oxidase**. In contrast to uricosuric drugs, allopurinol causes a decrease in uric acid excretion and a corresponding increase in the urinary excretion of hypoxanthine. In addition, allopurinol increases reutilization of hypoxanthine and

xanthine for nucleotide and nucleic acid synthesis via inhibition of **hypoxanthine-guanine phosphoribosyltransferase**. The resultant increase in nucleotide concentration leads to increased feedback inhibition of *de novo* purine synthesis. By lowering both serum and urine concentrations of uric acid below its solubility limits, allopurinol prevents or decreases urate deposition, thereby preventing the occurrence or progression of both **gouty arthritis** and **urate nephropathy**.

Allopurinol is administered orally. Most of the drug is rapidly converted to its active metabolite, **oxypurinol**, in the liver. Oxypurinol has a half-life of about 20 hours; most of this metabolite is excreted unchanged in the urine.

About 25% of patients are unable to tolerate allopurinol because of its adverse effects, which include nausea, vomiting, hepatitis, skin rashes, and other forms of **hypersensitivity**. Because allopurinol inhibits the catabolism of **azathioprine** and **mercaptopurine**, doses of these drugs may need to be reduced if allopurinol is given concurrently with either of them.

DRUGS FOR TREATING GOUT ATTACKS

Indomethacin

In patients with acute gout, a potent anti-inflammatory drug is given for the rapid relief of pain. Although **indomethacin** (see above) is widely used for this purpose, other NSAIDs are often effective when used in an adequate dosage. If these drugs do not provide relief or cannot be tolerated by the patient, **colchicine** can be given orally or parenterally.

Colchicine

Colchicine was traditionally used to treat acute gout, but it is less frequently used today because of its unpleasant side effects, which include nausea, vomiting, diarrhea, and abdominal cramps. The drug is believed to act by **disrupting microtubules** and **inhibiting the motility** of inflammatory leukocytes and thereby blocking their ability to cause urate crystal-induced joint inflammation. Colchicine is rapidly absorbed after oral administration. It is partly metabolized in the liver, and the drug and its metabolites are excreted by the biliary and fecal route. If colchicine treatment causes the adverse effects noted above, treatment should be stopped to avoid more serious toxicity.

SUMMARY OF IMPORTANT POINTS

■ NSAIDs act primarily by inhibiting COX and the synthesis of prostaglandins. The drugs exhibit varying degrees of analgesic, anti-inflammatory, and antipyretic activity. Most of them also inhibit platelet aggregation. Long-term use of NSAIDs can lead to renal or hepatic toxicity.

■ Nonselective COX inhibitors include acetaminophen, aspirin, ibuprofen, indomethacin, ketoprofen, ketorolac, and naproxen. Except for acetaminophen, the agents in this group can cause gastric irritation and bleeding, and their long-term use can lead to peptic ulcers.

■ Acetaminophen is an effective analgesic and antipyretic agent, but it lacks significant anti-inflammatory and antiplatelet activity. A minor metabolite of acetaminophen is a potentially hepatotoxic quinone. This quinone metabolite is normally inactivated by conjugation with glutathione, but toxic doses of acetaminophen can deplete glutathione and cause fatal liver failure.

■ Acetylcysteine, a sulfhydryl compound that conjugates and inactivates the quinone metabolite of acetaminophen, is used as an antidote for acetaminophen hepatotoxicity.

■ Low doses of aspirin have potent antiplatelet effects because they acetylate and irreversibly inhibit platelet COX. Low doses of aspirin also produce analgesic and antipyretic effects, but higher doses are needed to counteract inflammation.

■ High therapeutic doses of aspirin can cause tinnitus. Toxic doses cause hyperventilation and respiratory alkalosis, followed by metabolic acidosis. In cases of severe aspirin toxicity, sodium bicarbonate can be given to counteract acidosis and increase urinary excretion of salicylic acid.

■ Ibuprofen, ketoprofen, and naproxen are potent NSAIDs that are widely used as analgesic, antipyretic, and anti-inflammatory agents. Ketorolac is a potent analgesic that can be given orally or parenterally. To avoid hematologic toxicity, ketorolac use should be limited to a few days.

■ Indomethacin is a potent COX inhibitor that can be used to treat moderate to severe acute inflammatory conditions. It is also used to cause closure of the ductus arteriosus in infants.

■ Celecoxib, the first and only selective COX-2 inhibitor now available, is a potent analgesic, antipyretic, and anti-inflammatory drug. Its incidence of GI bleeding and peptic ulcers is lower than that of nonselective COX inhibitors. Increased risk of cardiovascular events for celecoxib and all nonaspirin NSAIDs is now a concern with chronic administration.

■ DMARDs are agents capable of slowing the progression of joint erosions in patients with RA. These drugs have a slow onset of action and can cause considerable toxicity. DMARDs act by inhibiting the proliferation and activity of lymphocytes and polymorphonuclear leukocytes.

■ Methotrexate, the most widely used and effective DMARD, can be combined with other drugs in this class for enhanced activity. It is generally well tolerated and can be used effectively for many years.

■ Etanercept, infliximab, and adalimumab are DMARDs that bind to and inactivate TNF. Abatacept decreases T-cell activation. Anakinra blocks the biologic activity of IL-1 by competitively inhibiting IL-1 binding to IL-1RI. These drugs are administered intermittently by injection and appear to benefit many patients with RA, but all carry the risk of increased infections.

■ Other DMARDs include gold salts, glucocorticoids, leflunomide, hydroxychloroquine, sulfasalazine, and penicillamine.

■ Gout is caused by hyperuricemia and the deposition of urate crystals in joints. Uricosuric drugs (e.g., probenecid and sulfinpyrazone) increase uric acid excretion, whereas allopurinol inhibits uric acid formation. These drugs are used to prevent gout attacks.

■ Acute gout is treated with an NSAID (e.g., indomethacin) or colchicine. Colchicine inhibits the motility of leukocytes and thereby prevents their migration into joints and their ability to cause urate crystal-induced joint inflammation.

Review Questions

1. Aspirin is often used in low doses to prevent platelet aggregation by inhibiting the synthesis of which substance?
   (A) leukotriene
   (B) prostacyclin (prostaglandin I_2 [PGI_2])
   (C) thromboxane A_2
   (D) arachidonic acid
   (E) phospholipase A_2

2. Acetaminophen is a potent analgesic and antipyretic NSAID, but differs from other agents in that it has no anti-inflammatory action. Which of the following reasons explains this unique aspect of acetaminophen?
   (A) the distribution of acetaminophen does not reach peripheral sites of inflammation
   (B) acetaminophen it is not an inhibitor of the COX enzyme
   (C) anti-inflammatory doses of acetaminophen are too high and toxic
   (D) it is selective for a newly discovered isozyme of COX
   (E) acetaminophen undergoes significant first-pass metabolism

3. Which of the following agents augments the physiologic concentration of IL-1Ra proteins in the treatment of RA?
   (A) adalimumab
   (B) leflunomide
   (C) etanercept
   (D) infliximab
   (E) anakinra

4. With respect to antigout therapy, inhibition of tubulin polymerization into microtubules is important given the role of which process in which aspect of the disease?
   (A) leukotriene synthesis
   (B) uric acid production
   (C) kidney reabsorption of uric acid
   (D) leukocyte migration
   (E) plasma binding of uric acid

5. A 45-year-old obese male with a history of alcohol abuse and hypertension presents with complaints of joint swelling and pain. His urate excretion rate is 950 mg/day. Which of the following agents is the best treatment for his condition?
   (A) probenecid
   (B) allopurinol
   (C) piroxicam
   (D) sulfinpyrazone
   (E) colchicine

Answers and Explanations

1. **The correct answer is C:** thromboxane A_2. Aspirin binds irreversibly to COX enzymes in platelets and, because the platelets do not have a nucleus and cannot synthesize new COX protein, the effect of aspirin persists until the platelet is taken out of circulation. Thromboxane A_2 produces vasoconstriction and promotes the formation of clots, therefore aspirin can prevent clot formation and coronary thrombosis. Answer (B), prostacyclin (prostaglandin I_2 [PGI_2]), is also inhibited by aspirin because it is a COX product, but the particular enzyme to synthesize PGI_2 is not found in platelets. The other agents are not affected by aspirin administration.

2. **The best answer is D:** it is selective for a newly discovered isozyme of COX. This isozyme, called COX-3, appears to be a splice variant of COX-1 (from the same gene, but with different posttranscriptional processing of the RNA). It is also sometimes mentioned that the peroxide formation at sites of inflammation inhibits the activity of acetaminophen, but this may be less of a factor now that COX-3 is recognized. Answers (A) through (C) are not correct and answer (E) is not true to a greater degree than other NSAIDs that do have anti-inflammatory action.

3. **The correct answer is E:** anakinra. Anakinra, a recombinant form of the human IL-1Ra protein, blocks the biologic activity of IL-1 by competitively inhibiting IL-1 binding to the IL-1RI. Answer (A), adalimumab, is a human IgG1 monoclonal antibody specific for human TNF. Answer (B), leflunomide, is an immunosuppressive drug that inhibits mononuclear and T-cell proliferation. Answer (C), etanercept, is a protein formed by recombining human p75 TNF receptors with Fc fragments of human IgG1. Answer (D), infliximab, is a chimeric human-murine (mouse) monoclonal antibody that inactivates TNF and is approved for the treatment of Crohn's disease and RA.

4. **The correct answer is D:** leukocyte migration. The invasion of leukocytes (macrophages, and so on) into the joint capsule and subsequent release of inflammatory cytokines is a key process in the progression of gout. The agent that disrupts tubulin formation is colchicine. Other processes given as answers are not important with regard to colchicine action.

5. **The correct answer is B:** allopurinol. The two main strategies for treating gout are to increase the excretion of uric acid with a uricosuric agent (probenecid or sulfinpyrazone) or decrease the production of uric acid by inhibiting xanthine oxidase with allopurinol. The 24-hour rate of uric acid excretion provides a guideline for which therapy to use: less than 800 mg, use a uricosuric because there is too little excretion of uric acid; and more than 800 mg, use allopurinol because there is too much uric acid being made.

SELECTED READINGS

Bieber, J.D., and R.A. Terkeltaub. Gout: on the brink of novel therapeutic options for an ancient disease. Arthritis Rheum 50:2400–2414, 2004.

Canter, P.H., B. Wider, and E. Ernst. The antioxidant vitamins A, C, E and selenium in the treatment of arthritis: a systematic review of randomized clinical trials. Rheumatology 46:1223–1233, 2007.

Lin, J., D. Ziring, S. Desai, S. Kim, M. Wong, et al. TNFalpha blockade in human diseases: an overview of efficacy and safety. Clin Immunol 126:13–30, 2008.

Kutzing, M.K., and B.L. Firestein. Altered uric acid levels and disease states. J Pharmacol Exp Ther 324:1–7, 2008.

Schönthal, A.H., T.C. Chen, F.M. Hofman, S.G. Louie, and N.A. Petasis. Celecoxib analogs that lack COX-2 inhibitory function: preclinical development of novel anticancer drugs. Expert Opin Investig Drugs 17:197–208, 2008.

Warner, T.D., and J.A. Mitchell. COX-2 selectivity alone does not define the cardiovascular risks associated with non-steroidal anti-inflammatory drugs. Lancet 371:270–273, 2008.

VI

ENDOCRINE PHARMACOLOGY

CHAPTER 31

Hypothalamic and Pituitary Drugs

OVERVIEW

The hypothalamus and pituitary gland constitute an important neuroendocrine system that regulates growth, reproduction, metabolic rates, and other important body functions. The pituitary gland is divided into two major lobes: the adenohypophysis (anterior lobe) and the neurohypophysis (posterior lobe). Various hormones are secreted by each of these lobes and by the hypothalamus.

Adenohypophysis and Hypothalamus

The adenohypophysis secretes six hormones: (1) **corticotropin** (adrenocorticotropic hormone, ACTH); (2) **somatotropin** (growth hormone); (3) **follicle-stimulating hormone** (FSH); (4) **luteinizing hormone** (LH); (5) **thyrotropin** (thyroid-stimulating hormone, TSH); and (6) **prolactin**. The actions of these **anterior pituitary hormones** are summarized in Figure 31–1.

The secretion of anterior pituitary hormones is controlled by several hormone-releasing and hormone-inhibiting factors that are formed in the hypothalamus. These **hypothalamic hormones** include the following: (1) **corticotropin-releasing hormone**; (2) **growth hormone–releasing hormone** (GHRH); (3) **somatostatin** (growth hormone–inhibiting hormone); (4) **gonadotropin-releasing hormone** (GnRH); (5) **thyrotropin-releasing hormone** (TRH); and (6) **prolactin-inhibiting hormone** (PIH). Evidence also suggests the presence of one or more prolactin-releasing factors. The various hypothalamic hormones are secreted by the arcuate and other hypothalamic nuclei, and they are transported to the anterior pituitary via the hypophysioportal circulation.

The anterior pituitary hormones are transported to their target organs via the systemic circulation. In the target organs, they stimulate growth, development, and the secretion of other hormones, which both activate specific functions in various organs and exert negative feedback inhibition of the corresponding hypothalamic and pituitary hormones.

Neurohypophysis

The neurohypophysis secretes **oxytocin** and **vasopressin.** These **posterior pituitary hormones** are synthesized in the cell bodies of neurons in the supraoptic and paraventricular nuclei of the hypothalamus. The hormones are transported down the nerve axons to their endings in the posterior pituitary, where they are released in response to electrical activity in the nerve terminals.

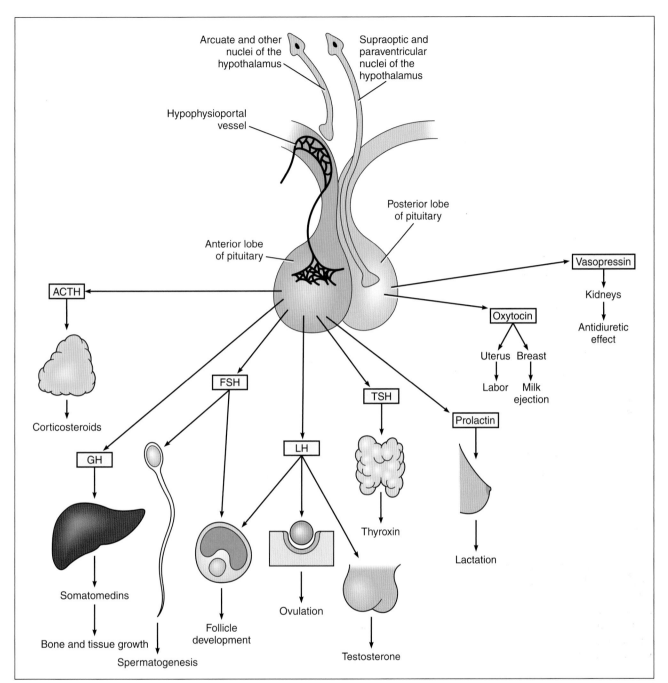

Figure 31–1. Relationships between hypothalamic hormones, pituitary hormones, and target organs. Numerous hormone-releasing and hormone-inhibiting factors formed in the arcuate and other hypothalamic nuclei are transported to the anterior pituitary by hypophysioportal vessels. In response to hypothalamic hormones, the anterior pituitary secretes the following: corticotropin, which evokes corticosteroid secretion by the adrenal cortex; growth hormone (GH), which elicits production of insulin-like growth factors (IGF) by the liver; follicle-stimulating hormone (FSH), which stimulates spermatogenesis and facilitates ovarian follicle development; luteinizing hormone (LH), which elicits testosterone secretion by the testes, facilitates ovarian follicle development, and induces ovulation; thyroid-stimulating hormone (TSH), which stimulates thyroxin secretion by the thyroid gland; and prolactin, which induces breast tissue growth and lactation. The posterior pituitary hormones, which are formed in the supraoptic and paraventricular nuclei, are transported by nerve axons to the posterior lobe, where they are released by physiologic stimuli. Oxytocin induces milk ejection by the breast and stimulates uterine contractions during labor. Vasopressin increases water and sodium reabsorption by the kidneys.

Uses of Hypothalamic and Pituitary Hormones

Hypothalamic and pituitary hormones are used for both diagnostic and therapeutic purposes. Hypothalamic hormone–releasing factors are helpful in assessing the functional capacity of the anterior pituitary to secrete particular pituitary hormones. Anterior pituitary hormones are used to evaluate the functional capacity of their target organs, to stimulate hypofunctional target organs, and to provide replacement therapy in hormone deficiency states. Posterior pituitary hormones are used therapeutically to activate specific physiologic functions.

All of the hypothalamic and pituitary hormones are peptides or small proteins that are extensively degraded in the gut following oral administration. For this reason, most of these hormones are administered parenterally. A few of them are available as a spray for intranasal administration.

ANTERIOR PITUITARY HORMONES

Corticotropin and Related Drugs

Corticotropin is a 39-amino-acid peptide that is released from the anterior pituitary in response to corticotropin-releasing hormone stimulation. Corticotropin then stimulates the adrenal cortex to produce cortisol, aldosterone, and adrenal androgens by increasing the activity of the enzyme that converts cholesterol to pregnenolone and is the rate-limiting enzyme in corticosteroid production.

Corticotropin Preparations

Two corticotropin preparations are available for clinical use: porcine **corticotropin** and a synthetic form of human corticotropin called **cosyntropin.** Cosyntropin contains the first 24 amino acids of human corticotropin, which are the ones necessary for its biologic activity. Cosyntropin is preferable for clinical use because it produces fewer allergic reactions.

Cosyntropin is used in two diagnostic tests. First, it is used to distinguish **congenital adrenal hyperplasia** from **ovarian hyperandrogenism.** Second, and more commonly, it is used to diagnose **adrenal insufficiency** in a test that measures plasma cortisol levels before and after a cosyntropin injection. Cosyntropin increases cortisol levels in healthy individuals but fails to increase cortisol levels in persons with adrenal insufficiency. Then to distinguish primary adrenal insufficiency from secondary adrenal insufficiency, endogenous plasma corticotropin concentrations are measured. In patients with primary adrenal insufficiency, corticotropin concentrations are high because of the lack of negative feedback inhibition of the hypothalamus and pituitary gland by the adrenal corticosteroids. In patients with secondary adrenal insufficiency, corticotropin concentrations are low because of inadequate production of corticotropin by the pituitary gland.

Corticotropin-Releasing Hormone

Corticorelin ovine triflutate is a preparation containing recombinant ovine corticotropin-releasing hormone. Intravenous administration of this preparation stimulates secretion of corticotropin and cortisol in normal subjects. Corticorelin is used as a diagnostic test to determine whether the excessive levels of cortisol that occur in persons with Cushing's syndrome are caused by excessive corticotropin secretion from a pituitary adenoma or by excessive secretion of cortisol by an adrenal tumor.

Growth Hormone and Related Drugs

Growth hormone (somatotropin), a large peptide that contains 191 amino acids, is produced by the anterior pituitary and has both direct and indirect actions on target organs.

Growth hormone acts directly to stimulate lipolysis and antagonize insulin to elevate blood glucose levels. Most of the effects of growth hormone, however, are mediated by **insulin-like growth factors** (IGF), which are peptides produced in the liver and cartilage. The IGF stimulate skeletal growth, amino acid transport, protein synthesis, nucleic acid synthesis, and cell proliferation.

The secretion of growth hormone is stimulated by GHRH and is inhibited by somatostatin. Several preparations of growth hormone, GHRH, and somatostatin are available for use in the diagnosis and treatment of **growth disorders** associated with excessive or inadequate secretion of growth hormone.

Growth Hormone Preparations

Growth hormone preparations obtained from animal sources are not active in humans. In the past, growth hormone obtained from human cadavers was used to treat patients with **growth hormone deficiency and short stature**, but some of the patients subsequently developed Creutzfeldt-Jakob disease. This fatal disease, as with mad cow disease and kuru, is characterized by spongiform encephalopathy and is thought to be transmitted by unconventional neurotoxic agents called prions.

Today, two biosynthetic growth hormone preparations are available for treatment of growth hormone deficiency. One that is identical to human growth hormone is called **somatropin recombinant.** The other, a human growth hormone analogue that contains one additional amino acid, is called **somatrem.** These preparations have been used to treat children with a variety of growth disorders including growth hormone deficiency, Turner syndrome, chronic renal failure, Prader-Willi syndrome, and cystic fibrosis. Growth hormone preparations have been clearly shown to improve height velocity and final height in these conditions. Children who received craniospinal irradiation for treatment of a childhood malignancy are less responsive to growth hormone replacement than children with idiopathic growth hormone deficiency and they have a tendency to enter puberty at an earlier age. These children may respond to supraphysiologic doses of growth hormone preparations and suppression of early puberty using a gonadotropin releasing hormone analogue (see below). Somatropin and somatrem are usually administered subcutaneously once daily to persons with growth hormone deficiency. Growth hormone deficiency is often accompanied by other pituitary hormone deficiencies, which should also be treated with appropriate hormones.

Growth Hormone–Releasing Hormone Preparations

Sermorelin, a synthetic analogue of GHRH, is available for use in a test to determine whether **growth hormone deficiency** is secondary to **hypothalamic insufficiency** or to **pituitary insufficiency.** In this test, plasma levels of growth hormone are measured before and after a single injection of sermorelin. A normal response indicates that the pituitary is capable of secreting growth hormone and that the patient's growth hormone deficiency is caused by hypothalamic insufficiency.

Sermorelin has orphan drug status for the treatment of growth hormone deficiency and the treatment of weight loss associated with acquired immunodeficiency syndrome (AIDS).

Growth Hormone–Inhibiting Hormone Preparations

Somatostatin (growth hormone–inhibiting hormone) inhibits growth hormone secretion, but it also exerts effects on several endocrine glands, including the pancreas, and this limits its therapeutic usefulness. Scientists searching for somatostatin preparations that were more selective for growth hormone inhibition discovered **octreotide**, a somatostatin analogue that consists of 8 amino acids. In comparison with somatostatin, octreotide is 45 times more potent in inhibiting growth hormone secretion but only 2 times as potent in inhibiting insulin secretion by the pancreas.

Octreotide is used to treat patients with **acromegaly.** This endocrine disorder, which is caused by excessive growth hormone secretion, is characterized by acral enlargement and soft tissue overgrowth of the hands and feet, coarsening of facial features, thickening and oiliness of the skin, and increased sweating. It is often accompanied by numerous other metabolic and endocrine abnormalities. Octreotide also has been used successfully in the treatment of several **neoplastic diseases,** including **carcinoid syndrome, pituitary adenomas that secrete thyrotropin,** and **tumors that produce vasoactive intestinal polypeptide.**

Octreotide is usually administered subcutaneously every 8 hours. A sustained-release preparation for intramuscular administration has also been developed. Adverse effects of octreotide treatment include nausea, vomiting, abdominal cramps, steatorrhea (excessive fat in the feces), and gallstones.

In patients with acromegaly, the use of **cabergoline** (see below) and other dopamine agonists can reduce circulating levels of growth hormone, IGF, and prolactin. These drugs are particularly useful in the treatment of persons with elevated growth hormone and prolactin secretion.

Growth Hormone Receptor Antagonist

Pegvisomant is a pegylated analogue of growth hormone that acts as a growth hormone receptor antagonist in target organs and thereby normalizes serum IGF-I concentrations in 97% of persons with acromegaly. **Pegylation** (addition of polyethylene glycol to the molecule) significantly increases the half-life of peptide drugs. Pegvisomant improves signs and symptoms of growth hormone excess in persons with acromegaly, including patients who were wholly or partially resistant to somatostatin analogues such as octreotide. In one study, pegvisomant reduced serum IGF levels and finger ring size in a dose-dependent manner while improving symptoms of tissue swelling, arthralgia, headache, perspiration, and fatigue. The drug appears to have a good safety profile, but liver function tests should be regularly monitored.

Gonadotropins and Related Drugs

The pituitary secretes two gonadotropins, namely, FSH and LH, in response to pulsatile stimulation by GnRH. The frequency and amplitude of the GnRH pulses at a particular time determine which gonadotropin is secreted. In females, FSH stimulates ovarian follicle maturation, whereas LH assists FSH in follicle development, induces ovulation, and stimulates the corpus luteum to produce progesterone and androgens. In males, FSH stimulates spermatogenesis, whereas LH stimulates Leydig's cells in the testes to produce testosterone.

Gonadotropin Preparations

Several gonadotropin preparations are available for the treatment of infertility and hypogonadism. One of them contains both FSH and LH, is called **menotropins** (human menopausal gonadotropin), and is obtained from the urine of menopausal women. Another primarily contains LH, is called **chorionic gonadotropin** (human chorionic gonadotropin); it is produced by the placenta and isolated from the urine of pregnant women.

In women with **infertility** caused by failure to ovulate, menotropins and chorionic gonadotropin are used sequentially. A dose of menotropins is administered each day for 9 to 12 days to stimulate maturation of the ovarian follicle. On the day after the last dose is given, a single dose of chorionic gonadotropin is administered to induce ovulation. In men with **hypogonadotropic hypogonadism,** menotropins therapy is used to stimulate spermatogenesis. In prepubertal boys with **cryptorchidism** (undescended testes) and hypogonadism, chorionic gonadotropin is administered to stimulate testosterone production and descent of the testes.

Gonadotropin-Releasing Hormone Preparations

Two classes of drugs target pituitary receptors for gonadotropin-releasing hormone: the GnRH agonists and the GnRH antagonist called abarelix.

The GnRH agonists include **gonadorelin, goserelin, leuprolide,** and **nafarelin.** Gonadorelin is a synthetic version of natural GnRH, and the other preparations are synthetic GnRH analogues. As with natural GnRH, these synthetic drugs affect the release of gonadotropins. The way in which they are administered determines their effects on the body. **Pulsatile administration** mimics the natural secretion of GnRH and is used therapeutically to stimulate the release of FSH and LH from the anterior pituitary. In contrast, continuous administration of GnRH agonists leads to downregulation of GnRH receptors and decreased secretion of FSH and LH. GnRH agonists are used in this manner to suppress gonadotropin stimulation of target organs.

Gonadorelin has a half-life of about 5 minutes. Unlike the other GnRH preparations, gonadorelin can be administered in a pulsatile manner via a portable infusion pump that injects a small bolus of the drug subcutaneously every 60 to 120 minutes. In women with infertility caused by **hypothalamic amenorrhea,** pulsatile treatment for 10 to 20 days is given to induce ovulation. Ovulation rates exceeding 90% are achieved by this method, and most women become pregnant within 6 months of therapy. Gonadorelin is also used diagnostically to evaluate the functional capacity of the gonadotropin-secreting cells of the pituitary. For this purpose, plasma gonadotropin concentrations are measured before and after a single dose of gonadorelin is injected.

Goserelin, leuprolide, and nafarelin are administered continuously and act to down-regulate pituitary GnRH receptors and thereby reduce gonadotropin secretion. By suppressing gonadotropin secretion, these GnRH analogues reduce testosterone levels in males and estrogen levels in females. This, in turn, decreases testosterone stimulation of the prostate gland and estrogen stimulation of the breast and uterus. For this reason, the GnRH analogues are effective in the treatment of precocious puberty in boys or girls and in the treatment of prostate cancer, breast cancer, and endometriosis in adults.

Nafarelin is used to manage endometriosis in women and central precocious puberty in children. It is administered as a nasal spray. Leuprolide and goserelin are administered as pellets that slowly release the drug following subcutaneous implantation. They are used to treat advanced prostate cancer, breast cancer, and endometriosis. Because these drugs cause a transient increase in testosterone levels when treatment of prostate cancer is begun, they should be given in combination with a testosterone antagonist (e.g., flutamide or bicalutamide) until testosterone levels fall. These drugs can cause a number of adverse effects because of decreased sex steroid levels, including hot flashes. Nafarelin, leuprolide, and goserelin have half-lives of about 3 hours.

Gonadotropin-Releasing Hormone Antagonist

Abarelix is the newest development in the treatment of advanced prostate cancer. It is a synthetic decapeptide that blocks GnRH receptors and thereby reduces pituitary secretion of LH and FSH, leading to reduced secretion of testosterone. More than 90% of men achieved medical castration, defined as a serum testosterone level less than 50 ng/dL, 4 weeks after a single intramuscular injection of abarelix. Although testosterone levels can increase in some patients over time, about 75% of men maintained testosterone levels below 50 ng/dL for 1 year. Unlike GnRH agonists, abarelix does not cause a transient increase in testosterone levels and concurrent treatment with testosterone antagonists is not necessary. A small percentage of men experienced an immediate hypersensitivity reaction following abarelix administration. The drug appears to be suitable for treating advanced symptomatic prostate cancer in men who are not good candidates for GnRH agonists and who refuse surgical castration.

Thyrotropin and Related Drugs

Thyrotropin (thyroid-stimulating hormone, TSH) is secreted in response to stimulation of the anterior pituitary by thyrotropin-releasing hormone (TRH). A preparation of recombinant human TSH is used to increase thyroid gland uptake of radioactive iodine in the diagnosis of various thyroid conditions and in the follow-up evaluation of thyroid cancer patients. A preparation of TRH called **protirelin** is employed in the diagnosis of central hypothyroidism caused by inadequate secretion of TSH. For this purpose, protirelin is injected and then the blood level of TSH is measured and compared with that of normal subjects.

Prolactin and Related Drugs

Prolactin contains 198 amino acids and acts on the mammary gland to stimulate tissue growth and promote lactation (milk production) in the presence of adequate levels of estrogens, progestins, and other hormones. Prolactin does not have any current clinical use.

The secretion of prolactin is inhibited by prolactin-inhibiting hormone (dopamine) and is stimulated by hypothalamic prolactin-releasing factors. Excessive prolactin secretion causes hyperprolactinemia and often leads to galactorrhea (excessive milk production), hypogonadism, and infertility. In some cases, hyperprolactinemia occurs secondary to prolactin-secreting pituitary adenomas.

Both the idiopathic and secondary forms of hyperprolactinemia can be treated with a dopamine agonist such as cabergoline or bromocriptine. Each drug mimics the action of PIH and thereby reduces prolactin secretion. In patients with prolactin-secreting adenomas, treatment with either drug also produces a significant reduction in tumor size.

Bromocriptine and cabergoline are both ergot alkaloid derivatives. The pharmacologic properties of bromocriptine, a drug that is also used to treat Parkinson's disease, are described in Chapter 24. In comparison with bromocriptine, cabergoline appears to be more effective and better tolerated in patients with hyperprolactinemia. Cabergoline selectively activates dopamine D_2 receptors in the pituitary gland and thereby suppresses the secretion of prolactin. It is also useful in persons with a mixed **growth hormone and prolactin-secreting pituitary adenoma.** The drug has an elimination half-life of about 65 hours, which provides a long duration of action. The most common adverse effects of cabergoline are nausea, headache, and dizziness.

POSTERIOR PITUITARY HORMONES

Oxytocin and vasopressin are 9-amino-acid peptides that are released from the posterior pituitary in response to specific physiologic stimuli (see Fig. 31–1).

Oxytocin and Related Drugs

Oxytocin is a hormone that increases the strength of uterine contractions and causes milk ejection (milk let-down) by contracting myoepithelial cells that line the ducts of the breast. The hormone is released via a reflex that is triggered by dilation of the uterine cervix, uterine contractions, or breast suckling. During late pregnancy, the uterus becomes highly sensitive to the actions of oxytocin owing to an increased number of oxytocin receptors. The sensitivity of the uterus is enhanced by estrogen and is inhibited by progesterone.

Synthetic oxytocin has several uses in obstetrics. The drug is given intravenously to induce or enhance uterine contractions during **labor**, and it is injected intramuscularly to **prevent postpartum uterine hemorrhage** by causing the uterine muscle to contract. In addition, a nasal spray preparation of oxytocin is available to **stimulate milk let-down in nursing mothers.** The spray is inhaled 2 to 3 minutes before breastfeeding. Adverse reactions to oxytocin are uncommon. They include cardiac arrhythmias, central nervous system stimulation, excessive uterine contraction, and hyponatremia.

Use of synthetic oxytocin is contraindicated in instances of fetal distress, abnormal fetal presentation, prematurity, or cephalopelvic disproportion.

Preterm labor is defined as labor that begins before completion of the 37th week of gestation and is associated with adverse neonatal outcomes. Atosiban is a peptide of 9 amino acids that acts as a competitive antagonist of oxytocin. It has been approved in European countries for treatment of preterm labor, but a recent analysis of clinical trials shows that atosiban did not reduce the incidence of preterm birth or improve neonatal outcome compared to placebo. In fact, atosiban was associated with lower birth weights and more maternal adverse effects than placebo, and atosiban appeared to increase neonatal mortality if used before the 28th week of gestation (see Simhan and Caritis, 2007).

Vasopressin and Related Drugs

Vasopressin (arginine vasopressin) is secreted by the posterior pituitary in response to a decrease in extracellular fluid volume or an increase in plasma osmotic pressure. The hormone interacts with two types of **vasopressin receptors** to exert its antidiuretic and vasoconstrictive effects.

The renal actions of vasopressin are mediated by V_2 **receptors** via production of cyclic adenosine monophosphate. Activation of V_2 receptors increases water reabsorption by the kidney by causing the insertion of water channels (aquaporins) in the luminal membranes of renal tubule cells in the collecting ducts. This action expands extracellular fluid volume and concentrates the urine. For this reason, vasopressin is also called **antidiuretic hormone**.

A deficiency of pituitary vasopressin secretion leads to **diabetes insipidus**, a condition characterized by excessive water excretion (polyuria) and increased water intake (polydipsia). Diabetes insipidus is usually treated with **desmopressin**, a long-acting synthetic analogue of vasopressin. This agent has potent antidiuretic activity but causes less vasoconstriction than natural vasopressin. Desmopressin solutions are available for injection and as a nasal spray that is used to prevent nocturnal urine production and enuresis in patients with diabetes insipidus. Desmopressin overdosage can result in dilutional hyponatremia.

Desmopressin is also used in treating children with **nocturnal enuresis**. This condition is often caused by a nocturnal diuresis volume that exceeds the functional bladder capacity. Not all children with nocturnal enuresis respond to desmopressin therapy, but it has been helpful in many cases. The factors that determine responsiveness to desmopressin are still being investigated.

Vasopressin causes vasoconstriction in several vascular beds by stimulating V_1 **receptors** in vascular smooth muscle. An injectable vasopressin preparation is used to control **bleeding caused by esophageal varices or colonic diverticula**. It should be used cautiously in persons with coronary artery disease. Desmopressin is also used for its vasoconstrictive effect, and it is employed in treating a variety of **hemorrhagic conditions**, including von Willebrand disease, mild hemophilia A, and congenital or drug-induced platelet function defects.

SUMMARY OF IMPORTANT POINTS

- Cosyntropin is a synthetic corticotropin analogue used to diagnose adrenal insufficiency, whereas corticorelin ovine triflutate is a corticotropin-releasing hormone used as a diagnostic test to distinguish adrenal and pituitary origins of Cushing's syndrome.

- Recombinant somatropin and somatrem are growth hormone preparations used to treat growth hormone deficiency in children with a low growth rate.

- Octreotide is a synthetic growth hormone–inhibiting hormone (somatostatin) analogue used in the treatment of acromegaly, carcinoid syndrome, pituitary adenomas that secrete thyrotropin, and tumors that secrete vasoactive intestinal polypeptide.

- Pegvisomant is a growth hormone analogue and growth hormone receptor antagonist used to treat acromegaly.

- Menotropins and chorionic gonadotropin are human gonadotropin preparations used to induce ovulation in infertile women. Chorionic gonadotropin is also used to stimulate spermatogenesis in men with hypogonadotropic hypogonadism and to treat cryptorchidism in prepubertal boys.

- Gonadorelin is a gonadotropin-releasing hormone (GnRH) preparation administered in pulsatile fashion to induce ovulation in women with hypothalamic amenorrhea.

- Goserelin and leuprolide are synthetic GnRH preparations administered continuously to suppress gonadotropin secretion in children with precocious puberty and in adults with prostate cancer, breast cancer, and endometriosis.

- Nafarelin is a GnRH preparation administered as a nasal spray to treat precocious puberty in children and endometriosis in women.

- Abarelix is a GnRH antagonist that reduces gonadotropin and gonadal steroid secretion, and is used to treat advanced prostate cancer.

- Dopamine agonists, cabergoline and bromocriptine, are used to suppress prolactin secretion in women with hyperprolactinemia. This condition is often associated with galactorrhea, hypogonadism, and infertility. Cabergoline may also reduce excessive growth hormone secretion in some persons with acromegaly and hyperprolactinemia.

- Oxytocin, which stimulates uterine contractions at term, is used to induce or augment labor, to prevent postpartum uterine hemorrhage, and to stimulate milk let-down in nursing women.

- Desmopressin is a synthetic vasopressin analogue that retains the antidiuretic activity of the natural hormone but lacks the vasoconstrictive effect. It is administered parenterally and intranasally to treat diabetes insipidus resulting from deficient pituitary vasopressin secretion. Synthetic vasopressin is used to control gastrointestinal bleeding by causing vasoconstriction.

Review Questions

1. Which drug is used to reduce secretion of gonadotropins and gonadal steroids in children with precocious puberty?
   (A) cabergoline
   (B) menotropins
   (C) leuprolide
   (D) gonadorelin
   (E) octreotide

2. Which drug for treating acromegaly acts by blocking receptors for growth hormone?
   (A) pegvisomant
   (B) somatropin
   (C) octreotide
   (D) sermorelin
   (E) cabergoline

3. By which mechanism does cabergoline relieve symptoms of hyperprolactinemia in persons with a prolactin-secreting pituitary adenoma?
   (A) blocking prolactin receptors
   (B) blocking receptors for prolactin releasing hormone
   (C) a cytotoxic effect on pituitary adenoma cells
   (D) activating receptors for prolactin-inhibiting hormone
   (E) stimulating the breakdown of prolactin

4. Which drug acts to block receptors for gonadotropin-releasing hormone in persons with advanced prostate cancer?
   (A) goserelin
   (B) abarelix
   (C) leuprolide
   (D) octreotide
   (E) pegvisomant

5. Octreotide is correctly described by which of the following statements?
   (A) It is identical to naturally occurring somatostatin.
   (B) It is used to treat growth hormone deficiency.
   (C) It is administered orally.
   (D) It is a more potent inhibitor of growth hormone secretion than is somatostatin.
   (E) It contains more than 100 amino acids.

Answers and Explanations

1. **The answer is C:** leuprolide. Leuprolide is an agonist at pituitary receptors for gonadotropin-releasing hormone (GnRH). When administered continuously, rather than in a physiologically pulsatile manner, leuprolide and other GnRH agonists cause down-regulation of GnRH receptors, leading to decreased secretion of gonadotropins (luteinizing hormone [LH] and follicle-stimulating hormone [FSH]). This action reduces secretion of gonadal steroids and thereby slows the onset of puberty in children with precocious puberty.

2. **The answer is A:** pegvisomant. Pegvisomant represents a new approach to treating acromegaly. It acts by blocking receptors for growth hormone and thereby reduces the formation of insulin-like growth factors (IGF) that mediate the growth-stimulating and other effects of growth hormone. Other drugs used to treat acromegaly act by reducing growth hormone secretion (octreotide and cabergoline).

3. **The answer is D:** activating receptors for prolactin-inhibiting hormone. Prolactin secretion is ordinarily restrained by tonic secretion of prolactin-inhibiting hormone (PIH or dopamine). Cabergoline and bromocriptine are dopamine receptor agonists that act to mimic the effect of endogenous prolactin-inhibiting hormone and thereby reduce excessive prolactin secretion in persons with prolactin-secreting pituitary adenomas.

4. **The answer is B:** abarelix. Abarelix is a gonadotropin-releasing hormone (GnRH) antagonist that blocks pituitary receptors for GnRH and thereby inhibits gonadotropin secretion in men with advanced prostate cancer. Unlike the GnRH agonists (e.g., leuprolide and goserelin), abarelix does not cause a transient increase in gonadotropin secretion when the drug is first given.

5. **The answer is D:** It is a more potent inhibitor of growth hormone secretion than is somatostatin. Octreotide only contains 8 amino acids and is not identical to somatostatin (answers A and E). It is not administered orally (answer C), and it is not used to treat growth hormone deficiency (answer B). In fact, octreotide is used to treat acromegaly caused by excessive growth hormone secretion.

SELECTED READINGS

Colao, A., M. Filippella, R. Pivonello, C. Di Somma, A. Faggiano, et al. Combined therapy of somatostatin analogues and dopamine agonists in the treatment of pituitary tumours. Eur J Endocrinol 156:S57–S63, 2007.

Franchini, M. The use of desmopressin as a hemostatic agent: a concise review. Am J Hematol 82:731–735, 2007.

Simhan, H.N., and S.N. Caritis. Prevention of Preterm Delivery. New Engl J Med 357:477–487, 2007.

Zaffanello, M., L. Giacomello, M. Brugnara, and V. Fanos. Therapeutic options in childhood nocturnal enuresis. Minerva Urol Nefrol 59:199–205, 2007.

CHAPTER 32

Thyroid Drugs

CLASSIFICATION OF THYROID DRUGS

Thyroid Hormone Preparations
- Levothyroxine (LEVOXYL, SYNTHROID)
- Liothyronine (CYTOMEL)

Antithyroid Agents
Thioamide Drugs
- Methimazole (TAPAZOLE)
- Propylthiouracil (PTU)

β-Adrenoceptor Antagonists
- Propranolol (INDERAL)

Other Antithyroid Agents
- Potassium Iodide Solution
- Sodium Iodide I-131 (^{131}I)

OVERVIEW

The thyroid gland synthesizes and secretes **triiodothyronine** (T_3) and **tetraiodothyronine** (T_4, thyroxine). **Thyroid hormones** are necessary for normal growth and development and timely sexual maturation. They affect every organ system and have a crucial role in metabolic processes, including those involved in the synthesis and degradation of essentially all other hormones. Thyroid hormones also augment sympathetic nervous system function, primarily by increasing the number of adrenoceptors in target tissues.

Thyroid Hormone Secretion

As discussed in Chapter 31, the secretion of thyroid hormones is initiated by a hypothalamic hormone called **thyrotropin-releasing hormone** (TRH), which increases secretion of an anterior pituitary hormone called **thyroid-stimulating hormone** (TSH, or thyrotropin). TSH is the prime regulator of iodide uptake and thyroid hormone formation by the thyroid gland. It fulfills this role by inducing the expression of three genes involved in iodide uptake and hormone production: (1) the sodium/iodide symporter that transports iodide into the thyroid gland, (2) thyroglobulin, and (3) thyroperoxidase. The secretion of TRH and TSH is regulated, in turn, by feedback inhibition of their secretion by T_4 and T_3 (Fig. 32–1).

Thyroid hormones are synthesized in a process that involves the uptake and organification of **iodide** and the subsequent coupling of iodotyrosine residues of **thyroglobulin.** These steps are depicted in Figure 32–2.

After iodide is actively transported into thyroid follicle cells, it diffuses across the cells to the apical membrane, where it is oxidized and attached to tyrosine residues of thyroglobulin. This process is called iodide organification. The iodinated tyrosine residues, monoiodotyrosine and diiodotyrosine are then coupled to form T_3 and T_4. Iodide organification and the coupling reactions are catalyzed by thyroperoxidase.

Thyroglobulin is stored as colloid in the follicular lumen. During the release of thyroid hormones, thyroglobulin reenters the follicular cell by endocytosis and undergoes proteolysis. The release of T_4 and T_3 is stimulated by TSH via the formation of cyclic adenosine monophosphate in thyroid follicular cells.

T_4 accounts for about 80% of the hormones secreted by the thyroid, and T_3 accounts for the remainder. These hormones are transported to target organs by thyroid-binding globulin, thyroid-binding prealbumin, and albumin. In peripheral tissues, some of the T_4 is converted to T_3 and reverse T_3 (rT_3) by 5′-deiodinase and 5-deiodinase, respectively. T_3 is about five times more active than T_4, whereas rT_3 in completely inactive. For this reason, the deiodinase enzymes have an important role in controlling the level of thyroid activity. The rate of conversion of T_4 to T_3 is also affected by a variety of other hormones, nutrients, and disease states. T_3 and rT_3 are eventually metabolized by deiodinase and sulfotransferase reactions to diiodothyronine sulfate.

When T_3 enters the nucleus of target cell, it binds to specific receptors that activate gene transcription, leading to increased synthesis of proteins necessary for growth, development, and **calorigenesis** (heat production).

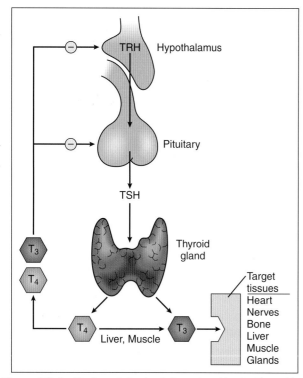

Figure 32–1. The hypothalamic-pituitary-thyroid axis. Thyroid hormone synthesis is initiated by the release of thyroid-releasing hormone (TRH) from the hypothalamus, which stimulates the pituitary to release thyroid-stimulating hormone (TSH). TSH acts on the thyroid gland to increase iodide uptake and the synthesis of thyroid hormones, T_4 and T_3. T_4 is converted to T_3 in liver and muscle. T_3 activates thyroid receptors in target tissues. Both T_4 and T_3 exert feedback inhibition of TRH and TSH secretion.

THYROID DISORDERS

Normal thyroid function, or **euthyroidism**, is maintained via feedback inhibition of TSH secretion so as to keep the plasma concentration of free (circulating or unbound) T_4 within a narrow range. Abnormally low or high T_4 and T_3 levels result in clinical manifestations of hypothyroidism or hyperthyroidism, respectively.

Hypothyroidism is characterized by low T_4 levels, and leads to impaired growth and development and decreased metabolic activity. In contrast, **hyperthyroidism** is due to high T_4 levels, leading to hyperactivity of organ systems (particularly the nervous and cardiovascular systems) and an increased metabolic rate.

Thyroid disorders are relatively common. In many cases, patients seek medical attention because they notice a diffuse or nodular thyroid gland enlargement (**goiter**) or suffer from other manifestations of abnormal thyroid function. Thyroid disorders are diagnosed primarily on the basis of their clinical manifestations and plasma T_4 and TSH levels. In most cases, TSH levels are abnormally high in persons with hypothyroidism and low in persons with hyperthyroidism.

Hypothyroidism

In infants and children, hypothyroidism causes irreversible mental retardation and impairs growth and development. In adults, hypothyroidism is associated with impairment of physical and mental activity and with slowing of cardiovascular, gastrointestinal, and neuromuscular functions. Hypothyroid patients may complain of lethargy, cold intolerance, weight gain, and constipation. The skin may become coarse, dry, and cold. Eventually, hypothyroidism causes **myxedema**, which is described as a dry, waxy swelling of the skin with nonpitting edema. **Myxedema coma** is characterized by hypothermia, hypoglycemia, weakness, stupor, and shock and is the end stage of long-standing, untreated hypothyroidism.

Many patients with mild hypothyroidism have a T_4 level within the normal range. As the disease progresses, however, the T_4 level usually falls below normal.

The most common cause of hypothyroidism in adults is **autoimmune thyroiditis (Hashimoto's disease)**. Other causes include thyroid surgery or radioactive iodine (RAI) treatment for hyperthyroidism; dietary iodine deficiency; and thyroid hypoplasia or enzymatic defects. Pituitary or hypothalamic dysfunction can cause secondary hypothyroidism.

Several types of drugs can induce thyroid disorders. Lithium inhibits the release of thyroid hormones by the thyroid gland (see Fig. 32–1) and can cause hypothyroidism by this mechanism. Amiodarone is an iodine-containing antiarrhythmic drug that can cause either hypothyroidism or hyperthyroidism through a variety of mechanisms that alter multiple thyroid functions.

The treatment for all forms of hypothyroidism is replacement therapy with a thyroid hormone preparation.

Hyperthyroidism

Manifestations of hyperthyroidism, or **thyrotoxicosis**, can include nervousness, emotional lability, weight loss despite an increased appetite, heat intolerance, palpitations, proximal muscle weakness, increased frequency of bowel movements, and irregular menses.

Most cases of hyperthyroidism are associated with overproduction of thyroid hormones by the thyroid gland, as indicated by the finding of increased RAI uptake. Excessive thyroid hormone production can result from excessive TSH, as occurs in patients with **TSH-secreting pituitary adenomas**, or it can result from gland stimulation by thyroid antibodies, as occurs in patients with **Graves' disease.**

Graves' disease results from the formation of antibodies directed against the TSH receptor on the surface of thyroid cells. These antibodies stimulate the receptor in the same manner as TSH, resulting in overproduction of thyroid hormones. Graves' disease is characterized by hyperthyroidism, thyroid enlargement, and exophthalmus (abnormal protrusion of the eyeball). Exophthalmus results from stimulation of orbital muscles by thyroid antibodies.

Excessive thyroid hormone production also occurs in persons with thyroid nodules that are independent of pituitary gland control. **Inflammatory thyroid disease (subacute thyroiditis)** can cause a transient form of hyperthyroidism that is caused by the release of preformed thyroid hormone from thyroid follicles.

Three treatment modalities are used in hyperthyroidism: antithyroid agents, surgery, and RAI treatment. The goals of therapy are to eliminate excessive thyroid hormone production and to control the symptoms of hyperthyroidism.

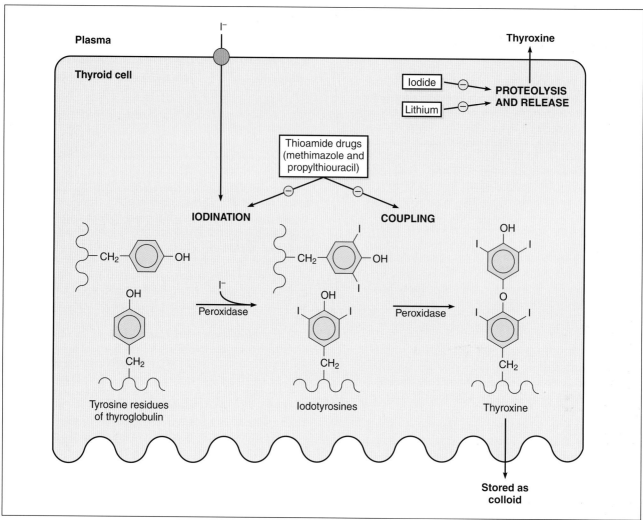

Figure 32–2. **Thyroid hormone synthesis and sites of drug action.** Iodide is accumulated by thyroid follicular cells by the sodium/iodide symporter. Thyroperoxidase catalyzes the iodination of tyrosine residues of thyroglobulin and the coupling of iodotyrosines to form triiodothyronine (T_3) and tetraiodothyronine (T_4, thyroxine). Thyroglobulin is stored as colloid in thyroid follicles and undergoes proteolysis to release T_4 and T_3 when stimulated by thyroid-stimulating hormone (TSH) or thyrotropin. Thioamide drugs inhibit the synthesis of thyroid hormones by inhibiting iodination and coupling of tyrosine residues. Elevated iodide concentrations and lithium inhibit the release of thyroid hormones.

The choice of treatment depends on the type and severity of hyperthyroidism and on the individual characteristics of the patient. Antithyroid agents are primarily used for the short-term treatment of hyperthyroidism, either to induce remission of Graves' disease or to control the symptoms of hyperthyroidism before thyroid surgery or RAI treatment. Surgery or RAI treatment can permanently cure hyperthyroidism. Either of these treatment modalities, however, often results in chronic hypothyroidism, which necessitates life-long thyroid hormone replacement therapy.

THYROID HORMONE PREPARATIONS

Synthetic levothyroxine is widely considered the drug of choice for thyroid hormone replacement in persons with hypothyroidism (Box 32-1). Thyroid hormones obtained from animal glands were used to treat thyroid disorders before the availability of synthetic hormones, but animal thyroid

preparations are no longer recommended by endocrinologists because of their variable composition and stability, and their potential to cause allergic reactions to animal proteins contained in these preparations.

The synthetic thyroid hormone preparations include **levothyroxine** (T_4), **liothyronine** (T_3), and **liotrix** (a mixture containing T_4 and T_3 in a ratio of 4:1). A recent analysis of controlled trials concluded that combined T_4 and T_3 was not superior to T_4 alone with respect to fatigue, depression, quality of life, or any other symptom of hypothyroidism, and liotrix is not currently recommended by most endocrinologists for treatment of hypothyroidism. The pharmacologic and pharmacokinetic properties of levothyroxine and liothyronine are shown in Table 32–1.

Levothyroxine

PHARMACOKINETICS. The oral bioavailability of levothyroxine is about 80%. Different brands and generic formulations of levothyroxine vary in hormone content and bioavailability,

BOX 32-1.　A CASE OF LETHARGY AND WEIGHT GAIN

CASE PRESENTATION: A 42-year-old woman complains to her health care provider of gaining 10 pounds over the last 6 months and of having a low energy level despite getting plenty of sleep. She has also had more trouble than usual with constipation and dry skin, and she has wanted to keep her home warmer than do other members of her family. On physical exam, her temperature is 97.3° F, her skin is dry, and she is found to have an enlarged thyroid gland (goiter). Laboratory tests are ordered and show that her TSH is 20 mU/L (normal is 0.4 to 5.5 mU/L), her free T_4 is 0.6 ng/dL (normal is 0.8 to 2.7 ng/dL), and her thyroperoxidase antibody level is 150. She is started on a low dose of levothyroxine and instructed to have a TSH level obtained in 6 weeks.

CASE DISCUSSION: The patient's enlarged thyroid and thyroid auto-antibodies are consistent with chronic autoimmune thyroiditis (Hashimoto's thyroiditis). Her symptoms and lab values are indicative of mild hypothyroidism. Her treatment goals are to relieve her symptoms and normalize her TSH level. The serum TSH concentration is the primary test used to evaluate replacement therapy in persons with hypothyroidism. This test is very sensitive to minute changes in free T_4 levels. A twofold change in the free T_4 level can cause a 100-fold change in the TSH level. In patients who have had their dose or brand of levothyroxine changed, the TSH level should be measured after 2 to 3 months. When the optimum replacement dose has been attained, clinical and lab monitoring should be performed every 6 to 12 months or whenever there is a change in the patient's status.

TABLE 32-1.　Pharmacologic and Pharmacokinetic Properties of Levothyroxine (T_4) and Liothyronine (T_3)

Property	Levothyroxine	Liothyronine
Relative potency	1	4
Oral bioavailability	80% (variable)	95%
Elimination half-life	7 days	1 day
Daily doses	1	1–3

wide range of doses to accommodate individualized therapy based on clinical and laboratory data. Therapy is usually begun with a lower dose, particularly in elderly patients and those with long-standing hypothyroidism. The dose is then increased at monthly intervals until a full replacement dose is achieved. A gradual increase in the dose prevents excessive stress on the cardiovascular and other organ systems and thereby causes fewer adverse reactions. Children usually require higher doses per kilogram of body weight than do adults.

The steady-state maintenance dose of levothyroxine is determined on the basis of the patient's clinical response, TSH levels, and T_4 levels. Many clinicians consider the TSH level to be the most sensitive test for determining thyroid replacement dosage. An elevated TSH level indicates that the levothyroxine dose is not sufficient. The expected range of T_4 levels in patients receiving thyroid replacement therapy is higher than that in healthy individuals, because a higher level of T_4 is required in patients to maintain adequate T_3 levels in the absence of endogenous T_3 production by the thyroid gland.

Levothyroxine is also the drug of choice for **suppressive therapy** in patients with **thyroid nodules**, **diffuse goiters**, or **thyroid cancer.** In these conditions, levothyroxine acts to suppress TSH production and reduce stimulation of abnormal thyroid tissue. Suppressive therapy thereby reduces goiter size and thyroid gland volume.

Myxedema coma is a medical emergency that requires intravenous administration of a loading dose of levothyroxine or liothyronine followed by smaller maintenance doses.

ADVERSE EFFECTS. Thyroid hormone preparations rarely cause adverse reactions if dosing is appropriate and is carefully monitored during the initial treatment of hypothyroidism and periodically thereafter. Excessive doses produce symptoms of hyperthyroidism.

INTERACTIONS. Aluminum hydroxide, cholestyramine, ferrous sulfate, and sucralfate are among the drugs that interfere with the absorption of levothyroxine. These drugs should be administered 2 hours before or after levothyroxine is administered. Estrogens, androgens, and glucocorticoids can alter thyroid-binding globulin and total T_4 and T_3 levels, but free T_4 and TSH levels usually remain normal in patients taking these steroid hormones. For this reason, the dosage of levothyroxine usually does not need to be adjusted in persons who are taking steroid hormones.

and formulations should not be substituted for one another without monitoring T_4 and TSH levels. Food also affects the bioavailability of levothyroxine, and it is now recommended that levothyroxine be taken at the same mealtime each day in order to obtain consistent blood levels. Because the half-life of levothyroxine is about 7 days, once-daily administration of the drug produces little fluctuation in plasma hormone levels. Because about 35% of T_4 is converted to T_3 in peripheral tissues, levothyroxine administration produces physiologic levels of both T_4 and T_3.

INDICATIONS. Levothyroxine is the drug of choice for **thyroid hormone replacement** in patients with **hypothyroidism**, because it is chemically stable, nonallergenic, and can be given orally once a day. Levothyroxine administration produces a stable pool of T_4 that is converted to T_3 at a steady and consistent rate. Levothyroxine tablets are available in a

Liothyronine

As shown in Table 32–1, liothyronine (T_3) is more potent than levothyroxine (T_4) and has a higher oral bioavailability. It is seldom used in the treatment of hypothyroidism, however, because it has several disadvantages. Liothyronine has a much shorter half-life than levothyroxine, and multiple daily doses may be needed to obtain a smooth response during hormone replacement therapy. Liothyronine does not increase plasma T_4 levels, so it is difficult to monitor the response to treatment. Liothyronine also causes more adverse cardiac effects and is more expensive than levothyroxine.

ANTITHYROID AGENTS

Antithyroid agents used in the treatment of hyperthyroidism include thioamide drugs, β-adrenoceptor antagonists, iodide salts, and radioactive iodine.

The thioamide drugs inhibit the synthesis of thyroid hormones, whereas sufficient doses of iodide salts inhibit the release of these hormones. The β-blockers are used to control the cardiovascular symptoms of hyperthyroidism until definitive treatment becomes effective. The β-blockers, the corticosteroids, some thioamide derivatives (see below), and some iodinated contrast agents (e.g., **ipodate**) also inhibit the peripheral conversion of T_4 to T_3. Because of this action, ipodate is being investigated for the treatment of acute thyrotoxicosis.

Thioamide Drugs

The thioamide drugs include **methimazole** and **propylthiouracil** (PTU).

Drug Properties

MECHANISMS. As discussed earlier in this chapter, the synthesis of thyroid hormones requires oxidation of trapped iodide, formation of iodotyrosines, and the coupling of iodotyrosines to form T_3 and T_4. Methimazole and PTU inhibit thyroperoxidase-catalyzed steps in this process (see Fig. 32–1). In addition, PTU (but not methimazole) inhibits the conversion of T_4 to T_3 in peripheral tissues. The contribution of this action to the therapeutic efficacy of PTU is uncertain, however, because PTU and methimazole appear to be therapeutically equivalent.

PHARMACOKINETICS. The thioamide drugs are well absorbed from the gut following oral administration. They are actively concentrated in the thyroid gland, which may account for their relatively long duration of action despite having relatively short half-lives. The thioamide drugs are extensively metabolized before undergoing renal excretion.

INDICATIONS. In patients with **Graves' disease**, a thioamide drug can be used in an attempt to induce remission or as a means to control symptoms before surgery or RAI treatment. The effects of thioamide drugs are delayed because it takes about 4 to 8 weeks of therapy before the glandular hormone stores are depleted and circulating hormone levels start to return to the normal range. At this time, doses can be gradually tapered at monthly intervals to achieve the desired steady-state thyroid hormone level. If the objective is long-term remission of Graves' disease, patients usually remain on the drug for 12 to 24 months. About 45% of patients will eventually obtain a permanent remission. The mechanisms responsible for remission are uncertain but may involve a reduction in the thyroid-stimulating activity of thyroid antibodies or an alteration of the immunologic defect that stimulated antibody production. Persons with persistent thyroid-stimulating antibodies have a higher incidence of relapse than do persons without persistent antibodies.

ADVERSE EFFECTS. Pruritic maculopapular **rash**, arthralgia, and fever occur in up to 5% of persons treated with a thioamide drug. Less frequently, a lupus erythematosus-like syndrome, hepatitis, or gastrointestinal distress is reported.

Many patients experience benign and transient **leukopenia**, with a white blood cell count of less than 4000/μL. This condition does not appear to be associated with the more severe **agranulocytosis** that sometimes occurs and is characterized by a granulocyte count of less than 250/μL. Severe agranulocytosis usually develops during the first 3 months of therapy and can be prevented by advising patients to stop treatment and immediately contact their physician if they experience fever, malaise, sore throat, or other flu-like symptoms.

Methimazole and PTU exhibit cross-sensitivity in about 50% of patients. For this reason, patients who have experienced a major adverse reaction should not be switched to the other drug.

Specific Drugs

Although methimazole and PTU appear to be clinically equivalent, they have minor differences. The plasma half-lives of methimazole and PTU are about 7 and 2 hours, respectively. Either drug, however, can be administered once or twice a day. Unlike methimazole, PTU inhibits the peripheral conversion of T_4 to T_3. Nevertheless, the clinical effects of the drugs are primarily related to inhibition of hormone synthesis and depletion of glandular stores.

About 70% of PTU is bound to plasma proteins. Methimazole is not bound to plasma proteins, and it readily crosses the placenta and appears in breast milk. Contrary to older studies, which indicated that PTU crosses the placenta less readily, newer evidence indicates that fetal blood concentrations of PTU are greater than maternal blood concentrations. Hence, both drugs must be used cautiously during pregnancy.

β-Adrenoceptor Antagonists

Thyroid hormones and the sympathetic nervous system act synergistically on cardiovascular function. This explains why increased levels of thyroid hormones cause tachycardia, palpitations, and arrhythmias. β-Adrenoceptor antagonists (e.g., **propranolol**) are used to reduce cardiovascular stimulation associated with hyperthyroidism. They act immediately and are particularly useful during **severe acute thyrotoxicosis (thyroid storm)**. They are also used to control symptoms of hyperthyroidism in patients awaiting either surgery or a response to RAI treatment.

Other Antithyroid Agents

Iodide Salts

Iodide salts are contained in **potassium iodide solutions**, such as **saturated solution of potassium iodide** and **Lugol's solution.** They are used on a short-term basis to treat patients with acute thyrotoxicosis, to prepare patients for thyroid surgery, and to inhibit the release of thyroid hormones following RAI treatment. Iodide salts can also be used to competitively block RAI uptake by the thyroid gland in the event of a nuclear reactor accident or other accidental exposure to toxic levels of RAI.

When administered in sufficient doses, iodide salts act immediately to inhibit the release of thyroid hormones from the thyroid gland. Plasma hormone levels then gradually decline as the circulating hormones are degraded. Patients with hyperthyroidism usually obtain symptomatic improvement within 2 to 7 days after starting iodide therapy. This effect is limited to several weeks, however, because the thyroid gland eventually escapes from the inhibitory effects of iodide salts. A thioamide drug can be used concurrently with iodide salts to further inhibit thyroid function and to provide a longer-lasting antithyroid effect.

In patients scheduled for thyroid surgery, a potassium iodide solution is usually administered preoperatively for 7 to 14 days to reduce the size and vascularity of the thyroid gland. As an adjunct to RAI treatment, potassium iodide is given 3 to 7 days following the administration of RAI.

The adverse effects of iodide salts are usually mild and can include skin rashes and other hypersensitivity reactions, salivary gland swelling, metallic taste, sore gums, and gastrointestinal discomfort.

Radioactive Iodine

Radioactive iodine is usually administered as a colorless and tasteless solution of **sodium iodide I 131** (^{131}I). The isotope is rapidly absorbed from the gut and concentrated by the thyroid gland. In the gland, it emits β-particles that destroy thyroid tissue. The particles have a tissue penetration of 2 mm, and the isotope has a half-life of 8 days. As thyroid tissue is destroyed, the circulating thyroid hormone levels gradually return to normal over several weeks.

β-Adrenoceptor antagonists are used to control symptoms of hyperthyroidism while the patient is awaiting the response to RAI treatment. Methimazole or PTU can be used if β-blockers alone are not adequate to control these symptoms. Pretreatment with thioamide drugs before RAI treatment, however, appears to reduce the cure rate and cause a higher incidence of posttreatment recurrence or persistence of hyperthyroidism. For this reason, thioamide drugs should be withdrawn several days before RAI treatment and reinstituted several days after it.

Iodide salts are used after RAI treatment to inhibit radioactive thyroid hormone release. They should not be used before RAI treatment, however, because nonradioactive iodide would compete with ^{131}I for uptake by the thyroid gland.

Treatment with RAI is absolutely contraindicated in pregnant women, because it destroys fetal thyroid tissue.

SUMMARY OF IMPORTANT POINTS

■ The thyroid gland synthesizes and secretes T_3 and T_4.

■ The steps in thyroid hormone synthesis include active iodide uptake by the thyroid gland, incorporation of iodide into tyrosine residues of thyroglobulin, and coupling of iodotyrosines to form T_3 and T_4. The secretion of T_3 and T_4 is modulated by TSH and by TRH.

■ The thyroid hormones, which activate cytoplasmic receptors, are translocated to the cell nucleus. In the nucleus, they activate gene transcription and thereby increase the metabolic rate and accelerate a wide range of cellular activities required for normal growth and development and for the maintenance of normal metabolism.

■ Levothyroxine (synthetic T_4) is the drug of choice for all forms of hypothyroidism. It has a long half-life (7 days) and can be administered orally once a day.

■ Liothyronine (synthetic T_3) is more potent than levothyroxine and has a higher oral bioavailability. It has a shorter half-life, however, and may need to be given several times a day.

■ Methimazole and PTU are thioamide drugs that inhibit thyroperoxidase-catalyzed steps in the synthesis of thyroid hormone. PTU also inhibits the peripheral conversion of T_4 to T_3. The onset of action of these drugs is delayed because of the time required to deplete glandular stores of thyroid hormone.

■ In patients with Graves' disease, methimazole or PTU is used in an attempt to induce remission or as a means to control symptoms before surgery or RAI treatment.

■ β-Adrenoceptor antagonists are used to control the cardiovascular symptoms of hyperthyroidism in patients who are suffering from acute thyrotoxicosis, are awaiting surgery, or are awaiting a response to RAI treatment.

■ The iodide salts in potassium iodide solutions act rapidly to inhibit the release of thyroid hormones from the thyroid gland. They produce symptomatic improvement in 2 to 7 days as circulating levels of thyroid hormones decline. Potassium iodide solutions are used to control symptoms of acute thyrotoxicosis, to reduce the vascularity and size of the thyroid gland before surgery, and to inhibit thyroid hormone release following RAI treatment.

■ RAI (^{131}I) is concentrated by the thyroid gland and emits β-particles that destroy thyroid tissue. It is used in the treatment of Graves' disease and other forms of hyperthyroidism. RAI treatment is absolutely contraindicated in pregnant women.

Review Questions

1. A man is given a drug to reduce thyroid gland size and vascularity before surgical thyroidectomy. Which mechanism is responsible for its use in this setting?
   - (A) inhibition of the sodium/iodide symporter
   - (B) inhibition of thyroperoxidase
   - (C) inhibition of TSH secretion
   - (D) inhibition of thyroid hormone release
   - (E) destruction of thyroid tissue

2. A woman with weight loss, nervousness, heat intolerance, and exophthalmus receives a drug that may induce a remission in her disease. Which serious adverse effect has been associated with this medication?
   - (A) gastrointestinal bleeding
   - (B) thromboembolism
   - (C) agranulocytosis
   - (D) hepatic failure
   - (E) esophageal ulcer

3. After total thyroidectomy, a woman is placed on a drug whose oral bioavailability is about 80%. Which attribute is correctly associated with this drug?
   - (A) partly converted to T_3 in the body
   - (B) administered several times a day
   - (C) the most potent thyroid hormone available
   - (D) has a half-life of about 1 day
   - (E) iron supplements increase its bioavailability

4. After exposure to radioactive fallout containing ^{131}I, which agent could be administered to prevent destruction of thyroid tissue?
   - (A) liothyronine
   - (B) methimazole
   - (C) propranolol
   - (D) potassium iodide
   - (E) levothyroxine

Answers and Explanations

1. **The answer is D:** inhibition of thyroid hormone release. Potassium iodide reduces the release of thyroid hormone and is given before thyroid surgery to reduce the size and vascularity of the gland and thereby facilitate surgical removal. It does not inhibit TSH secretion, inhibit the sodium/iodide symporter, or reduce synthesis of thyroid hormones.

2. **The answer is C:** agranulocytosis. Thioamide drugs are associated with leukopenia and, rarely, agranulocytosis, and patients should be carefully monitored for these conditions. These drugs do not typically cause hepatic failure, gastrointestinal bleeding, esophageal ulcers, or thromboembolism.

3. **The answer is A:** partly converted to T_3 in the body. Levothyroxine is the drug of choice for thyroid replacement therapy. After absorption, about 35% of levothyroxine is eventually converted to triiodothyronine. Levothyroxine is administered once a day, has a half-life of 7 days, and is not as potent as liothyronine (synthetic T_3). Its absorption is reduced by iron and aluminum salts.

4. **The answer is D:** potassium iodide. Potassium iodide would compete with radioactive iodide for uptake by the thyroid gland. Sufficient doses of potassium iodide can prevent destruction of the thyroid gland after exposure to [131]I.

SELECTED READINGS

Devdhar, M., Y.H. Ousman, and K.D. Burman. Hypothyroidism. Endocrinol Metab Clin North Am 36:595–615, 2007.

Nayak, B., and S.P. Hodak. Hyperthyroidism. Endocrinol Metab Clin North Am 36:617–656, 2007.

Nygaard, B. Hyperthyroidism. Am Fam Physician 76:1014–1016, 2007.

CHAPTER 33

Adrenal Steroids and Related Drugs

CLASSIFICATION OF ADRENAL STEROIDS AND RELATED DRUGS

Adrenal Steroid Drugs
Mineralocorticoids

- Fludrocortisone (FLORINEF)

Glucocorticoids

- Cortisone and Hydrocortisone
- Dexamethasone (DECADRON)[a]
- Prednisone (PREDNISONE INTENSOL) [b]
- Desoximetasone (TOPICORT)[c]

Adrenal Androgens

- Dehydroepiandrosterone (DHEA)

Adrenal Steroid Inhibitors
Corticosteroid Synthesis Inhibitors

- Aminoglutethimide (CYTADREN)

- Ketoconazole (NIZORAL)
- Metyrapone (METOPIRONE)

Corticosteroid Receptor Antagonists

- Mifepristone (MIFEPREX)
- Spironolactone (ALDACTONE)

[a]Also betamethasone (DIPROLENE), budesonide (RHINOCORT), and triamcinolone (ARISTOCORT).
[b]Also prednisolone (PRELONE) and methylprednisolone (MEDROL).
[c]Also desonide (TRIDESILON), fluticasone (FLONASE), fluocinonide (FLUONEX), ciclesonide (OMNARIS), and clobetasol (CLOBEVATE).

OVERVIEW

The adrenal glands are situated on top of the kidneys (as obvious from their name) and are essential for life. The adrenal glands are composed of two major parts; the adrenal cortex and the adrenal medulla, also called chromaffin tissue due to its brightly staining characteristics. The adrenal medulla produces epinephrine (adrenaline) as its main hormone and is an integral part of the sympathetic nervous system (see Chapter 5). This chapter describes the drugs that serve as replacements or alter the effects of steroid hormones produced by the adrenal cortex.

SYNTHESIS AND SECRETION OF ADRENAL STEROIDS

The adrenal cortex occupies about 90% of the adrenal gland, consists of three layers, and produces three types of steroid hormones, or **adrenocorticosteroids.** These hormones are classified as **mineralocorticoids, glucocorticoids,** and **adrenal androgens.** The mineralocorticoids are primarily produced in the outer layer (zona glomerulosa), whereas the glucocorticoids and adrenal androgens are produced in the middle layer (zona fasciculata) and inner layer (zona reticularis), respectively.

The major pathways for mineralocorticoid, glucocorticoid, and androgen biosynthesis are shown in Figure 33–1. Also shown is the site of action of drugs that inhibit **adrenocorticoid** synthesis. In humans, **aldosterone** is the major mineralocorticoid, **cortisol** is the major glucocorticoid, and **dehydroepiandrosterone (DHEA)** is the major adrenal androgen.

The regulation of corticosteroid secretion is depicted in Figure 33–2. The secretion of cortisol and adrenal androgens is primarily controlled by **corticotropin (ACTH)** secreted by the pituitary gland, whereas the secretion of aldosterone is chiefly regulated by the **renin-angiotensin system**. Various types of physical and mental stress are powerful activators of corticotropin-releasing hormone secretion, leading to increased

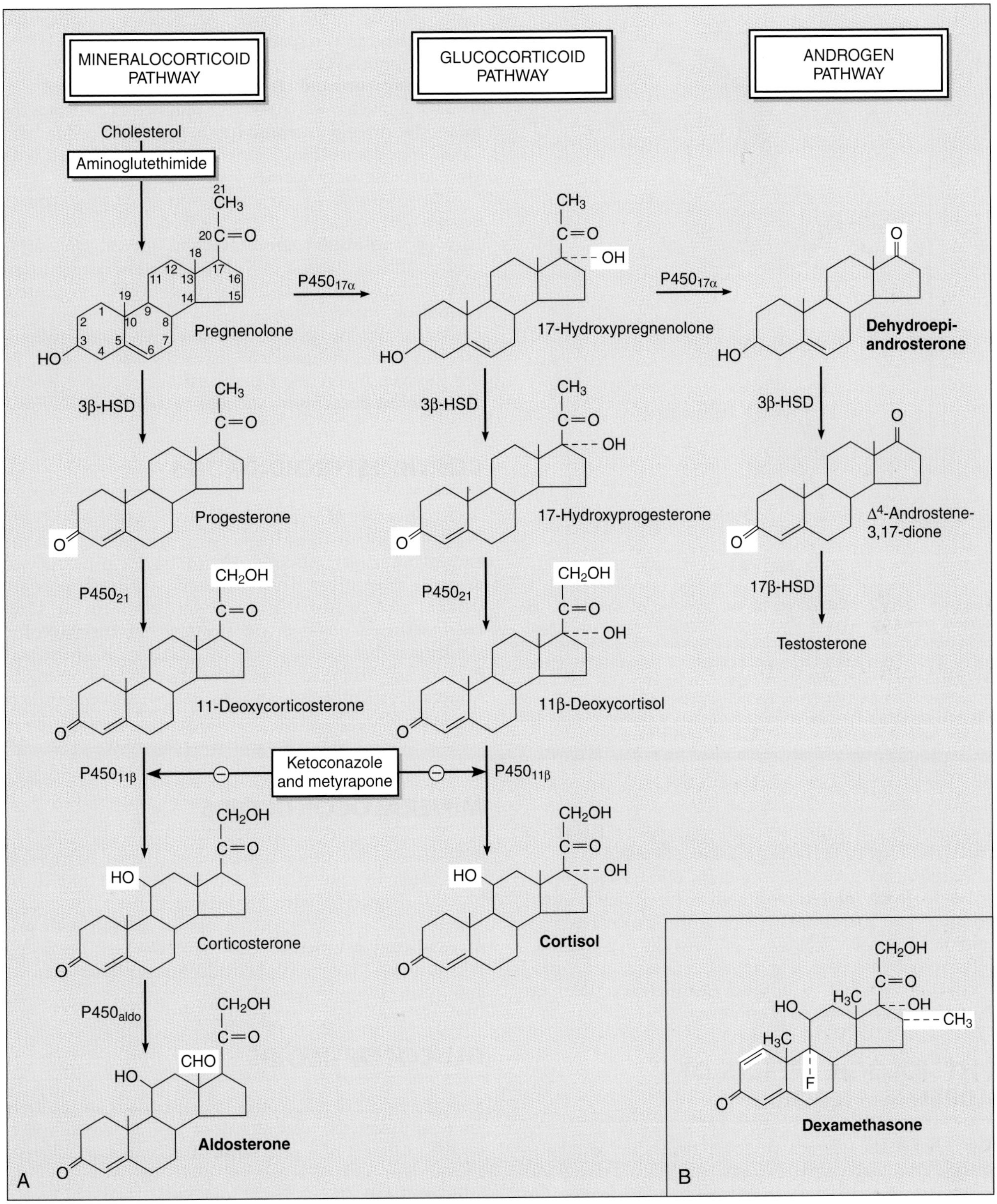

Figure 33-1. Biosynthetic pathways for adrenal steroids. (A) Major pathways for mineralocorticoid, glucocorticoid, and androgen biosynthesis are shown. Important enzymes include 3β-hydroxysteroid dehydrogenase (3β-HSD), steroid 21-hydroxylase ($P450_{21}$), steroid 11β-hydroxylase ($P450_{11\beta}$), aldosterone synthase ($P450_{aldo}$), steroid 17α-hydroxylase ($P450_{17\alpha}$), and 17β-hydroxysteroid dehydrogenase (17β-HSD). The structural changes produced by each reaction are unshaded. Aminoglutethimide blocks the synthesis of all adrenal steroids by inhibiting the conversion of cholesterol to pregnenolone. Ketoconazole and metyrapone inhibit $P450_{11\beta}$. The most common defect causing congenital adrenal hyperplasia is $P450_{21}$ deficiency. (B) The structure of dexamethasone is shown by the inset in lower right corner. In the synthetic steroids, glucocorticoid potency is enhanced by the introduction of a double bond at the 1,2 position or the introduction of a hydroxyl or methyl group at the 16 position. Both glucocorticoid and mineralocorticoid activities are increased by a fluorine substitution at the 9 position.

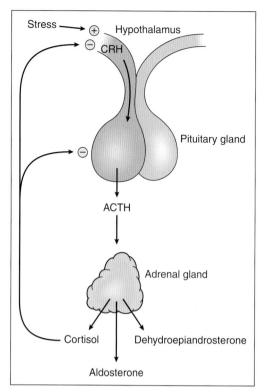

Figure 33–2. Regulation of the secretion of cortisol by the adrenal cortex. Stress and other stimuli increase the release of corticotropin-releasing hormone (CRH) from hypothalamic paraventricular nuclei, and CRH is carried by hypophysioportal vessels to the anterior pituitary, where it stimulates the release of corticotropin (ACTH). Corticotropin acts on the adrenal cortex to increase the release of adrenal steroids, although the release of aldosterone is primarily regulated by the renin-angiotensin system. Cortisol exerts feedback inhibition on the hypothalamus and pituitary to inhibit the release of CRH and corticotropin.

corticotropin and cortisol production. Cortisol exerts several effects that increase the body's **resistance to stress**.

As shown in Figure 33–2, cortisol and other glucocorticoids act as **feedback inhibitors** of both corticotropin-releasing hormone and corticotropin. This is why exogenously administered glucocorticoids can suppress the hypothalamic-pituitary-adrenal axis and inhibit endogenous cortisol production, leading to **adrenal insufficiency** when the exogenous glucocorticoid is withdrawn.

PHYSIOLOGIC EFFECTS OF ADRENAL STEROIDS

The adrenal steroids act on target tissues by binding to specific cytoplasmic steroid receptors, which are then translocated to the cell nucleus, a common mechanism for all steroid hormones (see Fig. 3–4 in Chapter 3). In the nucleus, the activated receptors stimulate the transcription of specific genes and thereby increase the translation of specific proteins. These actions lead to the various **metabolic** and **anti-inflammatory effects** of glucocorticoids, which are described below. In the renal tubules, activation of the mineralocorticoid receptor stimulates the synthesis of sodium channels and the sodium-potassium adenosine

triphosphatase that are needed for **sodium reabsorption**. This mechanism is responsible for the salt-retaining effects of mineralocorticoids.

The **glucocorticoid receptor** has a high affinity for cortisol but a much lower affinity for aldosterone, whereas the **mineralocorticoid receptor** has a high affinity for both aldosterone and cortisol. This enables cortisol to exert both glucocorticoid and mineralocorticoid actions.

Glucocorticoids induce enzymes involved in **gluconeogenesis** (the formation of glucose from amino acids) and have an **anti-insulin effect**. For this reason, glucocorticoid insufficiency can lead to **hypoglycemia** during stress. Glucocorticoids also activate enzymes involved in **protein catabolism**, thereby increasing the supply of amino acids needed for gluconeogenesis. Glucocorticoids **stimulate lipolysis** and inhibit the uptake of glucose by adipose tissue. By this mechanism, excessive glucocorticoid levels can lead to **abnormal fat distribution** and **muscle wasting** (see below).

CORTICOSTEROID DRUGS

A large number of semisynthetic glucocorticoid drugs are available; they are most frequently employed to attain the anti-inflammatory effects produced by supra-physiologic doses of these drugs. Less commonly, corticosteroids are used as replacement therapy in the treatment of **adrenal insufficiency** and in the treatment of **adrenogenital syndromes** that produce excessive quantities of adrenal androgens and insufficient quantities of other corticosteroids. **Mineralocorticoids** are primarily used as replacement therapy in persons with adrenal insufficiency. The properties of selected corticosteroids are listed in Table 33–1.

MINERALOCORTICOIDS

Aldosterone, the major mineralocorticoid in humans, is not suitable for clinical use due to the potential for electrolyte disturbances. **Fludrocortisone** is a mineralocorticoid that is used as replacement therapy in patients with **primary adrenal insufficiency (Addison's disease)**. The drug's salt-retaining potency is about 20 times greater than its anti-inflammatory potency.

GLUCOCORTICOIDS

A large number of glucocorticoid preparations are available for oral, parenteral, inhalational, or topical administration for the treatment of a wide range of inflammatory, allergic, autoimmune, and other disorders. Whenever possible, **topical** or **inhalational** administration is preferred because it is usually well tolerated and avoids most systemic adverse effects. Topical administration is widely used in the treatment of allergic or inflammatory conditions affecting the skin (see below), mucous membranes, or eyes. For example, topical ocular glucocorticoids are used to treat acute uveitis (inflammation of the iris, ciliary body, or choroid). Glucocorticoids are given by inhalation to treat allergic rhinitis, aspiration pneumonia, asthma, and other respiratory conditions (see Chapter 27).

TABLE 33-1. Pharmacologic Properties of Corticosteroids

Drug*	Route of Administration	Duration of Action (Hours)	Mineralocorticoid (Salt-Retaining) Potency	Glucocorticoid (Anti-inflammatory) Potency
Short-acting Drugs				
Hydrocortisone (cortisol)	Oral, parenteral, or topical	8–12	1	1
Cortisone	Oral, parenteral, or topical	8–12	0.8	0.8
Fludrocortisone	Oral	8–12	200	10
Intermediate-acting Drugs				
Methylprednisolone	Oral, parenteral, or topical	12–36	0.5	5
Prednisone	Oral	12–36	0.7	3.5
Triamcinolone	Oral, parenteral, or topical	12–36	0	5
Long-acting Drugs				
Betamethasone	Oral, parenteral, or topical	24–72	0	30
Dexamethasone	Oral, parenteral, or topical	24–72	0	30

*Fludrocortisone is classified as a mineralocorticoid; the other drugs are classified as glucocorticoids.

CLASSIFICATION. The glucocorticoids are usually classified according to their **potency and duration of action** (see Table 33–1). When given systemically, the duration of action of glucocorticoids is primarily determined by their potency at the glucocorticoid receptor, rather than by their elimination half-life. This is because the highly potent drugs evoke a longer-lasting **stimulation of gene transcription** than do less potent glucocorticoids. The potency of specific topical corticosteroids is discussed under the treatment of dermatologic conditions (see below).

LOW POTENCY, SHORT-ACTING GLUCOCORTICOIDS. Cortisol, the major glucocorticoid in humans, is called **hydrocortisone** when used as a pharmaceutical. Hydrocortisone and cortisone have a duration of action of 8 to 12 hours, have equal glucocorticoid and mineralocorticoid effects, and are the preferred glucocorticoids when **replacement therapy** is needed for patients with **adrenal insufficiency**. These drugs are also used as anti-inflammatory agents, but more potent glucocorticoids are often preferred for treating most inflammatory, allergic, and autoimmune disorders.

Medium Potency, Intermediate-acting Glucocorticoids

Prednisone, prednisolone, methylprednisolone, and triamcinolone are the glucocorticoids used most often for systemic treatment. In the body, **prednisone** is rapidly **converted to prednisolone**, a substance that is itself available as a drug. The intermediate-acting glucocorticoids have a duration of action of 12 to 36 hours and are often used to treat cancer, inflammation, allergy, and autoimmune disorders.

High Potency, Long-acting Glucocorticoids

Betamethasone and dexamethasone are stereoisomers that differ only in the configuration of a methyl group. Betamethasone is available for systemic use, and it is also used in the topical treatment of a number of skin disorders, including psoriasis, seborrheic or atopic dermatitis, and neurodermatitis. Dexamethasone is used in diagnostic dexamethasone suppression tests and in the treatment of a variety of neoplastic, infectious, and other inflammatory conditions that require the use of a potent and long-acting drug. Budesonide is a long-acting glucocorticoid that is administered by inhalation.

Anti-inflammatory Effects

The anti-inflammatory effects of glucocorticoids are primarily attributable to their multiple actions on several types of leukocytes (Fig. 33–3). First, glucocorticoids suppress the activation of T lymphocytes by interleukins and nuclear factor *kappa*B (NF-κB), a **transcription factor** for pro-inflammatory cytokine genes. Second, they suppress the production of cytokines by activated helper T cells. Cytokines play a major role in inflammation by recruiting and activating eosinophils and by stimulating antibody production by B cells. Glucocorticoids inhibit the production of pro-inflammatory cytokines by **increasing the transcription** of a gene for a protein that blocks NF-κB, as above.

Third, glucocorticoids decrease the release of various chemical mediators of inflammation, including histamine, prostaglandins, leukotrienes, and other substances from mast cells, eosinophils, and inflamed tissue. They decrease the synthesis of prostaglandins and leukotrienes by increasing the **transcription of lipocortin** which inhibits phospholipase A, the first step in the eicosanoid pathway (Chapter 26).

Fourth, glucocorticoids **stabilize lysosomal membranes** of neutrophils and prevent the release of catabolic enzymes (e.g., acid phosphatase) from these organelles; this limits cytotoxic effects of inflammation. Finally, glucocorticoids cause vasoconstriction and decrease capillary permeability by increased synthesis of lipocortin leading to **decreased prostacyclin** by the mechanism outlined above. They also decrease the synthesis of pro-inflammatory cytokines and other substances released from eosinophils in blood vessels as noted above, and both actions **reduce the vasodilation and plasma extravasation** that are the signs of inflammation.

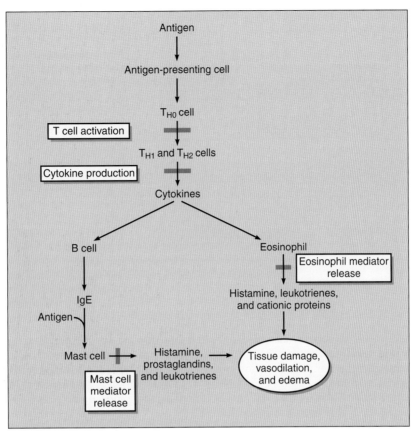

Figure 33-3. Anti-inflammatory actions of glucocorticoids. During the inflammatory process, undifferentiated helper T cells (T$_{H0}$) become activated T cells (T$_{H1}$ and T$_{H2}$) and produce cytokines. In addition to stimulating antibody production by B cells, cytokines recruit and activate eosinophils. Glucocorticoids act by suppressing T-cell activation, suppressing cytokine production, and preventing mast cells and eosinophils from releasing various chemical mediators of inflammation, including histamine, prostaglandins, leukotrienes, and other substances that cause tissue damage, vasodilatation, and edema. Glucocorticoids have additional anti-inflammatory effects that are described in the text. IgE = immunoglobulin E.

Glucocorticoids also have multiple effects on **circulating leukocytes**. Pharmacological doses of glucocorticoids suppress lymphoid tissue and reduce the number of circulating lymphocytes. They also reduce the concentration of circulating eosinophils, basophils, and monocytes while at the same time increasing the concentration of erythrocytes, platelets, and polymorphonuclear leukocytes.

INDICATIONS. Glucocorticoids are used for the diagnosis and treatment of adrenal diseases and for the treatment of a diverse group of nonadrenal disorders.

INFLAMMATION, ALLERGY, AND AUTOIMMUNE DISORDERS. The glucocorticoids are frequently used to **suppress inflammation and immune dysfunction** associated with diseases affecting almost every organ in the body. Glucocorticoids counteract inflammation evoked by physical trauma, extreme temperatures, noxious chemicals, radiation damage, and microbial pathogens. They also suppress inflammation caused by allergic and autoimmune reactions and other disease states. Examples of diseases treated with corticosteroids include systemic **lupus erythematosus, autoimmune thrombocytopenia purpura, polyarteritis nodosa, multiple sclerosis, ulcerative colitis, and polymyositis.**

Several glucocorticoids, including **beclomethasone**, are available for nasal inhalation or oral inhalation to treat **allergic rhinitis or asthma**, respectively. Inhaled glucocorticoids are often first-line therapy for these disorders, and their administration and use are described in Chapter 27. **Ciclesonide** is a newer agent also indicated for "hayfever" or allergic rhinitis.

For corneal inflammation and keratitis, many glucocorticoids are available in eyedrops, including a new combination of **loteprednol** and the antibiotic **tobramycin** (ZYLET). There are also combinations for the treatment of superficial bacterial infections of the external auditory canal ("swimmers ear") containing **hydrocortisone** and **neomycin** (CORTISPORIN).

Cancer

Because of their lymphotoxic effects, glucocorticoids are used in the treatment of **lymphocytic leukemias and lymphomas** (see Chapter 45). Dexamethasone is a long-acting glucocorticoid used in combination with other drugs to prevent emesis during cancer chemotherapy.

Respiratory Distress Syndrome

Betamethasone is used to prevent respiratory distress syndrome in premature infants. It acts by promoting fetal lung maturation in the same manner as endogenous cortisol

does. Betamethasone is used because it is not highly protein bound and will readily enter the placental circulation.

Adrenal Insufficiency

In primary adrenal insufficiency (**Addison's disease**), all regions of the adrenal cortex are destroyed. This gives rise to deficiencies in cortisol and aldosterone and to a reduction in androgen secretion. **Secondary adrenal insufficiency** has several causes, but it most commonly results when steroid drugs are used for a prolonged time, thereby suppressing the hypothalamic-pituitary-adrenal axis. Secondary disease is characterized by low levels of cortisol and androgens but normal levels of aldosterone.

Acute adrenal insufficiency (**adrenal crisis, addisonian crisis**) is a medical emergency that must be treated promptly with intravenously administered hydrocortisone for up to 48 hours. Once the patient's condition is stabilized, long-term oral hydrocortisone treatment can be instituted.

In the treatment of **chronic adrenal insufficiency**, hydrocortisone is administered orally in a manner that mimics the circadian secretion of cortisol by the normal adrenal gland, with two thirds of the daily dose given in the morning and one third given in the evening. If hyperkalemia is still present after the oral hydrocortisone dose is stabilized, the addition of a mineralocorticoid to the treatment regimen is usually required. A single daily dose, given in the morning, of **fludrocortisone** is often used for this purpose.

Congenital Adrenal Hyperplasia

Congenital adrenal hyperplasia (CAH) refers to a group of disorders caused by specific enzyme deficiencies that **impair the synthesis of cortisol and aldosterone**. Impaired synthesis leads to a compensatory increase in corticotropin secretion by the pituitary and results in adrenal hyperplasia. Because of the enzyme deficiencies, the steroid biosynthetic pathway **shifts** to the production of adrenal androgens, thereby resulting in virilization (masculinization) and pseudohermaphroditism in female children, and precocious development of secondary sex characteristics, including the genitals (macrogenitosomia), in male children. The most common defect is **21-hydroxylase deficiency**, which accounts for 90% of cases of CAH. The second most common defect is **11β-hydroxylase deficiency**, which accounts for 9% of cases. CAH is treated by giving **hydrocortisone** to suppress the secretion of corticotropin. **Fludrocortisone** can be given to provide additional mineralocorticoid activity for salt-losing patients with CAH.

Cushing's Syndrome

Adrenocortical hyperfunction (Cushing's syndrome), which is caused by excessive levels of circulating corticotropin, is treated with surgery, irradiation, and adrenal steroid inhibitors (Box 33-1). Cushing's syndrome most often results from a **pituitary adenoma** that produces excessive quantities of corticotropin, leading to adrenal hyperplasia and excessive cortisol production. Other causes of Cushing's syndrome include adrenal adenomas, adrenal carcinomas, and ectopic corticotropin (ACTH)-secreting tumors.

The diagnosis of Cushing's syndrome is often based on the free cortisol level in urine samples and on the results of testing with dexamethasone. In the **low-dose dexamethasone suppression test**, a single dose of dexamethasone is given

---

BOX 33–1. THE CASE OF THE MOON-FACED MAN

CASE PRESENTATION: A 49-year-old man, with a history of cigarette smoking, notices recent weight gain of about 15 pounds in the last few months. He is puzzled by this as he watches his diet and gets moderate exercise in his job as construction foreman. His wife says that his face is looks "puffy" and he has stretch marks on his stomach. Upon questioning by his physician, he admits to feeling tired lately, and physical examination reveals a small fatty hump on his back. The physician orders a low-dose dexamethasone suppression test, which results in no change of the man's elevated levels of cortisol; a similar finding is found after a high-dose dexamethasone test. Given the history of smoking, imaging studies including chest x-rays and CT scans are done and reveal small cell (oat cell) carcinoma of the lungs. He is prescribed metyrapone to treat Cushing's syndrome and told he has less than a year to live.

CASE DISCUSSION: Pituitary adenomas cause most cases of Cushing's syndrome, and benign tumors of the pituitary gland. This form of the syndrome, known as "Cushing's disease," affects women five times more frequently than men. Corticotropin (ACTH) can also be produced outside ("ectopic") the pituitary from benign or malignant tumors. In many cases, small oat cell lung tumors are the cause; more frequently in men than women. More rarely, an abnormality of the adrenal glands, most often an adrenal tumor, causes Cushing's syndrome. In the case of the moon-faced man, both suppression tests came back with no change in the elevated cortisol levels, suggesting that a pituitary adenoma was not the cause. Many cancer cells secrete excess levels of adrenal cortical hormones, including cortisol and adrenal androgens. Given the patient's history of smoking, it is likely his Cushing's syndrome was related to an ectopic ACTH-producing tumor. Metyrapone inhibits the synthesis of glucocorticoids by inhibiting the 11β-hydroxylase enzyme that catalyzes the final step in the glucocorticoid pathway. Metyrapone is occasionally used to treat Cushing's syndrome in patients who are refractory to other treatments and are not candidates for surgery, as in this case. An alternative is aminoglutethimide, which inhibits the conversion of cholesterol to pregnenolone, an early and rate-limiting step in adrenal steroid biosynthesis.

---

orally at 11:00 PM, and cortisol levels in plasma are measured at 8:00 AM the following morning. In healthy individuals, dexamethasone will suppress corticotropin secretion by the pituitary and cause plasma cortisol levels to be under 5 μg/dL. In persons with Cushing's syndrome, dexamethasone will not suppress corticotropin secretion, so the cortisol

level will usually exceed 10 µg/dL. The **high-dose dexamethasone suppression test** can be used to differentiate adrenal hyperplasia from other causes of hyperadrenocorticism.

Cushing's syndrome is usually treated by surgical excision of the pituitary adenoma or the hyperplastic adrenal glands. Patients must receive hydrocortisone parenterally in large doses during the surgical procedure. The dose is then gradually tapered to normal replacement levels.

Dermatologic Conditions

Corticosteroids are often used to treat a wide range of dermatologic conditions, including atopic (contact) and seborrheic **dermatitis**, **pruritus** (itching) from various causes, **psoriasis**, **sunburn**, and a number of other conditions. Topical corticosteroids are grouped according to their relative anti-inflammatory potency (high, medium, and low). Low-potency drugs are preferred for treating areas with thinner skin (e.g., the face, eyes) and intertriginous areas where skin is folded or overlapped. Low- to medium-potency steroids can be used on the ears, trunk, arms, legs, and scalp. Medium- to very high-potency drugs may be needed to treat disorders in areas of thicker skin (e.g., the palms and soles).

The type of lesion influences the choice of vehicle for drug administration. Ointments are preferred to treat disorders involving dry, cracked, scaly, or hardened skin. Lotions and creams are best for treating moist, weeping lesions or conditions with intense inflammation. Lotions and gels are usually more convenient for applying steroids to hairy areas.

Low-potency topical steroids include hydrocortisone, which is available without prescription for treating minor allergic reactions (e.g., insect bites). Other low-potency topical steroids include desonide and dexamethasone. **Medium-potency topical steroids** include triamcinolone and fluticasone. Desoximetasone and fluocinonide are **high-potency steroids,** whereas betamethasone dipropionate and clobetasol are **very high-potency steroids.**

Other Disorders

Glucocorticoids are used to treat **hypercalcemia**, and they are the drugs of choice for managing **sarcoidosis** (a systemic granulomatous disorder). Glucocorticoids are also used as immunosuppressant drugs to prevent **organ graft rejection** (see Chapter 45).

Systemic Administration and Pharmacokinetics

Glucocorticoids are highly lipid soluble and are well absorbed from the gut after oral administration. In the circulation, the glucocorticoids are highly bound to corticosteroid-binding globulin and albumin. Glucocorticoids are oxidized by cytochrome P450 enzymes and conjugated with sulfate or glucuronide in the liver before undergoing renal excretion.

Glucocorticoids are administered orally to treat **allergic reactions**, **autoimmune disorders**, **neoplastic diseases**, and many other conditions. For acute disorders, glucocorticoids are often more effective when they are initially given in large doses that are gradually tapered over several days until treatment is discontinued. For severe autoimmune and inflammatory disorders (e.g., systemic lupus erythematous and polymyositis with dermatomyositis), large doses of prednisone must be given daily for several months until a remission is achieved, and then the dose is slowly tapered and continued for 1 to 2 years or longer. In some conditions, it may be possible to convert the patient to **alternate-day therapy**, in which all or most of the dose is given on alternate days. This dosage schedule appears to reduce the severity of adverse effects and produces less suppression of the hypothalamic-pituitary-adrenal axis by allowing more time for recovery between doses.

Glucocorticoids are administered parenterally to treat **acute adrenal crises**, **acute allergic reactions, and similar emergencies.** In some cases, the drugs are given intravenously. In other cases, they are given intramuscularly, either as a rapidly absorbed solution or as a slowly absorbed drug suspension (depot preparation). Depot preparations are useful in providing a sustained level of the drug for several weeks, as is sometimes necessary in the treatment of a severe allergic reaction.

Adverse Effects

Administration of supraphysiologic doses of glucocorticoids for more than 2 weeks produces a series of tissue and metabolic changes that resemble Cushing's syndrome. The face becomes rounded and puffy ("moon face") as fat is redistributed to the face and trunk from the extremities. Fat accumulation in the supraclavicular and dorsocervical areas contributes to the development of a "buffalo hump." Increased hair growth (hirsutism), weight gain, and muscle wasting and weakness are often observed. Dermatologic changes can include acne (steroid acne), bruising, and thinning of the skin.

Other metabolic and physiologic changes caused by glucocorticoid administration include **hyperglycemia, glucose intolerance**, and **hypertension**. Some changes, such as sodium retention, potassium loss, and hypertension, are more common when cortisone or hydrocortisone is used because these drugs have greater mineralocorticoid activity than do other glucocorticoids.

Glucocorticoids increase bone catabolism and antagonize the effect of vitamin D on calcium absorption, thereby contributing to the development of **osteoporosis** (see Chapter 36). Glucocorticoids also have several effects on the central nervous system. They alter the mood in some persons and can cause **euphoria or psychosis**. Large doses of glucocorticoids stimulate gastric acid and pepsin production and may thereby exacerbate peptic ulcers. Glucocorticoids can also reduce the secretion of thyroid-stimulating hormone and follicle-stimulating hormone by the pituitary gland.

Long-term use of glucocorticoids can cause posterior subcapsular **cataracts** and **glaucoma**, and it can mask the symptoms and signs of mycotic and other infections. In children, long-term use can cause growth retardation.

For the above reasons, glucocorticoids should be avoided or used with caution in patients with psychoses, peptic ulcers, heart diseases, hypertension, diabetes, osteoporosis, and certain infections.

ADRENAL ANDROGENS

Dehydroepiandrosterone (DHEA) is the major androgen secreted by the adrenal cortex. Smaller quantities of **androstenedione** and **testosterone** are also secreted by the adrenal gland.

Dehydroepiandrosterone is an extremely weak androgen, but it is partly converted to testosterone in the body. In humans,

studies show that the production of DHEA by the adrenal gland **declines in a linear fashion** after the age of 20 years. In animals, studies indicate that DHEA protects against the development of diabetes mellitus, immune disorders, and cancer. DHEA also appears to prevent weight gain and prolong life in some species. For these reasons, the use of DHEA supplements has been adopted uncritically by the alternative medicine/health store culture. Although some evidence suggests beneficial effects of DHEA in the elderly and other people, much remains to be learned about the clinical utility of this steroid.

Because DHEA is a weak androgen, it should not be used by men with prostate cancer.

CORTICOSTEROID SYNTHESIS INHIBITORS

Figure 33–1 shows the sites of action of three inhibitors of corticosteroid synthesis: aminoglutethimide, metyrapone, and ketoconazole.

Aminoglutethimide

Aminoglutethimide inhibits the conversion of cholesterol to pregnenolone, an early and rate-limiting step in adrenal steroid biosynthesis. Because the synthesis of all steroids is reduced by aminoglutethimide, it has been used in the treatment of **breast cancer** and **malignant adrenocortical tumors.** It also has been used in combination with metyrapone (see "Metyrapone") to treat **Cushing's syndrome.**

Metyrapone

Metyrapone inhibits the synthesis of glucocorticoids by **inhibiting the 11β-hydroxylase** enzyme that catalyzes the final step in the glucocorticoid pathway. As a result of this action, the steroid biosynthetic pathway is shifted to the production of adrenal androgens. Metyrapone is occasionally used to treat **Cushing's syndrome** in patients who are refractory to other treatments and are not candidates for surgery. Metyrapone is also sometimes used in tests of adrenal function and for preparing patients for surgery.

Ketoconazole and Fluconazole

Ketoconazole and fluconazole are antifungal drugs that inhibit several cytochrome P450 enzymes involved in steroid biosynthesis, including 11β-hydroxylase. When used in the treatment of **Cushing's syndrome,** the drugs can lower the amount of cortisol to the normal range for some patients. They also inhibit androgen synthesis, however, and may cause gynecomastia in male patients.

CORTICOSTEROID RECEPTOR ANTAGONISTS

Spironolactone

Spironolactone is a synthetic steroid that competes with aldosterone for the mineralocorticoid (aldosterone) receptor in the renal tubules. It is used as a **potassium-sparing diuretic** (see Chapter 13) and as an agent for the treatment of hyperaldosteronism. Spironolactone is the drug of choice for **primary hyperaldosteronism** caused by bilateral adrenal hyperplasia, whereas surgery is the treatment of choice for hyperaldosteronism caused by an aldosterone-producing adenoma. **Secondary hyperaldosteronism** associated with heart failure, Bartter's syndrome, and other conditions may also be improved by the administration of spironolactone.

Mifepristone

Mifepristone is an antagonist at both progesterone and glucocorticoid receptors (see Chapter 34). It has been studied for the treatment of **Cushing's syndrome** and appears to be effective in reversing the effects of **hyperadrenocorticism.**

SUMMARY OF IMPORTANT POINTS

■ The adrenal gland secretes mineralocorticoids (primarily aldosterone), glucocorticoids (primarily cortisol), and adrenal androgens (primarily dehydroepiandrosterone).

■ Mineralocorticoids have salt-retaining activity. They include fludrocortisone, a short-acting drug that is used to supplement hydrocortisone (cortisol) treatment in patients with adrenal insufficiency.

■ Glucocorticoids increase gluconeogenesis, protein and lipid catabolism, and the body's resistance to stress. They reduce inflammation by inhibiting the migration of leukocytes and the production and release of cytokines, prostaglandins, leukotrienes, and other mediators of inflammation. They also stabilize lysosomal membranes and cause vasoconstriction.

■ Glucocorticoids are chiefly used as anti-inflammatory and immunosuppressive drugs in the treatment of a wide range of allergic, inflammatory, and autoimmune disorders. They are also used as replacement therapy in the treatment of primary adrenal insufficiency (Addison's disease) and congenital adrenal hyperplasia.

■ Glucocorticoids include short-acting drugs (cortisone and hydrocortisone), intermediate-acting drugs (methylprednisolone, prednisone, and triamcinolone), and long-acting drugs (betamethasone and dexamethasone).

■ In comparison with cortisol, most synthetic glucocorticoids have increased glucocorticoid potency and decreased mineralocorticoid potency.

■ Glucocorticoids are generally administered topically to treat skin, mucous membrane, and ocular disorders and by inhalation to treat allergic rhinitis and asthma.

■ Topical steroids for treating dermatologic conditions include desonide (low potency), triamcinolone and fluticasone (medium potency), desoximetasone (high potency), and clobetasol (very high potency).

■ In patients with acute allergic reactions, glucocorticoids are initially given in large doses. The doses are rapidly tapered and eventually discontinued. In patients with severe autoimmune and inflammatory diseases, large doses of prednisone or other glucocorticoids may be required for several months. Alternate-day therapy is preferred for their long-term administration.

■ Adverse effects of glucocorticoids include fat accumulation in the face and trunk, muscle wasting, skin changes, glucose intolerance, potassium depletion, osteoporosis, hypertension, and cataracts.

■ Aminoglutethimide, metyrapone, and ketoconazole inhibit various steps in corticosteroid biosynthesis and are occasionally used to diagnose and treat adrenal hyperplasia.

Review Questions

1. After receiving a low dose of dexamethasone, a patient is found to have a plasma cortisol level of 20 µg/dL the next morning. Which disorder is most likely in this patient?
   (A) congenital adrenal hyperplasia
   (B) chronic adrenal insufficiency
   (C) 11β-hydroxylase deficiency
   (D) Cushing's syndrome
   (E) pituitary insufficiency

2. A boy experiences a moderately severe reaction to a wasp sting. Which method of corticosteroid administration is appropriate for this patient?
   (A) continuous high dose therapy for several weeks
   (B) continuous low dose therapy for several weeks
   (C) gradually increasing doses over several days
   (D) gradually decreasing doses over several days
   (E) intermittent every-other-day therapy until symptoms resolve

3. A patient with Addison's disease continues to have hyperkalemia despite receiving adequate replacement doses of hydrocortisone (cortisol). Which drug should be added to the treatment regimen to reduce serum potassium levels?
   (A) dexamethasone
   (B) fludrocortisone
   (C) triamcinolone
   (D) prednisone
   (E) aldosterone

4. The long-term administration of large doses of prednisone will cause the least reduction in the secretion of which hormone?
   (A) cortisol
   (B) corticotropin
   (C) corticotropin-releasing hormone
   (D) aldosterone

5. A woman has developed a moderately severe contact dermatitis reaction to a cosmetic preparation on her face and eyes. Which topical corticosteroid would be most suitable for treating this condition?
   (A) desonide
   (B) prednisone
   (C) clobetasol
   (D) fluocinonide
   (E) deosoximetasone

Answers and Explanations

1. **The answer is D:** Cushing's syndrome. In healthy persons, a dose of dexamethasone should suppress cortisol secretion the next morning and cortisol levels should be <5 µg/dL. In this case, the patient's cortisol level was elevated, suggesting the presence of Cushing's syndrome. Congenital adrenal hyperplasia, chronic adrenal insufficiency, 11β-hydroxylase deficiency, and pituitary insufficiency are all associated with decreased cortisol secretion.

2. **The answer is D:** gradually decreasing doses over several days. For the treatment of acute allergic reactions, the most effective regimens are those in which glucocorticoids are given in large doses initially and then gradually tapered over 5 to 7 days. This produces the most rapid improvement in symptoms while causing relatively little adrenal suppression.

3. **The answer is B:** fludrocortisone. Fludrocortisone is approximately 100 times more potent as a mineralocorticoid than is cortisol and is the most potent mineralocorticoid available for clinical use. It acts to increase sodium retention and potassium excretion, thereby lowering serum potassium levels. Aldosterone (A), an endogenous mineralocorticoid, is not available as a drug. Dexamethasone (A), triamcinolone (C), and prednisone (D) are potent glucocorticoids that would cause excessive glucocorticoid effects in a person already receiving adequate doses of hydrocortisone.

4. **The answer is D:** aldosterone. Exogenous administration of glucocorticoid drugs causes feedback inhibition of the secretion of corticotropin-releasing hormone, corticotropin, cortisol, and cortisone. Secretion of the mineralocorticoid, aldosterone, is primarily under the influence of the renin-angiotensin axis and is not suppressed greatly by exogenous glucocorticoid administration.

5. **The answer is A:** desonide. Desonide is a low-potency topical corticosteroid appropriate for treating conditions of the face and eyes. Prednisone (B) is not administered topically. Clobetasol (C) is a medium-potency topical steroid, and fluocinonide (D) and desoximetasone (E) are high-potency topical steroids. Medium- to high-potency steroids are used on areas of the body with thicker skin than on the face and eyes.

SELECTED READINGS

Berris, K.K., A.L. Repp, and M. Kleerekoper. Glucocorticoid-induced osteoporosis. Curr Opin Endocrinol Diabetes Obes 14(6):446–450, 2007.

Diez, J.J., and P. Iglesias. Pharmacological therapy of Cushing's syndrome: drugs and indications. Mini Rev Med Chem 7(5):467–480, 2007.

Jacob, S.E., and M.P. Castanedo-Tardan. Pharmacotherapy for allergic contact dermatitis. Expert Opin Pharmacother 8(16):2757–2774, 2007.

Langan, R.C., P.B. Gotsch, M.A. Krafczyk, and D.D. Skillinge. Ulcerative colitis: diagnosis and treatment. Am Fam Physician 76(9):1323–1330, 2007.

Soloway, R.D., and A.T. Hewlett. The medical treatment for autoimmune hepatitis through corticosteroid to new immunosuppressive agents: a concise review. Ann Hepat 6(4):204–207, 2007.

CHAPTER 34

Drugs Affecting Fertility and Reproduction

CLASSIFICATION OF DRUGS AFFECTING FERTILITY AND REPRODUCTION

Estrogens
- Estradiol[a]
- Conjugated Equine Estrogens (PREMARIN)

Progestins
- Medroxyprogesterone (PROVERA)[b]
- Norethindrone (AYGESTIN)[c]

Antiestrogens
- Clomiphene (CLOMID, SEROPHENE)
- Raloxifene (EVISTA)
- Tamoxifen (NOLVADEX)
- Anastrozole (ARIMIDEX)
- Letrozole (FEMARA)

Antiprogestins
- Mifepristone (MIFEPREX)

Androgens
- Danazol (DANOCRINE)
- Testosterone (TESTEX, ANDROGEL)
- Methyltestosterone (ANDROID, TESTRED, VIRILON)

Antiandrogens
- Flutamide (EULEXIN)[d]
- Finasteride (PROPECIA, PROSCAR)
- Dutasteride (AVODART)

[a]Also ethinyl estradiol and mestranol.
[b]Also hydroxyprogesterone, megestrol (MEGACE), and progesterone (PROMETRIUM).
[c]Also desogestrel, drospirenone, levonorgestrel, norelgestromin, norethynodrel, and norgestimate.
[d]Also bicalutamide (CASODEX) and nilutamide (NILANDRON).

OVERVIEW

Human reproduction involves a cascade of hormonal secretions, beginning with the secretion of gonadotropin-releasing hormone (GnRH) from the hypothalamus. As described in Chapter 31, GnRH stimulates the pituitary to release two gonadotropins: follicle-stimulating hormone (FSH) and luteinizing hormone (LH). These gonadotropins then stimulate the production of **steroids** and gametes by the ovary in the female and by the testis in the male.

The three categories of steroids secreted by the gonads are (1) **estrogens**, which include **estradiol, estrone**, and **estriol**; (2) **progestins**, which include **progesterone**; and (3) **androgens**, which include **testosterone.** Estrogens, progesterone, and testosterone are produced in both males and females, but the relative amounts and patterns of secretion differ markedly between the sexes. Females primarily secrete estrogens and progesterone, whereas males primarily produce testosterone.

Biosynthesis of Gonadal Steroids

As shown in Figure 34–1, **pregnenolone** is the precursor to progesterone. It is also the precursor to dehydroepiandrosterone and androstenedione (two androgens secreted by the adrenal gland and discussed in Chapter 33) and to testosterone (the major androgen in males). The adrenal and gonadal androgens are converted to estrogens by **aromatase,** an enzyme that forms the aromatic A-ring necessary for the selective high-affinity binding of estradiol, estrone, and estriol to **estrogen receptors.**

In females, ovarian **thecal cells** secrete small quantities of testosterone. In males, about 95% of testosterone is produced by **Leydig's cells** in the testes, and the remainder is derived from the **adrenal cortex.** Testosterone is synthesized in the testes by the same pathways as in the ovaries. Testosterone is subsequently converted to **dihydrotestosterone** (DHT) by **5α-reductase** in the prostate, hair follicles, and skin. In the plasma, testosterone is

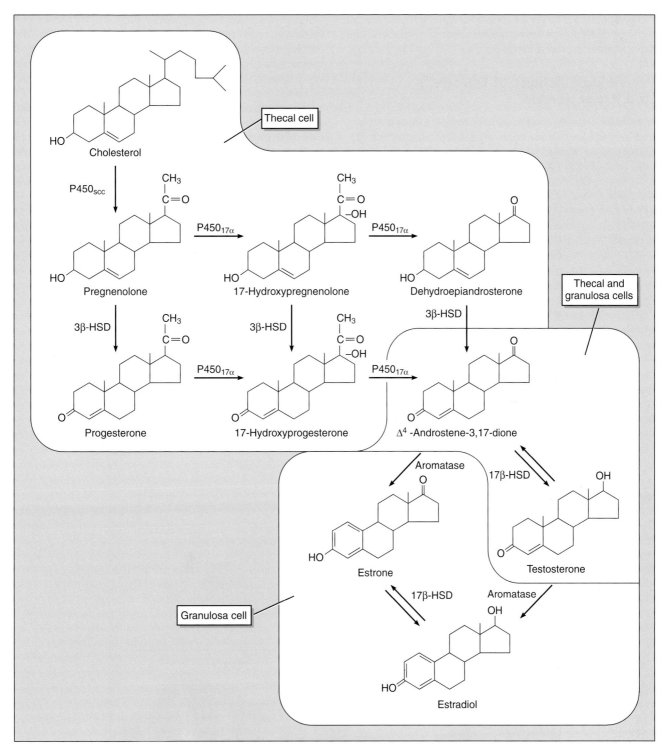

Figure 34–1. Biosynthesis of sex steroids. In the ovary, pregnenolone is converted to androstenedione and testosterone in thecal cells. These steroids are then converted to estrone and estradiol in granulosa cells. Enzymes involved in these steps include the cholesterol side-chain cleavage enzyme (P450$_{scc}$), steroid 17α-hydroxylase (P450$_{17α}$), 3β-hydroxysteroid dehydrogenase (3β-HSD), 17β-hydroxysteroid dehydrogenase (17β-HSD), and aromatase. Estrone and estradiol are partly converted to estriol by other enzymes. After ovulation, the major product of thecal cells is progesterone, owing to the development of a relative deficiency of 17α-hydroxylase activity.

primarily bound to sex steroid–binding globulin. In the liver, it is converted to androstenedione and other metabolites, including sulfate and glucuronide conjugates. About 90% of these metabolites are excreted in the urine.

Although both testosterone and DHT activate **androgen receptors**, DHT has greater receptor affinity and forms a more stable receptor-ligand complex than testosterone. If DHT formation is inhibited, this significantly reduces androgenic stimulation of the prostate gland and hair follicles. The androgen receptor located in target cells interacts with response elements in target genes and thereby stimulates protein synthesis in the same manner as other gonadal steroids.

Physiologic Actions of Estrogens and Progesterone

In females, estrogens and progesterone have multiple actions and interactions that are necessary for reproductive activity. Estrogens are formed in the **granulosa cells** of the ovary,

whereas progesterone is primarily produced by the **corpus luteum** in response to LH secretion. Estrogens promote the development and growth of the fallopian tubes, uterus, and vagina, as well as secondary sex characteristics such as breast development, skeletal growth, and axillary and pubic hair patterns.

The pattern of hormonal changes occurring during the **menstrual cycle** is depicted in Figure 34–2. During the **follicular phase** of the cycle, ovarian follicles are recruited and a dominant estrogen-secreting follicle develops. Estrogen

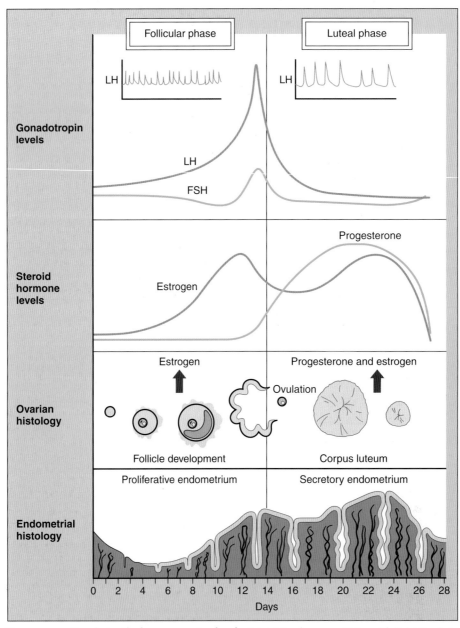

Figure 34–2. **Hormone secretion during the human menstrual cycle.** Luteinizing hormone (LH) and follicle-stimulating hormone (FSH) are released in a pulsatile manner from the pituitary gland in response to the pulsatile secretion of gonadotropin-releasing hormone (GnRH) from the hypothalamus. FSH stimulates ovarian follicle development and the secretion of estrogen during the follicular phase of the cycle. After ovulation, the corpus luteum produces both estrogen and progesterone during the luteal phase. Estrogen decreases FSH and LH secretion during most of the cycle (feedback inhibition) while provoking the mid-cycle LH and FSH surge that triggers ovulation. Progesterone decreases the frequency of hypothalamic GnRH pulses and the frequency of pulsatile LH and FSH secretion (*inset in top panel*). During the luteal phase, progesterone increases the amount of LH released (pulse amplitude). Estrogen stimulates the proliferation of the endometrium during the follicular phase, whereas progesterone causes the endometrium to become more vascular and secretory during the luteal phase.

levels gradually increase, whereas progesterone levels remain very low. A surge of LH is released at mid-cycle in response to positive estrogen feedback to the pituitary gland, and this LH surge triggers ovulation. During the **luteal phase** of the cycle, the follicle becomes the *corpus luteum* (literally "yellow body") that secretes both estrogen and progesterone in response to LH. Together, these hormones prepare the uterus for implantation of a fertilized egg as the endometrium becomes more vascular and secretory. If pregnancy does not occur, the corpus luteum ceases to produce estrogen and progesterone, resulting in menstruation. If pregnancy occurs, the placenta produces human chorionic gonadotropin, which maintains the production of progesterone by the corpus luteum. After about 3 months, the placenta becomes the predominant source of progesterone. This hormone serves to maintain pregnancy and prevents endometrial sloughing and miscarriage.

Estrogens have a number of other actions that are important in reproduction and other bodily functions. They sensitize the myometrium to oxytocin at parturition, and this facilitates labor. They stimulate protein synthesis in the brain and may thereby affect mood and emotions. Estrogens influence the distribution of body fat and thereby contribute to the development of feminine body contours. They enhance blood coagulation by increasing the synthesis of clotting factors, and they prevent osteoporosis by inhibiting bone resorption. In males and females, estrogens are responsible for epiphyseal closure, which halts linear bone growth.

Estrogens and progestins have different effects on serum lipoprotein levels. Estrogens decrease the levels of **low-density lipoprotein (LDL) cholesterol** and **lipoprotein(a)** while increasing the levels of **high-density lipoprotein (HDL) cholesterol**. In contrast, progestins produce a dose-related increase in LDL levels and a decrease in HDL levels.

Progesterone and other progestins increase basal body temperature by 0.5° C to 0.8° C (1.0° F to 1.5° F) at ovulation and throughout the luteal phase. They also affect the emotional state and have mild mineralocorticoid (salt-retaining) properties. Some of the synthetic progestins have other effects that are attributed to their androgenic activity (see below).

Physiologic Actions of Testosterone

LH stimulates testosterone synthesis in **Leydig's cells**, whereas FSH promotes spermatogenesis by **Sertoli's cells** in the seminiferous tubules. These cells provide an environment rich in testosterone, which is necessary for germ cell development. Sertoli's cells also produce a protein called **inhibin**, which acts in concert with DHT as a feedback regulator of FSH secretion by the pituitary.

Testosterone is responsible for the development of secondary sex characteristics in males during puberty. These include growth of the larynx, thickening of the vocal cords, and growth of facial, axillary, and pubic hair. In addition to stimulating growth of the penis, scrotum, seminal vesicles, and prostate gland, testosterone stimulates and maintains sexual function in males. Testosterone and other androgens also do the following: increase lean body mass; stimulate

skeletal growth; accelerate epiphyseal closure; increase sebaceous gland activity and sebum production, thereby contributing to the development of acne in both sexes; increase the production of erythropoietin in the kidneys; and decrease the levels of HDL cholesterol.

ESTROGENS AND PROGESTINS

An estrogen or progestin preparation can be used alone for the treatment of various disorders, or the two preparations can be used in combination for **hormone replacement therapy** (HRT) in postmenopausal women or for **contraception** in women of childbearing age.

Estrogens

Drug Properties

CHEMISTRY. The natural estrogens include **estradiol** and **conjugated estrogens**. Estradiol is an 18-carbon steroid with an aromatic A-ring (see Fig. 34–1). **Conjugated equine estrogens** are sulfate esters of **estrone** and **equilin** and can be obtained from the urine of pregnant mares. **Ethinyl estradiol** and **mestranol** are synthetic derivatives of estradiol.

PREPARATIONS. Micronized estradiol is an orally administered estradiol preparation that has good bioavailability. Also available are vaginal estradiol tablets and a vaginal ring that slowly releases estradiol.

Ethinyl estradiol and **mestranol** are modified by the addition of an ethinyl group to estradiol, which reduces first-pass metabolism, increases the half-life to about 20 hours, and results in greater oral potency compared with native estradiol. These agents are primarily used in estrogen-progestin contraceptives. **Conjugated equine estrogens** are hydrolyzed to **estrone** and **equilin** before absorption from the gut. They undergo relatively little first-pass metabolism and are converted in the liver to sulfate and glucuronide conjugates that are excreted in the urine. Estrone is also available in a rapidly absorbed formulation for intramuscular administration.

Several long-acting formulations of estradiol are available for transdermal or intramuscular administration. **Transdermal estradiol systems** slowly release the drug for absorption through the skin. These preparations are formulated for twice-weekly or weekly application. **Estradiol cypionate** and **estradiol valerate** are long-acting esters of estradiol that are slowly absorbed following intramuscular administration and provide effective plasma concentrations of estradiol for several weeks.

Following their absorption, the natural estrogens are highly bound to sex steroid–binding globulin, are widely distributed, and are concentrated in fat. They undergo enterohepatic cycling, in which conjugated metabolites are excreted in the bile and converted to free estrogens by intestinal bacteria. The free estrogens are then reabsorbed into the circulation. As with estrone and equilin, estradiol is metabolized in the liver to sulfate and glucuronide conjugates, and these conjugates are primarily excreted in the urine, with small amounts excreted in the feces.

INDICATIONS. Estrogen preparations are used in the treatment of **primary hypogonadism**, including cases caused by surgical oophorectomy, menopause, and other causes. Micronized estradiol, transdermal estradiol, and conjugated equine estrogens are primarily used for **HRT** (see below) in postmenopausal women. New low-dose and ultra-low-dose preparations are available containing 0.3 mg conjugated estrogens or 0.5 mg estradiol, respectively. Combination estrogen-progestin preparations contain ethinyl estradiol or mestranol. These preparations are often used for **oral contraception** and for the treatment of **acne vulgaris** and **dysmenorrhea.**

ADVERSE EFFECTS. Estrogens occasionally cause breast tenderness, headache, edema, nausea, vomiting, anorexia, and changes in libido. These effects are less likely to occur in women using the lower-dose preparations now recommended for HRT.

The more serious adverse effects of estrogens include **hypertension, thromboembolic disorders,** and **gallbladder disease.** The hypertensive effect of estrogens has been partly attributed to increased angiotensinogen synthesis and formation of angiotensin II, whereas thromboembolic complications result from increased hepatic synthesis of clotting factors. Estrogens increase cholesterol excretion in the bile, accounting for their tendency to cause gallstones.

Estrogens are contraindicated during pregnancy and should be avoided in women with uterine fibroids. Estrogens should be used with great caution in women with hepatic diseases, endometriosis, thromboembolic diseases, or hypercalcemia.

Progesterone and Its Derivatives

Progesterone is the primary natural progestin in mammals. Progesterone undergoes extensive first-pass metabolism following oral administration and has a short plasma half-life. To extend the oral bioavailability and half-life, esters of progesterone have been developed. These include **megestrol, hydroxyprogesterone caproate,** and **medroxyprogesterone acetate.** Megestrol is administered orally, whereas hydroxyprogesterone caproate is administered as a long-acting intramuscular preparation. Medroxyprogesterone acetate can be given either orally or intramuscularly. Following their absorption, the progesterone esters are bound to albumin in the circulation. The esters are converted to several hydroxylated metabolites and to pregnanediol glucuronide in the liver, and these metabolites are excreted in the urine.

Progesterone esters are used to suppress ovarian function in the treatment of **dysmenorrhea, endometriosis,** and **uterine bleeding.** In this setting, the progesterone derivatives produce feedback inhibition of gonadotropin secretion by the pituitary gland. In **HRT** (see below), the progesterone esters are used in combination with estrogens to decrease the incidence of estrogen-induced irregular bleeding and to prevent uterine hyperplasia and endometrial cancer.

Synthetic Progestins

Synthetic progestins are primarily used as **oral contraceptives** (see below), but they are also used to treat **dysmenorrhea, endometriosis,** and **uterine bleeding** in the same manner as the progesterone esters.

Most of the synthetic progestins are derivatives of 19-nortestosterone (testosterone without a methyl group on carbon-19) and have varying degrees of estrogenic, antiestrogenic, and androgenic activity. The drugs contain substitutions that increase their oral bioavailability and duration of action. Their half-lives range from 7 to 24 hours, whereas the half-life of progesterone is only about 5 minutes.

Two classes of 19-norprogestins have been developed: **estranes** and **gonanes.** The estranes include **norethindrone** and **norethynodrel,** whereas the gonanes include **levonorgestrel, desogestrel,** and **norgestimate.** Desogestrel and norgestimate have improved progestational selectivity and lessened androgenic activity. **Drospirenone** is a spironolactone derivative with antiandrogenic effects (see below).

Hormone Replacement Therapy

Menopause refers to the cessation of menstruation that occurs in most women between the ages of 45 and 55. Before menopause, the supply of eggs in a woman's ovaries declines and ovulation becomes irregular. The ovarian follicles fail to develop and secrete normal amounts of estrogen. When estrogen levels are no longer sufficient to suppress FSH secretion by the pituitary gland, FSH levels rise. When FSH levels are above 40 mIU/mL, a woman is said to be in menopause.

Although estrogens can be used alone for HRT in women who have had a hysterectomy, estrogen should be used in combination with a progestin for women with a uterus. This is because giving estrogen alone increases the risk of endometrial cancer in these women.

Therapeutic Effects

Studies consistently show that estrogens relieve symptoms of menopause in up to 90% of women. These symptoms include hot flashes or flushes that consist of alternating chills and sweating accompanied by nausea, dizziness, headache, tachycardia, and palpitations (Box 34-1). Episodes of these symptoms often occur several times a day, but night sweats are particularly common. These symptoms occur in association with surges in GnRH and gonadotropins that result from the lack of estrogen feedback inhibition. The gonadotropin surges alter hypothalamic thermoregulatory centers, leading to the symptoms described earlier in this paragraph.

Estrogens also relieve other menopausal symptoms, including urogenital, vulvar, and vaginal atrophy, and they protect against osteoporosis. Estrogens may improve mood and reduce cognitive difficulties, possibly secondary to improved sleep.

Although some epidemiologic studies suggest that HRT reduces the risk of cardiovascular disease, some recent clinical trials of estrogen replacement in postmenopausal women have reached the opposite conclusion. The **Nurses' Health Study** was an observational study of a cohort of women that obtained information about the relationship between cardiovascular disease and lifestyle, lipid levels, and HRT. This study concluded that HRT decreased the risk of coronary artery disease and that women with the highest risk of cardiovascular disease obtained the greatest benefit from HRT. This study has the same

BOX 34-1. A CASE OF HOT
FLASHES AND LOSS OF SLEEP

CASE PRESENTATION: A 50-year-old woman complains to her health care provider of episodes of hot flashes that occur mostly at night accompanied by sweating and interrupted sleep. She has also noticed vaginal dryness and feeling slightly depressed. Her periods have been increasingly infrequent over the past year. She suspects that she is entering menopause and asks about HRT. The woman has been healthy throughout her adult life and adheres to a good diet and a regular exercise program. Her mother developed osteoporosis after menopause and the patient is concerned about maintaining healthy bones. She does not have a family history of premature cardiovascular disease or of reproductive tract cancer. Her physical exam and laboratory tests are normal and she is scheduled for a bone density determination. She is started on a low dose of oral estrogen and a vaginal estrogen cream along with cyclic medroxyprogesterone. Her bone density will be monitored and appropriate therapy provided. She is encouraged to maintain a high level of calcium intake and to increase her vitamin D supplementation. This case is continued in Chapter 36.

CASE DISCUSSION: Menopause is defined as the absence of menstruation for 12 consecutive months and is caused by cessation of estrogen production by the ovaries. Common symptoms of menopause include hot flashes, mood swings, sleeplessness, vaginal dryness, and urinary incontinence. Many women experience irregular periods and other symptoms of menopause for several months preceding menopause. Tachycardia, depression, and other symptoms of estrogen withdrawal may also occur. Low doses of estrogens control most menopausal symptoms, and vaginal estrogen preparations effectively relieve vaginal atrophy. Clinical trials have been more confusing than helpful with respect to HRT and the risk of cardiovascular disease and cancer. In some cases, trials involving older women with heart disease have been erroneously extrapolated to healthy younger women. The latest analysis of trials suggests that hormonal replacement may protect against long-term cardiovascular disease, but may increase short-term risk in some women. For most healthy menopausal women, short-term HRT is a relatively safe and effective method of controlling menopausal symptoms and may provide some long-term cardiovascular benefits.

limitations as all cohort observational studies, and it has been postulated that the women who sought HRT were also more likely to adopt a healthy lifestyle that reduced their risk of heart disease.

The **Postmenopausal Estrogen/Progestin Interventions** study was a randomized, prospective trial of HRT in 875 women between the ages of 45 and 64. It demonstrated beneficial effects of HRT on risk factors for heart disease by showing that HRT reduced cholesterol and fibrinogen levels. The relatively short duration of the trial (3 years) was not sufficient to determine long-term effects of HRT on morbidity and mortality.

The **Heart and Estrogen-Progestin Replacement Study** was the first trial to investigate the effects of HRT in older postmenopausal women with **existing heart disease**. This study found a lack of benefit of HRT on fatal or nonfatal myocardial infarction. In fact, the study found that women were at an increased risk of myocardial infarction during the first year of HRT, although the risk of myocardial infarction decreased in subsequent years. After an additional 3 years of study, no significant differences were noted in cardiovascular outcomes between women on HRT and those not receiving HRT. This trial has been criticized because women in the study were already receiving cardioprotective medications and were allowed to begin or change statin therapy during the study. Also, the average age of women in the study was 67, which is well above the age when women enter menopause.

The **Women's Health Initiative** included a randomized trial of more than 16,000 women who received **conjugated equine estrogen** plus **medroxyprogesterone acetate** or a placebo. After 5 years, the study was halted because the data showed that women receiving HRT had increased risk of **coronary artery disease, stroke**, and **pulmonary embolism.** HRT, however, reduced the risk of **colorectal cancer** and **hip fractures**. Another arm of this study looked at the effect of estrogen by itself in women without a uterus. This study was stopped when it was reported that estrogen increased the risk of stroke but did not affect the incidence of coronary artery disease in these women. The Women's Health Initiative study has been criticized for the older age of the participants.

More recently, a trial conducted by the Women's Health Initiative in younger and generally healthier 50- to 59-year-old women found that that both estrogen alone and estrogen and progestin in combination provided **cardioprotective effects** with a reduction in coronary events and total mortality. Considering that neither aspirin nor statins have shown a statistically significant reduction in coronary heart disease in younger menopausal women, it is remarkable that estrogen may in fact reduce the risk of heart disease in these women (see Lobo, 2007).

In summary, low-dose estrogen preparations are still a very useful treatment for relieving menopausal symptoms in younger menopausal women. Estrogens also protect against osteoporosis and certain cancers and may reduce the risk of cardiovascular disease in younger women. The role of estrogens in older women remains uncertain. Older women with existing heart disease should not be placed on estrogen therapy. Other medications are available to prevent osteoporosis in menopausal women.

Treatment Considerations

Most women with an intact uterus should begin HRT with a combination of a progestin and a low-dose estrogen. Doses should be titrated to provide symptom relief without causing side effects such as headache, nausea, weight gain, breast tenderness, or vaginal bleeding. After 2 or 3 years of therapy, the dose of estrogen can be gradually reduced to the lowest level required to prevent hot flashes and other symptoms.

Estrogens can be administered using a wide variety of dosage forms and routes of administration, enabling women to try alternative preparations and determine which one is most effective and tolerable for them. Oral tablets are convenient and relatively inexpensive, whereas transdermal skin patches require less frequent administration. Women who suffer mainly vulvovaginal symptoms may prefer a vaginal cream, tablet, or ring. Other options include intramuscular injections and subcutaneously implanted pellets.

Hormone replacement therapy can be given as cyclic or continuous hormonal therapy. In cyclic therapy, estrogen is given for 25 days, a progestin (e.g., medroxyprogesterone) is given for the last 10 to 13 days of estrogen treatment, and then no therapy is given for 5 to 6 days. In continuous therapy, estrogen is given every day, and a progestin is added for the first 10 to 13 days of each month. The addition of a progestin suppresses endometrial hyperplasia and diminishes the risk of endometrial cancer.

CONTRACEPTIVES

Contraceptives are drugs or devices used to prevent conception (the onset of pregnancy, as indicated by the implantation of the blastocyst in the endometrium or the formation of a visible zygote). Some contraceptives act locally in the reproductive tract. These include agents that kill sperm (**spermicides**), devices that prevent sperm from reaching and fertilizing the ovum (**condoms** and **diaphragms**), and **intrauterine devices** that prevent implantation of the blastocyst. Other contraceptives are administered orally or parenterally. **Oral contraceptives** contain female sex hormones that act primarily by preventing ovulation. Most of the oral contraceptives contain both an estrogen and a progestin, whereas two products contain only a progestin. Progestin-only contraceptives are also available for administration as **long-acting subdermal implants, intramuscular injections,** or **intrauterine devices.** Table 34–1 lists the estrogen and progestin components of selected hormonal contraceptive preparations.

Estrogen-Progestin Contraceptives

Drug Properties

CLASSIFICATION. The combination estrogen-progestin oral contraceptives are classified as monophasic, biphasic, or triphasic, based on their progestin content. **Monophasic contraceptives** contain the same amount of progestin throughout the administration cycle, whereas **biphasic and triphasic contraceptives** increase the amount after the first third of the cycle (Fig. 34–3). The amount of progestin is increased in the biphasic and triphasic preparations to mimic the naturally occurring ratio of estrogen to progestin during the menstrual cycle. The estrogen content is constant in all monophasic and biphasic contraceptives and in most triphasic contraceptives.

MECHANISMS AND PHARMACOLOGIC EFFECTS. The estrogen-progestin contraceptives act primarily by feedback inhibition of GnRH secretion from the hypothalamus, leading to decreased gonadotropin secretion and inhibition of ovulation. The estrogen component is believed to reduce FSH secretion and the selection and maturation of the dominant follicle, whereas the progestin component inhibits the mid-cycle LH surge required for ovulation. Neither the estrogen nor the progestin dose used in oral contraceptives is sufficient to prevent ovulation by itself, but used together they act synergistically to suppress ovulation. Other effects that contribute to contraception include delayed maturation of the endometrium, which prevents implantation of the blastocyst, and the development of viscous cervical mucus, which retards sperm motility. The actions on the endometrium and cervical mucus are believed to be the mechanisms of estrogen-progestin preparations used for emergency (postcoital) contraception.

ADMINISTRATION. Estrogen-progestin preparations for **oral contraception** are usually packaged as 21 tablets that are administered once a day, beginning on day 5 of the menstrual cycle. Some preparations also include 7 inert pills that can be taken for the remainder of the cycle. The tablets are packaged in a calendar format to facilitate proper utilization. An "extended-cycle" preparation is now available for continuous daily administration for 84 days followed by 7 days of inactive tablets. This preparation contains ethinyl estradiol and levonorgestrel and allows for withdrawal bleeding only 4 times a year, whereas other estrogen-progestin oral contraceptives result in 13 withdrawal bleeding episodes a year. The extended-cycle preparation is as effective as 28-day cycle products. Whether the longer exposure to hormones could increase the risk of adverse effects (e.g., thromboembolism) has not been determined.

Estrogen-progestin preparations are also used to treat **acne vulgaris** and produce a significant improvement in facial acne lesions. They are also useful in managing **dysmenorrhea,** a condition characterized by episodic pain that is believed to result from a local increase in uterine prostaglandins. The release of prostaglandins is a reaction to the ischemia caused by vasoconstriction of small arteries in the uterine wall at the time of menstruation. For this condition, oral contraceptives are started a number of days before the onset of menstruation. Nonsteroidal anti-inflammatory drugs (e.g., ibuprofen and naproxen) can be used instead, especially by women desiring to maintain the ovulatory cycle.

Other estrogen-progestin contraceptives include a transdermal skin patch (see below) and a long-acting, injectable preparation containing estradiol cypionate and medroxyprogesterone acetate.

ADVERSE EFFECTS. Table 34–2 lists the common adverse effects resulting from estrogen or progestin excess or deficiency. Less frequent effects of oral contraceptives include **hypertension, thromboembolic complications,** and **gallstones.**

TABLE 34–1. Estrogen and Progestin Components of Selected Hormonal Contraceptive Preparations

Preparations	Estrogen	Progestin
Monophasic Oral Contraceptives		
BREVICON, GENORA 0.5/35, LOESTRIN, NORINYL, NORLESTRIN, OVCON	Ethinyl estradiol	Norethindrone
DEMULEN	Ethinyl estradiol	Ethynodiol
DESOGEN, ORTHO-CEPT	Ethinyl estradiol	Desogestrel*
YASMIN	Ethinyl estradiol	Drospirenone
LO/OVRAL, OVRAL	Ethinyl estradiol	Norgestrel
LEVLEN, NORDETTE, SEASONALE, SEASONIQUE	Ethinyl estradiol	Levonorgestrel
ORTHO-NOVUM 1/50	Mestranol	Norethindrone
Biphasic Oral Contraceptives		
MIRCETTE, ORTHO-NOVUM 10/11	Ethinyl estradiol	Norethindrone
Triphasic Oral Contraceptives		
ORTHO-NOVUM 7/7/7, TRI-NORINYL	Ethinyl estradiol	Norethindrone
TRI-LEVLEN, TRIPHASIL	Ethinyl estradiol	Norgestrel
ORTHO TRI-CYCLEN	Ethinyl estradiol	Norgestimate
Progestin-Only Oral Contraceptives		
MICRONOR, NOR-Q-D		Norethindrone
Contraceptive Implant		
NORPLANT		Levonorgestrel
Intrauterine Contraceptive		
MIRENA		Levonorgestrel
Injectable Contraceptives		
LUNELLE	Estradiol cypionate	Medroxyprogesterone acetate
DEPO-PROVERA		Medroxyprogesterone acetate
Transdermal Contraceptive		
ORTHO EVRA	Ethinyl estradiol	Norelgestromin
Vaginal Ring Contraceptive		
NUVARING	Ethinyl estradiol	Etonogestrel*
Emergency (Postcoital) Contraceptive		
PLAN B		Levonorgestrel

*Etonogestrel is the active metabolite of desogestrel.

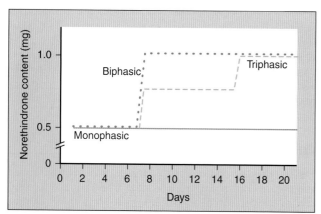

Figure 34–3. **Progestin (norethindrone) content in typical monophasic, biphasic, and triphasic oral contraceptives.** Monophasic preparations contain the same amount of progestin throughout the administration cycle. Biphasic and triphasic preparations increase the progestin content in a stepwise fashion after the initial part of the cycle. The amount of estrogen is constant in all monophasic and biphasic contraceptives and in most triphasic contraceptives. Some triphasic contraceptives contain a slightly greater amount of estrogen in the middle of the cycle.

Oral contraceptives have been associated with an increased risk of **stroke, myocardial infarction, deep vein thrombosis,** and other thromboembolic complications. The increased risk of thromboembolism in healthy women using preparations containing a low dose of estrogen (<50 μg of ethinyl estradiol) is extremely small. Smokers over 35 years of age have a greater risk of thromboembolic complications from oral contraceptives and should use other forms of contraception. Healthy nonsmokers who are 35 to 44 years old may continue to use oral contraceptives, according to the American College of Obstetricians and Gynecologists. A contraceptive skin patch containing ethinyl estradiol and norelgestromin (ORTHO EVRA) has been found to produce a greater systemic exposure to these steroids and to cause a greater incidence of venous thromboembolism, and possibly other thromboembolic disorders, compared to oral administration of these steroids.

Contraceptives containing estrogen should be used with caution in women with gallbladder disease. They are contraindicated in women with thromboembolic disease or a history of myocardial infarction or coronary artery disease. They are also contraindicated in women with active liver

TABLE 34–2. Common Adverse Effects of Oral Contraceptives

Effects of Estrogen Excess

Breast enlargement
Dizziness
Dysmenorrhea
Edema
Headache
Irritability
Nausea and vomiting
Weight gain (cyclic)

Effects of Progestin Excess

Acne
Depression
Fatigue
Hirsutism
Libido change
Oily skin
Weight gain (noncyclic)

Effects of Estrogen Deficiency

Atrophic vaginitis
Continuous bleeding
Early- or mid-cycle bleeding
Hypomenorrhea
Vasomotor symptoms

Effects of Progestin Deficiency

Dysmenorrhea
Hypermenorrhea
Late-cycle bleeding

disease, breast cancer, or carcinoma of the reproductive tract. The relationship between oral contraceptive use and cancer remains controversial. Epidemiologic studies suggest that oral contraceptives decrease the incidence of **ovarian and endometrial cancer.** Although use of the high-dose estrogen preparations has been associated with an increased risk of **breast cancer,** the risk associated with newer low-dose preparations is much lower. Oral contraceptives have also been associated with a low risk of hepatic adenoma.

The progestin component of oral contraceptives can cause adverse effects that can be attributed to excessive androgenic activity. The androgenic side effects of progestins include **acne, hirsutism, increased libido,** and **oily skin. Norgestrel** is one of the most androgenic progestins, whereas **desogestrel** is one of the least androgenic. **Norethindrone** appears to have an intermediate androgenic potency. **Drospirenone** is a newer progestin that is derived from spironolactone (see Chapter 13). Drospirenone is an **aldosterone antagonist** with a weak **antiandrogenic effect.** It lowers blood pressure by reducing salt and water retention, and a contraceptive containing this progestin has improved tolerability with respect to weight gain, mood changes, and acne in comparison with contraceptives containing other progestins.

INTERACTIONS. Carbamazepine, phenytoin, and other drugs that increase the hepatic metabolism of oral contraceptives may reduce the plasma levels of contraceptive steroids and lead to contraceptive failure. Antibiotics, including penicillins and tetracyclines, can eradicate intestinal flora involved in the enterohepatic cycling of contraceptive steroids and

thereby diminish their effectiveness. Estrogens can inhibit the metabolism and potentiate the effects of cyclosporine, antidepressants, and glucocorticoids. Estrogens increase the synthesis of vitamin K–dependent clotting factors and may thereby antagonize the effect of warfarin. Estrogens also appear to increase the hepatotoxicity of dantrolene.

Progestin-Only Contraceptives

The progestin-only contraceptives include **norethindrone** products that are administered orally (sometimes called minipills), subdermal implants and intrauterine devices that slowly release **levonorgestrel,** and long-acting intramuscular injections of **medroxyprogesterone acetate.**

The systemic progestin-only contraceptives may prevent pregnancy through several mechanisms. They act on the hypothalamus to decrease the frequency of the GnRH pulse generator and thereby blunt the mid-cycle LH surge that produces ovulation. Progestin-only pills thicken and decrease the amount of cervical mucus, making it more difficult for sperm to penetrate. Progestins also create a thin, atrophic endometrium that is hostile to implantation of the blastocyst. Intrauterine devices are believed to prevent pregnancy by producing localized effects on the endometrium.

The progestin-only contraceptives are particularly suited for women who smoke, older women, and women in whom an estrogen is contraindicated. The estimated failure rates, however, are slightly higher with perfect use of progestin-only contraceptives than with perfect use of estrogen-progestin products (rates of 0.5% and 0.1%, respectively). Progestin-only contraceptives are associated with frequent spotting and amenorrhea and with an increased risk of ectopic pregnancy. An irregular or unpredictable menstrual cycle is one of the most common reasons that women stop using these preparations. Unlike the estrogen-progestin preparations, the progestin-only preparations must be taken daily without interruption to prevent pregnancy.

A preparation containing levonorgestrel (PLAN B) is also available for use as an emergency or **postcoital contraceptive** in women who have not been taking another contraceptive. A single dose of this preparation is taken within 72 hours of intercourse, followed by a second dose 12 hours later. Use of an emergency contraceptive routinely causes nausea and vomiting and may require administration of an antiemetic agent (e.g., promethazine). It can also cause headache, dizziness, leg cramps, and abdominal cramps. A urine pregnancy test can be used to verify the prevention of pregnancy.

Other Contraceptives

Other types of contraceptives are particularly useful for short-term contraception in women who cannot take oral contraceptives while breastfeeding or for other reasons. These nonhormonal contraceptives include spermicides and barrier devices (e.g., condoms and diaphragms).

Most spermicides contain nonoxynol-9, a detergent that disrupts the cell membrane of the sperm. Spermicides increase the contraceptive efficacy of condoms and other barrier methods. They are moderately effective and well tolerated, although they can cause local irritation in some women.

ANTIESTROGENS

Antiestrogens include the estrogen receptor antagonists and the estrogen synthesis inhibitors (aromatase inhibitors). The estrogen receptor antagonists are nonsteroidal drugs that bind to estrogen receptors and exert tissue-specific antagonist or partial agonist effects. Examples are clomiphene, tamoxifen, and raloxifene. These drugs contain the structural elements required for estrogen receptor binding and weak agonist activity, but they also possess a substituted ethylamine moiety that is responsible for their estrogen antagonist effect.

Clomiphene

Drug Properties

PHARMACOKINETICS. Clomiphene is well absorbed after oral administration. It undergoes hepatic biotransformation and biliary excretion, and it is mostly eliminated in the feces. Its long elimination half-life of about 5 days is caused by extensive plasma protein binding, enterohepatic cycling, and accumulation in fatty tissues.

MECHANISMS AND INDICATIONS. Clomiphene is a weak estrogen agonist and a moderate estrogen antagonist. It is used to treat **anovulatory infertility**, including infertility associated with **polycystic ovary disease**. Clomiphene blocks estrogen receptors in the hypothalamus and pituitary and prevents estrogen's feedback inhibition of gonadotropin secretion (Fig. 34–4). This increases FSH and LH secretion, which induces ovarian follicle development and ovulation.

Suitable patients for clomiphene therapy often have an anovulatory disorder dating back to puberty but have a functional hypothalamic-pituitary-ovarian axis. Clomiphene is less successful in women who have reduced estrogen levels, and it is unlikely to benefit women with FSH levels at or above 40 mIU/mL or women with absent or resistant ovarian follicles.

Clomiphene treatment is usually begun on or about the fifth day of the cycle after the start of uterine bleeding and continues for 5 days. Ovulation is expected 5 to 10 days after the last dose of clomiphene and can be detected by monitoring basal body temperature, urinary LH secretion, plasma progesterone levels, or endometrial histology. However, only about 15% of women achieve pregnancy with clomiphene therapy. Aromatase inhibitors have recently been used to treat infertility and appear to have a better pregnancy rate (see below).

ADVERSE EFFECTS. About 5% to 7% of women treated with clomiphene have multiple births (twins in the vast majority of cases). The risk of multiple births is reduced if women are started on a lower dose of clomiphene. The dose can then be increased each cycle until ovulation occurs.

Tamoxifen

Drug Properties

PHARMACOKINETICS. Tamoxifen is administered orally, and it is well absorbed from the gut. It is then converted to a number of metabolites in the liver. Some of the minor metabolites

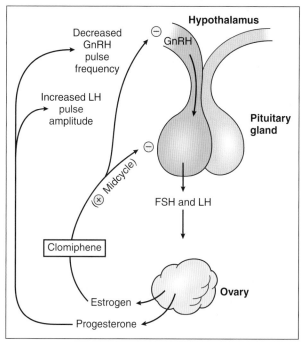

Figure 34–4. The hypothalamic-pituitary-ovarian axis. Follicle-stimulating hormone (FSH) and luteinizing hormone (LH) are released from the pituitary gland in response to gonadotropin-releasing hormone (GnRH) produced by hypothalamic neurons. During the follicular phase of the menstrual cycle, FSH stimulates the development of an ovarian follicle and the secretion of estrogen. Estrogen increases the synthesis of LH but inhibits its release until midcycle, when a surge in LH is accompanied by a smaller surge in FSH secretion, leading to ovulation. During the luteal phase, progesterone produced by the corpus luteum feeds back to the hypothalamus to decrease the frequency of GnRH pulses while acting on the pituitary to increase the amplitude of LH secretion. Together, these actions produce less frequent LH pulses of greater amplitude. Clomiphene inhibits estrogen feedback and thereby increases gonadotropin secretion in anovulatory women.

(e.g., 4-hydroxytamoxifen) have greater affinity for the estrogen receptor than tamoxifen does. The terminal elimination half-life of tamoxifen is about 7 days. Tamoxifen undergoes enterohepatic cycling and biliary excretion in the same manner as clomiphene.

MECHANISMS AND INDICATIONS. Tamoxifen has both estrogenic and antiestrogenic properties. In breast tissue, it acts as an estrogen receptor antagonist. It is primarily used to prevent or treat **breast cancer** in patients with tumor cells that are estrogen receptor–positive. In the treatment of breast cancer, it is typically used as adjuvant therapy in combination with surgery or other chemotherapy. Tamoxifen inhibits the proliferation of breast cancer cells and may thereby contribute to the eradication of micrometastases. In cases of advanced or metastatic breast cancer, tamoxifen can be used alone for palliative treatment.

ADVERSE EFFECTS. Tamoxifen can cause nausea, vomiting, hot flashes, vaginal bleeding, and menstrual irregularities. It can stimulate proliferation of endometrial cells, and some evidence suggests that it increases the risk of endometrial cancer.

Raloxifene

Raloxifene is called a **selective estrogen receptor modulator**. Raloxifene acts in a manner similar to tamoxifen by producing estrogen-like effects on bone and lipid metabolism while antagonizing the effects of estrogen on breast tissue. Unlike tamoxifen, however, raloxifene also acts as an estrogen antagonist in uterine tissue.

Raloxifene is primarily indicated for the prevention of **osteoporosis** in postmenopausal women. The effect of raloxifene on total body bone mineral density is similar to that of conjugated estrogens or alendronate. The effect of raloxifene on bone mineral density of the lumbar spine, however, may be less than that of these other drugs. The effect of estrogens on bone metabolism is discussed in greater detail in Chapter 36.

The effect of raloxifene on serum lipoproteins differs from the effect of estrogens. Raloxifene decreases the levels of total cholesterol, LDL cholesterol, and lipoprotein(a). Unlike estrogens, raloxifene does not increase the level of HDL cholesterol. The effect of raloxifene on cardiovascular disease requires further evaluation.

Aromatase Inhibitors

Breast cancer is often hormonally responsive—including breast cancer classified as estrogen, progesterone, or both—receptor positive. This type of breast cancer has responded to a variety of efforts to decrease estrogen levels (e.g., ovariectomy) or to inhibit estrogen effects, such as with estrogen antagonists. These interventions lead to decreased tumor mass, delayed progression, and improved survival in many patients.

In postmenopausal women, estrogens are derived from adrenal androgens, primarily testosterone and androstenedione, that are converted to estrogens in peripheral tissues and in cancer tissue itself by the enzyme **aromatase** (see Fig. 34–1). **Anastrozole** and **letrozole** are nonsteroidal aromatase inhibitors that reduce circulating levels of estrogen and are indicated as first-line treatments for locally advanced or **metastatic breast cancer** in postmenopausal women. By lowering estrogen levels, these drugs may halt progression of estrogen-sensitive breast cancer. Anastrozole and letrozole are well absorbed after oral administration and have long half-lives of about 2 days. The aromatase inhibitors are well tolerated but can cause hot flashes, nausea, headache, vaginal bleeding, and back pain.

Recently, letrozole has been used to treat infertility in anovulatory women, either alone or in combination with gonadotropins. Letrozole appears to result in better pregnancy rates than clomiphene.

ANTIPROGESTINS

Mifepristone is a synthetic steroid compound that acts as a progesterone receptor antagonist when progesterone is present. In the absence of progesterone, it acts as a partial agonist. It is also a competitive antagonist at the glucocorticoid receptor (see Chapter 33). Mifepristone is approved for **medical termination of pregnancy** through 49 days of gestation. It causes breakdown of the decidua (the endometrium of the pregnant uterus), leading to detachment of the blastocyst from the endometrium.

Mifepristone is administered as a single dose that is followed by a prostaglandin (e.g., misoprostol) 48 hours later to stimulate uterine contractions (see Chapter 26). Mifepristone has good oral bioavailability. Following absorption, the drug is highly bound to plasma proteins, which contributes to its long half-life of about 22 hours. Mifepristone is metabolized in the liver, is excreted in the bile, undergoes enterohepatic cycling, and is eventually excreted in the feces.

The major adverse effects of mifepristone include anorexia, nausea, vomiting, abdominal pain, fatigue, and heavy uterine bleeding.

ANDROGENS

Testosterone and Methyltestosterone

When given orally, testosterone undergoes extensive first-pass metabolism, and it must be given by other routes to achieve effective blood levels. **Methyltestosterone** can be given orally, but it is seldom used because long-term use can cause hepatic damage and liver failure.

Gels and skin patches are available for transdermal administration of testosterone, and long-acting esters of testosterone (e.g., testosterone cypionate) provide effective plasma levels for several weeks after intramuscular injection. A **buccal system** (STRIANT) has been developed that adheres to the gum or inner cheek and provides a sustained release of testosterone for absorption through the buccal mucosa throughout the day. All of these preparations can be used to treat **hypogonadism** caused by primary testicular failure or occurring secondary to pituitary insufficiency. In patients with hypopituitarism, testosterone should be given in combination with growth hormone to obtain a maximal effect on skeletal growth. In these patients, the androgen is added to the treatment regimen at the time of puberty, and the dosage is gradually increased. Testosterone therapy may also benefit older men with testosterone deficiency by preventing osteoporosis and improving overall quality of life.

Testosterone is occasionally used in **gynecologic disorders.** It is sometimes combined with estrogens for **HRT** in postmenopausal women who experience endometrial bleeding when only an estrogen is used.

Anabolic Steroids

Testosterone and its derivatives increase muscle mass and strength when used in a weight-training program. Anabolic steroids are synthetic derivatives of testosterone that have more anabolic than androgenic activity. The ratio of anabolic activity to androgenic activity for testosterone is 1:1, whereas the ratio for some synthetic androgens is as high as 3:1. Examples of androgenic steroids include oxandrolone and stanozolol. Tetrahydrogestrinone is a potent androgenic "designer drug" developed to escape detection in the urine. It is not approved by the U.S. Food and Drug Administration and cannot be legally marketed.

Anabolic steroids have been used by athletes to **increase body mass, strength,** and **physical performance.** This type of use has been banned by sports organizations. The large doses of anabolic steroids often used for this purpose can lead to a number of adverse effects, including **tendon rupture**, hepatic dysfunction or failure, cholestatic jaundice, increased aggressiveness, psychotic symptoms, acne, decreased testicular size and function, and impotence. In adolescents, androgenic drugs can cause **closing of epiphyses** and premature cessation of growth. In women, excessive use of androgens can cause masculinization, hirsutism, deepening of the voice, and menstrual irregularities (see also Chapter 25).

Danazol

Danazol is a synthetic steroid that has antiestrogenic activity and weak androgenic activity. It is used in the treatment of several gynecologic disorders because of its ability to cause feedback inhibition of pituitary gonadotropin secretion and decreased secretion of estrogen. In women with **heavy menstrual bleeding**, danazol treatment leads to endometrial atrophy and reduced menstrual loss. It appears to be more effective than other medical therapies for this condition. Danazol has also been used in treating **endometriosis**, a condition characterized by the presence of endometrial tissue outside the endometrial cavity. Danazol causes atrophy of ectopic endometrial tissue and may relieve the symptoms of disease, though analysis of clinical trials found that danazol does not improve fertility in subfertile women with this condition. By suppressing estrogen production, danazol also decreases the growth of abnormal breast tissue, making it useful in the treatment of **fibrocystic breast disease.**

Danazol is also used to treat **hereditary angioedema**, a disorder caused by deficiency of an inhibitor of the activated first component of complement (a cascade of plasma proteins involved in immunity to pathogens). Danazol prevents attacks of hereditary angioedema in both males and females by increasing levels of first-component esterase inhibitor. The mechanisms by which the drug increases these levels are unknown.

Common adverse effects of danazol include mild hirsutism, oily skin, acne, and menstrual irregularities. The drug can also cause hypercholesterolemia, hepatotoxicity, and thromboembolic events, including stroke. Danazol is teratogenic and should not be given to pregnant women.

ANTIANDROGENS

Several types of androgen antagonists have been developed and used in the treatment of prostate disorders, male pattern baldness, and other conditions. These drugs act through a variety of mechanisms, including inhibition of LH secretion, testosterone synthesis, and DHT synthesis, and antagonism of androgen receptors.

Gonadotropin-Releasing Hormone Analogues

When a GnRH analogue is administered in a continuous rather than a pulsatile fashion, it reduces LH secretion by the pituitary and thereby reduces testosterone production by the testes.

The GnRH analogues include **leuprolide**, an agent discussed in Chapter 31. Leuprolide has been successfully used in the treatment of inoperable **prostate cancer.** Because leuprolide increases the production of LH and testosterone when it is first administered, the drug is sometimes given in combination with an androgen receptor antagonist (e.g., flutamide). Combined androgen blockade with a GnRH analogue and an androgen receptor antagonist (see below) has been shown to significantly prolong the progression-free period and the length of survival in men with advanced prostate cancer.

Androgen Receptor Antagonists

Flutamide, bicalutamide, and **nilutamide** are nonsteroidal agents that compete with testosterone for the androgen receptor. These drugs are used in combination with a synthetic GnRH analogue to treat inoperable **prostate cancer.** Adverse effects of these drugs include nausea, gynecomastia, impotence, hot flashes, and hepatitis.

Cyproterone is a steroidal androgen receptor antagonist that has orphan drug status in the United States. It is being used to treat **hirsutism** in women and to reduce **excessive sex drive** in men.

5α-Reductase Inhibitors

Finasteride and **dutasteride** are synthetic testosterone derivatives that block 5α-reductase and decrease the synthesis of DHT in the prostate gland, skin, and other target tissues. The drugs are administered orally, undergo hepatic metabolism, and are eliminated in the feces. Finasteride has a half-life of about 8 hours, and it reduces DHT synthesis for about 24 hours.

Finasteride and dutasteride are used to treat symptomatic **benign prostatic hyperplasia**. The drugs reduce prostate volume and can retard the progression of benign prostatic hyperplasia. In men with benign prostatic hyperplasia, they improve urinary flow and decrease the risk of urinary retention. The reductase inhibitors are sometimes used in combination with an α-adrenoceptor antagonist, such as tamsulosin (see Chapter 9). Finasteride is also used for the treatment of **male pattern baldness.**

The adverse effects of finasteride and dutasteride include impotence and decreased libido, but these effects occur in only a few men and tend to decrease over time.

SUMMARY OF IMPORTANT POINTS

■ Estradiol preparations include skin patches for transdermal administration, micronized estradiol for oral administration, and estradiol cypionate and estradiol valerate for intramuscular administration.

■ Conjugated equine estrogens are sulfate esters of estrone and equilin. They are used for HRT in postmenopausal women and to treat other forms of hypogonadism.

■ In menopausal women, estrogens relieve vasomotor symptoms and protect against osteoporosis. Recent clinical trials suggest estrogens may prevent cardiovascular disease in healthy, younger menopausal women but may increase cardiovascular disease in older women.

■ Ethinyl derivatives of estradiol (ethinyl estradiol and mestranol) have higher oral bioavailability and longer half-lives than estradiol. They are used primarily in oral contraceptives.

■ Progesterone derivatives (e.g., medroxyprogesterone acetate) are primarily used in combination with estrogens in HRT to reduce endometrial hyperplasia and the risk of endometrial cancer. They are also used to suppress ovarian function in the treatment of dysmenorrhea, endometriosis, and uterine bleeding.

■ Synthetic progestins, including norethindrone, are primarily used in contraceptives, including combination estrogen-progestin contraceptives and progestin-only contraceptives.

■ Norgestrel is the most androgenic progestin, desogestrel is one of the least androgenic, and drospirenone has antiandrogenic and anti-mineralocorticoid activity.

■ Hormonal contraceptives act primarily by inhibiting gonadotropin secretion and ovulation. They also affect mucus viscosity, sperm transport, and endometrial histology.

■ Contraceptives have been associated with an increased risk of hypertension, thromboembolic disorders, and gallstones. The risk of thromboembolism is substantially reduced with preparations containing low doses of estrogen.

■ Some progestin-only contraceptives are administered as long-acting implants or injections, and others are given as oral tablets. Adverse effects include frequent spotting and amenorrhea.

■ Tamoxifen, an antiestrogen primarily used to treat breast cancer, is given in combination with surgery and other chemotherapy.

■ Anastrozole and letrozole, aromatase inhibitors that decrease estrogen synthesis, are used to treat breast cancer in postmenopausal women.

■ Clomiphene is an antiestrogen used to treat anovulatory infertility. By reducing estrogen feedback inhibition of gonadotropin secretion, clomiphene increases gonadotropin secretion and stimulates ovulation.

■ Raloxifene is a selective estrogen receptor modulator that acts as an estrogen antagonist in breast and uterine tissue. The drug produces estrogen-like effects on bone metabolism and reduces the risk of osteoporosis.

■ Mifepristone is an antiprogestin used for medical termination of intrauterine pregnancy.

■ Testosterone preparations are primarily used to treat hypogonadism.

■ Flutamide and other androgen receptor antagonists are used to treat prostate cancer, often in combination with a GnRH agonist (e.g., leuprolide).

■ Finasteride and dutasteride are 5α-reductase inhibitors that block the formation of DHT. They are used to treat benign prostatic hypertrophy and male pattern baldness.

Review Questions

1. A woman is placed on a drug that has antiestrogen effects on uterine and breast tissue. This drug is primarily used for which indication?
   (A) breast cancer
   (B) osteoporosis
   (C) menopausal symptoms
   (D) endometriosis
   (E) contraception

2. A progestin is included in regimens for HRT to prevent which of the following adverse effects?
   (A) breast cancer
   (B) endometrial cancer
   (C) myocardial infarction
   (D) stroke
   (E) elevated cholesterol levels

3. A man is taking a nonsteroidal drug that that competes with testosterone for its binding sites. Which adverse effect is most likely to occur in persons taking this drug?
   (A) breast tenderness
   (B) alopecia
   (C) glaucoma
   (D) deep vein thrombosis
   (E) hot flashes

4. A woman is placed on daily administration of a single hormone that decreases sperm penetration of cervical mucus. Which adverse effect is associated with this agent?
   (A) venous thromboembolism
   (B) irregular menstrual cycles
   (C) hot flashes
   (D) breast enlargement
   (E) hypertension

5. A woman is placed on a contraceptive that lowers her blood pressure and does not cause acne. Receptors for which hormone are blocked by this drug?
   (A) aldosterone
   (B) estrogen
   (C) progestin
   (D) gonadotropin
   (E) glucocorticoid

Answers and Explanations

1. **The answer is B:** osteoporosis. Raloxifene has antiestrogen effects on breast and uterine tissue but estrogenic effects on bone, and it is used to prevent osteoporosis. It is not used to treat breast cancer, menopausal symptoms, endometriosis, or for contraception.

2. **The answer is B:** endometrial cancer. Postmenopausal women receiving HRT should receive a progestin for 10 to 13 days each month to suppress endometrial hyperplasia that would otherwise be produced by unopposed estrogen therapy. A progestin is not required in women who have had a hysterectomy. Inclusion of a progestin will not prevent (A) breast cancer, (C) myocardial infarction, (D) stroke, or (E) elevated cholesterol levels.

3. **The answer is E:** hot flashes. Bicalutamide, flutamide, and nilutamide are androgen receptor antagonists that prevent feedback inhibition of hypothalamic GnRH secretion in men, leading to hot flashes. The drugs do not cause (A), breast tenderness, (B) alopecia, (C) glaucoma, or (D) deep vein thrombosis.

4. **The answer is B:** irregular menstrual cycles. Progestin contraceptives act in part by thickening cervical mucus and decreasing sperm penetration. An irregular or unpredictable menstrual cycle is one of the main reasons women discontinue progestin-only contraceptives. Progestins do not typically cause (A) venous thromboembolism, (C) hot flashes, (D) breast enlargement, or (E) hypertension.

5. **The answer is A:** aldosterone. Drospirenone is a progestin that antagonizes androgen and aldosterone receptors. It lowers blood pressure by decreasing salt and water retention, but it does not block estrogen, progestin, gonadotropin, or glucocorticoid receptors.

SELECTED READINGS

Battaglioli, T., and I. Martinelli. Hormone therapy and thromboembolic disease. Curr Opin Hematol 14:488–493, 2007.

Benagiano, G., C. Bastianelli, and M. Farris. Hormonal contraception: state of the art and future perspectives. Minerva Ginecol 59:241–270, 2007.

Edelstein, D., M. Sivanandy, S. Shahani, and S. Basaria. The latest options and future agents for treating male hypogonadism. Expert Opin Pharmacother 8:2991–3008, 2007.

Foidart, J.M., J. Desreux, A. Pintiaux, and A. Gompel. Hormone therapy and breast cancer risk. Climacteric 10:54–61, 2007.

Lobo, R.A. Postmenopausal hormones and coronary artery disease: potential benefits and risks. Climacteric 10:21–26, 2007.

Shapiro, S. Recent epidemiological evidence relevant to the clinical management of the menopause. Climacteric 10:2–15, 2007.

CHAPTER 35

Drugs for Diabetes Mellitus

CLASSIFICATION OF ANTIDIABETIC AGENTS

Insulin Preparations — see Table 35–1

Sulfonylurea Drugs
- Glipizide (GLUCOTROL)[a]

Meglitinide Drugs
- Repaglinide (PRANDIN)
- Nateglinide (STARLIX)

Alpha-glucosidase Inhibitors
- Acarbose (PRECOSE)
- Miglitol (GLYSET)

Biguanide
- Metformin (GLUCOPHAGE)

Thiazolidinediones
- Pioglitazone (ACTOS)
- Rosiglitazone (AVANDIA)

Amylin Analogue
- Pramlintide (SYMLIN)

Incretin Mimetics
- Exenatide (BYETTA)
- Sitagliptin (JANUVIA)

[a]Also glimepiride (AMARYL) and glyburide (DIABETA, MICRONASE).

OVERVIEW

Pancreatic Hormones

The hormones secreted by the endocrine pancreas are produced in clusters of cells called **islets of Langerhans.** These islets contain at least three types of cells. The alpha cells produce glucagon while the beta cells produce insulin and amylin, and the delta cells secrete somatostatin. Insulin promotes the uptake, utilization, and storage of glucose and thereby lowers the plasma glucose concentration, whereas glucagon increases the hepatic glucose output and blood glucose concentration. **Diabetes mellitus** (diabetes) results from inadequate insulin secretion or insulin activity that is not sufficient to maintain normal blood glucose concentrations.

Insulin

As shown in Box 35-1, **proinsulin** is converted to **insulin** and **C peptide.** Insulin consists of two peptide chains (the A chain and the B chain), which are linked by two disulfide bridges. Although both insulin and C peptide are released in response to rising glucose concentrations, the physiologic role of C peptide remains unknown.

Secretion

Insulin secretion has meal-stimulated and basal components. Insulin release is activated by the rise in blood glucose concentration that follows the digestion and absorption of carbohydrates (Fig. 35–1A and 35–1B). Insulin is released at the rate of 1 Unit (U) per 10 g of dietary carbohydrate, and it usually peaks within 1 hour of eating. Insulin promotes the uptake and storage of glucose and other ingested nutrients, and the postprandial (post-meal) plasma concentrations of both insulin and glucose return to preprandial (pre-meal) levels within 2 hours. Basal secretion, which usually ranges from 0.5 to 1 U of insulin per hour, serves to retard hepatic glucose output during the postabsorptive state.

Physiologic Effects

Insulin is sometimes referred to as the "storage hormone" because it promotes formation of glycogen, triglycerides, and protein while inhibiting their breakdown.

Insulin has several important actions on the **liver,** the organ that normally serves as the major source of blood glucose to supply the brain in the fasting state. The liver provides blood glucose through the processes of gluconeogenesis (the formation of glucose from amino acids) and glycogenolysis (the breakdown of glycogen). Insulin

BOX 35–1.   STRUCTURES OF PROINSULIN AND INSULIN MOLECULES

Preproinsulin is synthesized in the rough endoplasmic reticulum of pancreatic β cells, and proinsulin is formed by enzymatic cleavage of this precursor molecule. Proinsulin is then transported to the Golgi apparatus and converted to insulin and C peptide (connecting peptide) by the removal of four amino acids (dipeptide linkage). Insulin and C peptide are packaged in storage granules until released in equimolar amounts in response to rising glucose concentrations.

Insulin consists of a 21-amino-acid A chain and a 30-amino-acid B chain linked by two disulfide bridges.

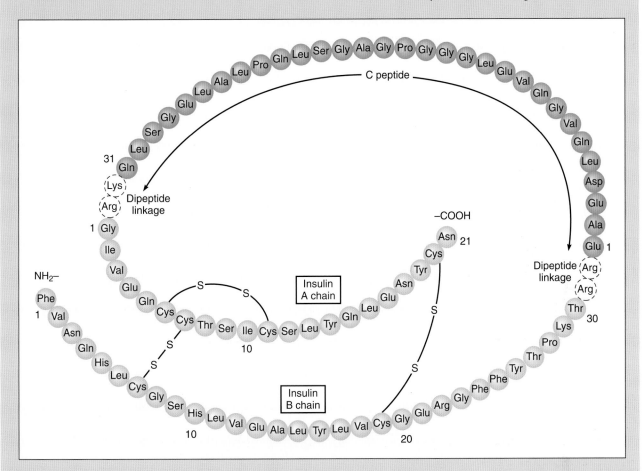

Differences in the amino acid composition of insulins are shown in the following table.

	Chain Position				
Type of Insulin	A-21	B-3	B-28	B-29	B-30
Human insulin	Asparagine	Asparagine	Proline	Lysine	Threonine
Insulin aspart	Asparagine	Asparagine	Aspartate	Lysine	Threonine
Insulin lispro	Asparagine	Asparagine	Lysine	Proline	Threonine
Insulin glulisine	Asparagine	Lysine	Proline	Glutamate	Threonine
Insulin glargine	Glycine	Asparagine	Proline	Lysine	Threonine[a]
Insulin detemir	Asparagine	Asparagine	Proline	Lysine[b]	None

[a]Two additional arginine residues are attached to threonine at B-30.
[b]A 14-carbon fatty acid chain is attached to this amino acid and threonine is omitted at B-30.

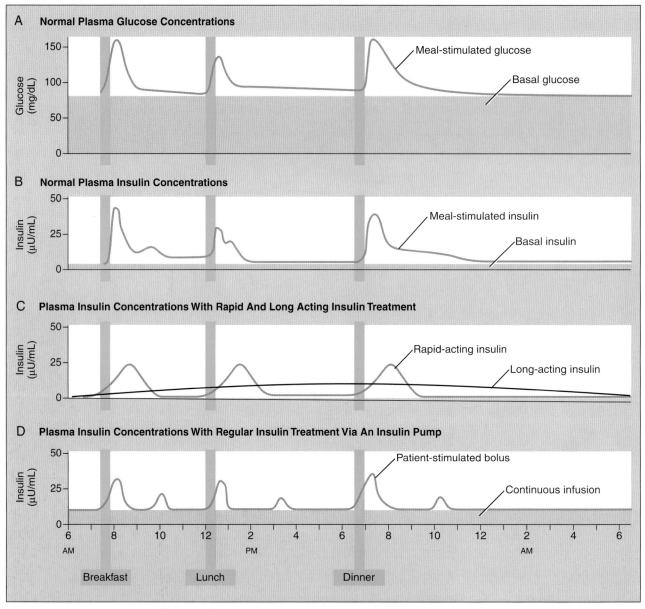

Figure 35–1. **Time course of plasma glucose and insulin concentrations.** (**A**) Plasma glucose concentrations result from hepatic glucose output in the fasting state and the digestion and absorption of carbohydrates after meals. (**B**) Plasma insulin levels result from a basal level of insulin secretion throughout the day and glucose-stimulated secretion after meals. (**C**) Insulin levels resulting from daily injections of long-acting insulin to provide the basal insulin requirement and pre-meal injections of rapid-acting insulin to control postprandial glycemia in type 1 diabetics. (**D**) Insulin levels obtained with an insulin pump. The pump delivers a constant infusion of regular insulin to fulfill the basal insulin requirement, and the patient activates small bolus injections of insulin before meals, snacks, and bedtime.

stimulates enzymes involved in glycogen synthesis while inhibiting glycogenolytic and gluconeogenetic enzymes, thereby reducing glucose output by the liver.

Insulin promotes the uptake of glucose by **skeletal muscle** and **adipose tissue** by activating a glucose transporter in these tissues called GLUT 4. Skeletal muscle and adipose tissue are dependent on insulin for glucose uptake, whereas the brain can utilize blood glucose in the absence of insulin. By promoting glucose uptake, insulin facilitates the metabolism of glucose to provide energy for skeletal muscle contraction, and it stimulates glycogen synthesis. In adipose tissue, insulin increases the conversion of glucose to fatty acids for storage as triglyceride. It also promotes the uptake

and esterification of fatty acids and inhibits lipolysis (the conversion of triglyceride to fatty acids). In skeletal muscle, insulin inhibits protein catabolism and amino acid output.

Mechanisms of Action

Insulin binds to **insulin receptors** located in the plasma membrane of target cells, which are primarily cells of the liver, skeletal muscle, and adipose tissue. Stimulation of insulin receptors activates a **tyrosine kinase** and leads to the phosphorylation of serine residues of target proteins. The phosphorylated proteins alter the synthesis or activity of enzymes involved in metabolic processes. Activation of tyrosine kinase also increases the insertion of glucose transporter molecules into cell membranes of muscle and fat tissue.

Glucagon

Glucagon is produced by alpha cells of the pancreas in response to decreased blood glucose concentrations. It activates glycogenolysis and gluconeogenesis and increases hepatic glucose production. Patients with diabetes continue to produce glucagon, and the imbalance between glucagon and insulin is one factor that contributes to the metabolic derangements of this disease. Glucagon is available in a formulation for subcutaneous injection that is used to counteract hypoglycemic reactions in patients with diabetes.

Diabetes Mellitus

Classification

Diabetes mellitus (diabetes) is characterized by elevated basal and postprandial blood glucose concentrations and affects about 20 million people in the United States. The two major forms of diabetes are type 1 and type 2, with the latter accounting for about 85% of cases of diabetes.

Type 1 diabetes usually has its onset before 30 years of age, with a median onset of 12 years of age. It is believed to be an autoimmune disease that is triggered by a viral infection or other environmental factor. The resulting destruction of pancreatic beta cells leads to severe insulin deficiency and excessive production of ketones, causing **ketonemia** and **ketoacidosis.** Persons with type 1 diabetes require exogenous insulin for survival.

Type 2 diabetes (Box 35-2) is a heterogeneous disease that usually has its onset after the patient reaches 30 years of age and is often associated with a significant degree of **insulin resistance** and **obesity.** Insulin resistance can be caused by the presence of insulin antibodies or by defects in insulin receptors and signal transduction mechanisms in target organs. Patients with type 2 diabetes are less susceptible to developing ketonemia and ketoacidosis than are type 1 patients. Most patients with type 2 diabetes have normal or elevated concentrations of insulin and do not require exogenous insulin for survival. Type 2 diabetes is usually treated with oral antidiabetic medications in combination with dietary modifications and exercise, but some patients benefit from insulin treatment.

Additional forms of diabetes include **gestational diabetes**, which has its onset during pregnancy, and **secondary diabetes**, which occurs in association with other endocrine disorders or with exposure to drugs or chemical agents that are toxic to the pancreas.

Pathophysiology

The early manifestations of diabetes are metabolic abnormalities resulting from lack of insulin, whereas the long-term complications of diabetes result in part from nonenzymatic glycosylation of proteins, primarily in the cardiovascular system, leading to endothelial and cardiac dysfunction, atherosclerosis, and other problems. The percentage of **glycosylated hemoglobin** (hemoglobin A1c) is used as a clinical marker of long-term control of glycemia in diabetics.

BOX 35–2. A CASE OF POSTPRANDIAL HYPERGLYCEMIA

CASE PRESENTATION: A 52-year-old man with an 8-year history of type 2 diabetes is concerned that his diabetes is not well controlled. He has started a regular exercise program and has lost 12 pounds. His A1c level is now 8.0%, down from 8.4% at the previous determination. He is already taking maximal doses of metformin and glipizide and has been taking insulin glargine every evening for the past 3 months. His self-monitored blood glucose values show that his fasting blood glucose (FBG) values are fairly good, but his postprandial glucose (PPG) values are often high after breakfast and lunch, ranging from 158 to 230 mg/dL (normal < 140). His evening PPG values are usually acceptable. Based on these findings, his health care provider suggests that he reduce carbohydrate intake at breakfast and lunch or add a rapid-acting insulin preparation prior to these meals. After considering his diet and activity level, the man decides to use insulin aspart before breakfast and lunch and to adjust the dose based on PPG values.

CASE DISCUSSION: Self-monitored blood glucose (SMBG) is one of the most effective tools available to assist patients in achieving optimal glycemic control and target A1c levels. However, studies show that a large percentage of diabetics fail to follow recommended guidelines for SMBG. Obstacles to the effective use of SMBG include patient denial and unwillingness to adopt changes indicated by SMBG data, lack of patient confidence in their ability to use SMBG data, and the cost, inconvenience, and physical discomfort of SMBG. It is no surprise that patient education is the largest factor determining successful use of SMBG.

Blood glucose monitors enable patients to obtain a record of glucose levels on which to base dietary and treatment decisions. Pre- and post-meal glucose values can be used to guide the selection and adjustment of insulin therapy. Rapid-acting insulins such as insulin aspart and insulin lispro can help patients control PPG levels, while long-acting insulins such as insulin glargine and insulin detemir can improve FBG values and overall glycemic control.

The **acute metabolic abnormalities** that occur in untreated diabetes result from decreased glucose uptake by muscle and adipose tissue, increased hepatic output of glucose, increased catabolism of proteins in muscle tissue, and increased lipolysis and release of fatty acids from adipose tissue. A reduction in glucose utilization combined with an increase in hepatic glucose production leads to hyperglycemia. Hyperglycemia can then cause glycosuria (glucose in the urine), osmotic diuresis, polyuria (excessive urine formation), and polydipsia (excessive water intake). These derangements lead to dehydration and the loss of calories and weight. For these reasons, diabetes has been described as "starvation in the midst of plenty."

In patients with type 1 diabetes, the absence of insulin accelerates lipolysis, and this leads to increased production of ketones (acetoacetic acid, acetone, and β-hydroxybutyric acid) in the liver. When the body becomes unable to metabolize these ketones, the keto acids are excreted in the urine. These derangements ultimately lead to ketoacidosis, acetone breath, abnormal respiration, electrolyte depletion, vomiting, coma, and death. Insulin deficiency also leads to increased catabolism of proteins and increased loss of nitrogen in the urine.

The **long-term complications** of diabetes include microvascular complications, such as **nephropathy** and **retinopathy**; macrovascular complications, such as **cerebrovascular disease**, **coronary artery disease**, and **peripheral vascular disease**; and neuropathic complications, such as **sensory, motor, and autonomic neuropathic disorders**.

Although all of the complications of diabetes contribute significantly to morbidity, the most prevalent cause of death is coronary artery disease. Patients with diabetes often develop **hypertension** and **dyslipidemia**, characterized by a decrease in the high-density lipoprotein (HDL) cholesterol level and an increase in the triglyceride level. Furthermore, diabetes appears to be a risk factor for coronary artery disease that is independent of other risk factors such as smoking, hypertension, and dyslipidemia. For these reasons, patients with diabetes should exercise regularly, adhere closely to dietary guidelines, and comply with pharmacologic interventions to control hypertension and dyslipidemia and to achieve near-normal blood glucose concentrations.

INSULIN PREPARATIONS

Insulin preparations are used to treat all patients with type 1 diabetes and about one third of patients with type 2 diabetes. Insulin is also used to treat pregnant women with gestational diabetes.

For many years, therapeutic insulin was obtained from pork and beef pancreas. More recently, **human insulin** has been produced by expression of the human insulin gene in *Escherichia coli* or yeast using recombinant DNA technology. Human insulin is less likely than pork or beef insulin to elicit insulin antibodies leading to insulin resistance, and it is less likely to cause allergic reactions or lipodystrophy at injection sites. The latest innovation in insulin therapy has been the development of **human insulin analogues** that overcome some of the limitations of native human insulin as a therapeutic agent. These analogues have improved pharmacokinetic properties and result in more physiological insulin levels and better control of hyperglycemia without causing as much hypoglycemia as native human insulin preparations. The insulin analogues are discussed below.

The concentration of insulin preparations is expressed as the number of units of insulin per milliliter of solution or suspension. The United States Pharmacopeia (USP) defines 1 unit (U) as the amount of insulin needed to decrease the blood glucose concentration by a defined amount in a fasting rabbit. The insulin preparations used by most diabetics contain 100 U/mL. Regular insulin is also available in a concentrated preparation containing 500 U/mL for use by persons with insulin resistance who require more than 100 U as a single injection.

ADMINISTRATION AND ABSORPTION

Insulin is usually injected subcutaneously or is administered by continuous subcutaneous infusion with an insulin pump. Insulin preparations for inhalation are also available. Insulin absorption is most rapid from an abdominal injection site and is progressively slower from sites on the arm, thigh, and buttock. Because repeated injections at the same site can contribute to tissue reactions (lipodystrophy) that affect the rate of insulin absorption, patients should be taught to rotate injection sites within a particular anatomic area. Newer, silicone-covered needles are painless and have reduced patient aversion to insulin injections.

Based on their onset and duration of action, insulin preparations are classified as short-acting, rapid-acting, intermediate-acting, and long-acting (Table 35–1).

Rapid-Acting Insulin

Three rapid-acting preparations are now available to control postprandial glycemia. **Insulin lispro**, **insulin aspart,** and **insulin glulisine** are human insulin analogues with amino acid substitutions in the B chain as shown in Box 35-1. These modifications reduce aggregation of insulin molecules and enable more rapid absorption after subcutaneous injection compared to regular insulin. An ideal insulin for pre-meal administration would have an onset of action in 10 to 20 minutes, peak at 1 hour, and have a duration of action less than 3 hours. Hence, the rapid-acting insulin analogues are well suited or this purpose. Because the hypoglycemic effect of these insulins begins 10 to 20 minutes after subcutaneous injection, patients can easily coordinate insulin injections and mealtimes. These insulins are often used as part of a regimen that includes a long-acting insulin to provide basal insulin requirements.

Short-Acting Insulin

Regular insulin (insulin injection USP) has a slower onset and a longer duration of action than the rapid-acting insulin analogues after subcutaneous administration. It can also be given intravenously to treat diabetic ketoacidosis. Regular insulin consists of insulin hexamers crystallized around a zinc molecule. After subcutaneous injection, the hexamers dissociate into dimers and monomers that are absorbed into the circulation. Because of the time required for this process, the onset of action of regular insulin occurs 30 to 60 minutes after an injection and the duration of action is 5 to 8 hours. For this reason, regular insulin is not ideally suited to control

TABLE 35-1.	Onset of Action, Peak Effect, and Duration of Action of Insulin Preparations Following Subcutaneous Administration or Inhalation		
Type of Insulin	**Onset**	**Peak**	**Duration**
Rapid-Acting			
Insulin aspart	10–20 minutes	40–50 minutes	3–5 hours
Insulin lispro	15–30 minutes	30–90 minutes	3–5 hours
Insulin glulisine	20–30 minutes	30–90 minutes	1–2.5 hours
Short-Acting			
Regular insulin	30–60 minutes	2–5 hours	5–8 hours
Intermediate-Acting			
Isophane (NPH) insulin	1–2 hours	4–12 hours	18–24 hours
Long-Acting			
Insulin glargine	1–1.5 hours	None	20–24 hours
Insulin detemir	1–2 hours	6-8 hours	up to 24 hours
Inhaled Insulin			
Human insulin liquid	5–10 minutes	1 hour	5–10 hours

NPH = neutral protamine Hagedorn.

postprandial glycemia. It is often absorbed too slowly to prevent postprandial hyperglycemia, while causing hypoglycemia later, thereby necessitating a snack and contributing to weight gain. Hence, a rapid-acting insulin preparation is usually more effective for pre-meal use and may contribute to a greater reduction in A1c levels than regular insulin.

Intermediate-Acting Insulin

NPH (neutral protamine Hagedorn) insulin is the only intermediate-acting insulin still available for human use, though a veterinary formulation of pork insulin zinc suspension recently became available to treat diabetic dogs. NPH insulin consists of particles of insulin combined with zinc and protamine that slowly dissolve after subcutaneous injection, enabling sustained absorption and blood levels. NPH is more prone to erratic absorption and intrapatient variability than the long-acting insulin analogues, and it must be gently rolled or inverted before each use to ensure uniform dosage. However, it offers a lower-cost alternative to insulin analogues to meet basal insulin requirements, especially in type 2 diabetics.

Long-Acting Insulins

Long-acting insulin preparations are used to provide basal levels of insulin and facilitate control of glycemia throughout the day. These preparations are formulated to slowly release insulin for absorption into the circulation following a subcutaneous injection. With the withdrawal of extended insulin zinc suspension (**Ultralente**) from the market, the only long-acting insulins currently available are insulin glargine and insulin detemir.

Insulin glargine contains amino acid substitutions in the A and B chains that enable it to be slowly released and absorbed after subcutaneous injection. It is formulated as a solution at a pH of 4, but it is less soluble at body pH and it forms microprecipitates after subcutaneous injection. These precipitates slowly release insulin glargine for absorption over a 24-hour period, providing a relatively constant

hypoglycemic effect over this time period. Hence, it does not exhibit a peak effect (see Table 35–1). Insulin glargine is administered subcutaneously once or twice daily. It is often used in combination with a rapid-acting insulin given at mealtimes and is suitable for both type 1 and type 2 diabetics, with little risk of hypoglycemia.

Insulin detemir is a solution of recombinant human insulin that has been chemically modified by deletion of threonine at B-30 and the attachment of a 14-carbon fatty acid chain to the amino acid at B-29 (see Box 35-1). After subcutaneous injection, it reversibly binds to albumin in the extracellular and vascular spaces through its fatty acid chain, and then it is slowly released from albumin for absorption and distribution to target tissues. Insulin detemir provides a consistent duration of action of about 24 hours with little intrapatient variability. In clinical studies, insulin detemir improved glycemic control with little or no weight gain and a reduced risk of hypoglycemia compared to NPH insulin. Insulin detemir is administered once or twice daily to meet basal insulin requirements.

Inhaled Insulin

A liquid form of human insulin is available for administration with an electronic device that senses a patient's inhalation velocity and delivers the insulin when inhalation velocity is optimal. This device can be set to administer the desired dose in 1-U increments. Inhaled insulin has a rapid onset of action and a duration of action of 5 to 10 hours. Inhaled insulin is primarily used in place of short- or rapid-acting insulin. Clinical studies show that inhaled insulin is as effective as injectable formulations and is well tolerated, but its ultimate role in therapy is yet to be determined.

OTHER ANTIDIABETIC AGENTS

A growing number of agents are now available to treat diabetes. Most of these drugs are only employed in treating type 2 diabetes, but an amylin analogue is used for both type 1 and type 2 diabetes (see below). The various antidiabetic drugs can be divided into two major groups known as the **hypoglycemic agents** and the **antihyperglycemic agents**.

Hypoglycemic drugs act primarily by increasing **insulin secretion**, and excessive doses can cause plasma glucose concentrations to fall below the normal range. The hypoglycemic drugs include the sulfonylurea compounds and the meglitinide drugs.

Antihyperglycemic drugs act to prevent or reduce hyperglycemia, but they do not typically cause hypoglycemia. This growing class of drugs includes metformin, the α-glucosidase inhibitors, the thiazolidinediones, the incretin mimetics, and an amylin analogue.

The pharmacologic properties, metabolic effects, and therapeutic effects of antidiabetic drugs are shown in Table 35–2, Table 35–3, and Figure 35–2.

Hypoglycemic Drugs

Sulfonylurea Drugs

The sulfonylurea drugs were the first oral antidiabetic agents. The original sulfonylureas, such as tolbutamide, are no longer used because of their lower potency and their greater tendency to cause side effects. The second-generation drugs, which are at least 100 times more potent than first-generation drugs, include **glimepiride**, **glipizide**, and **glyburide**.

PHARMACOKINETICS. The sulfonylurea drugs are administered orally and undergo varying degrees of hepatic metabolism followed by renal and biliary elimination of the metabolites.

MECHANISMS AND PHARMACOLOGIC EFFECTS. Sulfonylurea drugs act primarily by increasing the secretion of insulin and secondarily by decreasing the secretion of glucagon.

Sulfonylureas increase the release of insulin from pancreatic beta cells by inhibiting **adenosine triphosphate (ATP)-sensitive potassium channels** in the plasma membrane. The potassium channel contains a pore-forming subunit through which potassium moves out of the cell and a subunit that functions as the sulfonylurea receptor. When a sulfonylurea drug binds to this receptor, it closes the potassium channel. This prevents potassium efflux and leads to beta cell depolarization, influx of calcium, and activation of the secretory machinery that releases insulin. Sulfonylureas increase the pulsatile secretion of insulin by increasing the amount of insulin secreted during each pulse, but they have no effect on basal secretion.

The decrease in glucagon secretion appears to result from the increased secretion of insulin and pancreatic somatostatin evoked by sulfonylurea drugs. Both insulin and somatostatin are known to inhibit the release of glucagon from pancreatic alpha cells. This action tends to normalize the ratio of insulin to glucagon in diabetics. Sulfonylurea drugs may also increase insulin sensitivity in patients with type 2 diabetes.

In contrast to some of the antihyperglycemic drugs, sulfonylureas do not have beneficial effects on lipoprotein levels, and their use has been associated with weight gain.

INDICATIONS. A sulfonylurea drug can be used alone to treat type 2 diabetes that is not controlled with dietary restrictions, exercise, and weight reduction. A sulfonylurea can also be given in combination with metformin, and this combination may provide better control of blood glucose concentrations while causing fewer adverse reactions.

ADVERSE EFFECTS. Hypoglycemia, the most common adverse effect of sulfonylurea drugs, can result from skipping or delaying meals, inadequate ingestion of carbohydrate, excessive doses, or renal or hepatic disease. Other adverse effects include skin rashes (which occur in up to 3% of patients), nausea, vomiting, and cholestasis. Less commonly, sulfonylureas cause hematologic reactions such as leukopenia, thrombocytopenia, and hemolytic anemia.

INTERACTIONS. Health care providers should be aware that sulfonylureas can interact with many other drugs. Although the clinical significance of many of these interactions is usually minimal, dosage adjustments may be required. Thiazide diuretics, corticosteroids, estrogens, thyroid hormones, phenytoin, and other drugs decrease the effectiveness of sulfonylureas and may necessitate a dosage increase.

Angiotensin-converting enzyme inhibitors, sulfonamides, salicylates and other nonsteroidal anti-inflammatory drugs, gemfibrozil, and alcohol are among the agents that can increase the hypoglycemic effect of sulfonylureas. Excessive ingestion of alcohol by patients treated with sulfonylureas or insulin can cause significant hypoglycemia. A disulfiram-like reaction can also result when alcohol is taken with sulfonylureas. Diabetics should be counseled to use alcohol moderately and to limit consumption to about 2 oz (60 mL) of distilled beverage per day.

SEPCIFIC DRUGS. The second-generation sulfonylurea drugs consist of glimepiride, glipizide, and glyburide. Glyburide is called glibenclamide in some countries.

Sulfonylurea therapy usually begins with a low dose, given once a day. The dose is then increased every 1 to 2 weeks until adequate glycemic control is achieved, side effects occur, or the maximal dose is reached. The absorption of glipizide is slowed by food and it should be ingested 30 minutes before breakfast, but glyburide and glimepiride can be taken with breakfast. The second-generation sulfonylureas have a duration of action of about 24 hours, which is considerably longer than their plasma half-lives. Many patients require only a single daily dose of a sulfonylurea to control glycemia, but if larger doses are required they should be divided and given twice daily. Clinical studies have found that these drugs have similar efficacy in the treatment of type 2 diabetes.

Meglitinide Drugs

Repaglinide and **nateglinide** are meglitinide compounds that are rapidly absorbed and promptly produce a hypoglycemic effect. These drugs are intended to be taken before meals to control postprandial glycemia. Repaglinide and nateglinide increase the amount of insulin released by pancreatic beta cells during and immediately after a meal by inhibiting ATP-sensitive potassium channels in the same manner as sulfonylurea compounds. These drugs control

TABLE 35–2. Pharmacologic Properties of Oral Antidiabetic Drugs

Drug	Hypoglycemia	Hyperinsulinemia	Lactic Acidosis	Gastrointestinal Symptoms
Acarbose	No	No	No	Yes (frequent)
Metformin	No	No	Yes (rare)	Yes (frequent)
Repaglinide	Yes	Yes	No	Yes (uncommon)
Sulfonylureas	Yes	Yes	No	Yes (rare)
Pioglitazone	No	No	No	No

TABLE 35–3. Metabolic Effects of Oral Antidiabetic Drugs

Drug	GLYCEMIC EFFECTS			LIPID EFFECTS			Body Weight
	FPG	PPG	A1c (%)	LDL	HDL	TG	
Acarbose	→ or ↓	↓	↓0.3–1.0	→	→	↓	→ or ↓
Metformin	↓	↓	↓1.5–2.0	↓	↑	↓	→ or ↓
Repaglinide	→	↓	Unknown	→	→	→	→
Glipizide	↓	↓	↓1.5–2.0	→	→	→ or ↓	↑
Pioglitazone	↓	↓	↓0.8–1.8	→ or ↑	↑	↓	→ or ↑

A1c = glycosylated hemoglobin; HDL = high-density lipoprotein cholesterol level; FPG = fasting plasma glucose concentration; LDL = low-density lipoprotein cholesterol level; PPG = postprandial glucose concentration; TG = triglyceride level; → = unchanged; ↓ = decreased; ↑ = increased.

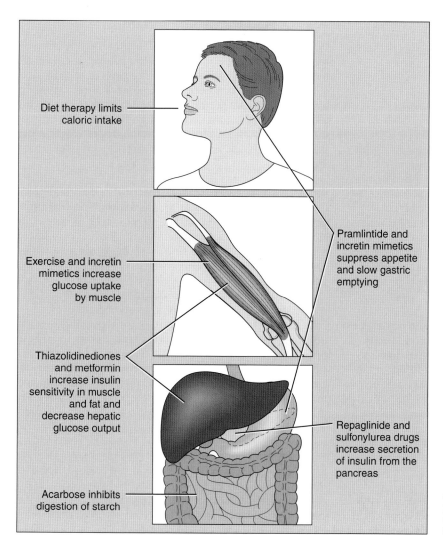

Diet therapy limits caloric intake

Exercise and incretin mimetics increase glucose uptake by muscle

Thiazolidinediones and metformin increase insulin sensitivity in muscle and fat and decrease hepatic glucose output

Acarbose inhibits digestion of starch

Pramlintide and incretin mimetics suppress appetite and slow gastric emptying

Repaglinide and sulfonylurea drugs increase secretion of insulin from the pancreas

Figure 35–2. Therapeutic effects of diet, exercise, and drugs used in the treatment of patients with type 2 diabetes. If these treatment measures are not adequate, insulin can be used to control glycemia.

postprandial glycemia and cause an overall decline in blood glucose concentrations and A1c levels.

Repaglinide and nateglinide can be taken anytime from 30 minutes before a meal right up to mealtime. They achieve peak effectiveness in about 1 hour, which coincides with the time when postprandial glucose concentrations are rising toward their peak. Repaglinide and nateglinide are completely metabolized and inactivated by the liver in about 3 to 4 hours. For this reason, their duration of action is relatively short, and insulin concentrations return to basal levels before the next meal.

Repaglinide and nateglinide are indicated as first-line drugs to treat type 2 diabetes in conjunction with diet and exercise. They are particularly useful for patients whose meal schedules vary from day to day, a factor that increases their risk of hypoglycemic reactions to sulfonylureas. Repaglinide and nateglinide can also be used in combination with metformin when either agent alone does not adequately control postprandial glycemia. They should not be used with other oral antidiabetic drugs or with insulin.

The primary adverse effect of meglitinide drugs is **hypoglycemia**. Hypoglycemic reactions are not often serious, but they have caused 1.4% of patients to discontinue their use of repaglinide. This is about half the rate of discontinuation attributed to hypoglycemic reactions in patients taking sulfonylureas. Mild hypoglycemia can be treated with oral glucose and severe hypoglycemia with intravenous D50W (50% dextrose in water) followed by a more dilute dextrose solution infusion.

Antihyperglycemic Drugs
Metformin

CHEMISTRY AND PHARMACOKINETICS. Metformin is the only **biguanide** type of oral antidiabetic medication currently available in the United States. Another biguanide, **phenformin**, was removed from the market in the 1970s because of an unacceptable risk of fatal lactic acidosis (see below).

The immediate-release formulation of metformin is administered orally from two to three times a day and is eliminated by renal excretion of the parent compound. Its duration of action is about 18 hours. A sustained-release metformin preparation is given as a single daily dose with the evening meal.

MECHANISMS AND PHARMACOOGIC EFFECTS. Metformin has several actions that result from increasing the number or affinity of insulin receptors in peripheral tissues. It reduces hyperglycemia partly by decreasing **hepatic glucose output**, resulting in increased glycogen stores. It also decreases glucose absorption from the gut and increases glucose uptake and utilization in skeletal muscle and adipose tissue. Unlike sulfonylureas, metformin does not stimulate insulin secretion or cause hypoglycemia or weight gain. Metformin often has a favorable effect on plasma lipid levels and can decrease body weight in some patients (see Table 35–3).

INDICATIONS. Metformin is a first-line drug for the treatment of type 2 diabetes. It may be particularly appropriate for obese patients with insulin resistance and for patients with hyperlipidemia, and it may lead to loss of weight. Metformin often controls hyperglycemia in patients who do not adequately respond to a sulfonylurea drug. Metformin can be used alone, or it can be used in combination with a sulfonylurea for patients who fail to respond appropriately to single-drug therapy. For this purpose, metformin is available in combination products containing metformin and either glyburide or glipizide.

ADVERSE EFFECTS. The most common adverse effects of metformin are gastrointestinal disturbances. **Diarrhea** occurs in up to 30% of patients and causes about 4% of them to stop taking metformin. Unlike phenformin, metformin does not bind to mitochondria or interfere with glucose oxidation, and it causes **lactic acidosis** rarely (in only 3 cases per 100,000 patient years of use). Patients with renal or hepatic disease, alcoholism, or a predisposition to metabolic acidosis should not be treated with metformin, however, because they are at increased risk of lactic acidosis.

INTERACTIONS. Metformin has few drug interactions, though cimetidine can inhibit the drug's metabolism and elevate its plasma concentrations.

Thiazolidinediones

CHEMISTRY AND PHARMACOKINETICS. Pioglitazone and rosiglitazone are members of the thiazolidinedione class of antihyperglycemic agents. Pioglitazone is taken once daily, and rosiglitazone is taken once or twice daily. These drugs are well absorbed from the gut and can be taken with or without food. Both pioglitazone and rosiglitazone are almost entirely metabolized by the liver. Two metabolites of pioglitazone have pharmacologic activity, but metabolites of rosiglitazone are inactive.

MECHANISMS AND PHARMACOLOGIC EFFECTS. The thiazolidinedione drugs act as agonists at the **peroxisome proliferator–activated receptor-gamma** (PPAR-γ), which is found in adipose tissue, skeletal muscle, and the liver. Hence, these drugs have a mechanism similar to the fibric acid drugs used to treat hyperlipidemia, which activate PPAR-α (see Chapter 15).

Activation of PPAR-γ increases transcription of insulin-responsive genes that control glucose and lipid metabolism, leading to increased insulin sensitivity and decreased insulin resistance in patients with type 2 diabetes. These drugs increase the sensitivity of peripheral tissues to insulin by about 60%. Specifically, thiazolidinediones increase the number of GLUT 4 glucose transporters in cell membranes of muscle and adipose tissue, which increases the uptake and utilization of glucose in these tissues. Pioglitazone and rosiglitazone also suppress hepatic glucose output.

The thiazolidinediones tend to lower serum triglyceride levels and increase HDL cholesterol levels. Rosiglitazone, however, may also increase low-density lipoprotein (LDL) cholesterol, and it may cause weight gain. Pioglitazone did not produce any consistent effect on LDL cholesterol levels.

INDICATIONS. Thiazolidinedione drugs are indicated as an adjunct to diet and exercise for the management of type 2 diabetes, and they can be used in combination with metformin. However, their future role in treating diabetes is uncertain because of their association with heart failure and myocardial infarction (see below). Clinical studies indicate that these drugs decrease plasma glucose concentrations by 40 to 80 mg/dL and decrease insulin requirements by 5% to 30%. The glucose-lowering effects of pioglitazone and rosiglitazone do not occur quickly, and their maximal effectiveness does not occur until 4 to 6 weeks after initiating treatment or increasing doses.

ADVERSE EFFECTS. Pioglitazone and rosiglitazone can cause **edema** and increase plasma volume, and they should not be used in persons with heart failure. Recent analyses of clinical trials have found that these drugs increase the **risk of developing heart failure** in type 2 diabetics, and some studies found that rosiglitazone also increases the risk of **myocardial infarction** and death. These drugs have not been associated with hepatic failure, but **liver function tests** should be performed periodically as a precaution.

α-Glucosidase Inhibitors

MECHANISMS AND PHARMACOLOGIC EFFECTS. The digestion of dietary starch and disaccharides (e.g., sucrose) is dependent on the action of **α-glucosidase,** an enzyme located in the brush border of the intestinal tract. This enzyme converts oligosaccharides and disaccharides to glucose and other monosaccharides. **Acarbose** and **miglitol** competitively inhibit this enzyme and delay the digestion of starch and disaccharides. This action decreases the rate of glucose absorption and lowers postprandial blood glucose concentrations, thereby reducing postprandial hyperglycemia. Studies have shown that acarbose and miglitol reduce A1c levels, although the reduction is usually less than that obtained with other oral antidiabetic drugs (see Table 35–3).

INDICATIONS AND PHARMACOKINETICS. Acarbose and miglitol are used in the treatment of type 2 diabetes, usually in combination with another oral antidiabetic agent. Acarbose and miglitol should be administered with the first bite of a meal. Acarbose is not absorbed systemically and it is eliminated in the feces, whereas miglitol is partly absorbed from the gut. Both drugs, however, act locally to inhibit α-glucosidase in the gastrointestinal tract.

ADVERSE EFFECTS AND INTERACTIONS. The most common side effects of acarbose and miglitol are increased **flatulence** and **abdominal bloating**. These reactions probably result from the delivery of greater amounts of carbohydrate to the lower intestinal tract, where they exert an osmotic attraction for water and are metabolized by bacteria. These drugs do not inhibit lactase or cause lactose intolerance.

Acarbose can increase the oral bioavailability of metformin and cause a decrease in iron absorption. Miglitol can decrease absorption of ranitidine and propranolol.

If concurrent administration of insulin or a sulfonylurea drug results in hypoglycemia in patients taking acarbose, this complication should be treated with glucose (dextrose)

rather than sucrose, because sucrose requires α-glucosidase activity for digestion.

INCRETIN MIMETICS

Incretins are intestinal hormones that are released in response to glucose and lipids derived from nutrients. Levels of these hormones are low in the fasting state but increase rapidly after ingestion of food. The incretins include glucose-dependent insulinotropic polypeptide and glucagon-like peptide-1 (GLP-1). These peptides have antihyperglycemic effects that include stimulation of glucose-dependent insulin secretion by the pancreas, increased uptake of glucose by muscle and adipose tissue, decreased secretion of glucagon, slowed gastric emptying, increased satiety, and decreased food intake. Because these effects would be beneficial to diabetics, drugs have been developed that mimic the effects of endogenous incretins.

GLP-1 is not well suited for therapeutic use because it is rapidly degraded by dipeptidyl peptidase-4 (DPP-4) and has a half-life of only 2 minutes. **Exenatide** is a GLP-1 mimetic derived from Gila monster saliva that resists degradation by DPP-4 and has a half-life of 12 to 14 hours. It is administered subcutaneously twice daily within 60 minutes of the morning and evening meals. Clinical trials found that giving exenatide in combination with a sulfonylurea drug, metformin, or both, resulted in greater improvement in A1c values and decreased body weight in type 2 diabetics compared to treatments without exenatide. Exenatide may cause mild to moderate nausea, and it has it as been associated with pancreatitis, particularly in persons with hypertriglyceridemia or gallstones. Patients taking exenatide should be instructed to report any episode of severe abdominal pain that might be a symptom of pancreatitis.

Sitagliptin is a DPP-4 inhibitor that is suitable for once-daily oral administration. Oral doses cause greater than 80% inhibition of DPP-4, resulting in a twofold increase in plasma GLP-1 levels. Clinical trials found that sitagliptin increased plasma insulin levels and reduced postprandial glucose levels in type 2 diabetics. It also caused a dose-dependent reduction of A1c levels. In one study, 45% of patients taking the highest dose achieved A1c levels below 7%. Sitagliptin is indicated to improve glycemic control in type 2 diabetics as monotherapy or in combination with metformin or a thiazolidinedione drug. Sitagliptin has been well tolerated and has not caused hypoglycemia or other significant adverse effects. **Vildagliptin** is another DPP-4 inhibitor that is currently under review by the U.S. Food and Drug Administration.

AMYLIN ANALOGUE

Amylin is a pancreatic hormone that is co-secreted with insulin by pancreatic beta cells in response to increased blood glucose levels. Amylin reduces the rate of rise of blood glucose after a meal by several mechanisms. It slows gastric emptying, thereby retarding digestion and absorption of nutrients, and it suppresses glucagon secretion and glucose output by the liver. Amylin also reduces appetite by an effect on the appetite centers in the brain. Because secretion of both insulin and amylin is impaired in diabetics, administration of amylin may improve glycemic control and lead to weight loss in these persons.

Pramlintide acetate is a synthetic analogue of human amylin that is approved for use in patients with **type 1** or **type 2 diabetes** who are being treated with insulin. It exerts an antihyperglycemic effect in these patients by slowing the rate at which food is delivered from the stomach to the intestines, and it reduces the rate of rise of plasma glucose for about 3 hours after a meal. However, the overall absorption of ingested carbohydrates is not changed. Pramlintide also reduces caloric intake and may lead to weight loss.

Pramlintide is given **subcutaneously** at mealtimes and is indicated for type 1 and type 2 diabetics who use mealtime insulin and have failed to achieve optimal glucose control. Co-administration of insulin and pramlintide increases the risk of **hypoglycemia**, and patients should begin treatment with low doses of pramlintide that are gradually increased over time. Pramlintide may also cause **nausea, vomiting, anorexia, headache**, and other adverse effects. It should be discontinued if recurrent hypoglycemic episodes or significant nausea occurs.

MANAGEMENT OF DIABETES

Type 1 Diabetes

All patients with type 1 diabetes require insulin therapy to achieve a high degree of glycemic control. Clinical trials have found that achieving and maintaining near-normal blood glucose concentrations in patients with type 1 diabetes reduces the incidence of nephropathy, neuropathy, and retinopathy and may lower the risk of cardiovascular disease.

Objectives of Insulin Therapy

The specific objectives of insulin therapy are to maintain the **fasting plasma glucose concentration** below 140 mg/dL (normal is <100 mg/dL); to maintain the **2-hour postprandial glucose concentration** below 175 mg/dL (normal is <140 mg/dL); and to maintain the **A1c concentration** below 7% (normal is 4%–6%). The A1c concentration provides a cumulative indication of overall glycemic control and may directly relate to the extent to which glycosylation of tissue proteins contributes to the microvascular and other complications of diabetes.

Insulin Requirements and Dosing Schedules

In patients with type 1 diabetes, multiple daily injections of insulin are required to obtain acceptable control of glycemia without causing hypoglycemia. The total amount of insulin required by most of these patients is 0.5 to 1 U/kg/day. This amount, however, usually decreases during the "honeymoon phase" of diabetes (during the first several months after the initial episode of illness).

The preferred regimens for most patients with type 1 diabetes consist of one or two injections of a **long-acting insulin analogue** to meet the basal insulin requirement

and multiple injections of **rapid-acting insulin** at mealtimes to control postprandial glycemia (see Fig. 35–1). The subcutaneous **insulin pump** is an option for patients who are sufficiently motivated to properly use and maintain the device. Some studies show that insulin pump therapy improves glycemic control and reduces rates of hypoglycemia compared to multiple daily injections. However, there have also been reports of pump failures and hypoglycemic episodes when these devices fail or are not used properly. **Inhaled insulin** offers a needle-free alternative that may be used in place of rapid-acting insulin at mealtimes. Inhaled insulin could be advantageous to patients with injection site reactions, needle aversion, or who have difficulty using injectable insulin. **Pramlintide**, an amylin analogue, may be useful in patients who have failed to achieve optimal glucose control with insulin therapy alone.

Diabetic Ketoacidosis

Diabetic ketoacidosis is a common and life-threatening complication of type 1 diabetes, with a mortality as high as 6% to 10%. It is the most common cause of death in children with type 1 diabetes. Diabetic ketoacidosis can also occur in type 2 diabetics, particularly those who are hospitalized for other medical or surgical conditions. Therapy must be individualized, based on the clinical and laboratory status of the patient. **Intravenous fluids** are given to restore fluid volume that has been depleted by osmotic diuresis and vomiting. A **continuous intravenous infusion of insulin** is given to decrease the plasma glucose concentration at a rate of 50 to 100 mg/dL/hour. Intravenous administration of **potassium chloride** is usually required to counteract hypokalemia that results from the correction of dehydration and acidosis. **Dextrose** (glucose) should be added to the intravenous infusion when glucose levels fall to 250 mg/dL, because hyperglycemia is usually corrected more rapidly than is acidosis. Insulin should be continued until acidosis is resolved and the plasma bicarbonate level is above 15 mEq/L.

Type 2 Diabetes

Treatment of type 2 diabetes rests on a foundation of a nutritious diet and appropriate exercise. Dietary recommendations should attempt to limit calories and saturated fat. Overweight patients should be encouraged to exercise and lose weight in an attempt to improve glycemic control, reduce insulin resistance, and lower plasma lipid levels. If nonpharmacologic measures are inadequate, as indicated by fasting blood glucose concentrations exceeding 140 mg/dL or A1c concentrations exceeding 7%, the next step is usually to add an oral antidiabetic medication.

Metformin, sulfonylureas, and meglitinide drugs are considered first-line drugs for type 2 diabetes. In obese patients with type 2 diabetes who have insulin resistance or hyperlipidemia, metformin is a logical choice to begin drug therapy, because it lowers elevated lipid levels and does not cause weight gain. Metformin can be combined with a sulfonylurea or meglitinide drug, or with an α-glucosidase inhibitor (e.g., acarbose) when metformin alone does not adequately control blood glucose levels. An incretin mimetic can also be used with metformin. These combinations can be tailored for individual patients based on their metabolic profiles and body weight.

Insulin can be used to treat type 2 diabetes when other drugs are not effective or not tolerated. The insulin regimens used to treat type 2 diabetes are usually less complicated than those used to treat type 1 diabetes. Patients with type 2 diabetes are less susceptible to ketoacidosis, and most of them have significant endogenous insulin production. Hence, the insulin requirement is often less than 20 U/day. Insulin therapy is usually started with a single daily dose of a long-acting insulin analogue. Giving a single dose at bedtime may be adequate for patients who experience only early morning hyperglycemia. Some patients also benefit from using a rapid-acting insulin analogue before meals to control postprandial glycemia (see Box 35-2). Inhaled insulin is another option for type 2 diabetics.

SUMMARY OF IMPORTANT POINTS

■ All patients with type 1 diabetes require insulin. Most patients with type 2 diabetes can be managed with diet, exercise, and oral antidiabetic drugs. Oral antidiabetic drugs have no role in the treatment of type 1 diabetes.

■ Insulin increases glucose uptake by muscle and fat, decreases hepatic glucose output, and controls postprandial glycemia.

■ Type 1 diabetes is typically treated with a long-acting insulin to meet basal insulin requirements and a rapid-acting insulin at mealtimes to control post-prandial glycemia. Alternatively, an insulin pump can be used to provide basal and mealtime injections of insulin

■ Insulin lispro, insulin aspart, and insulin glulisine are rapid-acting insulin preparations. Insulin glargine and insulin detemir are used as long-acting insulins.

■ Oral antidiabetic drugs include hypoglycemic agents (sulfonylureas and meglitinides) and antihyperglycemic agents (α-glucosidase inhibitors, metformin, and thiazolidinediones, incretin mimetics, and an amylin analogue).

■ Sulfonylurea (glipizide, glyburide, and glimepiride) and meglitinide drugs (repaglinide and nateglinide) increase insulin release from pancreatic β cells. Hypoglycemia is the main side effect of these drugs.

■ Acarbose and miglitol inhibit α-glucosidase and slow digestion and absorption of glucose.

■ Metformin, pioglitazone, and rosiglitazone decrease hepatic glucose output and increase insulin sensitivity in muscle and fat.

■ Metformin, sulfonylureas, and meglitinides are first-line drugs for the treatment of type 2 diabetes. Metformin can be used alone or in combination with most other antidiabetic agents.

■ Incretin mimetics (exenatide and sitagliptin) increase insulin secretion, increase glucose uptake by muscle and adipose tissue, and exert other antihyperglycemic effects in type 2 diabetics. Pramlintide is an amylin analogue that slows gastric emptying and the rate of rise of plasma glucose and is used in type 1 and 2 diabetics taking insulin.

Review Questions

1. A woman takes an orally administered drug 30 minutes before each meal and must eat at that time to prevent hypoglycemia. Which mechanism is responsible for the therapeutic effect of this drug?
   (A) closing of potassium channels
   (B) slowed gastric emptying
   (C) inhibition of α-glucosidase
   (D) inhibition of DPP-4
   (E) insertion of glucose transporters in cell membranes

2. A type 1 diabetic injects a medication at mealtimes that slows gastric emptying. Which adverse effect may result from this treatment?
   (A) increased appetite
   (B) nausea and anorexia
   (C) flatulence and bloating
   (D) weight gain
   (E) increased risk of heart failure

3. A woman takes an agent that activates PPAR-γ. Which effect is produced by this drug?
   (A) increased insulin secretion
   (B) lowered HDL cholesterol levels
   (C) increased serum triglyceride levels
   (D) insertion of glucose transporters in adipose tissue
   (E) weight loss

4. A diabetic injects an insulin preparation that forms microprecipitates in subcutaneous tissue. Which structural modification is found in this insulin analogue?
   (A) addition of a 14-carbon fatty acid chain
   (B) transposition of proline and lysine
   (C) substitution of aspartate for another amino acid
   (D) substitution of glutamate and lysine for other amino acids
   (E) addition of two arginine residues

5. A woman is placed on a drug that increases insulin sensitivity and typically results in a loss of body weight. Which adverse effect commonly results from taking this medication?
   (A) increased risk of heart failure
   (B) increased triglyceride and LDL cholesterol levels
   (C) diarrhea
   (D) lactic acidosis
   (E) hypoglycemia

Answers and Explanations

1. **The answer is A:** closing of potassium channels. The meglitinide drugs such as repaglinide are taken 30 minutes before meals to control postprandial glycemia in type 2

diabetics. Unlike α-glucosidase inhibitors that are taken with meals, meglitinide drugs can cause hypoglycemia. Meglitinide drugs increase insulin secretion in the same manner as sulfonylureas by inhibiting ATP-sensitive potassium channel in pancreatic beta cells. This leads to closing of potassium channels, membrane depolarization, and insulin secretion. Option B (slowed gastric emptying) is caused by an amylin analogue (pramlintide) and by incretin mimetics such as exenatide. Option C (inhibition of α-glucosidase) is the mechanism of acarbose and miglitol. Option D (inhibition of dipeptidyl peptidase-4) is produced by sitagliptin, and Option E (insertion of glucose transporters in cell membranes) may result from pioglitazone administration.

2. **The answer is B:** nausea and anorexia. Pramlintide is an amylin analogue that slows gastric emptying and the delivery of carbohydrates to the intestines. It is used in both type 1 and type 2 diabetics who use insulin, and its side effects include nausea, vomiting, and anorexia.

3. **The answer is D:** insertion of glucose transporters in adipose tissue. The thiazolidinediones such as pioglitazone activate the PPAR-γ and increase expression of the GLUT 4 glucose transporter in adipose tissue and muscle. These agents tend to raise HDL cholesterol and lower triglyceride levels. They may cause weight gain in some persons.

4. **The answer is E:** addition of two arginine residues. Insulin glargine is formulated as a solution that forms microprecipitates after subcutaneous injection. It contains a glycine substitution and the addition of two arginine residues to the terminal amino acid of native insulin.

5. **The answer is C:** diarrhea. Metformin increases insulin sensitivity and, unlike many other antidiabetic drugs, it may result in loss of weight. The most common side effect of metformin is diarrhea. It does not increase risk of heart failure and only rarely causes lactic acidosis. It tends to increase HDL cholesterol levels while reducing LDL cholesterol and triglyceride levels.

SELECTED READINGS

Bell, D.S. Insulin therapy in diabetes mellitus. Drugs 67:1813–1827, 2007.

Bloomgarden, Z.T. The Avandia debate. Diabetes Care 30:2401–2408, 2007.

Crotty, S., and S.L. Reynolds. The new insulins. Pediatr Emerg Care 23: 903–905, 2007.

Deacon, C.F., R.D. Carr, and J.J. Holst. DPP-4 inhibitor therapy: new directions in the treatment of type 2 diabetes. Front Biosci 13:1780–1794, 2008.

Kurtzhals, P. Pharmacology of insulin detemir. Endocrinol Metab Clin North Am 36:14–20, 2007.

Lago, R.M., P.P. Singh, and R.W. Nesto. Congestive heart failure and cardiovascular death in patients with prediabetes and type 2 diabetes given thiazolidinediones. Lancet 370:1129–1136, 2007.

CHAPTER 36

Drugs Affecting Calcium and Bone

CLASSIFICATION OF DRUGS AFFECTING CALCIUM AND BONE

Calcium and Vitamin D
- Ergocalciferol (CALCIFEROL, DELTALIN)[a]
- Calcium Carbonate and Calcium Citrate

Bisphosphonates
- Alendronate (FOSAMAX)[b]
- Pamidronate (AREDIA)[c]

Parathyroid Hormone and Related Drugs
- Teriparatide (FORTEO)
- Cinacalcet (SENSIPAR)

Other Agents
- Calcitonin (CALCIMAR, OSTEOCALCIN)
- Estrogen
- Raloxifene (EVISTA)
- Plicamycin (MITHRAMYCIN)
- Strontium Ranelate (PROTELOS)
- Sodium Fluoride (KARIDIUM, LURIDE)

[a]Also alfacalcidol, calcifediol (CALDEROL), and calcitriol (CALCIJEX, ROCALTROL).
[b]Also ibandronate (BONIVA), tiludronate (SKELID), and risedronate (ACTONEL).
[c]Also zoledronic acid (ZOMETA).

OVERVIEW

The strength and the structure of bone depend on the presence of calcium salts deposited on bone matrix proteins. Normal bone is constantly undergoing remodeling via demineralization and mineralization processes. During remodeling, bone calcium is in a dynamic equilibrium with ionized calcium in extracellular fluid. Bone mineralization tends to increase as the extracellular calcium concentration rises, and demineralization tends to increase as this concentration falls. The proper extracellular calcium concentration is required for normal function of nerves and muscles, blood coagulation, enzyme activities, and other physiologic functions.

Calcium and Bone Metabolism

Control of the extracellular calcium concentration depends on hormonal regulation of the absorption and excretion of calcium, as well as on the exchange of ionized calcium with bone. As shown in Figure 36–1, the hormones involved in regulation include **vitamin D**, **parathyroid hormone** (PTH), and **calcitonin**.

Vitamin D stimulates calcium absorption by increasing the synthesis of a calcium-binding protein that mediates the gastrointestinal absorption of calcium. Vitamin D also stimulates bone resorption and the closely coupled process of bone formation.

The PTH has four actions that increase the extracellular calcium concentration. First, it stimulates resorption of calcium by renal tubules. Second, it decreases resorption of phosphate by renal tubules. This decreases the extracellular phosphate concentration, which in turn tends to increase the extracellular calcium concentration. Third, PTH stimulates the hydroxylation of vitamin D in the kidneys (Fig. 36–2). Fourth, PTH increases bone resorption by stimulating osteoclast activity, which enables bone calcium to enter the extracellular pool.

Calcitonin is released in response to increased plasma calcium levels, and it acts to inhibit bone resorption and thereby decreases plasma calcium levels. The physiologic significance of calcitonin is unclear, because normal calcium balance is maintained in the absence of calcitonin in persons who undergo thyroidectomy.

Bone remodeling (Fig. 36–3) consists of a sequence of events involving the dynamic interaction of **osteoclasts** (bone-resorbing cells) and **osteoblasts** (bone-forming cells). The recruitment and activation of osteoclasts are mediated by compounds released from osteoblasts and peripheral leukocytes called **bone cell cytokines**. The cytokines include **interleukins, tumor necrosis factor**, and **colony-stimulating factors**. After the osteoclasts are activated, they adhere to the bone surface and release hydrogen ions and proteases to break down the bone. The destroyed bone releases growth factors that increase osteoblast production and decrease osteoclast

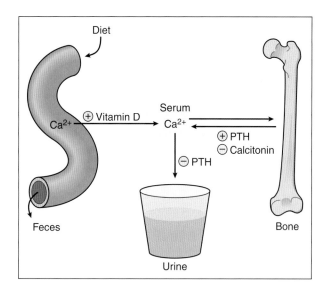

Figure 36-1. Calcium and bone metabolism. Vitamin D facilitates calcium absorption from the gut. Parathyroid hormone (PTH) decreases calcium excretion in the urine but increases phosphorus excretion (not shown). Endogenously secreted PTH increases bone resorption (and also bone formation), whereas calcitonin decreases bone resorption.

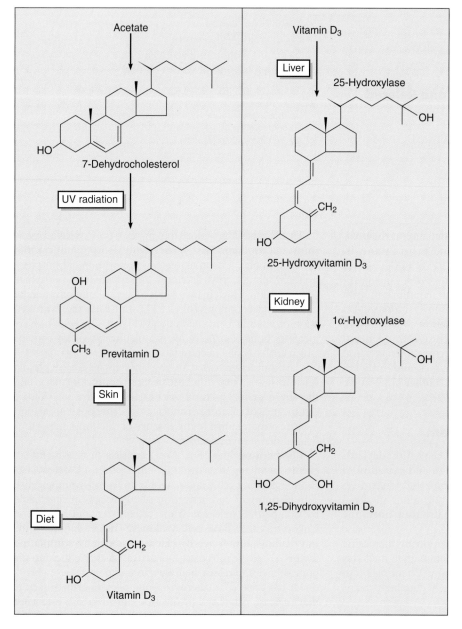

Figure 36-2. Synthesis of vitamin D. Vitamin D_3 (cholecalciferol) can be synthesized in the human body from acetate through a pathway that requires ultraviolet (UV) radiation. Diet and vitamin supplements also provide vitamin D_3, which is activated by specific hydroxylation steps in the liver and kidneys to form 1,25-dihydroxyvitamin D_3 (calcitriol).

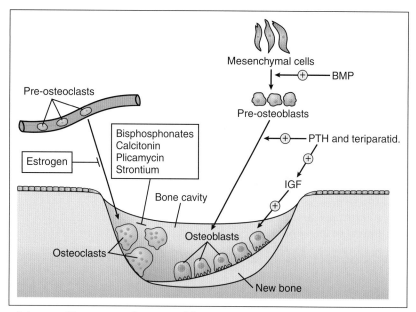

Figure 36-3. Effects of drugs and hormones on bone remodeling. Bone remodeling consists of two phases, bone resorption followed by bone formation. In the first phase, growth factors induce circulating pre-osteoclasts to differentiate to osteoclasts and attach to bone. Osteoclasts erode the mineral and matrix of bone surfaces, creating small cavities. In phase two, bone morphogenetic protein (BMP) and other factors induce mesenchymal cells to differentiate into pre-osteoblasts. Under the influence of PTH, pre-osteoblasts become osteoblasts and are further stimulated by insulin-like growth factor (IGF) to fill the cavities with new bone matrix that is subsequently mineralized. Short-term intermittent administration of teriparatide mimics the effect of PTH on bone formation and increases bone mass, but continuous long-term administration of these hormones increases bone resorption.

activity. The osteoblasts then lay down new bone in the cavity created by osteoclasts. The entire remodeling process takes about 100 days on average. Trabecular bone undergoes more remodeling than cortical bone (25% vs. 3% annually).

The balance between **bone resorption** and **bone formation** is usually maintained until the third or fourth decade of life, when a slow, age-related imbalance begins and favors resorption over formation. Hormonal and nutritional deficiencies can also contribute to this imbalance.

Bone Disorders

Osteoporosis, the most common bone disorder, is characterized by a gradual reduction in bone mass that weakens the bone and leads to the occurrence of fractures with minimal trauma. The disorder is frequently classified as postmenopausal, senile, or secondary to other diseases. **Vertebral fractures** are the most frequent type of fractures seen in patients with **postmenopausal osteoporosis**, a disorder caused primarily by estrogen deficiency. **Hip, humerus, pelvis, and vertebral fractures** occur in patients with **senile osteoporosis**, a disorder primarily resulting from advanced age; this disorder is a major cause of immobility, morbidity, and mortality in the elderly. In the United States, the annual cost of osteoporotic hip fractures alone is currently about $10 billion, and the cost is projected to rise to $240 billion by the year 2040 if more effective methods of prevention and treatment are not discovered and implemented (Box 36-1).

Paget's disease of bone, or **osteitis deformans**, is the second most common bone disorder. Characterized by excessive bone turnover, it causes bone deformities, pain, and fractures. Its cause is unknown.

Osteomalacia is characterized by abnormal mineralization of new bone matrix. The condition has numerous causes, the most common of which include vitamin D deficiency, abnormal vitamin D metabolism, phosphate deficiency, and osteoblast dysfunction. In children, osteomalacia usually results from vitamin D deficiency and is called **rickets**. This disorder is uncommon today because of vitamin D–supplemented foods and sun exposure. In adults, factors such as aging, malabsorption, chronic renal impairment, and use of phenytoin or other **anticonvulsant drugs** can interfere with vitamin D absorption, metabolism, or target organ response and result in osteomalacia.

Calcium and Vitamin D Supplements

An adequate intake of calcium and vitamin D is essential for optimal bone formation in children and to prevent osteoporosis in adults.

In the United States, two thirds of women 18 to 30 years of age and three fourths of women over 30 years of age have an inadequate calcium intake, and this predisposes them to osteoporosis. All persons, regardless of age or gender, should meet the recommendations of the National Institutes of Health for daily calcium intake (Table 36–1). These recommendations can be met by ingesting calcium-rich foods, which are primarily dairy products, and taking oral calcium supplements if dietary intake is inadequate. By ingesting optimal amounts of calcium and vitamin D, young adults may be able to increase their bone mass and older adults can decrease the rate of bone loss.

In one clinical study, nursing-home residents who were given 800 IU of vitamin D_3 and 1200 mg of calcium were

BOX 36–1 A CASE OF LOW BONE DENSITY

CASE PRESENTATION: A healthy 50-year-old woman has returned to her physician to assess hormone replacement therapy. She recently entered menopause and has been taking a low dose of oral estrogen and a vaginal estrogen cream along with cyclic medroxyprogesterone to relieve menopausal symptoms for the past 3 months. The treatment has reduced hot flashes and sleep disruption, but she still has an occasional episode. Because her mother suffered from osteoporosis and hip fracture, the woman asks about preventive therapy. She has been taking an adequate amount of calcium and has increased her intake of vitamin D. Her physician arranges for a BMD test, which reveals that her BMD T-score is −2 (normal is greater than −1). Based on her T-score and family history of osteoporosis, her physician suggests that she begin therapy with alendronate. She will be scheduled for a follow-up BMD in 6 months.

CASE DISCUSSION: BMD typically increases until about age 35 and then levels off until menopause. After menopause, BMD usually undergoes a sharp decline, and the risk of fractures increases with age. BMD is often determined using dual energy x-ray absorptiometry. The T-score compares a woman's BMD in grams per square centimeter with that of healthy young adults. The T-score is calculated as (patient's BMD − average young adult BMD) divided by 1 standard deviation of young adult BMDs. A normal T-score is greater than −1, whereas scores of −1 to −2.5 indicate low bone mass (osteopenia) and a risk of developing osteoporosis. Scores less than −2.5 indicate osteoporosis. Treatment guidelines recommend that women with risk factors receive preventive therapy if their T-score is less than −1.5. The risk factors include a previous fragility fracture, a family history of fracture, cigarette smoking, and low body weight (<127 lb). Hence, the woman meets the criteria for preventive treatment, and a bisphosphonate drug is usually selected for this purpose. If this treatment does not improve her BMD, teriparatide therapy might be considered.

TABLE 36–1. Calcium Intake Recommended by the National Institutes of Health Consensus Panel

Age Group	Daily Calcium Intake (mg)
Infants	
0–6 months	400
7–12 months	600
Children	
1–5 years	800
6–10 years	800–1200
Adolescents and Young Adults	
11–24 years	1200–1500
Men	
25–65 years	1000
>65 years	1500
Women	
25–50 years	1000
>50 years (postmenopausal) Taking estrogens	1000
Not taking estrogens	1500
>65 years	1500
Pregnant and nursing	1200–1500

Calcium

PHARMACOKINETICS. Calcium absorption from the gut is incomplete, even with consumption of adequate amounts of vitamin D. Only about 30% of calcium is absorbed from milk and other dairy products, and calcium absorption from supplements is often less than 30%. To enhance absorption, calcium tablets should be taken between meals.

The absorption of **calcium carbonate** requires stomach acid, whereas the absorption of **calcium citrate** does not. Because elderly persons can have decreased stomach acid secretion, they tend to benefit more from using calcium citrate.

INDICATIONS. In addition to their role in the prevention and treatment of **osteoporosis**, calcium and vitamin D are also the primary treatment for hypocalcemia. For this purpose, calcium can be given orally or intravenously.

ADVERSE EFFECTS AND INTERACTIONS. The most common adverse effect of calcium supplements is constipation. This is best managed by ingesting adequate amounts of fruits and vegetables. Calcium should not be taken with fiber laxatives, because they decrease calcium absorption. Calcium can decrease the absorption of ciprofloxacin, fluoride, phenytoin, and tetracycline, so calcium supplements should be taken at least 2 hours before or after taking these drugs.

Vitamin D

CHEMISTRY AND PHARMACOKINETICS. Vitamin D is a fat-soluble substance similar to cholesterol. The form of the vitamin that is obtained from the diet and can be synthesized in skin exposed to ultraviolet radiation is called **vitamin D₃**, or **cholecalciferol**. It is a relatively inactive precursor of

found to have an increase in bone density and a decrease in the incidence of hip and nonvertebral fractures in comparison with nursing-home residents who were given placebos. In another study, administration of vitamin D_3 was found to decrease the incidence of vertebral and peripheral fractures in women with previous fractures.

1,25-dihydroxyvitamin D$_3$, which is called **calcitriol,** and is the most active form of the vitamin in the human body. The formation of calcitriol involves hydroxylation of vitamin D$_3$ at the 25 position in the liver to form **calcifediol** (25-hydroxycholecalciferol), which is then hydroxylated at the 1 position in the kidneys to form calcitriol (see Fig. 36–2). PTH stimulates the renal hydroxylation of vitamin D. The roles of PTH and vitamin D in calcium metabolism and homeostasis are described above.

VITAMIN D PREPARATIONS. Several vitamin D preparations are available for use as nutritional supplements to prevent vitamin D deficiency. Many preparations contain vitamin D obtained from fish oil. Specific vitamin D compounds are available to treat vitamin D deficiency and related disorders, including calcifediol and calcitriol.

INDICATIONS. Vitamin D preparations are used for the following indications: to prevent and treat vitamin D deficiency and **vitamin D–dependent rickets,** to treat **familial hypophosphatemia** (vitamin D–resistant rickets), to treat **hypocalcemia** caused by **hypoparathyroidism,** to treat **postoperative and idiopathic tetany,** and to prevent vitamin D deficiency in persons with **chronic renal failure.** Persons, including the elderly, with inadequate dietary vitamin D intake and low sun exposure should take oral vitamin D supplements to develop and maintain skeletal mass and prevent osteoporosis. Patients with **chronic renal failure** must be treated with calcitriol because they lack the 1α-hydroxylase enzyme required to synthesize the active form of vitamin D (see Fig. 36–2).

ADVERSE EFFECTS AND INTERACTIONS. Excessive doses of vitamin D can cause hypercalcemia and hypercalciuria. Cholestyramine inhibits vitamin D absorption, and phenytoin and barbiturates can induce enzymes that metabolize vitamin D and thereby lead to vitamin D deficiency.

PHARMACOLOGIC AGENTS

Most of the drugs used in treating bone disorders inhibit bone resorption by osteoclasts. These agents include the bisphosphonate drugs, calcitonin, estrogen and raloxifene, and plicamycin. In contrast, teriparatide stimulates bone formation by osteoblasts. Strontium appears to have a dual mechanism, acting to inhibit bone resorption while increasing bone formation.

Bisphosphonates

A number of bisphosphonate compounds are available to treat several disorders of calcium metabolism and bone. These compounds can be classified according to their ability to inhibit bone resorption. The original bisphosphonate, etidronate, is the least potent inhibitor of bone resorption. It is no longer used extensively because its long-term administration caused osteomalacia. Second-generation bisphosphonates, such as **alendronate, pamidronate, risedronate,** and **tiludronate,** are about 100-fold more potent than

etidronate, and third-generation drugs, such as **ibandronate** and **zoledronic acid,** are almost 1000-fold more potent than etidronate.

Drug Properties

CHEMISTRY. Bisphosphonate drugs are pyrophosphate analogues in which the phosphorus-oxygen-phosphorus group is replaced with a phosphorus-carbon-phosphorus moiety that is resistant to enzymatic hydrolysis.

PHARMACOKINETICS. Pamidronate and zoledronic acid are given intravenously, but other bisphosphonates are administered orally and ibandronate can be given orally or intravenously. Less than 5% of orally administered bisphosphonates are absorbed when taken on an empty stomach, and absorption is further reduced by food, certain drugs, and liquids other than water. Hence, patients are advised to take bisphosphonates with a full glass of water 30 minutes before ingesting anything else in the morning. Once absorbed, about half of the drug is deposited in bone, and the remainder is excreted in the urine.

The bisphosphonates adsorb to hydroxyapatite and become a permanent part of the bone structure. They are slowly released from bone during bone remodeling, and the terminal half-life appears to be greater than 10 years.

MECHANISMS AND PHARMACOLOGIC EFFECTS. Bisphosphonates prevent bone resorption by inhibiting osteoclast activity. The most important mechanism is probably the prevention of the attachment of osteoclasts to bone. Bisphosphonates also decrease the metabolic activity of osteoclasts and their ability to resorb bone. For example, tiludronate decreases tyrosine phosphatase activity in osteoclasts, which appears to cause their detachment from bone surfaces. Tiludronate treatment also reduces activity of the proton pump by which osteoclasts secrete hydrogen ions that participate in bone resorption.

INDICATIONS. Bisphosphonate compounds are used in the management of a variety of disorders, including **osteoporosis, Paget's disease of bone, hypercalcemia,** and **osteolytic bone lesions of metastatic cancer.** As discussed below, the various compounds have different uses.

ADVERSE EFFECTS. Orally administrated bisphosphonates can cause esophageal erosion, but this can be prevented by remaining upright after swallowing these drugs. The bisphosphonate compounds produce varying degrees of gastrointestinal distress. Pamidronate causes more gastric irritation than other bisphosphonates and is not currently available in an oral formulation. Alendronate and risedronate seldom cause gastric distress except when high doses are used to treat Paget's disease. Occasionally, alendronate causes mild and transient nausea, dyspepsia, constipation, or diarrhea.

INTERACTIONS. The bisphosphonates have few interactions with other drugs. Calcium supplements and antacids decrease the absorption of bisphosphonates and should be taken at least 2 hours before or after a bisphosphonate compound.

Specific Drugs

Alendronate was the first bisphosphonate to be approved for the treatment of osteoporosis, and it appears to be effective in all forms of this disorder, including glucocorticoid-induced osteoporosis. Clinical trials in women with postmenopausal osteoporosis indicate that alendronate prevents bone loss and is more effective than calcium supplements or calcitonin therapy in producing a sustained increase in bone mass. A study of women with low bone mass and preexisting vertebral fractures found that alendronate reduced new vertebral fractures by 47% over a 3-year period. Alendronate is available as oral tablets that can be administered once daily (5 or 10 mg) or once weekly (35 or 70 mg). The lower doses are indicated for prevention of osteoporosis, and the higher doses are used for treatment of established osteoporosis.

Ibandronate, risedronate, and tiludronate are also indicated for the prevention and treatment of osteoporosis in postmenopausal women. Ibandronate is currently the only bisphosphonate available in formulations for once-daily and once-monthly administration.

Alendronate, pamidronate, risedronate, and tiludronate are approved for the treatment of **Paget's disease of bone**. Before treatment, imaging and laboratory studies usually show evidence of increased bone turnover (remodeling), bone hypertrophy, and abnormal bone structure. By inhibiting abnormal osteoclast activity in patients with this disease, the bisphosphonates help to normalize biochemical indices of bone remodeling and restore normal bone structure. Patients who are symptomatic or who require orthopedic surgery are candidates for bisphosphonate therapy. Treatment should be initiated as early as possible to halt disease progression. Tiludronate given once daily is usually effective in 3 months, whereas other bisphosphonate compounds may require 6 months to be effective. If a relapse occurs, another course of treatment can be given after a 6-month interval.

In patients with **bone cancer**, bisphosphonates are useful in the management of **osteolytic bone disease** and resulting **hypercalcemia**. Intravenous administration of **pamidronate** or **zoledronic acid** is the most effective treatment for hypercalcemia associated with cancer. Bisphosphonate treatment inhibits bone resorption, reduces the tumor burden in bone, decreases bone pain, and reduces the risk of fractures in patients whose cancer has metastasized to bone. For example, pamidronate reduces skeletal complications in women with stage IV breast cancer with bone metastases. In men, pamidronate inhibits the adhesion of prostate carcinoma cells to bone, and **zoledronic acid** prevents bone loss and increases bone mineral density (BMD) in patients with prostate cancer.

Estrogen and Raloxifene

Estrogen reduces bone resorption primarily by regulating various bone cell cytokines. Estrogen inhibits the production of interleukin-1, tumor necrosis factor, and granulocyte macrophage colony-stimulating factor by peripheral blood monocytes, and the secretion of interleukin-6 and colony-stimulating factors by osteoblasts. These actions decrease the formation and activation of osteoclasts, which in turn slows the bone loss that occurs in postmenopausal women.

Estrogen is often employed to relieve menopausal symptoms such as hot flashes, but the low doses of estrogen usually employed for this purpose may not provide sufficient protection against bone loss. However, the beneficial effects of estrogen may supplement other treatments used to prevent osteoporosis.

Raloxifene is a **selective estrogen receptor modulator** that mimics the effects of estrogen on bone but does not increase the risk of thromboembolic events. Raloxifene increases BMD in postmenopausal women and decreases **vertebral fractures** in women with osteoporosis. Although raloxifene activates estrogen receptors in bone, it has antiestrogen effects in other tissues and can cause or intensify **hot flashes** and other symptoms of estrogen withdrawal in menopausal women. Estrogen preparations and raloxifene are discussed in greater detail in Chapter 34.

Calcitonin

CHEMISTRY AND PHARMACOKINETICS. Calcitonin is a peptide hormone secreted by the parafollicular cells of the thyroid gland. It is not reliably absorbed from the gut and must be administered parenterally or by nasal inhalation. **Salmon calcitonin** has been available for a number of years, and **recombinant human calcitonin** is also available. Salmon calcitonin is 50 to 100 times more potent than human calcitonin.

MECHANISMS AND EFFECTS. Calcitonin binds directly to receptors on osteoclasts and increases cyclic adenosine monophosphate levels. When given on a short-term basis, calcitonin inhibits osteoclast activity, decreases bone resorption, lowers serum calcium concentrations, and reduces bone pain. When given on a long-term basis, calcitonin may decrease bone formation and its long-term effects on bone mass are uncertain.

INDICATIONS. Because of its ability to inhibit osteoclast activity and decrease bone turnover, calcitonin is used to treat **osteoporosis, Paget's disease of bone**, and **hypercalcemia**.

In patients with osteoporosis, calcitonin treatment has been shown to increase bone mass at multiple sites in the body during treatment of up to 2 years duration. Calcitonin treatment is usually reserved for women who cannot tolerate other treatments. Studies indicate that calcitonin increases the BMD in the spine but has variable effects on the BMD in the hips. Patients with osteoporosis can be treated with either subcutaneous or intranasal calcitonin. In those who have had fractures, treatment in the immediate postfracture period appears to be particularly useful because of the drug's ability to reduce bone pain. Patients taking calcitonin should be advised of the importance of adequate calcium and vitamin D intake during calcitonin therapy.

In patients with Paget's disease, calcitonin is administered subcutaneously or intramuscularly every 1 to 3 days. The nasal spray is not used for this indication. Calcitonin treatment inhibits osteoclast activity and reduces markers of abnormal bone turnover, such as serum alkaline phosphatase activity and urine hydroxyproline levels. Alleviation of bone pain usually occurs 2 to 8 weeks after calcitonin therapy has begun.

Hypercalcemia can be treated with subcutaneous or intramuscular injections of calcitonin. The injections are administered every 12 hours until a satisfactory response occurs.

Plicamycin

Plicamycin is a cytotoxic antibiotic that is a potent osteoclast inhibitor and may block the action of PTH. Plicamycin inhibits bone resorption and is used to treat **hypercalcemia** and **hypercalciuria** that are caused by malignant tumors and are not responsive to conventional therapy. It is also used to treat **Paget's disease of bone**.

Plicamycin is administered by intravenous infusion and causes numerous adverse effects, including myelosuppression, coagulation disorders, and frequent nausea and vomiting.

Teriparatide

Anabolic agents such as teriparatide are the newest type of drug available to treat osteoporosis. In contrast to drugs that inhibit bone resorption, the anabolic agents increase bone formation and have the potential to reverse bone loss (see Fig. 36–3). Several types of anabolic agents are currently being developed.

Teriparatide is a recombinant form of human PTH that consists of the 34 biologically active amino acids of the hormone. The skeletal effects of teriparatide depend on the frequency and duration of administration. Short-term subcutaneous administration of teriparatide stimulates new bone formation on trabecular and cortical bone surfaces by preferentially stimulating osteoblastic activity more than osteoclastic activity. In human studies, teriparatide increased markers of bone formation, skeletal mass, and bone strength. In contrast, long-term exposure to excessive amounts of PTH as occurs in hyperparathyroidism can stimulate bone resorption more than bone formation and have a detrimental effect on the skeleton.

Clinical trials of teriparatide in postmenopausal women and hypogonadal men with osteoporosis found that the drug increased vertebral and femoral neck BMD, while reducing the risk of vertebral and nonvertebral fractures. Teriparatide is indicated for the treatment of **postmenopausal women** with osteoporosis who are at **high risk for bone fracture**. These include women with a history of osteoporotic fracture, women who have multiple risk factors for fracture, and women who are intolerant of other therapy. Teriparatide is also indicated to increase bone mass in **hypogonadal men** who are at high risk for fracture, such as those having gonadotropin-releasing hormone therapy for prostate cancer. Cessation of teriparatide therapy may be followed by a rapid loss of bone. To preserve the benefits of treatment, teriparatide should be followed by a bisphosphonate or other antiresorptive agent.

Teriparatide increases the incidence of **osteosarcoma** in rats and should not be prescribed for persons who are at increased risk of osteosarcoma, including those with Paget's disease of bone and those with unexplained elevations of serum alkaline phosphatase (a marker of bone turnover).

Strontium

Strontium ranelate represents a new treatment option for the prevention of osteoporosis. Following oral administration, strontium is laid down on the surface of newly formed bone where it decreases osteoclastic activity and reduces bone resorption. At the same time, strontium induces the differentiation of pre-osteoblasts to osteoblasts and increases markers of bone formation. Overall, strontium increases bone mass and strength. Clinical trials found that strontium ranelate reduced the risk of new vertebral fractures by about 25% and nonvertebral fractures by 15%. Strontium may cause minor gastrointestinal problems but does not appear to have any serious adverse effects.

Fluoride

Sodium fluoride is used to prevent tooth decay and dental caries, a condition in which localized destruction of calcified tissue on the tooth surface is followed by enzymatic lysis of organic material and the development of cavities. After oral administration, fluoride is stored in bone and teeth where it replaces the hydroxyl group in calcium phosphate salts (hydroxyapatite) so as to form fluoroapatite. Fluoroapatite deposited on the tooth surface is more resistant to erosion than is hydroxyapatite. Fluoride has been added to the drinking water supply in many localities as a method of caries prevention, and it can be applied directly to the tooth surface as a gel or rinse. Liquid and chewable sodium fluoride formulations are available to provide fluoride to infants and children.

Fluoride also has potential application in the treatment of osteoporosis. It increases bone crystal size and decreases its solubility so as to render bone more resistant to resorption. Fluoride also prolongs the bone remodeling cycle and increases bone formation. Unfortunately, the use of fluoride is limited by its tendency to cause excessive hardening of bone (osteosclerosis) and by the formation of demineralized bone. One study found that fluoride did not reduce osteoporotic fractures. Fluoride may also cause gastrointestinal distress and interfere with calcium and magnesium absorption.

MANAGEMENT OF CALCIUM AND BONE DISORDERS

Osteoporosis

The prevention of osteoporosis rests on a foundation of lifelong calcium and vitamin D intake in an amount that is sufficient to maximize bone formation during development and to sustain bone mass during adulthood. Weight-bearing exercise reduces bone loss and helps improve strength and balance. Endogenous estrogen in women and testosterone in men also reduce bone resorption. After menopause, the absence of estrogen accelerates bone loss in women. Although all postmenopausal women are at risk of developing osteoporosis, BMD measurements are being used increasingly to identify those who are at greatest risk.

In most postmenopausal women, osteoporosis can be prevented by ensuring an adequate intake of calcium and vitamin D, exercising, and taking antiresorptive agents when required to maintain BMD. Bisphosphonates are often used for this purpose because they can be taken orally, have proven efficacy, and exhibit a low incidence of adverse effects. Teriparatide and other agents can be effective in women with very low or rapidly decreasing BMD measurements, women who have had fractures, and women who are at an increased risk of developing osteoporosis because they require chronic corticosteroid therapy or because they had natural or surgical menopause at an early age.

Paget's Disease of Bone

The goals of treating patients with Paget's disease are to control bone pain and to prevent progressive bone deformity and other manifestations of the disease. **Calcitonin** or a bisphosphonate drug such as zoledronic acid is usually employed for this purpose, and the combination of calcitonin and a bisphosphonate may be useful in more severe cases. Plicamycin is reserved for the treatment of patients who fail to respond to other drugs.

Hypercalcemia

The treatment of hypercalcemia depends on the etiology and severity of the condition. The major causes of hypercalcemia are hyperparathyroidism and cancer.

Saline diuresis is usually the preferred method of managing acute hypercalcemia that is severe enough to cause symptoms. A saline infusion is used for this purpose, which serves to increase renal calcium excretion and to counteract the dehydration that often accompanies hypercalcemia. A **loop diuretic** (e.g., furosemide) can be added to the saline infusion, and this will further enhance calcium excretion.

Bisphosphonates are useful in the treatment of hypercalcemia associated with cancer. Calcitonin is usually used to supplement other treatments for hypercalcemia, and plicamycin is useful if other therapeutic agents and procedures fail. As a last resort, intravenous phosphate infusions can be used to control hypercalcemia, but these infusions place the patient at considerable risk for acute hypocalcemia, hypotension, renal failure, and tissue calcification.

Cinacalcet has been approved both for treatment of **hyperparathyroidism** in adult patients with chronic kidney disease who are on dialysis and for treatment of **hypercalcemia** in patients with **parathyroid cancer**. The drug acts to increase the sensitivity of calcium-sensing receptors in the parathyroid gland to extracellular calcium, leading to decreased secretion of PTH and lowering of serum calcium levels. It appears to be safe and effective for these conditions.

SUMMARY OF IMPORTANT POINTS

■ The extracellular calcium concentration is regulated by vitamin D, PTH, and calcitonin. Vitamin D increases calcium absorption from the gut; PTH increases calcium reabsorption from renal tubules and increases bone resorption; and calcitonin decreases bone resorption.

■ A life-long intake of adequate amounts of calcium and vitamin D is essential for optimal bone formation and maintenance and for the prevention of osteoporosis.

■ Vitamin D is converted to its most active form, calcitriol, by hydroxylation in the liver and kidneys.

This active form must be supplied to patients with renal impairment. Dietary vitamin D is essential to prevent rickets in children.

■ Osteoporosis, the most common bone disorder, is characterized by a gradual loss of bone mass that leads to skeletal weakness and fractures.

■ Osteoporosis can be treated with a bisphosphonate drug, calcitonin, teriparatide, estrogen, raloxifene, or strontium ranelate. Most drugs reduce osteoclast activity and bone resorption. Teriparatide stimulates bone formation, while strontium appears to have a dual mechanism of action.

■ Bisphosphonates are also used to treat Paget's disease of bone, hypercalcemia, and osteolytic bone lesions associated with cancer.

■ Calcitonin reduces osteoclast activity and is used to treat Paget's disease of bone and hypercalcemia.

Review Questions

1. A 52-year-old postmenopausal woman is placed on a drug that decreases osteoclast activation but may intensify hot flashes. Which drug was most likely given to this patient?
   (A) alendronate
   (B) strontium ranelate
   (C) calcitonin
   (D) raloxifene
   (E) teriparatide

2. A woman with osteolytic bone cancer is treated with a drug that reduces the serum calcium level. Which drug is indicated for this purpose?
   (A) calcitonin
   (B) ibandronate
   (C) calcitriol
   (D) zoledronic acid
   (E) cinacalcet

3. A woman with a BMD T-score of −3 is given daily subcutaneous injections to increase bone formation. Which effect is most likely produced by this treatment?
   (A) increased absorption of dietary calcium
   (B) increased serum levels of vitamin D
   (C) decreased activation of osteoclasts
   (D) increased activation of osteoblasts
   (E) adsorption of the drug to bone

4. A man suffers from bone pain and deformities and is placed on a drug that increases cyclic adenosine monophosphate levels in osteoclasts. Which beneficial effect may result from this treatment?
   (A) increased serum alkaline phosphatase activity
   (B) decreased urine hydroxyproline levels
   (C) increased bone turnover
   (D) increased serum calcium levels
   (E) increased osteoblast activity

5. A woman is placed on a drug that adsorbs to hydroxy-apatite and remains in bone for years. Which effect most likely results from this treatment?
   (A) increased bone formation
   (B) decreased bone resorption
   (C) increased differentiation of pre-osteoclasts
   (D) increased formation of insulin-like growth factor I
   (E) increased formation of osteoblasts

Answers and Explanations

1. The answer is D: raloxifene. Raloxifene stimulates estrogen receptors in bone and reduces osteoporotic fractures. It acts as an estrogen antagonist in breast and other tissues and can increase the incidence and severity of estrogen withdrawal symptoms such as hot flashes.

2. The answer is D: zoledronic acid. Zoledronic acid is a potent bisphosphonate drug that prevents bone loss and reduces hypercalcemia in persons with malignancies. It is not indicated for the prevention and treatment of osteoporosis.

3. The answer is D: increased activity of osteoblasts. Teriparatide (and strontium ranelate) stimulate bone formation by promoting differentiation of pre-osteoblasts to osteoblasts. Teriparatide is given subcutaneously, whereas strontium ranelate is given orally. Teriparatide does not increase absorption of calcium (Option A), increase serum levels of vitamin D (Option B), decrease activity of osteoclasts (Option C), or adsorb to bone (Option E).

4. The answer is B. decreased urine hydroxyproline levels. The man most likely has Paget's disease of bone and was treated with calcitonin. Calcitonin decreases bone resorption and markers of abnormal bone turnover such as urine hydroxyproline levels. Calcitonin decreases, rather than increases, serum alkaline phosphatase activity (Option A), and it decreases, rather than increases, bone turnover (Option C). Calcitonin decreases, rather than increases, serum calcium levels (Option D). Calcitonin does not increase osteoblast activity (Option E).

5. The answer is B: decreased bone resorption. The woman received a bisphosphonate drug, such as alendronate. These drugs adsorb to bone and inhibit osteoclast activity, thereby decreasing bone resorption. Bisphosphonate drugs do not increase bone formation, differentiation of pre-osteoclasts, formation of insulin-like growth factors, or formation of osteoblasts (Options A, C, D, and E).

SELECTED READINGS

Canalis, E., A. Giustina, and J.P. Bilezikian. Mechanisms of anabolic therapies for osteoporosis. New Engl J Med 35:95–916, 2007.

Devogelaer, J.P., and D.H. Manicourt. Zoledronic acid for treatment of Paget's disease of bone. Expert Opin Pharmacother 8:2863–2869, 2007.

Silverman, S.L., and M. Maricic. Recent developments in bisphosphonate therapy Semin Arthritis Rheum 37:1–12, 2007.

Stevenson, M., S. Davis, M. Lloyd-Jones, and C. Beverley. The clinical effectiveness and cost-effectiveness of strontium ranelate for the prevention of osteoporotic fragility fractures in postmenopausal women. Health Technol Assess 11:1–134, 2007.

Stresing, V., F. Daubiné, I. Benzaid, H. Mönkkönen, and P. Clézardin. Bisphosphonates in cancer therapy. Cancer Lett 257:16–35, 2007.

CHEMOTHERAPY

CHAPTER 37

Principles of Antimicrobial Chemotherapy

OVERVIEW

Chemotherapy can be defined as the use of drugs to eradicate pathogenic organisms or neoplastic cells in the treatment of infectious diseases or cancer. Chemotherapy is based on the principle of **selective toxicity.** According to this principle, chemotherapeutic drugs inhibit functions in invading organisms or neoplastic cells that differ qualitatively or quantitatively from functions in normal host cells. The chemotherapeutic drugs include antimicrobial drugs (introduced in this chapter and discussed further in Chapters 38–43), antiparasitic drugs (discussed in Chapter 44), and antineoplastic drugs (discussed in Chapter 45).

Antibiotics and Chemotherapy

The **antimicrobial drugs** can be subclassified as **antibacterial, antifungal, and antiviral agents.** These agents include natural compounds, called antibiotics, as well as synthetic compounds produced in laboratories. An **antibiotic** is a substance that is produced by one microbe and inhibits the growth or viability of other microbes. The earliest use of antibiotics was probably in the treatment of skin infections with **moldy bean curd** by the ancient Chinese. The development of modern antibiotics can be traced to the work of **Louis Pasteur**, who observed that the in vitro growth of one microbe was inhibited when another microbe was added to the culture. Pasteur called this phenomenon **antibiosis** and predicted that substances derived from microbes would someday be used to treat infectious diseases.

Several decades later, **Alexander Fleming** observed that the growth of his staphylococcal cultures was inhibited by a *Penicillium* contaminant. Fleming postulated that the fungus produced a substance, which he called **penicillin**, and that this substance inhibited the growth of staphylococci. His observations eventually led to the isolation and use of penicillin for treating bacterial infections. The discovery of penicillin stimulated the discovery and development of many other antibiotics, the use of which has revolutionized the treatment of infectious diseases.

Synthetic drugs have also provided major advances in the treatment of infectious diseases and cancer. During the Renaissance, **Paracelsus** used **mercury compounds** for the treatment of syphilis. In the late 19th and early 20th centuries, **Paul Ehrlich** pioneered the search for selectively toxic compounds. After many failed attempts, he discovered **arsphenamine** (SALVARSAN), an arsenical compound for the treatment of syphilis. Ehrlich, who became known as the father of chemotherapy, also studied bacterial stains as potential antimicrobial agents. He reasoned that a stain's selective affinity for bacteria could be coupled with an inhibitory action to halt microbial metabolism and thereby destroy invading organisms. This concept led to the discovery of **sulfonamides**, drugs that were originally derived from a bacterial stain called PRONTOSIL. The sulfonamides were the first effective drugs for the treatment of systemic bacterial infections, and their development accelerated the search for other antimicrobial agents.

CLASSIFICATION OF ANTIMICROBIAL DRUGS

Antimicrobial drugs are usually classified on the basis of their site and mechanism of action and are subclassified on the basis of their chemical structure. The antimicrobial drugs include **cell wall synthesis inhibitors**, **protein synthesis inhibitors**, **metabolic and nucleic acid inhibitors**, and **cell membrane inhibitors**. The sites of action of these drugs are depicted in (Figure 37–1), and their mechanisms of action, pharmacologic properties, and clinical uses are described in subsequent chapters.

ANTIMICROBIAL ACTIVITY

The antimicrobial activity of a drug can be characterized in terms of its bactericidal or bacteriostatic effect, its spectrum of activity against important groups of pathogens, and its concentration- and time-dependent effects on sensitive organisms.

Bactericidal or Bacteriostatic Effect

A **bactericidal drug** kills sensitive organisms so that the number of viable organisms falls rapidly after exposure to the drug (Figure 37–2). In contrast, a **bacteriostatic drug** inhibits the growth of bacteria but does not kill them.

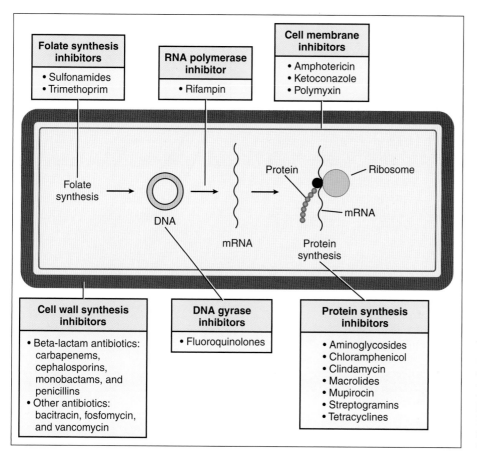

Figure 37–1. Sites of action of antimicrobial drugs. Antimicrobial drugs include cell wall synthesis inhibitors, protein synthesis inhibitors, metabolic and nucleic acid inhibitors (e.g., inhibitors of folate synthesis, DNA gyrase, and RNA polymerase), and cell membrane inhibitors.

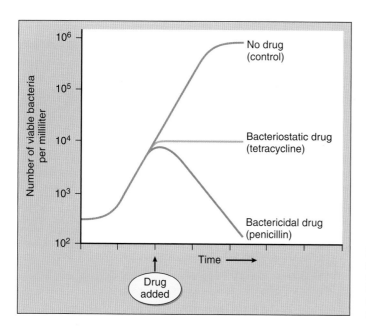

Figure 37–2. In vitro effects of bactericidal and bacteriostatic drugs. In the absence of an antimicrobial drug, bacteria exhibit logarithmic growth in a broth culture. The addition of a bacteriostatic drug (tetracycline) inhibits further growth but does not reduce the number of bacteria. The addition of a bactericidal drug (penicillin) reduces the number of viable bacteria.

For this reason, the number of bacteria remains relatively constant in the presence of a bacteriostatic drug, and immunologic mechanisms are required to eliminate organisms during treatment of an infection with this type of drug. (The same principle applies to a drug that kills or inhibits the growth of fungi and is referred to as a **fungicidal drug** or a **fungistatic drug**, respectively.)

A bactericidal drug is usually preferable to a bacteriostatic drug for the treatment of most bacterial infections. This is because bactericidal drugs usually produce a more rapid microbiologic response and more clinical improvement and are less likely to elicit microbial resistance. Bactericidal drugs have actions that induce lethal changes in microbial metabolism or block activities that are essential for microbial viability. For example, drugs that inhibit the synthesis of the bacterial cell wall (e.g., **penicillins**) prevent the formation of a structure that is required for the survival of bacteria. At the same time, penicillins activate autolytic enzymes that destroy bacteria. In contrast to bactericidal drugs, bacteriostatic drugs usually inhibit a metabolic reaction that is needed for bacterial growth but is not necessary for cell viability. For example, **sulfonamides** block the synthesis of folic acid, which is a cofactor for enzymes that synthesize DNA components and amino acids.

Drugs that reversibly inhibit bacterial protein synthesis (e.g., **tetracyclines**) are also bacteriostatic, whereas drugs that irreversibly inhibit protein synthesis (e.g., **streptomycin**) are usually bactericidal.

Some drugs can be either bactericidal or bacteriostatic, depending on their concentration and the bacterial species against which they are used.

Antimicrobial Spectrum

The spectrum of antimicrobial activity of a drug is the primary determinant of its clinical use. Antimicrobial agents that are active against a single species or a limited group of pathogens (e.g., gram-positive bacteria) are called **narrow-spectrum drugs**, whereas agents that are active against a wide range of pathogens are called **broad-spectrum drugs**. Agents that have an intermediate range of activity are sometimes called **extended-spectrum drugs**.

If the specific pathogen that is responsible for an infection is known, a narrow-spectrum drug is the logical choice to treat the infection. This is because a broad-spectrum drug is more likely to cause superinfection by eradicating organisms that make up the normal flora of the gut or respiratory tract. In cases in which an infection is serious and the responsible pathogen is not yet known, however, a broad-spectrum bactericidal drug (e.g., imipenem) is often used for initial treatment.

Concentration- and Time-Dependent Effects

Antimicrobial drugs exhibit various concentration- and time-dependent effects that influence their clinical efficacy, dosage, and frequency of administration. Examples of these effects are the **minimal inhibitory concentration** (MIC), the **concentration-dependent killing rate** (CDKR), and the **postantibiotic effect** (PAE).

The MIC is the lowest concentration of a drug that inhibits bacterial growth. Based on the MIC, a particular strain of bacteria can be classified as susceptible or resistant to a particular drug (see below).

An example of a CDKR is shown in (Figure 37–3A). Some **aminoglycosides** (e.g., tobramycin) and some **fluoroquinolones** (e.g., ciprofloxacin) exhibit a CDKR against a large group of gram-negative bacteria, including *Pseudomonas aeruginosa* and members of the family Enterobacteriaceae. In contrast, **penicillins** and **other β-lactam antibiotics** usually do not exhibit a CDKR.

After an antibacterial drug is removed from a bacterial culture, evidence of a persistent effect on bacterial growth may exist. This effect (see Fig. 37–3B) is called the PAE.

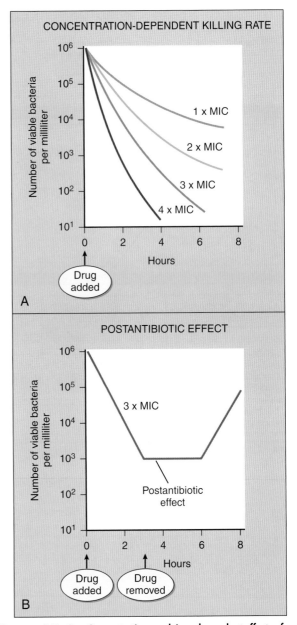

Figure 37–3. **Concentration- and time-dependent effects of antimicrobial drugs. (A)** When an aminoglycoside (e.g., tobramycin) is added to a culture of a gram-negative bacterium (e.g., *Escherichia coli*), it will exhibit a concentration-dependent killing rate. In this example, 10^6 bacteria were incubated with different concentrations of tobramycin, ranging from one to four times the minimal inhibitory concentration (MIC). **(B)** When tobramycin is removed from the culture, bacterial growth continues to be inhibited for several hours.

Most bactericidal antibiotics exhibit a PAE against susceptible pathogens. For example, penicillins show a PAE against gram-positive cocci, and aminoglycosides show a PAE against gram-negative bacilli. Because aminoglycosides exhibit both a CDKR and a PAE, treatment regimens have been developed in which the entire daily dose of an aminoglycoside is given at one time. Theoretically, the high rate of bacterial killing produced by these regimens would more rapidly eliminate bacteria, and the PAE would prevent any remaining bacteria from replicating for several hours after the drug has been eliminated from the body.

MICROBIAL SENSITIVITY AND RESISTANCE

Laboratory Tests for Microbial Sensitivity

Microbial sensitivity to drugs can be determined by various means, including the **broth dilution test**, the **disk diffusion method (Kirby-Bauer test)**, and the **Etest method**. These laboratory procedures are described in Box 37–1.

Either the broth dilution test or the Etest method can be used to determine the MIC of a drug, which is the lowest drug concentration that prevents visible growth of bacteria. On the basis of the MIC, the organism is classified as having **susceptibility**, **intermediate sensitivity**, or **resistance** to the drug tested. These categories are based on the relationship between the MIC and the peak serum concentration of the drug after administration of typical doses. In general, the peak serum concentration of a drug should be 4 to 10 times greater than the MIC in order for a pathogen to be susceptible to a drug (see below). Pathogens with intermediate sensitivity may respond to treatment with maximal doses of an antimicrobial drug.

Microbial Resistance to Drugs

Origin of Resistance

Resistance can be innate or acquired. Acquired drug resistance arises from mutation and selection or from the transfer of plasmids that confer drug resistance.

MUTATION AND SELECTION. Microbes can spontaneously mutate to a form that is resistant to a particular antimicrobial drug. These mutations occur at a relatively constant rate, such as 1 in 10^{12} organisms per unit of time. If the organisms are exposed to an antimicrobial drug during this time period, the sensitive organisms may be eradicated, enabling the resistant mutant to multiply and become the dominant strain (Figure 37–4A).

The probability that mutation and selection of a resistant mutant will occur is increased during the exposure of an organism to suboptimal concentrations of an antibiotic, and it is also increased during prolonged exposure to an antibiotic. This observation has obvious implications for antimicrobial therapy. Laboratory tests should be used to guide the selection of an antimicrobial drug, and the dosage and duration of therapy should be appropriate for the type of infection being treated. Whenever possible, the bacteriologic response to drug therapy should be verified by culturing samples of appropriate body fluids.

TRANSFERABLE RESISTANCE. Transferable resistance usually results from bacterial conjugation and the transfer of plasmids (extrachromosomal DNA) that confer drug resistance (see Fig. 37–4B). Transferable resistance, however, can also be mediated by transformation (uptake of naked DNA) or transduction (transfer of bacterial DNA by a bacteriophage). Bacterial conjugation enables a bacterium to donate a plasmid containing genes that encode proteins responsible for resistance to an antibiotic. These genes are called **resistance factors**. The resistance factors can be transferred both within a particular species and between different species, so they often confer **multidrug resistance**. The various species need not all be present during the period in which the antibiotic is administered. Studies have shown that resident microflora of the human body can serve as reservoirs for resistance genes, allowing the transfer of these genes to organisms that later invade and colonize the host.

Several genes responsible for drug resistance have been cloned, and the factors that control their expression are being studied. In the future, drugs that block the expression of these genes may find use as adjunct therapy for infectious diseases. For example, it may be possible to develop antisense nucleotides that block the transcription or translation of genes that encode proteins responsible for drug resistance.

Mechanisms of Resistance

The three primary mechanisms of microbial resistance to an antibiotic are (1) inactivation of the drug by microbial enzymes, (2) decreased accumulation of the drug by the microbe, and (3) reduced affinity of the target macromolecule for the drug. Examples of drugs affected by these mechanisms are provided in Table 37–1.

Inactivation of the drug by enzymes is an important mechanism of resistance to β-lactam antibiotics, including the penicillins. This form of resistance results from bacterial elaboration of β-lactamase enzymes that destroy the β-lactam ring. Resistance to aminoglycosides (e.g., gentamicin) is partly caused by the elaboration of drug-inactivating enzymes that acetylate, adenylate, or phosphorylate these antibiotics.

Decreased accumulation of an antibiotic can result from **increased efflux** or **decreased uptake** of the drug. Both of these mechanisms contribute to the resistance of microbes to tetracyclines and fluoroquinolones. Increased drug efflux is often mediated by membrane proteins that transport antimicrobial drugs out of bacterial cells. Some of these transport proteins are similar to, or indistinguishable from, human **P-glycoprotein**, a glycoprotein that transports antineoplastic drugs out of human cancer cells and thereby confers resistance to the drugs (see Chapter 45). Compounds that inhibit these transport proteins are being investigated as potential therapeutic agents to reduce drug resistance. Decreased uptake of antimicrobial drugs can result from altered bacterial **porins**. Porins are membrane proteins containing channels through which drugs and other compounds enter bacteria. Resistance to penicillins by gram-negative bacilli is partly caused by altered porin channels that do not permit penicillin entry.

Reduced affinity of target macromolecules for antimicrobial drugs is a common mechanism of drug resistance. It is partly responsible for resistance to cell wall synthesis inhibitors, protein synthesis inhibitors, DNA gyrase inhibitors, and RNA polymerase inhibitors (see Table 37–1). This type of drug resistance often results because of bacterial mutation, followed by the selection of resistant mutants during exposure to an antimicrobial drug. Altered target affinity has been the most difficult form of drug resistance to counteract by pharmacologic agents.

BOX 37–1. LABORATORY DETERMINATION OF MICROBIAL SENSITIVITY TO ANTIBIOTICS

Microbial sensitivity to drugs can be determined by various means, including the broth dilution test, the disk diffusion method, and the Etest method.

Broth Dilution Test

Tubes that contain a nutrient broth are inoculated with equal numbers of bacteria and serially diluted concentrations of an antibiotic. After incubation, the minimal inhibitory concentration (MIC) is identified as the lowest antibiotic concentration that prevents visible growth of bacteria. On the basis of the MIC, the organism is classified as having susceptibility, intermediate sensitivity, or resistance to the drug tested. In the following example, the MIC is 1 μg/mL, and the organism is susceptible to the drug.

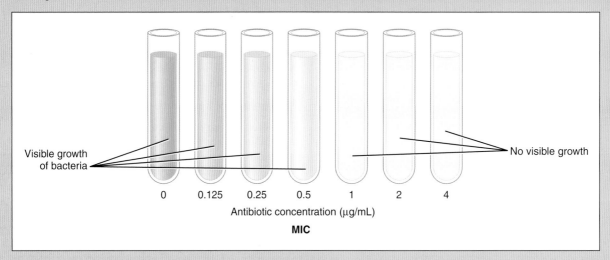

Disk Diffusion Method (Kirby-Bauer Test)

Each disk used in the disk diffusion method is impregnated with a different antibiotic. The disks are placed on agar plates seeded with the test organism. During the incubation period, the antibiotic diffuses from the disk and inhibits bacterial growth. After incubation, the zone inhibited by each antibiotic is measured. The zone diameter for each antibiotic is compared with standard values for that particular antibiotic. The organism is thereby determined to be susceptible, intermediate, or resistant to the various antibiotics tested.

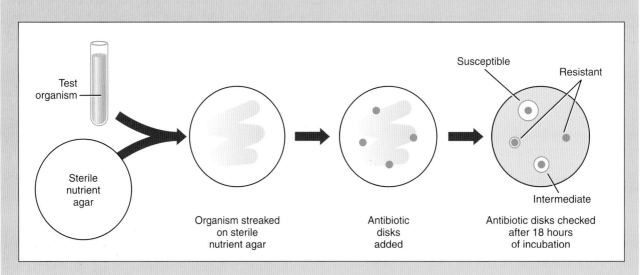

(Continued)

BOX 37-1. LABORATORY DETERMINATION OF MICROBIAL SENSITIVITY TO ANTIBIOTICS—cont'd

Etest Method

The Etest strip is a proprietary device that uses a diffusion method to determine the MIC of an organism. The device is a plastic strip that is impregnated with a gradient of antibiotic concentrations. After the strip is placed on an agar culture of the organism, the culture is incubated. During incubation, a tear-shaped zone of inhibition is formed. The point of intersection between the zone of inhibition and the scale displayed on the strip is the MIC. In the following example, the MIC is 0.125 μg/mL.

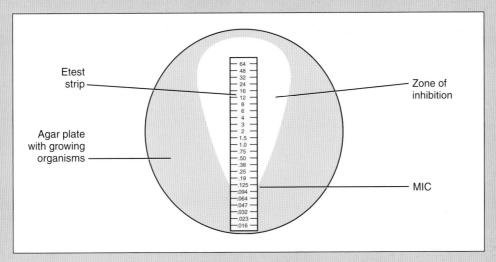

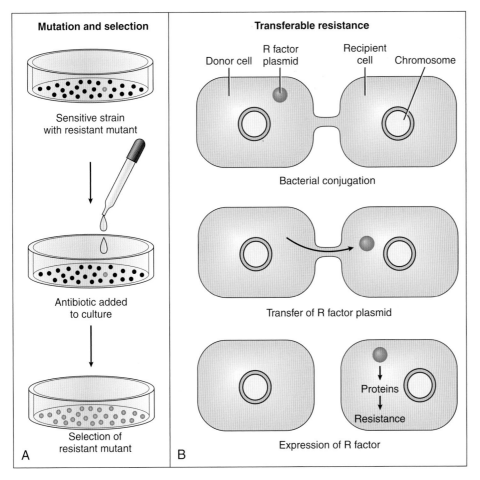

Figure 37-4. Acquired resistance to antimicrobial drugs can arise by mutation and selection or by transferable resistance. (A) Exposure of an organism to an antibiotic can result in the selection of a resistant mutant. **(B)** The most common mechanism of transferable resistance is bacterial conjugation and exchange of plasmids containing resistance factors.

TABLE 37-1. Mechanisms of Microbial Resistance

Mechanism	Examples
Inactivation of the drug by microbial enzymes	Inactivation of aminoglycosides by acetylase, adenylate synthetase, and phosphorylase enzymes
	Inactivation of penicillins and other β-lactam antibiotics by β-lactamase enzymes
Decreased accumulation of the drug by the microbe	Decreased uptake of β-lactam antibiotics due to altered porins in gram-negative bacteria
	Decreased uptake and increased efflux of fluoroquinolones
	Decreased uptake and increased efflux of tetracyclines
Reduced affinity of the target macromolecule for the drug	Reduced affinity of DNA gyrase for fluoroquinolones
	Reduced affinity of folate synthesis enzymes for sulfonamides and trimethoprim
	Reduced affinity of ribosomes for aminoglycosides, chloramphenicol, clindamycin, macrolides, or tetracyclines
	Reduced affinity of RNA polymerase for rifampin
	Reduced affinity of transpeptidase and other penicillin-binding proteins for penicillins and other β-lactam antibiotics

SELECTION OF ANTIMICROBIAL DRUGS

The selection of an antimicrobial agent for the treatment of a particular infection is based on the type of infection, the status of the patient, and the pharmacologic properties of the available drugs.

Host Factors

Host factors that influence the choice of a drug include pregnancy, drug allergies, age and immune status, and the presence of renal impairment, hepatic insufficiency, abscesses, or indwelling catheters and similar devices.

Most antimicrobial drugs cross the placenta and can thereby affect the fetus. For example, administering tetracyclines to a woman during **pregnancy** can cause permanent staining of her offspring's teeth. Penicillins and cephalosporins, however, cause very little fetal toxicity and can be safely administered to pregnant women who are not allergic to these drugs.

Many individuals are allergic to one or more antimicrobial drugs. Penicillins are the most common cause of drug allergy (see Chapter 38).

The patient's **immune status** is an important factor determining the success of antimicrobial therapy. **Advanced age, diabetes, cancer chemotherapy,** and **human immunodeficiency virus (HIV) infection** are among the more common

causes of impaired immunity. Immunocompromised individuals should be treated with larger doses of bactericidal drugs and may require a longer duration of therapy than do immunocompetent individuals.

Antibiotic access to **abscesses** is poor, so the concentration of an antibiotic in an abscess is usually lower than surrounding tissue. Moreover, immune responses to abscesses are impaired. For these reasons, abscesses must be surgically drained before they can be cured.

Foreign bodies, such as **indwelling catheters,** provide sites where microbes can become covered with a glycocalyx coating that protects them from antibiotics and immunologic destruction.

Many antibiotics are excreted unchanged by the kidneys, and lower doses must be used if the patient has significant **renal impairment.** Less commonly, **hepatic insufficiency** may require dosage adjustment for antimicrobial drugs that are extensively metabolized in the liver. For example, neonates cannot metabolize chloramphenicol, so their dosage of this drug per kilogram of body weight must be lower than the dosage given to older children or adults.

Antimicrobial Activity

Antimicrobial agents can be selected on the basis of laboratory test results (described earlier) or knowledge of the most common organisms causing various types of infections and the drugs of choice for these organisms (empiric considerations). Empiric therapy is often used initially to treat serious infections until test results are available. Empiric therapy is also used to treat minor upper respiratory tract infections and urinary tract infections because of the predictability of causative organisms and their sensitivity to drugs. In these situations, the cost of microbial culture and drug sensitivity testing is not usually justified.

The current drugs of choice for the treatment of infections caused by specific bacterial pathogens are listed in Table 37-2.

Pharmacokinetic Properties

The pharmacokinetic parameters of antibiotics that influence their selection for a particular use include their oral bioavailability, peak serum concentration, distribution to particular sites of infection, routes of elimination, and elimination half-life. An ideal antimicrobial drug for ambulatory patients would have good oral bioavailability and a long plasma half-life so that it would need to be taken only once or twice a day.

As described previously, the peak serum concentration of an antimicrobial drug should be several times greater than the MIC of the pathogenic organism for the drug to eliminate the organism. This is partly because the tissue concentrations of a drug are often lower than the plasma concentration. The relationship between the plasma concentration of a typical antimicrobial drug and the drug's MIC for several organisms is shown in (Figure 37-5). The urine concentration of an antimicrobial drug can be 10 to 50 times the peak serum concentration. For this reason, infections of the urinary tract can be easier to treat than are infections at other sites.

TABLE 37–2. Antimicrobial Drugs Most Often Used for the Treatment of Infections Caused by Selected Bacteria

Bacteria	Antimicrobial Drugs
Gram-Positive Cocci	
Enterococcus species	Penicillin G or ampicillin plus gentamicin; vancomycin plus gentamicin; quinupristin + dalfopristin, linezolid, daptomycin, tigecycline
Staphylococcus aureus	Penicillin G (if sensitive), nafcillin, oxacillin, vancomycin, quinupristin + dalfopristin, linezolid, daptomycin, tigecycline
Streptococcus pyogenes	Penicillin G or V, a cephalosporin, a macrolide, clindamycin
Viridans group streptococci	Penicillin G + gentamicin; vancomycin
Streptococcus pneumoniae	Penicillin G (if sensitive), a cephalosporin II or III, amoxicillin + clavulanate, an advanced fluoroquinolone, azithromycin, telithromycin
Gram-Positive Bacilli	
Bacillus anthracis (anthrax)	Ciprofloxacin ± clindamycin and rifampin; doxycycline
Clostridium difficile (diarrhea, pseudomembranous colitis)	Metronidazole, oral vancomycin
Clostridium perfringens, C. tetani	Penicillin G
Corynebacterium diphtheriae	A macrolide, penicillin G
Listeria monocytogenes	Ampicillin, gentamicin
Gram-Negative Cocci	
Moraxella catarrhalis	Amoxicillin + clavulanate, a cephalosporin II or III, a macrolide
Neisseria gonorrhoeae	Ceftriaxone, spectinomycin, a fluoroquinolone
Neisseria meningitides	Penicillin G, a cephalosporin II or III, chloramphenicol
Gram-Negative Bacilli	
Bacteroides species (anaerobes)	Metronidazole, penicillin + β-lactamase inhibitor, clindamycin, chloramphenicol, penicillin G (oropharyngeal strains)
Bordetella pertussis (whooping cough)	A macrolide, trimethoprim-sulfamethoxazole
Helicobacter pylori (peptic ulcer disease)	Tetracycline, clarithromycin, amoxicillin, metronidazole, bismuth compounds, proton pump inhibitors
Haemophilus influenzae	Amoxicillin + clavulanate, a cephalosporin II or III, azithromycin, a fluoroquinolone
Pseudomonas aeruginosa	An aminoglycoside, ceftazidime, a fluoroquinolone, aztreonam, a carbapenem, piperacillin + tazobactam
Most Enterobacteriaceae (*E. coli; Klebsiella, Proteus, Serratia, Enterobacter, Citrobacter, Providencia* species and others)	A cephalosporin II or III, an aminoglycoside, piperacillin + tazobactam, a carbapenem, aztreonam, a fluoroquinolone, trimethoprim + sulfamethoxazole (urinary tract infections)
Salmonella and *Shigella* species, *Campylobacter jejuni* (bacterial diarrhea)	A fluoroquinolone, ceftriaxone (*Salmonella*), ampicillin + sulbactam (*Shigella*)
Yersinia pestis (plague); *Francisella tularensis* (tularemia)	Streptomycin, a tetracycline, chloramphenicol
Actinomycetes	
Nocardia asteroides, N. brasiliensis	Trimethoprim-sulfamethoxazole
Chlamydiae, Ehrlichiae, Rickettsiae	A macrolide or a tetracycline antibiotic
Spirochetes	
Borrelia burgdorferi (Lyme disease)	Doxycycline, amoxicillin, a cephalosporin II or III
Borrelia recurrentis (relapsing fever)	A tetracycline, penicillin G
Treponema pallidum (syphilis, yaws)	Penicillin, a tetracycline

Sites of infection that are not readily penetrated by many antimicrobial drugs include the central nervous system, bone, prostate gland, and ocular tissues. The treatment of meningitis requires that drugs achieve adequate concentrations in the cerebrospinal fluid. Some antibiotics (e.g., penicillin G) penetrate the blood–cerebrospinal fluid barrier when the meninges are inflamed, but the aminoglycosides do not. For this reason, aminoglycosides can be given intrathecally for the treatment of meningitis. Because antimicrobial drug concentrations are low in bone, patients with osteomyelitis must usually be treated with antibiotics for several weeks to produce a cure. The prostate gland restricts the entry of some antimicrobial drugs because the drugs have difficulty crossing the prostatic epithelium and because prostatic fluid has a low pH. These characteristics favor the entry and accumulation of weak bases (e.g., trimethoprim) and tend to exclude the entry of weak acids (e.g., penicillin).

The route of elimination affects both the selection and the use of antimicrobial drugs. Drugs that are eliminated by renal excretion are more effective for urinary tract infections than are drugs that are largely metabolized or undergo biliary excretion. Antibiotics that are eliminated by the kidneys (e.g., the aminoglycosides) can accumulate in patients whose renal function is compromised, however, so their dosage must be reduced in these patients.

Adverse Effect Profile

Any antimicrobial drug can cause mild to severe adverse effects, but the incidence of these effects varies greatly among different classes of drugs. For this reason, it is important to

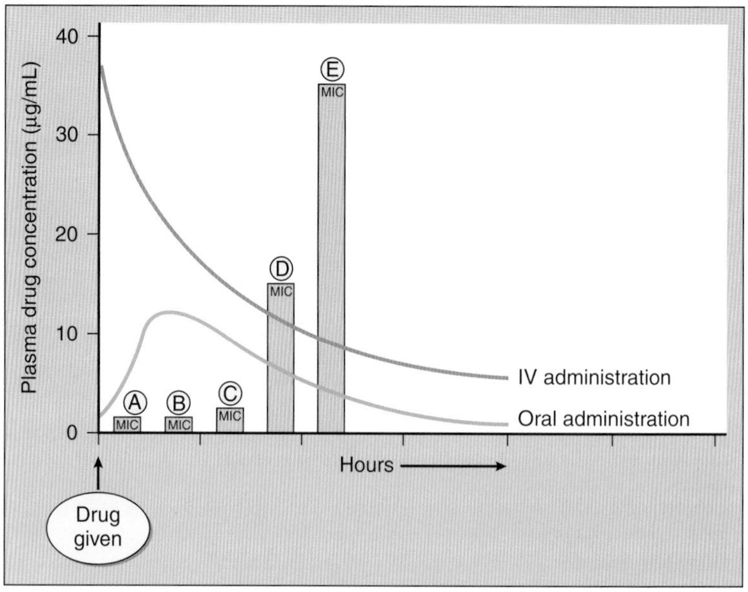

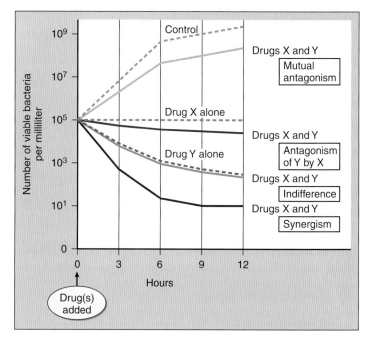

Figure 37–5. Relationship between the plasma concentration of a typical antimicrobial drug and the drug's minimal inhibitory concentration (MIC) for five bacterial organisms. The curves represent typical plasma concentrations over time after intravenous (IV) or oral administration of the drug. Each bar represents the MIC of a particular organism: *Streptococcus pneumoniae, Staphylococcus aureus,* and *Escherichia coli* (shown as **A**, **B**, and **C**, respectively, in this example) are susceptible to the drug; *Enterobacter* species (shown as **D**) are intermediate in sensitivity; and *Pseudomonas aeruginosa* (shown as **E**) is resistant.

Figure 37–6. Comparison of several possible interactions of two antimicrobial drugs combined in vitro. Curves show the results when cultures containing 10^5 bacteria per milliliter are incubated with no drug (control), with drug X alone, with drug Y alone, and with a combination of drugs X and Y. In this example, drug X is bacteriostatic, whereas drug Y is bactericidal. In an antagonistic interaction, the combined effect is less than the effect of either drug alone. In an indifferent interaction, the combined effect is similar to the greatest effect produced by either drug alone. In a synergistic interaction, the combined effect is greater than the sum of the independent effects.

consider the probable risk-to-benefit ratio when selecting drugs for treatment. The β-lactam and macrolide antibiotics cause a relatively low incidence of organ system toxicity and are often used to treat minor infections, including infections in pregnant women. In contrast, the aminoglycosides cause a relatively high incidence of severe adverse effects and are usually reserved for the treatment of serious or life-threatening infections.

COMBINATION DRUG THERAPY

When antimicrobial drugs are given in combination, they can exhibit antagonistic, additive, synergistic, or indifferent effects against a particular microbe (Figure 37-6). The

relationship between two drugs and their combined effect is as follows: **antagonistic** if the combined effect is less than the effect of either drug alone; **additive** if the combined effect is equal to the sum of the independent effects; **synergistic** if the combined effect is greater than the sum of the independent effects; and **indifferent** if the combined effect is similar to the greatest effect produced by either drug alone.

Treatment of Infections Caused by a Single Species

Some bacteriostatic drugs (e.g., chloramphenicol or tetracycline) are antagonistic to bactericidal drugs. Bactericidal drugs are usually more effective against rapidly dividing bacteria, and their effect is reduced if bacterial growth is slowed by a bacteriostatic drug.

Most infections caused by a single microbial species are treated with a single drug. This is because monotherapy usually is less expensive, equally or more effective, and less toxic than is combination therapy. A few situations occur in which combination therapy is preferable.

If two bactericidal drugs that act by two different mechanisms are given in combination, they tend to exhibit additive or synergistic effects against susceptible bacteria (Table 37–3). For example, penicillins, which are cell wall synthesis inhibitors, often show additive or synergistic effects with aminoglycosides, which are protein synthesis inhibitors, when they are used in combination against a gram-negative bacillus such as *P. aeruginosa*. These drugs also show additive or synergistic effects against many enterococci and staphylococci.

A few antimicrobial agents exhibit synergistic activity against some or all of the bacteria that are sensitive to the drugs. For example, sulfamethoxazole and trimethoprim inhibit sequential steps in bacterial folate synthesis and exhibit synergistic activity against many strains of organisms that are resistant to either drug alone.

Treatment of Mixed Infections

Mixed infections (i.e., infections caused by more than one microbial species) are usually treated with more than one drug. For example, an intra-abdominal infection can be caused by the combination of an aerobic gram-negative bacillus and an anaerobic gram-negative bacillus, such as *Escherichia coli* and *Bacteroides fragilis*, respectively. This type of infection can be treated with an aminoglycoside (active against aerobic bacilli) plus either metronidazole or clindamycin (active against anaerobic bacilli). Urethritis caused by a mixed infection with *Neisseria gonorrhoeae* and

TABLE 37–3. In Vitro Activity of Antimicrobial Drug Combinations

Synergistic Combinations
- Aminoglycoside plus ampicillin used against enterococci
- Aminoglycoside plus penicillin G used against enterococci
- Aminoglycoside plus broad-spectrum penicillin used against gram-negative bacilli
- Aminoglycoside plus cephalosporin used against gram-negative bacilli
- Amphotericin B plus flucytosine used against *Cryptococcus neoformans*
- Antistaphylococcal penicillin plus aminoglycoside used against staphylococci
- Antistaphylococcal penicillin plus rifampin used against staphylococci
- Reverse transcriptase inhibitor plus protease inhibitor used against human immunodeficiency virus

Antagonistic Combinations
- Aminoglycoside plus chloramphenicol used against members of the family Enterobacteriaceae
- Broad-spectrum penicillin plus chloramphenicol used against *Streptococcus pneumoniae*
- Broad-spectrum penicillin plus imipenem used against gram-negative bacilli

Chlamydia trachomatis can be treated with a cephalosporin such as ceftriaxone (active against gonococci) plus a tetracycline (active against chlamydiae).

Empiric Treatment of Serious Infections

More than one antibiotic is often used to treat patients with a serious infection until the causative organism can be identified and its sensitivity to antimicrobial drugs can be determined. For example, the initial treatment of serious nosocomial (hospital-acquired) infections can include the use of penicillin or vancomycin (active against staphylococci) in combination with an aminoglycoside or a cephalosporin (active against gram-negative bacilli).

Prevention of Antibiotic Resistance

As discussed in Chapter 40, tuberculosis is always treated with more than one drug. This is because about 1 in 10^6 *Mycobacterium tuberculosis* organisms will mutate to a resistant form during treatment with a single drug. The rate of mutation to a form that is resistant to two drugs is the product of the individual drug resistant rates, or about 1 in 10^{12} organisms. Because fewer than 10^{12} organisms are usually present in a patient with tuberculosis, it is unlikely that a resistant mutant will emerge during combination therapy.

PROPHYLACTIC THERAPY

The prevention of infections requires the sterilization of diagnostic and surgical instruments, the use of disinfectants to reduce environmental pathogens in hospitals and clinics, and the disinfection of skin and mucous membranes before invasive procedures. In some cases, antimicrobial drugs are also administered prophylactically either to reduce the incidence of infections associated with surgical and other invasive procedures or to prevent disease transmission to close contacts of infected persons. Recommendations for prophylaxis are summarized in (Table 37–4).

Prevention of Infection Caused by Invasive Procedures

Antibiotics are used to prevent **endocarditis** in persons with a history of valvular heart disease, such as mitral valve prolapse and rheumatic heart disease. These individuals are at risk of developing acute bacterial endocarditis caused by viridans and other streptococci that can be acquired during dental, oral, or upper respiratory tract procedures and surgery. Amoxicillin is currently considered the drug of choice, but endocarditis can be prevented by using an alternative drug (e.g., clindamycin, cephalexin, azithromycin, or clarithromycin).

Antibiotics are routinely used to prevent **wound and tissue infections** that can be acquired during a wide range of surgical procedures. The choice of antibiotic depends on the most likely sources of bacterial pathogens during a particular procedure. The skin is the most common source of pathogens, especially staphylococci, during most types of surgery. The

TABLE 37-4. Prophylactic Use of Antimicrobial Drugs

Prevention of infection during invasive procedures
- To prevent **endocarditis** in persons with a history of valvular heart disease, administer amoxicillin or other antibiotic prior to dental, oral, or upper respiratory tract procedures.
- To prevent **wound and tissue infections** in persons who will undergo surgery, administer a single dose of cefazolin (active against staphylococci and oral anaerobic organisms) or a single dose of cefoxitin or cefotetan (active against aerobic or anaerobic enteric bacilli).

Prevention of disease transmission in persons at increased risk
- To prevent **influenza type A**, give oseltamivir or zanamivir.
- To prevent **malaria**, give chloroquine or mefloquine.
- To prevent **meningococcal disease**, give rifampin.
- To prevent **tuberculosis**, give isoniazid.

gastrointestinal tract is also an important source of pathogens when surgical procedures involve the gastrointestinal system. Surgery to repair contaminated wounds (e.g., gunshot or knife wounds) presents the most severe requirements for prophylaxis because of the greater number and variety of bacteria that are often associated with this type of trauma.

Prevention of Disease Transmission

Antimicrobial drugs are occasionally used to prevent the transmission of a highly contagious disease, such as **meningococcal infection**, from an infected person or insect vector to an exposed individual. Drugs are also used to prevent **malaria** in persons who are traveling to regions of the world where malaria is endemic and to prevent **influenza type A** and **tuberculosis** in certain groups at increased risk for these diseases. Prophylactic drugs are discussed more thoroughly in subsequent chapters.

SUMMARY OF IMPORTANT POINTS

■ Antibiotics, which are substances produced by one microbe, are capable of inhibiting the growth or viability of other microbes. Antimicrobial drugs include cell wall synthesis inhibitors, protein synthesis inhibitors, metabolic and nucleic acid inhibitors, and cell membrane inhibitors.

■ Antimicrobial drugs can be characterized as bactericidal (able to kill microbes) or bacteriostatic (able to slow the growth of microbes). They can also be characterized as narrow-spectrum, broad-spectrum, or extended-spectrum, based on their range of antimicrobial activity.

■ Laboratory tests used to determine microbial sensitivity to drugs include the broth dilution test, the disk diffusion method (Kirby-Bauer test), and the Etest method. The broth dilution test and E test method are used to determine the MIC, which is the lowest drug concentration that inhibits microbial growth in vitro.

■ Acquired microbial resistance arises by mutation and selection or by transfer of genes encoding resistance factors. The most common mechanism of transferable resistance is bacterial conjugation and exchange of plasmids containing resistance factors.

■ The mechanisms responsible for microbial resistance to a drug include inactivation of the drug by microbial enzymes, decreased accumulation of the drug by the microbe, and reduced affinity of the target macromolecule for the drug.

■ The selection of an antimicrobial drug for treating a particular infection requires consideration of host factors (pregnancy, drug allergies, age and immune status, and the presence of concomitant diseases) and drug characteristics (antimicrobial activity, pharmacokinetic properties, adverse effect profile, cost, and convenience).

■ Combination drug therapy is generally used for the treatment of mixed infections, the empiric treatment of serious infections, and the prevention of antibiotic resistance. In some cases, combination therapy with synergistic drugs is used for the treatment of infections caused by a single microbial species.

■ Antibiotic prophylaxis is used to prevent infections during surgical and other invasive procedures and to prevent the transmission of infectious diseases to persons at increased risk.

Review Questions

For each numbered description, select the corresponding term from the lettered choices.

1. A cell membrane constituent that transports chemotherapeutic drugs out of a target cell.
   (A) plasmid
   (B) porin
   (C) resistance factor
   (D) β-lactamase
   (E) P-glycoprotein

2. The continued suppression of bacterial growth after an antibiotic is eliminated from the body.
   (A) bacteriostatic
   (B) postantibiotic effect
   (C) time-dependent killing
   (D) concentration-dependent killing
   (E) synergistic effect

3. The combined antibacterial effect of two drugs is greater than the sum of their individual effects.
   (A) mutual antagonism
   (B) indifference
   (C) synergism
   (D) supranormal
   (E) competition

4. The most frequent mechanism of transferable drug resistance.
   (A) transduction
   (B) transformation
   (C) transmission
   (D) conjugation
   (E) mutation and selection

5. An antibiotic diffusion method for determining the MIC of an antibiotic.
   (A) Etest strip method
   (B) broth dilution method
   (C) disk diffusion method
   (D) growth rate method
   (E) turbidity method

Answers and Explanations

1. **The answer is E:** P-glycoprotein. The P-glycoprotein is a cell membrane protein that pumps antibiotics and other drugs out of mammalian and microbial cells. It prevents accumulation of drugs in target cells and is one of the mechanisms that confer resistance to chemotherapeutic agents.

2. **The answer is B:** postantibiotic effect (PAE). The PAE refers to a period of time during which bacterial growth continues to be inhibited after an antibiotic has been removed from a bacterial culture or eliminated from the body. The PAE increases the effective duration of action of antimicrobial agents and enables less-frequent dosing of some antibiotics.

3. **The answer is C:** synergism. A synergistic effect occurs when the combined effect of two drugs is greater than the sum of their individual effects. Several antibiotic combinations show synergism against susceptible organisms, such as gentamicin and ampicillin against enterococci.

4. **The answer is D:** conjugation. Transferable drug resistance refers to the acquisition of genes conferring resistance from other bacteria. Most commonly, this occurs by bacterial conjugation and exchange of plasmids containing resistance factors. Transformation and transduction are less common mechanisms of transferring drug resistance.

5. **The answer is A:** Etest strip. The Etest strip is a semiquantitative antibiotic diffusion device for determining the MIC of an antibiotic. It is based on visualization of the point of intersection between the zone of bacterial growth inhibition and the concentration scale on the test trip. The Etest method is more convenient and economical than broth dilution methods.

SELECTED READINGS

Briken, V. Molecular mechanisms of host-pathogen interactions and their potential for the discovery of new drug targets. Curr Drug Targets 9:150–157, 2008.
Shakil, S., R. Khan, R. Zarrilli, and A.U. Khan. Aminoglycosides versus bacteria—a description of the action, resistance mechanism, and nosocomial battleground. J Biomed Sci 15:5–14, 2008.
Zinner, S.H. Antibiotic use: present and future. New Microbiol 30:321–325, 2007.

Inhibitors of Bacterial Cell Wall Synthesis

CLASSIFICATION OF CELL WALL SYNTHESIS INHIBITORS

Narrow-Spectrum Penicillins
- Penicillin G and Penicillin V

Penicillinase-Resistant Penicillins
- Nafcillin (UNIPEN)[a]

Extended-Spectrum Penicillins
- Amoxicillin (AMOXIL) and Ampicillin (OMNIPEN)
- Piperacillin (PIPRACIL) and Ticarcillin (with Clavulanate as TIMENTIN)

β-Lactamase Inhibitors
- Clavulanate (with Amoxicillin as AUGMENTIN)[b]

First-Generation Cephalosporins
- Cefazolin
- Cephalexin (KEFLEX)

Second-Generation Cephalosporins
- Cefprozil (CEFZIL) and Cefaclor (CECLOR)
- Cefuroxime (CEFTIN, ZINACEF)[c]

Third-Generation Cephalosporins
- Ceftriaxone (ROCEPHIN)[d]
- Cefdinir (DURICEF) and Cefpodoxime (VANTIN)

Fourth-Generation Cephalosporin
- Cefepime (MAXIPIME)

Monobactam
- Aztreonam (AZACTAM)

Carbapenems
- Imipenem (with Cilastatin as PRIMAXIN)[e]

Other Bacterial Cell Wall Synthesis Inhibitors
- Bacitracin
- Fosfomycin (MONUROL)
- Vancomycin

[a]Also oxacillin (BACTOCILL), dicloxacillin (DYNAPEN), and cloxacillin.
[b]Also sulbactam (with ampicillin as UNASYN) and tazobactam (with piperacillin as ZOSYN).
[c]Also cefoxitin (MEFOXIN), cefotetan (CEFOTAN), cefonicid, and cefmetazole.
[d]Also cefotaxime (CLAFORAN), ceftazidime (CEPTAZ), and ceftizoxime (CEFIZOX).
[e]Also doripenem (DORIBAX), ertapenem (INVANZ), and meropenem (MERREM).

OVERVIEW

A large group of antimicrobial drugs, including the β-lactam antibiotics, inhibit the synthesis of the bacterial cell wall. The penicillins were the first antibiotics to be discovered, and their development inaugurated the modern era of antimicrobial chemotherapy.

Cell Envelope

Two components of the cell envelope that are found in both gram-positive and gram-negative bacteria are the **cytoplasmic membrane** and the **cell wall.** The cell wall is much thicker in gram-positive bacteria than it is in gram-negative bacteria. The envelope of each gram-negative bacterium also has an **outer membrane** that is not found in other types of bacteria. The cell envelope components are illustrated in Figure 38–1.

Cytoplasmic and Outer Membranes

The cytoplasmic membrane is a trilaminar membrane. It contains various types of **transport proteins**, which facilitate the uptake of a wide variety of substrates used by bacteria, and it also contains several enzymes required for the synthesis of the cell wall. These enzymes, whose functions are described later in this chapter, are collectively known as **penicillin-binding proteins** (PBPs).

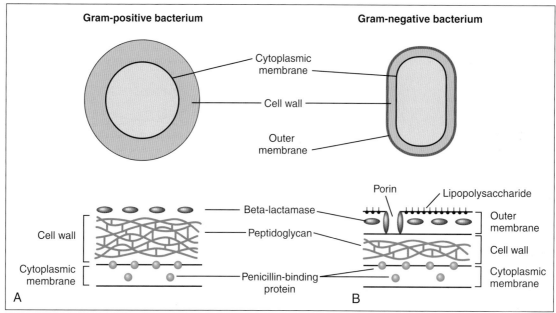

Figure 38–1. **Comparison of the cell envelopes of gram-positive and gram-negative bacteria. (A)** The gram-positive bacterium has a thick cell wall but does not have an outer membrane. β-Lactamases are located in the outer portion of the cell wall. Penicillin-binding proteins are found in the cytoplasmic membrane. **(B)** The gram-negative bacterium has a thin cell wall. It also has an outer membrane that contains lipopolysaccharide and protein channels called porins.

The outer membrane of gram-negative bacteria is also a trilaminar membrane. It contains species-specific forms of a complex **lipopolysaccharide** and various types of protein channels called **porins.** One portion of lipopolysaccharide (the lipid A portion) is the **endotoxin** responsible for gram-negative sepsis. This endotoxin activates immunologic mechanisms that lead to fever, platelet aggregation, increased vascular permeability, and other adverse effects on tissues. Porins allow ions and other small hydrophilic molecules to pass through the outer membrane, and they are responsible for the entry of several types of antibiotics. Acquired alterations in porin structure can lead to microbial resistance to antibiotics, such as is the case with resistance to imipenem.

The bacterial cytoplasmic membrane is the target of two peptide antibiotics, **daptomycin** and **polymyxin**. These drugs act directly on the cell membranes to increase membrane permeability and thereby cause the cytoplasmic contents to leak out of the cell. The properties and uses of these antibiotics are discussed in Chapter 40.

Cell Wall

The cell wall consists primarily of **peptidoglycan,** a polymer constructed from repeating disaccharide units of **N-acetylglucosamine** (GlcNAc) and **N-acetylmuramic acid** (MurNAc). Each disaccharide is attached to others through glycosidic bonds. Each molecule of MurNAc has a peptide containing two molecules of D-alanine and a pentaglycine side chain (Fig. 38–2). The strands of peptidoglycan in the cell wall are cross-linked by a transpeptidase reaction in which the glycine pentapeptide of one strand is attached to the penultimate D-alanine molecule of another strand. During this reaction, the terminal D-alanine is removed.

The cell wall maintains the shape of the bacterium and protects it from osmotic lysis if it is placed in a hypotonic medium. Without a cell wall, the bacterium is unprotected. This is why inhibition of cell wall synthesis by antimicrobial drugs is usually bactericidal. Because a cell wall is not found in higher organisms, antimicrobial drugs can inhibit its formation without harming host cells. The cell wall is synthesized during bacterial replication, and drugs that inhibit cell wall synthesis are more active against rapidly dividing bacteria than they are against bacteria in the resting or stationary phase. For the same reason, the effectiveness of cell wall inhibitors is usually reduced by concurrent administration of bacteriostatic antibiotics that slow the growth of bacteria.

SITES OF DRUG ACTION

β-Lactam Drugs

The β-lactam antibiotics bind to a group of bacterial enzymes, the **PBPs.** These enzymes are anchored in the cytoplasmic membrane and extend into the periplasmic space. The PBP are responsible for the assembly, maintenance, and regulation of the peptidoglycan portion of the bacterial cell wall. Some of the PBP have **transpeptidase** activity, whereas others have carboxypeptidase and transglycosylase activity.

The β-lactam antibiotics form a covalent bond with PBPs and thereby inhibit the catalytic activity of these enzymes. Inhibition of some PBPs prevents **elongation** or **cross-linking of peptidoglycan** (see Fig. 38–2), whereas inhibition of other PBPs leads to the bacterium's **autolysis** or to its change to a **spheroplast** or a **filamentous form.**

Each bacterial species has a set of unique PBPs to which particular β-lactam antibiotics bind with varying affinities.

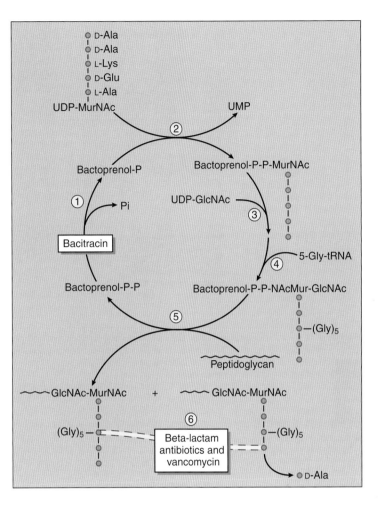

Figure 38–2. Sites of action of bacterial cell wall synthesis inhibitors. The bacterial cell wall consists primarily of peptidoglycan, a polymer constructed from repeating disaccharide units of N-acetylglucosamine (GlcNAc) and N-acetylmuramic acid (MurNAc). Numbers indicate the steps involved in the synthesis of the cell wall of *Staphylococcus aureus*. In step 1, bactoprenol pyrophosphate (bactoprenol-P-P) is dephosphorylated to regenerate the carrier molecule, bactoprenol phosphate (bactoprenol-P). In step 2, uridine diphosphate-MurNAc (UDP-MurNAc) is added. In steps 3 and 4, UDP-GlcNAc and a glycine pentapeptide (5-Gly-tRNA) are added. In step 5, the disaccharide peptide is transferred to the peptidoglycan growth point. In step 6, the cross-linking of peptidoglycan strands is catalyzed by transpeptidase, a type of penicillin-binding protein. In this reaction, a glycine of one strand forms a peptide bond with the penultimate D-alanine of an adjacent strand, and the terminal D-alanine is released. Bacitracin blocks step 1 and β-lactam antibiotics and vancomycin block step 6 by different mechanisms. Fosfomycin (not shown) inhibits enolpyruvyl transferase, the enzyme that catalyzes the condensation of UDP-GlcNAc with phosphoenolpyruvate to synthesize UDP-MurNAc.

This partly accounts for the variation in the sensitivity of different organisms to β-lactam antibiotics.

Other Drugs

Bacitracin and **fosfomycin** inhibit cell wall peptidoglycan synthesis by blocking specific steps in the formation of the disaccharide precursor, MurNAc-GlcNAc. As shown in Figure 38–2, bacitracin inhibits the dephosphorylation of bactoprenol pyrophosphate, which is the carrier lipid required for regeneration of bactoprenol phosphate, the active carrier of the disaccharide precursor. Fosfomycin inhibits enolpyruvyl transferase, the enzyme that catalyzes the condensation of uridine diphosphate–GlcNAc (UDP-GlcNAc) with phosphoenolpyruvate to synthesize UDP-MurNAc. **Vancomycin** binds tightly to the D-alanyl-D-alanine portion of the peptidoglycan precursor and prevents bonding of the penultimate D-alanine to the pentaglycine peptide during cross-linking of peptidoglycan strands.

β-LACTAM ANTIBIOTICS

The β-lactam antibiotics include penicillins, cephalosporins, carbapenems, and a monobactam antibiotic.

Penicillins

Penicillins were the first antibiotics to be isolated from microorganisms and used to treat bacterial infections. Alexander Fleming is credited with the discovery of penicillin, but he was unable to isolate the substance in sufficient purity and quantity for clinical use. Later, E. B. Chain and H. W. Florey, working in England, obtained enough penicillin to establish its clinical effectiveness. The production of sufficient quantities of penicillin for widespread use around the world was made possible by advances in microbial fermentation technology in the United States.

Penicillins can be grouped according to their antimicrobial activity. Narrow-spectrum penicillins include **penicillin G** and **penicillin V**. Penicillinase-resistant penicillins include **dicloxacillin** and **nafcillin**. Extended-spectrum penicillins include **amoxicillin**, **ampicillin**, **piperacillin**, and **ticarcillin**.

CHEMISTRY. The penicillins consist of a β-lactam ring fused to a thiazolidine ring, with an R group that is unique for each antibiotic (Fig. 38–3). The **natural penicillins** isolated from strains of *Penicillium* were originally assigned letter designations because their chemical structures could not be identified at that time. Penicillin G and penicillin V are the only natural penicillins still used today, and they are classified

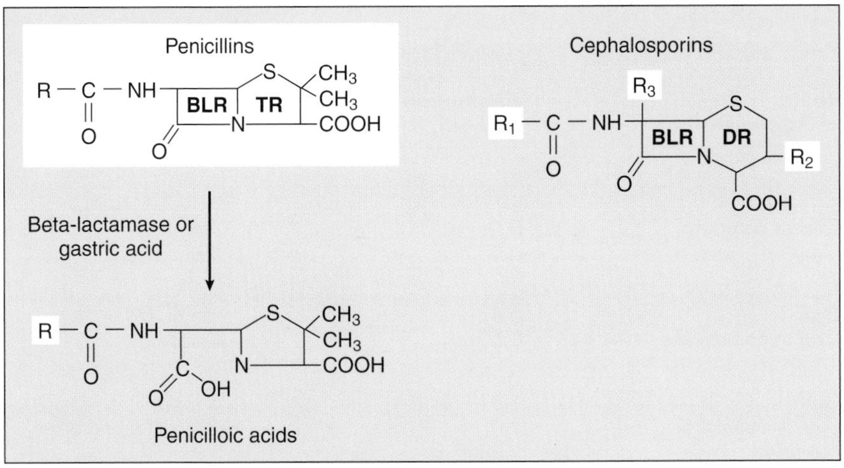

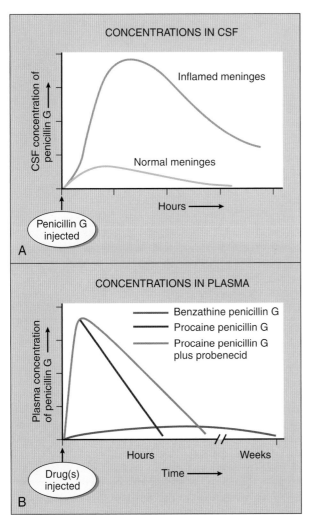

Figure 38-3. Structures of β-lactam drugs. Penicillins contain a β-lactam ring (BLR) and a thiazolidine ring (TR), whereas cephalosporins contain a BLR and a dihydrothiazine ring (DR). β-Lactamases hydrolyze the BLR and convert penicillins to penicilloic acids, which may react with body proteins to form antigens. β-Lactamases convert cephalosporins to inactive cephalosporanic acids (not shown).

Figure 38-4. Pharmacokinetics of penicillin G preparations. (A) When penicillin G is administered to patients with normal meninges, the concentration in cerebrospinal fluid (CSF) remains low, but when it is administered to patients with meningitis, the CSF concentration is much higher because meningeal inflammation increases meningeal permeability to penicillin G. **(B)** Administration of benzathine penicillin G produces low plasma concentrations of the drug for several weeks. Administration of procaine penicillin G produces higher plasma concentrations for about 24 hours. Probenecid inhibits the renal excretion of penicillin G, prolongs its half-life, and increases its plasma concentrations.

as narrow-spectrum drugs. **Semisynthetic penicillins** are produced by substituting a different R group for the R group of a natural penicillin. The penicillinase-resistant penicillins have a large, bulky R group that protects them from hydrolysis by staphylococcal β-lactamase.

PHARMACOKINETICS. The route of administration of penicillins depends on the stability of the drugs in gastric acid. **Acid-stable penicillins**, which include amoxicillin, dicloxacillin, and penicillin V, are effective when given orally. In contrast, **acid-labile penicillins**, which include piperacillin and ticarcillin, must be administered parenterally. Penicillin G has intermediate sensitivity to gastric acid and can be given orally in large doses, but penicillin V has better acid stability and oral bioavailability.

The penicillins are widely distributed to organs and tissues except the central nervous system. Because penicillins readily penetrate the cerebrospinal fluid when the meninges are inflamed (Fig. 38–4), they can be administered intravenously for the treatment of meningitis.

Most penicillin antibiotics are eliminated primarily by active renal tubular secretion and have short half-lives of about 0.5 to 1.3 hours (Table 38–1). A few penicillins (e.g., ampicillin and nafcillin) are excreted primarily in the bile. The renal tubular secretion of penicillins is inhibited by **probenecid**, a drug that competes with penicillins for the organic acid transporter located in the proximal tubule. Probenecid has been used to slow the excretion and prolong the half-life of penicillin G (see Fig. 38–4).

Penicillin G is available in two long-acting forms for intramuscular administration, **procaine penicillin G** and **benzathine penicillin G**. Penicillin G is slowly released from these two preparations for absorption into the circulation following an intramuscular injection. Benzathine penicillin G provides low plasma concentrations of the drug for several weeks, whereas procaine penicillin G produces higher plasma concentrations of penicillin for about 24 hours (see Fig. 38–4B).

SPECTRUM AND INDICATIONS. Table 38–2 outlines the spectrum and major clinical uses of penicillins.

The **narrow-spectrum penicillins**, penicillins G and V, are used to treat infections caused by sensitive strains

TABLE 38–1. **Pharmacokinetic Properties of Selected Bacterial Cell Wall Synthesis Inhibitors***

Drug	Route of Administration	Elimination Half-Life (Hours)	Primary Route of Elimination
β-Lactam Antibiotics			
Narrow-spectrum penicillins			
— Penicillin G	Oral or parenteral	0.5	Renal (TS)
— Penicillin V	Oral	1.0	Renal (TS)
Penicillinase-resistant penicillins			
— Dicloxacillin	Oral	0.6	Renal (TS)
— Nafcillin	Oral or parenteral	0.5	Biliary
Extended-spectrum penicillins			
— Amoxicillin	Oral	1.0	Renal (TS)
— Ampicillin	Oral or parenteral	1.0	Renal (TS) and biliary
— Piperacillin and ticarcillin	Parenteral	1.2 to 1.3	Renal (TS)
First-Generation Cephalosporins			
— Cefazolin	Parenteral	2.0	Renal (TS)
— Cephalexin	Oral	0.5	Renal (TS)
Second-Generation Cephalosporins			
— Cefotetan	Parenteral	4.0	Renal (TS)
— Cefoxitin	Parenteral	0.8	Renal (TS)
— Cefprozil	Oral	1.3	Renal (TS)
— Cefuroxime	Oral or parenteral	1.7	Renal (TS)
Third- and Fourth-Generation Cephalosporins			
— Cefdinir	Oral	1.7	Renal (TS)
— Cefotaxime	Parenteral	1.6[†]	Renal (TS)
— Ceftazidime	Parenteral	1.8	Renal (GF)
— Ceftriaxone	Parenteral	8.0	Biliary
— Cefepime	Parenteral	2.0	Metabolized
Monobactam			
— Aztreonam	Parenteral	1.7	Metabolized
Carbapenems	Parenteral	1.0 to 1.2	Renal (TS)
Other Bacterial Cell Wall Synthesis Inhibitors			
— Bacitracin	Topical	NA	NA
— Fosfomycin	Oral	6.0	Renal (GF)
— Vancomycin	Oral or parenteral	6.0	Renal (GF)

*Values shown are the mean of values reported in the literature.
†For cefotaxime, the value shown is the half-life of the metabolite.
GF = glomerular filtration; NA = not applicable; TS = tubular secretion.

of streptococci (including pneumococci), meningococci, and spirochetes (e.g., *Treponema pallidum*). For example, penicillin G is used to treat group A **streptococcal infections** and to treat **syphilis**. Penicillin G is also active against *Clostridium perfringens*, the cause of **gas gangrene**, and other pathogens. Most staphylococci and gonococci and some strains of pneumococci are now resistant to penicillin G.

The **penicillinase-resistant penicillins** (e.g., dicloxacillin and nafcillin) were developed to treat penicillin-resistant strains of **staphylococci** that elaborate penicillinase (β-lactamase). These penicillins are not active against most other species of penicillinase-producing bacteria. Nafcillin is usually preferred when parenteral administration is required, whereas dicloxacillin can be given orally for less severe infections.

The penicillinase-resistant drugs are used to treat serious staphylococcal infections, such as acute endocarditis and osteomyelitis, as well as skin and soft tissue infections. Staphylococci that are resistant to these penicillins are often designated **methicillin-resistant *Staphylococcus aureus*(MRSA)** because methicillin was the original drug in this class. Methicillin is seldom used today, however, because of its greater toxicity and tendency to cause interstitial nephritis. Bacteria that are resistant to methicillin are also cross-resistant to nafcillin and all other penicillinase-resistant penicillins. Most strains of methicillin-resistant *Staphylococcus aureus* are also resistant to cephalosporins.

The **extended-spectrum penicillins** can be subdivided into the **aminopenicillins** (amoxicillin and ampicillin) and the **antipseudomonal penicillins** (piperacillin, ticarcillin, and others).

The aminopenicillins are active against many streptococci, some strains of enterococci, and a limited number of gram-negative bacilli. Amoxicillin and ampicillin are often combined with a β-lactamase inhibitor (described below), and drug products containing amoxicillin and **clavulanate** (AUGMENTIN) or ampicillin and **sulbactam** (UNASYN) are

TABLE 38-2. Major Clinical Uses of Selected Bacterial Cell Wall Synthesis Inhibitors

Drug	Infections	Major Pathogens
Penicillins		
Penicillin G	Syphilis	*Treponema pallidum*
	Endocarditis	Viridans streptococci, enterococci
	Meningitis	Meningococci
	Pneumonia	Pneumococci
	Various	Streptococci
Penicillin V	Pharyngitis	*Streptococcus pyogenes*
Nafcillin, oxacillin	Osteomyelitis, endocarditis, pneumonia, skin/soft tissue	*Staphylococcus aureus*
Amoxicillin ± clavulanate	Otitis, upper respiratory tract, pneumonia, skin/soft tissue, urinary tract	Pneumococci, streptococci, staphylococci, *Haemophilus influenzae, Moraxella catarrhalis, E. coli, Pasteurella multocida*
Ampicillin ± sulbactam	Meningitis	*Listeria monocytogenes*
	Decubitus and diabetic foot ulcers	Gram-positive and anaerobic organisms
	Endocarditis	Streptococci, enterococci
	Lyme disease	*Borrelia burgdorferi*
Piperacillin ± tazobactam	Intra-abdominal, skin/soft tissue, pneumonia, and other	Aerobic and anaerobic organisms, including *Pseudomonas aeruginosa*
Cephalosporins		
Cephalexin	Skin and soft tissue infections	Streptococci, staphylococci
Cefazolin	Perioperative prophylaxis	Staphylococci, *E. coli*
Cefotetan	Intra-abdominal, gynecologic, biliary tract	Aerobic and anaerobic bacilli
Cefdinir, cefprozil, cefuroxime axetil	Respiratory tract, skin/soft tissue	Pneumococci, *Haemophilus influenzae, Moraxella catarrhalis*
Ceftriaxone	Gonorrhea,* urinary tract, otitis, meningitis, pneumonia, Lyme disease	Gonococci, pneumococci, meningococci, *Borrelia burgdorferi, H. influenzae,* other gram-negative bacilli
Ceftazidime	Urinary tract, pneumonia, others	*Pseudomonas aeruginosa*
Cefepime	Intra-abdominal, urinary tract, pneumonia, skin/soft tissue	Drug-resistant gram-negative bacilli, including *Citrobacter* and *Enterobacter* species
Carbapenems	Intra-abdominal, meningitis, febrile neutropenia	Aerobic, anaerobic, and drug-resistant gram-negative bacilli
Monobactam (aztreonam)	Urinary tract, gynecologic, intra-abdominal, skin, lungs, and others	Aerobic, gram-negative bacilli
Vancomycin	Bone and joint, skin and soft tissue, pneumonia, septicemia, endocarditis, and others	Methicillin-resistant staphylococci, enterococci, and others
Bacitracin	Skin and eye	Staphylococci, streptococci
Fosfomycin	Lower urinary tract	*E. coli, Enterococcus faecalis,* others

*Also cefpodoxime as a single oral dose.

widely used to treat infections caused by β-lactamase–producing bacteria.

Amoxicillin can be used alone to treat respiratory tract infections caused by sensitive bacteria, including **otitis media**, **sinusitis**, **bronchitis**, and community-acquired **pneumonia**. Many strains of *Haemophilus influenzae* and *Moraxella catarrhalis*, however, produce penicillinase, and infections caused by these organisms should be treated with amoxicillin-clavulanate. In addition, many strains of *Streptococcus pneumoniae* (pneumococci) have become increasingly resistant to amoxicillin, necessitating the use of larger doses to treat upper respiratory infections caused by this organism. For this reason, two formulations of amoxicillin-clavulanate have been developed to provide higher plasma levels of these drugs for longer periods of time. A sustained release tablet containing 1000 and 62.5 mg of amoxicillin and clavulanate, respectively, is given twice daily for treatment of **adult respiratory tract infections** caused by drug-resistant pneumococci, *H. influenzae*, or *M. catarrhalis*. A liquid suspension providing 90 and 6.4 mg/kg/day of amoxicillin-clavulanate is available to treat children with **otitis media** (Box 38–1) due to resistant strains of pneumococci, *H. influenzae*, or *M. catarrhalis*. For

infections not caused by resistant organisms, the usual dose of amoxicillin is 30 to 45 mg/kg/day in two divided doses.

Amoxicillin-clavulanate is also indicated for treating **bite wound infections** because it is active against the common pathogens causing bite wounds, including *Pasteurella multocida* and *Staphylococcus aureus*. Amoxicillin alone is used for prophylaxis of bacterial endocarditis in persons with heart valve defects.

Ampicillin is active against *Listeria monocytogenes* and is used to treat meningitis and other infections caused by this organism. It is also used in combination with **sulbactam** (a β-lactamase inhibitor) to treat infections caused by penicillinase-producing strains of bacteria, including bite wounds and diabetic foot ulcers. Ampicillin can be combined with an **aminoglycoside** (e.g., gentamicin) for the treatment of serious enterococcal infections, such as enterococcal endocarditis. Other uses for ampicillin and amoxicillin are listed in Table 38–2.

The **antipseudomonal penicillins** (e.g., **piperacillin**) are active against a broad spectrum of gram-positive and gram-negative aerobic and anaerobic bacteria, including some strains of *Pseudomonas aeruginosa*. Piperacillin combined with a β-lactamase inhibitor, tazobactam, is effective for the

BOX 38-1. A CASE OF COUGH, NASAL CONGESTION, AND IRRITABILITY

CASE PRESENTATION: A previously healthy 18-month-old infant is brought to her pediatrician with cough, nasal congestion, and irritability. Examination reveals a temperature of 39° C and redness and bulging of the tympanic membrane under pneumatic otoscopy, suggesting acute otitis media. Because of the possibility of an infection caused by pneumococci with intermediate penicillin resistance, she is placed on amoxicillin at a dose of 90 mg/kg/day in three divided doses for 10 days. Her mother is instructed to contact the pediatrician if the infant does not respond to treatment.

CASE DISCUSSION: Otitis media is a common infection of infants and children. Distinguishing acute otitis media (AOM) from otitis media with effusion is important because antibiotics are seldom indicated for the latter condition. An important diagnostic criterion is the position of the tympanic membrane, which is usually bulging in AOM and in a neutral or retracted position in otitis media with effusion.

Antibiotic treatment of AOM is mandatory in children less than 2 years of age to decrease inflammation in the middle ear and eustachian tube, particularly during the first episode. Amoxicillin is a good choice because of its superior penetration in the middle ear. *Streptococcus pneumoniae* with intermediate penicillin resistance necessitates an amoxicillin dosage of 90 mg/kg per day. In recurrent AOM with β-lactamase–producing *Haemophilus influenzae* or *Moraxella catarrhalis*, amoxicillin should be combined with clavulanic acid, or an oral cephalosporin or azithromycin may be used. In children over 2 years of age with AOM, antibiotic administration may be postponed a few days to counteract overuse of antibiotics and increased bacterial resistance. In such cases, children are given topical otic and systemic analgesics for a few days until either the infection resolves or antibiotic treatment is instituted.

treatment of patients with intra-abdominal, skin and soft tissue, lower respiratory tract, complicated urinary tract, and gynecologic infections as well as febrile neutropenia. In some cases, piperacillin and ticarcillin are given in combination with an aminoglycoside antibiotic.

BACTERIAL RESISTANCE. As shown in Table 38–3 there are three primary mechanisms by which bacteria exert resistance to penicillins and other β-lactam antibiotics: inactivation of the drugs by **β-lactamase** enzymes, reduced affinity of PBPs for the antibiotics, and decreased entry of the drugs into bacteria through outer membrane **porins.** In some bacteria, resistance can be caused by a combination of these effects.

The production of β-lactamases is the predominant cause of bacterial resistance to penicillins and other β-lactam antibiotics. These enzymes cleave the amide bond in the β-lactam ring and thereby inactivate the antibiotic (see Fig. 38–3). β-Lactamases are expressed by both chromosomal and plasmid genes. Some β-lactamases are constitutive, whereas others can be induced by β-lactam antibiotics. In gram-positive bacteria, β-lactamases are secreted as exoenzymes and act extracellularly. β-Lactamases remain in the periplasmic space in gram-negative bacteria where they attack the antibiotic before it can bind to PBP.

The β-lactamases are classified in two ways. The **functional** or **biochemical classification** of Bush-Jacoby-Medeiros contains four groups of β-lactamases (groups 1 to 4). The **molecular classification** based on amino acid sequences includes classes A through D, with A and C found most frequently in bacteria. Functional **group 1 β-lactamases** are enzymes that hydrolyze cephalosporins (cephalosporinases) and correspond to molecular **class C.** Group 2 β-lactamase enzymes correspond to molecular **classes A and D** and includes penicillinases, cephalosporinases, and carbapenemases. These enzymes are derived from the original β-lactamase genes called *TEM* and *SHV.* **Class A enzymes** are the only β-lactamases that are inhibited by **clavulanic acid, sulbactam,** or **tazobactam.**

Group 3 β-lactamases are metallo (zinc) enzymes that correspond to molecular **class B.** Group 3 enzymes hydrolyze most penicillins, cephalosporins, and carbapenems (but not monobactams) and are not inhibited by clavulanate. **Group 4 β-lactamases** are penicillinases that are not inhibited by clavulanate. These β-lactamases do not yet have a molecular classification.

The staphylococci were the first major group of bacterial pathogens to acquire β-lactamases that rendered them resistant to penicillin G. Later, many gonococci and other gram-negative bacteria acquired β-lactamases. Resistance of *H. influenzae* to amoxicillin and other penicillins is primarily caused by these enzymes. Many strains of Enterobacteriaceae, including *E. coli* and *Klebsiella pneumoniae,* have acquired plasmid-mediated *TEM* and *SHV* β-lactamases. In recent years, **extended-spectrum β-lactamases** have emerged and spread globally. Extended-spectrum β-lactamases are derivatives of common *TEM* and *SHV* genes, whose amino acid substitutions enable them to hydrolyze a wider range of substrates, including the third-generation cephalosporins.

Resistance caused by decreased affinity of PBPs for β-lactam drugs is also a growing problem. Gram-positive bacteria are innately resistant to aztreonam because their PBPs do not bind to this drug. Resistance of other bacteria to penicillins can be acquired when the structure of PBPs is altered in a manner that reduces the affinity of PBPs for the drugs. This mechanism has been responsible for the emergence of pneumococci that are resistant to penicillin G and of staphylococci that are resistant to methicillin.

TABLE 38–3. Bacterial Resistance to β-Lactam Antibiotics

Mechanism	Examples
Inactivation of the drug by β-lactamase enzymes	Resistance of gonococci and staphylococci to penicillin G
	Resistance of gram-negative bacteria to carbapenems, extended-spectrum penicillins, cefoxitin, and other cephalosporins
	Resistance of *Haemophilus influenzae* to amoxicillin and other penicillins
Reduced affinity of PBPs for the drug	Resistance of enterococci to cephalosporins
	Resistance of gram-positive bacteria to aztreonam
	Resistance of meningococci, pneumococci, and streptococci to penicillin G
	Resistance of staphylococci to methicillin
Decreased entry of the drug into bacteria through outer membrane porins	Resistance of gram-negative bacteria to various β-lactam antibiotics
	Resistance of *Pseudomonas aeruginosa* to imipenem

PBP = penicillin-binding protein.

Many gram-negative bacteria are innately resistant to penicillins because porins in their outer membrane are impermeable to these drugs. This is also an important mechanism of acquired resistance to penicillins, as in the case of *P. aeruginosa* resistance to imipenem.

ADVERSE EFFECTS. Penicillins are a common cause of **drug-induced hypersensitivity reactions**. However, it has been determined that true penicillin allergy occurs in only 7% to 23% of patients who give a history of penicillin allergy. Hypersensitivity reactions occur when penicillin is degraded to penicilloic acid and other compounds that combine with body proteins to form antigens that elicit antibody formation.

An immediate hypersensitivity reaction, which is a type of reaction mediated by immunoglobulin E, can lead to urticaria (hives) or anaphylactic shock. Other types of hypersensitivity reactions can lead to serum sickness, interstitial nephritis, hepatitis, and various skin rashes. Hepatitis is more common with antistaphylococcal and extended-spectrum penicillins and is usually reversible when use of the drug is discontinued. Ampicillin is particularly likely to cause a maculopapular skin rash in patients with certain viral infections, such as mononucleosis. This reaction is mediated by sensitized lymphocytes, and its incidence in ampicillin-treated patients with mononucleosis is over 90%.

Penicillin allergy can be confirmed by the use of commercial preparations of penicillin antigens. These preparations contain the major or minor antigenic determinants of penicillin that are formed in the body during penicillin degradation. These preparations are injected intradermally and cause erythema at the injection site in allergic persons. The preparations should be administered by personnel who are prepared to provide treatment for anaphylactic shock in the event that the patient develops a severe hypersensitivity reaction following the injection.

Except for hypersensitivity reactions, the penicillins are remarkably nontoxic to the human body and produce very few other adverse effects. High concentrations of penicillins can be irritating to the central nervous system and elicit seizures in patients who have received very large doses of these drugs. As with other antibiotics, penicillins can disturb the normal flora of the gut and produce diarrhea and superinfections with penicillin-resistant organisms, such as staphylococci and *Clostridium difficile*. Pseudomembranous colitis can occur in association with *C. difficile* superinfections.

β-Lactamase Inhibitors

Clavulanate, **sulbactam**, and **tazobactam** are β-lactam drugs that inhibit molecular class A β-lactamases. These drugs have no antimicrobial activity by themselves but serve as surrogate substrates for β-lactamases when given with a penicillin antibiotic. The current β-lactamase inhibitors do not inhibit class B, C, and D β-lactamases, but broad-spectrum β-lactamase inhibitors are now being developed.

The currently available penicillin–β-lactamase inhibitor combinations include **amoxicillin plus clavulanate** (AUGMENTIN), which is given orally, and three preparations that are administered parenterally: **ampicillin plus sulbactam** (UNASYN), **piperacillin plus tazobactam** (ZOSYN), and **ticarcillin plus clavulanate** (TIMENTIN). The major uses of these combinations are listed in Table 38–2.

Cephalosporins

The cephalosporins are one of the largest and most widely used groups of antibiotics. Based on differences in their antimicrobial spectrum, they have been divided into four generations. Table 38–2 lists examples of each. The first-generation cephalosporins are primarily active against gram-positive cocci and a limited number of gram-negative bacilli. Subsequent generations of cephalosporins have increased activity against gram-negative bacilli and less activity against some species of gram-positive cocci.

CHEMISTRY. The cephalosporins are semisynthetic drugs, most of which are derived from cephalosporin C, a substance obtained from a species of *Cephalosporium* discovered near a sewage outlet off the coast of Sardinia. Cephalosporins have a β-lactam ring and a dihydrothiazine ring (see Fig. 38–3). Unlike the penicillins, the cephalosporins have at least two R groups attached to the molecule, thereby enabling the synthesis of a greater number of derivatives with potentially useful properties. In **cephamycins**, a subcategory of cephalosporins that includes **cefotetan** and **cefoxitin**, there is a third R group that is attached to the β-lactam ring. By manipulating the structure of cephalosporins, it has been possible to obtain drugs with greater resistance to bacterial β-lactamases and with a wider range of antimicrobial activity.

PHARMACOKINETICS. Compared to penicillins, the cephalosporins are more stable in the body and are less likely to form antigens that evoke hypersensitivity reactions.

The route of administration depends on the particular cephalosporin being used. Some of the cephalosporins are given only orally; others are given only parenterally. **Cefuroxime** is one of the few cephalosporins available for use by both routes (as cefuroxime axetil for oral administration and cefuroxime sodium for parenteral administration). Some of the parenterally administered cephalosporins are used only intravenously; others are given either intravenously or intramuscularly.

The orally administered cephalosporins are well absorbed from the gut, and their bioavailability usually is not significantly affected by food. Most cephalosporins are excreted primarily by renal tubular secretion. Ceftriaxone is excreted primarily in the bile and has a much longer half-life than other cephalosporins.

SPECTRUM AND INDICATIONS. Tables 38–1 and 38–2 outline the spectrums and major clinical uses, respectively, of cephalosporins.

The **first-generation cephalosporins** have good activity against most streptococci and methicillin-sensitive staphylococci. They are also active against a few gram-negative enteric bacilli, including *E. coli* and *Klebsiella pneumoniae*. The orally administered drugs (e.g., **cephalexin**) are primarily used to treat skin and soft tissue infections caused by gram-positive cocci and to treat uncomplicated urinary tract infections caused by susceptible organisms. However, many strains of *E. coli* are now resistant to cephalexin. Parenterally administered **cefazolin** is used to treat more serious infections caused by these organisms and is widely employed for prophylaxis of surgical infections caused by staphylococci and aerobic gram-negative enteric bacilli.

In comparison with first-generation cephalosporins, the **second-generation cephalosporins** have similar activity against gram-positive cocci while demonstrating increased activity against gram-negative bacilli. For example, the second-generation drugs are active against many strains of *Hemophilus influenzae* and have been used to treat respiratory tract and other infections caused by this organism. Oral second-generation drugs, including **cefprozil** and **cefuroxime axetil**, are used to treat otitis media, particularly when it is caused by *H. influenzae* strains that are resistant to amoxicillin and other drugs. **Cefuroxime sodium**, a parenteral preparation, has been used as empiric therapy for patients with community-acquired pneumonia. **Cefotetan** is active against both aerobic and anaerobic gram-negative bacilli, including *Bacteroides fragilis*, and it is used to treat intra-abdominal, gynecologic, and biliary tract infections caused by these organisms. **Cefoxitin** has activity similar to that of cefotetan and is used for surgical prophylaxis of infections caused by gram-negative bacteria.

In comparison with second-generation cephalosporins, the **third-generation cephalosporins** have greater activity against a wider range of gram-negative organisms, including enteric gram-negative bacilli (Enterobacteriaceae), *H. influenzae*, and *M. catarrhalis*. In addition, **ceftazidime** is active against some strains of *P. aeruginosa*. Several third-generation drugs, including **cefpodoxime, cefotaxime,** and

ceftriaxone, are active against gonococci and have been used as a single-dose treatment for gonorrhea. Other clinical indications for third-generation drugs include otitis media, pneumonia, meningitis, intra-abdominal or urinary tract infections, and advanced Lyme disease.

Cefepime has been called a **fourth-generation cephalosporin** because it is active against many gram-negative bacilli, including *Citrobacter freundii* and *Enterobacter cloacae*, that are resistant to other cephalosporins. This is attributed to its more rapid penetration of bacteria, its ability to target multiple PBPs, and its lower affinity for several β-lactamases. Cefepime is resistant to plasmid-encoded β-lactamase and relatively resistant to inducible chromosomally encoded β-lactamase. It has been used in treating a variety of systemic infections, including intra-abdominal and urinary tract infections and pneumonia. However, a recent analysis of clinical trials found that cefepime is associated with **higher all-cause mortality** than are other β-lactam antibiotics, possibly due to drug-induced encephalopathy; thus its use should be carefully monitored.

Ceftobiprole is an investigational cephalosporin that has good activity against methicillin-resistant staphylococci and penicillin-resistant streptococci. It has completed Phase III clinical trials involving patients with skin and soft tissue infections or pneumonia. Ceftobiprole is approved for marketing in Canada and under review in the U.S.

BACTERIAL RESISTANCE. Bacteria acquire resistance to cephalosporins through the same three mechanisms by which they acquire resistance to penicillins (see Table 38–3). The cephalosporins are more resistant to β-lactamases than are the penicillins, and resistance to gram-negative β-lactamases increases with successive generations of cephalosporins. Many cephalosporins, however, are susceptible to the extended-spectrum β-lactamases. Some cephalosporins induce certain β-lactamase enzymes.

ADVERSE EFFECTS. The cephalosporins cause little toxicity to the host and have an excellent safety record. Although cephalosporins can elicit hypersensitivity reactions, the incidence of this is lower for cephalosporins than for penicillins. Cephalosporins exhibit some **cross-sensitivity** with penicillins, and about 5% of persons allergic to penicillin will also be allergic to cephalosporins. Persons who have had a mild hypersensitivity reaction to penicillin usually do not cross-react to a cephalosporin. However, a person who has had a severe hypersensitivity reaction to penicillin (e.g., an anaphylactic reaction) has a greater risk of cross-reacting and should usually not be given a cephalosporin.

A few cephalosporins can cause **platelet dysfunction and bleeding**, including cefotetan, cefmetazole, cefamandole, and cefoperazone. These cephalosporins can potentiate the effects of anticoagulants and antiplatelet drugs and thereby increase the risk of bleeding. These same cephalosporins can also produce a **disulfiram-like reaction** if they are taken with alcohol.

Monobactam

Aztreonam is a monocyclic β-lactam (monobactam) antibiotic. It is active against many aerobic gram-negative bacilli, including strains of *Enterobacter, Citrobacter, Klebsiella,* and

Proteus species as well as *P. aeruginosa.* Aztreonam is used to treat serious infections caused by susceptible organisms and is particularly useful for infections caused by multidrug-resistant strains of these organisms. The drug is administered intravenously and is extensively metabolized before undergoing renal excretion. Aztreonam can cause hypersensitivity reactions and thrombophlebitis. It only rarely shows cross-sensitivity with penicillins and cephalosporins, however, and can usually be used in persons allergic to other β-lactam antibiotics.

Carbapenems

Carbapenems are penicillin-like antibiotics in which the sulfur atom of the thiazolidine ring is replaced with a carbon atom. These agents are bactericidal to a wide range of gram-positive and gram-negative bacteria, including many aerobic and anaerobic gram-negative bacilli. **Imipenem** has high affinity for PBP-2, whereas **meropenem** binds to both PBP-2 and PBP-3. The greater affinity of meropenem for PBP-3 may account for its superior activity against *P. aeruginosa* and other gram-negative organisms. **Ertapenem** is a newer agent with good in vitro activity against extended-spectrum β-lactamase–producing organisms. **Doripenem** is a new ultra–broad-spectrum antibiotic that is particularly active against *Pseudomonas aeruginosa.*

Carbapenems are used to treat a wide range of systemic infections, including endocarditis, pneumonia, urinary tract, pelvic, skin and soft tissue, and intra-abdominal infections. They are particularly useful for infections caused by multidrug-resistant organisms and for mixed infections caused by aerobic and anaerobic enteric bacilli.

Carbapenems are administered intravenously. Imipenem is rapidly inactivated by renal dehydropeptidase and is available in a formulation containing a dehydropeptidase inhibitor called **cilastatin.** Other carbapenems are not susceptible to dehydropeptidase. The carbapenems are eliminated by renal tubular secretion that can be inhibited by probenecid. Dosage adjustments are required when these drugs are given to persons with renal impairment.

The carbapenems exhibit cross-sensitivity with penicillins and other β-lactam antibiotics and should not be administered to patients who are allergic to these drugs. Though generally well tolerated, they can cause seizures in patients with epilepsy. Less commonly, carbapenems may cause anemia, leukopenia, thrombocytopenia, and altered bleeding time.

OTHER BACTERIAL CELL WALL SYNTHESIS INHIBITORS

Vancomycin

Vancomycin is a glycopeptide antibiotic that is active against many **gram-positive cocci** and gram-positive **bacilli.** Vancomycin is active against some strains of **methicillin-resistant Staphylococcus aureus**, and it usually is the first choice for treating skin and soft tissue infections and other infections caused by these organisms. Vancomycin is also used to treat streptococcal and enterococcal infections caused by penicillin-resistant organisms, including endocarditis and necrotizing fasciitis. However, some strains

of staphylococci and enterococci have acquired resistance to vancomycin through mutations that alter the amino acid sequence of the cell wall pentapeptide containing D-alanine. Other glycoprotein antibiotics, such as **dalbavancin**, are currently undergoing clinical trials for treating methicillin-resistant *Staphylococcus aureus* infections (see Table 39–4).

Vancomycin is also active against *Bacillus, Clostridium,* and *Corynebacterium* species. Although it has been used to treat diarrhea and **pseudomembranous colitis** caused by *Clostridium difficile,* metronidazole is usually preferred for this infection.

Vancomycin is poorly absorbed from the gut and must be administered parenterally to treat systemic infections, though it is given orally to treat gastrointestinal *C. difficile* infections. Vancomycin is distributed to most body fluids and tissues, and it is excreted in the urine by the process of glomerular filtration. The half-life of vancomycin is normally about 6 hours (see Table 38–1), but the half-life is markedly prolonged in patients with renal failure.

Improvements in the manufacturing of vancomycin preparations have reduced the incidence of **nephrotoxicity** and **ototoxicity** associated with their use. Vancomycin, however, should be used cautiously with other nephrotoxic drugs, including aminoglycosides and amphotericin B. The ototoxic effects of vancomycin can include both **vestibular dysfunction** (ataxia, vertigo, nystagmus, and nausea) and **cochlear dysfunction** (tinnitus and hearing loss). Ototoxicity is usually caused by excessive serum concentrations and is reversible when these concentrations are reduced.

If vancomycin is infused at an excessive rate, it can cause hypotension and an **erythematous rash** on the face and upper body known as the **red neck** or **red man syndrome.**

Bacitracin

Bacitracin is an antibiotic derived from a *Bacillus subtilis* strain isolated from a girl named Tracy. The drug inhibits cell wall peptidoglycan synthesis by blocking the regeneration of bactoprenol phosphate, the lipid carrier molecule (see Fig. 38–2). Bacitracin is active against gram-positive cocci, including staphylococci and streptococci, and it is primarily used for the topical treatment of minor skin and ocular infections. It is often combined with polymyxin or neomycin in ointments and creams. Bacitracin is very nephrotoxic and is not used systemically.

Fosfomycin

Fosfomycin is a unique antibiotic that blocks one of the first steps in cell wall peptidoglycan synthesis, the formation of UDP-MurNAc. Fosfomycin is structurally similar to phosphoenolpyruvate. By irreversibly inhibiting the enzyme enolpyruvyl transferase, fosfomycin blocks the addition of phosphoenolpyruvate to UDP-GlcNAc and thereby prevents the synthesis of UDP-MurNAc.

Fosfomycin is active against enterococci and many gram-negative enteric bacilli, including *E. coli, Citrobacter* species, *Klebsiella* species, *Proteus* species, and *Serratia marcescens.* The drug is specifically approved for the treatment of

uncomplicated urinary tract infections caused by *E. coli* or *Enterococcus faecalis*. For this purpose, fosfomycin is administered orally as a single dose. The drug is excreted unchanged in the urine and feces and has a half-life of about 6 hours. Fosfomycin sometimes causes diarrhea but is otherwise well tolerated and is associated with few adverse effects.

SUMMARY OF IMPORTANT POINTS

■ β-lactam antibiotics, vancomycin, bacitracin, and fosfomycin are drugs that inhibit bacterial cell wall synthesis.

■ The β-lactam antibiotics inhibit the transpeptidase reaction that cross-links the peptidoglycan component of the cell wall. These antibiotics include penicillins, cephalosporins, aztreonam, and carbapenems.

■ A β-lactamase inhibitor (e.g., clavulanate, sulbactam, or tazobactam) is administered in combination with a β-lactam antibiotic to prevent degradation of the antibiotic by bacteria.

■ Narrow-spectrum penicillins (e.g., penicillin G) are primarily active against gram-positive cocci and spirochetes; penicillinase-resistant penicillins (e.g., dicloxacillin and nafcillin) are used to treat staphylococcal infections; and extended-spectrum penicillins (e.g., amoxicillin and ticarcillin) are active against various gram-negative bacilli.

■ Acid-stable penicillins (e.g., penicillin V, amoxicillin, and dicloxacillin) can be given orally, whereas acid-labile drugs (e.g., piperacillin and ticarcillin) must be given parenterally.

■ Most penicillins are eliminated primarily by renal tubular secretion, a process that is inhibited by probenecid. Two long-acting forms of penicillin G (procaine and benzathine penicillin G) are available for intramuscular administration.

■ Penicillins can elicit any of the four types of hypersensitivity reactions, including anaphylactic shock and other immediate hypersensitivity reactions mediated by immunoglobulin E.

■ Cephalosporins are semisynthetic antibiotics that are subdivided into four generations on the basis of their antimicrobial spectrum. The activity against gram-negative organisms increases from the first to the fourth generation.

■ Some cephalosporins (e.g., cefazolin) are eliminated by renal tubular secretion, whereas others (e.g., ceftriaxone) are eliminated in the bile. Ceftriaxone has a much longer half-life than other cephalosporins, enabling it to be used as single-dose treatment for certain infections, including gonorrhea.

■ Carbapenems (e.g., imipenem and meropenem) are active against a broad spectrum of bacteria including many strains resistant to other antibiotics. Aztreonam is a monobactam antibiotic that is active against aerobic gram-negative bacilli. It does not show cross-sensitivity with other β-lactam drugs.

■ Vancomycin is a glycopeptide antibiotic that is active against gram-positive organisms, including methicillin-resistant staphylococci, enterococci, and *Clostridium difficile*.

■ Bacitracin is used topically for infections caused by gram-positive cocci. Fosfomycin is administered as a single-dose treatment for uncomplicated urinary tract infections caused by *E. coli* or enterococci.

Review Questions

1. A woman with documented penicillin allergy is treated with a β-lactam antibiotic that rarely cross-reacts with penicillins. Her infection is most likely due to which organism?
   (A) *Staphylococcus aureus*
   (B) *Enterococcus faecium*
   (C) *Streptococcus pneumoniae*
   (D) *Pseudomonas aeruginosa*
   (E) *Bacillus anthracis*

2. A man is treated with a drug that is more resistant to extended-spectrum β-lactamases than are other β-lactam antibiotics. This drug should be avoided or used cautiously in persons with which condition?
   (A) myasthenia gravis
   (B) epilepsy
   (C) prolonged QT syndrome
   (D) deep vein thrombosis
   (E) diabetes mellitus

3. A boy is successfully treated for acute osteomyelitis due to methicillin-resistant staphylococci. Higher doses of the antibiotic that was most likely used in this patient may cause which adverse effect?
   (A) hepatitis
   (B) alopecia
   (C) hallucinations
   (D) hypertension
   (E) impaired hearing

4. A woman developed bleeding that required a reduction in her warfarin dose while being treated for a gallbladder infection. Which antibiotic was most likely responsible for this drug interaction?
   (A) aztreonam
   (B) ertapenem
   (C) cefotetan
   (D) cefotaxime
   (E) piperacillin-tazobactam

Answers and Explanations

1. **The answer is D:** *Pseudomonas aeruginosa.* The woman was most likely treated with aztreonam, a monobactam drug that rarely cross-reacts with penicillins. Cephalosporins and carbapenems cross-react with penicillins more frequently than does aztreonam. Aztreonam is active against gram-negative pathogens but not gram-positive organisms. Hence, her infection was most likely due to *P. aeruginosa.*

2. **The answer is B:** epilepsy. Carbepenems such as ertapenem and doripenem are more resistant to extended-spectrum β-lactamases than are other β-lactam drugs. Carbapenems may irritate brain tissue and lead to seizures, especially in persons with epilepsy. They are not associated with increased toxicity in persons with myasthenia gravis, prolonged QT syndrome, deep vein thrombosis, or diabetes mellitus.

3. **The answer is E:** impaired hearing. The boy was most likely treated with vancomycin, which is active against many strains of methicillin-resistant *Staphylococcus aureus.* Higher doses of this antibiotic may cause ototoxicity in the form of auditory or vestibular impairment. Higher doses of vancomycin do not typically cause hepatitis, alopecia, hallucinations, or hypertension.

4. **The answer is C:** cefotetan. Some cephalosporins, including cefotetan, may cause platelet dysfunction and bleeding and can potentiate the effects of antiplatelet drugs and anticoagulants. Cefotetan is active against aerobic and anaerobic organisms and is used to treat intra-abdominal and biliary tract infections.

SELECTED READINGS

Block, S.L., G.V. Doem, and M.A. Pfaller. Oral beta-lactams in the treatment of acute otitis media. Diagn Microbiol Infect Dis 57:338–348, 2007.

Gin, A., L. Dilay, J.A. Karlowsky, A. Walkty, E. Rubenstein, et al. Piperacillin-tazobactam: a beta-lactam/beta-lactamase inhibitor combination. Exper Rev Anti Infect Ther 5:365–383, 2007.

Lister, P.D. Carbapenems in the USA: focus on doripenem. Expert Rev Anti Infect Ther 5:793–809, 2007.

Loffler, C.A., and C. Macdougall. Update on the prevalence and treatment of methicillin-resistant *Staphylococcus aureus* infections. Expert Rev Anti Infect Ther 5:961–981, 2007.

Sader, H.S., and R.N. Jones. Cefdinir: an oral cephalosporin for the treatment of respiratory tract infections and skin and skin structure infections. Expert Rev Anti Infect Ther 5:29–43, 2007.

Yahav, D., M. Paul, A. Fraser, N. Sarid, and L. Leibovici. Efficacy and safety of cefepime: a systematic review and meta-analysis. Lancet Infect Dis 7:338–348, 2007.

Inhibitors of Bacterial Protein Synthesis

CLASSIFICATION OF INHIBITORS OF BACTERIAL PROTEIN SYNTHESIS

Drugs That Affect the 30S Ribosomal Subunit
Aminoglycoside and Related Antibiotics
- Gentamicin[a]
- Neomycin
- Streptomycin
- Spectinomycin (TROBICIN)

Tetracycline Antibiotics
- Doxycycline
- Minocycline
- Tetracycline
- Tigecycline (TYGACIL)

Drugs That Affect the 50S Ribosomal Subunit
Macrolide and Ketolide Antibiotics
- Azithromycin (ZITHROMAX)
- Clarithromycin (BIAXIN)

- Erythromycin
- Telithromycin (KETEK)

Other Antibiotics Binding the 50S Subunit
- Chloramphenicol
- Clindamycin (CLEOCIN)
- Quinupristin-Dalfopristin (SYNERCID)

Other Protein Synthesis Inhibitors
- Mupirocin (BACTROBAN)
- Linezolid (ZYVOX)

[a]Also amikacin (AMIKIN) and tobramycin (NEBCIN).

OVERVIEW

After the introduction of penicillin, scientists began an extensive search for antibiotics that could inhibit penicillin-resistant bacteria. A number of *Streptomyces* species were isolated from soil samples collected from all over the world, and these species eventually yielded several new classes of antibiotics, including the aminoglycosides, tetracyclines, and macrolides. Streptomycin, an aminoglycoside, was the first new antibiotic to be introduced through these efforts (Box 39–1).

Bacterial Protein Synthesis

Several classes of antibiotics act by selectively blocking one or more steps in the protein synthesis of bacteria (prokaryotes) while having relatively little effect on the protein synthesis of human and other eukaryotes. The selectivity for bacterial protein synthesis is due to differences in the structure and function of ribosomes in prokaryotic (bacterial) versus eukaryotic (mammalian) cells.

Each ribosome has two subunits. The **ribosome in prokaryotes** is composed of a 30S subunit and a 50S subunit (with S denoting the Svedberg unit of flotation, which forms the basis for the separation and isolation of ribosomal subunits from cell homogenates). In contrast, the **ribosome in eukaryotes** is composed of a 40S and a 60S subunit, and the proteins that initiate and carry out translation of messenger RNA (mRNA) in eukaryotic systems are more complex and function differently than the proteins of bacterial systems.

The basic steps in bacterial protein synthesis are illustrated in Figure 39–1. These steps include the binding of aminoacyl transfer RNA (tRNA) to the ribosome, the

CASE PRESENTATION: A 26-year-old man presents for evaluation of a painful lesion on his abdominal wall, which developed after he sustained an injury while playing basketball. There was a 4-day history of drainage from this abscess, which had increased in size and become more painful. His temperature is 38.5° C, and his pulse is 115 beats per minute. On examination, the lesion is tender and erythematous with a fluctuant area at the center. Purulent material was obtained by aspiration, and a culture yielded methicillin-resistant *Staphylococcus aureus* (MRSA) that was susceptible to clindamycin. The D-zone test was negative. Incision and drainage were performed on the lesion, and he was placed on oral clindamycin, 300 milligrams three times daily. The infection responded to a 7-day course of clindamycin therapy.

CASE DISCUSSION: The number of community-acquired MRSA infections has increased dramatically in the past 5 years. MRSA is now the most common pathogen isolated from skin and soft tissue infections in emergency departments. These infections may be managed by incision and drainage if systemic signs such as fever and tachycardia are absent. The optimal antibiotic therapy for these infections has not been established, but clindamycin, trimethoprim-sulfamethoxazole, and other oral agents are usually effective (see Table 39–4). Clindamycin susceptibility tests may be misleading because of the occurrence of inducible clindamycin resistance expressed by the *erm* gene (see text). The D-zone test can be used to detect this form of resistance. This test is positive if a D-shaped or blunted area of inhibition surrounds the clindamycin disk on a culture of the clinical isolate. In the present case, the D-zone test was negative, and the patient was effectively treated with clindamycin.

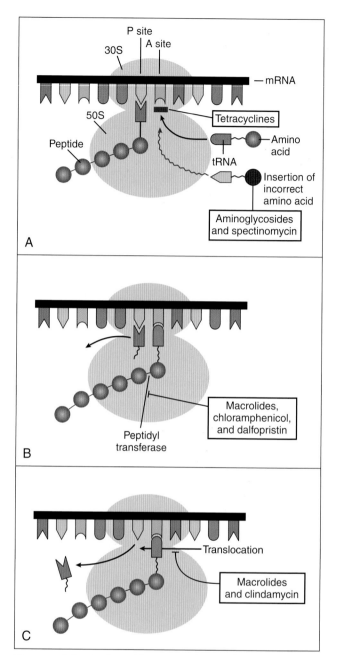

Figure 39–1. Bacterial protein synthesis and sites of drug action. The bacterial ribosome is composed of a 30S subunit and a 50S subunit. The steps in protein synthesis and translation of messenger RNA (mRNA) include the binding of aminoacyl transfer RNA (tRNA) to the ribosome, the formation of a peptide bond, and translocation. **(A)** Under normal circumstances, the nascent peptide is attached to the ribosome at the peptidyl site (P site), and the next aminoacyl tRNA binds to the acceptor or aminoacyl site (A site). Tetracyclines block aminoacyl tRNA from binding to the A site. Aminoglycosides and spectinomycin cause misreading of the genetic code, which leads to binding of the wrong aminoacyl tRNA and insertion of the wrong amino acid into the nascent peptide. **(B)** Macrolides, chloramphenicol, and dalfopristin block peptidyl transferase, the enzyme that catalyzes the formation of a peptide bond between the nascent peptide and the amino acid attached to the A site. **(C)** Macrolides and clindamycin block the translocation step in which the nascent peptide is transferred from the A site to the P site following the formation of a new peptide bond.

formation of a peptide bond, and translocation. Aminoacyl tRNA binds to the 30S ribosomal subunit, whereas peptide bond formation and translocation involve components of the 50S ribosomal subunit.

SITES OF DRUG ACTION

As shown in Figure 39–1, each type of antibiotic discussed in this chapter acts at a specific site on the ribosome to inhibit one or more steps in protein synthesis. Tetracyclines, aminoglycosides, and spectinomycin act at the **30S ribosomal**

subunit. Macrolides, chloramphenicol, dalfopristin, and clindamycin act at the **50S ribosomal subunit.**

Tetracyclines competitively block binding of tRNA to the 30S subunit and thereby prevent the addition of new amino acids to the growing peptide chain. This reversibility of this effect accounts for the bacteriostatic action of tetracyclines.

Aminoglycosides and **spectinomycin** also bind to the 30S subunit, where they interfere with the initiation of protein synthesis and cause misreading of the genetic code so that the wrong amino acid is inserted into the protein structure. These irreversible actions account for the bactericidal effects of these antibiotics.

Macrolides, chloramphenicol, and **dalfopristin** block peptidyl transferase, the enzyme that catalyzes the formation of a peptide bond between the new amino acid and the nascent peptide. **Macrolides** and **clindamycin** prevent translocation of the nascent peptide from the acceptor or aminoacyl site (A site) to the peptidyl site (P site) on the ribosome which, in turn, prevents binding of the next aminoacyl tRNA to the ribosome.

DRUGS THAT AFFECT THE 30S RIBOSOMAL SUBUNIT

Aminoglycosides

The aminoglycosides include **amikacin, gentamicin, neomycin, streptomycin,** and **tobramycin.** The properties and major clinical uses of these drugs are compared in Table 39–1 and 39–2.

CHEMISTRY AND PHARMACOKINETICS. Aminoglycoside antibiotics are composed of amino sugars linked through glycosidic bonds. The amino groups are highly basic and become extensively protonated and ionized in body fluids. For this reason, the aminoglycosides are poorly absorbed from the gut and must be administered parenterally for the treatment of systemic infections. Occasionally, they are administered orally to treat gastrointestinal infections such as neonatal necrotizing enterocolitis. They are also administered topically to treat infections of the skin, mucous membranes, and ocular tissues.

Because of their highly ionized nature, aminoglycosides do not penetrate tissue cells significantly, and their volumes of distribution are similar to the extracellular fluid volume. Aminoglycosides also have poor penetration of the meninges, even when the meninges are inflamed, and intrathecal administration may be required to treat meningitis.

The aminoglycosides are not metabolized. They are excreted primarily by renal glomerular filtration, with little tubular reabsorption. The renal clearance of aminoglycosides is approximately equal to the creatinine clearance, because creatinine is also filtered at the glomerulus but is not secreted or reabsorbed significantly by the tubules. Because the clearance of aminoglycosides is proportional to the glomerular filtration rate, the dosage of aminoglycosides must be reduced in patients with renal impairment. In most cases, this is accomplished by increasing the interval between doses.

The plasma concentrations of aminoglycosides are routinely measured to ensure adequate dosage and to minimize toxicity. The peak concentration is found about 30 minutes after completing an intravenous infusion of an aminoglycoside, whereas the trough concentration is found immediately before administration of the next dose. Optimal peak and trough concentrations have been established and can be used to guide dosage adjustments for individuals receiving the standard regimen of three daily doses given at 8-hour intervals. For example, therapeutic concentrations of gentamicin and tobramycin are usually between 4 and 8 mg/L. A peak concentration above 12 mg/L or a trough concentration above 2 mg/L is considered toxic and indicates the need to reduce the dosage of gentamicin or tobramycin. Therapeutic concentrations of amikacin are between 16 and 32 mg/L, and the toxic peak and trough concentrations are above 35 mg/L and above 10 mg/L, respectively.

SPECTRUM AND INDICATIONS. The aminoglycosides are highly active against a wide range of **aerobic gram-negative bacilli,** and these antibiotics are now the most commonly used agents worldwide in the treatment of gram-negative bacterial infections. Gram-negative organisms have become increasingly resistant to β-lactam antibiotics and fluoroquinolones. Consequently, aminoglycosides have undergone resurgence in use.

Of the five aminoglycosides listed in Table 39–2, streptomycin is the least toxic, but it is also the least active against most gram-negative bacilli. Streptomycin is primarily used to treat tuberculosis and infections caused by *Yersinia pestis* (plague) and *Francisella tularensis* (tularemia).

Tobramycin is the most active aminoglycoside against many strains of *P. aeruginosa*, whereas gentamicin is usually more active against members of the family Enterobacteriaceae (*Escherichia coli*, *Klebsiella* spp. and others). Gentamicin is also used in combination with a penicillin to treat serious enterococcal, staphylococcal, or viridans group streptococcal infections. Amikacin is more resistant to bacterial enzymes that inactivate aminoglycosides, and it is active against some strains resistant to gentamicin and tobramycin.

BACTERIAL RESISTANCE. Resistance to aminoglycosides is primarily caused by **inactivation of the drugs by bacterial enzymes** that conjugate the drugs with acetate, phosphate, or adenylate. Resistance to aminoglycosides can also be caused by **decreased binding** of the drugs to the 30S ribosomal subunit or to **decreased uptake** of the drugs by porins in bacterial membranes (Table 39–3). Both plasmid and chromosomal genes are involved in resistance to aminoglycosides.

ADVERSE EFFECTS. The most serious adverse effects of aminoglycosides are **nephrotoxicity** and **ototoxicity.** The risk of toxicity is related to the dosage and duration of treatment and varies with the specific drug. Irreversible toxicity can occur, even after use of the drug is discontinued, but serious toxicity is less likely if the offending drug is discontinued at the earliest sign of dysfunction.

Aminoglycosides are the most common cause of **drug-induced renal failure.** When the drugs accumulate in proximal tubule cells, they can cause **acute tubular necrosis.** Aminoglycosides also cause **glomerular toxicity.** These effects impair renal function and lead to a rise in plasma

TABLE 39-1.	Pharmacokinetic Properties of Bacterial Protein Synthesis Inhibitors*			
Drug	**Route of Administration**	**Oral Bioavailability**	**Elimination Half-Life (Hours)**	**Primary Route of Elimination**
Aminoglycoside and Aminocyclitol Antibiotics				
Amikacin	IV	NA	2.5	Renal excretion
Gentamicin	IV or topical	NA	1.5	Renal excretion
Neomycin	Topical	NA	NA	NA
Streptomycin	IM	NA	2.0	Renal excretion
Tobramycin	IV or topical	NA	2.5	Renal excretion
Spectinomycin	IM	NA	2.0	Renal excretion
Tetracycline Antibiotics				
Doxycycline	Oral or IV	90%	20.0	Fecal and renal excretion
Minocycline	Oral or IV	95%	20.0	Biliary and renal excretion
Tetracycline	Oral or IV	70%	10.0	Renal excretion
Macrolide and Ketolide Antibiotics				
Azithromycin	Oral or IV	37%	12.0	Biliary excretion
Clarithromycin	Oral	62%	5.0	Biliary and renal excretion
Erythromycin	Oral, IV, or topical	35% ± 25%	2.0	Biliary excretion
Telithromycin	Oral	60%	10.0	Biliary and renal excretion
Other Antibiotics				
Chloramphenicol	Oral, IV, or topical	95%	3.0	Hepatic metabolism; renal excretion
Clindamycin	Oral, IV, or topical	95%	2.5	Hepatic metabolism; renal, biliary, and fecal excretion
Linezolid	Oral or IV	100%	6	Hepatic metabolism; renal excretion
Mupirocin	Topical	NA	NA	NA
Quinupristin-dalfopristin	IV	NA	0.8 and 0.4†	Hepatic metabolism; biliary excretion

*Values shown are the mean of values reported in the literature.
†The half-lives for quinupristin and dalfopristin are 0.8 and 0.4 hours, respectively. The drugs are given in combination.
IM = intramuscular; IV = intravenous; NA = not applicable.

concentrations of the aminoglycosides. The elevated drug concentrations can further impair renal function and contribute to ototoxicity. Hence, it is important to monitor renal function and plasma aminoglycoside concentrations and to adjust the aminoglycoside dosage accordingly. Increasing the interval between doses to 24 hours or longer in persons with impaired renal function decreases the likelihood of toxicity.

Ototoxicity is associated with the accumulation of aminoglycosides in the **labyrinth** and **hair cells of the cochlea**, and has been attributed to activation of caspase-dependent apoptosis (programmed cell death) in hair cells. Patients can experience both **vestibular and cochlear toxicity**. Manifestations of vestibular toxicity include dizziness, impaired vision, nystagmus, vertigo, nausea, vomiting, and problems with postural balance and walking. Cochlear toxicity is characterized by tinnitus and hearing impairment and can lead to irreversible deafness. Often, a delay occurs between drug administration and the onset of symptoms, so many hospitalized patients are ambulatory before signs of toxicity appear.

The aminoglycosides vary in their tendency to cause cochlear or vestibular toxicity. Amikacin produces more cochlear toxicity (deafness), whereas gentamicin and streptomycin cause more vestibular toxicity. Tobramycin appears to cause similar degrees of cochlear and vestibular toxicity.

Neomycin is the most nephrotoxic aminoglycoside, and its use is limited to topical treatment of **superficial infections**. Neomycin is available in ointments and creams in combination with bacitracin and polymyxin. These **triple-antibiotic** preparations have been shown to prevent infections after minor skin trauma. Bacitracin provides gram-positive coverage, polymyxin provides gram-negative coverage, and neomycin is active against both gram-positive and gram-negative organisms. Neomycin can elicit hypersensitivity reactions, especially with long-term administration, and products containing only bacitracin and polymyxin are also available.

Aminocyclitol

Spectinomycin has an aminocyclitol structure that is similar to the structure of aminoglycoside drugs. As with the aminoglycosides, spectinomycin acts at the 30S ribosomal subunit. Spectinomycin is an alternative to ceftriaxone to

TABLE 39–2. Major Clinical Uses of Selected Bacterial Protein Synthesis Inhibitors

Drug	Infections
Aminoglycosides	
Streptomycin	Plague, tularemia, drug-resistant tuberculosis
Gentamicin, tobramycin, and amikacin	Serious infections due to aerobic gram-negative bacilli, including *Pseudomonas aeruginosa* and many Enterobacteriaceae species
Tetracycline antibiotics	Lyme disease, Rocky Mountain spotted fever, ehrlichiosis, granuloma inguinale, brucellosis, cholera, relapsing fever, peptic ulcer disease due to *H. pylori*, chlamydial urethritis, acne, MRSA
Erythromycin	Respiratory tract infections due to streptococci, pneumococci, *Legionella pneumophila, Mycoplasma pneumoniae,* or *Chlamydia pneumoniae*
Azithromycin, clarithromycin	Respiratory tract infections due to organisms sensitive to erythromycin, *Haemophilus influenzae,* or *Moraxella catarrhalis, Mycobacterium avium-intracellulare*
Clarithromycin	Peptic ulcer disease due to *Helicobacter pylori*
Telithromycin	Community acquired pneumonia due to pneumococci, *Legionella, Chlamydia,* and other organisms
Chloramphenicol	Meningitis, brain abscess
Clindamycin	Streptococcal, staphylococcal, and anaerobic infections
Quinupristin-dalfopristin	Infections due to vancomycin-resistant *Enterococcus faecium*
Linezolid	Infections due to vancomycin-resistant *Enterococcus faecium,* streptococci, and methicillin-resistant staphylococci
Mupirocin	Impetigo due to streptococci, staphylococci; eradication of nasal colonization of MRSA

MRSA = methicillin-resistant *Staphylococcus aureus.*

TABLE 39–3. Bacterial Resistance to Protein Synthesis Inhibitors

Mechanism	Examples
Inactivation of the drug by bacterial enzymes	Inactivation of aminoglycosides by acetylase, adenylase, and phosphorylase enzymes Inactivation of chloramphenicol by acetyltransferase
Decreased binding of the drug	Decreased binding of aminoglycosides to the 30S ribosomal subunit Decreased binding of macrolides and clindamycin to the 50S ribosomal subunit
Decreased accumulation of the drug by bacteria	Active removal of macrolides from bacteria via membrane proteins Decreased uptake of aminoglycosides via porins in bacterial membranes Decreased uptake of tetracyclines via porins in bacterial membranes

treat **gonorrhea** caused by **penicillinase-producing gonococci.** Spectinomycin can cause nausea and produce pain at the site of injection.

Tetracyclines

CHEMISTRY AND PHARMACOKINETICS. The tetracycline antibiotics are four-ring anthracycline compounds produced by *Streptomyces* species. **Doxycycline**, **minocycline**, and **tetracycline** are semisynthetic derivatives of older tetracyclines, whereas **tigecycline** is a semisynthetic glycylcycline compound. The properties and clinical uses of these drugs are outlined in Tables 39–1 and 39–2.

The oral bioavailability of the tetracyclines varies from 70% for tetracycline to over 90% for doxycycline and minocycline. All tetracyclines bind divalent and trivalent cations, including calcium, aluminum, and iron. For this reason, their oral bioavailability is reduced if they are taken with foods or drugs containing these ions. Dairy products reduce the oral bioavailability of tetracycline but have little effect on the bioavailability of doxycycline and minocycline. None of the tetracyclines, however, should be taken with antacids or iron supplements.

The tetracycline drugs undergo minimal biotransformation and are excreted primarily in the urine and feces. Unlike other tetracyclines, doxycycline is not dependent on renal elimination, and doses do not need to be adjusted in persons with renal insufficiency.

SPECTRUM AND INDICATIONS. The tetracyclines are broad-spectrum, bacteriostatic drugs that inhibit the growth of many gram-positive and gram-negative organisms, rickettsiae, spirochetes, mycoplasmas, and chlamydiae.

Tetracyclines are the drugs of choice for **Rocky Mountain spotted fever** and other infections caused by *Rickettsia* species. They are also used for the treatment of two spirochetal infections, **Lyme disease** and relapsing fever, which are caused by *Borrelia burgdorferi* and *Borrelia recurrentis,* respectively. Tetracyclines are alternatives to macrolides to treat infections caused by *Mycoplasma pneumoniae.* For most **genital infections** caused by *Chlamydia trachomatis,* a 7-day course of oral doxycycline is effective. For pelvic inflammatory disease caused by chlamydiae, intravenous doxycycline may be necessary.

Tetracyclines are used in the management of **acne vulgaris** and may be the most effective drugs for the treatment of moderately severe acne. In this condition, antibiotics suppress the growth of *Propionibacterium acnes,* an organism found on the skin that can infect sebaceous glands. This organism converts sebum triglycerides to fatty acids, which then cause skin irritation and contribute to sebaceous gland inflammation and the formation of comedones. Minocycline is often used for the treatment of **acne** because of its excellent penetration of the skin. Doxycycline and minocycline have also been used to treat skin and soft tissue infections caused by methicillin-resistant *Staphylococcus aureus* (Table 39–4).

Tetracyclines are also used in the treatment of **brucellosis, ehrlichiosis,** and **granuloma inguinale.** Whereas oral rehydration therapy is the most important treatment modality for persons suffering from severe diarrhea caused by *Vibrio cholerae,* a tetracycline can be used to shorten the

TABLE 39-4. **Agents for Methicillin-Resistant *Staphylococcus aureus* Infections**

Drug	Infection	Clinical Response*	Adverse Effects
Oral Agents			
Clindamycin	Community-acquired SSTIs	Excellent if strains are susceptible	Diarrhea
Trimethoprim-sulfamethoxazole ± rifampin	Community-acquired SSTIs	Most strains are susceptible	Nausea, vomiting, rash, photosensitivity, thrombocytopenia
Doxycycline, minocycline	Community-acquired SSTIs	83% in one study	Nausea, vomiting, photosensitivity
Rifampin	Community-acquired SSTIs	Must combine with another antibiotic	Drug interactions, discoloration of body fluids, abnormal liver function
Parenteral Agents			
Vancomycin	SSTIs	67 to 87%	Flushing and hypotension
Linezolid†	SSTIs	89%	Thrombocytopenia, anemia, neutropenia
Linezolid	Nosocomial pneumonia	80%	Same as above
Linezolid	Bacteremia	56%	Same as above
Tigecycline	SSTIs	84% responded	Nausea, vomiting, photosensitivity
Daptomycin	SSTIs	75 to 83%	Potential muscle toxicity
Daptomycin	Bacteremia and endocarditis	44%	Same as above
Quinupristin-dalfopristin	SSTIs	Uncertain	Arthralgia, myalgia, gastrointestinal effects
Dalbavancin‡ Telavancin‡ Oritavancin‡	SSTIs	82 to 89%	Gastrointestinal effects

SSTIs = skin and soft tissue infections.
*Reported as cure rate, response rate, success rate, or survival rate.
†Can also be given orally.
‡Glycopeptides undergoing clinical trials.

course of **cholera** and reduce the risk of disease transmission to other persons. A tetracycline is included in some regimens to treat **peptic ulcers** caused by *Helicobacter pylori*.

BACTERIAL RESISTANCE. Although tetracyclines inhibit the growth of a wide range of bacteria, they are no longer used to treat infections caused by many common pathogens because strains of these organisms have become resistant. Resistance to tetracyclines is caused by the transmission of plasmids containing resistance factors by bacterial conjugation. The resistance factors include genes that express modified bacterial porins that do not permit uptake of the tetracyclines. Resistance can also result from increased drug efflux, altered target binding, and enzymatic inactivation. The practice of including tetracyclines in **animal feeds** to promote weight gain has contributed to the development and transmission of tetracycline resistance around the world.

ADVERSE EFFECTS. Tetracyclines can cause many adverse effects, including several that are potentially life-threatening. These effects, however, can be avoided in most cases by avoiding their use in susceptible patients.

Tetracyclines are concentrated in growing teeth and bone. Their use by pregnant women or children under 8 years of age can cause **discoloration of the teeth** and hypoplasia of the enamel. In affected children, yellow-brown or gray mottling of a significant portion of the enamel of the front teeth occurs and is cosmetically unattractive.

Tetracyclines can cause potentially severe **nephrotoxicity** and **hepatotoxicity** in the form of fatty degeneration. Both of these reactions are rare, but the fact that pregnant women are at increased risk of hepatotoxicity is another reason for not administering tetracyclines to this

population. Use of tetracyclines potentiates the nephrotoxicity of aminoglycosides and other nephrotoxic drugs and should be avoided in patients having treatment with these other drugs. Tetracyclines are slowly degraded in pharmaceutical preparations to products that are more nephrotoxic than the parent drug. For this reason, tetracycline preparations must be used or discarded by their expiration date.

Tetracyclines sometimes cause **photosensitivity** in individuals who are exposed to the sun during therapy. This adverse effect results from the absorption of ultraviolet radiation by the tetracycline following its accumulation in the skin. The activated drug then emits energy at a lower frequency that damages skin tissue, leads to erythema, and either exacerbates sunburn or causes a reaction similar to sunburn. Doxycycline is more frequently associated with photosensitivity than are tetracycline and minocycline.

Tigecycline

Tigecycline is a glycylcycline antibiotic that is a semisynthetic derivative of minocycline. This unique compound has increased affinity for the 30S ribosomal subunit and decreased susceptibility to resistance mechanisms that afflict other tetracyclines. Tigecycline is indicated for treatment of complicated **skin and soft tissue infections** caused by methicillin-sensitive and methicillin-resistant *Staphylococcus aureus*, *Escherichia coli*, *Enterococcus faecalis*, various streptococci, and *Bacteroides fragilis*. It is also approved for treating complicated **intra-abdominal infections** caused by various gram-positive and gram-negative organisms. The drug is given intravenously every 12 hours. Dose-related nausea and vomiting are the predominant adverse effects.

DRUGS THAT AFFECT THE 50S RIBOSOMAL SUBUNIT

Macrolide Antibiotics

The macrolides include **azithromycin**, **clarithromycin**, and **erythromycin**. The properties and major clinical uses of these drugs are compared in Tables 39–1 and 39–2.

CHEMISTRY AND PHARMACOKINETICS. Each macrolide antibiotic consists of a large 14-atom lactone ring with two attached sugars. Erythromycin is produced by *Saccharopolyspora erythraea* (formerly *Streptomyces erythreus*). Azithromycin and clarithromycin are semisynthetic derivatives of erythromycin that have improved pharmacokinetic properties and antibacterial activity.

Macrolides are usually administered orally, but erythromycin and azithromycin are available in intravenous formulations for the treatment of serious infections such as Legionnaire's disease. Erythromycin can be administered topically to treat acne. When given orally, the bioavailability of erythromycin is low and variable. Azithromycin and clarithromycin are reliably absorbed from the gut, have a greater degree of bioavailability, and achieve higher tissue concentrations (see Table 39–1). Erythromycin also has a shorter half-life than other macrolides and is administered two to four times a day. Clarithromycin is administered twice a day, and azithromycin is given once a day. The macrolides undergo variable degrees of hepatic metabolism and are excreted in the bile and urine.

SPECTRUM AND INDICATIONS. The macrolides are active against many gram-positive and gram-negative bacteria that cause upper **respiratory tract infections** and **pneumonia**, including group A streptococci, pneumococci, chlamydiae, *Mycoplasma pneumoniae*, and *Legionella pneumophila*. Azithromycin is also active against pathogens responsible for sinusitis, otitis media, and bronchitis. Macrolides have little activity against gram-negative bacteria such as *Klebsiella pneumoniae* that typically causes pneumonia in neonates, elderly persons, and chronic alcoholics.

As shown in Table 39–2, some macrolides are active against chlamydiae and are effective in treating pneumonia and genitourinary tract infections caused by *Chlamydia pneumoniae* and *C. trachomatis*, respectively. Indeed, azithromycin is an effective single-dose treatment for uncomplicated **chlamydial urethritis**. Either azithromycin or clarithromycin can be used to treat *Mycobacterium avium-intracellulare* infections, such as those occurring in patients with acquired immunodeficiency syndrome. Clarithromycin is the most active macrolide against *H. pylori*, an organism that is frequently associated with **peptic ulcer disease**. As discussed in Chapter 28, clarithromycin is used in combination with amoxicillin and a gastric acid inhibitor to treat this condition.

BACTERIAL RESISTANCE. Resistance to macrolide antibiotics has gradually increased over several decades. Acquired resistance to macrolides can result from decreased binding to the 50S ribosomal subunit, enzymatic inactivation, and increased **bacterial efflux**. Most strains of staphylococci are now resistant, and pneumococci are increasingly resistant to macrolides. **Pneumococci** expressing the **macrolide efflux (mef)-A transporter** are increasingly prevalent, and about 30% of pneumococcal isolates from all over the world are resistant to macrolides. **Staphylococcal resistance** is often associated with the *erm* gene, which is inducible by erythromycin and which confers resistance to macrolides, clindamycin, and quinupristin.

ADVERSE EFFECTS. The macrolides are largely devoid of serious toxicity. Their most common adverse effects are stomatitis, heartburn, nausea, anorexia, abdominal discomfort, and diarrhea. Erythromycin binds to receptors for **motilin**, a gastric hormone that activates duodenal and jejunal receptors to initiate peristalsis. Activation of these receptors by erythromycin causes uncoordinated peristalsis leading to anorexia, nausea, and vomiting. Azithromycin and clarithromycin have less affinity for motilin receptors and cause less gastrointestinal distress than erythromycin.

Large intravenous doses of erythromycin cause ototoxicity in the form of **tinnitus** or **impaired hearing**. The ototoxic effects usually subside when use of the macrolide is discontinued. Intravenously administered erythromycin is irritating to veins and can cause thrombophlebitis. Rarely, use of a macrolide causes cholestatic hepatitis, which is probably a form of hypersensitivity and is reversible. The estolate form of erythromycin causes this reaction more frequently than do other esters or erythromycin base.

DRUG INTERACTIONS. Erythromycin and clarithromycin inhibit **cytochrome P450 isozyme 3A4** (CYP3A4) and can elevate the plasma concentration of a large number of drugs metabolized by this isozyme. For example, concurrent administration of erythromycin or clarithromycin with carbamazepine can lead to serious, life-threatening **carbamazepine toxicity**, and this combination should usually be avoided. Erythromycin and clarithromycin also inhibit the metabolism of lovastatin and simvastatin, and concurrent administration of these macrolide and statin drugs can lead to elevated statin levels and rhabdomyolysis. In contrast, azithromycin has little effect on P450 drug metabolism and may be the preferred macrolide antibiotic for persons taking other drugs metabolized by CYP3A4.

Ketolide Antibiotic

Telithromycin is a ketolide antibiotic that is structurally similar to the macrolides. Compared to erythromycin, it is more stable to stomach acid and has increased ribosomal binding affinity. Telithromycin is also less susceptible to bacterial efflux pumps than the macrolide antibiotics. As with the macrolide antibiotics, telithromycin binds to the 50S ribosomal subunit and inhibits bacterial protein synthesis.

Telithromycin has good activity against *Streptococcus pneumoniae*, including multidrug-resistant strains of this organism, as well as *Chlamydia* and *Mycoplasma* species, *Haemophilus influenzae* and *Moraxella catarrhalis*. It is approved only for treatment of mild-to-moderate **community-acquired pneumonia** caused by these organisms.

Telithromycin is administered orally without regard to food and has an oral bioavailability of nearly 60%. Because of its relatively long half-life (10 hours), it is given once daily.

The most common adverse effects of telithromycin are diarrhea and nausea. A small percentage of patients taking the drug have shown elevated serum levels of hepatic enzymes and a small fraction of these persons have had **severe liver toxicity**. The drug also prolongs the **QT interval** of the electrocardiogram and should not be taken with drugs that prolong the QT interval or by persons with a congenitally prolonged QT interval. Telithromycin can cause life-threatening **respiratory failure** in persons with **myasthenia gravis** and is contraindicated in this condition. It can also impair visual accommodation and has caused temporary **loss of consciousness** in a few individuals. Patients should not drive a vehicle or engage in other dangerous activities while taking the drug.

Clindamycin

Clindamycin is a chlorinated derivative of lincomycin, an antibiotic that was isolated from a *Streptomyces* species found in soil near Lincoln, Nebraska. The two drugs are amino-sugar compounds that are structurally unrelated to other antibiotics. Because lincomycin is less active than clindamycin, it is no longer used.

Clindamycin is active against gram-positive cocci and anaerobic organisms such as *Bacteroides fragilis* and *Clostridium perfringens* (the cause of gas gangrene). It has gained importance as a treatment for infections caused by methicillin-resistant staphylococci and penicillin-resistant streptococci, including necrotizing fasciitis (Box 39–1).

Clindamycin can be administered orally, parenterally, or topically. It is generally well tolerated, but it is associated with a higher incidence of gastrointestinal superinfections caused by *Clostridium difficile* than other antibiotics. These superinfections can lead to **severe diarrhea** and life-threatening **pseudomembranous colitis.** In affected patients, the pseudomembrane can be observed during proctoscopic examination and consists of mucous, desquamated epithelial cells, and inflammatory cells. Persons who develop diarrhea during clindamycin therapy should discontinue use of the drug and be closely monitored for superinfection and colitis.

Chloramphenicol

Chloramphenicol is a nitrobenzene derivative unrelated to other antibiotics. Because chloramphenicol is highly lipophilic, it is well absorbed from the gut and achieves high concentrations in the central nervous system, even in the absence of inflamed meninges. This property contributes to the drug's effectiveness in the treatment of meningitis.

Chloramphenicol is metabolized partly by glucuronate conjugation, and the parent drug and metabolites are excreted in the urine. In neonates, the ability to conjugate the drug is decreased because of low levels of glucuronyl transferase. If doses of chloramphenicol are not reduced in neonates, plasma drug concentrations become excessive and may lead to **"gray baby" syndrome** characterized by ashen gray cyanosis, weakness, respiratory depression, hypotension, and shock.

Other adverse effects of chloramphenicol include two distinct forms of anemia. One form is a **reversible,** **dose-dependent anemia** caused by blockade of iron incorporation into heme due to inhibition of the enzyme **ferrochelatase.** Another form of anemia is a potentially fatal **aplastic anemia.** Aplastic anemia is rare, affecting 1 of 20,000 to 40,000 individuals who are exposed to the drug. Although the exact mechanism responsible for the anemia is unknown, a hypersensitivity mechanism is suspected. Because safer antibiotics are now available, little justification exists for the use of chloramphenicol for most infections.

Chloramphenicol is a broad-spectrum antibiotic that is active against pneumococci, meningococci, and *H. influenzae*, which are the most common pathogens causing **meningitis.** Chloramphenicol has also been used to treat *Salmonella* and *Bacteroides* infections. The drug can be either bacteriostatic or bactericidal, depending on the organisms and the drug concentration. Chloramphenicol treatment is usually reserved for treating meningitis and other infections caused by organisms that are resistant to other drugs and for infections in persons who are allergic to less toxic antibiotics.

Quinupristin-Dalfopristin

Quinupristin and dalfopristin are the only **streptogramin** antibiotics currently available. They are administered intravenously, are partly converted to active metabolites, and are extensively distributed to tissues except the central nervous system. About 75% of the drugs are excreted in the bile.

Quinupristin and dalfopristin act synergistically to inhibit bacterial protein synthesis when administered as a preparation containing 30 parts of quinupristin and 70 parts of dalfopristin. Quinupristin and dalfopristin bind separate sites on the 50S ribosomal subunit and form a ternary complex with the ribosome. Quinupristin prevents the addition of new amino acids to the nascent peptide chain by inhibiting the **synthesis of aminoacyl transfer-RNA.** Dalfopristin blocks peptide bond formation by inhibiting **peptidyl transferase** in the same manner as chloramphenicol.

Quinupristin and dalfopristin are bactericidal against susceptible strains of staphylococci and streptococci, but are bacteriostatic against *Enterococcus faecium*. Given in combination, the drugs are active against many gram-positive bacteria, including multidrug-resistant staphylococci, penicillin resistant pneumococci, and vancomycin-resistant *E. faecium*. The combination has been used to treat bacteremia, pneumonia, and skin and soft tissue infections caused by these organisms. For example, it has been successfully employed in cases of bacteremia, peritonitis, endocarditis, and aortic graft infections caused by vancomycin-resistant organisms.

Quinupristin-dalfopristin can cause inflammation of veins, arthralgia, myalgia, diarrhea, and nausea. A few cases of elevated serum transaminase levels have been reported.

Other Protein Synthesis Inhibitors

Linezolid is a synthetic **oxazolidinedione** compound. It binds to the 23S RNA component of the 50S ribosomal subunit and prevents formation of the 70S initiation complex required for bacterial protein synthesis. Because of its unique mechanism, cross-resistance with other classes of antibiotics is unlikely.

Linezolid is active against aerobic gram-positive bacteria. It is bacteriostatic against enterococci and staphylococci, and bactericidal against most strains of streptococci. Linezolid is indicated for the treatment of infections caused by **vancomycin-resistant *E. faecium*, pneumonia** caused by methicillin-sensitive and **methicillin-resistant *Staphylococcus aureus***, and **skin and soft tissue infections** caused by methicillin-sensitive or methicillin-resistant staphylococci, *S. pyogenes*, or *S. agalactiae*. The drug is administered intravenously for serious infections, such as necrotizing fasciitis and pneumonia, and can be given orally for mild to moderate skin and soft tissue infections. Its oral bioavailability is approximately 100%, and it is widely distributed. About 70% of linezolid is metabolized, and the remainder is excreted unchanged in the urine.

Linezolid may cause **thrombocytopenia** in patients with renal insufficiency or during prolonged therapy. It is a weak inhibitor of monoamine oxidase and may cause **serotonin toxicity** when combined with a selective serotonin reuptake inhibitor such as fluoxetine. Patients taking this combination of drugs should be closely monitored.

Mupirocin is an antibiotic obtained from *Pseudomonas fluorescens*. It contains an epoxide side chain similar in structure to the amino acid isoleucine. The drug competes with isoleucine for binding to isoleucyl transfer-RNA synthetase and prevents formation of **isoleucyl transfer RNA**, thus preventing bacterial protein synthesis. Because of its unique mechanism of action, it does not exhibit cross-resistance with other antimicrobial drugs.

Mupirocin is active against most staphylococci, including many strains that are resistant to methicillin. It also inhibits most β-hemolytic streptococci, including *S. pyogenes*. Mupirocin is the first effective topical therapy for **impetigo**, a skin disease caused by streptococci and staphylococci. In cases of impetigo, it is applied as a cream to affected areas three times a day for 5 days. Mupirocin is also used to eradicate **nasal colonization of methicillin-resistant staphylococci** in infected patients and in health care workers. This reduces the risk of spreading infection during institutional outbreaks of this pathogen.

■ Most tetracyclines are excreted primarily in the urine, but doxycycline is excreted by other routes and can be used without dosage adjustment in patients with renal failure.

■ Macrolides, which are active against most pathogens causing respiratory tract infections, are used to treat otitis media and pneumonia caused by pneumococci, chlamydiae, *M. pneumoniae*, and *L. pneumophila*. Azithromycin is particularly effective against *H. influenzae*, whereas clarithromycin is active against *H. pylori* and can be used in the treatment of peptic ulcer disease.

■ Telithromycin is a ketolide antibiotic active against pathogens causing community-acquired pneumonia. It may cause liver toxicity, QT prolongation, and respiratory failure in myasthenia gravis.

■ Clindamycin, which is active against gram-positive cocci, is useful in treating infections caused by gram-positive cocci and anaerobes that are resistant to penicillin and other drugs. It causes a higher incidence of pseudomembranous colitis than do other antibiotics.

■ Chloramphenicol is used to treat meningitis when other antibiotics cannot be used. It rarely causes aplastic anemia.

■ Quinupristin-dalfopristin and linezolid are active against gram-positive cocci, including methicillin and vancomycin-resistant staphylococci and vancomycin-resistant enterococci.

■ Mupirocin is active against streptococci and staphylococci. It is administered topically to treat impetigo and to eradicate nasal carriers of methicillin-resistant staphylococci.

SUMMARY OF IMPORTANT POINTS

■ Inhibitors of bacterial protein synthesis act by selectively binding to components of the 30S or 50S ribosomal subunits. Aminoglycosides, tetracyclines, and spectinomycin inhibit 30S ribosomal function. Macrolides, clindamycin, chloramphenicol, and dalfopristin inhibit 50S ribosomal function.

■ Aminoglycosides are poorly absorbed from the gut and do not penetrate the central nervous system. They are excreted unchanged in the urine. Aminoglycosides are active against many aerobic gram-negative bacilli, including *P. aeruginosa*. These drugs often cause renal and otic toxicity.

■ Tetracyclines are broad-spectrum, bacteriostatic drugs are used to treat infections caused by rickettsiae, chlamydiae, mycoplasmas, and methicillin-resistant *S. aureus*. They are concentrated in growing teeth and bone and can cause permanent staining of teeth if administered during pregnancy or in children under 8 years of age.

Review Questions

1. A man with a skin infection due to methicillin-resistant *Staphylococcus aureus* is treated with an agent that binds 23S RNA. Which adverse effect is associated with this antibiotic?
   (A) myalgia and arthralgia
   (B) nystagmus and vertigo
   (C) thrombocytopenia
   (D) discoloration of body fluids
   (E) flushing and hypotension

2. An infant with meningitis due to *E. coli* is treated with an agent that causes nystagmus and vertigo. Which step in bacterial protein synthesis is inhibited by this antibiotic?
   (A) initiation
   (B) peptide bond formation
   (C) isoleucine transfer-RNA synthesis
   (D) peptide translocation
   (E) transfer-RNA binding to 30S subunit

3. A man being treated for chlamydial urethritis presents with severe erythema over his upper body after sun exposure. Which substance reduces the oral bioavailability of this antibiotic?
   (A) folic acid
   (B) ascorbic acid
   (C) vitamin B$_{12}$
   (D) gastric antacids
   (E) alcohol

4. A woman being treated with an orally administered drug for community-acquired pneumonia experiences syncopal episodes and is found to have a prolonged QT interval on the electrocardiogram. This antibiotic is contraindicated in persons with which disorder?
   (A) myasthenia gravis
   (B) epilepsy
   (C) hypertension
   (D) dyslipidemia
   (E) benign prostatic hyperplasia

5. A man with atypical pneumonia due to *Legionella pneumophila* is placed on an antibiotic that inhibits bacterial peptidyl transferase. Administration of large doses of this agent are typically associated with which adverse effect?
   (A) myalgia and arthralgia
   (B) renal impairment
   (C) ototoxicity
   (D) thrombocytopenia
   (E) aplastic anemia

Answers and Explanations

1. **The answer is C:** thrombocytopenia. Linezolid binds 23S RNA and prevents formation of the 70S initiation complex required for bacterial protein synthesis. It may cause bone marrow suppression leading to thrombocytopenia, anemia, or leukopenia. It is not associated with the other options.

2. **The answer is A:** initiation. Gentamicin and other aminoglycosides cause vestibular toxicity such as nystagmus and vertigo. These drugs bind the 30S ribosomal subunit and prevention formation of the initiation complex and cause misreading of messenger RNA.

3. **The answer is D:** gastric antacids. Chlamydial urethritis is often treated with doxycycline, an antibiotic that may cause phototoxicity in persons who are exposed to the sun during therapy. Antacids containing divalent and trivalent cations interfere with the absorption of tetracyclines and should not be administered concurrently with these antibiotics. The absorption of tetracyclines is not impaired by vitamins or alcohol.

4. **The answer is A:** myasthenia gravis. Telithromycin is used to treat community-acquired pneumonia and may prolong the QT interval leading to syncopal episodes due to ventricular tachycardia. The drug may cause muscle weakness and is contraindicated in myasthenia gravis. Telithromycin may be used in persons with epilepsy, hypertension, dyslipidemia, or benign prostatic hyperplasia.

5. **The answer is C:** ototoxicity. Legionnaire's disease is usually treated with a macrolide such as erythromycin. Large intravenous doses of this drug may cause reversible tinnitus and hearing loss. Myalgia and arthralgia (Option A) is associated with quinupristin-dalfopristin. Aminoglycosides may cause renal impairment (Option B). Linezolid may produce thrombocytopenia (Option D), while aplastic anemia is a rare effect of chloramphenicol (Option E).

SELECTED READINGS

Bonomo, R.A., P.S. Van Zile, Q. Li, K.M. Shermock, W.G. McCormick, et al. Topical triple-antibiotic ointment as a novel therapeutic choice in wound management and infection prevention: a practical approach. Expert Rev Anti Infect Ther 5:773–782, 2007.

Daum, R.S. Skin and soft-tissue infections caused by methicillin-resistant *Staphylococcus aureus.* N Engl J Med 357:380–390, 2007.

Drusano, G.L., P.G. Ambrose, S.M. Bhavnani, J.S. Bertino, A.N. Nafziger, et al. Back to the future: using aminoglycosides again and how to dose them optimally. Clin Infect Dis 45:753–760, 2007.

Martinez-Salgado, C., F.J. Lopez-Hernandez, and J.M. Lopez-Novoa. Glomerular nephrotoxicity of aminoglycosides. Toxicol Appl Pharmacol 223:86–98, 2007.

Rizzi, M.D., and K. Hirose. Aminoglycoside ototoxicity. Curr Opin Otolaryngol Head Neck Surg 15:352–357, 2007.

Vidal, L., A. Gafter-Gvili, S. Borok, A. Fraser, L. Leibovici, et al. Efficacy and safety of aminoglycoside monotherapy: systematic review and meta-analysis of randomized controlled trials. J Antimicrob Chemother 60:247–257, 2007.

CHAPTER 40

Quinolones, Antifolate Drugs, and Other Antimicrobial Agents

CLASSIFICATION OF QUINOLONES, ANTIFOLATE DRUGS, AND OTHER ANTIMICROBIAL AGENTS

Antifolate Drugs
- Sulfamethoxazole[a]
- Trimethoprim
- Trimethoprim-Sulfamethoxazole (BACTRIM, SEPTRA)

Fluoroquinolones
- Ciprofloxacin (CIPRO)[b]
- Levofloxacin (LEVAQUIN)[c]

Other Antibacterial Agents
- Nitrofurantoin (MACRODANTIN)

- Daptomycin (CUBICIN)
- Polymyxin B
- Rifaximin (XIFAXAN)

[a]Also sulfacetamide, sulfadiazine, and sulfisoxazole (GANTRISIN).
[b]Also norfloxacin (NOROXIN) and ofloxacin (FLOXIN).
[c]Also gatifloxacin (TEQUIN), gemifloxacin (FACTIVE), and moxifloxacin (AVELOX).

OVERVIEW

This chapter discusses several classes of antibacterial drugs that are often used in treating urinary tract and other infections, including the sulfonamides, trimethoprim, and the fluoroquinolones. Many of these drugs are synthetic compounds that affect the synthesis or metabolism of bacterial DNA.

ANTIFOLATE DRUGS

There are two types of antifolate drugs used in chemotherapy. Members of the first group, the sulfonamides, inhibit the synthesis of dihydrofolate in some bacteria and parasites. Members of the second group, the folate reductase inhibitors, block the action of dihydrofolate reductase and the formation of tetrahydrofolate in various organisms. This second group includes the following: pyrimethamine, which inhibits folate reduction in some protozoa, is primarily used to treat toxoplasmosis and malaria (see Chapter 44); methotrexate, which inhibits folate reduction in mammalian cells, is used in the treatment of neoplastic and autoimmune diseases (see Chapter 45); and trimethoprim, which selectively

blocks folate reduction in bacteria as described later in this chapter (see "Trimethoprim").

Mechanisms of Action

Bacterial synthesis of folate begins with the fusion of pteridine and p-aminobenzoic acid (PABA) to form **dihydrofolate**. This step involves the enzyme **dihydropteroate synthase.** Dihydrofolate is then converted to **tetrahydrofolate** by **folate reductase.**

In bacteria, the sulfonamides and trimethoprim inhibit sequential steps in the synthesis of folate (Fig. 40–1). The sulfonamides are structural analogues of PABA and competitively inhibiting dihydropteroate synthase. Hence, their effects can be counteracted by the administration of PABA. Trimethoprim inhibits bacterial folate reductase.

Mammals must obtain folic acid in their diet because they are unable to synthesize dihydrofolate. Once absorbed, dihydrofolate is converted to tetrahydrofolate and active folate derivatives (methyl, formyl, and methylene tetrahydrofolate) that donate single-carbon atoms during the synthesis of purine bases and other components of DNA (see Chapter 17). Although folate reductase is found in both microbial and mammalian cells, the affinity of trimethoprim for the

446

enzyme in bacteria is about 100,000 times greater than the affinity of the drug for the enzyme in mammalian cells.

Sulfonamides

In the 1930s, sulfanilamide was found to be the active metabolite of PRONTOSIL, a dye that had been developed in the search for bacterial stains with antimicrobial properties.

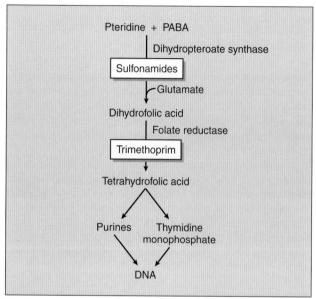

Figure 40–1. Mechanisms of action of antifolate drugs. Sulfonamides inhibit the action of dihydropteroate synthase and thereby block the synthesis of dihydrofolate. Trimethoprim inhibits the action of dihydrofolate reductase and thereby blocks the formation of tetrahydrofolate. PABA = p-aminobenzoic acid.

This discovery led to the synthesis and development of a large number of sulfonamide compounds to treat bacterial infections. Only a few of these are still used today.

CHEMISTRY AND PHARMACOKINETICS. The sulfonamides are benzene sulfonic acid amide derivatives. Most sulfonamides are adequately absorbed from the gut and are widely distributed to tissues and fluids throughout the body, including the cerebrospinal fluid. The half-lives of sulfonamides vary greatly (Table 40–1), but the most widely used compounds for treating human infections, such as **sulfisoxazole** and **sulfamethoxazole**, have half-lives ranging from 6 to 10 hours.

Sulfonamides are converted to inactive compounds by N-acetylation, and the parent drug and its metabolites are excreted in the urine. The acetylated metabolites are less soluble than the parent compound in urine, and they can precipitate in the renal tubules, causing **crystalluria**. Therefore, it is important for patients who are being treated with a sulfonamide to consume adequate quantities of water.

SPECTRUM, INDICATIONS, AND BACTERIAL RESISTANCE. The sulfonamides were the first drugs used in the treatment of systemic bacterial infections. They were once active against a wide variety of organisms, including streptococci, gonococci, meningococci, many gram-negative bacilli, and chlamydiae. Over the years, however, significant resistance to sulfonamides has developed in many bacterial species, and the antimicrobial spectrum of these drugs has been greatly reduced. Today, sulfonamides are primarily used to prevent or treat urinary tract infections (Table 40–2).

Sulfisoxazole or sulfamethoxazole can be used to prevent urinary tract infections or to treat uncomplicated infections of the urinary tract caused by susceptible organisms.

TABLE 40–1.	Pharmacokinetic Properties of Selected Antifolate Drugs, Fluoroquinolones, and Other Agents*			
Drug	**Route of Administration**	**Oral Bioavailability (%)**	**Elimination Half-Life (Hours)**	**Routes of Elimination**
Antifolate Drugs				
Sulfacetamide	Topical	NA	10	Metabolism; renal excretion
Sulfamethoxazole	Oral	≈100	10	Metabolism; renal excretion
Sulfisoxazole	Oral	≈100	6	Metabolism; renal excretion
Trimethoprim	Oral	≈100	10	Metabolism; renal excretion
Trimethoprim-sulfamethoxazole	Oral or IV	≈100	10	Metabolism; renal excretion
Fluoroquinolones				
Ciprofloxacin	Oral, IV, or topical	75	4	Metabolism; renal excretion
Levofloxacin	Oral or IV	99	8	Metabolism; renal excretion
Norfloxacin	Oral	35	3.5	Metabolism; renal excretion
Moxifloxacin	Oral	90	12	Metabolism; renal excretion
Gatifloxacin	Oral	96	7.5	Metabolism; renal excretion
Gemifloxacin	Oral	71	7	Metabolism, renal excretion
Other Antibacterial Drugs				
Nitrofurantoin	Oral	87	0.5	Metabolism; renal excretion
Polymyxin B	IV or topical	NA	5	NA
Daptomycin	IV	NA	9	Renal excretion

*Values shown are the mean of values reported in the literature.
NA = not applicable; IV = intravenous.

TABLE 40-2. Major Clinical Uses of Selected Fluoroquinolones, Antifolate Drugs, and Other Antibacterial Drugs

Drug	Major Clinical Uses
Fluoroquinolones	
Ciprofloxacin	Bacterial diarrhea; intra-abdominal infections; infections of the urinary tract, prostate, bone and joints, skin, and eye; anthrax exposure
Levofloxacin	Bronchitis and community-acquired pneumonia; infections of the urinary tract, prostate, skin, and eye
Gatifloxacin, gemifloxacin, moxifloxacin	Community-acquired pneumonia, sinusitis, bronchitis, tuberculosis
Norfloxacin	Urinary tract infections
Antifolate Drugs	
Trimethoprim-sulfamethoxazole	Urinary tract and prostatic infections; pulmonary infections caused by *Pneumocystis jiroveci (carinii)* and *Nocardia* species
Silver sulfadiazine	Burn infections, other skin infections
Sulfacetamide	Ocular infections
Other Antibacterial Drugs	
Nitrofurantoin	Lower urinary tract (bladder) infections
Polymyxin B	Superficial infections of skin and mucous membranes
Daptomycin	Infections due to methicillin- or vancomycin-resistant staphylococci or vancomycin-resistant enterococci

Sulfamethoxazole is usually administered in combination with trimethoprim (see "Trimethoprim-Sulfamethoxazole").

Sulfadiazine is available in the form of **silver sulfadiazine** ointment to prevent or treat **burn infections** and other superficial skin infections. The silver ions in this preparation have antibacterial activity and contribute to its utility in these infections.

Sulfacetamide is administered topically to treat blepharitis and conjunctivitis, **ocular infections** that are common throughout the world. It is also effective in treating **trachoma**, a highly contagious ocular infection that is caused by *Chlamydia trachomatis* and is prevalent in Asia and the Middle East.

ADVERSE EFFECTS. In some patients, sulfonamides cause skin rashes, which are hypersensitivity reactions that can remain mild or progress to a serious or life-threatening form, such as erythema multiforme or **Stevens-Johnson syndrome**. Other adverse effects of sulfonamides include crystalluria (discussed previously), gastrointestinal reactions, headaches, hepatitis, and hematopoietic toxicity. In persons with **glucose-6-phosphate dehydrogenase deficiency**, sulfonamides can cause **hemolytic anemia**.

Trimethoprim

Trimethoprim is a synthetic amino-pyrimidine drug. It is well absorbed from the gut and is widely distributed to tissues. After extensive hepatic metabolism, the remaining parent compound and metabolites are excreted in the urine.

Trimethoprim is a weak base and is concentrated in acidic prostate tissues and vaginal fluids via **ion trapping** (see Chapter 2). This makes trimethoprim useful in the treatment of bacterial prostatitis and vaginitis.

Trimethoprim is active against many aerobic gram-negative bacilli and a few gram-positive organisms. It is usually administered in combination with sulfamethoxazole to prevent or treat urinary tract infections (see "Trimethoprim-Sulfamethoxazole"), but it is occasionally used alone for these purposes. The adverse effects of trimethoprim include nausea, vomiting, and epigastric distress; rashes and other hypersensitivity reactions; hepatitis; and thrombocytopenia, leukopenia, and other hematologic disorders.

Trimethoprim-Sulfamethoxazole

PHARMACOKINETICS. Sulfamethoxazole and trimethoprim have synergistic activity against susceptible organisms and are available in fixed-dose combinations to treat bacterial infections. Sulfamethoxazole has been combined with trimethoprim because it has a similar half-life (10 hours). In vitro tests show that maximal synergistic activity occurs when the concentration of sulfamethoxazole is 20 times greater than the concentration of trimethoprim. To obtain plasma drug concentrations in a ratio of 20:1, the drugs are administered in a ratio of 5 parts of sulfamethoxazole to 1 part of trimethoprim. The 5:1 dose ratio produces a 20:1 plasma concentration ratio because trimethoprim has a greater volume of distribution than does sulfamethoxazole.

SPECTRUM AND INDICATIONS. Trimethoprim-sulfamethoxazole (TMP-SMX) exhibits bactericidal activity against some organisms that are not susceptible to either drug given alone. TMP-SMX is active against some members of the family **Enterobacteriaceae**, including strains of *Escherichia coli, Klebsiella pneumoniae, Proteus* species, and *Enterobacter* species. TMP-SMX is often used to prevent or treat **urinary tract** and **prostate infections** caused by these organisms. Because of increased bacterial resistance to TMP-SMX, it is not recommended for the empiric treatment of urinary tract infections in locations where greater than 30% of *E. coli* isolates are resistant to TMP-SMX. In these locations, fosfomycin, nitrofurantoin, or a fluoroquinolone drug can be used to treat these infections. TMP-SMX is not active against *Pseudomonas aeruginosa*, a common cause of urinary tract infections in hospitalized and nursing home patients.

TMP-SMX is also the drug of choice for treating pulmonary infections caused by *Pneumocystis jiroveci (carinii)* and *Nocardia asteroides*, which most often occur in immunocompromised patients. TMP-SMX is active against *Burkholderia cepacia* and some strains of *Haemophilus influenzae* and *Moraxella catarrhalis*.

TMP-SMX is active against some strains of *Salmonella* and *Shigella*, but other strains are resistant. Currently, a fluoroquinolone (see "Fluoroquinolones") is usually preferred to treat most infections caused by these organisms.

ADVERSE EFFECTS. The adverse effects of TMP-SMX are similar to those of the individual drugs. TMP-SMX can cause **megaloblastic anemia** in persons who have a low dietary intake of folic acid, but this adverse effect is uncommon.

FLUOROQUINOLONES

Fluoroquinolones have become increasingly important in the treatment of a wide range of infections because of their broad-spectrum bactericidal activity and attractive pharmacokinetic properties. The original fluoroquinolones, such as ciprofloxacin, are primarily active against gram-negative bacteria. Newer agents, such as levofloxacin, have good activity against both gram-positive and gram-negative organisms.

CHEMISTRY AND MECHANISMS. The original quinolone, nalidixic acid, had limited antimicrobial activity. Successive modification of its structure by the addition of a fluorine atom and other moieties resulted in a group of fluoroquinolones with increased affinity for DNA gyrase and improved antibacterial activity.

Fluoroquinolones inhibit two types of bacterial **DNA topoisomerase: Type II topoisomerase**, which is also called **DNA gyrase**, and **Type IV topoisomerase**. The topoisomerase enzymes are essential for maintaining DNA in a stable and biologically active form. DNA gyrase introduces **negative supercoils** (superhelical twists) into closed circular bacterial DNA. These negative supercoils eliminate the **positive supercoils** that occur ahead of the DNA replication fork during DNA replication. DNA replication cannot proceed without DNA gyrase activity. As shown in Figure 40–2, DNA gyrase produces supercoiling by breaking doubled-stranded DNA, moving another section of double-stranded DNA through the break, and then resealing the broken strands of DNA. DNA gyrase is a tetramer composed of two A and two B subunits. Fluoroquinolones selectively bind to the A subunits, which contain the catalytic site of the breaking and resealing reactions.

Type IV topoisomerase is responsible for separating the DNA of daughter chromosomes once DNA replication is completed. This process is called **decatenation**. In general, DNA gyrase is the primary target of fluoroquinolones in

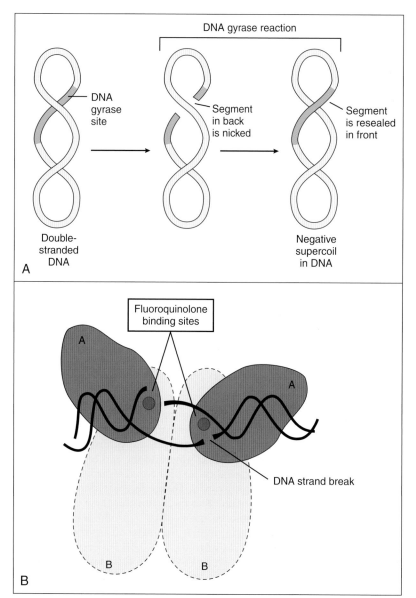

Figure 40–2. **Effect of fluoroquinolones on DNA gyrase. (A)** In the absence of fluoroquinolones, DNA gyrase catalyzes the formation of negative supercoils in the double-stranded DNA of bacteria. After both strands of one segment are nicked, the broken strands are passed across the other strands of DNA and then are resealed. This reaction requires energy in the form of adenosine triphosphate (ATP). **(B)** DNA gyrase is a tetramer composed of two A subunits and two B subunits. Fluoroquinolones inhibit DNA gyrase by binding to the catalytic sites on the A subunits. ATP binds to the B subunits.

gram-negative bacteria, whereas topoisomerase IV is the primary target in gram-positive organisms.

PHARMACOKINETICS. The pharmacokinetic properties of fluoroquinolones are shown in Table 40–1. Fluoroquinolones are usually given orally, and some (e.g., ciprofloxacin and levofloxacin) can also be administered intravenously. Ciprofloxacin has a half-life of 4 hours and is usually administered every 12 hours. Advanced fluoroquinolones (e.g., levofloxacin, gatifloxacin, gemifloxacin, and moxifloxacin) have half-lives ranging from 7 to 12 hours and are given once every 24 hours to treat most infections.

Fluoroquinolones are well absorbed from the gut, but, as with the tetracyclines, the fluoroquinolones chelate **divalent and trivalent cations**, including calcium, iron, magnesium, and zinc. Therefore, fluoroquinolones should be taken 2 hours before or 2 hours after ingesting foods and drugs containing these cations.

Fluoroquinolones are widely distributed to tissues, and their concentrations in the lungs, kidneys, liver, gallbladder, prostate, and female reproductive tissues are often 2 to 5 times greater than their plasma concentrations. Fluoroquinolones undergo varying degrees of hepatic biotransformation, and they are excreted unchanged in the urine, along with their metabolites. Norfloxacin is rapidly excreted in the urine and is indicated only for the treatment of urinary tract infections.

SPECTRUM AND INDICATIONS. Fluoroquinolones have **bactericidal activity** against a broad spectrum of gram-positive and gram-negative bacteria and acid-fast bacilli. Fluoroquinolones exhibit **concentration-dependent killing**, and it appears that maximal bacterial killing occurs when the ratio of the peak serum drug level to the organism's minimal inhibitory concentration is at least 10. Most fluoroquinolones have a long postantibiotic effect, with some organisms failing to resume growth for 2 to 6 hours after drug levels are no longer detectable. Because of their favorable properties, fluoroquinolones can be given orally to treat some infections that formerly required parenteral therapy with other drugs (see Table 40–2).

The original fluoroquinolones (e.g., **ciprofloxacin** and **ofloxacin**) have excellent activity against gram-negative bacteria and are used to treat infections caused by enteric gram-negative bacilli, gonococci, chlamydia, and *Pseudomonas aeruginosa*, including **urinary tract infections, prostatitis,** and **pelvic inflammatory disease.** Fluoroquinolones are used to treat **bacterial diarrhea** caused by *Campylobacter, Salmonella,* and *Shigella* species, as well as *Yersinia enterocolitica,* and they are effective in treating **traveler's diarrhea,** which is typically caused by enterotoxigenic strains of *E. coli.* Fluoroquinolones are used in combination with other drugs to treat intra-abdominal infections, bone and joint infections, skin infections, and patients with febrile neutropenia. Ciprofloxacin is also indicated to treat **anthrax** and for postexposure prophylaxis of inhalational anthrax, such as might occur in a **bioterrorism event.**

The "advanced generation" fluoroquinolones (**levofloxacin, moxifloxacin, gatifloxacin,** and **gemifloxacin**) have good activity against pneumococci while retaining activity against gram-negative organisms. These drugs are used to treat respiratory tract infections, including sinusitis and bronchitis caused by pneumococci, *H. influenzae,* or *M. catarrhalis*. They are also approved for the treatment of **community-acquired pneumonia** caused by pneumococci, *Chlamydia pneumoniae, Klebsiella pneumoniae, Mycoplasma pneumoniae,* and *Legionella pneumophila.* They are also active against mycobacteria and are used in the treatment of *Mycobacterium avium-intracellulare* infections and **drug-resistant tuberculosis.** Fluoroquinolones achieve high concentrations in neutrophils, and this contributes to their effectiveness in patients with mycobacterial infections.

Several fluoroquinolones (ciprofloxacin, gatifloxacin, levofloxacin, moxifloxacin) are available in formulations for topical ocular administration. These drugs have become the most commonly prescribed drugs for treating bacterial **corneal ulcers**.

BACTERIAL RESISTANCE. Resistance to fluoroquinolone drugs develops through two primary mechanisms: alterations in the target enzymes (topoisomerases) and alterations in drug access to the target enzymes. Alterations in bacterial DNA gyrase occur most commonly in gram-negative bacteria, whereas alterations in Type IV topoisomerase are more prevalent in gram-positive organisms. Resistance by DNA gyrase mutations is usually caused by decreased affinity of the A subunit of DNA gyrase for the drugs, but B subunit mutations can also lead to resistance. Topoisomerase IV mutations also lead to reduced fluoroquinolone binding affinity.

Resistance to fluoroquinolones can also occur through expression of membrane transport proteins or **efflux pumps** that actively transport a number of antibacterial agents out of bacterial cells, and thereby confer **multidrug resistance.** In addition, some gram-negative bacteria have decreased levels of **porins** in their outer membrane, resulting in decreased fluoroquinolone uptake by these bacteria.

ADVERSE EFFECTS AND INTERACTIONS. Fluoroquinolones are generally well tolerated, but they can cause serious adverse effects, including **tendonitis and tendon rupture.** Fluoroquinolones should not be prescribed to adolescents, young children, nursing mothers, and pregnant women. Fluoroquinolones have high affinity for cartilage and tendons, where they exert direct toxic effects on the tendon matrix and cause tendon cell death by activating apoptosis pathways (programmed cell death).

Other adverse effects of fluoroquinolones include **alterations in blood glucose** (hypoglycemia and hyperglycemia), seizures, **phototoxicity** (dermatitis after sun exposure), and **prolongation of the QT interval** (a measure of the time between the start of the **Q wave** and the end of the **T wave** in the heart's electrical cycle) of the electrocardiogram leading to ventricular tachycardia. These effects are more likely to occur in persons with other risk factors for these conditions.

Fluoroquinolones, particularly ciprofloxacin, norfloxacin, and ofloxacin, inhibit the metabolism of caffeine and theophylline by cytochrome P450 1A2. Patients taking these drugs should be advised to reduce their intake of caffeine to avoid excessive central nervous system stimulation, and theophylline doses may need to be reduced.

OTHER ANTIBACTERIAL DRUGS

Nitrofurantoin

Nitrofurantoin is a synthetic nitrofuran derivative. It is administered orally and is rapidly excreted in the urine. Because of its low plasma concentrations, its antibacterial activity is limited to the urinary bladder. Ingesting nitrofurantoin with food enhances its absorption and reduces the risk of gastrointestinal irritation.

Nitrofurantoin is bactericidal against gram-positive and gram-negative bacteria that commonly cause acute lower urinary tract infections, including *E. coli*, *Enterococcus faecalis*, *K. pneumoniae*, and *Staphylococcus saprophyticus*. Nitrofurantoin, however, is not active against *Proteus* species, *Serratia* species, or *P. aeruginosa*. Acquired microbial resistance to nitrofurantoin has generally not been a significant clinical problem.

Nitrofurantoin is usually well tolerated, but it can cause gastrointestinal irritation, nausea, vomiting, and diarrhea. To avoid these adverse effects, a **macrocrystalline formulation** of the drug is usually employed. The large drug crystals in this formulation dissolve slowly in the gut, producing less gastrointestinal distress than do other formulations. Less common adverse effects of nitrofurantoin include pulmonary fibrosis, hepatitis, and hematologic toxicity.

Daptomycin

Daptomycin is a **cyclic lipopeptide** that exerts a rapid bactericidal effect against most gram-positive organisms, including many drug-resistant strains. Its antibacterial effect results from insertion of the lipophilic daptomycin tail into the bacterial cell membrane, causing membrane depolarization and potassium efflux, and leading to the arrest of nucleic acid and protein synthesis and cell death.

Daptomycin is active against some strains of **methicillin-resistant *Staphylococcus aureus*** (MRSA), **vancomycin intermediate and resistant *S. aureus***, and **vancomycin-resistant enterococci**. Daptomycin has been approved for the treatment of MRSA skin and skin-structure infections that are a complication of surgery, diabetic foot ulcers, and burns. It has also been approved for MRSA bacteremia, but it should not be used for pneumonia. Daptomycin has limited efficacy in the lungs because it binds to lung surfactant. Other agents used to treat infections caused by drug-resistant, gram-positive organisms include quinupristin-dalfopristin, linezolid, and tigecycline (see Chapter 39).

Daptomycin is administered intravenously once a day. It is generally well tolerated but may cause muscle toxicity.

Polymyxin B

Polymyxin B is a drug often found in creams or ointments containing bacitracin, neomycin, or trimethoprim. The preparations are applied topically for skin and ocular infections.

Polymyxin B is a polypeptide antibiotic that interacts with the phospholipid component of bacterial cell membranes to disrupt cell membrane integrity and permit cytoplasmic components to leak out of the cell. Polymyxin is active against most gram-negative bacilli except *Proteus* species, but it produces considerable nephrotoxicity when given parenterally. Although the drug has been used to treat systemic infections caused by these organisms, safer drugs are now available for parenteral use.

Rifaximin

Rifaximin is a nonabsorbed, oral antibiotic derived from rifampin. It is used to treat **traveler's diarrhea** in patients 12 years of age or older. Traveler's diarrhea is usually a self-limited illness lasting several days that is acquired by drinking water or eating foods contaminated with various intestinal bacteria. The most common causes are enterotoxigenic or enteroaggregative strains of *E. coli*. Less commonly, strains of *Salmonella*, *Shigella*, *Campylobacter*, or other species are responsible. For mild to moderate traveler's diarrhea, nonprescription loperamide or bismuth subsalicylate usually relieve symptoms in less than 24 hours.

Rifaximin is active against noninvasive strains of *E. coli* and some *Salmonella* and *Shigella* species, but it is much less active against *Campylobacter jejuni* and *Yersinia enterocolitica*. The results of clinical trials indicate that rifaximin is about as effective as ciprofloxacin for traveler's diarrhea caused by *E. coli* but that it is not effective in patients with fever or blood in the stool, or in persons infected with *C. jejuni*. Rifaximin produces few adverse effects, but it is not currently recommended for pregnant women.

SUMMARY OF IMPORTANT POINTS

■ Sulfonamides and trimethoprim inhibit sequential steps in bacterial folic acid synthesis. Sulfonamides inhibit dihydropteroate synthase and the synthesis of dihydrofolate, whereas trimethoprim inhibits folate reductase and the formation of tetrahydrofolate.

■ The combination of sulfamethoxazole and trimethoprim (TMP-SMX) is primarily used to treat urinary tract infections, upper respiratory tract infections, and infections caused by *P. carinii* or *N. asteroides*.

■ Fluoroquinolones inhibit DNA gyrase and have bactericidal activity against a wide range of pathogens. Many fluoroquinolones, including ciprofloxacin, are used to treat a variety of infections, including urinary tract and gastrointestinal tract infections, bone and joint infections, skin infections, and anthrax exposure.

■ Advanced fluoroquinolones (e.g., levofloxacin) are also used to treat community-acquired pneumonia.

■ Because of the risk of arthropathy and osteochondrosis, fluoroquinolones are usually not used in children.

■ Nitrofurantoin is a urinary tract antiseptic that is effective in the treatment of uncomplicated urinary tract infections.

■ Polymyxin B is primarily used in combination with other drugs to treat superficial ocular and skin infections.

■ Daptomycin, a unique lipopeptide antibiotic, is used to treat infections caused by methicillin and vancomycin-resistant staphylococci and vancomycin-resistant enterococci.

Review Questions

1. A woman being treated for a urinary tract infection complains of heel pain and is found to have an inflamed Achilles tendon. Bacterial resistance to the agent causing this adverse effect may result from decreased binding to which cell constituent?
   (A) membrane phospholipid
   (B) RNA polymerase
   (C) folate reductase
   (D) topoisomerase
   (E) divalent cations

2. A man with a staphylococcal infection is placed on a drug that disrupts plasma membrane function. He should be monitored for which adverse effect?
   (A) muscle toxicity
   (B) tendinopathy
   (C) megaloblastic anemia
   (D) Stevens-Johnson syndrome
   (E) renal impairment

3. A man treated for a *Nocardia asteroides* infection subsequently develops hemolytic anemia. Which condition would predispose the patient to this adverse effect?
   (A) immunodeficiency
   (B) folate deficiency
   (C) glucose-6-phosphate dehydrogenase deficiency
   (D) iron deficiency
   (E) methionine deficiency

4. A woman with traveler's diarrhea is treated with an agent that is not absorbed from the gut. Which agent was most likely used for this condition?
   (A) ciprofloxacin
   (B) rifaximin
   (C) trimethoprim-sulfamethoxazole
   (D) daptomycin
   (E) nitrofurantoin

Answers and Explanations

1. **The answer is D:** topoisomerase. Tendonitis is most likely caused by fluoroquinolone drugs, which inhibit Type II topoisomerase (DNA gyrase). Fluoroquinolones bind divalent cations (Option E), but this effect is not related to the development of bacterial resistance. Bacterial resistance to daptomycin or polymyxin might result from decreased binding to membrane phospholipid (Option A). Decreased binding to folate reductase (Option C) could result in resistance to trimethoprim.

2. **The answer is A:** muscle toxicity. Methicillin-resistant Staphylococcus aureus infections may be treated with daptomycin, which binds to and disrupts bacterial plasma membranes. It may cause muscle toxicity and elevated creatine kinase levels. Tendinopathy (Option B) may be caused by fluoroquinolones, and megaloblastic anemia (Option C) most likely results from trimethoprim. Stevens-Johnson syndrome (Option D) is associated with sulfonamides, and renal impairment (Option E) may result from systemic polymyxin.

3. **The answer is C:** glucose-6-phosphate dehydrogenase deficiency. Nocardia infections are usually treated with trimethoprim-sulfamethoxazole. Sulfonamides may cause hemolytic anemia in persons with glucose-6-phosphate dehydrogenase deficiency. Trimethoprim-induced folate deficiency (Option B) may lead to megaloblastic anemia but not to hemolytic anemia. Immunodeficiency (Option A) predisposes to *Nocardia* infections but not to hemolytic anemia. Iron and thiamine deficiencies (Options D and E) are not specifically related to hemolytic anemia.

4. **The answer is B:** rifaximin. Rifaximin is a rifampin derivative that is not absorbed from the gut and is used to treat diarrhea caused by susceptible organisms. Ciprofloxacin (Option A) and trimethoprim-sulfamethoxazole (TMP-SMX) have also been used to treat traveler's diarrhea, but they are both well absorbed from the gut. Moreover, TMP-SMX is not a reliable therapy for this condition in many countries. Daptomycin and nitrofurantoin (Options D and E) are not used to treat traveler's diarrhea.

SELECTED READINGS

Brackett, C.C. Sulfonamide allergy and cross-reactivity. Curr Allergy Asthma Rep 7:41–48, 2007.

Haggerty, C.L., and R.B. Ness. Newest approaches to treatment of pelvic inflammatory disease: a review of recent randomized clinical trials. Clin Infect Dis 44:953–960, 2007.

Mehlhorn, A.J., and D.A. Brown. Safety concerns with fluoroquinolones. Ann Pharmacother, 41:1859–1866, 2007.

Micek, S.T. Alternatives to vancomycin for the treatment of methicillin-resistant *Staphylococcus aureus* infections. Clin Infect Dis 45:S184–S190, 2007.

Razavi, B., A. Apisamthanarak, and L.M. Mundy. *Clostridium difficile*: emergence of hypervirulence and fluoroquinolone resistance. Infection 35:300–307, 2007.

CHAPTER 41

Antimycobacterial Drugs

CLASSIFICATION OF ANTIMYCOBACTERIAL DRUGS

Drugs for Tuberculosis
- Isoniazid (NYDRAZID)
- Rifampin (RIFADIN)[a]
- Ethambutol (MYAMBUTOL)
- Pyrazinamide
- Streptomycin
- Amikacin (AMIKIN)

**Drugs for *Mycobacterium
avium-intracellulare* Infections**
- Azithromycin (ZITHROMAX)[b]

Drugs for Leprosy
- Dapsone
- Rifampin (RIFADIN)
- Clofazimine (LAMPRENE)
- Thalidomide (THALOMID)

[a]Also rifabutin (MYCOBUTIN) and rifapentine (PRIFTIN).
[b]Also clarithromycin (BIAXIN), ciprofloxacin (CIPRO), ethambutol (MYAMBUTOL), rifabutin (MYCOBUTIN), and amikacin (AMIKIN).

OVERVIEW

Tuberculosis (TB) claims a life every 10 seconds, and global mortality rates are increasing despite the use of chemotherapy. Apathy, poverty, and drug resistance are all contributing to our inability to fight this chronic disease. Effective treatment of TB now requires the use of increasingly complex drug regimens. Emerging drug discoveries could shorten treatment and combat drug resistance that helps make TB worthy of the moniker "The Great White Plague" (Shi et al., 2007). This chapter covers drugs used to treat TB, *Mycobacterium avium-intracellulare* infections, and leprosy.

MYCOBACTERIAL INFECTIONS

Mycobacteria are acid-fast bacilli that cause a variety of diseases, including TB, leprosy, and localized or disseminated *Mycobacterium avium-intracellulare* infections (Box 41–1).

Tuberculosis is caused by *Mycobacterium tuberculosis*. Atypical mycobacteria (e.g., *Mycobacterium kansasii* and members of the *M. avium-intracellulare* complex) can cause infections resembling TB. It is estimated that TB claims a life every 10 seconds. Worldwide mortality rates are climbing despite the use of chemotherapy. About one third of the world's population is latently infected with *M. tuberculosis*, with 9 million new cases and nearly 2 million deaths annually. In Western countries, the incidence of TB declined after the advent of effective drug therapy and improved public

health measures, but the emergence of highly drug-resistant organisms has posed new challenges to clinicians.

The goals of TB therapy are to kill tubercle bacilli rapidly, to prevent the emergence of drug resistance, to eliminate persistent bacilli and prevent relapse, and to prevent disease transmission. Isolation of patients with TB in single-person rooms is essential until sputum cultures are negative, and extended isolation may be required to prevent the spread of drug-resistant strains. At least 6 months of **multidrug therapy** is required to eradicate the pathogen. Because of the long duration of treatment and difficulties with patient adherence, **directly observed therapy** has been used in treating some patients. In directly observed therapy, a health care provider observes each drug administration to ensure adherence to the treatment regimen.

Since the 1980s, the prevalence of **multidrug-resistant TB** (MDR-TB) and **extreme drug-resistant TB** (XDR-TB) has been increasing at an alarming rate. MDR-TB is defined as resistance to at least isoniazid and rifampin, and XDR-TB is defined as MDR-TB plus resistance to fluoroquinolones and at least one of the injectable second-line drugs (amikacin, capreomycin, or kanamycin). The treatment of drug-resistant TB necessitates administration of second-line drugs that are less effective and more toxic than first-line drugs. Some cases of resistant TB may take up to 2 years of therapy to eradicate the pathogen, and many cases of drug-resistant TB are fatal.

***M. avium-intracellulare* infections** are seen most frequently in immunocompromised patients (e.g., those with

BOX 41–1. A CASE OF COUGH, NIGHT SWEATS, and LETHARGY

CASE PRESENTATION: A 42-year-old man is seen at a public health clinic. He complains of a productive cough, chills, fever, night sweats, loss of appetite, and feeling tired for the past month. He has a history of knife wounds and was jailed for 3 months after a barroom fight 2 years ago. His chest x-ray shows patchy infiltrates in both upper lobes, and a sputum sample is found to contain acid-fast bacilli. He is given a Mantoux tuberculin skin test, which is positive with a 15-mm induration 72 hours later. After completing lab work that will include a complete blood count, liver function tests, and chemistry profile, he will begin standard four-drug therapy for TB, because the incidence of multiple-drug resistant TB in his community is low. Liver function tests and a red-green color discrimination test will be conducted every 2 to 4 weeks throughout his treatment. The patient will be isolated until his sputum is negative for tubercle bacilli, and a public health nurse will visit him regularly to provide care and verify adherence to the treatment regimen.

CASE DISCUSSION: Tubercle bacilli are transmitted on microdroplets expelled by coughing from persons with active infections. Person-to-person transmission requires close contact with an active case and usually leads to a latent infection. Active infections typically occur months or years later when latent TB emerges due to decreased immune function, poor nutrition, physical stress, or other insults. The man in the present case has classic signs and symptoms of TB. The definitive diagnosis is based on finding acid-fast bacilli in sputum and a positive tuberculin test. Effective therapy will sterilize respiratory secretions in a few weeks or less, but eradication of persistent organisms from infected tissues requires lengthy exposure to antitubercular drugs. The prolonged therapy for this disease often leads to drug toxicity and emergence of drug-resistant organisms. There is an urgent need for new drugs that work more quickly to eradicate TB, and several promising agents are currently being developed.

AIDS) and often take the form of **pulmonary disease, lymphadenitis,** or **bacteremia.** In immunocompetent persons with chronic bronchitis or emphysema, exposure to *M. avium-intracellulare* can also result in pulmonary infections.

Leprosy, or Hansen's disease, is relatively common in many parts of the world. It results from infection of the skin and peripheral nervous system with *Mycobacterium leprae.* Because this organism grows so slowly, the disease exhibits a slow, progressive course over several decades. Contrary to popular opinion, leprosy is not highly contagious, and transmission of infection usually requires prolonged close contact with an infected individual. The disease occurs in two primary forms, **lepromatous leprosy** and **tuberculoid leprosy,** each of which has a characteristic pathophysiology and clinical presentation. If leprosy is not treated, it ultimately causes severe deformities and disabilities. Treatment of leprosy can require years of therapy with antimycobacterial agents, although the introduction of newer drugs has enabled the use of shorter courses of therapy for many patients.

DRUGS FOR MYCOBACTERIAL INFECTIONS

Drugs for Tuberculosis

Drugs initially used to treat most patients with TB are referred to as **first-line drugs.** They include **isoniazid, ethambutol,** and **pyrazinamide** (which are synthetic drugs), and **rifampin** and **streptomycin** (which are antibiotics). First-line drugs are discussed below, and some of their properties are shown in Table 41–1.

Second-line drugs are reserved to treat patients infected with organisms that are resistant to first-line drugs. They include **rifabutin** and **rifapentine** (other derivatives of rifamycin), **fluoroquinolone drugs** (see Chapter 40), **cycloserine, capreomycin, ethionamide, amikacin,** and **aminosalicylic acid.** Most of the second-line drugs are not discussed further in this chapter.

In persons who have had a relapse of TB after earlier treatment, the choice of drugs is guided by in vitro susceptibility of the infecting mycobacterial strain.

Isoniazid

After studies showed that nicotinic acid had a weak antitubercular effect, investigators tested many nicotinic acid derivatives. Isoniazid, also known as **isonicotinic acid hydrazide,** was found to be the most active derivative and subsequently became available for clinical use. The introduction of isoniazid in the early 1960s revolutionized the treatment of this disease.

PHARMACOKINETICS. Isoniazid is usually given orally and is well absorbed from the gut. The drug is widely distributed to tissues and reaches intracellular concentrations sufficiently high to be effective against organisms inside cells and caseous lesions.

Isoniazid is extensively metabolized, and the parent compound and its metabolites are excreted in the urine. The primary metabolite, **acetylisoniazid,** is formed by conjugation of acetate with isoniazid in a reaction catalyzed by acetyltransferase, an enzyme whose activity is genetically determined. **Slow acetylation** is an autosomal recessive trait, and persons with the slow phenotype are homozygous for the slow allele. Persons with the fast phenotype are either heterozygous or autosomal dominant. Because of the

TABLE 41-1. Pharmacokinetic Properties of Antimycobacterial Drugs*

Drug	Route of Administration	Oral Bioavailability	Elimination Half-Life	Routes of Elimination
Azithromycin	Oral	37%	12 hours	Biliary excretion
Ciprofloxacin	Oral or IV	75%	4 hours	Metabolism; renal excretion
Clarithromycin	Oral	62%	5 hours	Biliary and renal excretion
Clofazimine	Oral	55%	70 days	Biliary and fecal excretion
Dapsone	Oral	≈100%	28 hours[†]	Metabolism; renal excretion
Ethambutol	Oral	≈100%	3.5 hours	Metabolism; renal and fecal excretion
Isoniazid	Oral or IM	≈100%	2.5 hours[†]	Metabolism; renal excretion
Pyrazinamide	Oral	≈100%	9.5 hours	Metabolism; renal excretion
Rifabutin	Oral	16%	45 hours	Metabolism; renal and biliary excretion
Rifampin	Oral or IV	≈100%	2.75 hours	Metabolism; renal and biliary excretion
Streptomycin	IM	NA	2 hours	Renal excretion
Thalidomide	Oral	≈90%	6 hours	Metabolism; renal excretion

*Values shown are the mean of values reported in the literature.
†The half-lives of dapsone and isoniazid exhibit genetic variation.
IM = intramuscular; IV = intravenous; NA = not applicable.

different rates of acetylation of isoniazid, persons with the fast phenotype have lower plasma isoniazid concentrations than do persons with the slow phenotype (Fig. 41–1).

The prevalence of phenotypes varies from population to population. The slow phenotype predominates in some Middle Eastern populations, whereas the fast phenotype predominates in Japanese populations. In the United States, about half the population exhibits each phenotype.

A small amount of acetylisoniazid is converted to iso-nicotinic acid and **acetylhydrazine**. Investigators believe that acetylhydrazine is responsible for the **hepatic toxicity** of the drug.

MECHANISM. Isoniazid acts by inhibiting the synthesis of **mycolic acid**. This acid is the mycobacterial cell wall component responsible for the acid-fast staining property of mycobacteria.

Isoniazid is activated by mycobacterial **catalase-peroxidase**, an enzyme encoded by the **kat**G gene. The hydrazine moiety of isoniazid reduces the ferric component of catalase-peroxidase, and the reduced (ferrous) enzyme combines with oxygen to form an oxyferrous enzyme complex. This complex ultimately interacts with the target enzyme, a long-chain enoyl reductase involved in the **synthesis of mycolic acid**.

SPECTRUM AND INDICATIONS. Isoniazid is bactericidal against sensitive strains of M. tuberculosis and some strains of M. kansasii. It has little activity against M. avium-intracellulare and is not active against M. leprae or against most other bacteria.

Isoniazid is part of the standard four-drug regimen for TB for persons without known or suspected resistance to isoniazid (Table 41–2) These drugs are believed to kill different populations of TB bacilli, which include rapidly growing organisms and persistent nongrowing (stationary phase) bacteria. Isoniazid, together with rifampin and

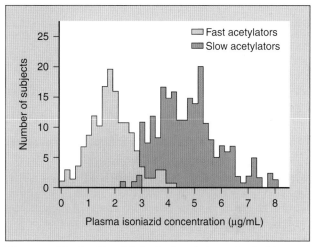

Figure 41-1. Bimodal distribution of plasma isoniazid concentrations. Plasma concentrations of isoniazid were measured 2 hours after the administration of a single 300-mg dose of isoniazid to each member of a general population of human subjects. Subjects with the fast acetylation phenotype showed lower plasma drug concentrations than did subjects with the slow acetylation phenotype.

pyrazinamide, eradicates rapidly growing organisms during the first 2 months of therapy. During the next 4 months of treatment, isoniazid and rifampin act against persistent bacteria that revert to actively growing forms.

Isoniazid is also given to treat **latent tuberculosis** (formerly called prophylaxis) in persons with a positive reaction to the tuberculin skin test and who meet one of the following criteria: human immunodeficiency virus (HIV) positive; recently infected (conversion from a negative to a positive tuberculin skin test in the past 2 years); chest x-ray study showing nonprogressive tuberculous disease; predisposing conditions including illicit injected drug use, diabetes mellitus, immunosuppression, or certain diseases. The preferred duration of treatment for latent TB is 9 months, but 6 months may be sufficient in

TABLE 41-2.	Regimens for Treating Mycobacterial Infections	
Situation	**Preferred Therapy**	**Alternative Therapy**
Prevention of tuberculosis in neonates and children <5 years of age who are exposed to tuberculosis	Isoniazid 10 mg/kg/day for 3 months	
Latent tuberculosis (formerly called prophylaxis)	Isoniazid for 9 months (adults: 5 mg/kg/day; children: 10 mg/kg/day)	Rifampin for 4 months (for isoniazid resistant strains)
Active Tuberculosis		
Isoniazid resistance <4%	Isoniazid, rifampin, pyrazinamide, and ethambutol for 6 months (up to 9 months for HIV-positive)	Isoniazid, rifampin, ethambutol for 9 months
Isoniazid resistance >4%	Rifampin, pyrazinamide, ethambutol ± a fluoroquinolone for 6 months	
Rifampin resistance	Isoniazid, ethambutol, and a fluoroquinolone for 18–24 months, with pyrazinamide for 2 months	
Isoniazid and rifampin resistance	A fluoroquinolone, pyrazinamide, ethambutol, and amikacin for 18–24 months	
Mycobacterium avium-intracellulare prophylaxis	Azithromycin weekly or clarithromycin twice daily	Rifabutin
M. avium-intracellulare treatment	Clarithromycin or azithromycin + ethambutol + rifabutin	Preferred therapy + ciprofloxacin and/or amikacin
Leprosy		
Tuberculoid	Dapsone + rifampin	
Lepromatous	Dapsone + rifampin + clofazimine	

HIV = human immunodeficiency virus.

some cases. Rifampin can be used for prophylaxis if isoniazid is contraindicated or if the mycobacterial strain is known to be resistant to isoniazid (see Table 41–2).

Isoniazid is given to prevent TB in neonates and children who have had close contact with persons in whom active TB was recently diagnosed.

BACTERIAL RESISTANCE. Resistance to isoniazid is increasingly prevalent. This resistance is mediated primarily by **mutations of the *kat*G gene**, which result in loss of the catalase-peroxidase enzyme required for activation of isoniazid.

ADVERSE EFFECTS. Isoniazid is fairly well tolerated by most patients, but it causes elevation of serum transaminase levels and potentially life-threatening **hepatitis** in some individuals. The risk of developing hepatitis during isoniazid therapy is low in persons under 35 years of age, is moderate in persons between 35 and 50 years of age, and is highest in persons over 50 years of age. Isoniazid treatment of latent TB (formerly called prophylaxis), however, appears to have a positive risk-benefit ratio in patients over 35 years of age if they are monitored appropriately for hepatotoxicity. Patients who have TB and are being treated with isoniazid should have their serum transaminase levels monitored periodically and should be told to inform their health care provider if they develop symptoms of hepatitis.

Isoniazid can also cause **peripheral neuritis**, with symptoms including paresthesias and numbness of the fingers and toes. This adverse effect is more likely to occur in individuals with the slow acetylator phenotype, because they have higher plasma concentrations of isoniazid. Peripheral neuritis is caused by a **pyridoxine (vitamin B$_6$) deficiency** resulting from direct inactivation of pyridoxine by the drug.

It can be prevented or treated by administering pyridoxine supplements to patients who are taking isoniazid.

In rare circumstances, isoniazid causes toxic encephalopathy or seizures. Hematologic abnormalities, such as granulocytosis, anemia, or thrombocytopenia, can occur.

Ethambutol

Ethambutol is a butanol derivative that has bacteriostatic activity against mycobacterial organisms. As shown in Table 41–2, it is used in combination with other drugs to treat TB or *M. avium-intracellulare* infections.

Ethambutol is administered orally, undergoes hepatic biotransformation, and is excreted in the urine and feces. The drug is generally well tolerated, but it can produce dose-dependent **optic neuritis** and **impaired red-green color discrimination.** It can also cause hyperuricemia, gout, hepatitis, and thrombocytopenia.

Pyrazinamide

Pyrazinamide is an important drug in TB therapy because of its more rapid bactericidal action and sterilizing effect compared to other agents. Including pyrazinamide in initial treatment regimens made it possible to reduce the treatment duration to 6 months, whereas other therapies required 9 to 12 months. Pyrazinamide is usually given in combination with isoniazid, rifampin, and ethambutol (see Table 41–2).

Pyrazinamide is a nicotinamide derivative that is converted to pyrazinoic acid by susceptible mycobacteria. Pyrazinoic acid inhibits the growth of *M. tuberculosis*, partly by lowering the ambient pH to a level at which the organism can no longer grow.

Pyrazinamide is given orally, is widely distributed to tissues, and is largely converted to pyrazinoic acid in the liver. A small amount of the drug is excreted unchanged in the urine, along with its metabolite. Adverse reactions to pyrazinamide include hyperuricemia, **gout**, hematologic toxicity, fever, **hepatitis**, and an increase in the serum iron concentration.

Rifampin

CHEMISTRY AND PHARMACOKINETICS. Rifampin (also known as rifampicin) is a derivative of the antibiotic called rifamycin that has improved pharmacokinetic properties compared to the natural antibiotic. Rifampin is rapidly absorbed after oral administration and is converted in the liver to an active metabolite, desacetylrifampin. The drug and its metabolite are widely distributed to tissues and fluids, including lung tissue, saliva, and peritoneal and pleural fluids. Rifampin undergoes significant enterohepatic cycling. It is primarily excreted in the feces via biliary elimination, but up to 30% is excreted in the urine.

MECHANISMS, SPECTRUM, AND INDICATIONS. Rifampin is a **broad-spectrum antibiotic** that has significant activity against many gram-positive, gram-negative, and acid-fast bacilli, including *M. tuberculosis, M. avium-intracellulare, M. kansasii,* and *M. leprae.* The drug acts by binding to the β subunit of DNA-dependent RNA polymerase. This prevents the enzyme from binding to DNA and thereby inhibits DNA transcription and RNA synthesis. Rifampin does not bind to the RNA polymerase of eukaryotic cells.

Rifampin is given prophylactically to prevent several types of diseases. It is used as an alternative to isoniazid for latent TB when resistance to isoniazid is known or suspected. It is used to prevent meningococcal disease in individuals who have had close contact with a *Neisseria meningitidis*-infected person or an asymptomatic meningococcal carrier. It is also given to individuals who have been exposed to *Haemophilus influenzae* type b and are at risk of transmitting infection to children 4 years of age or younger.

Rifampin is usually combined with isoniazid, ethambutol, and pyrazinamide to treat TB, and it can be combined with a sulfone (e.g., dapsone) or with clofazimine to treat leprosy (see below). Rifampin penetrates inflamed meninges and reaches levels in the cerebrospinal fluid that are 10% to 20% of levels in the serum. Hence, it can be used in the treatment of tubercular meningitis.

Rifampin is also used in combination with vancomycin and gentamicin to treat staphylococcal endocarditis, and it is occasionally used to treat *Legionella pneumophila* infections in combination with a macrolide or a fluoroquinolone drug.

BACTERIAL RESISTANCE. The major drawback of rifampin is the tendency for microbes to acquire resistance during exposure to the drug. Resistance is usually caused by the decreased affinity of RNA polymerase for rifampin. Because of the potential for the emergence of resistance during treatment, rifampin is never used alone to treat active infections.

ADVERSE EFFECTS AND INTERACTIONS. The adverse effects of rifampin are usually mild, but the drug can impair liver function, elevate serum bilirubin and transaminase levels, and cause **hepatitis.** Liver function tests should be conducted every 2 to 4 weeks during treatment, and rifampin should be discontinued if signs or symptoms of hepatic dysfunction become evident.

A **hypersensitivity reaction**, manifested as a flu-like illness with chills, fever, fatigue, and headache, develops in as many as 50% of persons taking rifampin. This reaction is more common in those who take large doses once or twice a week than in those who take smaller doses every day. High-dose intermittent therapy can also cause renal disease, leukopenia, and thrombocytopenia. Rifampin should be discontinued if purpura develops in persons taking the drug.

The consumption of alcohol by individuals who are taking rifampin appears to increase the risk of hepatitis. Rifampin can cause a reddish-orange to reddish-brown **discoloration of saliva, tears, and urine**. It can also cause permanent staining of soft contact lenses. Patients should be informed of these potential reactions.

Rifampin **induces cytochrome P450 isozymes** CYP1A2, CYP2C9, and CYP3A4 and can thereby accelerate the metabolism of other drugs and reduce their serum concentrations and therapeutic effectiveness. The affected drugs include macrolide antibiotics, benzodiazepines, calcium channel blockers, digoxin, estrogens, sulfonylureas, theophylline, and warfarin.

Rifabutin

As with rifampin, rifabutin **inhibits DNA-dependent RNA polymerase** in susceptible *Mycobacteria.* The drug is active against *M. avium-intracellulare* and most strains of *M. tuberculosis.*

Rifabutin is primarily used to prevent or treat *M. avium-intracellulare* disease in individuals who are HIV-positive or immunosuppressed. For the treatment of *M. avium-intracellulare* infections, rifabutin is administered in combination with azithromycin or clarithromycin plus ethambutol for a period of at least 16 weeks. Rifabutin is administered orally once a day with food to reduce gastrointestinal irritation. The drug is highly lipophilic, is widely distributed to tissues, and reaches substantial intracellular concentrations.

Streptomycin and Amikacin

Streptomycin and amikacin are aminoglycoside antibiotics used to treat TB in cases where resistance to other drugs is known or suspected. Amikacin is more active than streptomycin against some strains of *M. tuberculosis.* These drugs must be administered parenterally and are not as convenient as other drugs in the treatment of TB.

R207910

R207910 is the code name for diarylquinoline drug now in clinical trials for treatment of TB. The new drug **inhibits ATP synthase** in the organism. R207910 is attractive because of its long half-life and its extremely rapid bactericidal effect, and it is believed that it might shorten the duration of TB treatment to 2 months or less. It also appears to be well tolerated, and it is active against multidrug resistant strains of *M. tuberculosis.* If successful, it will be the first new type of drug for TB in four decades. Several other new drugs for TB are also undergoing clinical trials.

DRUGS FOR *MYCOBACTERIUM AVIUM-INTRACELLULARE* INFECTIONS

Drugs that are active against *M. avium-intracellulare* include **ethambutol** and **rifabutin** (described above); **azithromycin** and **clarithromycin** (described in Chapter 39); **ciprofloxacin** and other fluoroquinolones (described in Chapter 40); and **clofazimine** (see "Clofazimine").

Azithromycin, clarithromycin, or rifabutin can be used to prevent *M. avium-intracellulare* diseases in HIV-positive or immunosuppressed patients.

Multiple-drug therapy involving various combinations of azithromycin, ciprofloxacin, clarithromycin, ethambutol, amikacin, and rifabutin are used to treat *M. avium-intracellulare* disease. Clofazimine has been used as an alternative drug in regimens for HIV-positive or immunosuppressed patients with *M. avium-intracellulare* diseases.

DRUGS FOR LEPROSY

The treatment of leprosy requires the administration of antimycobacterial drugs for long periods of time, ranging from several months to a person's lifetime. The World Health Organization now recommends multidrug therapy for most persons with leprosy. Multidrug therapy has been shown to hasten the eradication of bacteria, to reduce the duration of active disease, and to prevent worsening of disabilities in persons with leprosy. In addition, multidrug therapy appears to reduce overall costs, increase patient compliance, and increase the motivation and availability of leprosy workers.

Sulfones

The sulfones have served as the foundation of drug therapy for leprosy for several decades. These compounds are related to the sulfonamides and have a similar mechanism of action. They inhibit the synthesis of folic acid by *M. leprae*, and they exhibit a bacteriostatic action against this organism.

Dapsone, or **diaminodiphenylsulfone**, is the sulfone that is most commonly used in the treatment of leprosy. It is given orally in combination with other drugs (see Table 41–2), is metabolized by acetylation, and is excreted in the urine. Adverse reactions are usually minimal, but dapsone can cause gastrointestinal disturbances, peripheral neuropathy, optic neuritis and blurred vision, proteinuria and nephrotic syndrome, lupus erythematosus-like syndrome, and hematologic toxicity. Individuals who have **glucose-6-phosphate dehydrogenase deficiency** may exhibit **hemolytic anemia** resulting from the oxidation of erythrocyte membranes by dapsone.

Rifampin

Rifampin (described previously) is the drug with the greatest bactericidal activity against *M. leprae*. For the treatment of leprosy, rifampin is usually combined with dapsone or with dapsone plus clofazimine. It is never used alone, because of the probability that organisms will become resistant to it during treatment.

Clofazimine

Clofazimine is a phenazine dye that has antimycobacterial and anti-inflammatory effects. The drug is bactericidal against *M. tuberculosis*, is bacteriostatic against *M. leprae*, and is active against *M. avium-intracellulare*. Clofazimine has little activity against other bacteria. In addition to its antimicrobial effects, the drug enhances the phagocytic activity of neutrophils and macrophages while reducing the motility of neutrophils and the ability of lymphocytes to transform.

The anti-inflammatory and immunologic effects of clofazimine may contribute to the drug's efficacy in the prevention and treatment of **erythema nodosum leprosum,** a Type II hypersensitivity reaction sometimes seen during or after the treatment of patients with lepromatous leprosy. This reaction is characterized by tender erythematous skin nodules that occur with inflammation of subcutaneous fat and acute vasculitis. Clofazimine appears to reduce the incidence of the reaction.

In patients with lepromatous leprosy, clofazimine is approved for use in combination with dapsone and rifampin. Clofazimine is usually combined with corticosteroids to treat leprosy that is complicated by erythema nodosum leprosum.

Clofazimine is slowly and incompletely absorbed from the gut, with an average bioavailability of about 55%. The highly lipophilic drug is primarily distributed to adipose tissue and reticuloendothelial cells, but it is accumulated by macrophages and can also concentrate in the liver, lungs, lymph nodes, spleen, and other tissues. The drug has a long half-life (about 70 days), and some of it remains in the body for years after therapy is discontinued. It is primarily excreted unchanged in the feces following biliary excretion.

Adverse effects of clofazimine include various forms of gastrointestinal distress (e.g., anorexia, nausea, vomiting, abdominal pain, and diarrhea); photosensitivity; skin discoloration or other dermatologic reactions; and discoloration of body secretions (sweat, tears, sputum, feces, and urine) during therapy. Because clofazimine can elevate hepatic enzyme levels and cause hepatitis, use of the drug is generally avoided in persons with hepatic disease.

Thalidomide

Thalidomide is a drug that was once banned because it caused phocomelia (congenital abnormalities of the limbs) in the offspring of women who took it during pregnancy. Subsequent investigations have shown that the drug has immunomodulating actions (see Chapter 45) that are beneficial in the management of several conditions. Thalidomide currently has orphan drug status in the United States and can be used to treat TB, leprosy, or erythema nodosum leprosum. The drug is often effective in alleviating the manifestations of erythema nodosum leprosum, possibly because of its ability to stimulate human T cells (particularly the CD8+ cell subset of T cells).

SUMMARY OF IMPORTANT POINTS

■ Tuberculosis and leprosy are chronic mycobacterial infections that often require treatment with multiple drugs for months or years. Combination drug therapy accelerates the eradication of bacteria and reduces the emergence of microbial drug resistance during therapy.

■ Most patients with TB are initially treated with a combination of isoniazid, rifampin, ethambutol, and pyrazinamide. Second-line drugs are used to treat TB caused by organisms resistant to first-line drugs.

■ Most patients with leprosy are treated with a combination of dapsone and rifampin or a combination of dapsone, rifampin, and clofazimine.

■ Isoniazid (isonicotinic acid hydrazide, or INH) is activated by catalase-peroxidase encoded by the *kat*G gene. It inhibits mycolic acid synthesis. The rate of acetylation of the drug exhibits genetic polymorphism, with some persons showing fast acetylation and some showing slow acetylation.

■ Isoniazid sometimes causes hepatitis; the risk is age related. The drug can also cause peripheral neuritis, an effect that results from drug-induced pyridoxine deficiency that can be prevented or treated with pyridoxine supplementation.

■ Rifampin is a semisynthetic antibiotic with broad-spectrum activity. It is used in the treatment of TB and leprosy, in the prevention of meningococcal and *H. influenzae* type b infections, and in the treatment of serious staphylococcal and *L. pneumophila* infections. Adverse effects of rifampin include hepatitis and discoloration of body fluids.

■ Pyrazinamide is a bactericidal drug that shortens the duration of therapy for TB.

■ Rifabutin, a semisynthetic antibiotic, is primarily used for the prevention and treatment of *M. avium-intracellulare* diseases in individuals who are infected with HIV or are immunosuppressed. Rifabutin is usually given in combination with azithromycin or clarithromycin and ethambutol.

■ Dapsone is a sulfone drug that forms the foundation of therapy for leprosy. It is used in combination with rifampin and clofazimine.

■ Clofazimine is a synthetic dye that has antimycobacterial and anti-inflammatory activity. As with rifampin, it can discolor body fluids.

Review Questions

1. Which of the drug regimens is recommended for treatment of latent TB?
   (A) rifampin for 6 months
   (B) isoniazid for 9 months
   (C) isoniazid and rifampin for 6 months
   (D) ethambutol for 6 months
   (E) isoniazid, rifampin, and ethambutol for 9 months

2. One of the drugs used to treat a man with leprosy causes orange-red colored urine. This drug inhibits the synthesis of which cell component?
   (A) mycolic acid
   (B) glycoproteins
   (C) membrane lipids
   (D) ribonucleic acid
   (E) folic acid

3. A woman being treated for a mycobacterial infection develops optic neuritis. This agent is used to treat infections caused by which organisms?
   (A) *M. leprae* and *M. tuberculosis*
   (B) *M. leprae* and *M. avium-intracellulare*
   (C) *M. tuberculosis* and *M. avium-intracellulare*
   (D) only *M. tuberculosis*
   (E) only *M. avium-intracellulare*

4. Mutations to the *kat*G gene may confer resistance to which agent?
   (A) isoniazid
   (B) pyrazinamide
   (C) amikacin
   (D) rifampin
   (E) ethambutol

5. Persons with a high acetyltransferase activity will have comparatively lower plasma levels of which drug?
   (A) pyrazinamide
   (B) rifabutin
   (C) amikacin
   (D) ethambutol
   (E) dapsone

Answers and Explanations

1. **The answer is B:** isoniazid for 9 months. Isoniazid is recommended for treating all persons with latent TB. If isoniazid is not tolerated, rifampin can be given for 4 months.

2. **The answer is D:** ribonucleic acid. Rifampin may color the urine orange-red. Rifampin prevents bacterial growth by inhibiting DNA-dependent RNA polymerase, the enzyme that synthesizes DNA. It does not affect the synthesis of mycolic acid, glycoproteins, membrane lipids, or folic acid.

3. **The answer is C:** *M. tuberculosis* and *M. avium-intracellulare.* Ethambutol may cause optic neuritis leading to impaired red-green color discrimination. This agent is used to treat TB and *M. avium-intracellulare* infections, but it is not active against *M. leprae.*

4. **The answer is A:** isoniazid. Isoniazid is activated by the enzyme catalase-peroxidase, which is expressed by the *kat*G gene in *M. tuberculosis*. Mutations to this gene may confer resistance to isoniazid, but not to other antimycobacterial drugs.

5. The answer is E: dapsone. Dapsone and isoniazid are metabolized by conjugation with acetate catalyzed by acetyltransferase. Genetic polymorphism gives rise to slow and fast acetylation phenotypes. Persons with the fast phenotype metabolize these drugs more rapidly and have lower levels of unmetabolized drug.

SELECTED READINGS

Sacchettini, J.C., E.J. Rubin, and J.S. Freundlich. Drugs versus bugs: in pursuit of the persistent predator *Mycobacterium tuberculosis*. Nat Rev Microbiol 6:41–52, 2008.

Shi, R., N. Itagaki, and I. Sugawara. Overview of anti-tuberculosis (TB) drugs and their resistance mechanisms. Mini Rev Med Chem 7:1177–1185, 2007.

Spielman, M.K. New tuberculosis therapeutics: a growing pipeline. J Infect Dis 196:S28–S34, 2007.

Zhang, Y. Advances in the treatment of tuberculosis. Clin Pharmacol Ther 82:595–600, 2007.

CHAPTER 42

Antifungal Drugs

CLASSIFICATION OF ANTIFUNGAL DRUGS

Polyene Antibiotics
- Amphotericin B (FUNGIZONE)[a]

Azole Derivatives
- Clotrimazole (LOTRIMIN, MYCELEX)[b]
- Fluconazole (DIFLUCAN)
- Itraconazole (SPORANOX)
- Ketoconazole (NIZORAL)
- Voriconazole (VFEND) and Posaconazole (NOXAFIL)

Allylamine Drugs
- Terbinafine (LAMISIL)[c]

Echinocandin Drugs
- Caspofungin (CANCIDAS)[d]

Other Antifungal Drugs
- Ciclopirox (LOPROX)
- Flucytosine (ANCOBON)
- Griseofulvin (FULVICIN)
- Tolnaftate (TINACTIN)

[a]Also nystatin (MYCOSTATIN) and natamycin (NATACYN).
[b]Also econazole (SPECTAZOLE).
[c]Also naftifine (NAFTIN) and butenafine (MENTAX).
[d]Also micafungin (MYCAMINE) and anidulafungin (ERAXIS).

OVERVIEW

Fungal Infections

Fungal infections can be divided into three groups: systemic mycoses, subcutaneous mycoses, and superficial mycoses.

Patients with **systemic mycoses** can present with signs and symptoms of **soft tissue infection**, **urinary tract infection**, **pneumonia**, **meningitis**, or **septicemia**. The diseases can be chronic and indolent or invasive and life-threatening. The systemic mycoses are most commonly caused by members of the genera *Aspergillus, Blastomyces, Candida, Coccidioides, Cryptococcus*, and *Histoplasma*. Some infections (e.g., **blastomycosis**, **coccidioidomycosis**, and **histoplasmosis**), which are endemic to certain geographic regions, are found in both immunocompetent and immunocompromised individuals. Other infections (e.g., **aspergillosis**, **candidiasis**, **cryptococcosis**, and **mucormycosis**) are more likely to occur in immunocompromised or debilitated patients, such as those receiving immunosuppressive drugs, those with indwelling catheters or prostheses, or those with acquired immunodeficiency syndrome (AIDS), diabetes, or chronic renal, hepatic, or cardiac diseases. These conditions either suppress cellular immunity or facilitate colonization and infection by fungi. For example, an increased

incidence is seen of invasive infections caused by *Aspergillus, Scedosporium*, and *Fusarium* species among recipients of hematopoietic stem cell transplants in the past decade.

Subcutaneous mycoses are often caused by puncture wounds contaminated with soil fungi. Examples of these infections are **chromomycosis**, **pseudallescheriasis**, and **sporotrichosis**.

Superficial mycoses are infections of the nails, skin, and mucous membranes, which are usually caused by dermatophytes or yeasts. The most common dermatophytes are *Epidermophyton, Microsporum*, and *Trichophyton*. Dermatophyte infections of the nails are referred to as **tinea unguium** or **onychomycosis**. Other dermatophyte infections include **tinea pedis** (athlete's foot), **tinea capitis** (ringworm of the scalp; Box 42–1), **tinea corporis** (ringworm of the body), and **tinea cruris** ("jock itch"). These infections usually present as a rash with pruritus (itching) and erythema. **Ringworm** is described as an annular, scaling rash with a clear center.

The most common yeasts causing superficial mycoses are *Candida albicans* and other *Candida* species. Affected patients may present with **thrush** (oral candidiasis), **vaginal candidiasis**, or *Candida* **infections of the axilla**, **groin**, and **gluteal folds** (including **diaper rash** in infants).

461

CASE PRESENTATION: A 5-year-old child is brought to his pediatrician after his mother noticed patches of hair loss and flaking skin on his scalp. Examination confirms diffuse scaling and hair loss without noticeable inflammation, and posterior cervical lymphadenopathy is present. Scrapings of scaly scalp and broken hairs mixed with 10% potassium hydroxide reveal fungal hyphae and spores under the microscope, and samples are obtained for culture in Sabouraud's dextrose agar. Because cultures may require several weeks to obtain positive growth, the boy is placed on ultra-microsized griseofulvin at a dose of 12 mg/kg/day for 6 weeks, with therapy to be continued 2 weeks after symptoms have resolved. Therapy will be evaluated after culture results are obtained.

CASE DISCUSSION: Tinea capitis is a dermatophyte infection of skin and hair on the scalp that is most common in prepubertal children, with the highest frequency from 3 to 7 years of age. *Trichophyton tonsurans* has been the most common fungus responsible for this infection in North America for several decades, but numerous other dermatophytes may cause the infection, including species that are primarily transmitted by humans (*T. tonsurans* and *T. violaceum*) or animals (*Microsporum canis*). The clinical presentation is variable, depending on the etiologic agent and other factors, but the diagnosis can be established by microscopic examination of skin and hair samples mixed with potassium hydroxide. Fungal culture is the most reliable diagnostic criteria, but results take several weeks to obtain. Griseofulvin is the standard therapy for tinea capitis, but higher doses must be utilized for successful treatment. For example, 10 to 15 mg/kg/day of ultra-microsized griseofulvin or 20 to 25 mg/kg/day of the microsized form for 6 to 8 weeks. Infections that do not respond to griseofulvin may be treated with fluconazole, itraconazole, or terbinafine.

Less common yeasts causing superficial mycoses include *Malassezia furfur* (also called *Pityrosporum orbiculare*) and *Malassezia ovalis* (also called *Pityrosporum ovale*). *M. furfur* causes **tinea versicolor** or **pityriasis versicolor**, a skin infection characterized by hypo- and hyperpigmented macules, typically in the shoulder girdle area. *P. ovale* and *M. furfur* cause **seborrheic dermatitis**, characterized by scaling and erythema on the ears, eyebrows, nose, and chest.

CLINICAL USES AND MECHANISMS OF ANTIFUNGAL DRUGS

Fungi are eukaryotic organisms whose growth is not inhibited by antibacterial drugs. Drugs that are selectively toxic to fungi have been discovered, however, and they are used to treat fungal infections in humans.

As shown in Table 42–1, drugs used in the treatment of systemic and subcutaneous mycoses include a polyene antibiotic (amphotericin B), several azole derivatives (fluconazole, itraconazole, ketoconazole, and voriconazole), an echinocandin drug (caspofungin), and flucytosine. The other drugs listed are used in the treatment of superficial mycoses. Amphotericin B tends to be used for treating severe mycoses, whereas the azoles are used for less severe infections. Newer antifungal agents (e.g., voriconazole and caspofungin) can be used to treat invasive *Candida* and *Aspergillus* infections. Flucytosine is usually administered in combination with amphotericin B for the treatment of systemic *Cryptococcus* or *Candida* infections.

Many antifungal drugs act by impairing **plasma membrane function** in fungal cells. The selective toxicity of these drugs is caused by the difference in the sterols found in fungal and mammalian cell membranes. Fungal cell membranes contain **ergosterol**, whereas mammalian cell membranes contain **cholesterol**. Some antifungal drugs bind to ergosterol and thereby increase plasma membrane permeability, whereas other drugs inhibit the synthesis of ergosterol (Fig. 42–1 and Table 42–1).

Polyene antibiotics selectively bind to ergosterol in fungal membranes. This action increases fungal plasma membrane permeability and allows the cytoplasmic contents to escape from the cell. The polyene drugs can also bind to cholesterol in mammalian cells, and this may account for their ability to produce kidney damage. **Ciclopirox** increases fungal cell membrane permeability by a different mechanism. It prevents amino acid transport into fungal cells, thereby altering membrane structure and allowing the escape of intracellular material.

The **allylamine drugs** and the **azole derivatives** block distinct steps in ergosterol biosynthesis, but these groups of drugs have little effect on cholesterol biosynthesis in humans. The allylamine drugs inhibit **squalene monooxygenase**, which converts squalene to squalene-2,3-oxide, the immediate precursor of lanosterol. The azoles inhibit **14-α-demethylase**, a cytochrome P450 enzyme that converts lanosterol to ergosterol.

The **echinocandin drugs** (e.g., caspofungin) represent a new class of antifungal agents that inhibit the synthesis of a **fungal cell wall** component, β-(1,3)-D-glucan. The fungal cell wall surrounds the plasma membrane and protects the cell from osmotic and mechanical stress.

Flucytosine, a pyrimidine antimetabolite, is the only antifungal drug that affects nucleic acid. Flucytosine is converted to **5-fluorouracil** (5-FU) in fungal cells by cytosine deaminase, an enzyme not found in mammalian cells. 5-FU is then incorporated into fungal RNA, and this inhibits fungal protein synthesis.

Griseofulvin acts by binding to fungal microtubules and thereby inhibiting microtubule function and mitosis. The mechanism of action of **tolnaftate** is unknown.

TABLE 42–1. Clinical Uses and Mechanisms of Antifungal Drugs

	CLINICAL USES			
Drug	Systemic and Subcutaneous Mycoses	Dermatophyte Infections	Superficial *Candida* Infections	Mechanisms
Polyene Antibiotics				
Amphotericin B	Yes	No	Yes	Binds ergosterol in fungal cell membrane; increases membrane permeability
Natamycin	No	No	Yes	Same as amphotericin B
Nystatin	No	No	Yes	Same as amphotericin B
Azole Derivatives				
Clotrimazole	No	Yes	Yes	Inhibits ergosterol synthesis
Econazole	No	Yes	Yes	Same as clotrimazole
Fluconazole	Yes	No	Yes	Same as clotrimazole
Itraconazole	Yes	Yes	Yes	Same as clotrimazole
Ketoconazole	Yes	Yes	Yes	Same as clotrimazole
Voriconazole	Yes	No	No	Same as clotrimazole
Allylamine Drugs				
Naftifine	No	Yes	No*	Inhibits ergosterol biosynthesis
Terbinafine	No	Yes	No*	Same as naftifine
Other Antifungal Drugs				
Caspofungin	Yes	No	No	Inhibits fungal cell wall synthesis
Ciclopirox	No	Yes	Yes	Increases fungal cell membrane permeability
Flucytosine	Yes	No	No	Inhibits nucleic acid synthesis
Griseofulvin	No	Yes	No	Inhibits microtubule function and mitosis
Tolnaftate	No	Yes	No	Unknown

*Naftifine and terbinafine have fungistatic activity against *Candida* but are not approved for the treatment of candidiasis.

DRUGS

Polyene Antibiotics

The polyene antibiotics are produced by various soil organisms of the family Streptomycetaceae. Examples are amphotericin A and B, natamycin, and nystatin. Each of these compounds consists of a macrolide (lactone) ring containing conjugated double bonds (polyene), with acidic and basic side groups. Because the acidic group and basic group are capable of donating or accepting a proton, respectively, the polyene drugs are **amphoteric**.

Amphotericin B has greater antifungal activity than does amphotericin A, which is not used clinically. Amphotericin B is the only polyene drug used to treat systemic and subcutaneous mycoses. The other polyene drugs are limited to topical application for the treatment of superficial mycoses.

Amphotericin B

PHARMACOKINETICS. The pharmacokinetic properties of amphotericin B are listed in Table 42–2. Amphotericin B is not absorbed from the gut and is available as a deoxycholate complex and as three **lipid formulations** for parenteral administration. The drug is also available in topical preparations for the treatment of superficial infections.

The dosage and route of parenteral treatment depend on the site and severity of the infection and on the immune status of the patient. Higher doses of amphotericin B are used to treat infections caused by more resistant fungi, especially

Aspergillus species, and lower doses are generally used to treat esophageal and urinary tract infections. Concentrations of the drug in cerebrospinal fluid are only 2% to 3% of those in plasma, reflecting that amphotericin B does not penetrate the blood-brain barrier very well. Nevertheless, the drug is usually administered intravenously to treat fungal meningitis and other systemic mycoses. Intrathecal administration or intraventricular administration with an Ommaya reservoir is usually reserved for extremely ill patients and those who do not respond to intravenous therapy.

Amphotericin B is extensively metabolized in the liver, and the metabolites are slowly excreted in the urine. The biotransformation pathways are not well understood. Amphotericin B has a biphasic half-life, with an initial half-life of about 24 hours and a terminal half-life of about 15 days.

SPECTRUM AND INDICATIONS. Amphotericin B is active against a wide variety of fungi (Table 42–3), and it has been the standard for comparison of other drugs in the treatment of serious fungal infections.

FUNGAL RESISTANCE. Although polyene antibiotics have been used to treat fungal infections for nearly 50 years, few reports have been issued of fungal resistance to these drugs. Fungi that do become resistant to polyenes have a reduced content of ergosterol in their cell membranes.

ADVERSE EFFECTS. Amphotericin B has been called "amphoterrible" and is probably the most toxic antibiotic in use today. It causes some degree of renal toxicity in about 80%

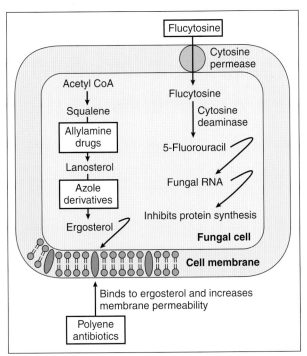

Figure 42-1. Mechanisms of action of antifungal drugs. The synthesis of ergosterol is inhibited by allylamine drugs and by azole derivatives. Amphotericin B and other polyene antibiotics bind to ergosterol in fungal cell membranes and increase membrane permeability. Ciclopirox increases membrane permeability by another mechanism (not shown). Flucytosine is accumulated by fungal cells and converted to 5-fluorouracil (5-FU). When 5-FU is incorporated into fungal RNA, protein synthesis is inhibited. Griseofulvin interferes with microtubule function and blocks mitosis (not shown). Caspofungin inhibits fungal cell wall synthesis (not shown).

of patients who receive it. Renal toxicity reduces the glomerular filtration rate and contributes to the development of hypokalemia and hypomagnesemia. It also leads to accumulation of creatinine and urea in the blood (azotemia). Electrolytes (especially sodium, potassium, and magnesium) should be monitored weekly during treatment and replacements administered as needed.

Lipid formulations of amphotericin B cause less renal toxicity and should be used in persons with renal impairment and those who are intolerant of the traditional deoxycholate formulation. These preparations include amphotericin B cholesteryl complex, amphotericin B lipid complex, and amphotericin B liposomal complex. The lipid formulations have unique pharmacokinetic characteristics that reduce renal drug concentrations and toxicity. Following intravenous administration, the lipid formulations are sequestered by cells of the reticuloendothelial system in the liver and spleen, which slowly release amphotericin B into the circulation over several days, resulting in lower but more sustained plasma levels of the drug.

In addition to causing nephrotoxicity, amphotericin B can cause acute liver failure, cardiac arrhythmias, and hematopoietic disorders such as anemia, leukopenia, and thrombocytopenia. The drug frequently causes less severe but unpleasant effects, including chills, fever, headache, nausea, and vomiting. The severity of these minor adverse effects can be lessened by pretreatment with corticosteroids, antipyretic drugs (e.g., acetaminophen), and antihistamine drugs.

Nystatin and Natamycin

Nystatin, which is active against *Candida* species, is available in various formulations, including the following: creams, ointments, and powders for mucocutaneous candidiasis; lozenges (troches) for oral candidiasis; orally administered tablets and suspensions for intestinal candidiasis; and vaginal tablets for vaginal candidiasis.

Natamycin is active against *Aspergillus, Candida, Fusarium,* and *Penicillium* species and is available as an ophthalmic suspension for the treatment of fungal blepharitis, conjunctivitis, or keratitis.

Azole Derivatives

The azole antifungal agents are synthetic drugs used in the treatment of various mycoses (see Table 42–1). These drugs possess a five-member ring containing two or three nitrogen atoms, which constitute the diazole and triazole compounds, respectively. The diazole compounds include **clotrimazole, econazole,** and **ketoconazole.** The triazole congeners include **fluconazole, itraconazole, posaconazole,** and **voriconazole.**

Drug Properties

PHARMACOKINETICS. The pharmacokinetic properties of azole antifungal drugs are compared in Table 42–2. Some azoles are applied topically to treat superficial fungal infections, whereas others are given orally to treat the more stubborn superficial mycoses (e.g., onychomycosis). Several of the azole drugs are given orally to treat systemic or subcutaneous mycoses. Fluconazole and voriconazole can also be administered intravenously to treat serious infections.

Most azole drugs are well absorbed from the gut. The absorption of ketoconazole and itraconazole requires the presence of gastric acid, so other drugs that reduce gastric acid should not be administered concurrently. Azoles are widely distributed to tissues and body fluids, but only fluconazole achieves significant concentrations in the cerebrospinal fluid (about 50% of concentrations in the plasma). For this reason, only fluconazole is used in the prophylaxis and treatment of **fungal meningitis**.

The azole derivatives undergo considerable hepatic biotransformation, and the parent compound and metabolites are excreted in the urine and feces.

SPECTRUM AND INDICATIONS. Azole drugs can be either fungistatic or fungicidal, depending on the particular organism and the drug concentration. The drugs are active against a wide range of fungi (see Table 42–3) and serve as alternatives to amphotericin B for the treatment of systemic and subcutaneous mycoses. Azoles are also active against most **dermatophytes** that cause tinea infections, including *Epidermophyton floccosum, Microsporum canis, M. gypseum, Trichophyton mentagrophytes, T. rubrum,* and *T. tonsurans.* Azoles also inhibit the growth of **yeasts**, including *Candida* and *Malassezia* species. The specific uses of particular azole drugs are discussed later (see "Specific Drugs").

TABLE 42-2. Pharmacokinetic Properties of Antifungal Drugs*

Drug	Route of Administration	Oral Bioavailability	Elimination Half-Life	Routes of Elimination
Polyene Antibiotics				
Amphotericin B	Topical, IV, intrathecal, or intraventricular	NA	24 hours or 15 days†	Metabolism; renal excretion
Natamycin	Topical ocular	NA	NA	NA
Nystatin	Oral or topical	None	NA	NA
Azole Derivatives				
Clotrimazole	Topical	NA	NA	NA
Econazole	Topical	NA	NA	NA
Fluconazole	Oral or IV	95%	35 hours	Renal excretion
Itraconazole	Oral	55%	60 hours	Biliary, fecal, and renal excretion
Ketoconazole	Oral or topical	Highly variable	8 hours	Biliary and fecal excretion
Voriconazole	Oral or IV	96%	Dose dependent	Metabolism, renal excretion
Allylamine Drugs				
Naftifine	Topical	NA	2.5 days	Renal and fecal excretion
Terbinafine	Oral or topical	40%	12.5 days	Metabolism; renal excretion
Other Antifungal Drugs				
Caspofungin	IV	NA	11 hours	Metabolism
Ciclopirox	Topical	NA	NA	NA
Flucytosine	Oral	82%	3.5 hours	Renal excretion
Griseofulvin	Oral	Variable	16 hours	Metabolism; renal excretion
Tolnaftate	Topical	NA	NA	NA

*Values shown are the mean of values reported in the literature.
†For amphotericin B, the values represent the initial and terminal half-life, respectively.
NA = not applicable; IV = intravenous.

TABLE 42-3. Causes and Management of Selected Systemic and Subcutaneous Mycoses

Mycosis	Pathogens	Treatments
Aspergillosis	*Aspergillus fumigatus*	Voriconazole, caspofungin, or both; amphotericin B
Blastomycosis	*Blastomyces dermatitidis*	Itraconazole or amphotericin B
Candidiasis	*Candida albicans, C. glabrata, C. parapsilosis, C. tropicalis, C. krusei*	Fluconazole, voriconazole, amphotericin B ± flucytosine, or caspofungin
Coccidioidomycosis*	*Coccidioides immitis*	Itraconazole or fluconazole (mild to moderate disease); amphotericin B (severe disease); fluconazole for meningitis
Cryptococcosis	*Cryptococcus neoformans*	Amphotericin B + flucytosine followed by fluconazole for meningitis; fluconazole or amphotericin B for nonmeningeal infections
Fusariosis	*Fusaria* species	Voriconazole
Histoplasmosis	*Histoplasma capsulatum*	Itraconazole for moderate disease; amphotericin B for severe disease and meningitis
Mucormycosis	*Absidia, Rhizopus,* and *Rhizomucor* species	Amphotericin B
Pseudallescheriasis	*Pseudallescheria boydii*	Voriconazole, itraconazole, or miconazole, with surgery
Sporotrichosis	*Sporothrix schenckii*	Itraconazole, fluconazole, or saturated potassium iodide solution

*No treatment needed for uncomplicated pulmonary infection in normal host (valley fever).

ADVERSE EFFECTS AND INTERACTIONS. Azole derivatives are usually well tolerated, but systemic administration can cause skin rash, elevated hepatic enzyme levels, hepatic injury, hematopoietic toxicity, or gastrointestinal distress (nausea, vomiting, and diarrhea). Because azoles inhibit cytochrome P450 3A4, their concurrent use with other drugs may cause drug interactions. Drugs whose metabolism is inhibited by the azoles include 3-hydroxy-3-methylglutaryl–coenzyme A (HMG-CoA) reductase inhibitors, some benzodiazepines, quinidine, and warfarin. The dosage of these drugs may need to be reduced during concurrent azole therapy.

Specific Drugs

Itraconazole is particularly useful in the treatment of blastomycosis and histoplasmosis, and it is widely used to treat **onychomycosis** (fungal infection of the nails). For

onychomycosis, the drug is often administered orally three times a week. This procedure is called pulse dosing.

Fluconazole achieves excellent penetration of the cerebrospinal fluid. It is useful in the prevention of **cryptococcal meningitis** in patients with AIDS, and it is effective as follow-up therapy in patients whose cryptococcal meningitis has been successfully treated with amphotericin B. Based on the results of clinical studies, fluconazole is probably the drug of choice to prevent the relapse of cryptococcal meningitis. Fluconazole is also used to treat mucocutaneous (oropharyngeal and esophageal) and disseminated **candidiasis**. Because the drug is excreted in the urine, it is effective in patients with urinary tract infections caused by *Candida* species. A single dose of fluconazole can eradicate acute **vaginal candidiasis**.

Voriconazole and **posaconazole** have been called **second-generation triazoles** because of their enhanced activity against *Aspergillus* and *Candida* species. Against *Candida* species, voriconazole is 60 to 100 times more potent than fluconazole, and it is active against non-albicans *Candida* species that are inherently resistant to fluconazole, such as *C. krusei*. In one study, voriconazole demonstrated better fungicidal activity against *Aspergillus fumigatus* than did amphotericin B, and voriconazole is active against some *Aspergillus* species that are inherently resistant to amphotericin B. Voriconazole has also demonstrated clinical efficacy in a wide variety of systemic fungal infections, including **invasive aspergillosis**, **esophageal candidiasis**, and **invasive candidiasis**. It has also been used to treat infections caused by *Cryptococcus*, *Fusaria*, *Coccidioides*, and *Pseudallescheria* species. Moreover, voriconazole appears to have additive activity with caspofungin in the treatment of invasive aspergillosis.

Although voriconazole is administered intravenously to treat serious fungal infections, patients can be switched to oral voriconazole as they improve because the oral bioavailability of the drug is approximately 96%.

Voriconazole is usually well tolerated. The most common adverse effects are **visual disturbances**, such as altered perception of light, abnormally colored vision (chromatopsia), and photophobia. These events are usually mild and transitory. Elevated serum levels of hepatic enzymes, primarily alanine aminotransferase and aspartate aminotransferase, occurred in 12% to 20% of patients treated with voriconazole and are the dose-limiting adverse effect of this drug. These elevations are usually transitory and reversible, but a few cases of **hepatic failure** and death have been reported. Hence, hepatic enzymes should be routinely monitored during voriconazole therapy.

Ketoconazole is available in oral and topical formulations. The oral drug is less widely used than itraconazole or fluconazole, because it has a greater potential for drug interactions, does not effectively penetrate the cerebrospinal fluid, and has lower activity against most fungi. Topical formulations are useful for treating **seborrheic dermatitis**.

Clotrimazole is available in topical formulations for treatment of the following: *Candida* **infections** of the mouth, throat, vagina, and vulva; *M. furfur* infection of the skin (tinea versicolor); and **dermatophyte infections** of the skin (e.g., tinea pedis and tinea cruris). Econazole is also available in topical formulations for the treatment of *Candida* and dermatophyte infections of the skin. These and other topical drugs are not effective for the treatment of dermatophyte infections of the scalp (tinea capitis) or nails (tinea unguium, or onychomycosis).

Several other azole derivatives not discussed in this chapter are available for the treatment of vaginal candidiasis and other superficial fungal infections.

Allylamine Drugs

Naftifine and **terbinafine** are allylamines that inhibit ergosterol synthesis (see Fig. 42–1). Although they are primarily used to treat superficial dermatophyte infections, they are also fungistatic against *Candida* species.

Both drugs are available in topical formulations, and terbinafine is also available for oral administration. Terbinafine is often administered orally once a day to treat **onychomycosis**. Fingernail infections usually require 6 weeks of therapy, whereas toenail infections can require 12 weeks of treatment.

Naftifine and terbinafine are well tolerated and rarely cause serious adverse effects.

Echinocandin Drugs

The echinocandin drugs are a new class of large, cyclic hexapeptide compounds with lipid side chains that inhibit **fungal cell wall synthesis**. The fungal cell wall is a rigid structure located just outside the plasma membrane that protects fungal cells from osmotic and mechanical stress. The fungal cell wall is composed of chitin and various glucans and glycoproteins. The echinocandin drugs inhibit the synthesis of the cell wall component known as β-**(1,3)-D-glucan** by noncompetitive inhibition of the β-(1,3)-D-glucan synthase enzyme complex. Inhibition of glucan synthesis leads to disruption of the fungal cell wall and cell death. Mammalians do not have cell walls, and inhibition of glucan synthesis has no direct effect on human hosts.

Caspofungin is the first echinocandin drug to be approved in the United States. It is a semisynthetic derivative of pneumocandin, a fermentation product of *Glarea lozoyensis*. Caspofungin has excellent activity against **Candida species** and good activity against **Aspergillus species**. It is highly active against *Candida albicans*, *C. glabrata*, *C. tropicalis*, and *C. krusei*, including strains that are resistant to azole compounds. Clinical trials have shown that caspofungin is very effective in treating esophageal, oropharyngeal, and invasive candidiasis (74%–96% response rate). In one study, caspofungin was moderately effective in treating invasive aspergillosis (45% response rate). Most patients in this study had already failed treatment with amphotericin B or azole drugs.

Caspofungin produces few adverse effects. The most common problems have been headache, fever, phlebitis at the site of drug administration, and abnormal liver function tests. Compared with amphotericin B, caspofungin has been very well tolerated. Because of its poor oral bioavailability, it must be administered intravenously. Caspofungin has a long half-life and is administered once daily.

Micafungin and **anidulafungin** are newer echinocandin drugs that are approved for prophylaxis and treatment of certain candidal infections.

Other Antifungal Drugs

Flucytosine

Flucytosine is a fluorinated pyrimidine analogue that is used orally to treat severe fungal infections. The drug is accumulated by fungal cells and is converted to its active metabolite, 5-FU, by cytosine deaminase. The metabolite is incorporated into fungal RNA, and this interferes with fungal protein synthesis (see Fig. 42–1). Unlike fungal cells, human cells lack cytosine deaminase and are unable to activate the drug.

Fungal resistance to flucytosine can result from mutations in genes encoding cytosine deaminase, cytosine permease, or enzymes that incorporate 5-FU into fungal RNA. Because drug resistance develops rapidly when flucytosine is given alone, the drug is administered in combination with amphotericin B. This combination produces a synergistic effect against *Candida* and *Cryptococcus* species and is effective in the treatment of pneumonia, meningitis, endocarditis, or septicemia caused by these organisms.

The adverse effects of flucytosine are usually mild. In some patients, however, hematologic toxicity and cardiopulmonary arrest have occurred.

Griseofulvin

Griseofulvin is a fungistatic antibiotic derived from *Penicillium griseofulvum*. It is active against numerous dermatophytes, including *Epidermophyton floccosum*, *Microsporum audouinii*, *M. canis*, *M. gypseum*, *Trichophyton rubrum*, *T. tonsurans*, and *T. verrucosum*, but it is not active against *Candida* or other fungi. Griseofulvin is the standard treatment for **tinea capitis**, which is most often caused by *Trichophyton tonsurans* (see Box 42–1).

Griseofulvin is a lipophilic drug that is not very soluble in water, and its absorption is increased when it is taken with a high-fat meal. To enhance its dissolution in the gut, microsized (microcrystalline) and ultra-microsized forms of the drug are utilized. The ultra-microsized formulation of griseofulvin is almost completely absorbed. The drug is deposited in keratin precursor cells of the skin, hair, and nails, where it disrupts microtubule function and inhibits the mitosis of susceptible dermatophytes. The infected cells are gradually exfoliated and replaced by noninfected tissue. After being metabolized in the liver, griseofulvin is excreted in the urine as inactive metabolites. Some infections respond to griseofulvin therapy in 2 to 8 weeks, but persistent nail infections may require 3 to 6 months of treatment.

Griseofulvin is usually well tolerated, but it can cause dizziness, headache, insomnia, and rarely gastrointestinal bleeding, hepatitis, skin rash, or leukopenia. Griseofulvin **induces cytochrome P450 3A4** and can reduce plasma concentrations of warfarin, oral contraceptives, and barbiturates that are taken concurrently.

Ciclopirox

Ciclopirox is an N-hydroxypyridinone compound that is active against dermatophytes, *C. albicans*, and *M. furfur*. It is applied topically twice a day to treat skin infections caused by these organisms. A lacquer formulation (nail polish) is available for topical treatment of mild onychomycosis.

Tolnaftate

Tolnaftate is a nonprescription thiocarbamate drug used to treat tinea versicolor and mild dermatophyte infections of the skin. The drug is usually applied twice daily to the affected areas for 2 to 6 weeks as a powder or cream. As with most other topical antifungal drugs, tolnaftate is not reliable for treating infections of the scalp or nail beds.

SUMMARY OF IMPORTANT POINTS

■ Polyene antibiotics (amphotericin B, nystatin) and ciclopirox increase the permeability of the fungal cell membrane. Azole derivatives and allylamine drugs inhibit synthesis of plasma membrane ergosterol, and caspofungin inhibits cell wall glucan synthesis.

■ Flucytosine is converted to 5-FU by fungal cells and is then incorporated into fungal RNA, where it inhibits protein synthesis. Flucytosine is used in combination with amphotericin B for cryptococcal meningitis and candidiasis.

■ Amphotericin B is used to treat severe systemic and subcutaneous mycoses, but it often causes chills, fever, nephrotoxicity, and other adverse effects. Lipid formulations have less toxicity and similar efficacy as nonlipid formulations.

■ Several azole derivatives are used to treat systemic mycoses. Itraconazole can be used to treat blastomycosis, coccidioidomycosis, histoplasmosis, and sporotrichosis. Fluconazole is used to treat candidiasis and cryptococcosis.

■ Voriconazole and caspofungin are used to treat invasive candidiasis and aspergillosis. Caspofungin inhibits the synthesis of a fungal cell wall component, β-(1,3)-D-glucan.

■ Superficial *Candida* infections can be treated with nystatin, azole derivatives, or ciclopirox.

■ Dermatophyte infections can be treated by topical or oral administration of an azole derivative or terbinafine; by oral administration of griseofulvin; or by topical administration of ciclopirox, naftifine, or tolnaftate.

■ Itraconazole and terbinafine are given orally to treat onychomycosis.

■ Griseofulvin interferes with microtubule function and blocks mitosis. It is given orally in treating tinea capitis and other dermatophyte infections.

Review Questions

1. After completing amphotericin B treatment for a cryptococcal infection, a man with HIV infection is placed on a drug to prevent relapse of his fungal infection. Which pharmacologic property is associated with this drug?
   (A) poor oral bioavailability
   (B) low cerebrospinal fluid concentrations
   (C) primarily excreted in the bile
   (D) long elimination half-life
   (E) must be given parenterally

2. A woman is given a drug that inhibits fungal cell wall synthesis. Which infection is most likely being treated in this patient?
   (A) tinea corporis
   (B) esophageal candidiasis
   (C) cryptococcal meningitis
   (D) blastomycosis
   (E) mucormycosis

3. After beginning oral therapy for onychomycosis, a woman develops a mild skin rash. This medication causes accumulation of which metabolite in fungal cells?
   (A) lanosterol
   (B) ergosterol
   (C) cholesterol
   (D) cytosine
   (E) β-(1,3)-D-glucan

4. A child with tinea capitis is treated with an agent that inhibits microtubule function in fungi. Which adverse effect most commonly results from this treatment?
   (A) diarrhea
   (B) constipation
   (C) nausea
   (D) blurred vision
   (E) insomnia

Answers and Explanations

1. **The answer is D:** long elimination half-life. Fluconazole is often used to prevent relapse in HIV-infected persons who have been treated with amphotericin B. Fluconazole has a high oral bioavailability, has a long half-life, and is excreted in the urine. Hence, the drug can be used to treat renal candidiasis. Fluconazole achieves high cerebrospinal fluid concentrations and is ideally suited for prophylaxis of cryptococcal meningitis.

2. **The answer is B:** esophageal candidiasis. The echinocandin drugs such as caspofungin are used to treat invasive *Candida* infections, including those resistant to other drugs. Caspofungin is not used to treat tinea infections, cryptococcal infections, blastomycosis, or mucormycosis.

3. **The answer is A:** lanosterol. The woman was most likely treated with itraconazole, which is prone to cause a skin rash in some people. Itraconazole inhibits a cytochrome P450 enzyme in fungal cells, 14-α-demethylase, that converts lanosterol to ergosterol, thereby leading to accumulation of lanosterol. Itraconazole causes depletion of ergosterol (Option B), whereas cholesterol (Option C) is primarily synthesized in mammalian cells. Azoles have no effect on cytosine or glucan metabolism.

4. **The answer is E:** insomnia. Griseofulvin is often used to treat tinea capitis and acts by inhibiting fungal cell microtubule function and mitosis. It may occasionally cause dizziness, headache, and insomnia, but is less likely to cause diarrhea, constipation, nausea, or blurred vision.

SELECTED READINGS

Scheinfeld, N. A review of new antifungals: posaconazole, micafungin, and anidulafungin. J Drugs Dermatol 6:1249–1251, 2007.

Schiller, D.S., and H.B. Fung. Posaconazole: an extended-spectrum triazole antifungal agent. Clin Ther 29:1862–1886, 2007.

Shao, P.L., L.M. Huang, and P.R. Hsueh. Recent advances and challenges in the treatment of invasive fungal infections. Int J Antimicrob Agents 30:487–495, 2007.

Zaoutis T., and T.J. Walsh. Antifungal therapy for neonatal candidiasis. Curr Opin Infect Dis 20:592–597, 2007.

CHAPTER 43

Antiviral Drugs

CLASSIFICATION OF ANTIVIRAL DRUGS

Drugs for Herpesvirus Infections
Nucleoside Analogues
- Acyclovir (ZOVIRAX)[a]
- Ganciclovir (CYTOVENE) and Cidofovir (VISTIDE)
- Trifluridine (VIROPTIC)

Other Drugs
- Foscarnet (FOSCAVIR)

Drugs for Human Immunodeficiency Virus Infection
Nucleoside and Nucleotide Reverse Transcriptase Inhibitors
- Zidovudine (AZT, RETROVIR)[b]
- Lamivudine (EPIVIR)[b]
- Emtricitabine (EMTRIVA)[b]
- Tenofovir (VIREAD)

Nonnucleoside Reverse Transcriptase Inhibitors
- Efavirenz (SUSTIVA)
- Nevirapine (VIRAMUNE)

Protease Inhibitors
- Atazanavir (REYATAZ)[c]

Fusion and Entry Inhibitors
- Enfuvirtide (FUZEON)
- Maraviroc (SELZENTRY)

Integrase Strand Transfer Inhibitor
- Raltegravir (ISENTRESS)

Drugs for influenza
- Amantadine (SYMMETREL) and Rimantadine (FLUMADINE)
- Oseltamivir (TAMIFLU) and Zanamivir (RELENZA)

Drugs for Other Viral Infections
- Ribavirin (VIRAZOLE)
- Interferon Alfa-2b (INTRON-A)

[a]Also famciclovir (FAMVIR), penciclovir (DENAVIR), and valacyclovir (VALTREX).
[b]Also abacavir (ZIAGEN), didanosine (VIDEX), and stavudine (ZERIT).
[c]Also fosamprenavir (LEXIVA, TELZIR), ritonavir (NORVIR), lopinavir with ritonavir (KALETRA), saquinavir (INVIRASE), and others.

OVERVIEW

Viruses are obligate intracellular parasites that use the host cell's metabolic pathways for reproduction. This limits the number of potential sites for antiviral drug action. Furthermore, antibacterial and antifungal drugs have little or no effect on viruses. Despite these obstacles, effective antiviral compounds have been developed for the treatment of some viral infections. These include herpesvirus infections, human immunodeficiency virus (HIV) infection, influenza, and hepatitis.

Most antiviral drugs, which are antimetabolites of endogenous nucleosides, prevent the replication of viral nucleic acid. Other antiviral drugs inhibit the entry, uncoating, or release and spread of the virus. Other targets for antiviral therapy are currently being investigated.

DRUGS FOR HERPESVIRUS INFECTIONS

All herpesviruses are DNA viruses. The most common examples are **herpes simplex virus** (HSV), **varicella-zoster virus** (VZV), and **cytomegalovirus** (CMV).

HSV frequently causes **herpes genitalis** (genital herpes infection), **herpes labialis** (infection of the lips and mouth),

469

or **herpetic keratoconjunctivitis** (infection of the cornea and conjunctiva). Less commonly, it causes **herpetic encephalitis,** a potentially fatal disease.

VZV is the cause of **chickenpox (varicella)** and **shingles (herpes zoster).** Chickenpox occurs primarily in young children. Shingles, which is reported more frequently in the elderly, results from activation of latent VZV in dorsal root ganglia. In patients with shingles, pain and skin lesions occur in areas where the virus travels peripherally along sensory nerves to the corresponding cutaneous or mucosal surfaces. The skin lesions eventually heal but can leave residual scars. Postherpetic neuralgia is a common and disabling complication of shingles.

CMV infections in immunocompetent individuals are usually asymptomatic. Symptomatic **CMV diseases,** such as **retinitis, esophagitis,** and **colitis,** are seen most often in immunocompromised patients, including those with HIV infection or acquired immunodeficiency syndrome (AIDS).

Numerous drugs are available to treat herpesvirus infections. With the exception of **foscarnet,** all of the drugs are nucleoside analogues.

Nucleoside Analogues

Drug Properties

CHEMISTRY AND MECHANISMS. Most of the nucleoside analogues used to treat herpesvirus infections contain a naturally occurring purine or pyrimidine base combined with a synthetic carbohydrate moiety.

The nucleoside analogues are prodrugs that are phosphorylated by viral and host cell kinases to form active triphosphate metabolites (Figure 43–1). In this process, the nucleoside analogues are initially converted to monophosphate metabolites by a virus-encoded thymidine kinase. The conversion occurs only in infected host cells, thereby contributing to the selective toxicity of the analogues. Host cell kinases subsequently convert the monophosphates to active triphosphate metabolites. The active metabolites then compete with endogenous nucleoside triphosphates and competitively inhibit viral DNA polymerase which, in turn, prevents the synthesis of viral DNA. Some nucleoside analogues (e.g., acyclovir) are incorporated into nascent viral DNA and cause DNA chain termination because they lack the 3′-hydroxyl group required for attachment of the next nucleoside (see Fig. 43–1). Other analogues (e.g., ganciclovir and penciclovir) inhibit viral DNA polymerase but do not cause DNA chain termination.

PHARMACOKINETICS AND INDICATIONS. The properties and clinical uses of individual drugs for herpesvirus infections are compared in Tables 43–1 and 43–2.

VIRAL RESISTANCE. The incidence of resistance to the nucleoside analogues varies with the drug and viral pathogen.

Resistance of HSV and VZV to acyclovir is not common, and resistant strains are usually less infective than are sensitive strains. Furthermore, most acyclovir-resistant HSV and VZV strains are not resistant to other nucleoside analogues or to foscarnet. Most acyclovir-resistant strains have been recovered from immunocompromised patients. Loss of thymidine kinase activity is the major cause of innate and acquired resistance to acyclovir.

Resistance of CMV to ganciclovir is a more serious clinical problem than is HSV resistance, but most ganciclovir-resistant CMV strains are sensitive to cidofovir and foscarnet. Loss of a virus-specific protein kinase is the major cause of resistance to ganciclovir.

Acyclovir, Famciclovir, and Valacyclovir

Acyclovir, famciclovir, and valacyclovir are nucleoside analogues that are effective in the treatment of various HSV and VZV infections (see Table 43–2). These drugs are not sufficiently active against CMV to be effective in treating CMV infections, but acyclovir and valacyclovir can be used for **prophylaxis of CMV infections,** such as in bone marrow and organ transplant recipients and in persons with HIV infection. All three drugs are available for oral use. In addition, acyclovir is available for intravenous and topical use.

The intravenous form of acyclovir is the most effective treatment for serious herpesvirus infections, including herpetic encephalitis and severe HSV and VZV infections in immunocompromised patients.

The topical form of acyclovir can be used to treat herpes genitalis and mild mucocutaneous infections in immunocompromised patients. In cases of herpes genitalis, however, the topical form is less effective than the oral form of acyclovir.

In its oral form, acyclovir has a relatively low bioavailability (22%). Valacyclovir, which was developed later than acyclovir, is a prodrug that is rapidly converted to acyclovir by intestinal and hepatic enzymes and is more completely absorbed than acyclovir. Because of its greater bioavailability (55%), valacyclovir requires less frequent administration than acyclovir. Famciclovir has the greatest bioavailability (80%) and is rapidly hydrolyzed to penciclovir following its absorption.

When acyclovir, famciclovir, or valacyclovir is given orally for the treatment of herpes genitalis, it prevents the replication of HSV and thereby reduces pain and other symptoms of acute infection. It also shortens the time to healing of lesions and reduces the amount of viral shedding. It does not eliminate the virus, and recurrent episodes of infection are common. Shorter courses of therapy are usually sufficient for these episodes, because recurrent infections are usually milder than the initial infection. Severe herpes genitalis may require **intravenous acyclovir** therapy.

When acyclovir, famciclovir, or valacyclovir is given orally for the treatment of **shingles,** it shortens the duration of acute illness, acute pain, and postherpetic pain (neuralgia). In patients with shingles, famciclovir and valacyclovir appear to be more effective than acyclovir. The newer drugs allow for less-frequent administration and provide higher serum drug levels because of their greater oral bioavailability. A new vaccine has been shown to reduce the incidence and severity of herpes zoster infections in older adults.

Acyclovir is available in an oral suspension for the treatment of children with chickenpox. The drug has a good safety record in this setting.

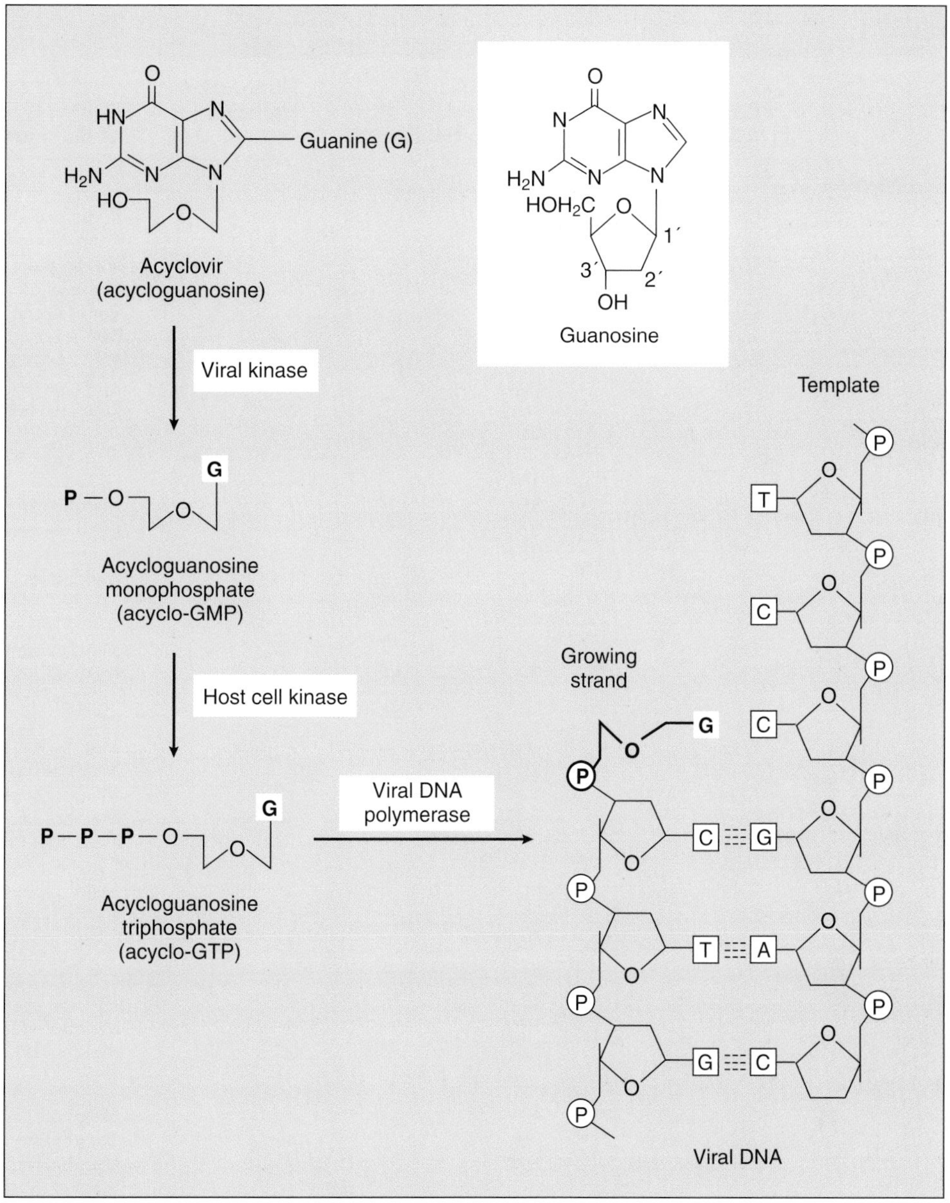

Figure 43–1. **Mechanisms of action of nucleoside analogues used in the treatment of viral infections.** Acyclovir and other nucleoside analogues are converted to active nucleoside triphosphates by viral and host cell kinases. These active nucleoside triphosphates compete with the corresponding endogenous nucleoside triphosphates and competitively inhibit viral DNA polymerase. Acyclovir and the nucleoside reverse transcriptase inhibitors (NRTIs) are incorporated into viral DNA and cause chain termination because they lack the 3'-hydroxyl group required to attach the next nucleoside. Ganciclovir and penciclovir do not cause chain termination.

Acyclovir, famciclovir, and valacyclovir are well tolerated when given orally, and they do not have significant interactions with other drugs. Gastrointestinal disturbances, headache, and rash are the most common side effects. Intravenous administration of acyclovir can produce phlebitis and reversible renal dysfunction.

Penciclovir

Penciclovir, the active metabolite of famciclovir, is now available in a topical cream formulation for the treatment of **herpes labialis.** In a study of patients with a history of frequent herpes labialis episodes, use of penciclovir was found to shorten the time to healing and the duration of pain by about a day. It also was found to decrease the duration of viral shedding.

Ganciclovir and Cidofovir

Ganciclovir and cidofovir are nucleoside analogues used to prevent and treat CMV diseases, including retinitis, esophagitis, and colitis. Both drugs are available for intravenous use, and ganciclovir is also available for oral use. Ganciclovir is usually given initially, whereas cidofovir is generally reserved for diseases that are resistant to ganciclovir or other drugs. Ganciclovir has a relatively low oral bioavailability, so oral administration is used only for long-term suppression of CMV retinitis. Cidofovir can be given intravenously for this purpose.

Ganciclovir is about 100 times more active against CMV than is acyclovir. Ganciclovir, however, produces a much

TABLE 43–1. **Pharmacokinetic Properties of Antiviral Drugs***

Drug	Route of Administration	Oral Bioavailability (%)	Elimination Half-Life (Hours)	Routes of Elimination
Drugs for Herpesvirus Infections				
Acyclovir	Oral, IV, or topical	22	3	Renal excretion
Cidofovir	IV	NA	2.5	Renal excretion
Famciclovir	Oral	80	2	Metabolism; renal and fecal excretion
Ganciclovir	Oral or IV	8	4	Renal excretion
Penciclovir	Topical	NA	NA	NA
Trifluridine	Topical ocular	NA	NA	NA
Valacyclovir	Oral	55	3	Renal excretion
Foscarnet	IV	NA	5	Renal excretion
Drugs for HIV Infection				
NRTI				
Didanosine	Oral	30	2	Metabolism; renal excretion
Lamivudine	Oral	85	6	Renal excretion
Stavudine	Oral	85	3.5	Renal excretion
Zidovudine	Oral or IV	65	1	Metabolism; renal excretion
NNRTI				
Efavirenz	Oral	50	65	Metabolism; fecal excretion
Nevirapine	Oral	92	30	Metabolism; fecal excretion
Protease inhibitors				
Atazanavir	Oral	Dose-dependent	7	Metabolism
Ritonavir	Oral	80	4	Metabolism; fecal excretion
Saquinavir	Oral	12	12	Metabolism; fecal excretion
Lopinavir	Oral	80	6	Metabolism; fecal excretion
Other drugs				
Enfuvirtide	Subcutaneous	NA	3	Metabolism
Maraviroc	Or	25	16	Metabolism
Raltegravir	Oral	Unknown	9	Fecal and renal excretion of glucuronide metabolite
Drugs for Influenza				
Oseltamivir	Oral	75	8	Metabolism, Renal excretion
Zanamivir	Nasal	NA	U	Metabolism; renal excretion
Drugs for Other Viral Infections				
Interferon alfa-2b	Subcutaneous	NA	7	Metabolism
Peginterferon alfa-2b	Subcutaneous	NA	40	Metabolism
Ribavirin	Inhalation or IV	NA	9.5	Metabolism; renal excretion

*Values shown are the mean of values reported in the literature.
HIV = human immunodeficiency virus; IM = intramuscular; IV = intravenous; NA = not applicable; NNRTI = nonnucleoside reverse transcriptase inhibitor; NRTIs = nucleoside reverse transcriptase inhibitor; U = unknown.

TABLE 43–2. **Use of Drugs for Treating Herpesvirus Infections**

Drug	Herpes Genitalis	Herpes Labialis	Herpetic Keratoconjunctivitis	Herpetic Encephalitis	Chickenpox	Shingles	Cytomegalovirus Diseases
Acyclovir	Yes	Yes	No	Yes	Yes	Yes	No[†]
Cidofovir	No	No	No	No	No	No	Yes*
Famciclovir	Yes	Yes	No	No	No	Yes	No
Foscarnet	Yes*	No	No	No	No	Yes*	Yes*
Ganciclovir	No	No	No	No	No	No	Yes
Penciclovir	No	Yes	No	No	No	No	No
Trifluridine	No	No	Yes	No	No	No	No
Valacyclovir	Yes	Yes	No	No	No	Yes	No[†]

*For treating patients with intolerance of or resistance to other drugs.
[†]Can be used for prophylaxis but not for treatment.

higher incidence of adverse effects than do acyclovir and famciclovir. The most common serious adverse effects of ganciclovir are leukopenia and thrombocytopenia. Severe myelosuppression is more likely if the drug is given concurrently with zidovudine. Other adverse effects of ganciclovir include retinal detachment, liver and renal dysfunction, rash, fever, and gastrointestinal disturbances.

Cidofovir sometimes causes nephrotoxicity, neutropenia, metabolic acidosis, and other serious adverse effects. About 25% of patients have discontinued cidofovir because of serious adverse effects. The drug is contraindicated in patients who are taking other nephrotoxic drugs, such as aminoglycosides or amphotericin B.

Trifluridine

Trifluridine is administered topically to treat ocular herpesvirus infections. It is the most widely used nucleoside analogue in patients with **herpetic keratoconjunctivitis** and **epithelial keratitis** (inflammation caused by infection of the cornea), and it is usually effective in treating infections that are not responsive to idoxuridine or vidarabine. The drug is generally well tolerated but can cause superficial ocular irritation and hyperemia.

Other Drugs for Herpesvirus Infections

Foscarnet is a pyrophosphate derivative that blocks the pyrophosphate-binding sites on viral DNA polymerase and prevents attachment of nucleotide precursors to DNA. Unlike the nucleoside analogues used to treat herpesvirus infections, foscarnet does not require activation by viral or host cell kinases.

Foscarnet is active against CMV, VZV, and HSV. It must be administered **intravenously** and is used to treat CMV retinitis in patients with AIDS and to treat acyclovir-resistant HSV infections and shingles. Foscarnet can be combined with ganciclovir to treat infections that are resistant to either drug alone.

Adverse reactions to foscarnet include renal impairment and acute renal failure, hematologic deficiencies, cardiac arrhythmias and heart failure, seizures, and pancreatitis. Renal toxicity can be minimized by administering intravenous fluids to induce diuresis before and during foscarnet treatment.

DRUGS FOR HUMAN IMMUNODEFICIENCY VIRUS INFECTION

Remarkable advances have been made in the treatment of HIV infection and AIDS. Many new drugs have been introduced, and the combined use of two or more drugs from different classes has been shown to markedly reduce viral loads and improve survival in many HIV-positive individuals. This type of multidrug treatment for HIV infection has been called **highly active antiretroviral therapy (HAART)**. Initially, HAART regimens were quite complicated and required multiple doses of several drugs throughout the day.

In recent years, emphasis has been placed on developing and using drug regimens that require only a few doses a day. This has been accomplished by developing longer-acting drugs and combination drug products.

Sites of Drug Action

HIV is an RNA **retrovirus**. Its replication and sites of drug action are depicted in Figure 43–2. Viral replication begins when **glycoprotein 120** on the surface of HIV-1 binds to the CD4 (cell differentiation-4) antigen on the surface of HIV-specific helper lymphocytes (CD4 cells). Binding of glycoprotein 120 to CD4 causes a conformational change in glycoprotein 120, enabling it to interact with the **chemokine co-receptor** (CCR5 or CXCR4) on the lymphocyte surface. These events expose a virus fusion protein, **glycoprotein 41**, which undergoes a conformational change so it can insert a hydrophobic tail into the host cell membrane and bind host cell integrins, leading to fusion of the viral and host cell membranes and transfer of the viral genome into the cytoplasm.

Once HIV enters the CD4 cell, viral RNA serves as a template to produce a complementary doubled-stranded DNA in a reaction catalyzed by viral **reverse transcriptase** (RNA-dependent DNA polymerase). The viral DNA then enters the host cell nucleus and is incorporated into the host genome in a reaction catalyzed by **HIV integrase**. Eventually, the viral DNA is transcribed and translated to produce large, nonfunctional polypeptides called **polyproteins.** These polyproteins are packaged into immature virions at the cell surface. An enzyme called **HIV protease** cleaves the polyproteins into smaller, functional proteins in a process called **viral maturation** as the virions are released into the plasma.

The drugs now available for treatment of HIV infection include those that inhibit fusion and entry, reverse transcriptase, integrase strand transfer, and protease.

Reverse Transcriptase Inhibitors

The two most important types of **reverse transcriptase inhibitors** are the **nucleoside reverse transcriptase inhibitors** (NRTIs) and the **nonnucleoside reverse transcriptase inhibitors** (NNRTIs). Small amounts of the NRTI are converted to their active triphosphate metabolites by host cell kinases. The triphosphate metabolites (nucleotides) compete with the corresponding endogenous nucleoside triphosphates for incorporation into viral DNA in the reaction catalyzed by reverse transcriptase. Once incorporated into DNA, the NRTIs cause DNA chain termination in the same manner as described earlier for acyclovir (see Fig. 43–1). The NRTIs also inhibit host cell DNA polymerase to varying degrees, and this may account for some of their toxic effects (e.g., anemia).

Unlike the NRTIs, the nonnucleoside drugs bind directly to reverse transcriptase and disrupt the catalytic site. Hence, the NNRTIs do not require phosphorylation for activity. Because they act by different mechanisms, the NRTIs and NNRTIs exhibit synergistic inhibition of HIV replication when they are given concurrently.

Tenofovir disoproxil fumarate, a diphosphonate diester of a nucleoside drug, is classified as a **nucleotide reverse transcriptase inhibitor** (a nucleotide being a phosphate

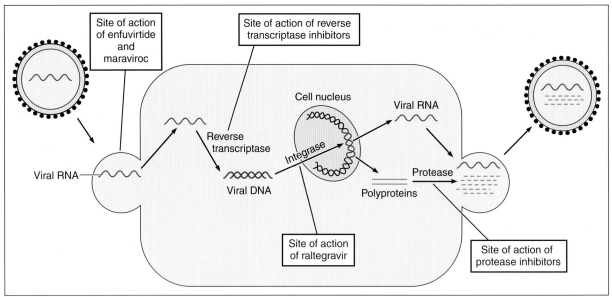

Figure 43-2. **Sites of action of drugs for human immunodeficiency virus (HIV) infection.** Enfuvirtide inhibits the fusion of HIV with host CD4 cell membranes. After the virus penetrates the host cell and becomes uncoated, the viral RNA is transcribed by reverse transcriptase to form viral DNA. Viral DNA is incorporated into the host genome in the cell nucleus by HIV integrase. The viral DNA is then transcribed to RNA. Viral RNA is incorporated into new virions and is translated to synthesize polyproteins. The polyproteins are cleaved into viral proteins by HIV protease as the new virions are released from the cell.

ester of a nucleoside). As a nucleotide prodrug, tenofovir disoproxil fumarate is hydrolyzed in the body to form tenofovir, and then tenofovir is converted to tenofovir diphosphate by CD4 cell kinases. Tenofovir diphosphate competes with deoxyadenosine 5'-triphosphate and is incorporated into viral DNA by reverse transcriptase, causing DNA chain termination. Hence, tenofovir is similar to the NRTI in its manner of activation and mechanism of action.

Nucleoside Reverse Transcriptase Inhibitors

The NRTIs were the first class of drugs developed for the treatment of HIV-positive individuals, and they are included in almost all HIV treatment regimens. Although all NRTIs have the same basic mechanism of action, different drugs in the class serve as antimetabolites of different purine and pyrimidine bases of DNA. For this reason, an NRTI is often more effective when it is given in combination with another NRTI than when it is given alone. As shown in Table 43–3, two NRTIs are usually combined with either an NNRTI or a protease inhibitor.

Drug Properties

CHEMISTRY AND PHARMACOKINETICS. The NRTIs are synthetic derivatives of naturally occurring nucleosides. Didanosine is a purine base congener, whereas lamivudine, stavudine, emtricitabine, and zidovudine are pyrimidine base congeners. All of the NRTIs can be given orally, and zidovudine can also be given intravenously. The NRTIs cross the blood-brain barrier and are distributed to the cerebrospinal fluid. The drugs are eliminated primarily by renal excretion, and renal impairment will prolong their plasma elimination half-life and may necessitate a reduction in dosage.

SPECTRUM AND INDICATIONS. The NRTIs are the foundation of chemotherapy for HIV infection. In addition to inhibiting the replication of human and animal retroviruses, some of the NRTIs have demonstrated activity against hepatitis B virus and Epstein-Barr virus.

VIRAL RESISTANCE. Resistance to NRTIs can develop during therapy and is more likely to occur in persons receiving single-drug therapy for 6 months or longer. Studies of zidovudine indicate that HIV type 1 (HIV-1) acquires resistance to the drug in a stepwise manner involving four or five specific mutations in the gene that encodes the reverse transcriptase enzyme. Because the virus undergoes frequent mutations, the only way to prevent resistance is to prevent HIV replication by using combination drug therapy. Resistance to lamivudine is associated with a mutation at codon 184 in the HIV reverse transcriptase gene. Reduced sensitivity of hepatitis B virus to lamivudine is related to mutations in the catalytic domain of hepatitis B virus DNA polymerase.

ADVERSE EFFECTS AND INTERACTIONS. As shown in Table 43–4, the NRTIs differ in their major toxicities and in their interactions with other drugs. Zidovudine produces bone marrow suppression and can cause anemia and neutropenia. Didanosine and stavudine can cause pancreatitis, and didanosine can also cause peripheral neuropathy. Abacavir is more likely to cause a hypersensitivity reaction, whereas tenofovir produces renal impairment in some patients.

Specific Drugs

Zidovudine, also known as **azidothymidine,** was the first NRTI to be developed, and it is still one of the most widely used drugs in this class. Zidovudine is most often combined today with lamivudine or emtricitabine. It is available in fixed-dose combination products with lamivudine and with

TABLE 43-3. Regimens for Initial Treatment of HIV Infection in Adults and Adolescents*
To construct an antiretroviral regimen, select one component from column A and one component from column B.

	COLUMN A NNRTI OR PI OPTIONS	COLUMN B DUAL NRTI OPTIONS
Preferred Components	NNRTI: efavirenz PI: atazanavir, fosamprenavir, or lopinavir; each in combination with ritonavir	abacavir + lamivudine or tenofovir + emtricitabine
Alternatives to Preferred Components	NNRTI: nevirapine PI: atazanavir, fosamprenavir, lopinavir, or saquinavir; each in combination with ritonavir	zidovudine + lamivudine or didanosine + (emtricitabine or lamivudine)

*Issued January 29, 2008. For details and updates, see http://AIDSinfo.nih.gov.
NRTI = nucleoside reverse transcriptase inhibitor; NNRTI = nonnucleoside reverse transcriptase inhibitor; PI = protease inhibitor.

TABLE 43-4. Most Important Adverse Effects and Interactions of Drugs for Human Immunodeficiency Virus (HIV) Infection

Drug	Adverse Effects and Interactions
NRTI	
All NRTI	Lactic acidosis, hepatic steatosis, and lipodystrophy (all higher with stavudine)
Abacavir	Hypersensitivity reactions
Didanosine	Pancreatitis, peripheral neuropathy, gastrointestinal intolerance
Stavudine	Pancreatitis, peripheral neuropathy
Tenofovir	Headache, gastrointestinal intolerance, renal impairment
Zidovudine	Headache, gastrointestinal intolerance, bone marrow suppression
NNRTI	
All NNRTI	Rash, drug interactions
Efavirenz	Neuropsychiatric reactions, teratogenic
Nevirapine	Hepatotoxicity, rash including Stevens-Johnson syndrome, induces metabolism of protease inhibitors and contraceptive steroids
Protease Inhibitors	
All protease inhibitors	Lipodystrophy (fat accumulation), hyperlipidemia, insulin resistance and diabetes, liver dysfunction and hepatitis; inhibit metabolism of other drugs including protease inhibitors, antiarrhythmic agents, opioids, and tricyclic antidepressants
Atazanavir	PR interval prolongation
Fosamprenavir	Gastrointestinal intolerance, rash
Lopinavir, ritonavir	Gastrointestinal intolerance
Other Drugs	
Enfuvirtide	Injection site reactions, hypersensitivity reactions
Maraviroc	Upper respiratory symptoms, possible hepatotoxicity
Raltegravir	Headache, diarrhea, nausea, vomiting

NRTI = nucleoside reverse transcriptase inhibitor; NNRTI = nonnucleoside reverse transcriptase inhibitor.

lamivudine and abacavir. Zidovudine and stavudine are not used together because they appear to be antagonistic.

Studies indicate that zidovudine treatment significantly reduces the incidence of **in utero transmission of HIV** from infected pregnant women to their offspring. To prevent transmission, zidovudine is administered from the 14th to the 34th week of gestation. Many authorities now recommend combination drug therapy for pregnant women with HIV infection.

Lamivudine, or **3-thiacytosine**, appears to cause fewer adverse effects than do other NRTIs. Lamivudine is often used in combination with zidovudine or stavudine. Combination therapy with these drugs produces a greater reduction in viral load than is obtained with single-drug therapy, and it also decreases the risk for emergence of

drug resistance. Lamivudine is also used in the treatment of **hepatitis B virus**.

Emtricitabine, or fluorothiacytidine, is a newer NRTI that is usually combined with zidovudine or **tenofovir.** A combination product containing emtricitabine and tenofovir intended for once-daily administration is under development.

Stavudine and **didanosine** are used as alternatives to first-line drugs, such as in cases where a first-line drug is not tolerated or when viral resistance occurs. For example, stavudine usually is used as a substitute for zidovudine in persons who cannot tolerate it or fail to respond to it. Didanosine, or **dideoxyinosine**, is mainly used in combination with lamivudine or emtricitabine plus a protease inhibitor.

Nonnucleoside Reverse Transcriptase Inhibitors

Drug Properties

The NNRTIs include efavirenz, nevirapine, and delavirdine. These drugs directly inhibit reverse transcriptase. Unlike NRTIs, NNRTIs do not require metabolic activation, and they are not incorporated into viral DNA. Delavirdine is no longer recommended for most patients with HIV infection because of its modest antiviral activity. Efavirenz is the preferred NNRTI for the initial treatment of patients with HIV infection.

PHARMACOKINETICS. The NNRTIs are administered orally and have good oral bioavailability (see Table 43–1). They are highly lipophilic, and the concentrations that they reach in the central nervous system are adequate for antiviral activity. The drugs are extensively metabolized before undergoing fecal and renal excretion.

ACTIVITY, INDICATIONS, AND VIRAL RESISTANCE. In vitro studies show that NNRTIs act synergistically with NRTIs and protease inhibitors against HIV. The NNRTIs are never used alone to treat patients with HIV infection, because viral resistance develops rapidly unless they are combined with other drugs.

Preferred and alternative treatment regimens are listed in Table 43–3.

ADVERSE EFFECTS AND INTERACTIONS. NNRTIs are moderately well tolerated. **Rash** is the most common side effect. In patients with a mild rash, the drugs can usually be continued or restarted. Patients should be monitored, however, because the rash can progress to Stevens-Johnson syndrome. Efavirenz is teratogenic in primates and should be avoided in pregnant women and women who may become pregnant. Efavirenz can also cause neuropsychiatric reactions. Drug interactions and other common adverse effects of NNRTIs are listed in Table 43–4.

Efavirenz

Efavirenz is the most potent NNRTI currently available. Unlike other NNRTIs, efavirenz can be taken once a day. For these reasons, it is the preferred NNRTI for initial treatment of most adult patients with HIV infection.

Nevirapine

Nevirapine is most often used in combination with two NRTIs (see Table 43–3). Nevirapine induces cytochrome P450 and accelerates the metabolism of certain drugs (see Table 43–4). In addition to skin rash, it can also cause hepatotoxicity.

Protease Inhibitors

HIV protease cleaves the **gag-pol** (group-specific antigen-polymerase) polyprotein to provide functional viral proteins and is essential for the **maturation** of the virus. Protease inhibitors bind the active site of the enzyme and inhibit proteolytic activity, resulting in production of immature, noninfectious viral particles.

Saquinavir, the first HIV protease inhibitor (PI), was approved in 1995, ushering in a new era in the treatment of HIV infection and AIDS. Other PIs were subsequently developed, including **lopinavir** and **ritonavir.** More recently, PIs that are better tolerated and have improved pharmacokinetic properties were introduced, including **atazanavir** and **fosamprenavir.**

Because ritonavir inhibits the metabolism of other PIs, it is often combined with other PIs to increase their plasma levels and duration, and this is known as **boosted therapy.** Ritonavir is used in combination with atazanavir, fosamprenavir, lopinavir, and saquinavir, and combination drug products are available (see Table 43–3).

Tables 43–1 and 43–4 compare information on the properties, effects, and interactions of selected PIs. Figure 43–2 shows the site of action of these drugs.

PHARMACOKINETICS. PIs are given orally and are extensively metabolized by cytochrome P450 enzymes before undergoing fecal excretion.

ACTIVITY, INDICATIONS, AND VIRAL RESISTANCE. PIs are synergistic with NRTIs and are often combined in treatment regimens. Administration of a PI and two NRTIs significantly reduces viral load, increases CD4 cells, and slows the clinical progression of disease and the emergence of drug resistance. Resistance to PIs is associated with the accumulation of mutations resulting in amino acid substitutions at 11 residue positions in the viral protease. Varying degrees of cross-resistance occur between different PIs, but cross-resistance between PIs and reverse transcriptase inhibitors is rare. The preferred PI and NRTI combinations are listed in Table 43–3.

ADVERSE EFFECTS AND INTERACTIONS. All PIs can cause lipid accumulation in tissues (lipodystrophy) and hyperlipidemia, insulin resistance and diabetes, elevated liver function tests, and drug interactions. Ritonavir appears to produce the highest incidence of adverse effects, whereas atazanavir is better tolerated that most other PIs and has a lower propensity to cause diarrhea, lipodystrophy, and hyperlipidemia.

PIs interact with a number of other drugs (see Table 43–4) via inhibition of cytochrome P450 enzymes. They have the greatest effect on drugs metabolized by the CYP3A4 isozyme, and they can cause a several-fold increase in the plasma concentration of these drugs and other PIs. The NNRTI nevirapine can induce the metabolism and decrease the therapeutic effect of PIs.

Fusion and Entry Inhibitors

Maraviroc and **enfuvirtide** are newer drugs that inhibit the fusion and entry of HIV. They are active against HIV strains that are resistant to reverse transcriptase and protease inhibitors, and they are approved for treatment of HIV infection caused by drug-resistant strains. In this setting, these drugs have been shown to decrease viral loads, increase CD4 cells, and improve symptoms.

Maraviroc is an **antagonist** of **chemokine co-receptor 5** (CCR5). Maraviroc binds to CCR5 and prevents interaction with HIV-1 glycoprotein 120 (see above) that is necessary for CCR5-tropic HIV-1 to enter cells. The drug does not bind CXCR4 and is only active against CCR5-tropic HIV strains. It has been shown to have a synergistic effect with enfuvirtide.

Enfuvirtide (T-20) is a large peptide that **binds to HIV glycoprotein 41** and thereby blocks the fusion process. Because of its peptide structure, enfuvirtide is not active when given orally and must be injected subcutaneously twice daily. This injection often causes injection site reactions, which can be minimized by rotating injection sites. Enfuvirtide is otherwise well tolerated and is approved for use in both adults and children. In clinical trials called TORO-1 and TORO-2 (T-20 vs. optimized Regimen only, 1/2), enfuvirtide was given to patients who had developed resistance to other antiretroviral drugs. In these studies, enfuvirtide—in combination with an optimized regimen of antiretroviral agents—caused a significantly greater decrease in viral loads and a significantly greater increase in CD4 cell counts than did the other antiretroviral agents given alone. Enfuvirtide appears to represent a valuable alternative to other anti-HIV drugs when drug resistance or intolerance occurs.

Integrase Strand Transfer Inhibitor

Integrase incorporates the viral DNA formed by reverse transcriptase into the DNA of CD4 cells through a multistep process. First, integrase removes the last nucleotide from both 3-prime ends of the viral DNA strand to enable formation of a preintegration complex between viral DNA, integrase, and other viral and host cell proteins. This complex is able to pass from the cell cytoplasm into the nucleus where integrase randomly incorporates viral DNA into the host chromosome by DNA strand transfer.

Raltegravir is the first **integrase strand inhibitor** to be approved for treating HIV infections. It appears that raltegravir prevents DNA strand transfer by binding divalent cations in the catalytic core of integrase that are required for interaction of the enzyme with host cell DNA.

Raltegravir has potent in vitro activity against wild-type and multidrug-resistant HIV strains, and it is approved for the treatment of HIV-1 infection in adult patients who have HIV-1 strains that are resistant to multiple antiretroviral agents and who show evidence of increased viral replication. Clinical trials found that raltegravir, when used in combination with other antiretroviral agents, decreased viral loads and increased CD4 cells in comparison with placebo.

Raltegravir is given orally twice daily without regard to food and its terminal half-life is about 9 hours. Headache, diarrhea, nausea, and vomiting were most common adverse effects in clinical trials. The drug is not a substrate for cytochrome P450 enzymes and does not appear to inhibit or induce these enzymes.

Treatment Considerations

The decision to initiate therapy for HIV infection is based on several considerations, including the patient's CD4 count (expressed in terms of the number of T cells per microliter [μL]), the patient's viral load (expressed in terms of the number of HIV **RNA copies per milliliter** [**mL**]), and whether the patient has clinical symptoms of disease.

Symptomatic patients should be offered treatment regardless of CD4 cell count and viral load. **Asymptomatic patients** with less than 200 CD4 cells/μL should be treated, and those with more than 200 but less than 350 cells/μL should be considered for treatment. For asymptomatic patients with more than 350 cells/μL, some clinicians recommend treatment if the viral load is more than 100,000 copies/mL.

Drug regimens for treating HIV infection in adults and adolescents are listed in Table 43–3. The preferred regimens for initial drug therapy consist of two NRTIs and either an NNRTI or a PI. The NNRTI-based regimens are the simplest to take, and the formulation containing tenofovir, emtricitabine, and efavirenz in a single pill allows for once-daily dosing. PI-based regimens usually include ritonavir, may be dosed once or twice daily, and generally require more pills in the regimen, although the pill burden associated with PI-based regimens has decreased over the years.

To determine the response to therapy, viral loads should be measured 2 to 8 weeks after beginning therapy and every 3 to 4 months thereafter. The time course of the response is highly variable. Viral suppression can take many months in patients with high viral loads.

The main reasons for changing medication after initiating therapy are treatment failure and drug toxicity. Treatment failure is indicated by increased viral loads and decreased CD4 cells. If the patient fails to respond to a drug regimen, the new regimen should include at least two new drugs. **Drug resistance testing** can provide useful information concerning the selection of alternative therapy. Alternative drug combinations are listed in Table 43–3. If dose-limiting or intolerable toxicity occurs, the clinician should choose alternative drugs that cause a lower incidence of the particular adverse effects experienced by the patient.

DRUGS FOR INFLUENZA

Because **influenza** is one of the most common causes of infectious disease-related deaths, efforts have been made to develop methods to prevent and treat illness caused by this RNA virus. Vaccines are the primary means of prevention, but neuraminidase inhibitors are useful for prophylaxis during outbreaks and can shorten the duration of illness in infected persons (Box 43–1).

Adamantanes

The adamantanes, **amantadine** and **rimantadine,** are synthetic tricyclic amine compounds that block the **M2 proton-selective ion channel** and prevent acidification of influenza type A virus and the fusion of viral membranes and endosomes required for **uncoating** and transfer of viral nucleic acid into the host cell cytoplasm.

Adamantanes have previously been used for prevention and treatment of influenza A, but not influenza B. However, the recent emergence of **resistant strains** has rendered these agents ineffective, and adamantanes are not currently recommended for prophylaxis and treatment of influenza in the United States. Whether influenza strains will evolve which are sensitive to these drugs is uncertain. Other drugs that target the M2 proton-selective ion channel are being developed.

CASE PRESENTATION: A 20-year-old student presents to the university health clinic complaining of chills, fever, sore throat, cough, chest discomfort, severe myalgia, and extreme tiredness that began about 12 hours ago. Examination reveals a temperature of 102° F, nonexudative pharyngitis, nasal discharge, and scattered rhonchi upon chest auscultation. A nasal aspirate is subjected to a rapid test for influenza nucleoproteins and is found to be positive. The patient is started on oseltamivir and acetaminophen and is sent to the clinic infirmary for bed rest. She is instructed to use an ear-loop face mask in the presence of others. Her symptoms improve over the next 48 hours, and she has an uneventful recovery.

CASE DISCUSSION: Influenza is a seasonal respiratory infection caused by influenza type A and type B viruses. Hand washing and influenza vaccines are the primary means of prevention, but the vaccines often fail to include strains that cause influenza outbreaks because vaccine strains must be selected many months before the next flu season begins. The presentation of influenza varies considerably, and it may be difficult to distinguish it from other upper respiratory infections. However, patients with influenza usually have a higher fever and more severe constitutional symptoms, such as myalgia, compared to those with other infections. The availability of rapid tests has improved diagnostic accuracy. These tests can be performed in as little as 10 minutes and usually cost less than $20 (US). The rapid diagnostic tests are highly specific but their sensitivity, typically 70% to 80%, is less than with viral culture methods that require more time and expense. Hence, clinical judgment is still important in diagnosing influenza. Treatment of influenza includes antipyretic agents such as acetaminophen, antiviral agents, and bed rest. Oseltamivir and zanamivir are the only drugs that are effective against current strains of influenza, and they are useful for both prophylaxis and treatment.

Neuraminidase Inhibitors

Oseltamivir and zanamivir inhibit the enzyme **neuraminidase (sialidase)** in **influenza A** and **B** viruses. These drugs were designed to bind to the active site of neuraminidase based on studies of its crystalline structure.

Neuraminidase catalyzes reactions that promote viral spreading and infection. First, neuraminidase catalyzes the **release of virions** from the surface of infected cells following viral replication. Secondly, neuraminidase inactivates respiratory tract mucus that would otherwise prevent **spreading of virions** through the respiratory tract. Neuraminidase accomplishes this by cleaving **sialic acid residues** attached to mucous proteins.

Oseltamivir and zanamivir are active against essentially all strains of influenza A and B viruses, and they are active against the H5N1 avian influenza virus. Although drug-resistant mutants may occur, such mutants are less virulent than their drug-sensitive predecessors and spread less easily. **Oseltamivir** can be used for either prophylaxis or treatment of influenza in patients who are at least 1 year of age. If administered within 48 hours after the onset of symptoms, it decreases **symptom severity** and reduces the **duration of illness.** For treatment of influenza, oseltamivir is administered orally twice a day for 5 days, and it is given once daily for prophylaxis. **Zanamivir** is administered as a nasal spray twice daily for treatment of influenza treatment in persons who are at least 7 years of age, and for prophylaxis in persons at least 5 years of age. Because it is administered intranasally, it should not be used by patients with underlying airway disease, such as asthma or emphysema.

The adverse effects of neuraminidase inhibitors are usually mild and transient, consisting of minor respiratory and gastrointestinal reactions.

DRUGS FOR HEPATITIS

Lamivudine inhibits the replication of **hepatitis B virus** and has been approved as the first orally effective drug for patients with hepatitis B virus. As discussed earlier in this chapter, the drug also inhibits the replication of HIV. Unlike HIV, which is an RNA virus, hepatitis B is a DNA virus. Lamivudine is active against hepatitis B virus because the replication of this virus depends on reverse transcription of an intermediate RNA. Reverse transcription produces a negative-sense strand of DNA. The negative-sense DNA then serves as a template for synthesis of positive-sense DNA.

Ribavirin is active against **hepatitis A** and **C viruses,** whereas **interferon-alfa** is active against **hepatitis B** and **C alfa viruses.** Hepatitis A and C viruses are both RNA viruses.

DRUGS FOR OTHER VIRAL INFECTIONS

Ribavirin

MECHANISM OF ACTION. Ribavirin is a synthetic guanosine analogue that acts by several mechanisms to inhibit the synthesis of viral nucleic acid. Ribavirin is activated by kinases that phosphorylate the drug. The active metabolites disrupt cellular **purine metabolism** by inhibiting inosine monophosphate dehydrogenase and thereby causing a deficiency of guanosine triphosphate. This deficiency, in turn, inhibits the synthesis of viral DNA and RNA. Unlike acyclovir and some reverse transcriptase inhibitors, ribavirin also inhibits the synthesis of host cell nucleic acid, and this may account for some of the toxicity of ribavirin.

PHARMACOKINETICS, SPECTRUM, AND INDICATIONS. Table 43–1 outlines the pharmacokinetic properties of ribavirin.

The drug is a **broad-spectrum antiviral** drug that is active in vitro against a wide range of RNA and DNA viruses. These include adenovirus, Colorado tick fever virus, Crimean-Congo hemorrhagic fever virus, Hantaan virus, hepatitis A and C viruses, herpesviruses, influenza A and B viruses, Lassa virus, measles virus, Muerto Canyon fever virus, mumps virus, respiratory syncytial virus, Rift Valley fever virus, and yellow fever virus.

Although ribavirin has been successfully used to treat infections caused by several of these viruses, the only indication approved by the U.S. Food and Drug Administration is for the treatment of **severe respiratory syncytial virus infection.** For the treatment of neonates with this type of infection, ribavirin is administered by aerosol, using a small-particle aerosol generator. Influenza has also been treated by aerosol administration, whereas most other viral infections have been treated by intravenous administration.

ADVERSE EFFECTS AND INTERACTIONS. When ribavirin is given by inhalation, it can cause serious pulmonary and cardiovascular effects, including apnea, pneumothorax, worsening of respiratory status, and cardiac arrest. When the drug is given intravenously, seizures can occur. Ribavirin is teratogenic in animals, and its use is contraindicated in pregnant or lactating women. Ribavirin antagonizes the antiviral effects of zidovudine and zalcitabine, so concurrent therapy with these drugs should be avoided.

Interferons

Interferons are now available through recombinant DNA technology for the treatment of several viral infections, as well as for the treatment of neoplasms and other conditions (see Chapter 45). The interferon preparations available today for treating viral and neoplastic diseases include several alpha interferons (alpha-2a, alpha-2b, and alpha-n3, and pegylated alpha-2b) and a type 1 interferon (alphacon-1). **Pegylated interferon alpha-2b** (peginterferon alpha-2b) consists of a covalent conjugate of recombinant alpha interferon with **polyethylene glycol**. Pegylation significantly increases the half-life (40 hours) and duration of action of the interferon. Therefore, this preparation is only given once a week for 1 year, rather than several times a week as are other interferon preparations.

CHEMISTRY AND MECHANISMS. The interferons are a group of naturally occurring proteins produced by host cells in response to a viral infection. The interferons have multiple immunomodulating effects and antiproliferative effects, and their most important mechanisms of action in the treatment of specific disorders are uncertain. The antiviral activity of interferons results in part from induction of proteins that inhibit viral penetration or uncoating, inhibit viral peptide elongation, or degrade viral messenger RNA (mRNA).

PHARMACOKINETICS, SPECTRUM, AND INDICATIONS. The alpha interferon preparations are active against **hepatitis viruses** and against some **papillomaviruses.** They are used in the treatment of hepatitis B, hepatitis C, non-A, non-B or non-C hepatitis (chronic, active hepatitis), genital warts (condyloma acuminatum), hairy cell leukemia, chronic myelocytic leukemia, Kaposi's sarcoma, renal carcinoma, malignant melanoma, and multiple myeloma.

Treatment with interferon produces clinical remission in some patients with **hepatitis B** or **hepatitis C** virus. Interferon preparations used in treating patients with hepatitis are interferon alpha-2a, interferon alpha-2b, and pegylated interferon alpha-2b. Except for pegylated interferon, the drugs are administered subcutaneously or intramuscularly three times a week for at least 12 months. In patients with hepatitis C virus, combination therapy with interferon and ribavirin produced a higher response rate than therapy with either drug alone. Some studies showed that pegylated interferon alpha-2b produced better results than conventional alpha-2b.

In clinical studies of chronic hepatitis B, interferon treatment was found to result in loss of hepatitis B antigens, normalization of serum aminotransferase activity, sustained histologic improvement, and a lower risk of progression of liver disease in about one third of the patients. AIDS patients with hepatitis B, however, responded poorly to interferon treatment.

Interferon-alpha is also effective in the treatment of **anogenital warts (condylomata acuminata)**, which are caused by several types of papillomavirus. For this infection, the interferon is injected directly into the lesions three times a week for 3 weeks, with a repeated course of treatment after 12 to 16 weeks.

ADVERSE EFFECTS. Interferons can cause many serious and unpleasant adverse effects, including hematologic toxicity, cardiac arrhythmias, changes in blood pressure, central nervous system dysfunction, gastrointestinal distress, chills, fatigue, headache, and myalgia.

SUMMARY OF IMPORTANT POINTS

- Acyclovir, famciclovir, penciclovir, and valacyclovir are nucleoside analogues used to treat HSV and VZV infections.

- Trifluridine is a nucleoside analogue used to treat herpetic keratoconjunctivitis.

- Cidofovir and ganciclovir are nucleoside analogues used for the prevention and treatment of CMV diseases (e.g., retinitis, esophagitis, and colitis).

- Valacyclovir is a prodrug that is converted to acyclovir in vivo. It has better oral bioavailability than acyclovir.

- Acyclovir, ganciclovir, and penciclovir are selectively phosphorylated to their monophosphate metabolites by viral kinases, and then host cell kinases convert them to triphosphates. Other nucleoside analogues, including those for treating HIV infection, are phosphorylated only by host cell kinases.

- Acyclovir and most NRTIs cause chain termination when they are incorporated into viral DNA. Ganciclovir and penciclovir inhibit viral DNA polymerase but are not incorporated into viral DNA.

■ Foscarnet is a nonnucleoside drug used to treat CMV retinitis and acyclovir-resistant HSV and VZV infections.

■ Drugs for HIV infection include agents that inhibit reverse transcriptase, HIV protease, integrase strand transfer (raltegravir), and HIV fusion (maraviroc and enfuvirtide). Drug combinations act synergistically to reduce viral loads, increase CD4 cells, and ameliorate symptoms. The most commonly used combinations consist of two NRTIs plus either a protease inhibitor or an NNRTI.

■ Frequently used NRTIs include zidovudine, tenofovir and lamivudine. Zidovudine can cause anemia and neutropenia.

■ Examples of PIs include lopinavir and ritonavir. Efavirenz is a frequently used NNRTI.

■ Some PIs and NNRTIs interact with other drugs via inhibition or induction of cytochrome P450 isozymes.

■ Oseltamivir and zanamivir, neuraminidase inhibitors that inhibit the release and spreading of influenza A and B virions, are used in prophylaxis and treatment of influenza.

■ Ribavirin is a broad-spectrum antiviral drug used to treat respiratory syncytial virus infection in neonates, and hepatitis C in combination with interferon-alpha.

■ Interferon-alfa is used to treat hepatitis B, hepatitis C, and anogenital warts. Lamivudine, an NRTI, is also used to treat hepatitis B.

Review Questions

1. A man with HIV infection is taking an agent that prevents viral maturation. Which adverse effect is typically associated with this type of drug?
   (A) anemia
   (B) pancreatitis
   (C) neuropsychiatric reactions
   (D) peripheral neuropathy
   (E) lipodystrophy

2. A patient with shingles receives a drug that is converted to penciclovir in the body. Which antiviral action is exerted by this agent?
   (A) blockade of purine biosynthesis
   (B) inhibition of DNA polymerase
   (C) inhibition of viral entry
   (D) DNA chain termination
   (E) prevention of viral maturation

3. A woman with an upper respiratory infection is treated with an agent that is administered by nasal inhalation. Which step in viral replication is prevented by this drug?
   (A) entry into host cells
   (B) uncoating of viral nucleic acid
   (C) replication of viral nucleic acid
   (D) maturation of viral proteins
   (E) release of progeny virions

4. A man with immunodeficiency syndrome being treated for a severe herpesvirus infection develops acute renal insufficiency and tachycardia. Which drug is he most likely receiving?
   (A) foscarnet
   (B) trifluridine
   (C) acyclovir
   (D) famciclovir
   (E) ganciclovir

Answers and Explanations

1. **The answer is E:** lipodystrophy. Protease inhibitors prevent viral maturation by preventing cleavage of polyproteins into functional proteins such as reverse transcriptase. Anemia (Option A) is most often caused by zidovudine. Pancreatitis (Option B) and peripheral neuropathy (Option D) are associated with didanosine and stavudine. Neuropsychiatric reactions (Option C) may be caused by efavirenz.

2. **The answer is B:** inhibition of DNA polymerase. The patient received famciclovir, which is converted to penciclovir in the body. The active triphosphate metabolite of penciclovir inhibits viral DNA polymerase, but it is not incorporated into nascent DNA to cause chain termination (Option D). Penciclovir has no direct effect on purine biosynthesis (Option A), viral entry (Option C), or viral maturation (Option E).

3. **The answer is E:** release of progeny virions. The woman most likely has influenza and was treated with zanamivir nasal spray. Zanamivir and oseltamivir inhibit viral neuraminidase and the release and spread of progeny virions. They do not affect entry into host cells (Option A), uncoating or replication of viral nucleic acid (Options B and C), or maturation of viral proteins (Option D).

4. **The answer is A:** foscarnet. Foscarnet is an alternative drug for treating herpesvirus infections due to strains that are resistant to nucleoside analogues such as acyclovir and ganciclovir. Foscarnet may cause renal failure, cardiac arrhythmias, hematologic deficiencies, and other adverse effects. Nucleoside analogues (Options B, C, D, and E) do not cause these adverse effects.

SELECTED READINGS

American Academy of Pediatrics Committee on Infectious Diseases. Antiviral therapy and prophylaxis for influenza in children. Pediatrics 119: 852–860, 2007.

Chacko, M., and J.M. Weinberg. Famciclovir for cutaneous herpesvirus infections: an update and review of new single-day dosing indications. Cutis 80:77–81, 2007.

Correll, T., O.M. Klibanov. Integrase inhibitors: a new treatment option for patients with human immunodeficiency virus infection. Pharmacotherapy 28:90–101, 2008.

Panel on Antiretroviral Guidelines for Adults and Adolescents. Guidelines for the use of antiretroviral agents in HIV-1-infected adults and adolescents. U.S. Department of Health and Human Services, January 29, 2008 (http://AIDSinfo.nih.gov)

CHAPTER 44

Antiparasitic Drugs

CLASSIFICATION OF ANTIPARASITIC DRUGS*

Drugs for Infections Caused by Lumen- and Tissue-Dwelling Protozoa
- Metronidazole (FLAGYL)
- Tinidazole (TINDAMAX)
- Paromomycin (HUMATIN)
- Diloxanide
- Iodoquinol (YODOXIN)
- Nitazoxanide (ALINIA)

Drugs for Infections Caused by Blood- and Tissue-Dwelling Protozoa
Drugs for Malaria
- Artesunate
- Artemether
- Chloroquine
- Primaquine
- Atovaquone with Proguanil (MALARONE)
- Artemether with Lumefantrine (COARTEM)
- Pyrimethamine with Sulfadoxine (FANSIDAR)

Drugs for Toxoplasmosis
- Spiramycin
- Pyrimethamine with Sulfadiazine

Drugs for Other Protozoan Infections
- Melarsoprol (ARSOBAL)
- Pentamidine (NEBUPENT)[a]

Drugs for Helminth Infections
Drugs for Nematode Infections
- Albendazole (ALBENZA)[b]
- Pyrantel pamoate
- Ivermectin (STROMECTOL)
- Diethylcarbamazine

Drugs for Trematode and Cestode Infections
- Praziquantel (BILTRICIDE)

Drugs for Ectoparasite Infestations
- Permethrin (ACTICIN)

[a]Also miltefosine, nifurtimox, and suramin.
[b]Also mebendazole and thiabendazole.
*Additional drugs are included in Table 44–1.

OVERVIEW

Endoparasitic infections are extremely common in many parts of the world, particularly in areas where the climate is warm and moist, the sanitation is poor, and insects and other vectors of disease are prevalent. In fact, billions of people in tropical and subtropical regions are infected with protozoa (single-cell organisms that dwell in the lumen, tissue, or blood) and helminths (worms, including nematodes, trematodes, and cestodes). Factors, such as immigration, an increase in the number of international travelers, and an increase in the number of individuals who have acquired immunodeficiency syndrome (AIDS) and are therefore at

greater risk for opportunistic infections, have all increased the probability that physicians will see endoparasitic infections that were rarely found in their usual patient population.

Since 1960, the introduction of new drugs has enabled remarkable advances in the chemotherapy of some endoparasitic infections. Albendazole and mebendazole have significantly improved the treatment of several intestinal nematode infections, whereas praziquantel has revolutionized the treatment of trematode and cestode infections. At the same time, metronidazole and tinidazole have provided more-effective and less-toxic drugs for the treatment of amebiasis, giardiasis, and trichomoniasis. The sites and mechanisms of action of selected antiparasitic drugs are depicted in Figure 44–1.

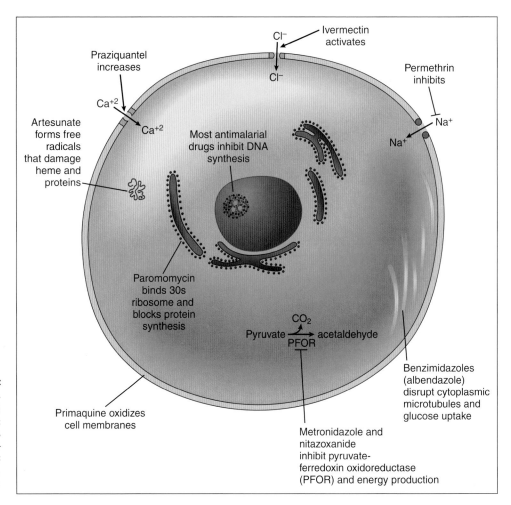

Figure 44-1. Sites of action and mechanisms of antiparasitic drugs. The sites and mechanisms of antiparasitic agents include cell membranes and ion channels, energy metabolism enzymes, cytoplasmic microtubules, DNA synthesis, ribosomal protein synthesis, and free radical damage.

Unlike endoparasitic infections, **ectoparasitic infestations** are caused by organisms that live on the skin or hair shafts of patients. The most common examples are the **lice** and **mites** that cause pediculosis and scabies, respectively.

Table 44–1 provides information about the causes and treatment of numerous protozoan infections, helminthic infections, and ectoparasitic infestations. The antiparasitic agents that are commonly used or represent pharmacologic advances are discussed in this chapter. In some cases, an antibacterial or antifungal agent (e.g., tetracycline or amphotericin B) is listed as either a preferred or alternative drug; these agents are discussed in earlier chapters. A detailed discussion of other agents listed in the table is beyond the scope of this chapter.

DRUGS FOR INFECTIONS CAUSED BY LUMEN- AND TISSUE-DWELLING PROTOZOA

Amebiasis, balantidiasis, cryptosporidiosis, giardiasis, and trichomoniasis are examples of infections caused by protozoan parasites that dwell in the lumen and tissues of their human hosts. Among the agents used to treat these infections are metronidazole, tinidazole, iodoquinol, and paromomycin (see Table 44–1).

Metronidazole

Drug Properties

CHEMISTRY AND PHARMACOKINETICS. Metronidazole is a nitroimidazole compound. It is well absorbed from the gut and is widely distributed to tissues and fluids throughout the body, including the liver and central nervous system (CNS). The drug is extensively metabolized before undergoing renal excretion. Metronidazole is usually administered orally, although an intravenous preparation is available for use in patients with severe infections.

SPECTRUM AND MECHANISMS. Metronidazole is active against several anaerobic protozoa that commonly cause infection. These include *Entamoeba histolytica* (the agent of amebiasis); *Giardia intestinalis* (*G. lamblia*); *Trichomonas vaginalis* (trichomoniasis); and *Balantidium coli* (balantidiasis). Metronidazole is also active against anaerobic bacteria, including *Bacteroides fragilis*, *Helicobacter pylori*, and *Clostridium difficile*.

A number of anaerobic organisms express **pyruvate-ferredoxin oxidoreductase**, an enzyme not found in mammalian cells, which is involved in energy production, carbon recycling, and other metabolic functions. In susceptible anaerobic protozoa, this enzyme transfers electrons to the nitro

TABLE 44–1. Causes and Treatment of Parasitic Infections and Infestations

Condition	Common Pathogens	Primary Drugs	Alternative Drugs
Intestinal Protozoan Infections			
Amebiasis	Entamoeba histolytica	Metronidazole or tinidazole followed by paromomycin or iodoquinol	Diloxanide
Balantidiasis	Balantidium coli	Tetracycline	Metronidazole
Cryptosporidiosis	Cryptosporidium parvum	Nitazoxanide*	Antidiarrheal medication
Dientamoeba infection	Dientamoeba fragilis	Iodoquinol	Tetracycline, metronidazole, or paromomycin
Giardiasis	Giardia intestinalis	Metronidazole or tinidazole	Nitazoxanide, paromomycin
Microsporidiosis	Encephalitozoon and Enterocytozoon species	Albendazole	Fumagillin
Extraintestinal Protozoan Infections			
Amebic meningoencephalitis	Naegleria fowleri	Amphotericin B; azithromycin	
Babesiosis	Babesia microti	Atovaquone + azithromycin	Clindamycin + quinine
Leishmaniasis	Leishmania species	Miltefosine	Amphotericin B, antimony drug, fluconazole (cutaneous infections)
Malaria	Plasmodium vivax or P. ovale	Primaquine + chloroquine	Primaquine + quinine and doxycycline
	Chloroquine-sensitive P. falciparum	Chloroquine (if sensitive)	Quinine + doxycycline; mefloquine; halofantrine
	Chloroquine-resistant P. falciparum	Quinine + doxycycline or FANSIDAR†; atovaquone + proguanil	Artesunate + mefloquine
Toxoplasmosis	Toxoplasma gondii	Pyrimethamine + sulfadiazine; spiramycin	Trimethoprim + sulfamethoxazole
Trichomoniasis	Trichomonas vaginalis	Metronidazole or tinidazole	
Trypanosomiasis (African sleeping sickness)	Trypanosoma brucei	Pentamidine (early disease); melarsoprol (late CNS disease)	Suramin
Trypanosomiasis, American (Chagas' disease)	Trypanosoma cruzi	Nifurtimox	Benznidazole
Intestinal Nematode Infections			
Ascariasis	Ascaris lumbricoides	Albendazole or mebendazole	Pyrantel pamoate
Capillariasis	Capillaria philippinensis	Mebendazole	Albendazole
Pinworm infection	Enterobius vermicularis	Albendazole or mebendazole	Pyrantel pamoate
Hookworm infection	Ancylostoma duodenale and Necator americanus	Albendazole or mebendazole	Pyrantel pamoate
Strongyloidiasis	Strongyloides stercoralis	Ivermectin	Thiabendazole
Whipworm infection	Trichuris trichiura	Albendazole	Mebendazole
Extraintestinal Nematode Infections			
Cutaneous larva migrans	Ancylostoma braziliense	Ivermectin	Albendazole
Guinea worm	Dracunculus medinensis	Surgical removal + metronidazole	Mebendazole
Filariasis, lymphatic	Wuchereria bancrofti; Brugia malayi and B. timori	Ivermectin	Diethylcarbamazine
Filariasis, cutaneous	Loa loa	Diethylcarbamazine	Ivermectin
River blindness	Onchocerca volvulus	Ivermectin + prednisone	
Trichinosis	Trichinella spiralis	Albendazole + prednisone	Mebendazole + prednisone
Trematode Infections			
Schistosomiasis	Schistosoma species	Praziquantel	Oxamniquine for S. mansoni
Chinese liver fluke	Clonorchis sinensis	Praziquantel	Albendazole
Sheep liver fluke	Fasciola hepatica	Triclabendazole	Bithionol
Lung fluke	Paragonimus westermani	Praziquantel	Bithionol
Cestode Infections			
Beef tapeworm	Taenia saginata	Praziquantel	Niclosamide
Pork tapeworm	Taenia solium	Praziquantel	Niclosamide
Cysticercosis	Larval T. solium	Albendazole for CNS disease + dexamethasone	Praziquantel
Dog tapeworm	Dipylidium canium	Praziquantel	Niclosamide
Dwarf tapeworm	Hymenolepis nana	Praziquantel	
Fish tapeworm	Diphyllobothrium latum	Praziquantel	Niclosamide

(Continued)

TABLE 44–1. Causes and Treatment of Parasitic Infections and Infestations*—cont'd

Condition	Common Pathogens	Primary Drugs	Alternative Drugs
Echinococcosis (hydatid disease)	Echinococcus granulosus	Aspiration + albendazole	
Ectoparasite Infestations			
Head lice, crabs	Pediculus humanus, Phthirus pubis	Permethrin	Lindane, malathion
Scabies (mites)	Sarcoptes scabiei	Permethrin	Lindane, oral ivermectin

*For patients with AIDS, nitazoxanide alone or paromomycin plus azithromycin may be prescribed.
†FANSIDAR contains pyrimethamine and sulfadoxine.
CNS = central nervous system.

group of metronidazole to form free nitro-radicals that attack DNA and proteins and thereby produce a cytotoxic effect.

INDICATIONS. Metronidazole, the drug of choice for **amebiasis, giardiasis,** and **trichomoniasis,** is also used as an alternative drug in the treatment of **balantidiasis.**

Patients with amebiasis can suffer from intestinal infection, with or without dysentery, hepatic abscesses, or other extraintestinal manifestations of disease. Metronidazole acts primarily as a tissue amebicide and is usually given in combination with a luminal amebicide (e.g., iodoquinol) to eradicate intestinal amebas.

Giardiasis causes abdominal discomfort and diarrhea in persons infected with the cyst form of *Giardia.* In the western United States, *Giardia* cysts are sometimes present in contaminated streams and ponds and are ingested by campers. The administration of metronidazole for 5 days usually cures the infection.

Trichomoniasis is a sexually transmitted disease that produces vaginitis in women but is usually asymptomatic in men. To prevent reinfection, it is important to treat patients and their sexual partners. Treatment can consist either of a single large dose of metronidazole or of smaller doses taken over a 7-day period.

Metronidazole is also used in the management of several disorders that are not caused by protozoa. For example, it is sometimes used in the treatment of patients with **dracunculiasis (guinea worm infection).** This infection is caused by *Dracunculus medinensis,* a nematode found in India, Pakistan, and parts of Africa. Although metronidazole is not curative, it reduces inflammation and facilitates manual removal of the worm. Metronidazole is considered the drug of choice for **enterocolitis** caused by *C. difficile,* and it is occasionally used to treat infections caused by other anaerobic bacteria. Metronidazole is available in gel or cream form for the topical treatment of **rosacea (acne rosacea),** a skin condition characterized by persistent erythema of the middle third of the face and other areas of the body.

ADVERSE EFFECTS AND INTERACTIONS. Metronidazole is usually well tolerated, but it causes considerable gastrointestinal discomfort in some persons. Other adverse effects include nausea, vomiting, a metallic taste, and transient leukopenia or thrombocytopenia. To reduce the gastrointestinal side effects, patients should take metronidazole with food.

Metronidazole increases the anticoagulant effect of warfarin, so the dosage of warfarin should be adjusted as necessary. Metronidazole also causes a disulfiram-like reaction with ethanol, so patients should avoid drinking alcohol while they are undergoing treatment.

Metronidazole has been shown to be mutagenic in bacteria and mammalian cell cultures. Although retrospective studies of women who took the drug during pregnancy failed to reveal an increased incidence of birth defects or cancer, it appears prudent to avoid prescribing the drug to women during their first trimester of pregnancy whenever possible.

Tinidazole

Tinidazole is a second-generation nitroimidazole similar to metronidazole but active against metronidazole-resistant strains of *Trichomonas vaginalis.* As with metronidazole it is indicated for the treatment of **trichomoniasis, giardiasis, intestinal amebiasis,** and **amebic liver abscess.** It is also active against *Helicobacter pylori* and anaerobic bacteria, including *Bacteroides fragilis,* and it is approved for treating bacterial vaginosis due to *Gardnerella vaginalis.*

In clinical trials, a single dose of tinidazole cured 93% of patients with giardiasis. In persons with symptomatic intestinal amebiasis, a 3-day course of tinidazole resulted in a cure rate of 86% to 93%, and 2 to 5 days of tinidazole cured 81% to 100% of those with amebic liver abscess. In general, tinidazole produced a higher cure rate in a shorter time period than did metronidazole.

Tinidazole is completely absorbed and widely distributed after oral administration. Its plasma half-life of about 13 hours is considerably longer than that of metronidazole (8 hours). Because it is metabolized by cytochrome P450 3A4, its serum concentrations can be affected by other drugs that inhibit or induce this enzyme. As with metronidazole, tinidazole can cause anorexia, nausea, and vomiting, as well as a bitter taste in the mouth, and it is contraindicated in the first trimester of pregnancy.

Iodoquinol, Paromomycin, Diloxanide, and Nitazoxanide

Iodoquinol, paromomycin, and diloxanide furoate act as luminal amebicides but not tissue amebicides. A luminal amebicide can be used alone to treat **asymptomatic carriers of *E. histolytica*,** but it must be used in combination with a tissue amebicide to treat patients with **amebic dysentery** or **liver abscess.** The preferred combination is usually tinidazole

or metronidazole followed by paromomycin or iodoquinol (see Table 44–1). Iodoquinol can also be used to treat infections with *Dientamoeba fragilis*, a lumen-dwelling protozoan parasite that causes **diarrhea** and **abdominal pain**.

Cryptosporidiosis is a diarrheal illness that may cause chronic diarrhea in immunocompromised persons and has been reported in up to 50% of patients with AIDS. **Nitazoxanide** is a new drug with broad-spectrum activity against many intestinal protozoa, including *Cryptosporidium parvum*. The drug is a noncompetitive inhibitor of **pyruvate-ferredoxin oxidoreductase** and is approved for treatment of **cryptosporidiosis** and **giardiasis** in immunocompetent persons. Further studies of nitazoxanide are needed in persons with AIDS. The drug is well tolerated, and a short course of treatment is usually effective. Antidiarrheal medications may also be helpful for these conditions.

DRUGS FOR INFECTIONS CAUSED BY BLOOD- AND TISSUE-DWELLING PROTOZOA

Babesiosis, leishmaniasis, malaria, toxoplasmosis, and trypanosomiasis are examples of infections caused by protozoan parasites that dwell in the blood and tissues of their human hosts.

Drugs for Malaria

Malaria, one of the most common infectious diseases in the world today, is believed to be responsible for more deaths than any other infectious disease. Four species of *Plasmodium* cause malaria: *Plasmodium falciparum, P. malariae, P. ovale,* and *P. vivax.* Most cases of malaria are caused by *P. falciparum* or *P. vivax.* The disease is spread via the bites of female *Anopheles* mosquitoes and is primarily found in tropical and subtropical areas. Malaria has largely been eliminated from industrialized countries in temperate regions, so most infections that are diagnosed in people residing in the United States are infections that were acquired during travel in other countries. Nevertheless, periodic outbreaks of mosquito-borne malaria still occur in the United States.

Malaria is transmitted when infected mosquitoes inject *Plasmodium* sporozoites into the blood of the human host (Figure 44–2). The sporozoites invade the liver, where they undergo schizogony (asexual multiplication) to form tissue schizonts. The multinucleated schizonts divide their cytoplasm to form thousands of merozoites in a process called **exoerythrocytic schizogony**. The merozoites are then released from the liver into the blood, where they infect erythrocytes and undergo **erythrocytic schizogony**. Additional merozoites are subsequently released into the blood by hemolysis.

The synchronous release of merozoites is responsible for the episodic fever observed in patients with malaria. During an infection with *P. falciparum* or *P. vivax,* the fever spikes every other day. The disease produced by *P. falciparum* (malignant tertian malaria) is more severe than that produced by *P. vivax* (benign tertian malaria), partly because *P. falciparum* causes a higher level of parasitemia and produces a

persistently higher temperature during the periods between fever spikes. Whereas both *P. vivax* and *P. ovale* have a persistent exoerythrocytic stage, *P. falciparum* and *P. malariae* do not. To eradicate this persistent stage and prevent the relapse of malaria, patients infected with *P. vivax* or *P. ovale* can be treated with primaquine.

Sites and Mechanisms of Action

Figure 44–2 shows the sites of action of drugs for malaria. Primaquine inhibits exoerythrocytic (hepatic) schizogony. In contrast, all of the other antimalarial agents inhibit erythrocytic schizogony.

The mode of action of **primaquine** is unclear, but the drug appears to act by forming quinoline-quinone intermediates that oxidize schizont membranes. These oxidizing intermediates may also be responsible for the hemolytic effect of the drug.

Chloroquine, mefloquine, and **quinine** are believed to inhibit nucleic acid synthesis or function during erythrocytic schizogony, although the exact mechanisms of action are unclear. Chloroquine may block the synthesis of nucleic acid, and it may also impair the ability of plasmodia to utilize hemoglobin. The selective toxicity of chloroquine can be partly explained by the drug's greater accumulation in infected erythrocytes than in uninfected cells. Quinine appears to form a complex with plasmodial DNA, thereby preventing replication and transcription.

Sulfadoxine is a sulfonamide that acts synergistically with **pyrimethamine** to inhibit the synthesis of folic acid in plasmodia and thereby prevent the synthesis of nucleic acid. The sulfonamides inhibit dihydrofolate formation, whereas pyrimethamine prevents dihydrofolate reduction.

Other drugs used in the treatment of malaria include **artesunate, atovaquone,** and **proguanil.** Proguanil acts by inhibiting folate reductase, and artesunate forms free radicals that damage heme and proteins.

Chloroquine, Quinine, and Quinidine

Quinine, a drug that had been used for centuries to treat malaria, was supplanted by chloroquine after World War II. Until the 1980s, when resistance to chloroquine became widespread, chloroquine remained the drug of choice. Now that drug resistance has severely curtailed the effectiveness of chloroquine, quinine is once again being used to treat malaria in many regions of the world. In addition, other drugs have been introduced.

The only areas where most *P. falciparum* organisms are sensitive to chloroquine are the Caribbean islands, the part of Central America that is west of the Panama Canal, and parts of North and West Africa and the Middle East. In these chloroquine-sensitive areas, chloroquine is still the drug of choice for both the prevention and the treatment of all types of malaria, although it must be used in combination with primaquine (see "Primaquine") to eradicate vivax or ovale malaria.

The most common adverse effects of chloroquine are gastrointestinal distress, nausea, and vomiting. Toxic doses can cause retinal damage and even blindness. In pregnant women, chloroquine should be used cautiously because fetal damage has been reported.

Patients with **chloroquine-resistant malaria** are usually treated with a combination of quinine sulfate plus either

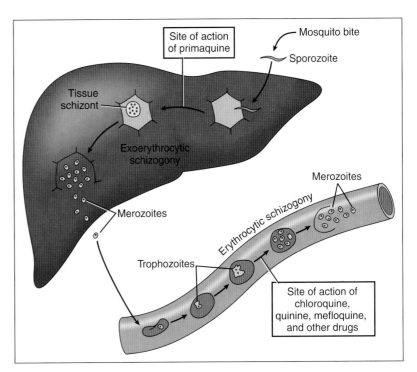

Figure 44-2. Sites of action of drugs for malaria. When a person is bitten by an infected mosquito, *Plasmodium* sporozoites enter the liver, form tissue schizonts, and undergo exoerythrocytic schizogony to produce merozoites. The merozoites that are released from the liver invade erythrocytes and form trophozoites that undergo erythrocytic schizogony. Some trophozoites develop into male and female gametocytes, which must subsequently pass back into a mosquito before they can develop into sporozoites and repeat the infection cycle. Primaquine blocks exoerythrocytic schizogony, whereas other antimalarial drugs inhibit erythrocytic schizogony.

doxycycline or pyrimethamine-sulfadoxine. Alternatives include atovaquone-proguanil and artesunate plus mefloquine.

Mefloquine

Mefloquine is a newer antimalarial drug that has been used for both the prevention and the treatment of chloroquine-resistant malaria. Because cure rates with chloroquine have dropped from almost 100% in the 1980s to 40% by 1995, mefloquine is now primarily used to prevent malaria in areas where chloroquine-resistant strains are prevalent. The drug is given orally, undergoes hepatic metabolism, has a half-life of about 14 days, and is eliminated via the bile and feces.

Mefloquine can cause a severe **neuropsychiatric syndrome** characterized by hallucinations, anxiety, confusion, seizures, and coma. It can also cause leukopenia and thrombocytopenia.

For patients who cannot tolerate mefloquine, doxycycline (see Chapter 39) can be used to prevent malaria in areas where chloroquine-resistant organisms are prevalent.

Primaquine

Primaquine is an 8-aminoquinoline derivative that is active against the exoerythrocytic stage of *P. vivax* and *P. ovale*. By eradicating tissue plasmodia, it prevents the reemergence of organisms from the liver and relapse of the infection. Primaquine must be used in combination with other drugs to treat infection with *P. vivax* or *P. ovale*, because primaquine is not active against the erythrocytic stage of these organisms.

Primaquine is converted to oxidizing quinoline-quinone intermediates in the body. These intermediates are believed to be responsible for the antimalarial effects and some of the toxic effects of the drug. In individuals who have **hereditary glucose-6-phosphate dehydrogenase**

(G6PD) deficiency, the intermediates may oxidize erythrocyte membranes and thereby cause red cell hemolysis and **hemolytic anemia**. This anemia occurs because G6PD is unable to generate sufficient quantities of reduced nicotinamide adenine dinucleotide phosphate to maintain glutathione in its reduced form and thereby prevent oxidation of erythrocyte membranes. Individuals who experience this type of hemolytic anemia are said to have **primaquine sensitivity**. A number of other drugs with oxidizing properties, including sulfonamides and sulfones, can also cause this reaction.

Pyrimethamine and Sulfadoxine

Pyrimethamine is a folate reductase inhibitor that is generally used in combination with a sulfonamide such as sulfadiazine or sulfadoxine. Pyrimethamine and sulfadiazine are used in the treatment of **toxoplasmosis** (a disease discussed in "Drugs for Toxoplasmosis"), whereas pyrimethamine and sulfadoxine are used in the treatment of **malaria**. Some resistance to pyrimethamine-sulfadoxine has been reported in parts of Southeast Asia, the Amazon Basin, sub-Saharan Africa, and Bangladesh.

The adverse effects of pyrimethamine-sulfadoxine include anorexia, nausea, vomiting, megaloblastic anemia, leukopenia, thrombocytopenia, hemolytic anemia, and Stevens-Johnson syndrome with epidermal necrolysis.

Proguanil and Atovaquone

Proguanil, or **chloroguanide**, is a biguanide derivative that acts as a **folate reductase inhibitor**. Sometimes combined with atovaquone to treat chloroquine-resistant malaria, it is available as a fixed-dose combination product.

Atovaquone is a naphthoquinone derivative that has a high level of activity against the erythrocytic stage of all *P. falciparum* strains, including the chloroquine-resistant strains.

The drug should be used in combination with doxycycline (see Chapter 39) or proguanil for the treatment of malaria, because studies indicate that a high rate of relapse occurs when atovaquone is used alone.

Atovaquone is also used in the treatment of *Pneumocystis jiroveci (carinii)* infections.

Artesunate and Artemether

The search for new agents to treat multidrug-resistant falciparum malaria led to the identification of **artemisinin** (*qinghaosu*) as the active ingredient of *Artemisia annua*, a plant used in traditional Chinese medicine for over 2 millennia. Two derivatives of artemisinin were subsequently found to have potent activity against the erythrocytic stages of malaria. These sesquiterpene derivatives are called **artemether** and **artesunate**. These drugs form carbon-centered free radicals that alkylate heme and proteins in malarial parasites and thereby inhibit erythrocytic schizogony.

Artemether and artesunate have been used effectively in the treatment of millions of cases of falciparum malaria in Southeast Asia, sub-Saharan Africa, and elsewhere. The drugs can be administered orally or parenterally. Artesunate can be combined with quinine or mefloquine.

Drugs for Toxoplasmosis

In immunocompetent individuals, *Toxoplasma gondii* infection is common but is rarely symptomatic. Even in cases in which it is symptomatic, treatment is not normally required.

In immunocompromised individuals and congenitally infected neonates, however, *T. gondii* can cause severe damage to many organs. For example, *T. gondii* frequently causes **ocular infections** and **encephalitis** in patients with AIDS and is the most common CNS disease found in these patients. *T. gondii* can cause encephalomyelitis, hydrocephaly, microcephaly, or chorioretinitis in the offspring of women who were infected for the first time during pregnancy. Women who were infected with *T. gondii* before pregnancy are not at risk of transmitting the infection to their offspring.

Although toxoplasmosis is usually treated with **pyrimethamine** plus **sulfadiazine**, this drug combination has some major drawbacks. First, it is not effective against *T. gondii* tissue cysts. Second, the use of pyrimethamine in combination with a sulfonamide drug sometimes induces **folate deficiency** and causes severe hematologic abnormalities and other adverse effects, even when the combination is given in normal doses and for short-term treatment. In patients with AIDS, high doses of pyrimethamine plus sulfadiazine are required to treat toxoplasmosis, and life-long maintenance therapy is often required to prevent reactivation of the disease. In an effort to prevent the adverse hematologic effects of pyrimethamine in these patients, **leucovorin** (folinic acid) can be added to the treatment regimen.

The toxic side effects of pyrimethamine plus sulfadiazine, however, preclude its administration in up to 40% of patients with AIDS. As an alternative, pyrimethamine can be given either with clindamycin or with dapsone.

Spiramycin is a macrolide antibiotic recommended for fetal infection resulting from acute maternal infection during pregnancy.

Drugs for *Pneumocystis jiroveci (carinii)* Infections

Because *Pneumocystis jiroveci*, formerly *Pneumocystis carinii*, has traditionally been classified as a protozoan parasite, it is discussed in this chapter. Results of several studies, however, support the argument that it is actually a fungus. In addition to causing pneumonia in premature and malnourished infants, the organism causes pneumonia and other diseases in immunocompromised persons, including those with AIDS.

The treatment of choice for *P. jiroveci* infections is **trimethoprim-sulfamethoxazole**, a drug combination discussed in Chapter 40. **Atovaquone** (an antimalarial agent discussed earlier in this chapter), and **pentamidine** are alternatives. Other alternatives include dapsone plus trimethoprim or pyrimethamine. Prednisone, a corticosteroid drug, is also administered to acutely ill patients to reduce pulmonary inflammation.

The antimicrobial agents used to treat *Pneumocystis* infections are also used for prophylaxis and for posttreatment suppression of this infection. Pentamidine is given intravenously for the treatment of *P. jiroveci* infections, but it is administered by inhalation to prevent pneumonia. The adverse effects of pentamidine include hematologic toxicity, ventricular tachycardia, edema, pancreatitis, bronchospasm, and Stevens-Johnson syndrome.

Drugs for Other Protozoan Infections

Pentamidine or **suramin**, either given alone or in combination with **melarsoprol**, is used to treat **African trypanosomiasis (sleeping sickness)**, a disease caused by *Trypanosoma brucei*. Pentamidine and suramin are used for the early stages of the infection. Melarsoprol is indicated for use in patients with late CNS manifestations of the disease. These drugs must be administered intravenously and can cause serious toxicity.

Nifurtimox is the drug of choice for the treatment of **American trypanosomiasis (Chagas' disease)**, a disease caused by *Trypanosoma cruzi*. The effectiveness of nifurtimox is limited. Giving interferon-gamma in combination with nifurtimox, however, appears to shorten the acute phase of the illness.

The causes and treatment of **babesiosis** and **leishmaniasis** are outlined in Table 44–1. **Miltefosine** is a new drug for treating **visceral leishmaniasis**, which is also known as **Kala azar** (black fever). Miltefosine is a phosphorylcholine ester of hexadecanol, a membrane-active phospholipid. Miltefosine inhibits key enzymes involved in the metabolism of **glycolipids** found on the surface of *Leishmania* species. It is well absorbed after oral administration and has a half-life of about 8 days. In the past, antimonial drug treatments for leishmaniasis had to be given parenterally for prolonged periods and they caused considerable toxicity. In contrast, miltefosine given orally for 28 days produced a 94% to 97% cure rate of visceral

leishmaniasis in children at the end of treatment and at 6 months follow-up. The most common adverse effects have been vomiting and diarrhea, but they were usually of brief duration and only mild to moderate in severity. A few patients experienced reversible hepatic and renal toxicity. Because of its high efficacy and relatively low toxicity, the availability of miltefosine appears to be a breakthrough in the treatment of visceral and other forms of leishmaniasis (Box 44–1).

DRUGS FOR INFECTIONS CAUSED BY HELMINTHS

Helminths can be classified as **nematodes (roundworms)**, **trematodes (flukes)**, and **cestodes (tapeworms)**. The most common parasites in these groups are listed in Table 44–1 and are responsible for infecting billions of people throughout the world. Effective drugs are available to treat most of the helminthic infections, but the cost of drug treatment is high. Fortunately, the World Health Organization and government agencies have sponsored mass treatment programs that appear to have had a significant impact on some helminthic infections, such as onchocerciasis (river blindness) and schistosomiasis.

Anthelmintic drugs usually act either by inhibiting metabolism in the parasite (as occurs when a benzimidazole drug is used) or by causing muscle paralysis of the parasite (as occurs when ivermectin, praziquantel, or pyrantel is used). The anthelmintic drugs kill the parasites without harming host cells, but the molecular basis for their selective toxicity is not entirely clear. In many cases, a single dose or a few doses of the drug are curative.

Drugs for Nematode Infections

Albendazole, Mebendazole, and Thiabendazole

CHEMISTRY AND PHARMACOKINETICS. Albendazole and related drugs are benzimidazole compounds. Albendazole has poor solubility in water. Only about 5% of an oral dose of the drug is absorbed from an empty stomach. Absorption is markedly improved, however, if the drug is taken with a high-fat meal. Albendazole is converted to albendazole sulfoxide by first-pass hepatic metabolism, and this metabolite accounts for the systemic anthelmintic activity of the drug. Sulfoxidation of albendazole also occurs in the intestinal tract. The level of albendazole in cerebrospinal fluid is about 40% of the level in plasma.

About 10% of mebendazole is absorbed from the gut, metabolized in the liver, and excreted in the urine. In contrast to mebendazole and other benzimidazoles, thiabendazole is well absorbed from the gut, and this may partly account for its higher incidence of adverse effects. Thiabendazole is completely metabolized before undergoing renal excretion.

MECHANISMS. The benzimidazoles bind to β-tubulin and thereby inhibit the polymerization of tubulin dimers to form cytoplasmic microtubules in parasites. This action impairs the uptake of glucose by these organisms and leads to depletion of glycogen stores and decreased production of

BOX 44–1. A CASE OF CUTANEOUS SORES

CASE PRESENTATION: A 42-year-old embassy official in Afghanistan presents to a medical clinic with spreading sores on his left cheek and both arms. The lesions, which developed at the site of insect bites he received several weeks earlier, now measure 2 to 2.5 centimeters in diameter. The sores are blistery in appearance with an indurated edge and a central ulceration. A biopsy of the lesions shows *Leishmania* amastigotes (the form of the parasite found in infected tissue), and an indirect immunofluorescence test is positive for *Leishmania*. After a discussion of treatment options, the patient is given oral miltefosine for 4 weeks. The treatment is well tolerated. However, there is a mild increase in serum aspartate aminotransferase and alanine aminotransferase levels during the first week of therapy, which resolves spontaneously. The lesions gradually improve during the course of therapy, and the skin is completely healed 4 months later.

CASE DISCUSSION: Leishmaniasis is a protozoan infection caused by a number of *Leishmania* species and which is usually transmitted by the bite of tiny female phlebotomine sandflies. The disease is found in many tropical and subtropical countries, ranging from the rainforests of Central and South America to the deserts of North Africa. It is found in India, Iraq, and Afghanistan, as well as in Mexico and southern Texas, and a few cases have been reported recently in northern Texas. Cutaneous leishmaniasis is the most common form of the disease and often heals spontaneously after several months. Visceral leishmaniasis, which may develop from cutaneous lesions, can cause life-threatening spleen and liver damage if not treated. Cutaneous leishmaniasis often begins with small erythematous lesions that develop weeks to months after a sandfly bite and gradually increase in size to several centimeters in diameter. Frequent use of insect repellant and sleeping under a bed net are the best methods of preventing sandfly bites and leishmaniasis. Relatively toxic antimony compounds requiring parenteral administration have been the main treatment for leishmaniasis until recently. Miltefosine is a new orally effective drug that appears to be well tolerated, though gastrointestinal disturbances are common and serum liver enzymes may be elevated by the drug.

adenosine triphosphate. Eventually the organisms are immobilized and die.

SPECTRUM AND INDICATIONS. Albendazole and mebendazole are primarily used to treat intestinal nematode infections, including **ascariasis**, **capillariasis**, **hookworm infection**, **pinworm infection**, and **whipworm infection**. For **trichinosis**, the anthelmintic drug is usually given in combination with a corticosteroid (e.g., prednisone) to relieve the inflammation.

As shown in Table 44–1, albendazole is also used to treat two cestode infections: **cysticercosis** and **echinococcosis**. For echinococcosis, surgical aspiration usually is used in conjunction with albendazole therapy. Treatment is not recommended for cysticercosis outside the CNS, which is benign. For cysticercosis in the CNS, albendazole or praziquantel can be effective along with a corticosteroid (e.g., dexamethasone) to control inflammation caused by cyst death.

Albendazole is also used to treat **microsporidiosis**, an infection caused by several species of intestinal protozoans.

PARASITIC RESISTANCE. Resistance to the benzimidazoles is now a worldwide problem in veterinary medicine, but it is not yet a significant problem in human medicine.

ADVERSE EFFECTS AND CONTRAINDICATIONS. The adverse effects of thiabendazole include anorexia, nausea, vomiting, paresthesias, delirium, and hallucinations. Albendazole and mebendazole are well tolerated and produce fewer adverse effects than thiabendazole does. The most common side effects of albendazole and mebendazole are mild gastrointestinal discomfort and constipation or diarrhea. The high doses of albendazole used to treat echinococcosis can cause hepatitis or hematologic toxicity. All of the benzimidazole drugs are contraindicated during pregnancy because of their potential to inhibit mitosis and impair fetal development.

Pyrantel

Pyrantel is a pyrimidine derivative. The drug activates nicotinic acetylcholine receptors in somatic muscles of nematodes and causes **depolarizing neuromuscular blockade**. A liquid suspension of pyrantel pamoate is administered to children and adults who have **ascariasis**, **hookworm infection**, or **pinworm infection**. The drug is poorly absorbed from the gut and acts primarily within the intestinal tract. It is usually well tolerated, but it can cause abdominal cramps, anorexia, diarrhea, and vomiting.

Ivermectin

CHEMISTRY AND PHARMACOKINETICS. Ivermectin is a semisynthetic derivative of avermectin, an antibiotic containing a macrocytic lactone obtained from *Streptomyces avermitilis*. The drug is well absorbed from the gut, undergoes hepatic biotransformation, and is excreted in the feces with an elimination half-life of about 25 hours.

MECHANISMS. Ivermectin increases the chloride permeability of invertebrate muscle cells. This hyperpolarizes the cell membrane and causes paralysis of the pharyngeal muscles in helminths. Ivermectin is believed to activate the **glutamate-gated chloride channel** in invertebrate tissue, but it has no effect on chloride ion permeability in mammalian tissue.

SPECTRUM AND INDICATIONS. Ivermectin is a broad-spectrum anthelmintic drug that is active against a wide range of nematodes. It has been used to treat a number of intestinal helminthic infections in domestic and companion animals. In humans, it is used to treat **strongyloidiasis**, **onchocerciasis**, and **cutaneous larva migrans**. Ivermectin has revolutionized the management of onchocerciasis. It is active against the microfilariae (skin-dwelling, first-stage larvae) of *Onchocerca volvulus*, even at a very low dosage. When a single dose is administered once a year, it can prevent the ocular form of onchocerciasis, which is called **river blindness**. Repeated treatment is necessary because the drug is not active against the adult parasites and only prevents the maturation of filarial offspring.

Ivermectin is active against all stages of the *Loa loa* parasite and is currently used as an alternative to diethylcarbamazine to treat **loiasis**, a disease that can cause both ocular and skin manifestations. Ivermectin is also active against the microfilariae of *Brugia malayi* and *Wuchereria bancrofti*, parasites that cause **lymphatic filariasis**. Studies show that low doses of the drug kill *W. bancrofti*, whereas higher doses are effective against *B. malayi*. Recently, ivermectin has also been used to treat scabies.

ADVERSE EFFECTS. Ivermectin is usually well tolerated and produces few adverse effects. Uncommonly, it causes constipation, diarrhea, dizziness, vertigo, or sedation.

Diethylcarbamazine

Diethylcarbamazine is a piperazine derivative that is administered orally and is well absorbed from the gut. The drug is partly metabolized and is primarily excreted in the urine. Although it has little activity against the larger nematodes (macrofilariae, such as the pinworm, hookworm, and whipworm), it is active against several microfilariae. Studies suggest that it acts in vivo by inhibiting prostaglandin I_2 (prostacyclin) and prostaglandin E_2, both in host endothelial cells and in filariae. These actions constrict blood vessels and increase aggregation of host granulocytes. Thus, diethylcarbamazine appears to augment the innate immune response to filarial infection.

The administration of diethylcarbamazine produces a rapid filaricidal effect, which sometimes leads to a severe host hypersensitivity response to the dying microfilariae. To prevent such reactions, patients are started on low doses, which are gradually increased as the parasites are eliminated. Otherwise, the drug is well tolerated.

Drugs for Trematode and Cestode Infections

Praziquantel

When praziquantel was introduced in the early 1970s, it revolutionized the treatment of **schistosomiasis**, a disease that can affect a wide range of organs, including the skin, liver, spleen, intestinal and urinary tracts, lungs, brain, and spinal cord. As shown in Table 44–1, it is now the drug of choice for infections caused by several other tissue flukes (trematodes) and tapeworms (cestodes).

CHEMISTRY AND PHARMACOKINETICS. Praziquantel is an orally effective isoquinoline derivative that is not related to any other antiparasitic drug. In patients taking praziquantel, the drug is widely distributed and enters the CNS. It undergoes some first-pass and systemic metabolism, and the parent drug and metabolites are excreted in the urine.

MECHANISMS. Each schistosome is surrounded by a tegument. Praziquantel acts to increase the calcium permeability of the tegument and thereby cause its depolarization. When the outer bilayer of the tegument is damaged, *Schistosoma* antigens that were previously hidden from host defenses are exposed. This enables host immune cells to move in and attack the schistosomes. Thus, praziquantel acts to facilitate host immunity to these flukes. The drug's mechanism of action in other flukes and in tapeworms is unknown but is thought to be similar to that in schistosomes.

SPECTRUM AND INDICATIONS. Praziquantel is active against most tissue flukes, including the Chinese liver fluke (*Clonorchis sinensis*), the lung fluke (*Paragonimus westermani*), and the various *Schistosoma* species that cause human infections. It is also active against the larval form of the pork tapeworm (the cause of cysticercosis) and against the adult forms of the pork, beef, fish, dog, and dwarf tapeworms.

For patients with **schistosomiasis** or **other fluke infections**, three doses of praziquantel are administered in a single day. For patients with **cysticercosis**, three doses of praziquantel are given each day for a period of 2 weeks. If manifestations of **neurocysticercosis** are present, corticosteroids are given before praziquantel treatment. For patients with **adult tapeworm infections**, a single dose of praziquantel is usually effective.

PARASITIC RESISTANCE. Despite intensive use of praziquantel for over 20 years, few cases of parasitic resistance to the drug have been documented.

ADVERSE EFFECTS. Adverse effects are uncommon but include abdominal discomfort, dizziness, drowsiness, and headache.

Other Drugs

Triclabendazole is the drug of choice for the treatment of **sheep liver fluke infection** (*Fasciola hepatica* infection). Bithionol is an alternative drug for the treatment of sheep liver fluke and **lung fluke infection** (*P. westermani* infection).

Oxamniquine is used as an alternative to praziquantel for *Schistosoma mansoni* infections, but it is not useful in treating infections caused by other *Schistosoma* species.

Niclosamide is an alternative to praziquantel for treating cestode infections.

Treatment Considerations

In Africa, Central and South America, and Asia, the use of anthelmintic drugs has evolved from the treatment of individuals to the treatment of populations. This has been possible because of the development of broad-spectrum agents that are effective in a single dose. Albendazole, mebendazole, ivermectin, and praziquantel are examples of drugs that have been successfully used as single-dose therapy to eradicate parasites in a large population.

In most parts of the United States, pinworm infection (enterobiasis) is the most common helminthic infection. It is acquired by ingesting eggs that are initially deposited by the female parasite on the perianal skin and are then transmitted to the mouth via unwashed fingers or fingernails. Contaminated clothing or bedding can also serve as a source of infection. Pinworm infection is often spread to family members, and outbreaks among children are common in day-care settings. For this reason, family members and other close contacts of the patient should be treated at the same time. In cases of pinworm infection, a dose of albendazole, mebendazole, or pyrantel should be followed 2 weeks later by a second dose of the same drug. In cases of whipworm, hookworm, or *Ascaris* infection, a single dose of an appropriate anthelmintic drug (see Table 44–1) is usually effective.

DRUGS FOR INFESTATIONS CAUSED BY ECTOPARASITES

The most common ectoparasites that cause illness in humans are **lice** and **mites**. These parasites cause **pediculosis** and **scabies**, respectively.

Permethrin is the treatment of choice for both types of infestation. The drug is a synthetic pyrethrin-like compound that blocks sodium currents in the neurons of parasites and thereby causes paralysis of the organisms. For pediculosis, a liquid preparation is applied in sufficient volume to saturate the hair and scalp, and then it is rinsed off after 10 minutes. For scabies, a permethrin cream is applied to the skin from head to toe, and it is left on the skin for at least 8 hours before it is washed off. For both types of infestation, a single treatment is usually effective, but it can be repeated in 1 week, if necessary. Resistance to permethrin has been increasing, and new drugs for ectoparasites are needed. Alternative drugs are listed in Table 44–1.

SUMMARY OF IMPORTANT POINTS

■ Metronidazole and tinidazole are the drugs of choice for treating symptomatic amebiasis, giardiasis, and trichomoniasis.

■ Primaquine is the only antimalarial drug that blocks exoerythrocytic schizogony. Chloroquine, quinine, and other antimalarial drugs inhibit erythrocytic schizogony.

■ Many strains of *P. falciparum* have become resistant to chloroquine.

■ Chloroquine is used to prevent malaria in geographic regions without chloroquine-resistant plasmodia. Mefloquine or doxycycline is used to prevent malaria in regions with chloroquine-resistant plasmodia.

■ Chloroquine is used to treat all types of malaria caused by chloroquine-sensitive plasmodia. In cases of vivax or ovale malaria, chloroquine is given in combination with primaquine. Primaquine is active against the persistent tissue phase of *P. vivax* and *P. ovale* and prevents relapses of malaria caused by these organisms.

■ Quinine sulfate is usually given in combination with doxycycline or pyrimethamine-sulfadoxine to treat malaria caused by chloroquine-resistant plasmodia.

■ Toxoplasmosis can be treated with pyrimethamine plus sulfadiazine.

■ Pentamidine or suramin with melarsoprol is used to treat African trypanosomiasis, whereas nifurtimox is used to treat American trypanosomiasis (Chagas' disease).

■ Miltefosine is a newer drug for treating cutaneous and visceral leishmaniasis (Kala azar).

■ Most anthelmintic drugs act either by inhibiting microtubule formation (as occurs when a benzimidazole drug is used) or by causing muscle paralysis of the parasite (as occurs when ivermectin, praziquantel, or pyrantel is used). Praziquantel exposes parasite antigens to host cell immune mechanisms.

■ Albendazole, mebendazole, and pyrantel are used to treat intestinal nematode infections.

■ Diethylcarbamazine and ivermectin are used to treat filarial nematode infections, including river blindness (onchocerciasis). Ivermectin is also used to treat strongyloidiasis and cutaneous larva migrans.

■ Praziquantel is the drug of choice for all forms of schistosomiasis and for most tissue fluke infections and tapeworm infections. Triclabendazole is used to treat sheep liver fluke infections.

■ Permethrin is the drug of choice for the treatment of lice and scabies.

Review Questions

1. A boy is treated with an agent that activates nicotinic acetylcholine receptors in a helminth. Which organism is most likely infecting this patient?
   (A) *Taenia solium*
   (B) *Ascaris lumbricoides*
   (C) *Schistosoma mansoni*
   (D) *Onchocerca volvulus*
   (E) *Trichinella spiralis*

2. A Peace Corps volunteer experiences severe anxiety and hallucinations while taking medication to prevent a protozoan infection. Which drug might be substituted for the offending agent?
   (A) doxycycline
   (B) nitazoxanide
   (C) miltefosine
   (D) primaquine
   (E) tinidazole

3. A susceptible population is treated with a drug to prevent an ocular filarial infection. The permeability of which ion is increased in the parasite by this treatment?
   (A) calcium
   (B) magnesium
   (C) potassium
   (D) sodium
   (E) chloride

4. A man with diarrhea is treated with a drug that inhibits pyruvate-ferredoxin oxidoreductase. He is most likely being treated for which infection?
   (A) whipworm infection
   (B) beef tapeworm infection
   (C) cryptosporidiosis
   (D) trypanosomiasis
   (E) strongyloidiasis

5. A young child with episodic fever is treated with a drug that causes free radical damage to heme and proteins. The child most likely has which infection?
   (A) trypanosomiasis
   (B) leishmaniasis
   (C) amebiasis
   (D) malaria
   (E) toxoplasmosis

Answers and Explanations

1. **The answer is B:** *Ascaris lumbricoides.* The boy received pyrantel, which activates nicotinic receptors in nematodes. It is used to treat ascariasis, pinworm infection, and hookworm infection. Pyrantel is not used to treat cestode, trematode, or filarial infections (Options A, C, and D), and it is not used to treat trichinosis (Option E).

2. **The answer is A:** doxycycline. Neuropsychiatric reactions are most likely to be caused by mefloquine in persons taking the drug for malaria prophylaxis. Doxycycline is a suitable alternative for adult patients. The other options are not effective for malaria prophylaxis or treatment.

3. **The answer is E:** chloride. Onchocerciasis is an ocular filiarial infection that may be prevented by annual administration of ivermectin, a drug that increases chloride permeability and causes hyperpolarization of nematode tissues. Ivermectin does not have any direct effect on sodium, potassium, calcium, or magnesium permeability (Options A through D).

4. **The answer is C:** cryptosporidiosis. Several antiprotozoan agents inhibit pyruvate-ferredoxin oxidoreductase, including metronidazole, tinidazole, and nitazoxanide. Nitazoxanide is used to treat giardiasis and cryptosporidiosis. These drugs are not used to treat intestinal helminth infections or trypanosomiasis.

5. **The answer is D:** malaria. The child is being treated with artesunate or artemether for malaria. These drugs are believed to inhibit erythrocytic schizogony by forming free radicals that damage heme and proteins unique to malarial parasites.

SELECTED READINGS

Aslam, S. and D.M. Musher. Nitazoxanide: clinical studies of a broad-spectrum anti-infective agent. Future Microbiol 2:583–590, 2007.

Beyrer, C., J.C. Villar, V. Suwanvanichkij, S. Singh, S.D. Baral, et al. Neglected diseases, civil conflicts, and the right to health. Lancet 370:619–627, 2007.

Chappuis, F., S. Sundar, A. Hailu, H. Ghalib, S. Rijal, et al. Visceral leishmaniasis: what are the needs for diagnosis, treatment, and control? Nat Rev Microbiol 5:873–882, 2007.

Checkley, A.M., and C.J. Whitty. Artesunate, artemether, or quinine in severe *Plasmodium falciparum* malaria? Expert Rev Anti Infect Ther 5:199–204, 2007.

Falagas, M.E., and I.A. Bliziotis. Albendazole for the treatment of human echinococcosis: a review of comparative clinical trials. Am J Med Sci 334:171–179, 2007.

CHAPTER 45

Antineoplastic and Immunomodulating Drugs

CLASSIFICATION OF ANTINEOPLASTIC AND IMMUNOMODULATING DRUGS

DNA Synthesis Inhibitors
Folate Antagonists
- Methotrexate, Pemetrexed (ALIMTA)

Purine Antagonists
- Cladribine, Clofarabine, Fludarabine, Mercaptopurine, Nelarabine, Thioguanine

Pyrimidine Antagonists
- Capecitabine (XELODA), Cytarabine, Floxuridine, Fluorouracil, Gemcitabine (GEMZAR)

Ribonucleotide Reductase Inhibitor
- Hydroxyurea

DNA Alkylating Drugs
Nitrogen Mustards
- Chlorambucil, Cyclophosphamide (CYTOXAN), Ifosfamide, Mechlorethamine, Melphalan

Nitrosourea Drugs
- Carmustine, Lomustine, Streptozocin

Platinum Compounds
- Cisplatin, Carboplatin, Oxaliplatin

Other DNA Alkylating Drugs
- Busulfan, Dacarbazine, Mitomycin

DNA Intercalating Drugs
- Bleomycin
- Doxorubicin (ADRIAMYCIN), Daunorubicin, Idarubicin
- Mitoxantrone, Dactinomycin

DNA Topoisomerase Inhibitors
- Etoposide, Teniposide
- Irinotecan, Topotecan

Mitotic Inhibitors
- Paclitaxel (TAXOL), docetaxel
- Vincristine (ONCOVIN), Vinblastine, Vinorelbine
- Ixabepilone

Monoclonal Antibodies
- Alemtuzumab, Bevacizumab, Cetuximab, Gemtuzumab Ozogamicin, Panitumumab, Rituximab, Trastuzumab, ^{90}Y-Ibitumomab, ^{131}I-Tositumomab

Protein Kinase Inhibitors
- Dasatinib, Erlotinib, Gefitinib, Imatinib, Lapatinib, Nilotinib, Sorafenib, Sunitinib

Antineoplastic mTOR Inhibitor
- Temsirolimus

Cytokines and Interferons
- Aldesleukin, Interferon alfa-2b

Immunomodulating Drugs
Microbial Products
- Cyclosporine, Sirolimus, Tacrolimus

Monoclonal Antibodies
- Basiliximab, Daclizumab, Muromonab-CD3, Palivizumab

Other Drugs
- Azathioprine, Prednisone
- Thalidomide

OVERVIEW

Cancer occurs when normal cells are transformed into neoplastic cells through alteration of their genetic material, leading to abnormal gene expression. This transformation usually results from genetic mutations that cause expression of oncogenes and inhibition of tumor suppressor genes. Oncogenes encode growth factors, many of which are kinases that activate regulatory proteins that promote cell division. For example, the cyclins are a group of proteins that activate cyclin kinases, leading to activation of enzymes that promote progress through the cell cycle of replication (Fig. 45–1). Some oncogenes express kinases that activate growth factor receptors, such as the epidermal growth factor receptor and the vascular endothelial growth factor receptor. In addition to their uncontrolled proliferation, neoplastic cells often invade previously unaffected organs through a process called metastasis. This process is dependent on angiogenesis, which is the formation of new blood vessels to support metastatic invasion and growth.

Increased understanding of the regulation of cancer cell proliferation has led to the development of drugs that target specific growth factors involved in this process, including agents that inhibit protein kinases and growth factor receptors involved in cell cycle kinetics and metastasis. Drugs that increase cancer cell apoptosis (programmed cell death) are being developed, and it may be eventually possible to develop agents that reverse the malignant transformation of cells.

Antineoplastic drugs can be divided into two broad categories: (1) **cytotoxic agents** that nonspecifically inhibit DNA replication or mitosis, and (2) **targeted anticancer drugs** that inhibit specific proteins involved in tumor cell growth. The introduction of new anticancer drugs has accelerated with the release of a growing number of **monoclonal antibodies** and a plethora of "small molecule" inhibitors of protein kinases linked to growth factor receptors. New cytotoxic agents have also contributed to the explosion of antineoplastic drugs. Significant advances in cancer biology will further accelerate the introduction of new drugs. Because of the growing number of similar antineoplastic agents, this chapter focuses on important examples of each class of anticancer drugs.

PRINCIPLES OF CANCER CHEMOTHERAPY

Uses and Goals of Treatment

Antineoplastic drugs are used to treat **hematologic cancers** that cannot be surgically excised, such as **leukemia** and **lymphoma**. They are also used in combination with surgery or radiation therapy to treat **solid tumors**. In patients with solid tumors that can be surgically removed, chemotherapy may eliminate micrometastases and prevent recurrence of the malignant growth. In patients with inoperable tumors, chemotherapy is often palliative rather than curative.

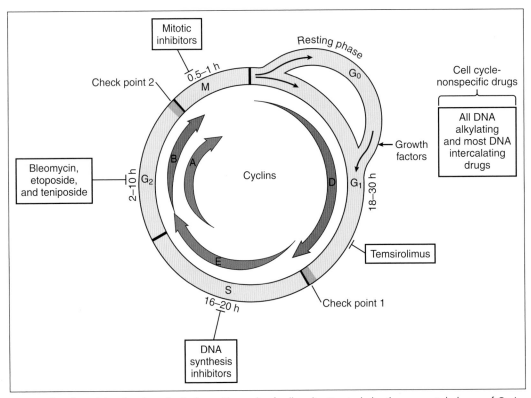

Figure 45–1. Cell cycle activity of antineoplastic drugs. The cycle of cell replication includes the sequential phases of G_1 (gap 1), S (DNA synthesis), G_2 (gap 2), and M (mitosis). Differentiated cells can enter a resting state called G_0. Growth factors may stimulate resting cells to reenter the cell cycle. Progress through the cycle is promoted by proteins called cyclins (A, B, D, E), which are controlled by cyclin-dependent kinases. Two check points, which often malfunction in cancer cells, control entry into the critical phases of DNA synthesis and mitosis. Cell cycle–specific drugs primarily act during the designated phase of the cycle. Cell cycle–nonspecific drugs act throughout the cell cycle.

Palliative therapy is intended to prolong life and reduce incapacitating symptoms.

Treatment Regimens and Schedules

Drug regimens for cancer chemotherapy are designed to optimize the synergistic effects of drug combinations while minimizing toxicity. The regimens often use drugs that have different toxicities and different mechanisms of action to maximize cytotoxic effects on tumor cells while sparing host tissue.

In the treatment of some types of cancer, specific drug regimens are used for induction of remission, consolidation therapy, and maintenance therapy. **Induction therapy**, such as that used in acute lymphocytic leukemia, seeks to produce a rapid reduction in the tumor cell burden and thereby produce a symptomatic response in the patient. **Consolidation therapy** seeks to complete or extend the initial remission, and it often uses a different combination of drugs than that used for induction. **Maintenance therapy** aims to sustain the remission as long as possible, and it can use less-frequent courses of chemotherapy and different classes of drugs than were used for induction and consolidation.

Cancer chemotherapy regimens are probably the most complicated form of drug therapy in use today. These regimens often employ multiple drugs administered as intermittent courses of therapy rather than as continuous therapy. Intermittent therapy allows the bone marrow and other normal host cells to recover between treatment courses and reduces the level of toxicity. The selection of drugs is largely based on **clinical trials** comparing the effectiveness of various drug combinations in patients with particular **stages of a specific type of cancer**, and the treatments for each stage of a particular cancer sometimes vary considerably. First-line drugs are used for the initial treatment of tumors, whereas other drugs are indicated for patients who have relapsed after first-line therapy. These regimens are continuously evolving with the introduction of new drugs and completion of new trials. The dosage and frequency of treatment are typically based on such factors as drug kinetics, tumor cell cycle kinetics, and drug toxicity.

Cell Cycle Specificity

The cytotoxic antineoplastic drugs can be classified as cell cycle–specific and cell cycle–nonspecific agents. As shown in Figure 45–1, the **cycle of cell replication** includes the G_1, **S**, G_2, and **M phases**. DNA is replicated during the S phase, and mitosis occurs during the M phase. Because early cytologists observed no activity between the S and M phases, they referred to the period before S as G_1 (gap 1) and to the period before M as G_2 (gap 2). It is now known that cells are actively preparing for DNA synthesis and mitosis during the G_1 and G_2 phases, respectively. **Cyclins** are growth factors that regulate the progression of cells through the cell cycle and are targets of new drug development. Examples of cyclins are shown in Figure 45–1.

Drugs that act during a specific phase of the cell cycle are called **cell cycle–specific drugs**, whereas drugs that are active throughout the cell cycle are called **cell cycle-nonspecific drugs**. Cell cycle–specific drugs include all DNA synthesis inhibitors and mitotic inhibitors. Cell cycle-nonspecific drugs include all DNA alkylating agents and most DNA intercalating agents.

Limitations of Cancer Chemotherapy

Most antineoplastic drugs have three major limitations: susceptibility to tumor cell resistance, production of host toxicity, and an inability to suppress metastasis. Newer drugs have had some success in overcoming these obstacles, though a cure for most cancers is yet to be developed.

Drug Resistance

Drug resistance is a major cause of cancer treatment failure. As with microbial drug resistance, tumor cell resistance can be innate or acquired. Acquired drug resistance can result from genomic mutations or abnormal gene expression as cancer cells continuously evolve. The mechanisms of tumor cell resistance include induction of drug efflux pumps, decreased affinity or overexpression of target enzymes, decreased drug activation or increased drug inactivation, altered expression of proapoptotic and antiapoptotic molecules, and increased tumor cell repair.

Drug resistance can occur through failure of the drug to reach its target because of drug efflux from tumor cells. Two important efflux pumps are the **P-glycoprotein** (Pgp) and the **multidrug-resistance protein** (MRP). Both pumps are members of the adenosine triphosphate–binding cassette family. Pgp is the product of the multidrug resistance-1 gene and acts to transport many naturally occurring drugs out of neoplastic cells, including anthracyclines, taxanes, and vinca alkaloids (Fig. 45–2). Induction of Pgp by antineoplastic drugs can lead to multidrug resistance.

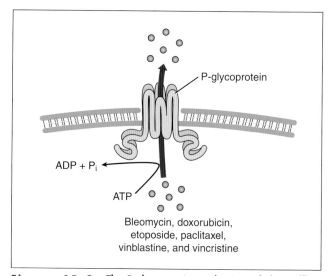

Bleomycin, doxorubicin, etoposide, paclitaxel, vinblastine, and vincristine

Figure 45–2. The P-glycoprotein mechanism of drug efflux. P-glycoprotein utilizes adenosine triphosphate to actively export bleomycin and many other naturally occurring antineoplastic drugs from the cell. Because some agents (e.g., verapamil) inhibit the P-glycoprotein pump and thereby allow antineoplastic drugs to stay in the cell, these agents are being studied as potential adjuncts to cancer chemotherapy. ADP = adenosine diphosphate; ATP = adenosine triphosphate.

MRP removes drugs from tumor cells after conjugation of drugs with glutathione. The drugs transported by MRP are similar to those transported by Pgp except that the taxane drugs are poorly transported by MRP. Several drugs that block both Pgp and MRP are undergoing clinical trials as antineoplastic drug enhancers.

Other examples of acquired drug resistance include **topoisomerase mutations** that convey resistance to topoisomerase inhibitors (e.g., etoposide). Resistance to methotrexate can occur through mutations in its target enzyme, dihydrofolate reductase, or through overexpression of the enzyme. Mutations in genes for tubulin or microtubule-associated proteins can cause resistance to the vinca alkaloids and taxane drugs. Finally, expression of **antiapoptotic proteins** (e.g., Bcl-2) can produce resistance to many drugs by interfering with the cell death signal induced by an antineoplastic agent.

Drug Toxicity

The most common toxicities of traditional antineoplastic drugs (Table 45–1) result from nonspecific inhibition of cell replication in the bone marrow, gastrointestinal epithelium, and hair follicles. Many antineoplastic drugs also stimulate the chemoreceptor trigger zone in the medulla and thereby elicit nausea and vomiting.

The **myelosuppression (bone marrow suppression)** produced by many antineoplastic drugs often results in **leukopenia** and **thrombocytopenia**, although **anemia** can also occur. Leukopenia predisposes patients to serious infections, whereas thrombocytopenia can lead to bleeding. The onset of leukopenia is delayed because of the time required to clear circulating cells before the effect that drugs have on precursor cell maturation in the bone marrow becomes evident. With many drugs, including **methotrexate, fluorouracil,** and **cyclophosphamide,** the leukocyte count reaches its nadir in about 7 days and recovery occurs in 2 to 4 weeks. Nitrosourea drugs (e.g., **carmustine**) produce a more delayed and long-lasting suppression of leukocyte production. **Bleomycin, cisplatin,** and **vincristine** produce less myelosuppression than do other antineoplastic drugs, so they are often used in combination with myelosuppressive drugs.

The **nausea** and **vomiting** caused by antineoplastic drugs range from mild to severe. Among the antineoplastic drugs, the most emetic are **cisplatin** and **carmustine.** Their adverse effects can be prevented or substantially reduced, however, by pretreatment with a combination of antiemetic drugs, including serotonin antagonists (e.g., **ondansetron**) and corticosteroids (e.g., **dexamethasone**). The antiemetics are discussed in greater detail in Chapter 28.

Alopecia is a cosmetically distressing but less-serious adverse effect of chemotherapy. It is generally reversible after treatment ends, although the hair might differ in texture and appearance from its previous condition.

Several antineoplastic drugs have characteristic organ system toxicities that appear unrelated to inhibition of cell division. For example, use of **doxorubicin** and other anthracyclines can cause **cardiotoxicity;** use of **cyclophosphamide** and **ifosfamide** can cause **hemorrhagic cystitis;** use of **cisplatin** can cause **renal toxicity;** use of **bleomycin** or **busulfan** can cause **pulmonary toxicity;** and use of **vincristine, paclitaxel,** and other vinca alkaloids and taxanes can cause **neurotoxicity.**

Agents have been developed to prevent some of these organ system toxicities. For example, **dexrazoxane** was developed to prevent anthracycline-induced cardiotoxicity. Another cytoprotective drug, **mesna,** was developed to prevent cyclophosphamide-induced hemorrhagic cystitis. Cisplatin-induced renal toxicity can be partly prevented by administering fluids, along with **mannitol** and **sodium thiosulfate.** Mannitol maintains renal blood flow and tubular function, whereas sodium thiosulfate inactivates the drug in the kidneys. No specific agents currently exist to prevent pulmonary toxicity and neurotoxicity; therefore, patients at risk should be closely monitored so that treatment can be discontinued if these toxicities develop.

DNA SYNTHESIS INHIBITORS

Most of the DNA synthesis inhibitors are analogues of purine or pyrimidine bases found in DNA or of folic acid. They act as antimetabolites to inhibit enzymes catalyzing various steps in DNA synthesis. The uses and adverse effects of selected inhibitors are listed in Table 45–1.

Folate Antagonists

Methotrexate

Nearly 50 years ago, methotrexate (MTX) was used successfully to induce remission in patients with acute childhood leukemia. Today, it is the most widely used antimetabolite in cancer chemotherapy, and it is also used as an immunosuppressive drug in the treatment of rheumatoid arthritis, lupus erythematosus, and other conditions (see Chapter 30).

CHEMISTRY AND MECHANISMS. The structures of MTX and folic acid are similar. MTX, however, has an amino group substituted for a hydroxyl group on the pteridine ring, and it also has an additional methyl group.

Methotrexate is actively transported into mammalian cells and inhibits dihydrofolate reductase, the enzyme that normally converts dietary folate to the tetrahydrofolate form required for thymidine and purine synthesis (Fig. 45–3).

PHARMACOKINETICS. MTX can be administered orally or parenterally. The oral bioavailability of the drug is dose-dependent. Low doses are completely absorbed, whereas higher doses undergo significantly less absorption. Because MTX does not penetrate the central nervous system (CNS), it must be administered intrathecally for the prevention or treatment of CNS disease.

Methotrexate is rapidly distributed throughout the total body water, and it is partly degraded in the intestine (by intestinal flora) and in the liver. The drug has a biphasic elimination pattern. It is primarily eliminated as the parent compound and metabolites in the urine. The terminal half-life reflects redistribution from tissues and "third space" fluids, such as ascites and pleural effusions.

TABLE 45-1. Major Clinical Uses and Adverse Effects of Antineoplastic Drugs

Drug	Major Clinical Uses	Acute Toxicity	Delayed Toxicity
DNA Synthesis Inhibitors			
Cladribine	Hairy cell leukemia, non-Hodgkin's lymphoma	Mild nausea and vomiting	Myelosuppression
Cytarabine	AML non-Hodgkin's lymphoma	Diarrhea, mild nausea and vomiting	Hepatotoxicity, gastrointestinal and oral ulcers, myelosuppression
Floxuridine	Colorectal and hepatic carcinoma	Diarrhea, mild nausea and vomiting	Alopecia, gastrointestinal and oral ulcers, myelosuppression
Fludarabine	CLL, non-Hodgkin's lymphoma	Mild nausea and vomiting	Myelosuppression
Fluorouracil	Breast, colorectal, gastric, and skin cancer	Diarrhea, mild nausea and vomiting	Alopecia, gastrointestinal and oral ulcers, myelosuppression
Gemcitabine	Pancreatic, bladder, and breast cancers	Mild nausea	Myelosuppression and lung cancers
Hydroxyurea	CML, sickle cell anemia	Mild nausea and vomiting	Myelosuppression
Mercaptopurine	AML, ALL, CML	Usually well-tolerated	Hepatotoxicity, myelosuppression
Methotrexate	ALL, breast cancer, non-Hodgkin's lymphoma, osteosarcoma, trophoblastic tumors	Diarrhea, nausea	Gastrointestinal and oral ulcers, hepatotoxicity, myelosuppression, renal toxicity
Pemetrexed	Colorectal cancer, non–small cell lung cancer	Nausea	Myelosuppression, lung and pancreatic cancers
Thioguanine	AML, ALL, CML	Usually well-tolerated	Myelosuppression
DNA Alkylating Drugs			
Busulfan	CML	Diarrhea, mild nausea and vomiting	Myelosuppression, pulmonary fibrosis
Carboplatin	Ovarian cancer	Moderate nausea and vomiting	Myelosuppression
Carmustine	Brain tumors, melanoma, myeloma, non-Hodgkin's lymphoma	Severe nausea and vomiting	Myelosuppression, pulmonary fibrosis, renal toxicity
Chlorambucil	CLL	Well tolerated	Myelosuppression, sterility
Cisplatin	Bladder, cervical, ovarian, and testicular cancer; melanoma, myeloma, non-Hodgkin's lymphoma	Acute renal failure, severe nausea and vomiting	Mild myelosuppression, ototoxicity, renal toxicity
Cyclophosphamide	Breast, lung, and ovarian cancer; CLL, ALL, myeloma, neuroblastoma, non-Hodgkin's lymphoma, sarcoma	Nausea and vomiting	Alopecia, hemorrhagic cystitis, myelosuppression, pulmonary fibrosis
Dacarbazine	Hodgkin's disease, melanoma, sarcoma	Severe nausea and vomiting	Alopecia, myelosuppression
Ifosfamide	Sarcoma, testicular cancer	Nausea and vomiting	Alopecia, hemorrhagic cystitis, myelosuppression, pulmonary fibrosis
Lomustine	Brain tumors, non-Hodgkin's lymphoma	Severe nausea and vomiting	Myelosuppression, pulmonary toxicity
Mechlorethamine	Hodgkin's disease, lymphoma	Mild nausea	Alopecia, myelosuppression
Melphalan	Breast and ovarian cancer, myeloma	Severe nausea and vomiting	Myelosuppression
Mitomycin	Bladder, breast, lung, pancreatic, cervical, and stomach cancer	Nausea and vomiting	Alopecia, myelosuppression, pulmonary and renal toxicity, stomatitis
Oxaliplatin	Colon cancer	Nausea and vomiting	Peripheral neuropathy, myelosuppression
Streptozocin	Carcinoid tumor, pancreatic islet cell tumor	Severe nausea and vomiting	Renal toxicity
DNA Intercalating Drugs			
Bleomycin	Cervical, head, neck, and testicular cancer; Hodgkin's and non-Hodgkin's lymphoma	Fever, mild nausea and vomiting	Alopecia, mild myelosuppression, mucocutaneous toxicity, pneumonitis, pulmonary fibrosis
Dactinomycin	Ewing's sarcoma, trophoblastic tumors, Wilms' tumor	Diarrhea, nausea and vomiting	Alopecia, myelosuppression, oral ulcers
Daunorubicin	ALL, AML	Nausea and vomiting	Alopecia, cardiotoxicity, mucosal ulcers, myelosuppression
Doxorubicin	ALL; bladder, breast, gastric, lung, ovarian, soft tissue, and thyroid cancer; myeloma, neuroblastoma	Nausea and vomiting	Alopecia, cardiotoxicity, mucosal ulcers, myelosuppression
Idarubicin	AML	Nausea and vomiting	Alopecia, cardiotoxicity, mucosal ulcers, myelosuppression

(Continued)

TABLE 45-1. **Major Clinical Uses and Adverse Effects of Antineoplastic Drugs—cont'd**

Drug	Major Clinical Uses	Acute Toxicity	Delayed Toxicity
Mitoxantrone	AML	Nausea and vomiting	Alopecia, cardiotoxicity, mucosal ulcers, myelosuppression
Mitotic Inhibitors			
Docetaxel	Breast and ovarian cancer, non–small cell lung cancer	Usually well-tolerated	Alopecia, myelosuppression, neurotoxicity
Paclitaxel	Breast and ovarian cancer; non–small cell lung cancer	Usually well-tolerated	Alopecia, myelosuppression, neurotoxicity
Vinblastine	Bladder, breast, ovarian, and testicular cancer; Hodgkin's and non-Hodgkin's lymphomas	Nausea and vomiting	Alopecia, myelosuppression, stomatitis
Vincristine	ALL; Hodgkin's and non-Hodgkin's lymphoma, lung cancer, myeloma, neuroblastoma, sarcoma	Usually well-tolerated	Alopecia, mild myelosuppression, peripheral neurotoxicity
Vinorelbine	Non–small cell lung cancer	Nausea and vomiting	Myelosuppression
Topoisomerase inhibitors			
Etoposide	Non-Hodgkin's lymphoma, small-cell lung cancer, testicular cancer, AML	Mild nausea and vomiting	Alopecia, myelosuppression
Irinotecan	Ovarian and colorectal cancer	Diarrhea, mild nausea and vomiting	Alopecia, myelosuppression
Teniposide	ALL, AML	Mild nausea and vomiting	Alopecia, myelosuppression
Topotecan	Lung and ovarian cancer	Mild nausea and vomiting	Alopecia, myelosuppression
Hormones and Hormone Antagonists			
Anastrozole, Letrozole	Breast cancer	Nausea and hot flashes	None
Flutamide	Prostate cancer	Nausea and vomiting	Impotence
Leuprolide	Prostate cancer	Nausea and vomiting	Hot flashes, gynecomastia
Prednisone	ALL, breast cancer, CLL, Hodgkin's and non-Hodgkin's lymphoma, myeloma	None	Hyperadrenocorticism
Tamoxifen	Breast cancer	Nausea and vomiting	Hot flashes, hypercalcemia
Protein Kinase Inhibitors			
Imatinib	Chronic myeloid leukemia	Nausea	Edema, rash, diarrhea, pain
Nilotinib	Chronic myeloid leukemia	Nausea	QT interval prolongation, arrhythmia
Erlotinib	Non–small cell lung cancer	Nausea	Rash, diarrhea, fatigue, dyspnea
Cytokines, Interferons, and Monoclonal Antibodies			
Aldesleukin	Colorectal cancer, melanoma, renal cell carcinoma	Varies with dosage and route of administration	Fluid retention, hematologic deficiencies, hypotension, neuropsychiatric effects, renal dysfunction, skin lesions
Bevacizumab	Colorectal cancer	None	Gastrointestinal bleeding and perforation, pulmonary hemorrhage
Cetuximab	Colon cancer	Nausea	Skin rash, allergic reactions
Interferon-alpha	CML, hairy cell leukemia, Kaposi's sarcoma	Flulike illness	Fatigue
Rituximab	Non-Hodgkin's lymphoma	Chills, fever, headache, nausea	Myelosuppression
Trastuzumab	Breast cancer	Chest pain, chills, dyspnea, fever, nausea, vomiting	Heart failure, pulmonary toxicity

ALL = acute lymphocytic leukemia; AML = acute myeloid leukemia; CLL = chronic lymphocytic leukemia; CML = chronic myeloid leukemia.

INDICATIONS. The use of MTX in the treatment of choriocarcinoma, a trophoblastic tumor, was the first demonstration of curative chemotherapy. Today, MTX has a variety of uses, including the treatment of trophoblastic tumors, breast cancer, non-Hodgkin's lymphomas, and osteosarcoma. It is also effective for treating acute lymphocytic leukemia and the meningeal metastases of a wide range of tumors.

ADVERSE EFFECTS. The bone marrow and gastrointestinal mucosa are the normal tissues most sensitive to MTX toxicity. Although myelosuppression is the primary dose-limiting toxicity of the drug, severe oral ulceration (stomatitis) can also occur and necessitate dosage reduction. Administration of a fully activated form of folic acid called **leucovorin (folinic acid)** can prevent these adverse reactions, but it cannot reverse them after they have occurred. Leucovorin rescue is normally used with high doses of MTX (doses exceeding 100 mg/m² body surface area). Assays for MTX in plasma are readily available, and drug level monitoring provides a useful guide to the duration of leucovorin administration.

Methotrexate can cause hepatotoxicity, especially with long-term low-dose therapy for psoriasis and rheumatoid

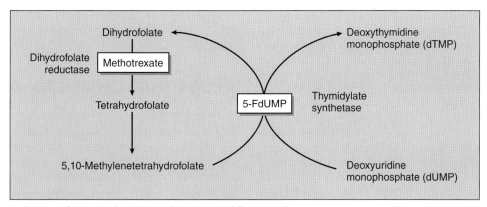

Figure 45-3. Inhibition of DNA synthesis by methotrexate and fluorouracil. Methotrexate inhibits dihydrofolate reductase and the conversion of dihydrofolate to tetrahydrofolate. This reduces the supply of 5,10-methylenetetrahydrofolate, a substance required for the synthesis of deoxythymidine monophosphate (dTMP). The conversion of deoxyuridine monophosphate (dUMP) to dTMP, a critical step in DNA synthesis, is catalyzed by thymidylate synthetase. This enzyme is inhibited by 5-fluorodeoxyuridine monophosphate (5-FdUMP), which is the active form of fluorouracil.

conditions. At high doses, MTX can **crystallize in the urine** and cause renal damage. To prevent renal toxicity, dosage reduction is necessary in persons with renal insufficiency.

Pemetrexed

Pemetrexed is a novel antifolate drug. It is rapidly metabolized to active polyglutamate forms that inhibit several tetrahydrofolate-dependent enzymes involved in the synthesis of purine and pyrimidine bases, including thymidylate synthase. Although the drug can cause considerable and even life-threatening toxicities when given alone, investigators found that these toxicities can be minimized by giving folic acid and vitamin B_{12} without impairing drug efficacy. Pemetrexed has broad antitumor activity, and initial studies found that it prolongs survival in patients with advanced colorectal cancer. Early clinical trials show that it is also active against non–small-cell lung cancer and pancreatic cancer. Neutropenia and other forms of bone marrow suppression are the primary adverse effects of pemetrexed.

Purine Analogues

The first purine analogue to be used in cancer chemotherapy was **mercaptopurine**, a drug introduced almost 60 years ago for the treatment of acute lymphocytic leukemia. Mercaptopurine and thioguanine are the thio analogues of the purine bases hypoxanthine and guanine, respectively. Both drugs are converted to nucleotides by the addition of ribose phosphate, a reaction catalyzed by **hypoxanthine guanine phosphoribosyltransferase**. Tumor cells may acquire resistance to these drugs by deleting this enzyme, and cross-resistance is usually observed between the two drugs. The active metabolites of mercaptopurine and thioguanine inhibit several steps in the biosynthesis of purine bases (adenine and guanine) and in purine recycling pathways that supply purine precursors, thereby impairing DNA synthesis.

Mercaptopurine and thioguanine are given orally, and their bioavailability is variable, incomplete, and reduced by food. Mercaptopurine is given with methotrexate to maintain remission in patients with acute lymphocytic leukemia.

Thioguanine is used to maintain remission in patients with acute lymphocytic and acute myeloid leukemia. Mercaptopurine is metabolized by **xanthine oxidase**, whereas thioguanine is degraded by other enzymes.

Mercaptopurine and thioguanine are usually well tolerated. Myelosuppression is generally mild with mercaptopurine but can be dose-limiting with thioguanine. Long-term mercaptopurine use can cause hepatotoxicity, and both drugs contribute to the development of other cancers (therapy-related cancer). Doses of mercaptopurine must be reduced by at least 50% in patients who are taking **allopurinol**, which inhibits xanthine oxidase and thereby elevates plasma levels of mercaptopurine. Allopurinol is often given to patients undergoing cancer chemotherapy because it inhibits the synthesis of uric acid and thereby prevents hyperuricemia and gout. Cancer chemotherapy places patients at risk for these problems because the destruction of cancer cells increases purine catabolism and uric acid formation.

Purine Nucleoside Analogues

Fludarabine and **cladribine** are halogenated purine nucleoside analogues whose triphosphate metabolites are incorporated into nascent DNA, causing DNA chain termination. Fludarabine is a highly active agent in the treatment of **chronic lymphocytic leukemia** and low-grade non-Hodgkin's lymphoma. Cladribine is primarily used for **hairy cell leukemia**. **Clofarabine** and **nelarabine** are new purine nucleoside antagonists for treating refractory or relapsed **acute lymphocytic leukemia**.

Pyrimidine Antagonists
Cytarabine, Fluorouracil, and Related Drugs

Cytarabine (cytosine arabinoside) and fluorouracil are commonly used pyrimidine antimetabolites. Cytarabine is composed of cytosine and the sugar arabinose. Fluorouracil is an analogue of thymine in which the methyl group is replaced by a fluorine atom. **Floxuridine** is the deoxyribonucleoside derivative of fluorouracil, whereas **capecitabine** is converted in the body to fluorouracil and its active metabolites.

The active triphosphate metabolite of cytarabine blocks DNA synthesis by several actions, including the inhibition of DNA polymerase and incorporation of the drug into nascent DNA, causing DNA chain termination. Cytarabine crosses the blood-brain barrier and reaches cerebrospinal fluid levels that are 40% to 50% of plasma levels. Fluorouracil has two active metabolites: 5-fluorodeoxyuridine monophosphate (5-FdUMP) and 5-fluorodeoxyuridine triphosphate (5-FdUTP). 5-FdUMP inhibits **thymidylate synthetase** and prevents the synthesis of thymidine, a major building block of DNA (see Fig. 45–3). 5-FdUTP is also incorporated into RNA by RNA polymerase and interferes with RNA function. When the drugs are given parenterally, they are extensively metabolized before undergoing renal excretion.

Cytarabine can be administered intravenously or subcutaneously and is used in combination with daunorubicin to treat **acute myeloid leukemia**. Fluorouracil is administered intravenously to treat solid tumors, especially breast, colorectal, and gastric tumors and squamous cell tumors of the head and neck. Regional delivery of the drug via the hepatic artery can produce a sustained response in patients whose colorectal cancer has metastasized to the liver. Topical application of fluorouracil is used to treat **actinic keratoses** and noninvasive **skin cancers**. Capecitabine is indicated for colorectal and breast cancer, whereas floxuridine is used in the treatment of colorectal and hepatic carcinoma.

The pyrimidine antimetabolites can cause nausea and vomiting, myelosuppression, and oral and gastrointestinal ulceration. Nausea and vomiting are usually mild. With fluorouracil, myelosuppression is more problematic after bolus injections, whereas mucosal damage is dose-limiting with continuous infusions. High doses of these drugs can damage the liver, heart, and other organs.

Gemcitabine

Gemcitabine, an S-phase specific inhibitor of DNA synthesis, is a fluorinated cytidine analogue. After conversion to gemcitabine diphosphate and triphosphate, these metabolites inhibit the synthesis of deoxynucleoside triphosphates and the incorporation of deoxynucleoside triphosphates into DNA. In addition, gemcitabine triphosphate itself is incorporated into DNA, causing DNA chain termination. The drug is indicated as a first-line treatment for **pancreatic carcinoma** and for use with cisplatin as first-line therapy for inoperable, non–small-cell lung cancer. Gemcitabine has also been used for biliary tract, gallbladder, breast, and ovarian cancer. As with other DNA synthesis inhibitors, gemcitabine can cause myelosuppression leading to anemia, leukopenia, and thrombocytopenia. It also causes alopecia and various gastrointestinal disturbances.

Ribonucleotide Reductase Inhibitor

Hydroxyurea inhibits ribonucleotide reductase, the enzyme that converts ribonucleotides to deoxyribonucleotides. It thereby stops DNA synthesis and causes cells to accumulate in the S phase of the cell cycle.

Hydroxyurea is given orally to treat chronic myelogenous leukemia, ovarian cancer, and melanoma. Hydroxyurea is also used in the management of **sickle cell anemia**. In this condition, hydroxyurea elevates the concentration of fetal hemoglobin and decreases the frequency of sickle cell crises. The dose-limiting toxicity of hydroxyurea is rapid-onset myelosuppression.

DRUGS THAT CROSS-LINK DNA

A DNA alkylating drug is an agent that cross-links DNA strands by forming covalent bonds between alkyl groups of the drug and guanine bases of DNA. The DNA alkylating drugs include nitrogen mustards, nitrosourea drugs, and several other agents. Platinum compounds (e.g., cisplatin) do not contain alkyl groups but cross-link DNA by forming intrastrand and interstrand covalent bonds with DNA bases.

Nitrogen Mustards

The nitrogen mustards are nitrogen analogues of the sulfur mustards that were used as chemical warfare agents in World War I. The cytotoxic effects of nitrogen mustards were discovered in the early 1940s, and the drugs were soon introduced into clinical use. They are considered the first effective antineoplastic drugs.

The nitrogen mustards are bifunctional alkylating agents that undergo spontaneous conversion to active metabolites in body fluids or are enzymatically converted to active metabolites in the liver. The strong electrophilic intermediates formed by these reactions attack the N7 nitrogen of guanine and thereby form covalent bonds with this base. Sequential attachment to two guanine residues results in cross-linking of DNA, and this prevents DNA replication and transcription (Fig. 45–4A). The alkylating drugs act throughout the cell replication cycle.

Cyclophosphamide and Ifosfamide

CHEMISTRY AND PHARMACOKINETICS. Cyclophosphamide and ifosfamide are prodrugs that must be converted to active metabolites by hepatic mixed-function oxidase (cytochrome P450) enzymes. The active alkylating metabolite of cyclophosphamide is thought to be phosphoramide mustard. Cyclophosphamide and ifosfamide are partly converted to acrolein, which is probably responsible for hemorrhagic cystitis, an adverse effect that sometimes occurs with use of these drugs. Both drugs can be administered intravenously; cyclophosphamide can also be given orally. Cyclophosphamide is completely absorbed after oral administration.

INDICATIONS. Cyclophosphamide is the most widely used nitrogen mustard because of its broad spectrum of activity. It is used in the treatment of acute and chronic lymphocytic leukemia; non-Hodgkin's lymphoma; breast, lung, and ovarian cancers; and a variety of other cancers (see Table 45–1). Because cyclophosphamide is a potent immunosuppressant, it is used in the management of rheumatoid disorders and autoimmune nephritis. It is also used in preoperative regimens for bone marrow transplantation.

Ifosfamide is primarily used to treat patients with sarcoma and patients with testicular cancer that is refractory to first-line treatments.

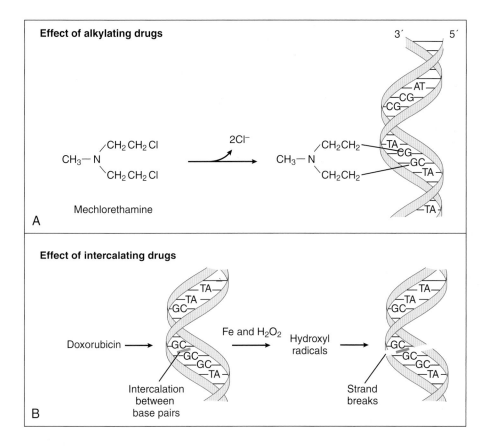

Figure 45-4. Mechanisms of action of DNA alkylating drugs and DNA intercalating drugs. **(A)** Mechlorethamine and other bifunctional alkylating drugs form electrophilic intermediates that attack the N7 nitrogen of guanine residues in DNA, thereby cross-linking DNA strands and preventing replication and transcription. **(B)** Doxorubicin and other anthracycline drugs intercalate between DNA base pairs. Anthracyclines are reduced to intermediates that donate electrons to oxygen to form superoxide. Superoxide then reacts with itself to make hydrogen peroxide, which is cleaved in the presence of iron to form the destructive hydroxyl radical that cleaves DNA.

ADVERSE EFFECTS. Adverse effects of cyclophosphamide and ifosfamide include alopecia, nausea, vomiting, myelosuppression, and hemorrhagic cystitis. Nausea and vomiting are usually mild when cyclophosphamide is given orally, but they can be severe when given intravenously. The dose-limiting toxicity of cyclophosphamide is myelosuppression, whereas that of ifosfamide is usually hemorrhagic cystitis. This type of cystitis is characterized by symptoms of urinary frequency and irritation and by blood loss from the bladder. Ingestion of large amounts of fluid and the administration of mesna, a sulfhydryl reagent, can significantly reduce the incidence of cystitis. Mesna binds to acrolein, the toxic metabolite that causes cystitis, and converts it to an inactive substance.

Chlorambucil, Mechlorethamine, and Melphalan

Chlorambucil, mechlorethamine, and melphalan are nitrogen mustards that act via the mechanisms described earlier.

Chlorambucil is orally administered, has selective cytotoxicity for lymphocyte cell lines, and is primarily used to manage **chronic lymphocytic leukemia**. It is well tolerated but can cause dose-limiting myelosuppression and sterility. Long-term therapy is associated with a high incidence of secondary acute leukemia.

Mechlorethamine is a highly reactive and vesicant drug that is rapidly and spontaneously converted to its alkylating intermediate in body fluids after it is given intravenously. Mechlorethamine is used for treating Hodgkin's and non-Hodgkin's lymphomas. Melphalan is a nitrogen mustard that is primarily used to treat multiple **myeloma** (plasma cell myeloma) and breast cancer.

Nitrosourea Drugs

The nitrosourea drugs include **carmustine** (*bis*-chloroethyl nitrosourea), **lomustine** (*cis*-chloroethyl nitrosourea), and a closely related methylnitrosourea called **streptozocin**.

CHEMISTRY AND MECHANISMS. The nitrosoureas are bifunctional alkylating drugs with structures similar to those of the nitrogen mustards. They spontaneously form active intermediates that cross-link DNA.

PHARMACOKINETICS. Nitrosoureas can be given orally or intravenously. They are highly lipophilic and reach cerebrospinal fluid concentrations that are about 30% of plasma concentrations. The drugs are extensively metabolized before renal excretion.

INDICATIONS. Because of their excellent CNS penetration, carmustine and lomustine have been used to treat brain tumors, such as astrocytomas. Both drugs are used to treat lymphomas, and carmustine is also used to treat melanoma and multiple myeloma. Streptozocin is used only to treat carcinoid tumor and pancreatic islet cell tumor (insulinoma).

ADVERSE EFFECTS. The nitrosoureas produce delayed and prolonged myelosuppression, with complete recovery taking 6 to 8 weeks. The thrombocytopenia caused by nitrosoureas usually occurs earlier and is more pronounced than the leukopenia produced by these drugs. Although all of the drugs cause nausea and vomiting, these effects are most pronounced with streptozocin treatment. Pulmonary damage occurs when high doses of nitrosoureas are used.

Platinum Compounds

CHEMISTRY AND MECHANISMS. The drugs cisplatin, carboplatin, and oxaliplatin are inorganic platinum derivatives. Cisplatin is converted to an active cytotoxic form by reacting with water to form positively charged, hydrated intermediates that react with guanine in DNA. This leads to the formation of intrastrand cross-links between neighboring guanine residues. The intrastrand links cause DNA to bend and distort the normal conformation of DNA and thereby impair its function. Carboplatin and oxaliplatin are believed to have a similar mechanism of action.

INDICATIONS. Cisplatin has efficacy against a wide range of neoplasms. It is given intravenously as a first-line drug for testicular, ovarian, cervical, and bladder cancers, and it is also useful in the treatment of melanoma and a number of other solid tumors. Carboplatin has a similar spectrum of activity, but it is approved only for ovarian cancer. Oxaliplatin is used in treating colon cancer.

ADVERSE EFFECTS. Cisplatin produces mild myelosuppression but can cause severe nausea, vomiting, and nephrotoxicity. Pretreatment with an antiemetic (e.g., **ondansetron**) will prevent or significantly reduce the severity of nausea and vomiting. The use of **mannitol** and **sodium thiosulfate** will decrease the severity of nephrotoxicity, an adverse effect associated with loss of potassium and magnesium, reduced glomerular filtration, and renal failure. Mannitol increases urine flow and can reduce binding of cisplatin to renal tubule proteins. Sodium thiosulfate accumulates in renal tubules and neutralizes the cytotoxicity of cisplatin. Renal damage caused by cisplatin is often slowly reversible.

Other DNA Alkylating Drugs

Busulfan

Busulfan is an alkyl sulfonate drug that acts as a bifunctional alkylating agent in the same manner as the nitrogen mustards act. After busulfan is administered orally, it is extensively metabolized. Its metabolites are then excreted in the urine.

Unlike other alkylating drugs, busulfan has greater activity against myeloid cells than against lymphoid cells. For this reason, it has been used in the management of **chronic myeloid leukemia**.

Busulfan causes mild nausea and vomiting and produces dose-limiting myelosuppression. It can also cause pulmonary fibrosis ("busulfan lung"), which occurs in about 4% of patients treated on a long-term basis with the drug. Pulmonary fibrosis usually has its onset about 3 years after treatment begins. It is characterized by a nonproductive cough, dyspnea, and a reticular pattern on chest x-ray film. No treatment has been successful, and the average survival after diagnosis is 5 months.

Dacarbazine

Dacarbazine is an atypical alkylating agent. The drug is converted to active intermediates that can alkylate DNA, although the exact mechanisms are uncertain. Ultimately, the drug inhibits DNA, RNA, and protein synthesis.

Dacarbazine is primarily used to treat Hodgkin's disease. Dacarbazine is administered intravenously and is part of the **ABVD regimen**, which consists of **ADRIAMYCIN** (doxorubicin), bleomycin, vinblastine, and dacarbazine.

Mitomycin

Mitomycin (mitomycin C) is an antineoplastic antibiotic that alkylates DNA and thereby causes strand breakage and inhibition of DNA synthesis. After the drug is administered parenterally, it is activated by hepatic reduction reactions to the active alkylating compound. Most of the drug is metabolized, but a small amount of it is excreted unchanged in the urine.

Mitomycin is primarily used in combination with vincristine as salvage therapy for breast cancer. It is also used in the treatment of non–small-cell lung cancer, pancreatic and stomach tumors, and superficial transitional cell carcinomas of the bladder. Although it is administered intravenously for most types of cancer, it is administered intravesically for bladder cancer.

Mitomycin produces delayed and prolonged myelosuppression that preferentially affects platelets and leukocytes. It can also cause severe pulmonary damage and a hemolytic uremic syndrome characterized by hemolytic anemia, renal dysfunction, and thrombocytopenia. Extravasation can result in severe necrosis.

DNA INTERCALATING DRUGS

The DNA intercalating drugs include the anthracycline drugs, bleomycin, and dactinomycin. These are some of the most widely used antitumor antibiotics. Several of the drugs have a broad spectrum of activity against hematologic cancers and solid tumors, whereas others have a more limited range of clinical uses.

Anthracycline Drugs

Daunorubicin, Doxorubicin, and Idarubicin

CHEMISTRY. Daunorubicin and doxorubicin are antibiotics obtained from *Streptomyces peucetius*, and idarubicin is a semisynthetic derivative. These drugs have a four-member anthracene ring with attached sugars. Two of the four rings are quinone and hydroquinone moieties that enable the compounds to accept and donate electrons and thereby promote the formation of free radicals. The anthracene ring accounts for the intense red color of the drug compounds.

MECHANISMS. Several mechanisms are responsible for the cytotoxicity of the anthracycline drugs: intercalation of DNA, inhibition of topoisomerase, and formation of free radicals. The drugs bind strongly to DNA by inserting themselves between paired bases of double-stranded DNA and thereby causing deformation and uncoiling of the DNA (see Fig. 45–4B). The anthracyclines cause DNA strands to break by interfering with the action of topoisomerase II (an enzyme discussed later in this chapter) and by forming free radicals. The anthracyclines undergo reduction (addition of electrons) to form highly destructive hydroxyl radicals that

produce DNA cleavage. The process appears to involve an iron-anthracycline complex that is strongly bound to DNA.

PHARMACOKINETICS. After intravenous administration, the anthracyclines are rapidly distributed to all body tissues except those of the CNS. They avidly bind to tissues and have large volumes of distribution and long half-lives. The drugs are extensively metabolized in the liver, and some metabolites are as pharmacologically active as the parent compounds.

INDICATIONS. Daunorubicin and idarubicin are agents used in induction and consolidation therapy for acute myeloid leukemia. Doxorubicin has a much broader spectrum of activity. It is one of the most active drugs against breast cancer, and it is also useful in the treatment of Hodgkin's disease, bladder cancer, ovarian cancer, gastric carcinoma, and other hematologic cancers and solid tumors (see Table 45–1).

ADVERSE EFFECTS. Among the adverse effects of anthracyclines are myelosuppression and cardiac damage, which are dose-limiting effects; nausea and vomiting, which are dose-related and may be moderate to severe; alopecia; and mucosal ulcerations. Extravasation of the drugs during intravenous infusion can lead to severe localized tissue ulceration and necrosis. These localized reactions can progress over many weeks, and no effective treatment for them currently exists. Hence, exceptional care and specialized training is required for proper administration of anthracycline drugs.

The anthracyclines cause both acute and chronic cardiotoxicity. Manifestations of acute toxicity include sinus tachycardia and ventricular premature beats. These cardiac rhythm disturbances often occur during the first 24 hours and are self-limited. Chronic toxicity leads to congestive cardiomyopathy and limits the cumulative dose of anthracycline that can be given to any patient. The cardiomyopathy appears to result from iron-catalyzed formation of free radicals. Information about this process has led to the development of a cardioprotective drug called **dexrazoxane**. Dexrazoxane is a potent chelator of ferric iron, and it is believed to act by disrupting the iron-anthracycline complex and thereby preventing reactive free radical formation. Dexrazoxane is primarily given to women with breast cancer who might benefit from continued doxorubicin therapy. Another method of preventing cardiotoxicity is to administer doxorubicin as a **liposomal complex** that is not taken up as much by cardiac tissue as is the free drug. This preparation is now approved for the treatment of Kaposi's sarcoma in patients with acquired immunodeficiency syndrome (AIDS), and it is expected to be used in the treatment of other solid tumors.

INTERACTIONS. Drugs that increase the toxicity of doxorubicin include cyclosporine, cyclophosphamide, and mercaptopurine. Verapamil can increase the cytotoxicity of doxorubicin and other anthracycline drugs by inhibition of the Pgp that transports anthracyclines out of cells.

Mitoxantrone

Mitoxantrone is a synthetic anthracene derivative that is primarily used in combination with cytarabine for induction of remission in patients with acute myeloid leukemia. The drug is administered intravenously. As with the anthracycline antibiotics, mitoxantrone intercalates DNA and produces DNA strand breaks, but it has much less potential for free radical formation. Partly for this reason, mitoxantrone causes less cardiotoxicity, less tissue damage after extravasation, and less nausea, vomiting, mucosal ulceration, and alopecia than do doxorubicin and other anthracycline antibiotics.

Other DNA Intercalating Drugs

Bleomycin

CHEMISTRY AND MECHANISMS. Bleomycin is a mixture of two peptides obtained from *Streptomyces verticillus*. The drug has its greatest effect on neoplastic cells in the G_2 phase of the cell replication cycle. Although bleomycin intercalates DNA, the major cytotoxicity is believed to result from iron-catalyzed free radical formation and DNA strand breakage. The iron-bleomycin complex binds to DNA, which reduces molecular oxygen to oxygen free radicals that cause single strands of DNA to break.

PHARMACOKINETICS. Bleomycin is administered intravenously, is widely distributed, and is primarily eliminated by renal excretion. The drug is inactivated in cells by aminohydrolase, whose low levels in skin and lung may partly account for the toxicity of bleomycin in these tissues.

INDICATIONS. Bleomycin has a broad range of activity and is one of the most widely used antitumor antibiotics. It is useful in Hodgkin's and non-Hodgkin's lymphomas, testicular cancer, and several other solid tumors. It is included in the ABVD regimen for Hodgkin's disease (Table 45–2).

ADVERSE EFFECTS. Bleomycin produces very little myelosuppression. For this reason, it is often combined with myelosuppressive drugs in treatment regimens. The most serious toxicities of bleomycin are pulmonary and mucocutaneous reactions. Patients taking the drug can develop pneumonitis that progresses to interstitial fibrosis, hypoxia, and death. It is important, therefore, to monitor patients carefully for manifestations of pulmonary toxicity, which include cough, dyspnea, rales, and pulmonary infiltrates noted on chest x-ray film. Mucocutaneous toxicity usually presents as mild stomatitis (inflammation of the oral mucosa), skin hyperpigmentation, erythema, and edema.

Dactinomycin

Dactinomycin (actinomycin D) intercalates DNA and thereby prevents DNA transcription and messenger RNA synthesis. The drug is given intravenously, and its clinical use is limited to the treatment of trophoblastic tumors, such as **choriocarcinoma**, and the treatment of pediatric tumors, such as **Wilms' tumor** and **Ewing's sarcoma**.

MITOTIC INHIBITORS

The mitotic spindle that separates the chromosomes during mitosis is made up of hollow tubules called microtubules. The microtubules are formed by the polymerization of the

TABLE 45–2. **Examples of Drugs Commonly Used in the Treatment of Selected Neoplastic Diseases**

Disease	Treatment
Hematologic Cancers	
Acute lymphocytic leukemia	Vincristine, prednisone, methotrexate, mercaptopurine, nelarabine, clofarabine
Acute myeloid (nonlymphocytic) leukemia	Cytarabine, daunorubicin, gemtuzumab ozogamicin, cladribine
Chronic lymphocytic leukemia	Chlorambucil or cyclophosphamide, prednisone, fludarabine, alemtuzumab
Chronic myeloid leukemia	Imatinib, dasatinib, nilotinib
Hodgkin's disease	Doxorubicin, bleomycin, vinblastine, dacarbazine
Multiple myeloma	Melphalan, cyclophosphamide, prednisone, bortezomib
Non-Hodgkin's and histiocytic lymphomas	Cyclophosphamide, doxorubicin, vincristine, prednisone, rituximab, ^{90}Y-ibitumomab, ^{131}I-tositumomab
Nodular (low-grade) lymphomas	Cyclophosphamide, vincristine, prednisone
Solid Tumors	
Bladder cancer	Cisplatin, doxorubicin
Brain tumors	Carmustine or lomustine, procarbazine, carboplatin, vincristine, etoposide
Breast cancer	Tamoxifen, aromatase inhibitors, trastuzumab, doxorubicin, cyclophosphamide, fluorouracil, paclitaxel, docetaxel, ixabepilone
Choriocarcinoma	For gestational use only: methotrexate; dactinomycin
Colorectal cancer	Fluorouracil, irinotecan, cetuximab, bevacizumab
Gastric cancer	Fluorouracil, doxorubicin, mitomycin
Lung cancer, non–small cell	Gemcitabine, cisplatin, vinorelbine, pemetrexed, docetaxel, gefitinib
Lung cancer, small cell	Cisplatin or carboplatin, etoposide, irinotecan
Malignant melanoma	Dacarbazine, carmustine, cisplatin
Ovarian cancer	Cisplatin, carboplatin, cyclophosphamide, doxorubicin, paclitaxel, docetaxel
Renal cell carcinoma	Aldesleukin, sorafenib, sunitinib, temsirolimus
Sarcoma	Doxorubicin, dacarbazine
Testicular cancer	Cisplatin, etoposide, bleomycin

structural protein called tubulin. During mitosis, microtubules are continuously assembled and disassembled by means of tubulin polymerization and depolymerization. As shown in Figure 45–5, antineoplastic drugs inhibit mitosis and cause metaphase arrest by interfering with microtubule function. The **vinca alkaloids** bind to tubulin and block tubulin polymerization, whereas the **taxanes** bind to tubulin and prevent depolymerization. By their action, the taxanes promote the formation of stable but nonfunctional microtubules. **Ixabepilone** is a semisynthetic analogue of epothilone B. It binds β-tubulin subunits and suppresses microtubule dynamics. The fact that microtubules also have important roles in nerve conduction and neurotransmission may explain why use of mitotic inhibitors can cause neurotoxicity.

Vinca Alkaloids

Vincristine and Vinblastine

CHEMISTRY AND PHARMACOKINETICS. Vincristine and vinblastine are natural alkaloids from the periwinkle plant. Despite their structural similarity and identical mechanisms of action, the two drugs have different antitumor activities and toxicities. The oral absorption of vincristine and vinblastine is unreliable, so the drugs are administered intravenously. Neither drug enters the CNS in significant amounts. Both drugs are extensively metabolized and undergo biliary excretion.

INDICATIONS. Vincristine is often used to treat hematologic cancers, including acute lymphocytic leukemia, Hodgkin's and non-Hodgkin's lymphomas, and multiple myeloma. It also is used in the treatment of some solid tumors (e.g., small-cell lung cancer, neuroblastoma, and sarcoma). Vinblastine is used for lymphomas and for bladder, breast, ovarian, and testicular cancers. Vinblastine is a component of the ABVD regimen for Hodgkin's disease (see Table 45–2).

ADVERSE EFFECTS. Vincristine produces dose-limiting neurotoxicity. It can cause a form of peripheral neuropathy that is usually distal and symmetric and affects both sensory and motor function. Suppression of deep tendon reflexes, which is often found, may be the earliest sign of neurotoxicity. Paresthesias of the hands and toes are also common. These adverse effects are usually reversible and do not justify discontinuation of vincristine therapy unless they are disabling. Cranial nerve damage can cause hoarseness, facial palsies, or jaw pain, whereas autonomic neuropathies can cause orthostatic hypotension, abdominal pain, and constipation. In contrast to vinblastine, vincristine usually causes little myelosuppression.

The major dose-limiting toxicity of vinblastine is myelosuppression. Vinblastine usually causes little neurotoxicity.

Vinorelbine

Vinorelbine is a new semisynthetic derivative of vinblastine. It has shown good activity against non–small-cell lung cancer and is being used as monotherapy for this disease.

Taxanes

CHEMISTRY AND PHARMACOKINETICS. The taxanes (taxoids) are plant alkaloids obtained from yew trees. In 1971, **paclitaxel** (TAXOL) was isolated from the bark of a slow-growing Pacific yew, *Taxus brevifolia*. Because the complex ring structure of

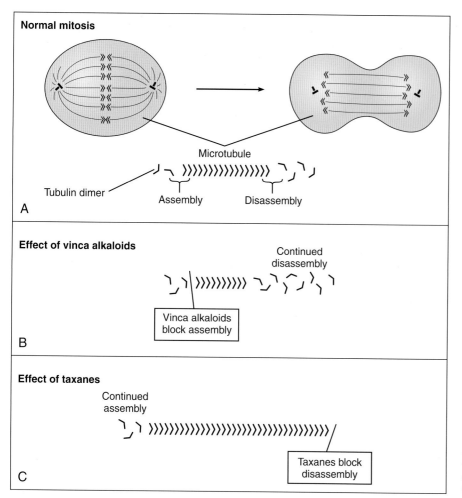

A

B

C

Figure 45-5. Mechanisms of action of mitotic inhibitors. **(A)** In normal mitosis, the mitotic spindle is formed by microtubules that continuously undergo assembly and disassembly as a result of tubulin polymerization and depolymerization, respectively. **(B)** Vincristine and other vinca alkaloids bind to tubulin and prevent the polymerization of tubulin dimers. **(C)** Paclitaxel and other taxanes bind to tubulin, stabilize the tubulin polymer, and thereby prevent depolymerization. As with vinca alkaloids, taxanes cause metaphase arrest.

paclitaxel cannot be synthesized easily and because harvesting the bark kills the tree, efforts were made to find a more renewable source of this compound. The search resulted in the discovery of **docetaxel**, which was isolated from the needles of the European yew, *Taxus baccata.*

Paclitaxel and docetaxel are given intravenously and are eliminated via metabolism and biliary excretion.

INDICATIONS. The taxanes have good activity against several types of cancer (see Table 45–1). Paclitaxel is indicated as first-line therapy for metastatic ovarian cancer, in combination with cisplatin; treatment of non–small-cell lung cancer; and treatment of metastatic breast cancer unresponsive to first-line therapy. Docetaxel is approved for locally advanced or metastatic breast cancer and for metastatic non–small-cell lung cancer after failure of cisplatin-based chemotherapy.

ADVERSE EFFECTS. The major dose-limiting toxicity of taxanes is myelosuppression, particularly neutropenia. Taxanes can also cause alopecia and neurotoxicity.

Ixabepilone

Ixabepilone is a new mitotic inhibitor for the treatment of metastatic or locally advanced breast cancer resistant to treatment with other drugs. In addition to direct antitumor

activity, it also appears to inhibit angiogenesis. Ixabepilone has low susceptibility to efflux transporters such as Pgp and MRP, and it is active against tumors resistant to taxanes, vinca alkaloids, and anthracyclines. The drug is given intravenously and is extensively metabolized before fecal and renal excretion.

TOPOISOMERASE INHIBITORS

The DNA topoisomerases are enzymes that serve to maintain the normal structural topology of DNA. These enzymes relieve the torsional strain that is caused by the unwinding of DNA during the replication or transcription of DNA strands. Topoisomerases work by producing strand breaks that permit the strands to pass through the gap before the breaks are resealed. **Topoisomerase I** breaks and reseals single-stranded DNA, whereas **topoisomerase II** breaks and reseals double-stranded DNA.

Drugs that inhibit topoisomerases cause permanent strand breaks by preventing the resealing of the nicked strands of DNA. The two groups of topoisomerase inhibitors are (1) the podophyllotoxins, which inhibit topoisomerase II; and (2) the camptothecin analogues, which inhibit topoisomerase I.

Podophyllotoxins

CHEMISTRY AND PHARMACOKINETICS. Podophyllin is a natural substance that is extracted from the mandrake or mayapple plant. Two semisynthetic derivatives of this substance, **etoposide** and **teniposide**, are used as antineoplastic drugs. Both drugs can be given intravenously. Although etoposide can also be given orally, its oral bioavailability varies greatly from patient to patient, so this route of administration can result in significant underdosing or overdosing. Etoposide is primarily eliminated unchanged in the urine, whereas teniposide is extensively metabolized in the liver.

INDICATIONS. Etoposide has a broad spectrum of activity against hematologic cancers and solid tumors. It is especially valuable in the treatment of testicular carcinoma, lung cancer, and non-Hodgkin's lymphoma. It also has value as a preoperative treatment for bone marrow transplantation. Because of its synergy with platinum compounds, etoposide is most frequently administered with cisplatin when it is used in combination therapy. Teniposide has a more limited spectrum of activity than etoposide, and it is primarily used to treat acute lymphocytic and acute myeloid leukemias.

ADVERSE EFFECTS. Etoposide and teniposide are fairly well tolerated, although they can produce alopecia, mild nausea and vomiting, and dose-limiting myelosuppression. They have also been associated with a low incidence of secondary nonlymphocytic leukemias.

Camptothecin Analogues

Camptothecin is an alkaloid obtained from *Camptotheca acuminata*. Although camptothecin is a potent inhibitor of topoisomerase I, it has relatively low clinical efficacy. **Irinotecan** and **topotecan** are synthetic camptothecin analogues that have greater clinical activity and less toxicity than the natural alkaloid and are given intravenously for the treatment of cancer. Irinotecan is rapidly metabolized to an active metabolite called SN-38 that has 250 to 1000 times greater antitumor activity than the parent compound. SN-38 is eliminated primarily in the bile, whereas topotecan undergoes renal excretion.

Irinotecan is approved for the treatment of **colorectal cancer** that has recurred or progressed following fluorouracil therapy. It is also active against lymphomas and breast, cervical, gastric, lung, and other tumors. Topotecan is active against glioma, sarcoma, and lung and ovarian tumors.

The dose-limiting toxicity of both camptothecin analogues is myelosuppression. Irinotecan produces diarrhea in a significant percentage of patients, and both drugs can cause alopecia and mild nausea and vomiting.

TARGETED ANTICANCER DRUGS

Protein Kinase Inhibitors

The protein kinase inhibitors have been among the most successful of the targeted anticancer drugs. These agents inhibit various kinases that phosphorylate tyrosine or serine and threonine residues of growth factor receptors and other regulatory proteins, and thereby impede pathways promoting malignant cell transformation and proliferation.

Imatinib, **dasatinib**, and **nilotinib** inhibit the **BCR-ABL tyrosine kinase** expressed by the **Philadelphia chromosome** in **chronic myeloid leukemia** cells (Fig. 45–6). BCR-ABL (breakpoint cluster region–Abelson) kinase is an oncoprotein resulting from a reciprocal chromosomal translocation (swap) between chromosomes 9 and 22 designated t(9;22). This swap inserts ABL from chromosome 9 adjacent to BCR on chromosome 22, forming the BCR-ABL fusion gene and leading to malignant transformation of hematopoietic stem cells. Inhibition of BCR-ABL reduces cell proliferation and induces apoptosis. Imatinib has produced remarkable rates of hematologic and cytogenetic remission in chronic myeloid leukemia and is a first-line treatment for this disease. Both dasatinib and nilotinib are effective in patients with imatinib-resistant tumors. Imatinib also inhibits **c-kit**, a tyrosine kinase stem cell receptor, and has been used to treat gastrointestinal stromal tumors associated with c-kit mutations.

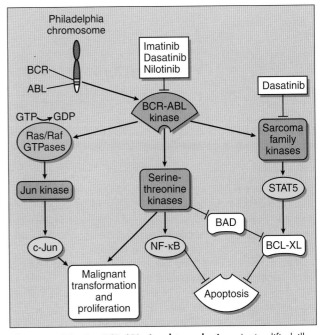

Figure 45–6. BCR-ABL signal transduction. A simplified illustration of pathways by which the BCR-ABL tyrosine kinase invokes malignant transformation and proliferation by activating small cytoplasmic GTPases (Ras and Raf) and various serine/threonine kinases, including the Jun kinase and sarcoma family kinases. The activated kinases stimulate transcription factors, including c-Jun, NF-κB (nuclear factor-kappa B), and STAT 5 (signal transducer and activator of transcription 5). Some of these factors increase expression of cyclins and other positive regulators of the cell cycle (Fig. 45–1). The activated kinases and transcription factors also modulate mitochondrial apoptotic regulators, including a proapoptotic caspase (BAD) and the antiapoptotic BCL-XL. Together, these effects lead to inhibition of apoptosis (programmed cell death) and promotion of cell replication. BCR-ABL also activates cytoskeletal regulators, leading to altered cell adhesion and motility (not shown). Imatinib and similar drugs inhibit BCR-ABL kinase and induce hematologic and cytogenetic remissions in patients with chronic myeloid leukemia. Dasatinib also inhibits sarcoma family kinases.

Erlotinib is a highly specific inhibitor of the tyrosine kinase associated with the epidermal growth factor receptor. It has been approved as a second-line therapy for **non–small-cell lung cancer** in patients who have failed at least one chemotherapy regimen. Clinical trials have shown that it produces modest increases in median survival time and 1-year survival compared with placebo. It is metabolized by cytochrome P450 3A4, and drugs that inhibit or induce this enzyme can alter plasma levels of erlotinib.

Sunitinib and **sorafenib** are newer drugs that inhibit multiple receptor tyrosine kinases, including VEGFR and c-kit. Both drugs are indicated for advanced **renal cell carcinoma**. Sunitinib is also approved for gastrointestinal stromal tumor, whereas sorafenib is also used to treat **hepatocellular carcinoma**. **Gefitinib** targets epidermal growth factor receptor and is approved for treating non–small-cell lung cancer. **Lapatinib** inhibits the kinase associated with the HER2/neu receptor in breast cancer cells.

A large number of other targeted anticancer drugs are currently under development, including agents that inhibit the proteosome, such as **bortezomib,** and drugs that target apoptosis inhibitors, such as the X-linked inhibitor of apoptosis protein and the B-cell lymphoma gene-2 (Bcl-2) protein. Bortezomib has recently been approved for treating **multiple myeloma**. Significant advances in cancer chemotherapy will likely result from the introduction of these and other targeted anticancer drugs.

Monoclonal Antibodies

Monoclonal antibodies are a growing class of targeted anticancer agents. The fragment antigen binding portion of a monoclonal antibody binds to a specific antigen on a particular type of cancer cell, leading to disruption of essential cancer cell processes. Some antibodies target growth factors or their receptors, while others release a cytotoxic drug or isotope, or enhance host immunity. Because of their protein structure, these agents must be given intravenously, and they are very expensive.

A nomenclature for monoclonal antibodies has been established. The names of monoclonal antibodies end in "mab" or "monab." The letters before mab indicate the source of the antibody: "o" for mouse, "u" for human, and "xi" for chimeric. An internal letter or syllable identifies the therapeutic use of the antibody, for example, "tu" for tumor, "vi" for virus, and "c" or "ci" for circulation. For example, rituximab is a chimeric human-murine antibody used in treating tumors. It was the first monoclonal antibody approved for cancer chemotherapy.

Rituximab, ^{90}Y-ibitumomab, and ^{131}I-tositumomab bind to the **CD20 antigen** found on the surface of over 90% of non-Hodgkin's lymphoma cells, as well as on normal B lymphocytes. CD20 is believed to regulate an early step in cell cycle initiation. Two of these agents release a toxic isotope that destroys cancer cells. These agents are used to treat relapsed or refractory B-cell **non-Hodgkin's lymphomas**.

Alemtuzumab binds to **CD52**, a cell surface glycoprotein found on all B and T lymphocytes and many other types of leukocytes, leading to cell lysis. It is indicated for the treatment of B-cell **chronic lymphocytic leukemia** in patients who have been treated with alkylating agents and who have failed fludarabine therapy.

Gemtuzumab ozogamicin is a unique monoclonal antibody conjugated with a **cytotoxic antitumor antibiotic** known as **calicheamicin.** The drug binds to the **CD33** antigen expressed by hematopoietic cells, resulting in formation of a complex that is internalized and sequestered in lysosomes, where calicheamicin is released. Calicheamicin then binds to DNA, resulting in double strand breaks and cell death. The drug is indicated for treatment of patients with CD33-positive **acute myeloid leukemia**.

Trastuzumab (Herceptin) is a recombinant human monoclonal antibody that binds to the extracellular domain of the **human epidermal growth factor-2 (HER2/neu) receptor**. The HER2 receptor is a tyrosine kinase and a member of the epidermal growth factor receptor family involved in stimulating cell proliferation. Trastuzumab is used to treat metastatic breast cancer in the 25% of women whose cancer cells overexpress HER2/neu. Trastuzumab is administered once a week, usually in combination with doxorubicin and paclitaxel. Its adverse effects include chills, fever, nausea, vomiting, chest pain, and dyspnea.

Cetuximab, bevacizumab, and **panitumumab** are monoclonal antibodies for the treatment of **colorectal cancer.** These agents bind the **epidermal growth factor receptor** expressed in many normal tissues and overexpressed in certain human cancers, particularly colon cancer. Overexpression of epidermal growth factor receptor is associated with unrestricted cell growth and a poor prognosis. Cetuximab is used to treat **colon cancer** in combination with irinotecan. Patients receiving this drug combination had better response rates and increased time to tumor progression than patients not receiving cetuximab. The most common adverse effect of cetuximab is an acne-like skin rash, whereas about 3% of patients experience hypersensitivity reactions during drug infusion. It is also approved for **head and neck cancer** in combination with radiation therapy.

Bevacizumab is a recombinant humanized antibody to **vascular endothelial growth factor** (VEGF). The drug prevents binding of VEGF to receptors on endothelial cells and thereby inhibits the formation of new blood vessels. It is the first VEGF **angiogenesis inhibitor** to be approved for cancer chemotherapy, and it is indicated for treating metastatic **colon cancer** and **non–small-cell lung cancer**. When bevacizumab is used in a fluorouracil regimen, it increases tumor response rates, progression-free survival time, and overall survival time in these patients. The drug can cause gastrointestinal bleeding and perforation, pulmonary hemorrhage, and other thromboembolic events.

CYTOKINES AND INTERFERONS

Interferons are endogenous proteins that increase the activity of various cytotoxic cells in the immune system. **Interferon alfa-2b (IFN alfa-2b)** directly suppresses cancer cell growth by inhibiting expression of oncogenes and reducing cancer cell proliferation. **IFN alfa-2b** is used to treat **Kaposi's sarcoma** in patients with AIDS, and it produces a clinical response in about 70% of persons with hairy cell leukemia or chronic myeloid leukemia. In myeloid leukemia, it causes a cytogenetic response (loss of the Philadelphia chromosome) in 30% of cases, which is considerably less than achieved with imatinib and other tyrosine kinase inhibitors. IFN alfa-2b is also used to treat bladder and renal carcinoma, malignant melanoma, and multiple myeloma.

IFN alfa-2b is administered intramuscularly. Its most common adverse effects include leukopenia, thrombocytopenia, a flulike syndrome, nausea or vomiting, tiredness, altered taste, and diarrhea.

Aldesleukin (interleukin-2 [IL-2]) is a lymphokine that activates IL-2 receptors and promotes B- and T-cell proliferation and differentiation. The antitumor effect of the drug is primarily caused by increased numbers of cytotoxic T cells that can recognize and destroy tumor cells without damaging normal cells. These cytotoxic cells include natural killer cells, lymphokine-activated killer cells, and tumor-infiltrating cells.

Aldesleukin is primarily used to treat metastatic **renal cell carcinoma**, but it also has activity against malignant melanoma and colorectal cancer. In about 20% of patients with renal cell carcinoma, it produces a good response, which in some cases persists for several years without further therapy.

In low doses, aldesleukin is fairly well tolerated and can be given as outpatient therapy. In higher doses, the drug can be very toxic. The most common dose-limiting toxicities are hypotension, fluid retention, and renal dysfunction. Other toxicities include a broad range of hematologic deficiencies, skin lesions, and neuropsychiatric changes. The toxicities are usually reversible and can be prevented or managed by giving corticosteroids before aldesleukin therapy and providing vigorous supportive care. Prolonged infusions of aldesleukin appear to be less toxic than high-dose bolus injections.

HORMONES AND THEIR ANTAGONISTS

Several types of hormone-dependent cancer (especially breast, prostate, and endometrial cancers) respond to treatment with their corresponding hormone antagonists. **Estrogen antagonists** are primarily used to treat breast cancer, whereas **androgen antagonists** are used to treat prostate cancer. **Corticosteroids** are particularly useful in treating lymphocytic leukemias and lymphomas.

The pharmacologic properties of estrogens, androgens, and their antagonists are described in Chapter 34, and those of corticosteroids are described in Chapter 33. The use of these drugs in cancer treatment is summarized in the following paragraphs.

Hormones Used in Breast Cancer

Breast cancer is usually estrogen-dependent and can be suppressed by the administration of estrogen antagonists. **Tamoxifen** is the antagonist used most widely. This drug can be given alone to prevent breast cancer in women who have a strong family history of the disease or are otherwise highly predisposed to developing it. Tamoxifen is often used

in combination with surgery and other chemotherapeutic drugs for the treatment of breast cancer. In women over 50 years of age, adjuvant use of tamoxifen was found to reduce the annual odds of recurrence by 30%. Long-term survival appears to be greater in women receiving both cytotoxic chemotherapy and tamoxifen.

Aromatase inhibitors that prevent estrogen synthesis, including **anastrozole** and **letrozole**, are a first-line therapy for certain forms of breast cancer in postmenopausal women. The actions and effects of these drugs are described in Chapter 34.

Hormones Used in Prostate Cancer

Prostate cancer cell proliferation is stimulated by androgens and suppressed by estrogens. Continuous administration of either a gonadotropin-releasing hormone agonist (e.g., **leuprolide**) or a gonadotropin-releasing hormone receptor antagonist (**abarelix**) can be used to inhibit luteinizing hormone secretion and testosterone production in men with advanced prostate cancer and thereby suppress cancer growth. Androgen antagonists (e.g., **flutamide**) can be used to further reduce testosterone stimulation of prostate carcinoma cells.

Corticosteroids

Corticosteroids (e.g., **prednisone**) are primarily used because of their lymphocytotoxic effects in the treatment of lymphocytic leukemias, lymphomas, and multiple myeloma. Corticosteroids are relatively well tolerated and do not produce myelosuppression or other serious organ damage in most patients. They are often combined with cytotoxic and targeted anticancer agents.

IMMUNOMODULATING DRUGS

Drugs that affect the immune system are called **immunomodulators**. Most of these drugs suppress immune mechanisms and are used to treat autoimmune diseases or to prevent **allograft rejection** following organ or bone marrow transplantation. In the latter case, these drugs act by inhibiting the immune response to the foreign antigens contained in an allograft, which is a graft of tissue between individuals of the same species but of disparate genotypes. A few drugs, including thalidomide and palivizumab, act to enhance host immunity and are used in treating cancer.

Monoclonal Antibodies

Daclizumab and **basiliximab** are monoclonal antibodies to the high-affinity **IL-2 receptor** that is expressed on activated T cells. These antibodies bind to the α-subunit of the receptor and prevent IL-2 binding. By this action, IL-2–mediated activation of lymphocytes is prevented, and the response of the immune system to antigens (e.g., those present in transplanted allografts) is impaired. Daclizumab and basiliximab are used in combination with cyclosporine and prednisone to prevent rejection of **renal transplants**.

Muromonab-CD3 is a monoclonal antibody to the CD3 glycoprotein that is part of the **T-cell antigen recognition receptor**. The antibody prevents antigen access to the receptor and thereby prevents T-cell activation. Muromonab-CD3 is used to treat **acute allograft rejection** in renal transplant patients. In addition, it is used to reverse bone marrow, cardiac, hepatic, kidney, and pancreatic transplant rejection episodes that are resistant to conventional drugs (e.g., cyclosporine).

Palivizumab is a human monoclonal antibody to the fusion protein of **respiratory syncytial virus**. It is approved for prevention of respiratory syncytial virus infection in infants with bronchopulmonary dysplasia and in **premature infants** whose gestational age is under 35 weeks. It is given as five monthly intramuscular doses.

Microbial Products

Cyclosporine, **tacrolimus**, and **sirolimus** are examples of immunosuppressants that are derived from microbes. Cyclosporine is a complex fungal polypeptide, whereas tacrolimus and sirolimus are macrolide antibiotics produced by *Streptomyces* species. Cyclosporine and tacrolimus inhibit the production and release of IL-2 that is required for activation of cytotoxic T lymphocytes in response to alloantigenic challenge. Specifically, cyclosporine and tacrolimus bind to intracellular proteins called immunophilins (cyclophilin and FK506-binding protein, respectively). The drug-immunophilin complex then binds the phosphatase enzyme called **calcineurin** and inhibits calcineurin-mediated transcription of the IL-2 gene.

Sirolimus, also called **rapamycin**, forms a complex with FK12-binding protein, which then inhibits a key regulatory kinase (**mammalian target of rapamycin** [mTOR]) involved in cytokine-driven T-cell proliferation (cell cycle progression).

Cyclosporine, tacrolimus, and sirolimus can be used to prevent rejection of organ transplants and are usually given in combination with corticosteroids or other drugs. For example, sirolimus is given in combination with cyclosporine and a corticosteroid (e.g., prednisone). Cyclosporine can also be used to treat **psoriasis** and severe autoimmune diseases that are resistant to other therapeutic agents, such as **rheumatoid arthritis** that does not respond to MTX. In addition to these indications, sirolimus and tacrolimus have been incorporated into vascular stents that slowly release the drugs to inhibit the proliferation of vascular smooth muscle cells and other vascular cells that otherwise cause restenosis of coronary arteries following stent placement. The use of drug-releasing stents has dramatically reduced the incidence of coronary restenosis in this setting.

Cyclosporine frequently causes nephrotoxicity, hypertension, hirsutism, gingival hyperplasia, and muscle tremor. Cyclosporine is metabolized by CYP3A4, a cytochrome P450 enzyme, and interacts with other drugs that inhibit or induce this enzyme. CYP3A4 inhibitors can increase the plasma levels and toxicity of cyclosporine, and these include erythromycin and other macrolide antibiotics, azole antifungal drugs, calcium channel blockers, and grapefruit juice. CYP3A4 inducers can decrease the plasma levels of cyclosporine, and these include carbamazepine, phenytoin, and rifampin.

Corticosteroids

Prednisone and other corticosteroids inhibit T-cell proliferation and the expression of genes encoding various cytokines. They are used with other immunosuppressive drugs to prevent organ transplant rejection and to prevent graft-versus-host disease in patients who have undergone bone marrow transplantation. Corticosteroids are frequently used to treat various autoimmune disorders, including lupus erythematosus and rheumatoid arthritis. Their anti-inflammatory actions are also very beneficial in these disorders (see Chapter 30).

Other Drugs
Azathioprine, Cyclophosphamide, and Methotrexate

In the body, azathioprine is converted to 6-mercaptopurine. As with methotrexate, 6-mercaptopurine acts by inhibiting DNA synthesis. Cyclophosphamide acts by alkylating DNA. Because these agents prevent the proliferation of B and T lymphocytes, they are used to prevent organ graft rejection and treat autoimmune disorders and collagen diseases. Cyclophosphamide and MTX are also used in the treatment of cancer (see previous).

Azathioprine is often given in combination with corticosteroids and cyclosporine or tacrolimus to patients with tissue transplants, and it is also useful in the treatment of patients with inflammatory bowel disease, rheumatoid arthritis, or lupus erythematosus. Cyclophosphamide is used primarily to treat lupus erythematosus and other autoimmune diseases and is usually given in combination with corticosteroids. MTX has anti-inflammatory effects that make it especially useful in the management of rheumatoid arthritis (see Chapter 30). It is also useful in the treatment of psoriasis and severe asthma.

Thalidomide

Thalidomide was once banned because of its potential to cause phocomelia and other congenital malformations. It was subsequently discovered to have immunomodulating effects, and it is now being used to treat cancer, recurrent aphthous ulcers (canker sores), tuberculosis, leprosy, erythema nodosum leprosum, and the AIDS-associated wasting syndrome (cachexia).

Thalidomide acts, in part, by inhibiting **angiogenesis**, the formation of new blood vessels. This action appears to account for its teratogenic effects, because the drug prevents vascular growth during fetal limb development. The antiangiogenesis actions of the drug and its analogues are now being evaluated in the treatment of cancer, and early trials are encouraging.

Thalidomide has both immunosuppressant and immunostimulant effects. It inhibits the production of IL-2, tumor necrosis factor-alpha, and other cytokines. Although thalidomide inhibits lymphocyte proliferation stimulated by alloantigens, some studies show that it stimulates CD8 cells in vitro. The mechanism of action of thalidomide in specific diseases continues to be investigated.

SUMMARY OF IMPORTANT POINTS

■ Most antineoplastic drugs inhibit DNA synthesis or disrupt DNA structure and function.

■ DNA synthesis inhibitors include folate antagonists (methotrexate and trimetrexate), purine antagonists (mercaptopurine, thioguanine, and others), pyrimidine antagonists (cytarabine, floxuridine, and fluorouracil), and a ribonucleotide reductase inhibitor (hydroxyurea).

■ DNA alkylating drugs that cross-link DNA include nitrogen mustards (cyclophosphamide and others), nitrosoureas (carmustine and others), and miscellaneous drugs (busulfan, dacarbazine, and mitomycin). Platinum compounds (cisplatin and others) also cross-link DNA strands.

■ DNA intercalating drugs include the anthracycline drugs (doxorubicin and others), bleomycin, and dactinomycin.

■ Inhibitors of mitosis include vinca alkaloids (vincristine and others) and taxane drugs (docetaxel and paclitaxel).

■ Topoisomerase inhibitors include podophyllotoxin drugs (etoposide and teniposide) and camptothecin analogues (irinotecan and topotecan).

■ Biologic response modifiers used in the treatment of cancer include IFN alfa-2b, aldesleukin, and monoclonal antibodies (bevacizumab, cetuximab, rituximab, and trastuzumab).

■ Myelosuppression is the dose-limiting toxicity of most antineoplastic drugs.

■ Doxorubicin and other anthracycline drugs produce cardiotoxicity; cyclophosphamide and ifosfamide cause hemorrhagic cystitis; bleomycin and busulfan produce pulmonary fibrosis; vincristine, docetaxel, and related drugs cause neurotoxicity; and cisplatin produces renal toxicity.

■ Hormonal agents are used to treat some cancers, especially estrogen antagonists to treat breast cancer, androgen antagonists to treat prostate cancer, and corticosteroids (e.g., prednisone) to treat lymphocytic leukemias and lymphomas.

■ Immunosuppressant drugs used to prevent organ transplant rejection or to treat autoimmune diseases include monoclonal antibodies (basiliximab, daclizumab, and muromonab-CD3), microbial products (cyclosporine, sirolimus, and tacrolimus), corticosteroids (e.g., prednisone), and cytotoxic drugs (e.g., azathioprine).

Review Questions

1. A woman being treated for breast cancer develops numbness and tingling in her hands and feet. She is most likely being treated with which drug?
   (A) cyclophosphamide
   (B) docetaxel
   (C) doxorubicin
   (D) vincristine
   (E) trastuzumab

2. A man being treated for testicular cancer experiences ototoxicity. The drug causing this adverse effect inhibits cancer growth by which mechanism?
   (A) folate antagonism
   (B) inhibition of tyrosine kinase
   (C) inactivation of epidermal growth factor receptors
   (D) cross-linking of DNA
   (E) formation of free radicals

3. A woman with leukemia responds to first-line therapy for her cancer by loss of the Philadelphia chromosome. Which adverse effect is most likely to occur in this patient?
   (A) rash
   (B) alopecia
   (C) constipation
   (D) myelosuppression
   (E) severe vomiting

4. A woman who has developed resistance to cytarabine is given a monoclonal antibody that releases a toxin. She is most likely being treated for which cancer?
   (A) breast cancer
   (B) ovarian cancer
   (C) acute myeloid leukemia
   (D) multiple myeloma
   (E) melanoma

5. Which drug forms a complex with a regulatory protein, resulting in inhibition of the mammalian target of rapamycin?
   (A) cyclosporine
   (B) prednisone
   (C) muromonab-CD3
   (D) sirolimus
   (E) azathioprine

Answers and Explanations

1. **The answer is B:** docetaxel. Drugs that inhibit microtubule function, such as docetaxel and vincristine, are associated with peripheral neurotoxicity. Docetaxel is often used to treat breast cancer, whereas vincristine is not. Cyclophosphamide, doxorubicin, and trastuzumab (Options A, C, and E) do not inhibit microtubule function.

2. **The answer is D:** cross-linking of DNA. The man is most likely receiving cisplatin, which may cause ototoxicity. Cisplatin forms interstrand and intrastrand cross-links with DNA bases and thereby prevents DNA replication.

3. **The answer is A:** rash. Among the most frequent adverse effects of imatinib are edema, rash, diarrhea, and pain. Imatinib is not likely to cause alopecia, myelosuppression, constipation, or severe vomiting.

4. **The answer is C:** acute myeloid leukemia. The patient is receiving gemtuzumab ozogamicin, which release a toxic antibiotic, calicheamicin, after binding to receptors on leukemic cells. This agent is not used to treat breast or ovarian cancer, melanoma, or myeloma.

5. The answer is D: sirolimus. Sirolimus and temsirolimus form complexes with regulatory protein, FK12-binding protein, resulting in inhibition of the mammalian target of rapamycin (mTOR), which is involved in proliferation of T lymphocytes and tumor cells. Sirolimus is used as an immunosuppressant to prevent organ transplant rejection. Temsirolimus causes G_1-phase growth arrest and is used to treat advanced renal cell carcinoma.

SELECTED READINGS

Feldman, D.R., G.J. Bosl, J. Sheinfeld, and R.J. Motzer. Medical treatment of advanced testicular cancer. JAMA 299:672–684, 2008.

Fornier, M.N. Ixabepilone, first in a new class of antineoplastic agents: the natural epothilones and their analogues. Clin Breast Cancer 7:757–763, 2007.

Gerber, D.E. Targeted therapies: a new generation of cancer treatments. Am Fam Physician 77:311–319, 2008.

Hiles, J.J., and J.M. Kolesar. Role of sunitinib and sorafenib in the treatment of metastatic renal cell carcinoma. Am J Health Syst Pharm 65:123–131, 2008.

Jordan, M.A., and K. Kamath. How do microtubule-targeted drugs work? An overview. Curr Cancer Drug Targets 7:730–742, 2007.

Sessions, J. Chronic myeloid leukemia in 2007. Am J Health Sys Pharm 64:S4–S9, 2007.

Shepard, H.M., P. Jin, D.J. Slamon, Z. Pirot, and D.C. Maneval. Herceptin. Handb Exp Pharmacol 181:183–219, 2008.

INDEX

Page numbers followed by b indicate material in boxes; page number followed by f indicate figures; and page number followed by t indicate table